FUNDAMENTALS OF
ONCOLOGY

FUNDAMENTALS OF ONCOLOGY

FOURTH EDITION, REVISED AND EXPANDED

Henry C. Pitot

McArdle Laboratory for Cancer Research
University of Wisconsin Medical School
Madison, Wisconsin

With a Contribution by
Daniel D. Loeb

McArdle Laboratory for Cancer Research
University of Wisconsin Medical School
Madison, Wisconsin

MARCEL DEKKER, INC.   NEW YORK · BASEL

ISBN: 0-8247-0650-1

This book is printed on acid-free paper.

Headquarters
Marcel Dekker, Inc.
270 Madison Avenue, New York, NY 10016
tel: 212-696-9000; fax: 212-685-4540

Eastern Hemisphere Distribution
Marcel Dekker AG
Hutgasse 4, Postfach 812, CH-4001 Basel, Switzerland
tel: 41-61-261-8482; fax: 41-61-261-8896

World Wide Web
http://www.dekker.com

The publisher offers discounts on this book when ordered in bulk quantities. For more information, write to Special Sales/Professional Marketing at the headquarters address above.

Current printing (last digit):
10 9 8 7 6 5 4 3 2 1

PRINTED IN THE UNITED STATES OF AMERICA

To Mary

Julie and Beth

Anita
Jeanne
Cathy
Henry
Michelle
Lisa
Patrice

Mom, Dad, and Big Anita

I am a cancer cell.

Of my earliest ancestry no evidence remains. When the earth's first creatures stirred the ancient seas, when the Pharaohs wrought the pyramids, when the medieval scribes laboriously recorded their philosophies, I was there. The ingenious Virchow, who recognized my stamp, marshaled the forces of science against me. Malicious, relentless, insidious I am, full of destruction, ripe for carnage, yet in my enduring frame I carry the secret of life. Study me, and you will bring into the light of day precious urns of wisdom long buried in the tomb of ignorance. For you I shall tell a wondrous tale of the beginning of things that are and are to be. Study me, know me, and you will hold the world in fief. Neglect me, and as surely as the fingers of the dawn grasp first the temples of the East, I will strike you dead.

Preface to the Fourth Edition

It has been some 15 years since the third edition of this text was published. The original purpose of the book was to replace notes in a course, "Introduction to Experimental Oncology," which has been given in the Department of Oncology at the University of Wisconsin–Madison for more than 25 years. The course has evolved from being primarily directed towards graduate students to one that includes more than 80% undergraduates, usually juniors and seniors in various sciences. The course has always been offered for two credits, but with the enormous increase in information in the field of oncology, it will likely be increased to three credits.

In this revision, four new chapters have been added and the other chapters significantly expanded. The genetics of neoplasia is now covered in two chapters, as is the stage of progression. Discussion of carcinogenesis in humans has also been expanded to two full chapters in addition to the chapter on the evaluation of risk of carcinogenic environmental agents. Finally, another chapter has been added in the area of host–tumor relationships, covering endocrine and stromal responses. Of necessity, the glossary has been somewhat expanded, as have the number of figures and tables. (We are very grateful to the authors and publishers who gave us permission to incorporate their work in this text. In addition, for instructors wishing to use this text in classes in oncology, we have developed an extended series of slide illustrations that may be found at our web site: http://mcardle.oncology.wisc.edu/pitot.+ Click on "Courses" and scroll down to "Oncology 401.")

As in the third edition, I have again cited references in the text. Although some of the third edition's references have been retained because of their usefulness, a larger number of new references have been added since the last edition than were in the third edition itself. Still, this fundamental text is not exhaustive in its treatment of the literature (although some students may think it is), but it presents reasonably representative samples of each of the topics and areas covered. My sincere apologies are extended to any colleagues whose work was not specifically cited. If there are other subjects in the field of oncology that should be covered in a basic text such as this, I would certainly appreciate receiving such information.

I would like to express my sincere appreciation to my colleague Dr. Daniel Loeb, who, after some arm-twisting, agreed to write the vast majority of Chapter 4, on viruses and cancer. This field has become much more complex since the third edition, and I felt need of an expert in the area. I am also grateful to other colleagues who read and made critical comments on the manuscript, especially Drs. Norman Drinkwater, the late Dr. James Miller, and Bill Sugden of the McArdle Laboratory; Dr. Lynn Allen-Hoffmann of the Department of Pathology at the University of Wisconsin–Madison; my son, Dr. Henry C. Pitot IV, and his colleagues in the Department of Oncology of the Mayo Clinic, Rochester, Minnesota; and Dr. Peter Duesberg of the University of California, Berkeley. In particular, I express my deepest thanks to Dr. Ilse Riegel for her invaluable help in editing and correcting the manuscript throughout all its stages. Our special appreciation and thanks go to Mrs. Mary Jo Markham and Mrs. Kristen Adler for their patient, enduring, and expert transcribing and typing of the manuscript and indexing the entire book. A special thanks is given to my colleague Dr. Yi-hua Xu, who aided us immensely in developing and digitizing figures.

Perhaps the greatest debt of gratitude in developing the fourth edition of this text is owed my wife and our children, who have endured the constant "working on the book" that kept me from spending more time with them. As the final corrections were being made to the text, our oldest daughter was diagnosed with metastatic breast cancer. Several years ago she gave me a small blackboard on which was written, "A teacher affects eternity; they can never tell where their influence stops." I can only hope and pray that these words are prophetic and that this text may play a small role in the ultimate control of cancer.

Henry C. Pitot

Preface to the Third Edition

Since the manuscript for the second edition of this text was completed, information regarding the science of oncology, in the human and the experimental animal as well as in the plant kingdom, has expanded in an astounding manner. The prediction of an earlier reviewer that this test would require constant updating has proven true many times over. Furthermore, for the sake of our students—the prime motivation for writing this text—a reasonably succinct survey of the field of experimental oncology and its applications to humans continues to be of primary importance in our basic instructional program.

In this revision of the text, a number of new chapters have been added. A new Chapter 5, concerned with hereditary factors in the causation of cancer, has been included. The discussion of human cancer has been divided into two chapters: Chapter 9 is concerned with the direct known causes and Chapter 10 with the scientific and societal considerations of human cancer. Finally, the chapter on the biochemistry of neoplasia (Chapter 10 in the second edition) has also been divided into two chapters, one dealing with the biochemistry of the neoplastic transformation in vivo (Chapter 12), the other with the biochemistry and molecular biology of the neoplastic transformation in vitro (Chapter 13).

At the suggestion of one of the reviewers of the second edition, we have cited the references in the text for the convenience of the reader. This has the disadvantage of a somewhat more formal presentation, but we hope that it will be useful to the student who wishes to study the field of experimental oncology in greater depth. This fundamental text is not exhaustive in its treatment of the literature but presents representative examples of each of the topics and areas covered. My apologies to any colleagues whose work was not specifically cited. If anyone feels strongly that additional references are needed, please communicate your suggestions to the author.

Again I would like to express my sincere appreciation to my colleagues at the McArdle Laboratory who read and made critical comments on the manuscript, especially Doctors Norman Drinkwater, Janet Mertz, James and Elizabeth Miller, Gerald C. Mueller, Van R Potter, Rex Risser, Jeffrey Ross, Bill Sugden, and Howard M. Temin, and to Dr. Paul Carbone of the

Wisconsin Clinical Cancer Center. In particular I would like to express my thanks to Dr. Ilse Riegel and Bette Sheehan for their invaluable help in editing and correcting the manuscript throughout all of its stages and my appreciation to Mary Jo Markham and Karen Denk for their patient and expert transcribing and typing. Finally, my thanks are extended to Carol Dizack for her expert artistry in drawing the figures added to this edition of the text and to Terrill P. Stewart for his photographic skills.

Henry C. Pitot

Preface to the Second Edition

In the few short years since the publication of the first edition of this text, a number of significant facts have been uncovered in the science of oncology. Many of these findings have been incorporated into the teaching of our basic course in experimental oncology through additional notes and lectures, and the revision of this text became a clear necessity.

In this revision we have maintained the same format as in the first edition but have altered the contents of most of the chapters, adding both figures and tables. In addition, the pathogenesis of cancer and the natural history of cancer in vivo have been divided into Chapters 6 and 8 respectively. Finally, Chapter 13 has been added to present some aspects of the basis for cancer chemotherapy. Although this chapter is not an attempt to discuss the various treatment modalities used in cancer therapy, the subject matter does introduce the student to the experimental basis for chemotherapy and also briefly discusses the methodology and rationale for the chemical therapies used today.

We have continued to utilize illustrative slides to supplement the lectures and text. Lectures by several of my clinical colleagues on the diagnosis, therapy, and psychosocial aspects of cancer continue to be significant components of our course.

Again I would like to express my sincere appreciation to a number of my colleagues at the McArdle Laboratory, especially Doctors Roswell Boutwell, James and Elizabeth Miller, Van R. Potter, Rex Risser, Bill Sugden, and Howard Temin, as well as others who have read and made critical comments on the manuscript. In particular, I would like to express my thanks to Dr. Ilse Riegel and Ms. Bette Sheehan for their invaluable help in collating, editing, and correcting the manuscript throughout all of its stages, and my appreciation to Ms. Karen Denk for her patient and expert typing. Finally, my thanks are again extended to Mr. John L. Shane for his continued artistic aid in drawing the new figures for this text.

Henry C. Pitot

Preface to the First Edition

The sensationalism and publicity directed toward the investigation, diagnosis, and treatment of cancer as a disease in the human being have reached a dramatic level in the United States. In part this is a result of the decision by the political administration of Richard M. Nixon to make the conquest of cancer a major goal of his office. Although it is not my desire nor is this the place to consider the ramifications of this decision and the subsequent difficulties that have arisen in its implementation, it is clear that cancer research received a "shot in the arm" of international proportions by political decisions at the beginning of this decade. The U.S. public, who have supported the National Cancer Plan through their taxes, have been repeatedly apprised of its existence and progress since its inception in 1970. Much has been written on the subject of cancer in the scientific literature as a direct result of the financial impetus given to research in oncology over the past decade. A variety of books and monographs on the general subject of cancer in humans and animals for both the scientist and the layman have appeared during this same period.

This text is not meant to be a popular account of the cancer problem. More than two decades ago, the Department of Oncology, which comprises the McArdle Laboratory for Cancer Research of the University of Wisconsin at Madison, initiated a graduate course in oncology. This course consisted of a series of lectures covering a variety of aspects of experimental oncology including chemical and biological carcinogenesis, host-tumor relationships, the natural history of cancer, and the biochemistry of cancer. In addition, within a few years of its inception, several lectures were given on the diagnosis and therapy of cancer in the human patient. The course was and always has been oriented primarily toward the graduate student in oncology rather than specifically for the medical student or postgraduate physician. In part as a result of the increased interest in cancer research by both graduate and undergraduate students and as part of the mechanism of self-evaluation of teaching programs, several years ago the McArdle Laboratory expanded its original course into three separate courses in experimental oncology. The first course in this series is open to all students and fellows at the University of Wisconsin, and the notes given to the students comprise the basis for this short text on the fundamentals of oncology.

During the course period, these notes are supplemented by several sessions in which slides are shown depicting a variety of examples both from human and animal neoplasms to illustrate many of the specific points presented in the text. A list of these slides can be made available to anyone interested, on written request to the author. In addition, at the end of the course several lectures are given to the students on the diagnosis and therapy of human cancer as well as on the psychosocial aspects and bioethics of human oncology.

It is the hope of those of us in the McArdle Laboratory involved in the teaching of this course that we can instill in our students the basic concepts of the science of this disease and thereby interest them in learning more about the mechanisms of neoplastic disease and the use of such knowledge toward the ultimate control of cancer in the human patient.

In particular, I would like to express my appreciation to my colleagues in the McArdle Laboratory, especially Drs. James and Elizabeth Miller, Van R. Potter, Ilse L. Riegel, Bill Sugden, Howard M. Temin, and others who have read and made critical comments on this manuscript at its earlier stages. My thanks also go to the several outside reviewers of the manuscript whose suggestions resulted in an increased number of illustrations and the addition of the epilogue, and to Mr. John L. Shane, whose artistic skill produced the drawings of the figures.

Henry C. Pitot

Contents

FUNDAMENTALS OF
ONCOLOGY

1

Cancer: Yesterday and Today

History tells us that disease has been a part of the living process on this planet for eons. In fact, it is clear that life as we know it, by its very nature, requires that disease processes exist. It is natural, then, that a thinking, reasoning human organism should concern itself with disease and its effects on individuals as well as populations. Diseases that are self-limiting and readily controlled by natural life processes present no major problem for humans, animals, or plants. Our concern is with diseases that are potentially life-threatening or morbidly debilitating.

Since the dawn of civilization there have always been a few disease entities of great concern to humans. As evidenced by biblical writings, the disease most feared and abhorred by the population of the western civilized world at that time was leprosy. Later, in the Middle Ages and the Renaissance in Europe, the dreaded disease was the bubonic plague, or "black death." During the last century, a major killer associated with considerable human suffering was the "white death," or tuberculosis. With the effective antimicrobial therapy developed in the twentieth century, infectious diseases now play a lesser role in "developed cultures" than in the past, although in relatively underdeveloped countries of the Third World, infectious diseases such as malaria and hookworm are still of paramount importance and concern. In modern times, however, especially during the last half of the twentieth century, the most feared disease is cancer. One of the more succinct descriptions emphasizing the impact of this fear was presented at a symposium on cancer in 1936 by Glenn Frank, President of the University of Wisconsin.

> But not all these tragic consequences together are the worst evil wrought by cancer. For *everybody* that is *killed* by the *fact* of cancer, multiplied thousands of *minds* are *unnerved* by the *fear* of cancer. What cancer, as an unsolved mystery, does to the morale of millions who may never know its ravages is incalculable. This is an incidence of cancer that cannot be reached by the physician's medicaments, the surgeon's knife, or any organized advice against panic. Nothing but the actual conquest of cancer itself will remove this sword that today hangs over every head.*

Although the United States was not the first country to proclaim the conquest of cancer as a national effort, the government's financial backing of cancer research during the 1970s provided the greatest single impetus in the history of this country to the scientific search for knowledge and understanding to control and eliminate cancer. In 1970, a special panel of consultants called together by the U.S. Senate submitted a "Report of the National Board of Consultants on the Conquest of Cancer" (1971); at that time, this was perhaps the best summary of the status of

*Quoted from the welcome by President Glenn Frank to participants in "A Symposium on Cancer," University of Wisconsin School of Medicine, Madison, Wisconsin, September 7–9, 1936. University of Wisconsin Press, Madison, 1938.

cancer as a disease and of cancer research in this country. This report showed that cancer is the primary health concern of the people of the United States. In several polls, approximately two-thirds of those questioned admitted fearing cancer more than any other disease. Of 200 million Americans living in 1970, some 50 million were destined to develop cancer, and approximately 34 million would die of the disease. According to the American Cancer Society (1993), about 85 million Americans living in 1993 will eventually develop cancer. About one-half of all deaths due to cancer occur prior to the age of 65, and cancer causes more deaths among children aged 1 to 14 than any other disease. About 20% of all deaths in this country are caused by cancer; it is second only to cardiovascular disease as the greatest killer of our population.

The committee of consultants that was convened in 1970 pointed out that in 1969 the budget of this country, on a per capita basis, provided $410 for national defense; $125 for the war in Vietnam; $19 for the space program; $19 for foreign aid; but only 89 cents for cancer research. During the same year, deaths from cancer were eight times the number of lives lost in all 6 years of the Vietnam War up to that time, 5½ times the number of people killed in automobile accidents in that year, and greater than the number of American servicemen killed in battle in all 4 years of World War II. Hodgson and Rice (1995) have indicated that the yearly cost to this nation's economy because of cancer is nearly $73 billion, with the cost of medical care of cancer patients being more than $18 billion per year. These figures do not take into account the costs in suffering, mental anguish, and psychosocial trauma that haunt both cancer patients and their families.

We do not yet understand the basic nature of cancer; however, we know a great deal more about the disease today than we did 50 years ago. In 1930, the medical cure rate for those afflicted with cancer was about one in five. Today, approximately two in five are cured, and the panel's findings and subsequent studies have demonstrated that this could be improved to almost one in two simply by better application of the knowledge that exists today. In fact, in 1982, the National Cancer Institute's SEER Program (see below) presented data to indicate that nearly 50% of white patients with cancer, excluding nonmelanoma skin cancer and carcinoma in situ (see Chapter 9), will survive to die of other diseases. Certain specific types of cancers that were 100% fatal prior to 1960 can now be cured in as many as 70% of the cases (see Chapter 16).

CANCER: YESTERDAY

In all likelihood, all multicellular organisms are afflicted or have the potential to be afflicted with the disease we call cancer. Paleopathologists have shown that cancerous lesions occurred in dinosaur bones long before the advent of *Homo sapiens* (Bett, 1957). In view of the numerous reports of spontaneous and induced cancers in plants and animals, vertebrates as well as invertebrates, it is probable that cancer has been with us for much of the evolutionary period of life on earth. Ancient Egyptians knew of the existence of cancer in humans, and in one papyrus, the Edwin Smith papyrus, a glyph clearly refers to a clinical cancer of the breast (Fig. 1.1). In addition, autopsies of mummies have shown the existence of bone tumors and the probability of other cancerous processes.

By the era of Hippocrates in the fourth century B.C., many types of cancers were clinically recognized and described, such as cancer of the stomach or uterus. Hippocrates felt that in many instances little could be done for the cancer patient and, more importantly, that it was to this disease that one of his cardinal rules, *Primum non nocere* (first do no harm), applied. Hippocrates coined the term *carcinoma*, which referred to tumors that spread and destroyed the patient. This was in contrast to the group he termed *carcinos*, which included benign tumors, hemorrhoids, and other chronic ulcerations. He proposed that cancer was a disease of an excess

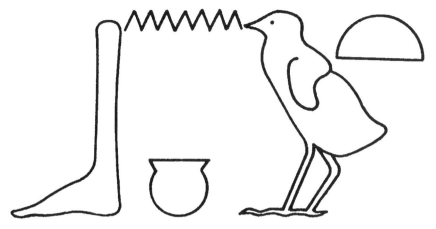

Figure 1.1 The hieroglyphic symbol for the word *tumor*, referring to the surgical treatment of cancer of the breast as described in the Edwin Smith papyrus, dated earlier than 1600 B.C. The reader is referred to Breasted's translation (1930) of the document for further information.

of black bile, which was manufactured by both the spleen and stomach but not the liver. This concept of the causation of cancer remained the predominant theory for almost 2000 years. Hippocrates as well as other physicians during the next two millennia tended not to treat ulcerated or deep-seated cancers, because "if treated, the patients die quickly; but if not treated, they hold out for a long time."

Almost 600 years later, Galen distinguished "tumors according to nature," such as enlargement of the breast with normal female maturation; "tumors exceeding nature," which included the bony proliferation occurring during the reuniting of a fracture; and "tumors contrary to nature," which today we may define as benign or malignant tumors (Chapter 2). This distinction, proposed some 1800 years ago, is still reasonably correct. Galen also suggested the similarity in gross outline between a crab and the disease we know today as cancer.

The concepts of Hippocrates and Galen dominated medical practice during the Middle Ages. With the advent of the Renaissance and during the seventeenth and eighteenth centuries, the "black bile" theory of the causation of cancer was disputed by a number of physicians (including Ramazzini), and the surgery of neoplasms became somewhat more extensive. Several treatises on mastectomies for breast cancer, including dissection of regional lymph nodes, were written. Ramazzini attributed the high occurrence of breast cancer among nuns to the celibate life of these women. This was the first example of occupation-associated cancer, an observation that has withstood the test of time. In addition, in 1761, John Hill of London suggested that tobacco in the form of snuff was a cause of nasal tumors or polyps.

It was not until the nineteenth century, however, that physicians and scientists began to study cancer systematically and intensively. The anatomist Bichat extended the principles of Galen, which had reigned supreme for more than 1600 years. Bichat (1821) described the anatomy of many neoplasms in the human and suggested that cancer was an "accidental formation" of tissue built up in the same manner as any other portion of the organism. Seventeen years later, Johannes Müller (1838) extended the findings of Bichat through the use of the microscope. Although the cellular theory was just being formulated during this period, Müller independently demonstrated that cancer tissue was made up of cells. At the time little was known about cell division, and Pasteur and others had not yet demonstrated the doctrine *Omnis cellula e cellula*, that is, "Every cell from a cell."

A student of Müller, Rudolf Virchow (1863), dramatically extended our descriptive knowledge of cancer; although he proposed a number of theories that were later disproved, he was the first to point out a relation between chronic irritation and some cancers.

Early in this rapid advance of our knowledge of cancer, two possible pathogenetic bases for the origin of cancer were proposed—that normal cells are converted to cancer cells, or that cancer cells exist from embryonic life but do not express themselves until later in the organism's existence. Müller (1838) supported the latter concept, as did Julius Cohnheim, who in 1877 advanced the "embryonal rest theory" of cancer. On the other hand, many pathologists, such as Laënnec, argued that a number of cancers resemble the normal tissues of the body and that "there are as many varieties of these as there are kinds of normal tissues." Laënnec did, however, recognize that a number of tumors bore no direct resemblance to any normal tissue found in the adult organism. Laënnec's studies supported the cellular theory (see above) and actually added to it the words *ejusdem naturae*, which, combined with the original statement, may be translated as "Every cell arises from a cell *of the same kind*" (cf. Shimkin, 1977).

In 1829, Recamier published *Recherches du Cancer*, in which he specifically introduced the term *metastases* and described clearly how cancer spreads by this method (Chapter 2). Another major advance was the demonstration by Waldeyer (1872) that metastases were the result of cell emboli. In addition, he was able to show that cells from primary cancers infiltrated blood and lymphatic vessels.

After major advances had been made in the knowledge of the biology of human cancer, experimental oncology emerged as a separate area of study. The first example of the successful transplantation of an experimental tumor was reported by Novinsky (1877), who succeeded in transplanting a nasal cancer from an adult dog to several puppies and then maintained the cancer in vivo for at least one or two generations. By 1900, some animal neoplasms had been carried through many generations of grafts with few alterations in the microscopic appearance of the cancers.

Students interested in a more detailed and readable discussion of some aspects of the history of the science of oncology are referred to Shimkin's *Contrary to Nature* (1977), which shows by extensive illustration and relatively complete documentation the development of oncology from ancient times to many of the major discoveries through 1975.

During the nineteenth century, many hypotheses of the origin and development of cancer were presented. In general, these hypotheses may be categorized as follows:

1. The irritation hypothesis
2. The embryonal hypothesis
3. The parasitic hypothesis

The first hypothesis encompassed what little was known at the time of the effects of chemical agents, mostly crude, and of radiation in the genesis of cancer. The relation of some ulcerations, both internal and external, to cancer appeared to support and strengthen this hypothesis. Cancers arising in old scars and those occurring after both acute and chronic injury were also cited in support of the irritation hypothesis.

Perhaps the most common example in support of the embryonal hypothesis is the nevus, or common mole of the skin. In most instances nevi are present from birth, and a very small percentage of such structures become cancerous. Many cancers that appear to resemble embryonic tissue, such as the teratoma (Chapter 2) occurring in the adult, also support this hypothesis.

Prior to the nineteenth century, Hippocrates' "black bile" theory of cancer causation served to inhibit any concepts of an infectious etiology of cancer. However, in view of the rapid advances in our understanding of infectious disease during the last century by Pasteur and numerous others, physicians and scientists have searched for an infectious origin of cancer during the last 100 years. Several reports appeared at the end of the nineteenth century, including that of Doven, who described a bacterium, *Micrococcus neoformans*, which he isolated from several neoplasms and believed to be the cause of all types of cancer (cf. Bett, 1957; Oberling, 1952). As it turned out, this organism was merely a common staphylococcus. It was not until the twentieth century that the infectious hypothesis became scientifically sound. Even with the dawn of this century, more than 50 years were to pass before proper scientific recognition was given to the parasitic hypothesis (see Chapter 4).

CANCER: TODAY

Today the demographics and statistics of cancer in the human race have become topics of great popular concern and study. An interesting prelude to the extensive statistical and epidemiologic investigations (Chapters 11 and 12) of human cancer was the book *The Mortality from Cancer Throughout the World*, by F. L. Hoffman (1915), which in part comprised a report to the Prudential Insurance Company of America on the "statistics" of cancer and its application to the life insurance industry. A number of the points raised by Hoffman in relation to the increase in cancer incidence seen in the world at that time, the mortality from cancer in different occupations, and the geographical consideration of cancer statistics have all proved to be major factors in our understanding of cancer as a disease in the human race today.

Incidence

The incidence of cancer in the human population may be defined as the rate of diagnosis of the disease in the human population. This can be expressed in a variety of ways, as demonstrated by several tables and figures in this chapter. For the student it is important to gain a clear understanding of the distinction between cancer incidence rates and cancer mortality rates, the latter being discussed later in this chapter. Cancer survival rates are related to cancer mortality rates by the success or failure of the therapy of the disease.

Table 1.1 lists the ten most common cancers in the world (excepting nonmelanotic skin cancer) in 1985 on the basis of estimates by the International Agency for Research on Cancer (Parkin et al., 1993; Pisani et al., 1993). The basis of these studies was an investigation of cancer incidence and mortality patterns in 23 geographical areas of the world, as depicted in Figure 1.2. In this worldwide survey, the crude cancer incidence rates (see below) for all (or most) of the countries in a given area were estimated and then the weighted average was calculated, where the weights are the populations of the individual countries as determined in 1985. Wherever possible, incidence rates were derived from population-based cancer registries or other reliable sources (Parkin et al., 1993). In countries in which no incidence data were available but mortality rates from cancer could be obtained, estimates of incidence were determined with a set of conversion factors (Parkin et al., 1993). Similarly, for countries or regions in which valid cause-specific mortality information is not available, mortality rates have been estimated from incidence data. For a given cancer site, mortality is empirically related to incidence by the following relationship:

$$M = I\,[k - S_i]$$

where S_i is the relative survival at year i of follow-up, while k is a constant depending on i. M and I are the mortality and incidence rates respectively (Pisani et al., 1993). Muir (1990) has also

Table 1.1 The Most Frequent Cancers Worldwide, 1985

	Males Number[a]		Females Number[a]		Both Sexes Number[a]	
	New Cases	Deaths	New Cases	Deaths	New Cases	Deaths
1. Lung / 1. Breast / 1. Lung	677	600	719	308	896	785
2. Stomach / 2. Cervix / 2. Stomach	472	384	437	203	755	620
3. Colon/rectum / 3. Colon/rectum / 3. Breast	331	191	347	203	719	308
4. Prostate / 4. Stomach / 4. Colon/rectum	270	166	283	236	678	394
5. Mouth/pharynx / 5. Lung / 5. Cervix	291	149	162	106	437	203
6. Liver / 6. Ovary / 6. Mouth/pharynx	195	187	143	96	413	272
7. Esophagus / 7. Mouth/pharynx / 7. Lymphoma	214	212	140	55	302	287
8. Bladder / 8. Corpus uteri / 8. Liver	182	82	219	185	315	312
9. Lymphoma / 9. Esophagus / 9. Esophagus	181	109	107	100	316	188
10. Leukemia / 10. Lymphoma / 10. Prostate	121	99	135	79	291	149
11. Larynx / 11. / 11. Bladder	121	62	—	—	243	113
12. / 12. / 12. Leukemia	—	—	—	—	217	178

[a] In thousands of cases.

Adapted from Pisani et al., 1993.

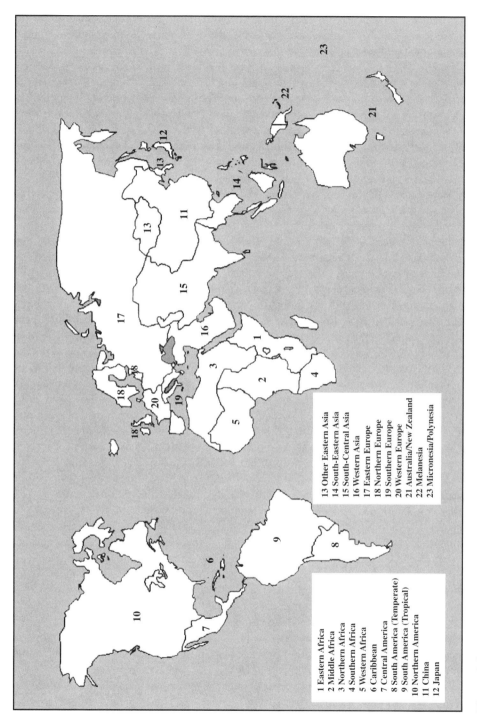

Figure 1.2 Map showing the 24 world areas studied by the International Agency for Research on Cancer (IARC) to obtain the data of Table 1.1. (Adapted from Pisani et al., 1999, with permission of authors and publisher.)

1 Eastern Africa
2 Middle Africa
3 Northern Africa
4 Southern Africa
5 Western Africa
6 Caribbean
7 Central America
8 South America (Temperate)
9 South America (Tropical)
10 Northern America
11 China
12 Japan

13 Other Eastern Asia
14 South-Eastern Asia
15 South-Central Asia
16 Western Asia
17 Eastern Europe
18 Northern Europe
19 Southern Europe
20 Western Europe
21 Australia/New Zealand
22 Melanesia
23 Micronesia/Polynesia

indicated that the expected increase in cancer in the world each year is approximately 6.4 million new cases. This number is almost equally divided between Third World countries and those that are more developed.

In the United States, the most accurate cancer incidence rates are those of the National Cancer Institute's Surveillance, Epidemiology, and End Results (SEER) program, now covering 12 geographic areas with population-based registries. These include the metropolitan areas of Atlanta, Detroit, New Orleans, Seattle–Puget Sound, and Oakland–San Francisco as well as the states of Connecticut, Iowa, New Jersey, New Mexico, Utah, and Hawaii and the Commonwealth of Puerto Rico. Several more population areas are due to be added to the SEER program in the near future. This program involves a sample of approximately 10% of the U.S. population and thus has a base analogous to that of the world incidence study seen in Table 1.1. While this is a very large sample of the U.S. population and has been shown to reflect trends in cancer statistics for the entire country, some race-, sex-, and site-specific differences in the magnitude of trends and levels of mortality occur in the SEER data as compared with those from the entire U.S. population (Frey et al., 1992).

On the basis of previous data from the SEER program, the American Cancer Society estimated that, in the United States in 1993, approximately 1.17 million new cases of cancer, excluding nonmelanoma skin cancer, would occur, essentially equally divided between males and females. For a child born in 1985, the probability at birth of developing cancer (excluding nonmelanotic skin cancer) at some time during its life span is about 33%. The probability for that individual of eventually dying of cancer is about 20% (Centers for Disease Control, 1986). In general, males have a higher age-specific incidence of cancer than females when all sites combined are considered. Even in the best-controlled epidemiological studies as exemplified by the SEER program, these data may be incomplete, since some cases of cancer are never diagnosed. The failure to diagnose cancer is related not only to the lack of contact of an individual with a physician but also to the frequent lack of interaction of a patient with the best methods of cancer diagnosis, found only in modern hospitals. Earlier studies (cf. Bauer et al., 1973) demonstrated that the likelihood of discovering an undiagnosed or incorrectly diagnosed case of cancer increases dramatically as the number of hospital admissions increases. Thus, as medical care for the U.S. population improves in efficiency and availability, it is hoped that the patient who seeks medical advice and has undiagnosed cancer will become a relative rarity in our society.

Except for cancer of the skin—the most common and, in most cases, the most curable of human cancers—75% of all cancers in humans in the United States occur in only ten anatomic sites: colon and rectum, breast, lung and bronchus, prostate, uterus, lymph organs, bladder, stomach, blood, and pancreas. In the U.S. male, one of the most common sites is the lung, accounting for 17% of such cancers in 1993 (American Cancer Society, 1993). A similarly common site of cancer incidence in the U.S. male is the prostate, which accounts for 27% of the 10 most common cancers. In the U.S. female, cancer of the breast accounts for 32% of these cancers; in both males and females in the United States, the incidence of cancer of the colon and rectum is approximately 13% of all cancers.

The age-specific incidence of cancer at the four most frequent sites for males and females as reported by the most recent SEER publication (Miller et al., 1992) is seen in Figure 1.3. In the male, the incidence of these cancers increases dramatically after age 40 and continues throughout life except for cancer of the lung and bronchus. The reason for this decline in men over age 80 has been speculated to be the result of either (1) the relatively low incidence of smoking in this group as young individuals, since smoking became most popular after the 1930s, or (2) the lethality of the disease and its greater incidence in the 60- to 80-year-old age range. The former explanation does not coincide with the study by Harris (1983), who reported that, in a representative sample of the U.S. population, maximum exposure to cigarette smoking probably oc-

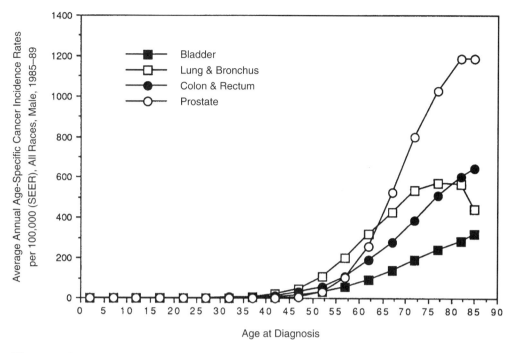

Figure 1.3A   Age-specific cancer incidence in U.S. males of all races based on incidence rates (1986–1988). Data obtained from the SEER study. (Miller et al., 1992.)

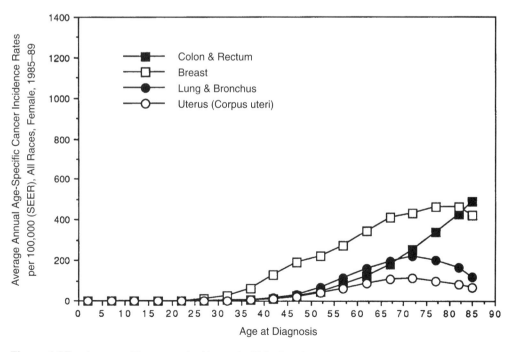

Figure 1.3B   Age-specific cancer incidence in U.S. females of all races based on incidence rates (1986–1988). Data obtained from the SEER study. (Miller et al., 1992.)

curred among men now in their seventh and eighth decades. In that study it was also postulated that the peak exposure to smoking probably occurred in women presently in their fifth and sixth decades; this would also conform with the decreasing incidence of lung cancer in females over age 70. Today, deaths from lung cancer exceed those from breast cancer in women (see below). The reason for the slight decrease in breast cancer and in cancer of the uterus at older ages is not readily apparent.

On a worldwide basis, the incidence of various types of potentially fatal cancers is somewhat different from that in the United States, as noted in Table 1.1, when compared with Figure 1.3. As in the United States, the total cancer burden in the world includes cancer of the lung and cancer of the breast as exhibiting the highest incidences in males and females, respectively. When all areas were considered together for both sexes, the most frequent cancer worldwide in 1980 was cancer of the lung (Table 1.1). Stomach cancer remains the most common cancer in some parts of the world, including Japan, China, other east Asian countries, and the former Soviet Union, and incidence rates still remain relatively high in both Europe and Latin America. Nevertheless, stomach cancer is declining in frequency almost everywhere in the world, with the estimated number of cases decreasing by 1.9% since the previous estimates in 1975. This is especially noteworthy since a population increase of 9.4% occurred during the same period. Unlike stomach cancer, lung cancer has been increasing in incidence between 1975 and 1980, by 11.8% in males and 16% in females worldwide. Thus, lung cancer is the most common fatal cancer in the human race as we approach the twenty-first century. Another striking finding from these data is that cancers of the breast and cervix, both limited to females, have a higher incidence than the two most common cancers in males—lung and stomach. Although it is possible that the increasing incidence of breast cancer worldwide may be the result of changes in the way the estimates are calculated (Parkin et al., 1993), cancer of the uterine cervix is also increasing, especially in underdeveloped nations, in which methods for early diagnosis are not as well developed as in the "developed" areas of the world.

In the United States, the most dramatic changes in the incidence of cancer also reflect those seen in the world. This is exemplified in Figure 1.4, showing the change in incidence of specific cancer types during the period 1950–1989. As seen from the figure, the most striking differences are again seen in cancer of the lung and bronchus, with the percentage change being greatest in females during this period. Among other cancers that increased dramatically during this period, non-Hodgkin's lymphomas, melanomas, and cancers of the kidney, testes, and prostate increased by more than 100%. The incidence of cancer of the breast, while increasing markedly during this period, has not seen a dramatic change like those indicated above. Not listed in the figure is the recent finding of the dramatic increases seen in the incidence of brain cancers in the period 1973–1985. The most dramatic increases during this period were noted for persons aged 75 to 79, 80 to 84, and 85 years and older, where the relative increases were 187%, 394%, and 501% respectively (Greig et al., 1990).

There are even more striking differences in the incidences of specific cancers in certain areas and countries of the world. The rates for a variety of cancers in the highest- and lowest-incidence areas are shown in Table 1.2. The incidence rates of some cancers may vary as much as 300-fold in different areas of the world. Such variability led some epidemiologists more than two decades ago, when this information first became available, to suggest that most cancers in humans are the result of environmental factors, since inherent genetic and related factors could not explain such large differences in incidence of specific cancers in various parts of the world (cf. Wynder and Gori, 1977).

Changes in the incidence of cancer may be due either to an absolute change in the incidence—resulting, for example, from some alteration in the environment or to better diagnostic methods—which give rise to an apparent increase in the incidence of a specific cancer. One ex-

Primary Site	Percent Change in Incidence 1950–1989

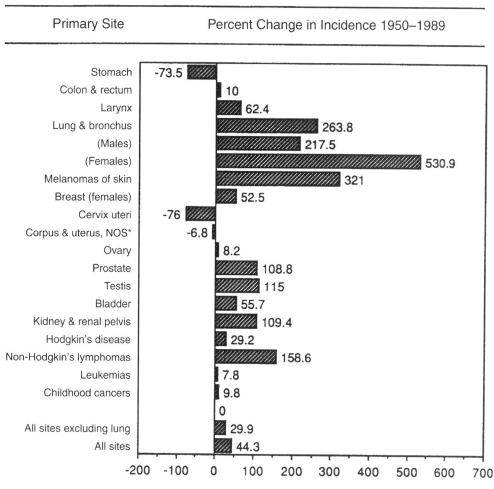

Figure 1.4 Percentage change in incidence of major potentially fatal cancers in the U.S. population for the period 1950–1989. (Miller et al., 1992.) *Not otherwise specified.

ample of the latter was described by Linos and associates (1981) for a bone marrow cancer, multiple myeloma. Although a number of incidence studies indicated that multiple myeloma had increased significantly in recent years in the United States, no such increase occurred in the population of a carefully monitored county in Minnesota over a 20-year period. Since no other study that reported increased incidence rates analyzed a well-defined population over a long period, it is likely that the increased incidence of multiple myeloma reported in several other parts of the country were the result of improved diagnosis. This factor is also important when one attempts to compare incidence, mortality, and survival rates over defined periods of time (see below).

Mortality Rates

Mortality rates from cancer are usually more easily obtained for statistical studies, and the data are usually more reliable, than incidence rates. However, in many developing countries, few or

Table 1.2 Incidence Rates for Common Cancers Among Males and Certain Cancers Among Females

Site of Origin of Cancer	High-Incidence Area	Sex	Cumulative Incidence in High-Incidence Area (%)[a]	Ratio of Highest to Lowest Rate[b]	Low-Incidence Area
Skin (chiefly nonmelanoma)	Australia, Queensland	Male	20	200	India, Bombay
Esophagus	Iran, northeast section	Male	20	300	Nigeria
Lung and bronchus	England	Male	11	35	Nigeria
Stomach	Japan	Male	11	25	Uganda
Cervix uteri	Columbia	Female	10	15	Israel: Jews
Prostate	United States: blacks	Male	9	40	Japan
Liver	Mozambique	Male	8	100	England
Breast	Canada, British Columbia	Female	7	7	Israel: non-Jews
Colon	United States, Connecticut	Male	3	10	Nigeria
Corpus uteri	United States, California	Female	3	30	Japan
Buccal cavity	India, Bombay	Male	2	25	Denmark
Rectum	Denmark	Male	2	20	Nigeria
Bladder	United States, Connecticut	Male	2	6	Japan
Ovary	Denmark	Female	2	6	Japan
Nasopharynx	Singapore: Chinese	Male	2	40	England
Pancreas	New Zealand: Maori	Male	2	8	India, Bombay
Larynx	Brazil, Sao Paulo	Male	2	10	Japan
Pharynx	India, Bombay	Male	2	20	Denmark
Penis	Parts of Uganda	Male	1	300	Israel: Jews

[a]By age 75 years, in the absence of other causes of death.
[b]At ages 35–64 years, standardized for age. At these ages, even the data from cancer registries in poor countries are likely to be reasonably reliable (although at older ages serious underreporting may affect the data).
From Doll and Peto, 1981, with permission of the authors and publisher.

no cancer mortality data are available. The methods utilized for mortality rates under such circumstances have been outlined by Pisani et al. (1993) in their estimates of worldwide mortality from major cancers, as noted in Table 1.1. As seen from the table, in a few instances, mortalities for cancer of the liver and esophagus are almost identical, indicating that the therapy of such cancers is mostly unsuccessful. The SEER program, which is carefully monitored, has made estimations of incidence and mortality rates in the population base of their continuing study. On the other hand, some studies of mortality rates that have been published do not reflect the SEER data (Frey et al., 1992) but rather consider data taken from a variety of sources, most notably death certificates and data from Health Departments in states where cancer is a reportable disease. The most notable of such studies was carried out by a number of individuals at the National Cancer Institute on data obtained through the National Center for Health Statistics, which in turn obtained data from individual counties throughout the country. These studies resulted in a series of maps, each relating the mortality of a specific cancer in each of the 3056 counties of the 48 contiguous states from 1950 to 1969 (cf. Fraumeni, 1983). This heroic effort led to a number of interesting findings, which potentially related certain environmental factors to unusual incidences of specific types of cancer. A number of these are discussed in a later chapter (Chapter 10). The United States was not unique in this form of study of cancer mortality within its own borders, in that England and Wales went through a similar exercise (Gardner, 1984), and the People's Republic of China carried out a similar but far more extensive study of cancer mortality rates within its borders for a number of different types of cancers.

Although the geographic distribution of cancer mortality within specific regions of a country has been studied, it is important to understand the overall cancer mortality within a single country. In the United States, the American Cancer Society has maintained annual studies of age-adjusted cancer death rates for selected anatomic sites for both males and females. The most recent extension of these studies is seen in Figure 1.5. For both males and females, the most dramatic increase over the years has been in the mortality from lung cancer. In fact, in 1988, the mortality rate for lung cancer in women surpassed that of breast cancer, previously the most fatal cancer in this sex in this country. In 1992, just under 20% of all deaths in developed countries can be attributed to tobacco usage in one form or another; however, this percentage is still rising (Peto et al., 1992). In 1995, there were over 2.1 million deaths due to tobacco usage in all developed countries, this figure extrapolating to an annual death rate of 3.4 million by the year 2025. During this time, Hirayama (1987) predicted that lung cancer mortality will decrease in most developed countries but continue to increase in Japan, so that it will exceed the lung cancer death rates in most European and North American developed countries.

Other trends in this chart are discussed below; however, it should be noted that whereas the data of Figure 1.5 reflect the entire population, certain segments of the population exhibit significantly different characteristics of cancer mortality and incidence. These include members of certain religious groups (Phillips et al., 1980) and nonsmokers (Enstrom, 1979a), who exhibit lower rates of both incidence and mortality for many types of cancer, especially lung in the latter case, as well as an increased incidence and mortality of cancer in patients of older age groups. However, it was recognized more than two decades ago that lung cancer mortality is rising among nonsmokers (Enstrom, 1979b). Several studies have proposed that this increase is due in large part to passive or involuntary exposure of nonsmokers to cigarette smoke (Vainio and Partanen, 1989; Woodward and McMichael, 1991). Figure 1.6 shows the mortality due to all cancers in several different age groups.

The mortality from cancer of individuals less than 45 years of age has been decreasing significantly during the past three decades. This decrease is probably the result of the greater efficacy of cancer therapy, especially drug therapy (Miller and McKay, 1984) for childhood cancer, as is discussed more extensively in Chapter 16.

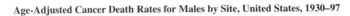

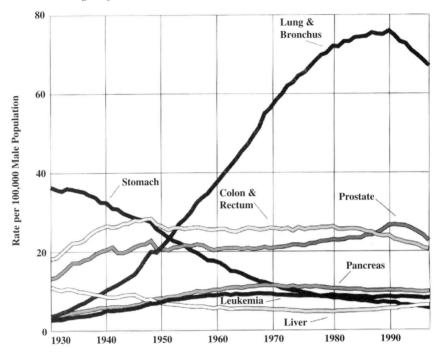

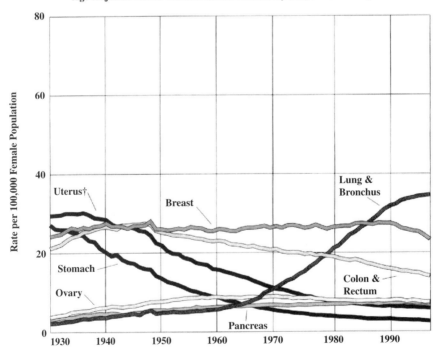

Figure 1.5 Cancer death rates by site in the United States from 1930 to 1990 in males and females. (American Cancer Society, 2001, with permission.)

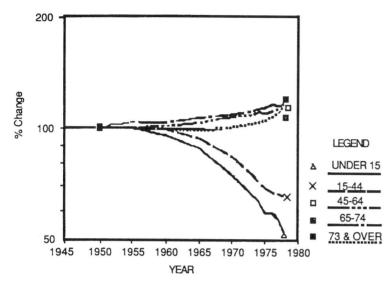

Figure 1.6   Cancer mortality by age group, all races, men and women in the United States between 1950 and 1980. The mortality rate in 1950 is taken as 100%. (Davis et al., 1990, with permission of authors and publisher.)

Although considerable financial and human effort has been expended, especially during the last two decades, in attempts to control and/or eradicate cancer in the U.S. population, it is clear that we are still a long way from achieving such goals. Recently, investigators both in this country (Bailar and Gornik, 1997) and abroad (Becker et al., 1989) have indicated that despite all the advances being made, the overall mortality for cancer has not improved significantly during the last decade, although, as shown in Figures 1.5 and 1.6, mortality rates have decreased in certain subsets of the population. The data presented in both of these publications are generally valid, but the crude overall data hide many advances that have been made. Furthermore, the preponderance of mortality due to lung cancer, now in both sexes, skews the data toward an unfavorable conclusion. Removal of this single, most preventable cause of human cancer from these statistics results in a stabilization or significant decrease in mortality rates from all other cancers over the last several decades (Holleb, 1986). Furthermore, more effective therapy of cancer has effectively delayed death in older patients from the more common cancers of the colon, breast, lung, and others but has not eliminated the inevitable (Mathé, 1986). In addition, as pointed out by these two investigators (Holleb, 1986; Mathé, 1986), early lesions in the development of human cancer are not considered in such statistical evaluations, although their treatment and control would clearly have an impact on the overall figures. Furthermore, Cole and Rodu (1996) have reviewed vital statistics from the United States Department of Health and Human Services as well as the SEER program for the period 1990 to 1995 in relation to overall age-adjusted cancer mortality rates. These authors found that the rate declined by about 4.2% in the United States during this period and proposed that the decline is due both to the effect of cancer prevention and to improved medical care and therapy of the disease. This decline in cancer mortality may be seen in greater detail in Figure 1.7, wherein the annual percentage change in cancer death rates in the United States from 1970 to 1995, broken into two time periods and related to major cancers as well as age, is seen. It should be noted that in virtually none of the specific types of neoplasms or age ranges has the change seen between 1990 and 1995 been significantly

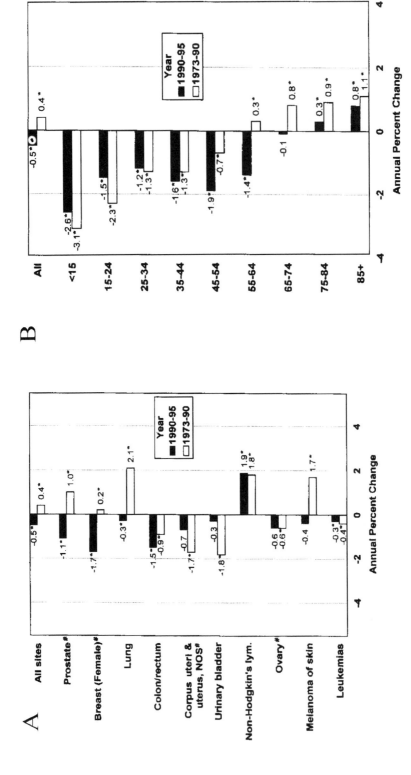

Figure 1.7 Annual percentage change in U.S. Cancer Death Rates for the top ten sites (A) and by age (B) for all races and genders except prostate and breast cancer as noted. *The annual percent change (APC) is significantly different from zero ($p < 0.05$). Death rates are age adjusted to the 1970 U.S. standard million population. NOS, not otherwise specified; lym, lymphoma. (Modified from Wingo et al., 1998, with permission of authors and publisher.)

greater than that between 1973 and 1990. Despite these various arguments, however, it is clear that hundreds of thousands of persons die from cancer in the United States, and millions in the entire world, each year. The decrease in the mortality of cancer in the young is laudable but does not make a major impact on the numerous deaths from this disease in the older age groups.

Survival Rates

In the early part of this century, relatively few cancer patients had any hope of long-term survival. In the 1930s less than 1 person in 5 remained alive 5 years after the initial treatment for the disease. This ratio increased to 1 in 4 during the next decade, and by the 1960s it was 1 in 3. At the present time it is estimated by the American Cancer Society (1994) that some 483,000 Americans, or 4 out of 10 patients diagnosed with potentially fatal cancer this year, will be alive 5 years after diagnosis. This increase in survival from the 1960s represents a total of almost 85,000 persons in 1994 by comparison. This number is termed the *observed* survival rate, which is an estimate of the proportion of the original group of patients who survive the selected length of time. The *expected* survival rate is that of a group similar to the patient group in such characteristics as age, sex, and race but free of the specific disease under study, in this case cancer (Ederer et al., 1961). The *expected* rate is related to factors such as death from heart disease, accidents, and diseases of old age. The *relative* survival rate is the ratio of the observed survival rate during a specific interval to the *expected* survival rate. Therefore, a relative survival rate of less than 100% indicates that, during the specified interval, mortality in the patient group was greater than that of persons in the general population free of disease under study comprising the expected survival rate group (Ederer et al., 1961). Many consider the relative survival rate a more accurate yardstick for measuring the results of cancer therapy (American Cancer Society, 1994). Another term that is used somewhat less frequently is the *prevalence* of cancer. This is defined as the number of existing cases of cancer in a given population at a specific time. It takes into account both incidence and survival and is important in planning for health care and other needs of cancer survivors (Polednak, 1997). In 1982 it was estimated that the prevalence of cancer was approximately 2% of the American population who had ever received a diagnosis of invasive cancer (Feldman et al., 1986). However, calculation of the prevalence of cancer is somewhat complex, and a number of assumptions must be made that may or may not be entirely valid (Coldman et al., 1992).

Increasing survival trends after the initial diagnosis of cancer have not been limited to the United States. In Sweden the 5-year relative survival increased from 34% to 47% in males and 49% to 57% in females between the periods 1960–64 and 1980–84 (Adami et al., 1989). During the period 1960–78, the observed and relative survival of cancer of the colon in Sweden decreased; but after 5 years of survival, there was essentially no change in the relative survival for the next 15 years (Adami, 1988). This relationship between 5- and 20-year relative survival rates is also true for most of the major human cancers, as seen in Figure 1.8. The two cancers that deviate most dramatically from the mean are prostate and breast cancer. The former deviation is probably owing to the relatively old age at which diagnosis is made, thus leading to relatively few 20-year survivors under any condition. In contrast, cancer of the breast in a significant number of cases remains latent for many years after treatment before reappearing at a later date (cf. Chapter 7).

Not all survival trends follow the general changes noted above. In the United States, young white patients ages 0 to 14 diagnosed with cancer, especially acute leukemia (Steinhorn and Ries, 1988), have shown dramatic increases in 5-year survival rates, but the survival of all black patients with cancer has not improved nearly as dramatically as that of white patients for the periods 1960–63 to 1980–85 (Table 1.3). As pointed out by Freeman and associates (Cummings

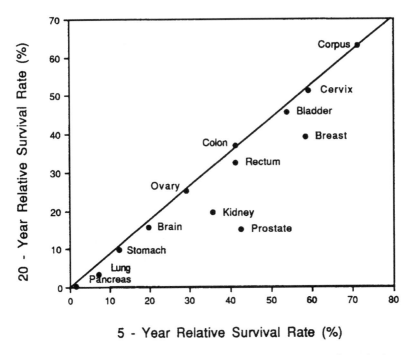

Figure 1.8 Relation between 5- and 20-year relative survival rates for major human cancers.

and Floyd, 1989), the major reason for this difference is not race but rather the economic and social conditions that place members of the black race in the United States at a marked disadvantage in health care compared with the white population. Blacks and whites of the same economic status exhibit the same level of survival from this disease. One may also see distinctive differences in the survival of patients with specific diseases such as Hodgkin's disease who are treated in major cancer centers as compared with those receiving treatment for the disease in other settings representative of the average population. When these two groups are compared with respect to the survival from Hodgkin's disease, the mortality rate among SEER patients in the

Table 1.3 5-Year Relative Rates (Percentages), All Sites Combined, Males and Females

Race	Year of Diagnosis				
	1960–63[a]	1970–73[a]	1974–76[b]	1977–79[b]	1980–85[b]
All races	38	42	48.9	49.2	49.8[c]
Whites	39	43	49.9	50.3	51.1[c]
Blacks	27	31	38.6	38.4	38.1
Whites, ages 0–14	28	45	55.0	61.2	65.2[c]

[a]Rates are based on End Results Group data from a series of hospital registries and one population-based registry.
[b]Rates are from the SEER Program. They are based on data from population-based registries in Connecticut, New Mexico, Utah, Iowa, Hawaii, Atlanta, Detroit, Seattle–Puget Sound, and San Francisco–Oakland. Rates are based on follow-up of patients through 1986.
[c]The difference in rates between 1974–76 and 1980–85 is statistically significant ($p < 0.05$).

average population was approximately 50% greater than that among patients treated at major cancer centers (Davis et al., 1987). Finally, another complicating factor is the risk of a second primary cancer after the diagnosis of cancer at the original site. Relative risks (observed:expected values) for the development of such cancers range from approximately 1.1 in a large study in Denmark (Storm et al., 1986) to almost 6 as reported from Japan by Okamoto et al. (1987). Further consideration of this complication appears later (Chapter 16).

Trends and Factors in Cancer Incidence, Mortality, and Survival

In general, the cancer death rates by site for males and females parallel the incidence rates (Figures 1.4 and 1.5), especially with cancers of the stomach, lung, pancreas, brain, liver, ovary, and several other sites. On the other hand, for certain types of cancer, the mortality rates have fallen dramatically during the past several decades. This is true for cancer of the uterus and cervix, where the overall death rate has decreased more than 70% over the past 40 years. This is probably due to the widespread use of the Pap test (Chapter 2) and early detection of cervical cancer. Mortality from colorectal cancer has fallen 29% for women and 6% for men during the past 30 years, while—as pointed out earlier—the mortality rate for cancer in children has declined 60% since 1950 primarily because of better methods of treatment. In some cancers, such as cancer of the stomach, there has been a steady decrease in both incidence and mortality in this country and in many others since the 1930s, although in Japan the decrease in mortality did not begin to occur until after 1955 (Coggon and Acheson, 1984). In contrast, not only in this country (Figures 1.3 to 1.5) but throughout the world, cancer of the lung has been increasing in both sexes.

Since 1978, in the age group 75 to 84, trends of cancer incidence have revealed significant increases in myeloma, a cancer of the bone marrow, as well as cancers of the breast and the brain (see above) (Davis et al., 1990). The reasons for such specific changes in incidence of the cancer mentioned—with the exception of tobacco abuse—are not entirely clear. However, such factors as diet, workplace conditions, and infectious disease may have played a role in this group during their younger years as well as in the population in general. These factors will be considered later in the text (Chapter 10).

Trends in relative survival rates in the United States for white males and females over the quarter century beginning in 1960 may be seen in Table 1.4. Survival rates in a number of different cancers have increased significantly even over the past 10 years; however, interpretation of cancer survival rates is difficult and subject to many variables, as pointed out by Enstrom and Austin (1977). Improvements in survival rates may be due to a number of factors including:

1. An increase in the proportion of cancers diagnosed at a controllable stage of development as a result of improved diagnostic techniques and of a better-informed public alerted to the danger signals of cancer and the benefits of early diagnosis
2. Improvements in surgical and supportive techniques, including the control of infectious diseases that complicate cancer
3. Improvements in radiotherapy, endocrine therapy, and chemotherapy

Specifically, for patients with lung cancer, Feinstein et al. (1985) pointed out that the enhanced survival from 1960 to 1977 was apparent rather than real, being the result of the use of new diagnostic imaging procedures to classify patients into specific "stages" of the disease more accurately. This effect has been called the "Will Rogers phenomenon" by these investigators. Cairns (1985) also pointed out that the apparent increase in survival for patients with cancer of the prostate was the result of better diagnosis, resulting in an actual increase in the number of patients reported with the disease but with no change in the actual death rate from the disease. Thus, a number of factors must be considered in determining the absolute or real survival rates of patients with cancer to obtain a clear picture of the efficacy of cancer therapy. Despite such factors, it is clear that there has been a steady though slow improvement in the survival rates of most types of cancers in the human (Table 1.4). Therefore, although the absolute numbers of cancers and cancer deaths are increasing in our society, owing primarily to one or two major types of cancer, significant advances have been made in the treatment of many types of cancer, as listed in Table 1.4.

Social and Economic Costs Resulting from Cancer

Especially significant and important to society in general in relation to this dread disease are the number of years of life lost and the cost to the individual and to society of the mortality and morbidity resulting from cancer. If a person is struck down by this disease in early or middle life, the remaining productivity of that individual's life is lost to society. When measured in dollars

Table 1.4   5-Year Relative Survival Rates (Percentage) By Selected Sites, White Males and Females

Site	Year of Diagnosis				
	1960–63[a]	1970–73[a]	1974–76[b]	1977–79[b]	1980–85[b]
All sites	39	43	49.9	50.3	51.1[c]
Oral cavity and pharynx	45	43	54.5	53.4	53.8
Esophagus	4	4	5.1	5.5	8.1[c]
Stomach	11	13	14.1	15.9	15.5[c]
Colon	43	49	50.0	52.4	55.2[c]
Rectum	38	45	48.4	50.3	52.9[c]
Liver	2	3	4.3	2.7	4.3
Pancreas	1	2	2.8	2.1	2.7
Larynx	53	62	66.1	67.5	68.2
Lung and bronchus	8	10	12.2	13.4	13.1[c]
Skin (melanoma)	60	68	79.2	80.8	81.0[c]
Breast (females)	63	68	74.6	74.7	76.3[c]
Cervix uteri	58	64	69.0	68.4	66.9
Corpus uteri	73	81	89.0	86.5	83.4[c]
Ovary	32	36	36.1	37.2	38.4[c]
Prostate gland	50	63	67.4	71.3	73.4[c]
Testis	63	72	78.4	87.5	91.4[c]
Urinary bladder	53	61	73.3	75.1	77.7[c]
Kidney and renal pelvis	37	46	51.3	50.0	52.4
Brain and nervous system	18	20	21.8	23.6	23.5[c]
Thyroid gland	83	86	91.9	92.0	93.3
Hodgkin's disease	40	67	71.5	72.8	75.7[c]
Non-Hodgkin's lymphoma	31	41	47.3	47.8	50.9[c]
Multiple myeloma	12	19	23.8	23.9	25.8[c]
Leukemia	14	22	34.0	35.8	34.2

[a]Rates are based on End Results Group data from a series of hospital registries and one population-based registry.
[b]Rates are from the SEER Program. They are based on data from population-based registries in Connecticut, New Mexico, Utah, Iowa, Hawaii, Atlanta, Detroit, Seattle–Puget Sound, and San Francisco–Oakland. Rates are based on follow-up of patients through 1986.
[c]The difference in rates between 1974–76 and 1980–85 is statistically significant ($p < 0.05$).

alone, such a loss in the United States was estimated to be nearly $25 billion per year about a decade ago (Hodgson and Rice, 1982). In 1990, a decade later, the National Cancer Institute estimated that the overall annual cost for cancer was $104 billion and in 2000, a total of $180.2 billion. Of this $105.2 billion, or almost three times the amount estimated in 1982 represented the mortality costs, which include the loss of productivity because of premature death (Brown, 1990). In 1985, it was estimated that cancer accounts for a little more that 10% of the total cost of disease in the United States and almost 21% of the cost of premature death or mortality in this country (Hodgson and Rice, 1995).

Although it is difficult to estimate the economic impact of cancer on society with a high degree of accuracy, it is possible through the use of statistical data compiled for the United States to determine the years of life lost as a result of premature death because of cancer. Tables 1.5 and 1.6 show the person-years of life lost (PYLL) in males and females because of premature death from cancer in the United States (Horm and Sondik, 1989) for the years 1970 and 1984. A comparison of the data between the two years indicates the dramatic increase in the social and economic burden of all cancers, several in particular. In 1984 the most costly cancer for women was cancer of the breast, resulting in over 760,000 PYLL among almost 40,000 women; this was an increase of almost 28% over the 1970 figure. These women died an average of 19.3 years earlier than expected. Some studies (Shapiro et al., 1982; Tabar et al., 1985) have indicated that the mortality from breast cancer can be reduced by 30% through mass screening programs. This would mean the prevention of almost 12,000 breast cancer deaths per year, or nearly 230,000 PYL that could be saved. Similarly, the PYLL to lung cancer in women in 1984 was almost triple that in 1970. In men, the toll of this cancer is considerably higher. In both

Table 1.5 Person-Years of Life Lost (PYLL) Due to Premature Deaths from Cancer in the United States, All Races, Males

Cancer Sites	Number of Deaths		PYLL	
	1970	1984	1970	1984
All sites	179,352	242,763	2,558,996	3,284,558
Oral cavity	5,495	5,764	79,810	87,527
Esophagus	4,442	6,312	62,308	90,091
Stomach	9,802	8,469	121,490	107,681
Colon and rectum	22,117	27,989	269,512	338,649
Pancreas	10,061	11,516	130,937	149,202
Lung	52,680	82,385	751,081	1,113,112
Skin (melanoma)	1,735	3,207	34,394	62,209
Breast	265	250	3,552	3,409
Prostate gland	17,249	25,400	156,281	228,597
Testis	760	401	26,693	14,343
Urinary bladder	6,257	6,600	66,853	66,762
Kidney	3,858	5,201	59,091	74,664
Brain and central nervous system	3,434	5,395	81,686	111,329
Hodgkin's disease	2,016	1,204	50,566	31,461
Non-Hodgkin's lymphoma	5,233	7,312	94,256	115,937
Multiple myeloma	2,340	3,737	30,269	46,449
Leukemia	8,128	9,378	174,139	166,464

Adapted from Horm and Sondik, 1989, with permission of authors and publisher.

Table 1.6 Person-Years of Life Lost (PYLL) Due to Premature Deaths from Cancer in the United States, All Races, Females

Cancer Sites	Number of Deaths		PYLL	
	1970	1984	1970	1984
All sites	150,023	210,687	2,744,672	3,596,723
Oral cavity	2,115	2,697	38,043	46,568
Esophagus	1,527	2,345	25,597	36,667
Stomach	6,218	5,777	88,216	83,364
Colon and rectum	23,807	29,521	345,751	406,293
Pancreas	7,824	11,638	116,015	165,817
Lung	12,323	36,180	238,254	643,889
Skin (melanoma)	1,411	2,170	32,507	48,556
Breast	29,647	39,470	593,498	760,102
Cervix uteri	6,547	4,564	146,261	105,899
Corpus uteri	5,468	5,965	88,100	89,563
Ovary	9,831	11,208	193,462	200,279
Urinary bladder	2,754	3,114	34,171	36,414
Kidney	2,245	3,210	41,219	53,273
Brain and central nervous system	2,593	4,471	72,197	104,476
Hodgkin's disease	1,394	756	38,683	21,561
Non-Hodgkin's lymphoma	4,359	7,174	81,976	116,135
Multiple myeloma	2,077	3,733	32,773	54,287
Leukemia	6,364	7,837	159,300	154,01

Adapted from Horm and Sondik, 1989, with permission of authors and publisher.

sexes, prevention of the disease by the cessation of tobacco abuse could save well over a million PYL every year (Horm and Sondik, 1989).

These statistics on cancer incidence, mortality, survival, and economic and social impact are critical to our understanding of the impact of this disease on our society. Obviously, these figures cannot take into account the morbidity and suffering, both mental and physical, caused by cancer. However, they do point out a variety of differences in the effects of this disease on males and females and in the types of cancers that are most common in our society and in other countries. Later in this text (Chapter 10), a consideration of the epidemiology of cancer includes explanations for the various statistics relative to specific neoplasms.

REFERENCES

Adami, H. O. Aspects of descriptive epidemiology and survival in colorectal cancer. Scand. J. Gastroen-terol. Suppl. *149*:6–20, 1988.

Adami, H. O., Sparén, P., Bergström, R., Holmberg, L., Krusemo, U. B., and Pontén, J. Increasing survival trend after cancer diagnosis in Sweden: 1960–1984. J. Natl. Cancer Inst., *81*:1640–1647, 1989.

American Cancer Society, Cancer Facts & Figures—2001. Atlanta: American Cancer Society, 2001.

Bailar, J. C. III, and Gornik, H. L. Cancer Undefeated. N. Engl. J. Med., *336*:1569–1574, 1997.

Bauer, F. W., Robbins, S. L., and Berg, J. W. An autopsy study of cancer patients. II. Hospitalizations and accuracy of diagnoses (1955 to 1965) Boston City Hospital. J. Am. Med. Assoc., *223*:299–301, 1973.

Becker, N., Smith, E. M., and Wahrendorf, J. Time trends in cancer mortality in the Federal Republic of Germany: progress against cancer? Int. J. Cancer, *43*:245–249, 1989.

Bett, W. R. Historical aspects of cancer. *In*: R. W. Raven (Ed.), Cancer, Vol. 1, Chap. 1, pp. 1–5. London: Butterworths, 1957.

Bichat, M. F. X. Anatomie Générale, Appliquée à la Physiologie et à la Medecine (nouvelle edition). Paris: Brosson, Gabon et Cie, 1821.

Breasted, J. H. The Edwin Smith Surgical Papyrus, Vol. 1, pp. 367, 403. Chicago: University of Chicago Press, 1930.

Brown, M. L. The national economic burden of cancer: an update. J. Natl. Cancer Inst., *82*:1811–1814, 1990.

Cairns, J. The treatment of diseases and the war against cancer. Sci. Am., *253*:51–59, 1985.

Coggon, D., and Acheson, E. D. The geography of cancer of the stomach. Br. Med. Bull., *40*:335–341, 1984.

Cohnheim, J. Vorlesungen Über Allgemeine Pathologie. Berlin: A. Hirschwald, 1877.

Coldman, A. J., McBride, M. L., and Braun, T. Calculating the prevalence of cancer. Stat. Med., *11*:1579–1589, 1992.

Cole, P., and Rodu, B. Declining cancer mortality in the United States. Cancer, *78*:2045–2048, 1996.

Cummings, C. C., and Floyd, J. D. (Eds.) Human Behavior and Cancer Risk Reduction. Proceedings of Working Conference on Unmet Research Needs, August 9–11, 1989. Atlanta: American Cancer Society, 1989.

Davis, S., Dahlberg, S., Myers, M. H., Chen, A., and Steinhorn, S. C. Hodgkin's disease in the United States: a comparison of patient characteristics and survival in the centralized cancer patient data system and the surveillance, epidemiology, and end results program. J. Natl. Cancer Inst., *78*:471–478, 1987.

Davis, D. L., Hoel, D., Fox, J., and Lopez, A. D. International trends in cancer mortality in France, West Germany, Italy, Japan, England and Wales, and the United States. *In*: D. L. Davis and D. Hoel (Eds.), Trends in Cancer Mortality in Industrial Countries. Ann. N.Y. Acad. Sci., Vol. 609, pp. 5–48, 1990.

Doll, R., and Peto, R. The Causes of Cancer. New York: Oxford University Press, 1981.

Ederer, F., Axtell, I. M., and Cutler, S. J. The relative survival rate: a statistical methodology. Monogr. Natl. Cancer Inst., *6*:101–121, 1961.

Enstrom, J. E. Cancer mortality among low-risk populations. CA, *29*:352–360, 1979a.

Enstrom, J. E. Rising lung cancer mortality among nonsmokers. J. Natl. Cancer Inst., *62*:755–760, 1979b.

Enstrom, J. E., and Austin, D. F. Interpreting cancer survival rates. The available data on survival are not a sensitive measure of progress in cancer control. Science, *195*:847–851, 1977.

Feinstein, A. R., Sosin, D. M., and Wells, C. K. The Will Rogers phenomenon. Stage migration and new diagnostic techniques as a source of misleading statistics for survival in cancer. N. Engl. J. Med., *312*:1604–1608, 1985.

Feldman, A. R., Kessler, L., Myers, M. H., and Naughton, M. D. The prevalence of cancer: Estimates based on the Connecticut Tumor Registry. N. Engl. J. Med., *315*:1394–1397, 1986.

Fraumeni, J. F., Jr. The face of cancer in the United States. Hosp. Pract., December, pp. 81–96, 1983.

Frey, C. M., McMillen, M. M., Cowan, C. D., Horm, J. W., and Kessler, L. G. Representatives of the surveillance, epidemiology, and end results program data: recent trends in cancer mortality rates. J. Natl. Cancer Inst., *84*:872–877, 1992.

Gardner, M. J. Mapping cancer mortality in England and Wales. Br. Med. Bull., *40*:320–328, 1984.

Greig, N. H., Ries, L. G., Yancik, R., and Rapoport, S. I. Increasing annual incidence of primary malignant brain tumors in the elderly. J. Natl. Cancer Inst., *82*:1621–1624, 1990.

Harris, J. E. Cigarette smoking among successive birth cohorts of men and women in the United States during 1900–80. J. Natl. Cancer Inst., *71*:473–478, 1983.

Hirayama, T. The problem of smoking and lung cancer in Japan with special reference to the rising trend in age-specific mortality rate by number of cigarettes smoked daily. Jpn. J. Cancer Res. (Gann), *78*:203–210, 1987.

Hodgson, T. A., and Rice, D. P. Economic impact of cancer in the United States. *In*: D. Schottenfeld and J. F. Fraumeni, Jr. (Eds.), Cancer Epidemiology and Prevention, 2nd ed. New York: Oxford University Press, 1995.

Hoffman, F. L. The Mortality from Cancer Throughout the World. Newark, NJ: The Prudential Press, 1915.

Holleb, A. I. Progress against cancer? A broader view. CA, *36*:243–244, 1986.

Horm, J. W., and Sondik, E. J. Person-years of life lost due to cancer in the United States, 1970 and 1984. Am. J. Public Health, *79*:1490–1493, 1989.

Linos, A., Kyle, R. A., O'Fallon, W. M., and Kurland, L. T. Incidence and secular trend of multiple myeloma in Olmstead County, Minnesota: 1965–77. J. Natl. Cancer Inst., *66*:17–20, 1981.

Mathé, G. Oncologists have lost a battle against cancer; biomedicine has not lost the war. Biomed. Pharmacother., *40*:370–371, 1986.

Miller, B. A., Ries, L. A. G., Hankey, B. F., Kosary, C. L., and Edwards, B. K. (Eds). Cancer Statistics Review: 1973–1989, NIH Pub. No. 92–2789. Washington, D.C.: National Cancer Institute, 1992.

Miller, R. W., and McKay, F. W. Decline in U.S. childhood cancer mortality. J.A.M.A., *251*:1567–1570, 1984.

Muir, C. S. Epidemiology, basic science, and the prevention of cancer: implications for the future. Cancer Res., *50*:6441–6448, 1990.

Müller, J. Ueber den feinern Bau und die Formen der krankhaften Geschwülste. Berlin: G. Reimer, 1838.

Novinsky, M. On the question of inoculation of malignant neoplasms (thesis). St. Peterburg: Yakov Trey, 1877.

Oberling, C. The Riddle of Cancer. New Haven, CT: Yale University Press, 1952.

Okamoto, N., Morio, S., Inoue, R., and Akiyama, K. The risk of a second primary cancer occurring in five-year survivors of an initial cancer. Jpn. J. Clin. Oncol., *17*:205–213, 1987.

Parkin, D. M., Pisani, P., and Ferlay, J. Estimates of the worldwide incidence of eighteen major cancers in 1985. Int. J. Cancer, *54*:594–606, 1993.

Peto, R., Lopez, A. D., Boreham, J., Thun, M., and Heath, C., Jr. Mortality from tobacco in developed countries: indirect estimation from national vital statistics. Lancet, *339*:1268–1278, 1992.

Phillips, R. L., Kuzma, J. W., and Lotz, T. M. Cancer mortality among comparable members versus nonmembers of the Seventh-Day Adventist Church. Reprinted from Banbury Report 4: Cancer Incidence in Defined Populations. Cold Spring Harbor, NY: Cold Spring Harbor Laboratory, 1980.

Pisani, P., Parkin, D. M., and Ferlay, J. Estimates of the worldwide mortality from eighteen major cancers in 1985. Implications for prevention and projections of future burden. Int. J. Cancer, *55*:891–903, 1993.

Pisani, P., Parkin, D. M., Bray, F., and Ferlay, J. Estimates of the worldwide mortality from 25 cancers in 1990. Int. J. Cancer, *83*:18–29, 1999.

Polednak, A. P. Estimating the prevalence of cancer in the United States. Cancer, *80*:136–141, 1997.

Recamier, J. C. A. Recherches sur le traitement du cancer, par la compression methodique simple ou combineé, et sur l'histoire générale de la même maladie. Paris: Gabon, 1829.

Report of the National Board of Consultants on the Conquest of Cancer. Washington, D.C.: U.S. Government Printing Office, 1971.

Shapiro, S., Venet, W., Strax, P., Venet, L., and Roeser, R. Ten-to fourteen-year effect of screening on breast cancer mortality. J. Natl. Cancer Inst., *69*:349–355, 1982.

Shimkin, M. B. Contrary to Nature. Washington, D.C.: U.S. Department of Health, Education, and Welfare, 1977.

Steinhorn, S. C., and Ries, L. G. Improved survival among children with acute leukemia in the United States. Biomed. Pharmacother., *42*:675–682, 1988.

Storm, H. H., Lynge, E., Osterlind, A., and Jensen, O. M. Multiple primary cancers in Denmark 1943–80; influence of possible underreporting and suggested risk factors. Yale J. Biol. Med., *59*:547–559, 1986.

Tabar, L., Fagerberg, C. J., Gad, A., et al. Reduction in mortality from breast cancer from mass screening with mammography. Lancet, *1*:829–832, 1985.

Vainio, H., and Partanen, T. Population burden of lung cancer due to environmental tobacco smoke. Mutat. Res., *222*:137–140, 1989.

Virchow, R. Die krankhaften Geschwülste. Berlin: A. Hirschwald, 1863.

Waldeyer, H. W. Die Entwickelung der Carcinome. Virchows Arch. Abt. A Pathol. Anat., *55*:67–159, 1872.

Wingo, P. A., Ries, L. A. G., Rosenberg, H. M., Miller, D. S., and Edwards, B. K. Cancer incidence and mortality, 1973–1995. Cancer, *82*:1197–1207, 1998.

Woodward, A., and McMichael, A. J. Passive smoking and cancer risk: the nature and uses of epidemiological evidence. Eur. J. Cancer, *27*:1472–1479, 1991.

Wynder, E. L., and Gori, G. B. Contribution of the environment to cancer incidence: an epidemiologic exercise. J. Natl. Cancer Inst., *58*:825–832, 1977.

2
The Language of Oncology

THE DEFINITION OF NEOPLASIA

As an illustration of the enigma that cancer has presented to physicians and scientists over the years, it was not until the 1920s that meaningful attempts were made to define cancer. In the ensuing half-century, a number of definitions of this biological phenomenon were proposed, mostly by physicians and scientists but more recently also by lay persons writing for the scientific press. Some definitions have been rather extensive and detailed, usually reflecting the author's basic experience and research interests; others have been of a more general character. To confuse the field further, clinicians, scientists, and lay persons have used such terms as *cancer*, *neoplasm*, *tumor*, and *malignancy* as if they were synonymous in every way (cf. Maugh and Marx, 1975). In this text we use the terms *neoplasm* and *neoplasia* for the basic disease process defined below. *Cancer* has come to be used almost exclusively to indicate a process that has the biological characteristics of a malignant neoplasm (see below). The term *malignancy* should also be limited to references to malignant neoplasms. Perhaps the greatest confusion is caused by the use of the word *tumor*. Since the Greco-Roman era, *tumor* has been used to denote a readily defined mass of tissue distinct from normal physiological growth. Thus, a scar, a healing bone fracture or callus, "proud flesh," a granuloma, a chronic abscess, or a parasitic mass are all tumors, but they are not neoplasms. Part of this confusion arises because several English pathologists employed the term *tumour* synonymously with *neoplasia* (cf. Walter and Israel, 1979; Willis, 1967). In this text, however, we do not use this last terminology.

Most of the definitions of neoplasia that have been proposed have common themes, but we use the definition modified from that originally proposed by the pathologist James Ewing (1940):

A neoplasm is a heritably altered, relatively autonomous growth of tissue.

This definition encompasses several concepts. The changes from normal exhibited by a neoplastic cell are heritable in that such characteristics are passed on from the neoplastic cell to its progeny. *Heritably altered* indicates alterations that are transmitted to all progeny in a heritable and irreversible manner. This characteristic does not *necessarily* imply that the heritable change is dependent on structural genomic alteration(s), since phenotypic characteristics are transmitted to the progeny of cells of a specific differentiated lineage without known qualitative genomic alterations—e.g., hepatocytes, intestinal crypt cells, neurons, etc. Autonomy indicates that a cancer is not subject to the "rules and regulations" that govern the individual cells and the overall cell interactions of the functional organism. The adverb *relatively* modifies *autonomous* to indicate that neoplasms are not completely autonomous. In many instances the autonomy that a neoplasm possesses may be quite subtle and relative only to the tissue from which it arose.

However, it should be emphasized that this phrase, *relatively autonomous*, is, together with the heritable nature of neoplasia, the most important aspect of the definition and characterizes a particular cell type as being neoplastic in the general sense. *Relative autonomy* is used here in the biological sense, but it is anticipated that one day we will understand it in the molecular sense; when we do, we will probably understand the mechanisms of the malignant process itself.

The next essential component of the definition is the term *growth*. Here this term may indicate the rate of cell division as modified by the rate of cell death (apoptosis, see below) or the rate of intracellular processes involved in the synthesis of macromolecules for use within the cell or for excretion by the cell. The actual *rate* of growth may be extremely low, differing little from that in the normal counterpart of the neoplasm; or, in the most serious cases, the rate may be extremely rapid, approaching that of the growth rate of embryonic tissue. In some instances, as with neoplasms of the small intestine or certain chronic leukemias (see below), the rate of growth of the neoplastic cell may even be less than that of its normal counterpart. Obviously, if the cells of a neoplasm do not proliferate to a point where the tumor is grossly or histologically recognizable, it is practically impossible to designate the cellular population as neoplastic. Thus, enhanced cell replication and/or decreased cell death becomes a part of the operational definition of neoplasia. Furthermore—from the results of a number of experiments and clinical observations—we recognize that neoplastic cells may exist for a lifetime in the host without ever undergoing demonstrable cell division (Chapter 10).

The final component of the definition is the term *tissue*, which stems from the fact that, at our present state of knowledge, cancer or neoplasia can be defined only in a multicellular organism. By this definition, unicellular organisms are free of the disease. In this sense cancer may be called "the curse of evolution."

The definition of neoplasia proposed by Ewing in the mid-1930s was that of a pathologist knowledgeable in the biology of cancer as expressed in vivo. Today, the in vivo system is still the basic reference for our definition of the neoplastic cell. On the other hand, with the recent advances of carcinogenesis in vitro, characteristics of the cancer cell as it grows in tissue culture have been described (Chapter 14). Although it is not yet possible to define the malignant cell in vitro without reference to its behavior in vivo, an ultimate goal of experimental oncology is to elucidate the molecular definition of the cancer cell regardless of its environment.

TYPES OF GROWTH (PLASIAS)

Hyperplasia

The term *hyperplasia* has been used to denote an increase in cell number. *Hypertrophy* indicates an increase in cell size but not in cell number. Although many neoplasms are characterized by hyperplasia, many normal tissues are also characterized by a dramatic increase in cell number. Embryonic tissue has perhaps the fastest rate of hyperplasia, but some adult tissues, especially those involved in certain metabolic functions—such as the crypt cells of the small intestine, cells of the bone marrow, and, to a lesser extent, the cells of the basal layer of the skin—are normally hyperplastic. In reactions such as wound healing and callus formation, hyperplasia is a normal process. Thus, hyperplasia may occur in cancer but is not a unique characteristic or even an absolute requirement of neoplasia.

Metaplasia

Metaplasia is a process in which one adult, differentiated cell type in a specific organ or organ structure is replaced by another differentiated cell type. In most instances the secondary or replacing cell type is not normally seen in the particular region in which the metaplasia occurs. Metaplasia may be either epithelial or mesenchymal and has been observed in a wide variety of reactive and neoplastic human tissues (Willis, 1962; Leube and Rustad, 1991). In recent years developmental biologists have referred to this process as "transdifferentiation," which refers to changes occurring not only in the adult but also in the developing fetus and newborn (Okada, 1986). Thus, as might be expected, the potential pathways of transdifferentiation are somewhat more complex, since the cells involved usually have a greater potential for differentiation. Okada points out that transdifferentiation is "principally an irreversible process." However, in the adult, the "operational reversibility" of metaplasia does occur (see below).

There are several known and presumed mechanisms of metaplasia. Lugo and Putong (1984) have proposed that the abnormal differentiation of metaplasia could occur by several pathways. These can be seen in Figure 2.1. Stem cell metaplasia results from the differentiation of immature, undifferentiated *stem cells*, which are present in tissues for the purpose of repairing and replacing mature cellular loss, along a new pathway leading to abnormal differentiation. This has generally been considered to be the mechanism most often involved in metaplasia, especially in epithelial metaplasia. A second possible pathway has been termed *direct metaplasia*, which was originally proposed by Virchow (1853) and is the result of normal, mature, differentiated cells being converted in the absence of cell division directly into another mature differentiated cell type. Finally, *indirect metaplasia* involves the formation of intermediate cells, which are still capable of proliferation and differentiation, differentiating into a new or abnormal cell type. Lugo and Putong (1984) have described several examples of these various types of metaplasia.

The most common example of *epithelial metaplasia* is in the change of columnar or pseudostratified columnar epithelium of the respiratory tract to squamous epithelium. This phenomenon is known as squamous metaplasia and may result from numerous stimuli, among which are chronic irritation and inflammation. In this particular example, the mechanism of metaplasia of respiratory epithelial cells is most commonly the result of stem cell metaplasia. However, studies by McDowell et al. (1979) suggested that metaplasia may arise from fully mature cells, such as mucus-secreting cells, which are still capable of cell division. But more recent findings have indicated that an indirect mechanism of metaplasia (Figure 2.1) may play a role in this process (Leube and Rustad, 1991).

In the respiratory epithelium, the stem cell normally gives rise to pseudostratified columnar epithelium, but in the presence of certain stimuli it may differentiate into squamous epithelium. The lack of vitamin A may be associated with such squamous metaplasia, since animals deficient in this vitamin show extensive squamous metaplasia of mucous columnar epithelium; treatment with vitamin A may reverse the squamous metaplasia. The appearance of mucous co-

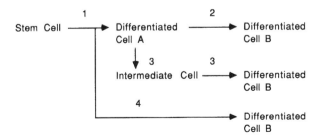

Figure 2.1   Scheme of potential pathways of metaplasia in a tissue composed of A cells to a tissue composition of B cells. (1) proliferation and differentiation; (2) the path of direct metaplasia; (3) indirect metaplasia; (4) stem cell metaplasia. (From Lugo and Putong, 1984, with permission.)

lumnar epithelium and its conversion to squamous epithelium by vitamin A deficiency, with its reversal to its original form when vitamin A is again added to the diet, is shown schematically in Figure 2.2. The mechanism of this metaplasia also appears to result from redifferentiation of certain stem cells (shown as small black nuclei along the basement membrane) of each of the epithelia. Because these epithelial cells are constantly being replaced by progeny of the stem cells, in the absence of vitamin A or in the presence of some chronic stimulus as yet undefined, the differentiation of the stem cell may be redirected to the more primitive squamous epithelium. In the presence of vitamin A or some other unknown environmental factor, normal differentiation of the stem cell may recur. It should be noted, however, that once a cell begins on the pathway of differentiation toward either a squamous cell or a columnar cell, the process appears to be irreversible, as predicted in the definition of transdifferentiation (see above). A further discussion of the effect of vitamin A on carcinogenesis may be found in Chapter 8.

Another interesting example of epithelial metaplasia induced by a specific experimental protocol is the differentiation of regenerating pancreatic cells into hepatocytes identical with those present in normal liver (Scarpelli and Rao, 1981). Rao and associates (1988) have demonstrated that adult rats maintained on a copper-deficient diet for several months and then returned to a normal diet exhibit an almost complete loss of pancreatic acinar cells and the development of multiple foci of hepatocytes during the recovery phase. Cossel (1984) has suggested that this metaplasia is the result of the redifferentiation of "intermediate" cells seen in the adult pancreas of mammals, including the human. By Cossel's thesis, this epithelial differentiation would be classified as indirect metaplasia (Figure 2.1).

Mesenchymal metaplasia, like epithelial metaplasia, may result from any of the mechanisms seen in Figure 2.1. Examples of the conversion of epithelial cells to mesenchymal cells, mesenchymal cells to epithelial cells, and mesenchymal cells of one differentiated form to that of another have been described (cf. Lugo and Putong, 1984). In fact, these authors have suggested that, under appropriate environmental circumstances, a given cell, by the process of metaplasia, may exhibit epithelial or mesenchymal characteristics regardless of the tissue of origin. Metaplasia may also occur in cell culture, since it is possible to alter the differentiated state experimentally by a variety of methods of cell biology (Blau, 1989). It is not surprising that metaplasia occurs in adult tissues under a variety of different circumstances.

SQUAMOUS METAPLASIA IN THE ABSENCE OF VITAMIN A

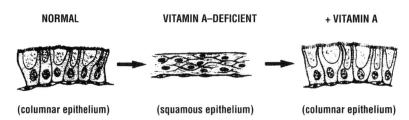

NORMAL   **VITAMIN A–DEFICIENT**   **+ VITAMIN A**

(columnar epithelium)   (squamous epithelium)   (columnar epithelium)

Figure 2.2 Artist's representation of the morphological changes occurring in the metaplasia of ciliated columnar epithelium to squamous epithelium in vitamin A–deficient animals and the subsequent redifferentiation of the squamous epithelium to columnar epithelium in the presence of vitamin A.

Dysplasia and Anaplasia

Robbins (1974) defined *dysplasia* as "an alteration in adult cells characterized by variation in their size, shape, and organization." More recently Rubin and Farber (1988) have defined dysplasia as being distinct from normal cell and tissue organization "by variations in the size and shape of the cells; by enlargement, irregularity, and hyperchromatism of the nuclei; and by disorderly arrangement of the cells within the epithelium." Furthermore, Walter and Israel (1979), as well as Rubin and Farber (1988), have pointed out that the term *dysplasia* has been used by some pathologists to designate abnormalities in the development of tissues, although not always strictly with reference to developmental disorders. Because this variation in definition may be somewhat confusing, we have chosen to use the term *anaplasia* in a manner similar to that utilized by Ritchie (1970). Anaplasia is characterized at two different biological levels: (1) intercellular relations and associations, as described below, and (2) alterations in intracellular macromolecular syntheses.

Positional or organizational anaplasia refers to the interrelations of cells in a specific tissue. Normally, there are distinct histological patterns in tissues. When positional anaplasia occurs, these distinct patterns are altered in that either cell organelles are arranged randomly with respect to one another in adjacent cells or the cells themselves are disarranged with respect to one another.

Cytological anaplasia is largely a function of increased or altered nucleic acid synthesis in growing tissues. This term usually refers to the staining characteristics of cells, especially with respect to basophilia and the nuclear/cytoplasmic ratio. Cytologic anaplasia may also be a function of the ploidy of the cell; it is seen normally in the placenta, in a callus, and occasionally in wound healing. Evidence by Therman et al. (1983) indicates that processes giving rise to different sizes and types of nuclei seen in the cytological anaplasia of neoplastic cells include endoreduplication, true endomitosis, and a sort of polytenization. All of these latter processes result in nuclear enlargement from increased DNA content. Cytological anaplasia is extremely important in the cytological diagnosis of malignancy (Pap test). However, it should be emphasized that, since normal tissues may exhibit cytological anaplasia as well as positional anaplasia, this phenomenon is not an absolute characteristic of malignancy.

Figure 2.3 is a conceptual drawing of both positional and cytological anaplasia. The artist's conception demonstrates that in positional anaplasia there is an alteration in the distribution in space of cell organelles within a specific tissue or epithelium or in the spatial relation of one cell or group of cells to another within a tissue. Cytological anaplasia is shown as a distortion of cellular architecture compared with the normal cell type and is characterized by intensified staining (denoted by the darkened nuclei) of the nucleus and cytoplasm of the cell. The student should be aware, however, that in many neoplasms both positional and cytological anaplasia occur simultaneously.

Another process, which histologically may be mistaken for cytological anaplasia, is a process of "controlled cell deletion" or programmed cell death occurring coincidentally with normal physiological processes within a tissue. Kerr et al. (1972) employed the term *apoptosis* to refer to this process, which plays a complementary but opposite role to mitosis in the regulation of animal cell populations. Specific morphological changes occur in cells undergoing apoptosis (Wyllie, 1981, 1988). The first of these involves a rapid loss of the volume of the cell as well as a condensation of the chromatin with subsequent fragmentation and phagocytosis by macrophages or a similar process by parenchymal cells. Figure 2.4A is an artist's conception of the formation and fate of apoptic cells of an epithelial parenchyma such as that of liver. In the lower portion of the figure are shown simple morphological changes occurring during necrosis, which involves an initial generalized swelling and subsequent dissolution of organelles with final rupture of plasma membranes (Corcoran et al., 1994).

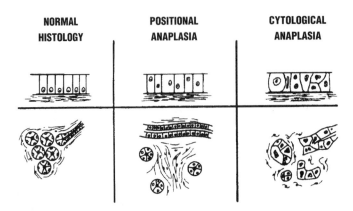

Figure 2.3 Artist's representation of positional and cytological anaplasia. In positional anaplasia (center), in a single layer of epithelium, the altered position of nuclei in relation to one another in adjacent cells is depicted, as well as the altered position of ducts and glands in a specific representative structure. Cytological anaplasia (right) is noted by the marked variation in nuclear size and staining characteristics, nucleolar size, and nuclear/cytoplasmic ratio. Normal histology is shown at the left.

   The apoptotic process in tissues is rapid, with complete disappearance of all phagocytosed cells within 4 hours (cf. Fesus et al., 1991). Apoptosis is to be distinguished both morphologically and biochemically from cell *necrosis*, which is cell death resulting from unphysiological external environmental toxic factors. While there is some overlap both in occurrence and characteristics, certain general differences between the two processes can be noted (Table 2.1). Apoptosis occurs spontaneously during embryological development and in a variety of normal tissues (cf. Wyllie, 1974). This process also occurs during involution of normal tissues, such as lactating breasts in rodents (Walker et al., 1989), as well as in hormone-induced cell death (Morris et al., 1984) and in the process of immunocyte-induced cell death (Wyllie, 1988). This process also occurs spontaneously in untreated malignant neoplasms but may be triggered in both normal and neoplastic cells by a variety of environmental agents including cytotoxic drugs (Schwartzman and Cidlowski, 1993) and promoting agents (Chapter 7). Apoptosis is a genetically directed program of cell death in contrast to necrosis, and there are distinctive morphological as well as molecular differences between the two processes (Table 2.1 and Chapter 7).
   As implied by the information in Table 2.1, the mechanism of apoptosis is significantly different from that of necrosis. A very important difference is the fact that gene expression is required for apoptosis, and the expression of a number of genes has now been implicated as a requirement for apoptosis in one or more tissue types (Schwartzman and Cidlowski, 1993; Hengartner, 2000). In neoplasms, apoptosis occurs spontaneously, although in a more haphazard and presumably autonomous manner than seen in normal tissues.

Neoplasia

We have defined a neoplasm, and thus neoplasia, as a heritably altered, relatively autonomous growth of tissue. In the next sections, as we consider the classification of neoplasms, certain contradictions may become apparent. It should be emphasized that all neoplasms, regardless of their biological behavior, are components of the disease classification of neoplasia. In this sense the terms *cancer* and *malignancy* may occasionally be incorrectly used synonymously with *neoplasm* or *neoplasia*. This may be done without reference to the biological behavior of the

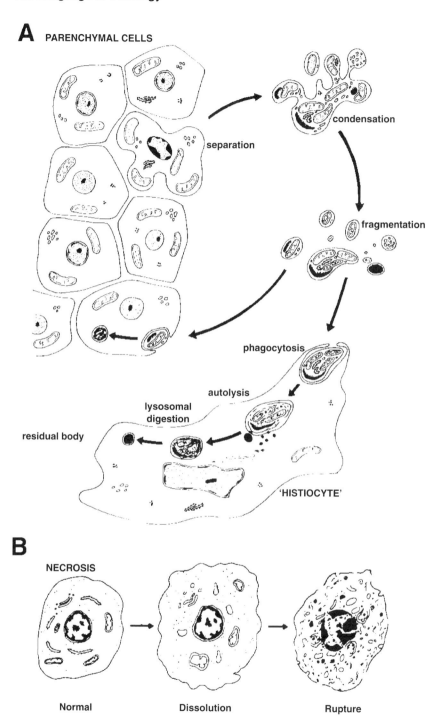

Figure 2.4 (A) Diagrammatic illustration of the morphological features of apoptosis of parenchymal cells of a glandular tissue. (Adapted from Kerr et al., 1972, with permission of authors and publisher.) (B) Diagram of parenchymal cell necrosis from a normal cell to the initial phase of generalized swelling progressing to a dissolution of organelles and final rupture of plasma membranes. (Adapted from Corcoran et al., 1994, with permission of authors and publisher.)

Table 2.1 General Differences between Apoptosis and Necrosis

Characteristics	Apoptosis	Necrosis
Stimuli	Physiological	Pathological (injury)
Occurrence	Single cells	Groups of cells
Reversibility	No (after morphological changes)	Yes (up to the point of no return)
Cytoplasmic organelles	Late-stage swelling	Very early swelling
Lysosomal enzyme release	Absent	Present
Nucleus	Convolution of nuclear outline and breakdown (karyorrhexis)	Disappearance (karyolysis)
Nuclear chromatin	Compaction in uniformly dense masses	Clumping not sharply defined
DNA breakdown	Internucleosomal	Randomized
Cell	Formation of apoptotic bodies	Swelling and later disintegration
Phagocytosis by other cells	Present	Absent
Exudative inflammation	Absent	Present
Scar formation	Absent	Present

Modified from Gerschenson and Rotello, 1992.

neoplasm, and for this reason the student must be on guard to ensure that the actual meanings of these terms are clear when they are used.

THE CLASSIFICATION OF NEOPLASMS

Behavioristic (Biological) Classification

Since our definition of neoplasia is presently based on the biological behavior of neoplasms, it is proper to make a classification on the basis of such behavior. However, in making this classification, it should be noted that all neoplasms that we are considering conform to the definition of Ewing. As we shall see, the distinction between benign and malignant neoplasms in the behavioristic classification has considerable usefulness in determining the prognosis in a specific patient but is of little use to the scientist who is studying the mechanisms of neoplasia at the molecular level.

The principal behavioristic characteristics of benign and malignant neoplasms are as follows:

	Benign	*Malignant*
1.	Usually encapsulated	Nonencapsulated
2.	Usually noninvasive	Invasive
3.	Highly differentiated	Poorly differentiated
4.	Rare mitoses	Mitoses relatively common
5.	Slow growth	Rapid growth
6.	Little or no anaplasia	Anaplastic to varying degrees
7.	No metastases	Metastases

The majority of the differences between benign and malignant neoplasms are relative. The critical difference between the two types is point no. 7, in that benign neoplasms by *definition* do not exhibit metastatic growth, whereas all malignant neoplasms have the potential for successful metastatic growth. A metastasis is defined as the secondary growth of a neoplasm, originating from a primary neoplasm and growing within the host organism in a location distant from the initial or primary site of neoplastic growth. As is shown in Chapter 7, there are various routes and mechanisms of metastases for malignant neoplasms.

Although there is little doubt from the literature that most pathologists and students of oncology define a malignant neoplasm by its ability to metastasize (Ackerman and de Regato, 1962; Bland-Sutton, 1911; Cappell, 1958; Hopps, 1964; Montgomery, 1965), the artificiality of this distinction from the viewpoint of the natural history of neoplasia will soon become evident. It is well known that a number of benign neoplasms may at some time during their natural history take on the behavior of a malignant neoplasm. This phenomenon, which is discussed later under the heading "Progression of Neoplasia" (Chapters 7, 9, and 10), was emphasized by Foulds (1965), who considered the behavioristic distinction between benign and malignant neoplasms to be essentially nonexistent. In the United States (Shubik et al., 1977; Huff et al., 1989) as well as internationally (Faccini et al., 1992), both benign and malignant neoplasms have been considered important in the determination of the carcinogenicity (Chapter 3) of a specific chemical agent. However, students of oncology have made the distinction between benign and malignant neoplasms presented here.

Histogenetic Classification

Although the behavioristic classification is one of the most commonly accepted segments of the nomenclature of neoplasms, the most important principle in the classification of neoplasms is their grouping according to the type of tissue from which the neoplasm has arisen (Table 2.2). Ritchie (1970) distinguished groups of neoplasms on the basis of their histogenetic origin as follows:

1. Epithelium
2. Connective tissue
3. Hemopoietic and immune systems
4. Nervous system
5. Multiple histogenetic cellular origin
6. Miscellaneous

This classification has considerable usefulness in itself, especially when considered with other aspects of the lesions, from both the diagnostic and the biological viewpoints. For example, it is very important to determine the region, origin, or tissue from which the neoplasm arose. In addition, other descriptive terms are often utilized in classifying or diagnosing a specific problem. Such descriptive terms as *papillary, cystic, follicular*, and others may relate to various histological characteristics of neoplasms of epithelial origin. In addition, some neoplasms have been named according to the individual first describing the lesion; examples are Ewing tumor of bone, Hodgkin disease of lymph tissue, and Wilms' tumor of the kidney.

The behavioristic and histogenetic classifications of neoplasms are presently the most widely used by both physicians and scientists alike. However, it is becoming increasingly evident, as our knowledge of histogenesis and differentiation increases, that a reevaluation, especially of the histogenetic classification, would be appropriate (Gould, 1986). Later in the text are discussions of various molecular markers of neoplasms that relate both to the definition of neoplasia and to the histogenesis of tissues from which such neoplasms arose. As such markers come to be more widely known and the ultrastructural techniques for cytological histogenesis become more widely used, the classification of neoplasia may evolve into the use of more molecular terminology.

Table 2.2 Examples of Neoplasms According to Histogenetic Classifications

Tissues of Origin	Benign	Malignant
Epithelial neoplasms		
Epidermis	Epidermal papilloma	Epidermal carcinoma
Stomach	Gastric polyp	Gastric carcinoma
Biliary tree	Cholangioma	Cholangiocarcinoma
Adrenal cortex	Adrenocortical adenoma	Adrenocortical carcinoma
Connective tissue neoplasms		
Fibrous tissue	Fibroma	Fibrosarcoma
Cartilage	Chondroma	Chondrosarcoma
Bone	Osteoma	Osteogenic sarcoma
Fat	Lipoma	Liposarcoma
Smooth muscle	Leiomyoma	Leiomyosarcoma
Skeletal muscle	Rhabdomyoma	Rhabdomyosarcoma
Neoplasms of hemopoietic and immune systems		
Lymphoid tissue	Brill-Symmers disease	Lymphosarcoma (lymphoma)
		Lymphatic leukemia
		Reticulum cell sarcoma
		Hodgkin disease
Thymus	Thymoma	Thymoma
Granulocytes		Myelogenous leukemia
Erythrocytes	Polycythemia vera	Erythroleukemia
Plasma cells		Multiple myeloma
Neoplasms of nervous system		
Glia	Astrocytoma	Glioblastoma multiforme
	Oligodendroglioma	
Meninges	Meningioma	Meningeal sarcoma
Neurons	Ganglioneuroma	Neuroblastoma
Adrenal medulla	Pheochromocytoma	Pheochromocytoma
Neoplasms of multiple histogenetic cellular origin		
Breast	Fibroadenoma	Cystosarcoma phylloides
Kidney		Wilms' tumor
Ovary, testis, etc.	Dermoid (benign teratoma)	
Miscellaneous neoplasms		
Melanocytes	Nevus	Melanoma
Placenta	Hydatidiform mole	Chorionepithelioma
Ovary	Granulosa cell tumor	Granulosa cell tumor
	Cystadenoma	Cystadenocarcinoma
Testis		Seminoma

After Ritchie, 1970, with permission of the publisher.

Nomenclature of Neoplasms and Its Embryonic Basis

In order to discuss the phenomenon of neoplasia, it is important that certain aspects of currently accepted nomenclature be understood. It should be noted, however, that there is no one system of nomenclature of neoplasms used worldwide; in this country, nomenclature has revolved around the use of the suffix *-oma*, which literally means "tumor." With some exceptions, words with this suffix do refer to neoplasms. An exception is the term *granuloma*, which is a nonneoplastic tumor of inflammatory tissue.

In the behavioristic classification, benign tumors may be named with a prefix that refers to the tissue from which the neoplasm arose and with the suffix *-oma*. For example, a benign neoplasm of fibrous tissue is called a *fibroma*; a benign neoplasm of cartilage, a *chondroma*; a benign neoplasm of glandular tissue, an *adenoma*; and so on. When one considers the malignant tumors, however, some other aspects of classification apply. Malignant neoplasms are divided into two general categories, depending on their embryonic origin. Figure 2.5 outlines some of the steps in the early development of a fertilized egg of higher vertebrate animals. After fertilization, the egg divides a number of times, giving rise to 2, 4, 8, 16, 32 cells, and so on; these then form a small spherical structure, termed the *blastula*, with a central cavity. Continued development of this structure to the *gastrula* involves an invagination of the cells of one part of the surface, giving rise to a small "ball within a ball," as diagrammed in a sectional view in Figure 2.5. At this stage it is possible for the embryologist to distinguish three different layers of cells. The outermost layer is termed the *ectoderm* and develops to give rise to the skin and its associated structures in the adult. The layer of invaginated cells is termed the *endoderm* and ultimately gives rise to the gastrointestinal tract and its associated structures. Between these two layers, a mass of cells forms in the gastrula, termed the *mesoderm*, giving rise in the adult to supporting structures such as bone, fat, muscle, blood, and so on. As can be seen from the figure, a malignant neoplasm arising from derivatives of the mesodermal (mesenchymal) embryonic germ layer is termed a *sarcoma*. If the neoplasm arises from tissues derived from embryonic ectoderm or endoderm, the term *carcinoma* applies to malignant neoplasms of such tissues. Thus, the term *adenocarcinoma*—of the stomach, pancreas, or breast—is appropriate for malignant neoplasms of the glandular epithelium of these organs. On the other hand, a *liposarcoma* may arise from the fat tissue of the breast, a *chondrosarcoma* from cartilage of the ribs, or an *osteogenic sarcoma* from the bony rib itself.

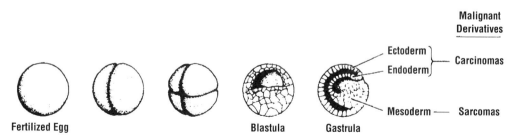

Figure 2.5 Developmental biology of the early fertilized egg and embryo of the vertebrate. At the developmental stage of gastrulation, the three germ layers (ectoderm, mesoderm, and endoderm) are clearly differentiated. Tissues derived from these different layers may give rise to malignant neoplasms, with the terminology based on their germ layer of derivation. See text for further details.

Several terms do not fit strictly into this type of nomenclature. The suffix *-blastoma* is used to denote certain types of neoplasms to indicate that the tissue has a primitive appearance that resembles embryonic structures. Examples of this situation are the neuroblastoma and the myoblastoma. In other examples the terminology is rather confusing. A highly malignant tumor that has the appearance of both a carcinoma and a sarcoma is termed a *carcinosarcoma*. This would indicate that the neoplasm was derived from two germ layers. Another condition, the "mixed" tumor of the salivary gland, which is definitely not a carcinosarcoma, was once thought to have this same embryonic derivation. It is now felt that the mixed tumor is probably a low-grade carcinoma, and the term *carcinosarcoma* should be reserved only for highly malignant, quite primitive tumors with the histological characteristics mentioned above.

The most common neoplasm of multiple-tissue origin is the *teratoma*, which is derived from all three germ layers. These neoplasms may be either benign or malignant in the behavioristic sense.

Table 2.2 lists a number of neoplasms classified according to the behavioristic and histogenetic methods. Although the rules of classification mentioned in this outline are reasonably inclusive, there are some exceptions in the designation of specific neoplasms, as can be seen from the table. For example, the melanoma is not a benign neoplasm but rather a highly malignant tumor of melanocytes. Although the term *hepatoma* suggests a benign neoplasm, it is malignant in almost all instances. As one's knowledge of experimental oncology increases, the specific exceptions to the rules become more familiar.

REFERENCES

Ackerman, L. V., and de Regato, J. A. Cancer—Diagnosis, Treatment, and Prognosis, p. 77. St. Louis: Mosby, 1962.

Bland-Sutton, J. Tumours—Innocent and Malignant: Their Clinical Characters and Appropriate Treatment, 5th ed., p. 8. London: Cassell, 1911.

Blau, H. M. How fixed is the differentiated state? Lessons from heterokaryons. Trends Genet., 5:268–272, 1989.

Cappell, D. F. Muir's Textbook of Pathology, 7th ed., p. 224. London: Edward Arnold, 1958.

Corcoran, G. B., Fix, L., Jones, D. P., Moslen, M. T., Nicotera, P., Oberhammer, F. A., and Buttyan, R. Apoptosis: Molecular control point in toxicity. Toxicol. Appl. Pharmacol., 128:169–181, 1994.

Cossel, L. Intermediate cells in the adult human pancreas. Contribution to the transformation of differentiated cells in vertebrates. Virchows Arch. [Cell Pathol.], 47:313–328, 1984.

Ewing, J. Neoplastic Disease: A Treatise on Tumors, 4th ed. Philadelphia: Saunders, 1940.

Faccini, J. M., Butler, W. R., Friedmann, J.-C., Hess, R., Reznik, G. K., Ito, N., Hayashi, Y., and Williams, G. M. International Federation of Societies of Toxicologic Pathologists (IFSTP) guidelines for the design and interpretation of the chronic rodent carcinogenicity bioassay. Exp. Toxicol. Pathol., 44:443–456, 1992.

Fesus, L., Davies, P. J. A., and Piacentini, M. Apoptosis: Molecular mechanisms in programmed cell death. Eur. J. Cell Biol., 56:170–177, 1991.

Foulds, L. Multiple etiologic factors in neoplastic development. Cancer Res., 25:1339–1347, 1965.

Gerschenson, L. E., and Rotello, R. J. Apoptosis: A different type of cell death. FASEB J., 6:2450–2455, 1992.

Gould, V. E. Histogenesis and differentiation: a re-evaluation of these concepts as criteria for the classification of tumors. Hum. Pathol., 17:212–215, 1986.

Hengartner, M. O. The biochemistry of apoptosis. Nature, 407:770–776, 2000.

Hopps, H. C. Principles of Pathology, 2nd ed., p. 311. New York: Appleton-Century-Crofts, 1964.

Huff, J. E., Eustis, S. L., and Haseman, J. K. Occurrence and relevance of chemically induced benign neoplasms in long-term carcinogenicity studies. Cancer Metast. Rev., 8:1–21, 1989.

Kerr, J. F. R., Wyllie, A. H., and Currie, A. R. Apoptosis: A basic biological phenomenon with wide-ranging implications in tissue kinetics. Br. J. Cancer, 26:239–257, 1972.

Leube, R. E., and Rustad, T. J. Squamous cell metaplasia in the human lung: molecular characteristics of epithelial stratification. Virchows Archiv. B Cell Pathol., 61:227–253, 1991.

Lugo, M., and Putong, P. B. Metaplasia. An overview. Arch. Pathol. Lab. Med., 108:185–189, 1984.

Maugh, T. H., II, and Marx, J. L. Seeds of Destruction—The Science Report on Cancer Research. New York: Plenum, 1975.

McDowell, E. M., Becci, P. J., Schürch, W., and Trump, B. F. The respiratory epithelium. VII. Epidermoid metaplasia of hamster tracheal epithelium during regeneration following mechanical injury. J. Natl. Cancer Inst., 62:995–1008, 1979.

Montgomery, G. L. Textbook of Pathology, Vol. 1, p. 95. Baltimore: Williams & Wilkins, 1965.

Morris, R. G., Hargreaves, A. D., Duvall, E., and Wyllie, A. H. Hormone-induced cell death. 2. Surface changes in thymocytes undergoing apoptosis. Am. J. Pathol., 115:426–436, 1984.

Okada, T. S. Transdifferentiation in animal cells: Fact or artifact? Dev. Growth Diff., 28(3):213–221, 1986.

Rao, M. S., Dwivedi, R. S., Subbarao, V., Usman, M. I., Scarpelli, D. G., Nemali, M. R., Yeldandi, A., Thangada, S., Kumar, S., and Reddy, J. K. Almost total conversion of pancreas to liver in the adult rat: A reliable model to study transdifferentiation. Biochem. Biophys. Res. Commun., 156:131–136, 1988.

Ritchie, A. C. The classification, morphology and behaviour of tumours. In: H. Flored (Ed.), General Pathology, 4th ed., Chap. 22, pp. 668–719. Philadelphia: Saunders, 1970.

Robbins, S. L. Pathologic Basis of Disease, pp. 106, 118. Philadelphia: Saunders, 1974.

Rubin, E., and Farber, J. L. Pathology. Philadelphia: Lippincott, 1988.

Scarpelli, D. G., and Rao, M. S. Differentiation of regenerating pancreatic cells into hepatocyte-like cells. Proc. Natl. Acad. Sci., U.S.A., 78:2577–2581, 1981.

Schwartzman, R. A., and Cidlowski, J. A. Apoptosis: the biochemistry and molecular biology of programmed cell death. Endocr. Rev., 14:133–151, 1993.

Shubik, P. General criteria for assessing the evidence for carcinogenicity of chemical substances: Report of the Subcommittee on Environmental Carcinogenesis, National Cancer Advisory Board. J. Natl. Cancer Inst., 58:461–464, 1977.

Therman, E., Sarto, G. E., and Buchler, D. A. The structure and origin of giant nuclei in human cancer cells. Cancer Genet. Cytogenet., 9:9–18, 1983.

Virchow, R. Das normale Knochenwachstum und die rachitische Störung desselben. Virchows Arch. Pathol. Anat., 5:409–507, 1853.

Walker, N. I., Bennett, R. E., and Kerr, J. F. R. Cell death by apoptosis during involution of the lactating breast in mice and rats. Am. J. Anat., 185:19–32, 1989.

Walter, J. B., and Israel, M. S. General Pathology, 5th ed., pp. 309–390. London: Churchill Livingstone, 1979.

Willis, R. A. The Borderland of Embryology and Pathology, 2nd ed., pp. 519–581. Washington, D.C.: Butterworth, 1962.

Willis, R. A. Pathology of Tumours, 4th ed. London: Butterworth, 1967.

Wyllie, A. H. Death in normal and neoplastic cells. J. Clin. Pathol., 27, Suppl. 7:35–42, 1974.

Wyllie, A. H. Cell death: A new classification separating apoptosis from necrosis. In: I. D. Bowen and R. A. Lockshin (Eds.), Cell Death in Biology and Pathology, pp. 9–34. London: Chapman & Hall, 1981.

Wyllie, A. H. Apoptosis. ISI Atlas of Science. Immunology, 1:192–196, 1988.

3
The Etiology of Cancer:
Chemical and Physical Agents

Our earliest knowledge concerning chemical carcinogenesis came from clinical observations in humans. In 1775, Percivall Pott, an eminent English physician and surgeon, described the occurrence of cancer of the scrotum in a number of his patients. The common history given by these individuals was their employment as chimney sweeps when they were young. On the basis of this observation, Pott, with remarkable insight, concluded (1) that the occupation of these men as young boys was directly and causally related to their malignant disease and (2) that the large amounts of soot to which they were exposed was the causative agent of the cancer. Strangely enough, Pott did not suggest avoidance of contact with soot as a means of prevention, although his report in 1775 apparently inspired the Danish Chimney Sweepers' Guild to rule 3 years later that its members should bathe daily. While the publication of Pott soon led other observers to attribute cancer of various sites to soot exposure, there was a relative lack of effective impact of his work on British public health practice during the succeeding century (Lawley, 1994). It was not until more than a century later that Butlin (1892) reported the relative rarity of scrotal cancer in chimney sweeps on the European continent compared with those in England. It appeared that the lower incidence of the disease on the continent was the result of frequent bathing and protective clothing.

The lesson from Pott's report has been a long time in the learning. One hundred years after his publication, the high incidence of skin cancer among certain German workers was traced to their exposure to coal tar, the chief constituent of the chimney sweeps' soot (cf. Miller, 1978). It was another 40 years before the disease was reproduced experimentally, and even today—more than 200 years after Pott's original scientific report of the association of soot and smoke products with cancer—many still disregard the obvious hazards of the carcinogenic products that result from the combustion of tobacco in cigarettes and of many of the organic fuels of the industrialized world.

Before we embark on a discussion of the causation of cancer, it again becomes important to add to our vocabulary. The term *carcinogen* has generally been used by oncologists to indicate an agent that causes cancer. However, as our knowledge of oncology increases, this simplistic definition is not sufficient. We have proposed the following definition to include most examples of agents that are carcinogens, at the same time excluding those agents that do not have a direct action on cells undergoing neoplastic transformation.

> A *carcinogen* is an agent whose administration to previously untreated animals leads to a statistically significant increased incidence of neoplasms of one or more histogenetic types as compared with that in appropriate untreated animals, whether the control animals have low or high spontaneous incidences of the neoplasms in question.

This definition includes the induction of neoplasms that are not usually observed, the earlier induction of neoplasms that are usually observed, and/or the induction of more neoplasms than are usually found. Although it would be important to distinguish between agents that induce neoplasms by direct action on the cells that become neoplastic and those that produce neoplasia by indirect actions in the animal as a whole, at present it is not always possible to do so. Some agents, such as immune suppressants, can increase the incidence of neoplasms in tissues previously exposed to carcinogens by indirect effects on the host. Where the action of a chemical in causing an increase in neoplasms is known to be indirect—mediated by its effect on the host—the agent should not be designated a carcinogen.

At this stage of our discussion, the above definition and a prolonged explanation may be confusing. Later in the text (Chapters 7 and 8) we consider the stages and modifying factors of the process of carcinogenesis. As we learn more of the process of carcinogenesis, the term *carcinogen* will be further refined in relation to general usage as well as in terms of specific chemicals.

CHEMICAL CARCINOGENESIS

One hundred and forty years after Dr. Pott's report of the association of soot from the combustion of coal with epidermal cancer of the scrotum, an experimental basis for Pott's clinical observation was reported. In 1915, the Japanese pathologists Yamagawa and Ichikawa described the first production of skin tumors in animals by the application of coal tar to the skin. These investigators repeatedly applied crude coal tar to the ears of rabbits for a number of months, finally producing both benign and, later, malignant epidermal neoplasms. Later studies demonstrated that the skin of mice was also susceptible to the carcinogenic action of such organic tars. During the next 15 years, extensive attempts were made to determine the nature of the material in the crude tars that caused malignancy. In 1932, Kennaway and associates reported the production of carcinogenic tars by pyrolysis of simple organic compounds consisting only of carbon and hydrogen (cf. Kennaway, 1955). In the early 1930s, several polycyclic aromatic hydrocarbons were isolated from active crude tar fractions. In 1930, the first synthetic carcinogenic chemical was produced. This compound, dibenz(a,h)anthracene (Figure 3.1), was tested for carcinogenic activity by painting it on the skin of mice and found to be a potent carcinogen. The isolation from coal tar and the synthesis of benzo(a)pyrene (3,4-benzpyrene) were achieved in 1932. The structures of several polycyclic aromatic hydrocarbons are given in Figure 3.1. Polycyclic hydrocarbons vary in their carcinogenic potencies; for example, the compound dibenz(a,c)anthracene has very little carcinogenic activity while, as noted above, the a,h isomer is carcinogenic (cf. Heidelberger, 1970). Among the more potent polycyclic aromatic hydrocarbon carcinogens yet described are 3-methylcholanthrene and 7,12-dimethylbenz(a)anthracene. The carcinogenic dibenzo(c,q)carbazole is also considered in this class of compounds, possessing a nitrogen in its central ring. Further on, other polycyclic aromatic hydrocarbons containing nitrogen, sulfur, and halogens are considered (Chapters 7 and 9). Benzo(e)pyrene is reportedly inactive in inducing skin cancer in mice but can serve to "initiate" the carcinogenic process (Chapter 7). Perylene is inactive as a chemical carcinogen, while chrysene may have slight carcinogenic activity in this system.

Polycyclic aromatic hydrocarbons, both carcinogenic and noncarcinogenic, are found ubiquitously in air, soil, and other places in our environment. Reportedly as much as 894 tons of benzo(a)pyrene are emitted into the air per year in the United States. Much of this is due to industrial and home combustion of carbon-containing materials, whereas natural fires contribute only about 1% (Zedeck, 1980). As expected, soil contents of carcinogenic polycyclic aromatic

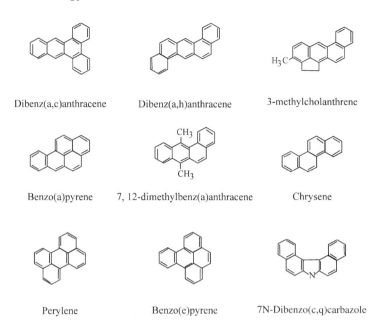

Dibenz(a,c)anthracene   Dibenz(a,h)anthracene   3-methylcholanthrene

Benzo(a)pyrene   7, 12-dimethylbenz(a)anthracene   Chrysene

Perylene   Benzo(e)pyrene   7N-Dibenzo(c,q)carbazole

Figure 3.1   Chemical structures of some carcinogenic polycyclic hydrocarbons.

hydrocarbons are much greater near cities and industrial areas than in rural and wilderness areas, with concentrations differing by as much as a thousandfold.

Because of the relatedness of the chemical structures of many carcinogenic polycyclic hydrocarbons, numerous studies have reported attempts to determine the molecular configuration(s) of these molecules that is (are) responsible for their carcinogenic activity. One of the earlier attempts was that of the Pullmans (cf. Pullman and Pullman, 1955), who utilized quantum mechanics and molecular orbital theory to determine reactivity of specific regions of carcinogenic polycyclic aromatic hydrocarbons. Reactivity indices were calculated for regions of the molecules termed the K and L regions (Figure 3.2). A K region is defined as the external corner of a phenanthrenic moiety in a polycyclic aromatic hydrocarbon, whereas an L region consists of a pair of opposed, open anthracenic "point" atoms (cf. Lowe and Silverman, 1984). If the calculated reactivity of the K region exceeds a certain limit, the chemical is expected to be carcinogenic unless the more active L region also exceeds its reactivity limit. In the latter case, the molecule will not be carcinogenic. The K and L regions for several polycyclic aromatic hydro-

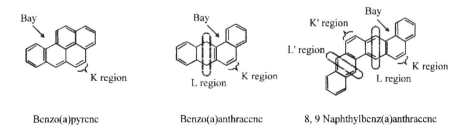

Benzo(a)pyrene   Benzo(a)anthracene   8, 9 Naphthylbenz(a)anthracene

Figure 3.2   Chemical structures of three carcinogenic polycyclic hydrocarbons exhibiting K and L regions.

carbons are noted in Figure 3.2. Although this early attempt at discovering a relationship between the structure of a chemical and its carcinogenic activity has not found general application because of numerous exceptions, much more extensive methods of relating structure and carcinogenic activity of polycyclic aromatic hydrocarbons have recently been developed through the use of computerized databases (Richard and Woo, 1990). In addition, as outlined below, the metabolism of polycyclic aromatic hydrocarbons is important for their carcinogenicity, and certain structural components of the molecule have been utilized in predicting carcinogenic activity (Jerina et al., 1982).

In 1935, Sasaki and Yoshida opened another field of chemical carcinogenesis by demonstrating that the feeding of the azo dye o-aminoazotoluene (2′,3-dimethyl-4-aminoazobenzene) (Figure 3.3) to rats resulted in the development of liver neoplasms. Kinosita (1936) later demonstrated that administration of 4-dimethylaminoazobenzene in the diet also caused neoplasms in the liver. A number of analogs of this compound were also prepared and tested for carcinogenic potential. An interesting correlation arising from all of these studies was the fact that the amino

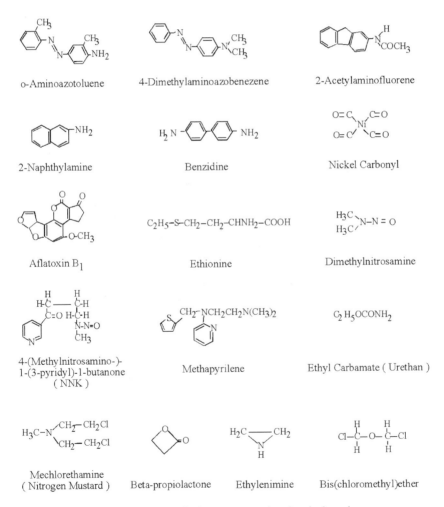

Figure 3.3 Chemical structures of other representative chemical carcinogens.

group of carcinogenic dyes usually had at least one methyl substituent, although o-aminoazotol-uene does not. Unlike the polycyclic aromatic hydrocarbons, the azo dyes generally did not act at the site of first contact of the compound with the organism but rather in a remote area, the liver. Painting of the skin with most azo dyes resulted in few or no tumors, and the oral adminis-tration of polycyclic aromatic hydrocarbons to rodents except in the neonatal period has gener-ally resulted in no hepatomas. Another important carcinogen that acts at remote sites is 2-acetylaminofluorene (Figure 3.3). In addition, the aromatic amines, 2-naphthylamine and benzi-dine, are carcinogenic for the urinary bladder in humans. The carcinogenic chemical ethyl car-bamate also appears to be a general "initiating agent" in the mouse (Chapter 6). Ethyl carbamate was in use in Japan from 1950 to 1975 as a cosolvent for dissolving water-insoluble analgesic drugs (Miller, 1991), but this practice was stopped after 1975. No systematic study of the inci-dence of cancer in this cohort has been made as yet. In addition, certain cytocidal drugs, such as the nitrogen mustards (Figure 3.3), which have been used to treat cancer in humans, are also known to be potent carcinogens (Chapter 11). The other three agents depicted on the bottom line of Figure 3.2 are also alkylating agents that are used industrially. Bis(chloromethyl)ether, a pop-ular intermediate in organic synthetic reactions, has been classified as carcinogenic to the human based on epidemiological as well as animal studies (Vainio et al., 1991).

Members of a number of other classes of compounds have been shown to be strong carcin-ogens and of potential importance in the genesis of neoplasia in the human being. The dialkylni-trosamines have the following general structure:

$$\begin{array}{c} R_1 \\ \diagdown \\ N-N=O \\ \diagup \\ R_2 \end{array}$$

in which R_1 and R_2 can be alkyl substituents or can be fused to yield a cyclic aliphatic substitu-ent. One of the structurally simplest nitrosamines, dimethylnitrosamine (Figure 3.3), is highly carcinogenic for the liver and kidney in rodents and for these and/or other tissues in all other mammals tested. Hepatic toxicity due to dimethylnitrosamine exposure occurred in humans working with this chemical at the time of its earliest industrial use. Subsequently, such exposure was eliminated by cessation of the industrial use of nitrosamines as solvents. Several investiga-tors (cf. Lijinsky, 1977; Magee and Swann, 1969; Mirvish et al., 1983) have shown in experi-mental animals that certain dietary components, especially in the presence of high levels of nitrite, may give rise to low levels

$$\begin{array}{c} R \qquad\qquad O \\ \diagdown \qquad \diagup\!\!\diagup \\ N-C \\ \diagup \qquad \diagdown \\ O=N \qquad\quad R' \end{array}$$

of nitrosamines or nitrosamides in the diet or in the stomach and induce neoplasia of the gas-trointestinal tract. The action of bacterial flora within the intestine may enhance the formation of these compounds. Furthermore, there is increasing evidence of an etiological role for endoge-nously formed N-nitroso compounds in the development of certain human cancers (Bartsch et al., 1990). The nitrosamine NNK (Figure 3.3) is produced in tobacco smoke from nicotine, a normal tobacco alkaloid (cf. Hecht, 1985). This is an extremely potent carcinogen to which all tobacco smokers are exposed and may play a role in the induction of tobacco-related cancers in the human. Methapyrilene was developed as an antihistamine but is a potent carcinogen in the rat (Mirsalis, 1987).

Another important environmental as well as experimental hepatocarcinogenic agent is aflatoxin B_1. This toxic substance is produced by certain strains of the mold *Aspergillus flavus*. Aflatoxin B_1 is one of the most potent hepatocarcinogenic agents known and has produced neoplasms in rodents, fish, birds, and primates. This agent is a potential contaminant of many farm products (for example, grain, peanuts) that are stored under warm and humid conditions for some time. Aflatoxin B_1 and related compounds may cause some of the toxic hepatitis and hepatic neoplasia seen in various parts of Africa and the Far East (Chapter 11).

Ethionine is an antimetabolite of the normal amino acid methionine. Farber (cf. 1963) was the first to show definitively that administration of ethionine in the diet for extended periods resulted in the development of liver cancer in rats. This was the first example of the direct interference with the metabolism of a normal metabolic constituent resulting in the development of cancer.

In addition to organic compounds such as those illustrated in Figures 3.1 and 3.3, a number of inorganic elements and their compounds have been shown to be carcinogenic in both animals and humans (IARC, 1973). Figure 3.4 shows a periodic classification of the elements with an indication of those elements that, in their elemental form or compounded with other elements, have been shown to be carcinogenic or possibly carcinogenic in humans, other animals, or both (Martell, 1981). This is not to say that all the elements of the table that have not been specifically shown to be carcinogenic should be considered noncarcinogenic. Many elements and their compounds have not yet been adequately tested for carcinogenicity in animals, and at this time there is no evidence that such elements exhibit effects in humans on the basis of epidemiological studies (Chapter 11). On the basis of epidemiological studies (Chapter 11), chromium and nickel are carcinogenic in both humans and experimental animals. However, several other elements have so far demonstrated carcinogenicity only in experimental animals. Exposure to several of these, including lead (Verschaeve et al., 1979) and beryllium (Kuschner, 1981), has been implicated as causes of cancer in humans, but as yet the data are not sufficient to demonstrate such an association unequivocally. On the other hand, arsenic and its derivatives present an

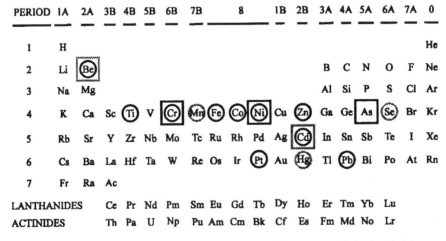

Figure 3.4 Periodic classification of the elements forming compounds having definite carcinogenic effects in the human (squares) or lower animals (circles). Dashed squares or circles around the symbols of some elements indicate that the compounds formed from them are suggestive of but not proven as to their carcinogenicity for humans or lower animals. (Adapted from Martell, 1981, with permission of the author and publisher.)

interesting paradox (Landrigan, 1981) in that there is essentially no experimental evidence to substantiate the carcinogenicity of this element and its compounds in lower animals, but the evidence for its carcinogenicity in humans is quite clear (Chapter 11).

One class of chemical carcinogens is different from those described thus far—the group of inert plastic and metal films or similar forms that cause sarcomas at the implantation site in some rodents (Brand et al., 1975). The implantation site is usually subcutaneous. At least one study indicated that the implantation of metal "films" did not induce neoplasms when they were implanted within the central nervous system (Bischoff and Bryson, 1976), although this may have been related to the relatively small size of the implants. Rats and mice are highly susceptible to this form of carcinogenesis, but guinea pigs appear to be resistant (Stinson, 1964). The carcinogenic properties of the implant are, to a large extent, dependent on its physical characteristics and surface area. Multiple perforations—each greater than a certain diameter (for example, 0.4 µm)—pulverization, or roughening of the surface of the implant (Ferguson, 1977) markedly reduced the incidence of neoplasms. Plastic sponge implants may also induce sarcomas subcutaneously, and in this instance the yield of tumors is dependent on the thickness of the sponge implant (Roe et al., 1967). The age of the animal upon implantation also affects the time from implantation until tumor development. Young rats first developed sarcomas at the site of implantation after nearly 1½ years, whereas older animals developed such neoplasms within 6 months after implantation of the material (Paulini et al., 1975).

The chemical nature of the implant is clearly not the critical factor in its ability to transform normal cells to neoplastic cells. Brand and associates (cf. Johnson et al., 1970) have studied this phenomenon for many years and have demonstrated a variety of kinetic and morphological characteristics of the process of "foreign-body tumorigenesis" in mice. These studies have shown that DNA synthesis occurs in the film-attached cell population throughout the preneoplastic phase and that preneoplastic cells may be identified well before neoplasms develop (Thomassen et al., 1978). More recently, Kirkpatrick and associates (2000), using a variety of plastics and metals as the subcutaneous implant, found that about one-third of the animals developed sarcomas in association with the implant by 2 years of age. Examination of the implants between 8 and 24 months after implantation revealed the presence of nonneoplastic proliferative lesions as well as preneoplastic lesions (Chapter 7), which may have served as precursors to the sarcomas. Brand has suggested that such "preneoplastic" cells may already be present in the normal tissue prior to implantation and that the implant appears to "create the conditions" required for carcinogenesis of these cells (Brand et al., 1975). Other possible mechanisms for this unique type of carcinogenesis are discussed later (Chapter 7), as well as its relation to specific human carcinogens (Chapter 11). An interesting but possibly unrelated observation is the demonstration by Hirono and associates (1983) of the carcinogenicity of sodium dextran sulfate in relation to its molecular weight. Only the polymer with a molecular weight of approximately 54,000, compared with polymers of 520,000 and 9500, induced colon cancer in rats when given orally.

While the epidemiological evidence that implants of prostheses in the human—such as seen with the repair of hernias, joint replacements, etc.—induce the formation of sarcomas is not substantial, there have been a number of isolated reports of neoplasms arising in association with such foreign bodies (Sunderman, 1989). A study in the rat of the carcinogenic potential of a number of materials used in such prostheses demonstrated a small increase in sarcomas in animals with certain metal alloy implants that contained significant amounts of cobalt, chromium, or nickel (Memoli et al., 1986). However, it is likely that in the human "foreign-body tumorigenesis" may be induced by certain types of asbestos fibers, wherein the dimensions of the fiber are directly related to its effectiveness as a carcinogenic agent (Chapter 11).

Chemical Carcinogenesis by Mixtures—Defined and Undefined

While most of this chapter concerns itself with the carcinogenic action of specific chemicals, it is relatively unusual that an individual is exposed to a single carcinogenic agent. Despite this fact, relatively few detailed studies on mixtures of carcinogenic chemicals have been carried out experimentally. The most common environmental mixtures are those seen in tobacco smoke and other combustion products, including engine exhaust and air pollution (Mauderly, 1993). Interactions between chemicals in mixtures may be additive, multiplicative, or inhibitory (Mumtaz et al., 1993). In the examples given above, however, the exact chemical nature of components in tobacco smoke or air pollution is not always known, nor are their amounts determined. Thus, one may be forced to deal with a mixture as if it were a single entity or, if the constituents are known, to treat the effects of the mixture in some empirical way usually related to the most potent component of the mixture.

Studies on the carcinogenic action of defined mixtures of chemicals are usually done with a knowledge of the carcinogenic effect of the chemicals involved. Warshawsky et al. (1993) demonstrated that extremely low levels of benzo[a]pyrene, which yielded no skin tumors on repeated application, resulted in a significant yield of neoplasms when added in the presence of five noncarcinogenic polycyclic aromatic hydrocarbons. In an earlier study, administration of two noncarcinogenic aminoazo dyes in the diet of the rat for a year resulted in the appearance of a variety of neoplasms (Neish et al., 1967). More recently, administration of three to five N-nitrosamines resulted in either an additive or synergistic carcinogenic effect of the combinations of the compounds given at low dose rates (Berger et al., 1987; Lijinsky et al., 1983). In contrast, administration of a mixture of 40 chemical carcinogens to rats for 2 years at 1/50 of the dose normally used to induce neoplasms in 50% of the animals and representing a wide variety of target sites resulted in significant tumor incidences only in the thyroid and liver (Takayama et al., 1989). In a more recent study, ingestion of a mixture of 20 pesticides given at "acceptable daily intake levels" was found to exert no effect on carcinogenesis in rat liver (Ito et al., 1994). While these are only a few examples, the toxicological study of complex mixtures, not only in the area of carcinogenesis, is a critical field in human health, as evidenced by disease resulting from tobacco smoke, engine exhaust, and other components of air pollution (Mauderly, 1993). One of the most important chemical mixtures associated with human neoplasia is that of diet.

Chemical Carcinogenesis by Diet

There is substantial evidence in the human to argue that many dietary components—including excess caloric intake (Osler, 1987; Lutz and Schlatter, 1992), excessive alcohol intake (IARC, 1987), and a variety of chemical contaminants of the diet including aflatoxin B_1 (Figure 3.2) (Gorchev and Jelinek, 1985; Lutz and Schlatter, 1992)—are carcinogenic (Chapter 11). Some general and specific studies have supported these views (Jensen and Madsen, 1988; Habs and Schmähl, 1980; Miller et al., 1994), whereas others have been more controversial (Willett and MacMahon, 1984; Pariza, 1984). Evidence for dietary factors associated with cancer incidence in animals is more substantial and serves to support much of the evidence relating environmental factors to increased cancer incidence in the human (Kritchevsky, 1988; Rogers et al., 1993).

Although a relative lack of "antioxidant micronutrients"—such as carotenoids, selenium, and the vitamins A, C, and E—has been implicated as a factor in the incidence of neoplastic development (Dorgan and Schatzkin, 1991), more studies are needed before the effectiveness of these agents in cancer prevention can be established unequivocally (Chapters 8 and 11). In contrast, experimental evidence that the lack of available sources of methyl groups can actually induce liver cancer in rats is well documented (Mikol et al., 1983; Ghoshal and Farber, 1984). This observation may be closely related to the earlier studies by Farber (1963) on the induction of liver cancer in rats by the administration of ethionine, which, indirectly, may cause a lack of available methyl groups in this tissue.

METABOLISM OF CHEMICAL CARCINOGENS IN RELATION TO CARCINOGENESIS

Although the discovery that polycyclic hydrocarbons and other chemical compounds could produce cancer gave hope that the complete understanding of the nature of neoplasia might be at hand, more than 60 years have elapsed since those findings appeared and we still seem to be a long way from such an understanding. The excretory metabolites of polycyclic hydrocarbons were found to be hydroxylated derivatives, which usually had little or no carcinogenic activity. Similarly, hydroxylation of the rings of the aromatic amine carcinogens, such as 2-acetylamino-fluorene (AAF) and 4-dimethylaminoazobenzene, usually resulted in a complete loss of activity. The enzymatic production of these more polar metabolites facilitated the further metabolism and excretion of the parent compounds.

The different classes of chemical carcinogens have no single common structural feature (Figures 3.1, 3.3, and 3.4). Thus, the complexity of the variety of chemicals capable of inducing cancer posed a striking dilemma in attempts to understand the mechanisms of action of these agents. The beginning of our present-day understanding of the solution to this dilemma was reported in 1947 by Elizabeth and James Miller, who first demonstrated that, during the process of hepatocarcinogenesis, azo dyes became covalently bound to proteins of the liver but not to proteins of the resulting neoplasms. Sorof and associates (1958) studied the proteins of liver that bind the dyes and demonstrated that azo dye–induced hepatomas did not contain the major dye-binding protein species, as evidenced by the technique of electrophoresis. Later studies with more highly differentiated hepatocellular carcinomas have shown the presence of the dye-binding proteins, but even in such lesions there was little or no binding of the dye to proteins of the neoplasm even when the carcinogens inducing those neoplasms were fed to animals bearing the transplanted cancers (Sorof et al., 1966). The initial studies of the Millers led them to suggest that the binding of carcinogens to proteins might lead to the loss or deletion of critical proteins for growth control (Chapter 11). The reader should recall that, at the time this hypothesis was proposed (1947), the molecular concept of the gene was in its infancy if understood at all.

As an extension of this work, Elizabeth Miller (1951) demonstrated the covalent binding of benzo(a)pyrene or some of its metabolites to proteins in the skin of mice treated with the hydrocarbon. Later Abell and Heidelberger (1962) showed the same phenomenon with another carcinogenic polycyclic hydrocarbon, 3-methylcholanthrene. These findings strongly suggested that a critical step in the induction of cancer by chemicals was the covalent interaction of some form of the chemical with proteins and possibly other macromolecules as well. Since the parent compound in all cases studied was incapable of covalent binding directly with macromolecules, the logical conclusion was that the interaction of the chemical with the macromolecule was the result of the metabolic action of the cell. Although a number of studies in the 1950s (cf. Weisburger and Weisburger, 1958) demonstrated that ring-hydroxylation was a major pathway in the metabolism of AAF, in 1960 the Millers and Cramer (Miller et al., 1960) reported that this compound was also metabolized by hydroxylation of the nitrogen of the acetylamino group. They isolated N-hydroxy-AAF from the urine of AAF-treated rats, and in subsequent investigations found this compound to be more carcinogenic that its parent, AAF. Furthermore, N-hydroxy-AAF also induced neoplasms that the parent compound was unable to induce, such as subcutaneous sarcomas at the site of injection. In animals (such as the guinea pig) that convert little of the AAF to its N-hydroxy derivative in vivo, cancer of the liver was not produced by feeding the parent compound. These findings strongly supported the suggestion that, at least in the case of AAF, the parent compound was not the direct carcinogen but rather that certain metabolic derivatives were the active components in the induction of neoplasia. These studies paved the way to further investigations of the activation of carcinogens by means of their metabolism by cellular enzymes (cf. J. A. Miller, 1970).

Figure 3.5 depicts a number of metabolic reactions involved in the "activation" of chemicals to forms that are directly involved with the induction of cancer. One may divide such metabolic functions into two general classes (cf. Goldstein and Faletto, 1993). Those involved in phase I metabolism (Figure 3.5) occur within the intracellular membrane system known as the endoplasmic reticulum. These reactions involve metabolism by cytochrome P-450 enzymes and their reductase. Generally these metabolic reactions convert the substrate to a more polar

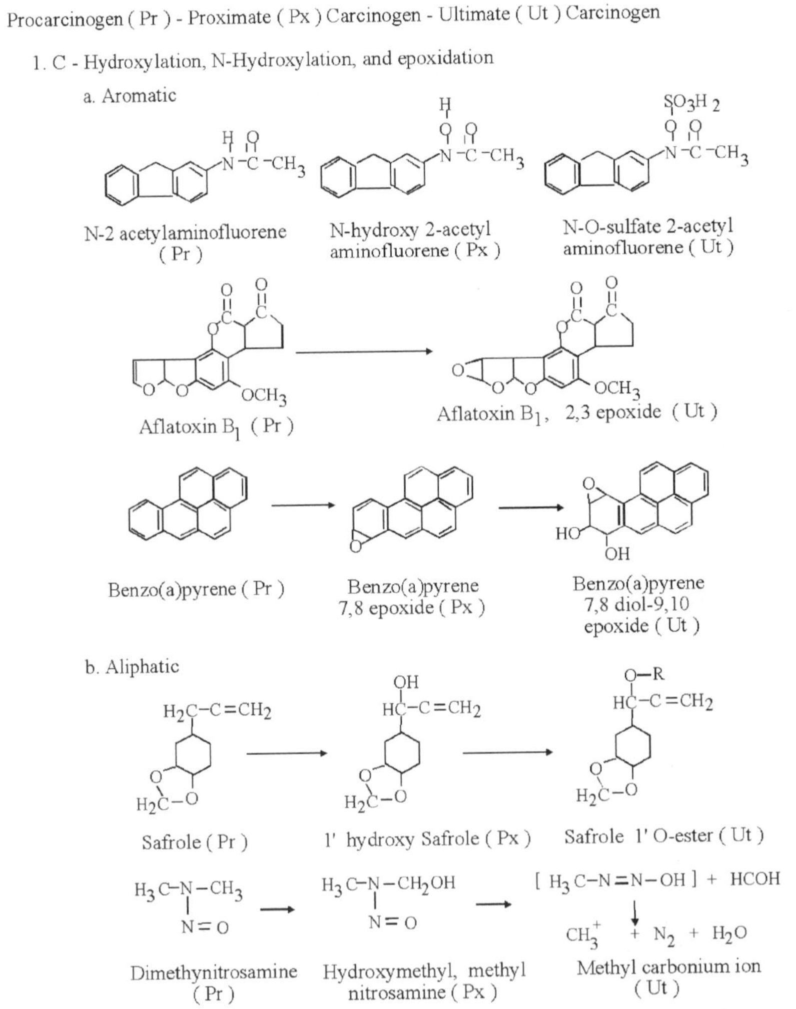

Figure 3.5 Structures of representative chemical carcinogens and their metabolic derivatives, the proximate and ultimate carcinogenic forms resulting from the action of phase I metabolism of procarcinogens.

A. Elimination (detoxification) reactions:

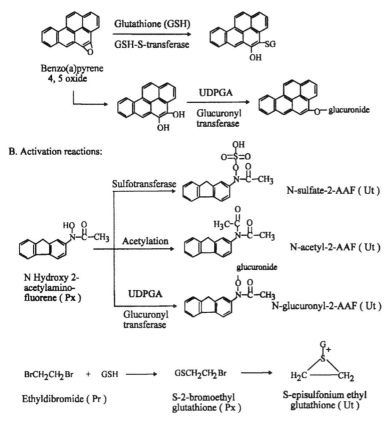

B. Activation reactions:

Figure 3.6 Structures of representative chemical carcinogens and their metabolic derivatives resulting from the action of phase II metabolism of procarcinogens.

compound through the insertion of molecular oxygen. Phase II metabolic reactions (Figure 3.6) involve mostly hydrolysis and conjugation and occur primarily, although not exclusively, in the extramembranous, cytosolic environment of the cell. This listing of xenobiotic metabolic reactions of the cell is not complete, a detailed consideration of these and other such reactions being beyond the scope of this text. The interested reader is referred to several pertinent references (Porter and Coon, 1991; Guengerich, 1992) for more complete coverage of this topic.

As noted in Figure 3.5, the N-hydroxylation of AAF can be followed by the esterification of the N-hydroxyl group, yielding a highly reactive compound capable of nonenzymatic reaction with nucleophilic sites on proteins and nucleic acids as well as comparable small molecules. The demonstration that the metabolism of AAF led to a highly reactive chemical prompted the Millers to propose that chemical carcinogens are—or are converted by their metabolism into—electrophilic reactants (chemicals with electron-deficient sites) that exert their biological effects by covalent interaction with cellular macromolecules, the most critical target probably being DNA (cf. Miller, 1978). Furthermore, utilizing the metabolism of AAF as a model, the Millers proposed that chemical carcinogens requiring metabolism for their carcinogenic effect be termed *procarcinogens*, whereas their highly reactive metabolites, such as the N-hydroxy AAF esters, were termed *ultimate carcinogens*. Metabolites intermediate between the procarcinogens and ultimate carcinogens, where such existed, were termed *proximate carcinogens*. The ultimate form of the carcinogen, that is, the form that actually interacts with cellular constituents and probably causes the neoplastic transformation, is the final product shown in most of the pathways seen in Figure 3.5. In some instances, however, the structure of the ultimate form of certain carcinogenic chemicals is still not clear. In other cases there may be more than one ultimate carcinogenic metabolite.

After the demonstration by the Millers of the critical significance of electrophilic metabolites in chemical carcinogenesis, a number of such ultimate forms—especially those of aromatic amines such as benzidene, naphthylamine and 4-aminobiphenyl—were described. However, the carcinogenic polycyclic hydrocarbons still posed a problem. As early as 1950, Boyland had proposed the formation of epoxide intermediates in the metabolism of these chemicals. However, it was not until 1970 that Jerina and associates detected the formation of such an intermediate in a biological system. Other investigations showed that epoxides of polycyclic hydrocarbons could react with nucleic acids and proteins in the absence of any metabolizing system. Surprisingly, K-region epoxides of a number of carcinogenic polycyclic hydrocarbons were weaker carcinogens than the parent hydrocarbons. Following this finding, scientific attention shifted to other reactive metabolites of these molecules. In 1974 Sims and associates proposed that a diol epoxide of benzo(a)pyrene was the ultimate form of this carcinogen. Subsequent studies by a number of investigators (Yang et al., 1976; see reviews: Conney, 1982; Harvey, 1981; Lowe and Silverman, 1984) have demonstrated that the structure of this ultimate form is (+)anti-benzo(a)pyrene-7,8-dihydrodiol-9,10-epoxide. A number of the metabolic reactions that benzo(a)pyrene may undergo in vivo are seen in Figures 3.5 and 3.6. As mentioned earlier, the 4,5-(K-region) epoxide of benzo(a)pyrene is less carcinogenic than the parent compound and markedly less carcinogenic than the diol epoxide. The reader is referred to the cited reviews for further discussion of the implications of such metabolic pathways.

One of the interesting ramifications of these findings is the importance of oxidation of the carbons of the "bay region" of potentially carcinogenic polycyclic hydrocarbons. Figure 3.2 shows the bay regions of benz(a)anthracene and benzo(a)pyrene. Analogous bay regions may easily be identified in the other structures seen in Figure 3.1. Jerina, Conney, and associates (for example, Levin et al., 1978), as well as others (cf. Conney, 1982), have proposed that epoxidation of a dihydro, angular benzo ring that forms part of a bay region of a polycyclic hydrocarbon forms the most likely ultimate carcinogenic form of the hydrocarbon. The bay region is the sterically hindered region formed by the angular benzo ring. Although the bay-region concept has not been tested with all known carcinogenic polycyclic hydrocarbons, it appears to be generally applicable. In addition, Cavalieri and Rogan (1992) have proposed that radical cations of polycyclic aromatic hydrocarbons formed by oxidation of the parent compound via the cytochrome P-450 pathway are also important intermediates in the formation of ultimate carcinogenic metabolites of these chemicals.

Although conjugation reactions usually inactivate chemical carcinogens and cause their rapid urinary excretion because of their water solubility, an interesting exception to this has recently been shown. Both haloalkanes and haloalkenes react with glutathione as catalyzed by glutathione S-transferase. As an example, the glutathione-dependent bioactivation of ethylene dibromide is seen in Figure 3.6. The proximate carcinogen, glutathione S-ethylbromide, spontaneously forms an episulfonium ion as the ultimate carcinogenic form. This highly reactive chemical alkylates DNA at the N^7 position of guanine (Koga et al., 1986). Cysteine S-conjugates of several haloalkenes as well as the glutathione conjugates are nephrotoxic as well as mutagenic (cf. Monks et al., 1990). While such halogenated aliphatics may induce neoplasia in several organs, the kidney is the predominant target organ; but the actual mechanism of the carcinogenic effect is not yet clear despite the observations noted above (Monks et al., 1990).

In addition to the electrophilic intermediates previously discussed that make up many if not all of the structures of the ultimate forms of chemical carcinogens, substantial evidence has also indicated that free radical derivatives of chemical carcinogens may be produced both metabolically and nonenzymatically during their metabolism (cf. Nagata et al., 1982). Free radicals carry no charge but possess a single unpaired electron, which makes the radical extremely reactive. That such forms may be important in the induction of the neoplastic transformation by chemicals comes from two lines of evidence. Several different molecules that inhibit the formation of free radicals, many of which are termed antioxidants, are capable of inhibiting the carcinogenic action of many chemical carcinogens (Ito and Hirose, 1987; Simic, 1988). Although there is no question that free radical intermediates are sometimes formed during the metabolism of chemical carcinogens (Guengerich, 1991), the evidence suggests that relatively specific metabolic reactions of a number of chemical carcinogens may proceed through free radical intermediates. Marnett (1981) has described the co-oxygenation of polyunsaturated fatty acids, especially arachidonic acid, with polycyclic aromatic hydrocarbons, leading to the formation of the diol epoxide (Figure 3.5). Such co-oxygenation occurs in the formation of prostaglandins, a series of hormones important in the normal homeostasis of the organism, from the polyunsaturated fatty acid arachidonic acid. The reaction involves the formation of a hydroperoxide by the incorporation of molecular oxygen (two atoms) at a double-bond position with the simultaneous formation of a ring peroxide. The peroxidase activity of the prostaglandin-synthesizing enzyme (synthetase) catalyzes the transfer of the free radical to another molecule with the formation of oxygen, as shown in Figure 3.7 to be the case with AAF. In the case of the 7,8-diol of benzo(a)pyrene (Figure 3.7), the peroxidase catalyzes the transfer of the free radical oxygen from the hydroperoxide to the hydrocarbon, forming an epoxide, which in this case is the ultimate form of the carcinogen. N-acetoxy AAF is also one of the ultimate forms of that carcinogen. This pathway of metabolic activation of carcinogens is not ubiquitous in all tissues but is more important in some than in others. Wise et al. (1984) demonstrated that the metabolic activation of 2-naphthylamine via the prostaglandin synthase reaction was quite marked in dog bladder but virtually nonexistent in the liver of this animal. This finding suggests that the carcinogenic action of 2-naphthylamine on bladder transitional epithelium involves primarily the co-oxygenation of the arylamine and polyunsaturated fatty acids in the prostaglandin synthetase reaction. Other chemical carcinogens, including nitrosamines (Bartsch et al., 1989) and nitro compounds (Conaway et al., 1991), may exhibit ultimate forms that are free radicals in nature.

Endogenous Free Radicals and Chemical Carcinogenesis

In addition to the formation of free radicals affecting the metabolism of exogenous procarcinogens, endogenous free radicals are also formed both as by-products of carcinogen metabolism and during normal metabolic reactions. Molecular oxygen (O_2) contains unpaired electrons and acts as the final pathway of electrons produced during metabolism. In such metabolic reactions oxygen is reduced by single electrons by processes depicted in Figure 3.8. The most reactive species that may be considered free radicals are the superoxide anion and the hydroxyl radical. Hydrogen peroxide is formed from the superoxide radical but itself is not a free radical. On the other hand, in the presence of trace amounts of metal ions, especially those of iron and copper, the hydroxyl free radical is formed from hydrogen peroxide (Bast et al., 1991). In addition to the reduction of oxygen in mitochondria, which is perhaps the largest source of these radicals, a process termed *redox cycling*, involving the one-electron reduction of a xenobiotic followed by

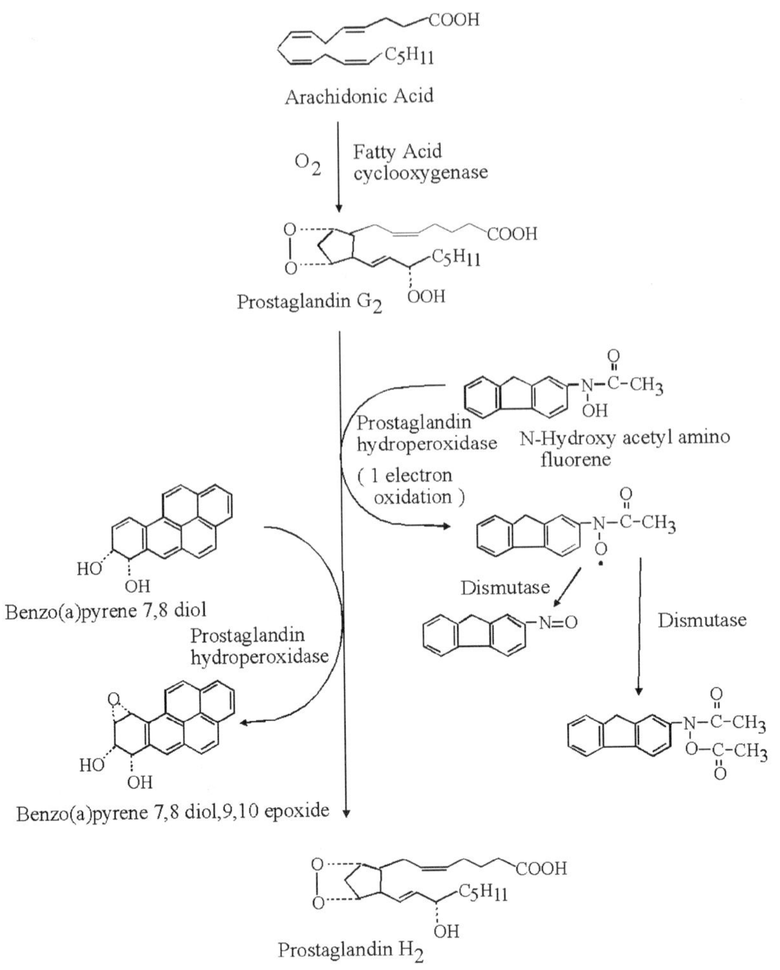

Figure 3.7 The metabolic activation of benzo(a)pyrene 7,8 diol and N-hydroxy 2-acetylaminofluorene during the peroxidation of arachidonic acid.

interaction with molecular oxygen and resulting in superoxide production and regeneration of the parent xenobiotic, also gives rise to reactive oxygen species (ROS) by a scheme noted in Figure 3.9. Free radicals of oxygen reduction, especially the hydroxyl radical, may abstract a hydrogen atom from lipids, leading to their peroxidation. Peroxidation of lipids having conjugated double bonds may lead ultimately to the formation of a variety of aldehydes, which are also capable of reacting with macromolecules (Bast and Goris, 1989). Two toxic aldehydes formed by this process are malonaldehyde and 4-hydroxy-2-nonanal. These aldehydes are mutagenic (Chung et al., 1993) and at least malonaldehyde has been reported to be carcinogenic for mouse skin (Shamberger et al., 1974). Epoxyaldehydes of hydroxynonanal can react with deoxyribonucleosides to form etheno adducts as seen in Figure 3.10 (Chung et al., 1996). In addition, reactive oxygen species may be involved in the alteration of signal transduction pathways (Chapter 7), and as noted later in this chapter in discussing the effects of ionizing radiation on living cells (Toyokuni, 1999).

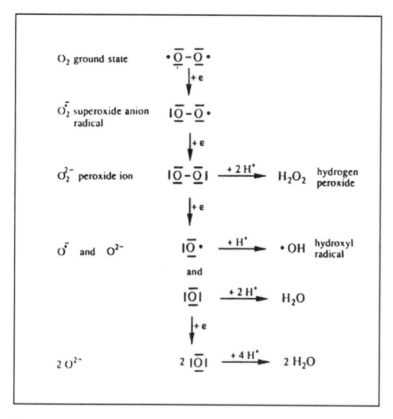

Figure 3.8 The univalent reduction of oxygen. (Adapted from Bast et al., 1991, with permission of authors and publisher.)

Some Conclusions

All of these studies taken together demonstrate that the majority of chemical carcinogens must be metabolized within the cell before they exert their carcinogenic effects. In this respect carcinogenesis by some chemicals becomes a "lethal synthesis" analogous to that of the earlier studies by Peters (1957), who coined the term with reference to fluoroacetate. Furthermore, this finding explains how a substance that is not carcinogenic for one species may be carcinogenic

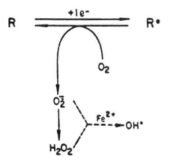

Figure 3.9 General scheme for redox cycling of xenobiotics (R) with generation of oxygen radicals. (Adapted from Ross, 1989, with permission of author and publisher.)

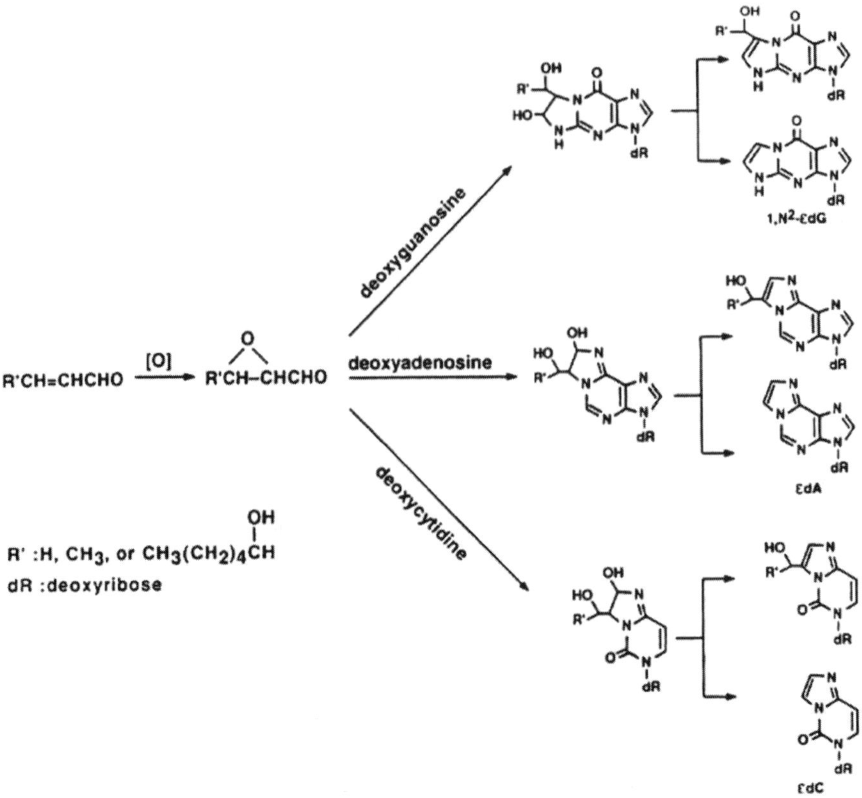

Figure 3.10 Formation of some etheno adducts from reactions of deoxyribonucleosides with epoxyaldehydes. (Adapted from Chung et al., 1996, with permission of authors and publisher.)

for another, the result depending on the metabolic capacities present within the species itself. This becomes extremely important for carcinogen testing in whole animals (see below).

Not all chemical carcinogens require intracellular metabolism to become ultimate carcinogens. Examples are the direct alkylating agents β-propiolacetone, nitrogen mustard, ethyleneimine, and bis(chloromethyl)ether (Figure 3.3), the latter having been shown to be carcinogenic for humans (Chapter 9). These chemicals have been termed *direct-acting* or *alkylating carcinogens* because of the highly reactive nature of their native structure, which itself is the ultimate carcinogenic form of that molecule.

Chemical Structure and Chemical Carcinogenesis

Knowledge of the metabolic activation of chemicals has dramatically advanced our understanding of carcinogenic mechanisms underlying the extreme diversity of chemical structures involved in cancer development. The relationship of chemical structure to carcinogenic activity plays a significant role in the potential identification and mechanism of potential chemical carcinogens. Computerized databases of carcinogenic and noncarcinogenic chemicals have been developed to relate structure to carcinogenic activity in a variety of carcinogens (Enslein et al., 1994; Rosenkranz and Klopman, 1994).

Using as a primary basis the results of rodent bioassays on more than 500 chemicals, Ashby and Paton (1993) have studied the influence of chemical structure on both the extent and the target tissue specificity of carcinogenesis for these chemicals. From analysis of the presence of potential electrophilic sites (DNA reactive), mutagenicity to *Salmonella*, and level of carcinogenicity to rodents (Chapter 13), these authors have developed a list of chemical structures that possess a high correlation with the development of neoplasia in rodent tests (Ashby et al., 1989; Tennant and Ashby, 1991). These "structural alerts" signify that a chemical having such structures should be examined closely for carcinogenic potential. These authors have developed a composite model structure indicating the various structural alerts that appear to be associated with DNA reactivity or carcinogenicity (Figure 3.11). The substantial database used to generate these structural alerts indicates the utility of this information for the identification of potential carcinogens and their mechanisms of their action in specific tissues. In addition, investigation of the metabolic activation of such functional groups during the carcinogenic process should provide insight into their role in the induction of cancer.

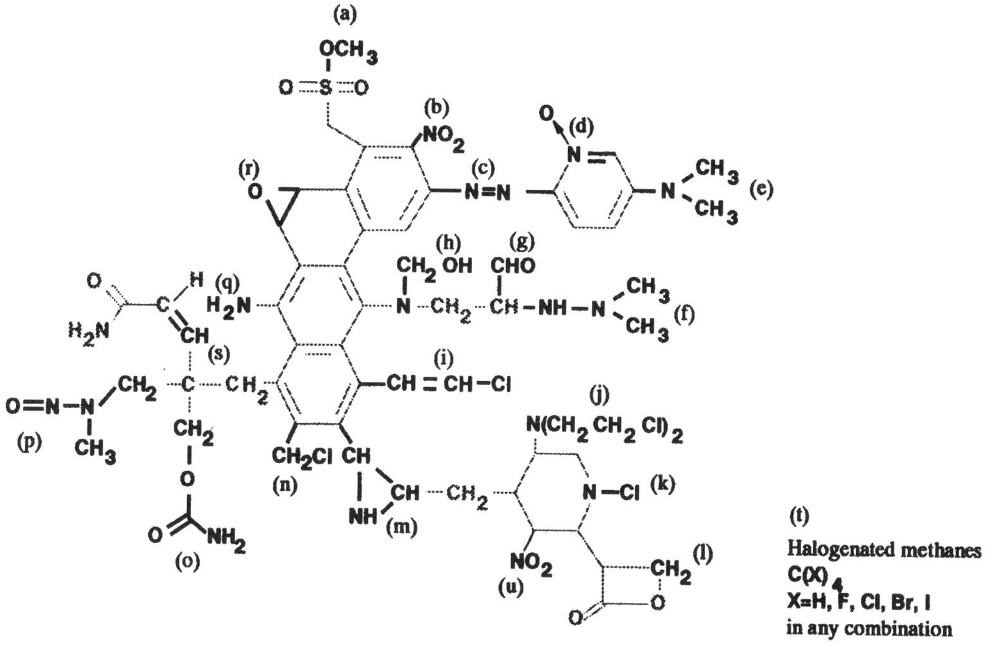

Figure 3.11 The substituents are as follows: (a) alkyl esters of either phosphonic or sulfonic acids; (b) aromatic nitro groups; (c) aromatic azo groups, not per se, but by virtue of their possible reduction to an aromatic amine; (d) aromatic ring, *N*-oxides; (e) aromatic mono- and dialkylamino groups; (f) alkyl hydrazines; (g) alkyl aldehydes; (h) *N*-methylol derivatives; (i) monohaloalkenes; (j) a large family of *N* and *S* mustards (ß-haloethyl); (k) *N*-chloramines (see below); (l) propiolactones and propiosultones; (m) aromatic and aliphatic aziridinyl derivatives; (n) both aromatic and aliphatic substituted primary alkyl halides; (o) derivatives of urethane (carbamates); (p) alkyl-*N*-nitrosamines; (q) aromatic amines, their *N*-hydroxy derivatives and the derived esters; (r) aliphatic and aromatic epoxides. The *N*-chloramine substructure (k) has not yet been associated with carcinogenicity, but potent genotoxic activity has been reported for it (discussed in Ashby et al., 1989). Michael-reactive a,ß-unsaturated esters, amides or nitriles form a relatively new class of genotoxin (e.g., acrylamide). However, the structural requirements for genotoxicity have yet to be established, and this structural unit is not shown in the figure. (Adapted from Tennant and Ashby, 1991, with permission of the authors and publisher.)

DNA, RNA, AND PROTEIN ADDUCTS RESULTING FROM THEIR REACTION WITH ULTIMATE CARCINOGENIC FORMS

One of the most intriguing problems that experimental oncologists have considered in the area of chemical carcinogenesis is the characterization of the covalent compounds resulting from reactions between the ultimate metabolite of a chemical carcinogen and a macromolecule. The structures of several different chemical carcinogens covalently bound or adducted to protein and nucleic acids are shown in Figure 3.12. For the detailed chemistry of the reactions involved in the formation of such adducts, students are referred to several of the references, especially those by the Millers (1970, 1978), Weisburger and Williams (1982), Hathway and Kolar (1980), and Dipple et al. (1985). Guanine is the nucleic acid base that has been found to react most avidly with the "ultimate" forms of chemical carcinogens. As noted in Figure 3.12, the reaction of the ultimate form of N-methyl-4-aminoazobenzene with polypeptides involves a demethylation of

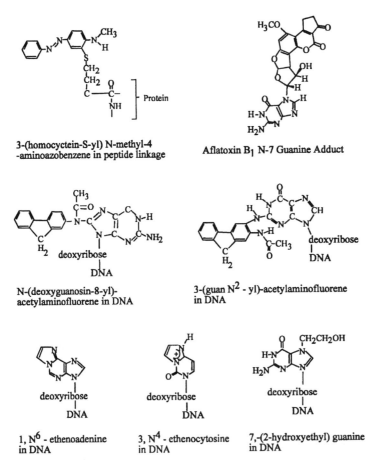

3-(homocyctein-S-yl) N-methyl-4
-aminoazobenzene in peptide linkage

Aflatoxin B$_1$ N-7 Guanine Adduct

N-(deoxyguanosin-8-yl)-
acetylaminofluorene in DNA

3-(guan N^2 - yl)-acetylaminofluorene
in DNA

1, N^6 - ethenoadenine
in DNA

3, N^4 - ethenocytosine
in DNA

7,-(2-hydroxyethyl) guanine
in DNA

Figure 3.12 Structures of some protein- and nucleic acid–bound forms of certain chemical carcinogens. The macromolecular linkages are shown schematically. Esters of 2-acetylaminofluorene react predominantly with the 8-position of guanine, whereas the epoxide of aflatoxin B$_1$ reacts primarily with the N-7 position of guanine. The ethano-adenine and ethanocytosine adducts result from the reaction of DNA with halogenated acetaldehydes or ultimate forms of vinyl chloride and related structures. 7,-(2-hydroxyethyl)guanine is a product of the reaction of ethylene oxide with DNA.

methionine and reaction of the electrophilic position ortho to the amino group of the azobenzene with the nucleophilic sulfur of methionine and subsequent loss of the methyl of methionine. Adducts formed with DNA, which in most instances are similar to those seen in RNA, exhibit stereospecific configurations as exemplified by the reaction of the epoxide of aflatoxin B_1 with N-7 position of guanine. AAF also reacts with guanine at the two positions of the DNA base, as shown. The formation of an additional ring structure in adenine and cytosine occurs with the ultimate form of the carcinogen vinyl chloride as well as related chemicals that exhibit the same ultimate form (Bolt, 1988). In contrast, ethylene oxide directly alkylates the N-7 position of guanine in DNA (Bolt et al., 1988). An interesting adduction occurs during the metabolism of 2-nitropropane that causes the formation of 8-aminoguanine, possibly from the spontaneous reaction with the highly reactive intermediate (NH_2^+) that is probably formed during the metabolism of the nitro group (Sodum et al., 1993).

Of the number of chemical carcinogens that adduct DNA by direct methylation, ethylation, or higher alkylations, several such agents are of considerable experimental and environmental significance. The positions alkylated by ethylating and methylating chemicals are noted in Figure 3.13, taken from the review by Pegg (1984). In this same discussion, Pegg described the relative proportions of methylated bases present in DNA after reaction with carcinogen-methylating agents (Table 3.1). The predominant adduct seen with methylating agents such as methylmethane sulfonate administered in vivo or in vitro is 7-methylguanine. In contrast, ethylation of DNA is predominantly in the phosphate backbone. Pegg has argued that the principal carcinogenic adduct is the O^6-alkylguanine. In contrast, Swenberg et al. (1984) reported that O^4-alkylthymine may be a more important adduct for carcinogenesis because it remains in the DNA for much more extended periods than the O^6-alkylguanine. The importance of the persistence of DNA adducts of ultimate carcinogens is discussed below.

Another common structural change in DNA is the hydroxylation of DNA bases. Such changes have been found in all four of the bases making up DNA (Marnett and Burcham, 1993), but the more commonly analyzed are 5-hydroxymethylthymine (Srinivasan and Glauert, 1990) and 8-hydroxyguanine (cf. Floyd, 1990). These hydroxylated bases have been found in DNA of target organs in animals exposed to chemical carcinogens, but they are also present in the DNA of organisms not subjected to any known carcinogenic agent (Marnett and Burcham, 1993). Estimates of a rate of endogenous depurination of DNA of 580 bases per hour per cell and DNA strand breaks at a rate of 2300 per hour per cell have been reported (Shapiro, 1981). These estimates are not incompatible with the presence of oxidative DNA lesions at a level of 10^6 per cell in the young rat and almost twice this in the old rat (cf. Table 3.6; Ames et al., 1993). Such oxidative damage is presumably due to free radical reactions occurring endogenously in the cell that are capable of producing activated oxygen radicals (cf. Floyd, 1990; Ames et al., 1993). Such oxidative reactions, occurring either as a result of an endogenous oxidative phenomenon or from the administration of exogenous chemical and radiation carcinogens, are presumably rapidly repaired by mechanisms discussed below. Thus, endogenous mutations are kept to a minimum.

Finally, structural changes in DNA of largely unknown character have been reported through the use of a unique technology known as ^{32}P-postlabeling (Reddy and Randerath, 1987). The outline of procedures used in this technology can be seen in Figure 3.14. After digestion of DNA to its constituent nucleotides, each nucleotide is labeled by using $g^{32}PO_4$-labeled ATP and a bacterial kinase, an enzyme that transfers the terminal phosphate of ATP to the available 5′ hydroxyl of the 3′ nucleotides to convert all of the nucleotides to a radioactive, biphosphorylated form. Nucleotides of the normal DNA bases are removed by appropriate chromatographic procedures, leaving only those nucleotides that contain structural adducts. Although this technique has been used to demonstrate adduction of DNA by a variety of known chemical carcinogens, equally if not more interesting is the fact that a number of adducts of unknown structure have

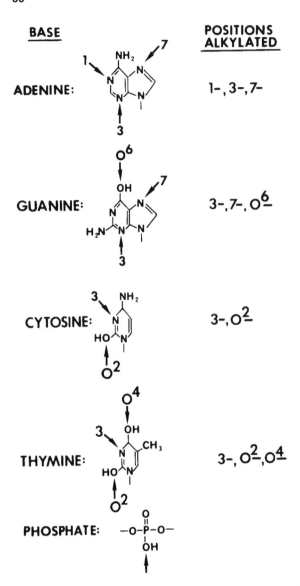

Figure 3.13 Sites of alkylation of DNA under physiological conditions. (From Pegg, 1984, with permission of the author and publisher.)

been discovered in living cells. Some of these structurally unknown DNA adducts, termed I-compounds (Li and Randerath, 1992), change with dietary modifications, drug administration (Randerath et al., 1992), and species and tissue differences (Li et al., 1990). I-compounds occur in human fetal tissues (Hansen et al., 1993), tend to increase with age and caloric restriction, but decrease in the liver during hepatocarcinogenesis (Randerath et al., 1991). Thus, the exact role if any of many DNA adducts of unknown structure in the process of carcinogenesis remains a question.

The mechanisms of inorganic chemical carcinogenesis have not been as well defined as those of organic chemicals. The interesting uniqueness of arsenic as a human carcinogen has not

Table 3.1 Relative Proportions of Methylated Bases Present in DNA After Reaction with Carcinogenic Alkylating Agents

	Percentage of Total Alkylation by:	
	Dimethylnitrosamine N-methyl-N-nitrosourea 1,2-dimethyl-hydrazine	Diethylnitrosamine N-ethyl-N-nitrosourea
1-Alkyladenine	0.7	0.3
3-Alkyladenine	8	4
7-Alkyladenine	1.5	0.4
3-Alkylguanine	0.8	0.6
7-Alkylguanine	68	12
O^6-Alkylguanine	7.5	8
3-Alkylcytosine	0.5	0.2
O^2-Alkylcytosine	0.1	3
3-Alkylthymine	0.3	0.8
O^2-Alkylthymine	0.1	7
O^4-Alkylthymine	0.1–0.7	1–4
Alkylphosphates	12	53

Adapted from Pegg, 1984, with permission of the author and publisher.

yet been adequately explained. On the other hand, chromate induces DNA crosslinks in vivo in possible association with active oxygen radicals (Tsapakos et al., 1981; Costa, 1991). While the mechanisms of cadmium carcinogenesis are also relatively unclear, nickel as a carcinogen both in animals and humans apparently may effect carcinogenesis by a variety of mechanisms, including alterations in the structure of DNA itself (Sunderman, 1989; Costa, 1991).

The best-known and structurally identified normal modification of DNA is the methylation of deoxycytidine residues by the transfer of a methyl group from S-adenosylmethionine by DNA methyltransferase (Holliday, 1989; Michalowsky and Jones, 1989). Such methylation results in the heritable expression or repression of specific genes in eukaryotic cells. When such methylation occurs during development, the expression or repression of specific genes may be "imprinted" by DNA methylation at various stages during development (Chapter 5; Barlow, 1993). Chemical carcinogens may inhibit this process by several mechanisms, including the formation of covalent adducts, single-strand breaks in the DNA, and the direct inactivation of the enzyme DNA S-adenosylmethionine methyltransferase, which is responsible for normal methylation (cf. Riggs and Jones, 1983). Therefore the inhibition of DNA methylation by chemical carcinogens may represent a further potential mechanism for carcinogenesis induced by chemicals. That such a mechanism may be important in hepatocarcinogenesis was reported by Mikol et al. (1983), wherein half of the animals receiving a defined diet devoid of methionine and choline developed hepatocellular carcinomas and cholangiomas when subjected to this regimen for 18 months. The methyl-deficient diet induces a drastic hypomethylation of hepatic nuclear DNA (Wilson et al., 1984).

From this brief survey, the student may appreciate that the role of structural adducts of DNA in carcinogenesis is not a simple matter of adduct = mutation = carcinogenesis. Defined adducts of known complete chemical carcinogens, as exemplified by those depicted in Figure 3.11, generally may be considered to have a significant role in carcinogenesis induced by their procarcinogenic forms. However, the role and function of structurally undefined adducts such as I-compounds in the carcinogenic process is not so clear, nor is there substantial evidence that

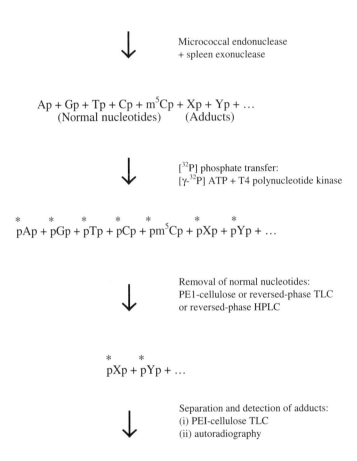

Carcinogen - adducted DNA

Maps of ^{32}P-labeled carcinogen-DNA adducts

Figure 3.14   The basic features of ^{32}P-postlabeling assay for carcinogen-adducted DNA. The ^{32}P-assay involves four steps: digestion of DNA, ^{32}P-labeling of the digestion products, removal of ^{32}P-labeled non-adduct components, and thin layer chromatography mapping of the [^{32}P] adducts. Asterisks indicate the position of the ^{32}P-label. (Modified from Gupta et al., 1982.)

such adduction leads directly to mutation. Finally, the inhibition of normal methylation of DNA may itself play a role, as yet undefined, in the carcinogenic process.

PERSISTENCE OF DNA ADDUCTS AND MUTAGENESIS

The extent to which DNA adducts occur as the result of the administration of chemical carcinogens depends on the overall metabolism of the chemical agent as well as the chemical reactivity of the ultimate metabolite. Once the adduct is formed, its continued presence in the DNA of the cell depends primarily on the ability of the cellular machinery to repair the structural alteration in the DNA, the mechanisms for which are discussed below.

Persistence of DNA Adducts

It is from many of the considerations noted above as well as the presumed critical nature of the adduct in the carcinogenic process that a working hypothesis has evolved which postulates that the extent of the formation of DNA adducts and their persistence in the DNA should correlate with the biological effect of the agent (Neumann, 1983). In accord with this hypothesis, several studies have correlated the persistence of DNA adducts occurring during chemical carcinogenesis with the high incidence of neoplasms in specific tissues (Table 3.2). Among the earliest of these studies was that of Goth and Rajewsky (1974), who demonstrated the relative persistence of O^6 ethylguanine in DNA of brain but not liver of animals administered ethylnitrosourea at 10 days of age. The rapid loss of the adduct in liver DNA contrasted with the seven times slower loss in DNA of the brain correlated with the appearance of neoplastic lesions in these tissues later in life. Swenberg and associates (1985) demonstrated an analogous situation in the liver, wherein administration of symmetrical dimethylhydrazine induced a high incidence of neoplasms of hepatic vascular endothelium but a very low incidence in parenchymal cells of this tissue. Examination of the same adduct, O^6-ethylguanine, demonstrated its rapid removal from the DNA of hepatocytes but much slower removal from the DNA of nonparenchymal cells in the liver, a large proportion of which are vascular endothelial cells. Similarly, Kadlubar and associates (1981) demonstrated that more guanine adducts of 2-naphthylamine persisted in bladder epithelium (urothelium) than in liver after administration of the carcinogen to dogs. The bladder, but not the liver, is a target for this carcinogen and, as discussed earlier, the metabolic activation of this chemical and other aromatic amines appears to be different in the two tissues (see above). When the susceptibility to carcinogenesis by diethylnitrosamine was investigated in the same tissue in two different species, only the DNA of hamster lung exhibited significant alkylation and the development of neoplasia.

While the correlations noted in Table 3.2 support the working hypothesis of the importance of specific adducts during the carcinogenic process, this is not the entire picture. Swenberg et al. (1984) demonstrated that the O^4-ethylthymine adduct but not the O^6-ethylguanine adduct is stable in liver parenchymal cells after the continuous exposure of rats to diethylnitrosamine. Furthermore, Müller and Rajewsky (1983) found that the O^4-ethylthymine adduct persisted in all organs after the administration of ethylnitrosourea to neonatal or adult rats. Later studies by Rajewsky and associates (1998) found that the O^6-ethylguanine adduct was removed from the DNA of specific genes in the mammary gland some 20 times faster than the O^6-methylguanine adduct. Persistence of DNA adducts of the carcinogenic trans-4-aminostilbene did not correlate with tissue susceptibility. While the liver and kidney exhibited the greatest burden and persistence of the adduct, and the ear duct glands of Zymbal the least adduct concentration, it is the latter tissue that is most susceptible to carcinogenesis by this agent (Neumann, 1983).

Despite these and other exceptions to the working hypothesis, our knowledge of the persistence of covalent adducts of DNA and carcinogenic chemicals in tissues has been utilized in attempts to quantitate the exposure of humans to carcinogenic chemicals and relate the potential risk of neoplastic development to such exposure. The occurrence of adducts of benzo(a)pyrene throughout the tissues of exposed animals at unexpectedly similar levels (Stowers and Anderson, 1985) further supports the rationale for the investigation of persistent DNA adducts as well as carcinogen-protein adducts in the human. Immunological and highly sensitive chromatographic technologies have been used to demonstrate the presence of persistent DNA adducts of several carcinogenic species (Perera et al., 1991; Shields and Harris, 1991). The detection of DNA adducts of carcinogenic polycyclic aromatic hydrocarbons has been demonstrated at relatively high levels in tissues, especially in blood cells of smokers and foundry workers, compared with nonexposed individuals (Perera et al., 1991). Huh et al. (1989) have demonstrated an increased level of O^4-ethylthymine in the DNA of liver from individuals with and without malignant neo-

Table 3.2 Organ and Species Specificity of Chemical Carcinogenesis in Relation to Persistence of Adducts in DNA

Species	Carcinogen	Tissue	DNA Adduct ($t_{1/2}$)	Neoplastic Development	Reference
Rat (neonates)	ENU	Liver	O^6EtG (30 h)	±	(Goth & Rajewsky, 1974)
Rat (neonates)	ENU	Brain	O^6EtG (220 h)	+++	
Rat	SDMH	Liver, hepatocytes	O^6MeG (~1.6 days)	±	(Swenberg et al., 1985)
Rat	SDMH	Liver, nonparenchymal cells	O^6MeG (>20 days)	+++	
Dog	2-NA	Liver	N-(dG-8-yl)-2-NA (~2 days)	0	(Kadlubar et al., 1981)
Dog	2-NA	Urothelium	N-(dG-8-yl)-2-NA (>20 days)	+++	
Hamster	DEN	Lung	O^6EtG (91 h)	+++	(Becker and Shank, 1985)
Rat	DEN	Lung	O^6EtG (undetectable)	0	

Key: ENU, ethylnitrosourea; SDMH, symmetrical dimethylhydrazine; DEN, diethylnitrosamine; 2-NA, 2-naphthylamine; O^6EtG, O^6 ethylguanine; N-(dG-8-yl)-2-NA, N-(deoxyguanosin-8-yl)-2-naphthylamine; O^6MeG, O^6 methylguanine; +++, high incidence of neoplasms; ±, occasional neoplasm; 0, no increased incidence of neoplasia above untreated controls.

plasms; however, a statistically significant increased level of ethylation of this base was noted in cancer patients as compared with controls. In a more recent study by Hsieh and Hsieh (1993), DNA adducts of aflatoxin B_1 were demonstrated in samples of human placenta and cord blood from patients in Taiwan, an area of high liver cancer incidence (Chapter 11). In addition to the determination of specific structural DNA adducts, the use of the ^{32}P-postlabeling assay to determine the presence of DNA adducts in human tissues has also been exploited (Beach and Gupta, 1992). As expected, a variety of adducts are found in both normal individuals and those potentially exposed to specific carcinogenic agents. In addition to DNA adducts, adducts of specific carcinogens with serum proteins have been demonstrated. Bryant et al. (1987) have shown a five- to sixfold greater level of hemoglobin adducts of 4-aminobiphenyl in smokers compared with nonsmokers. While this adduct has a finite lifetime, the chronic exposure to cigarette smoke dramatically increases the level of the adduct, suggesting the use of such determinations in estimating exposure to carcinogenic agents.

Thus, the persistence of macromolecular adducts of the ultimate forms of chemical carcinogens may be very important in the carcinogenic mechanism of such agents. However, as noted above, such persistence is only one factor in the complex process of cancer development.

Mutagenesis and Carcinogenesis

As noted above, the majority of chemical carcinogens must be metabolized within the cell before they exert their carcinogenic activity. In this respect, metabolism of some chemicals results in a bioactivation instead of elimination. Thus, metabolic capabilities may underlie how a substance that is not carcinogenic for one species may be carcinogenic for another. This becomes important for carcinogen testing in whole animals for both hazard identification and risk assessment. Such considerations impact directly on the choice of the most sensitive species or the species most similar to humans for these evaluations.

Since chemical carcinogens are reactive per se or are activated by metabolism to reactive intermediates that bind to cellular components including DNA, their electrophilic derivatives—which bound to a variety of nucleophilic (electron-dense) moieties in DNA, RNA, and protein—were considered the ultimate carcinogenic form of the compounds of interest (see above). Several lines of evidence indicate that DNA is the critical target for carcinogenesis. The first hint that DNA was the target for heritable alterations due to carcinogen administration was from the increased incidence of cancer in genetically prone individuals with defective ability to repair DNA damage—e.g., xeroderma pigmentosum, Bloom syndrome, Cockayne syndrome, etc. (Smith, 1991). The second major piece of evidence that DNA was the target of carcinogen action was the observation of carcinogen-induced mutations in specific target genes associated with neoplasia in a multitude of experimental systems. A comparison of DNA adduct formation with biologically effective doses of carcinogens with different potencies demonstrated that the level of DNA damage was relatively similar. Since covalent adducts in DNA could be derived from carcinogenic compounds, the mechanism by which mutations arise and their relationship to carcinogenesis was the next area to be examined in the quest for an understanding of cancer development.

The induction of mutations is due primarily to chemical or physical alterations in the structure of DNA that result in inaccurate replication of that region of the genome. The process of mutagenesis consists of structural DNA alteration, cell proliferation that fixes the DNA damage, and DNA repair that either directly repairs the alkylated base(s) or results in removal of larger segments of the DNA (cf. Naegeli, 1994). Electrophilic compounds can interact with the ring nitrogens, exocyclic amino groups, carbonyl oxygens, and the phosphodiester backbone of DNA (Chang et al., 1994). Carcinogenic agents that result in formation of bulky adducts often specifically react with sites in the purine ring. For example, aromatic amines bind to the C8 position of guanine, while the diol epoxide of polycyclic aromatic hydrocarbons binds to the N2 and N6 position of guanine (see above). The position of an adduct in DNA and its chemical and physical properties in that context dictate the type(s) of mutations induced (Essigmann and Wood, 1993). This indicates that different adducts can induce a distinct spectrum of mutations and additionally that any given adduct can result in a multitude of different DNA lesions. Confirming the need for metabolic activation of carcinogenic compounds to their ultimate reactive form it was demonstrated that, whereas 2-acetylaminofluorene itself is not mutagenic, its sulfate metabolite was highly mutagenic for transforming DNA (Maher et al., 1968). These findings led to the development of mutagenesis assays for the detection of chemical carcinogens from the premise that one could detect carcinogens in highly mutable strains of bacteria given exogenous liver microsomal preparations for in vitro metabolism of the test agent (Chapter 13). Cultured mammalian cells have also been developed for evaluation of the mutagenic action of potential carcinogenic agents. Compounds are evaluated in the presence (Michalopoulos et al., 1981) or absence (Li et al., 1991) of metabolic activation systems such as irradiated hepatic feeder layers or hepatic microsomes. The use of these in vitro screens of mutagenicity has permitted analysis of the mutational specificity of some carcinogens (Table 3.3). While the data shown in Table 3.3 were derived from bacterial mutagenesis studies, several other systems have also been utilized in attempts to determine mutagenic specificity of various agents (Essigmann and Wood, 1993).

Point mutations, frameshift mutations, chromosomal aberrations, aneuploidy, and polyploidization can be induced by chemicals with varying degrees of specificity that are, in part, dose-dependent. Mutagenesis can be the result of several different alterations in the physical and chemical nature of DNA. While alkylation of DNA with small alkyl groups or large bulky adducts can result in mutation, other processes may also be involved. Conformation of the DNA has a major impact on the potential mutagenic activity of a compound. This is best demonstrated by the related compounds 2-acetylaminofluorene and 2-aminofluorene, which both form bulky DNA adducts at guanine residues in DNA. The AAF adduct distorts the double helix, while the AF adduct remains outside the helix and does not distort the helix. The AAF adduct induces frameshift mutations, whereas that of AF induces primarily transversions (Bichara and Fuchs, 1985). Planar agents that can intercalate between the base pairs in DNA can effectively induce frameshift mutations by exacerbating slippage mispairing in repetitive sequences. In addition, agents that lie within the major or minor groove of DNA can perturb nucleosome formation and may alter DNA replication. Some of these agents are potential chemotherapeutic agents. Agents such as irradiation and topoisomerase inhibitors that induce double-strand breaks can also enhance mutagenesis (Eastman and Barry, 1992).

Several mechanisms of mutagenesis exist. The presence of certain alkylation products, such as the O-6 alkyl deoxyguanosine and the O-4 alkyl deoxythymidine, permits a degenerate

Table 3.3 A Comparison of the Mutagenic Spectrum of Aflatoxin B_1 (AFB$_1$), Benzo[a]pyrene Diolepoxide (BPDE), 2-Acetylaminofluorene (2-AAF), and Ethylnitrosourea (ENU)

Mutation	AFB$_1$	BPDE	2-AAF	ENU
GC to TA (transversion)	0.94	0.76	0.88	0.09
GC to AT (transition)	0.06	0.11	0.06	>0.77
GC to CG	0.00	0.13	0.06	—

Modified from Loechler, 1989 (AFB, BPDE, and 2-AAF) and Horsfall et al., 1990 (ENU).

base pairing able to base pair with the appropriate base as well as an inappropriate base. This can be demonstrated in vitro and in vivo as the induction of transition mutations after treatment with certain alkylating agents (Singer, 1986). Thus, methylating or ethylating agents result in mutations as a result of base mispairing. The active metabolites of compounds, such as polycyclic aromatic hydrocarbons and aromatic amines, form bulky DNA adducts that block DNA synthesis, resulting in a noncoding lesion. The synthetic machinery employs bypass synthesis to avoid the lethal impact of these unrepaired lesions (Friedberg, 1994). Under this condition, the most prevalent base, frequently deoxyadenosine (Shearman and Loeb, 1979), is inserted opposite the offending adducted nucleotide base. Thus, DNA binding and repair, induction of point mutations, and clastogenicity have proven useful as endpoints in the identification of potential carcinogens as well as biomarkers of carcinogen exposure (Chapter 13). The role of DNA repair in protection of the genome and in the induction of mutations is an essential component in the mutagenesis process (see below).

Not all chemical carcinogens require intracellular metabolism to become ultimate carcinogens. Examples of direct-acting mutagens include alkylating agents such as β-propiolactone, nitrogen mustard, ethyleneimine, and bis(chloromethyl)ether (Figure 3.3). Direct-acting carcinogens are typically carcinogenic at multiple sites and in all species examined. A number of the direct-acting alkylating agents, including some used in chemotherapy, are carcinogenic for humans (Chapter 11).

DNA REPAIR AND CARCINOGENESIS

The persistence of DNA adducts is the result, for the most part, of the failure of DNA repair, so that its structure returns to normal without evidence of alteration. The structural alterations that may occur in the DNA molecule as a result of interaction with reactive chemical species or directly with ultraviolet or ionizing radiation are considerable. A number of the more frequently seen structural changes in DNA are schematically represented in Figure 3.15. The reaction with chemical species produces adducts on bases, sugars, and the phosphate backbone. Bifunctional reactive chemicals may also cause the crosslinking of DNA strands through reaction with two opposing bases. Other structural changes, such as the pyrimidine dimer formation, are specific for ultraviolet radiation (see below), whereas double-strand DNA breaks are most commonly seen with ionizing radiation (see below). On the other hand, most of the remaining lesions demonstrated in Figure 3.15 may occur as a result of either chemical or radiation effects on the DNA molecule. In order to cope with so many structurally different types of DNA damage, a variety of mechanisms have evolved in living cells to deal with each of the types of damage shown in Figure 3.15. A summary of the types of DNA repair most commonly encountered in mammalian systems is given in Table 3.4.

Two types of damage-response pathways exist: one is the repair pathway and the other is a tolerance mechanism (Friedberg, 1994). In repair mechanisms, the DNA damage is removed, while tolerance mechanisms circumvent the damage without fixing it. Tolerance mechanisms are by definition error-prone. Certain repair mechanisms reverse the DNA damage; for example, by removal of adducts from bases and insertion of bases into AP sites. One example of direct reversal is the removal of small alkyl groups from the O^6 portion of guanine by alkyltransferases. Alkyltransferases directly transfer the alkyl (methyl or ethyl) group from the DNA base guanine to a cysteine acceptor site in the alkyltransferase protein (Pegg and Byers, 1992). In microorganisms, the intracellular concentration of the alkyltransferase protein is regulated by environmental factors, including the presence of the alkylating agents themselves. A similar adaptation may occur in certain mammalian tissues in response to DNA-damaging agents as well as treatments

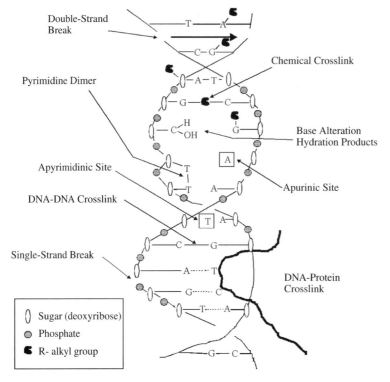

Figure 3.15 Schematic representation of chemical and radiation-induced lesions in DNA. (Adapted from Fry et al., 1982, with permission of the authors and publisher.)

causing an increase in cell proliferation. However, the increase in the alkyltransferase protein seen in mammalian tissues is much less than that in bacteria. In mammalian tissues, the level of the alkyltransferase protein is a major factor in the resistance of some cancer cells to certain chemotherapeutic agents (Chapter 20). Direct reversal of the premutational lesion by the alkyl-transferase reaction restores normal base pairing specificity.

Table 3.4 Types of DNA Repair

1. Direct reversal of DNA damage
   Alkyltransferases
2. Base excision repair
   Glycosylase and AP endonuclease
3. Nucleotide excision repair
   T-T, C-C, C-T repair
   "Bulky" adduct repair
4. Double-strand break repair
   Homologous recombination (HR)
   Nonhomologous DNA end joining (NHEJ)
5. Mismatch repair
   Repair of deamination of 5-Me cytosine
   Repair of mismatches in DNA due to defective repair, etc.

Modified from Myles and Sancar, 1989, and from Lieber, 1998.

The excisional repair of DNA may involve either the removal of a single altered base having a relatively low-molecular-weight adduct, such as an ethyl or methyl group, and is termed *base excision repair*, or the repair may involve a base with a very large bulky group adducted to it (nucleotide excision repair). The linkage of two bases seen in the dimerization of pyrimidines by ultraviolet light is also repaired by the latter pathway. This nucleotide excision pathway is represented diagrammatically in Figure 3.16.

Nucleotide excision repair in multicellular organisms involves a series of reactions noted in the figure. These include recognition of the damage, unwinding of the DNA, 3' and 5' sequential dual incisions of the damaged strand, repair synthesis of the eliminated patch, and final ligation. Each of these steps, as noted in the figure, involves a number of different proteins. In Table 3.5 may be seen a listing of the various proteins occurring in different fractions and their functions in the process of nucleotide excision repair (Petit and Sancar, 1999).

Other studies (cf. Sancar and Tang, 1993; Hanawalt, 1994) have also demonstrated that nucleotide excision repair in many instances occurs simultaneously with gene transcription. In fact, Hanawalt and associates showed earlier (cf. Bohr et al., 1987) that nucleotide excision repair occurred preferentially in genes that were actively being transcribed. For the final resynthesis of the segment of excised DNA, both the proliferating cell nuclear antigen (PCNA) as well as at least two different DNA polymerases (δ or ε) are needed to complete the repair process together with a ligase (Sancar, 1994).

Since animal cell DNA polymerases are not absolutely faithful in their replication of the template strand, there is the potential for a mutation to occur in the form of one or more mispaired bases during the process outlined above. This possibility is greater in the case of nucleotide excision repair as compared to simple base excision since a much longer base sequence is removed and resynthesized during the nucleotide excision mechanism. The existence and ultimate characterization of a number of the proteins involved in nucleotide excision repair has been the result of human diseases in which defects in this mechanism are known. In particular, the disease xeroderma pigmentosum is an autosomal recessive (Chapter 5) condition in which most patients are highly sensitive to exposure to ultraviolet light. Thus, on chronic exposure to sunlight, such individuals have a much greater risk of developing skin cancer than normal individuals. This fact emphasizes the potential importance of altered DNA repair in the development of neoplasia.

While the repair of adducts as indicated above involves several possible pathways, the repair of double DNA strand breaks is more complicated and as a result more prone to error than either the excisional or direct reversal pathways. Single-strand breaks may result from a variety of alterations by chemicals or radiation and, as noted above, during the repair process itself. Double-strand breaks in DNA are largely the result of ionizing radiation or high doses of alkylating carcinogens such as nitrogen mustard or polycyclic hydrocarbons, although even under normal conditions, transient double-strand DNA breaks occur as the result of the normal function of topoisomerases involved in the winding and unwinding of DNA and in antibody formation (Chapter 19).

In Figure 3.17 may be noted a schematic diagram of three forms of double-strand DNA repair. Recombinational repair or homologous recombination (HR) is more commonly seen in lower eukaryotes such as yeast while the nonhomologous end joining (NHEJ) pathway of double-strand DNA repair is more commonly seen in higher vertebrates (Van Dyck et al., 1999). The single-strand annealing pathway has not yet been well studied in higher vertebrates. While the exact mechanisms involved in each of these steps will not be considered in detail here, the interested reader is referred to more detailed references (Pastink and Lohman, 1999; Lieber, 1998; Featherstone and Jackson, 1999). In general, in the HR and NHEJ pathways, specific proteins interact with the open ends of the DNA, members of the Rad52 group genes in the case of HR

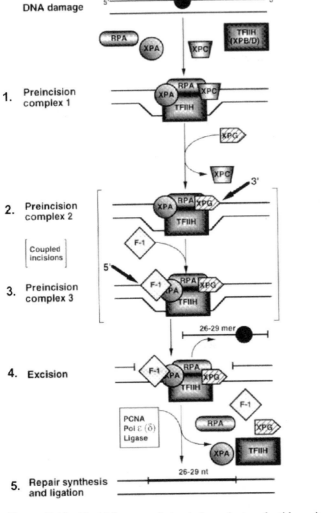

Figure 3.16 Model for transcription-independent nucleotide excision repair of DNA in humans. (1) The damage is first recognized in an ATP-independent step by the short-lived XPA·RPA complex. In a second, ATP-dependent step, the damaged DNA-bound XPA·RPA complex recruits XPC and TFIIH, to form the preincision complex 1 (PIC1). TFIIH possesses both 3′-5′ and 5′-3′ helicase activities, respectively through its XPB and XPD subunits and unwinds DNA by about 20 base pairs around the damage. (2) XPG binds the PIC1 complex while the molecular matchmaker XPC dissociates, leading to the more stable PIC2 excinuclease complex. (3) PIC2 recruits XPF·ERCC1 (F-1) to form PIC3. XPG makes the 3′ incision and F-1 makes the 5′ incision a fraction of a second later, in a concerted but asynchronous mechanism. (4) The excised damaged fragment is released by the excinuclease complex, leaving in place a postincision complex whose exact composition is still unclear. The proliferating cell nuclear antigen (PCNA) forms a torus around the DNA molecule associating with DNA polymerase δ and/or ε [Pol ε (δ)] (Tsurimoto, 1998) and a DNA ligase replacing the postincision complex with these repair synthesis proteins. (5) The gap is filled and the repair patch is ligated. (From Petit and Sancar, 1999, with permission of authors and publisher.)

Table 3.5 Proteins Involved in the Nucleotide Excision Repair Process in Humans

Fraction	Proteins	Sequence Motif	Activity of the Fraction	Role in Repair
XPA	XPA	Zinc finger	DNA binding	Damage recognition
RPA	p70	Zinc finger	XPA binding	Damage recognition
	p34		DNA binding	
	p11			
TFIIH	XPB	3′-5′ helicase	DNA-dependent ATPase	Formation of preincision complexes PIC 1-2-3
	XPD	5′-3′ helicase	Helicase	Transcription-repair coupling
	p62 (TFB1)		GTF	
	p52			
	p44 (SSL1)	Zinc finger	CAK	
	Cdk7	S/T kinase		
	CycH	Cyclin		
	p34	Zinc finger		
XPC	XPC		DNA binding	Molecular matchmaker
	HHR23B	Ubiquitin		Stabilization of PIC1
XPG	XPG		Nuclease	3′ incision
XPF	XPF		Nuclease	5′ incision
	ERCC1			

Key: GTF, general transcription factor; CAK, CDK-activating kinase.
Adapted from Petit and Sancar, 1999, with permission of authors and publisher.

(Van Dyck et al., 1999) and the Ku70 and Ku80 proteins in the NHEJ pathway (Featherstone and Jackson, 1999). A DNA-dependent protein kinase (DNA-PKcs) as well as the protein interacting with the DNA ligase (XRCC4) is involved in this mechanism. It should be noted—as indicated in the legend to the figure—however, that these mechanisms are quite error-prone and only under the best of circumstances result in a faithful recapitulation of the normal DNA sequence.

Double-strand breaks may occur at sites of single-strand DNA resulting from adduction of bulky molecules, preventing further polymerase action and subsequent endonuclease cleavage and resulting in double-strand breaks and potential chromosomal aberrations (Kaufmann, 1989).

Incorrectly paired nucleotides may occur in DNA as a result of DNA polymerase infidelity, formation and/or repair of apurinic and nucleotide excision sites, double-strand DNA repair, and metabolic modification of specific bases. Mismatch repair can be distinguished from nucleotide and base excision repair by several characteristics. Nucleotide and base excision repair generally involves the recognition of nucleotides/bases that have been chemically modified or fused to an adjacent nucleotide. In contrast, mismatch repair recognizes normal nucleotides which are either unpaired or paired with a noncomplementary nucleotide (cf. Fishel and Kolodner, 1995). Thus, mismatch repair may become involved in virtually any of the types of DNA repair seen in Table 3.4 with the possible exception of the direct reversal of DNA damage. The various combinations of gene products involved in several of the types of mismatch repair are seen in Figure 3.18. While the nomenclature of the various components varies depending on the phyla—e.g., eukaryotes, yeast, vertebrates—a functional similarity occurs throughout, most faithful in eukaryotes. As noted from the figure, recognition of the mismatch appears to be a major function of the MSH2 (hMSH2 in the human) while MSH3 and MSH6 are involved in the

(a) recombinational   (b) single-strand   (c) nonhomologous
     repair   annealing   end joining

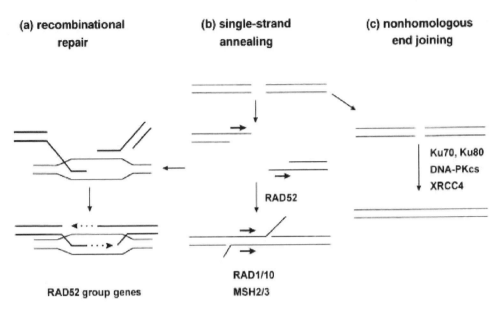

RAD52

RAD1/10
RAD52 group genes   MSH2/3

Ku70, Ku80
DNA-PKcs
XRCC4

Figure 3.17 Schematic representation of pathways involved in the repair of double-strand breaks in DNA. (a) The first step in recombinational repair is the formation of 3′ single-stranded tails by exonucle-olytic activity followed by invasion of a homologous undamaged donor sequence. Repair synthesis and branch migration lead to the formation of two Holliday junctions, i.e., a single DNA strand linking two double-stranded DNA molecules. Resolution of these intermediate structures results in the formation of two possible crossover and two possible noncrossover products (not shown). The fidelity of this repair is dependent on the exact complementation of the unaffected double-strand by the strands undergoing repair. (b) In the single-strand annealing pathway, exposures of regions of homology during resection of the 5′ ends allows formation of joint molecules. Repair of the double-strand break is completed by removal of nonhomologous ends and ligation. As a consequence, a deletion is introduced in the DNA. (c) Nonhomolo-gous end joining is based on religation of the two ends involving a complex of proteins, some of which are indicated in the figure and may involve the deletion and/or insertion of nucleotides. (Adapted from Pastink and Lohman, 1999, with permission of authors and publisher.)

specificity of binding itself (Fishel and Wilson, 1997). Thus, these complexes act as sensors of mismatch as well as other structural changes in the genome (Modrich, 1997; Li et al., 1996; cf. Fishel and Wilson, 1997). As in the case of other types of repair following the recognition and interaction with the mismatch repair proteins, the normal sequence is restored following removal of the mismatch DNA, resynthesis, and ligation (cf. Jiricny, 1998).

As an example of the importance of mismatch DNA repair, the extent of endogenous DNA damage and subsequent repair processes in normal human cells in vivo is seen in Table 3.6. With the possible exception of some single-strand break repair, all the other types of damage are those monitored by the mismatch repair mechanism and repaired under normal conditions. Obviously, a defect in this repair system may result in a dramatic increase in mutational events and in neo-plasia, as later discussions show (Chapter 5).

DNA Repair, Cell Replication, and Chemical Carcinogenesis

The persistence of DNA adducts in relation to the development of neoplasia in specific tissues (Table 3.2) and the differences in the repair of the adducts are critical factors in chemical car-cinogenesis. The removal of methyl, ethyl, and similar small alkyl radicals from individual bases

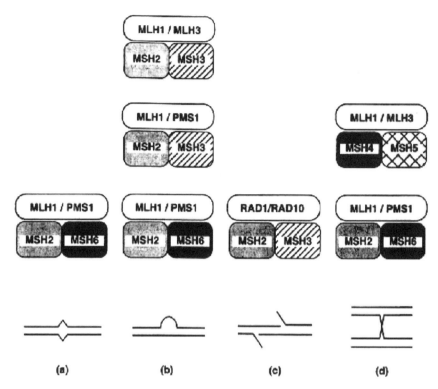

Figure 3.18 Combinational specificities of heterocomplexes of gene products of mismatch repair genes. (a) Base/base mispairs; (b) insertion/deletion mispairs; (c) 5′ tailed DNA structures generated by single-strand DNA annealing following recombination—e.g., HR; and (d) Holliday junctions. (Adapted from Nakagawa et al., 1999, with permission of authors and publishers.)

is to a great extent dependent on the presence of alkyltransferases (see above). While in some tissues, such as liver, it may be possible to increase the level of such enzymes in response to damage or hormonal or other influences, many tissues do not have an inducible repair mechanism. Furthermore, some adducts are extremely difficult if not impossible for the cell to repair. One example of a lesion, the 3-(deoxyguanosine-N^2-yl)-acetylaminofluorene adduct first described by Kriek and his associates (Westra et al., 1976), is depicted in Figure 3.12. This may in part account for the relatively wide spectrum of neoplasms inducible by this chemical carcinogen.

Of equal importance is the continuous damage to DNA that occurs within cells as a result of ambient mutagens, radiation, and endogenous processes including oxidation, methylation, deamination, and depurination. DNA damage induced by oxidative reactions (oxidative stress) is probably the source of most endogenous DNA damage. Ames et al. (1993) have estimated that the individual reactive "hits" in DNA per cell per day are of the order of 10^5 in the rat and 10^4 in the human as a result of endogenous oxidative reaction. Such reactions can produce alkylation through peroxidative reactions such as those described in Figure 3.7 or hydroxylation of bases and single-strand breaks (Figure 3.15). The end product of oxidative damage to DNA can also be interstrand crosslinks and double-strand breaks (cf. Demple and Harrison, 1994) with the potential for subsequent major genetic damage, as noted below. A more complete listing of the estimates of endogenous DNA damage and repair processes in the human is seen in Table 3.6. The data of this table emphasize the considerable degree and significant variation in types of DNA damage and repair that occur within each cell of the organism at a molecular level.

Table 3.6 Estimates of Endogenous DNA Damage and Repair Processes in Human Cells in Vivo

Type of Damage	Estimated Occurrences of Damage per Hour per cell[a]	Maximal Repair Rate, Base Pairs per Hour per Cell[a]
Depurination	1000	10^4 +
Depyrimidination	55	10^4 +
Cytosine deamination	15	10^4 +
Single-stranded breaks	5000	2×10^5
N^7-methylguanine	3500	Not reported
O^6-methylguanine	130	10^4
Oxidation products	120	10^5

[a] Might be higher or lower by a factor of 2.
Modified from data of the National Academy of Sciences, 1989.

Experimental studies in mammalian cells have demonstrated that active oxygen radicals may contribute to clastogenesis directly (Ochi and Kaneko, 1989) and indirectly through the production of lipid peroxides (Emerit et al., 1991). While methods for the repair of some types of oxidative damage—including base hydroxylation (Bessho et al., 1993) and single-strand breaks (Satoh and Lindahl, 1994)—do exist, such repair requires time and may be dependent on many other intracellular factors. Since the formation of a mutation occurs during the synthesis of a new DNA strand by use of the damaged template, cell replication becomes an important factor in the "fixation" of a mutation. The importance of the rate of cell division and DNA synthesis in carcinogenesis has been emphasized by several authors (Ames et al., 1993; Butterworth, 1991; Cohen and Ellwein, 1991). Thus, while many DNA repair mechanisms themselves may not be abnormal in neoplastic cells compared with their normal counterpart, a high rate of cell division will tend to enhance both the spontaneous and induced level of mutation through the chance inability of a cell to repair damage prior to DNA synthesis. An important pathway of DNA repair that is genetically defective in a number of hereditary and spontaneous neoplasms in the human (Umar et al., 1994) is the mismatch repair mechanism that corrects spontaneous and postreplicative base alterations and thus is an important pathway for avoidance of mutation in normal cells. Genetic defects in mismatch repair mechanisms lead to microsatellite DNA and instability, with subsequent alteration in the stabilization of the genome itself (Modrich, 1994). Enhanced mitogenesis may also trigger more dramatic genetic alterations including mitotic recombination, gene conversion, and nondisjunction. These genetic changes result in further progressive genetic alterations with a high likelihood of resulting in cancer. The types of mutational events, the numbers of such mutations, and the cellular responses to them thus become important factors in our understanding of the mechanisms of chemical carcinogenesis.

HORMONAL CARCINOGENESIS

The concept that hormones may be a causative factor(s) in the development of specific types of neoplasms was first pointed out by Beatson (1896), who at the end of the last century suggested a relation between breast cancer and the ovary. Within the past 40 years, this concept has been reinforced by data from several experimental systems, and within the past 15 years the role of hormones in the genesis of cancer in humans has become a subject of considerable interest.

The physiological role of hormones in maintaining the "internal milieu" (Bernard, 1878, 1879) is now a well-accepted scientific fact. That some cancers may result from an abnormal production internally or the excessive administration of specific hormones externally represents potentially interesting pathways of carcinogenesis, since the former indicates that the derangement of an organism's homeostatic mechanisms may result in the neoplastic transformation. Furth (1975) was emphatic in the propositions and demonstrations that disruption of the cybernetic relation between peripheral endocrine glands and the anterior pituitary may result in neoplasia of one or another of the glands involved. These cybernetic relations are depicted graphically in Figure 3.19 for a number of the more common peripheral endocrine-related organs and the pituitary. According to this hypothesis, interruption of any of the feedback relations may result in a neoplasm of the glands involved (cf. Clifton and Sridharan, 1975). One of the classic examples is the experimental transplantation of normal ovaries into the spleens of castrated rodents (Biskind and Biskind, 1944). This results in a break in the pituitary-gonadal hormone feedback loop, since estrogens produced by the ovary are carried by the splenic venous system to the liver, where they are metabolized and thus are prevented from entering the general circulation to suppress the pituitary production of gonadotropins (Figure 3.20). The excessive production of gonadotropins and their constant stimulus of the ovarian fragment in the spleen result ultimately in neoplasia of the ovarian implant.

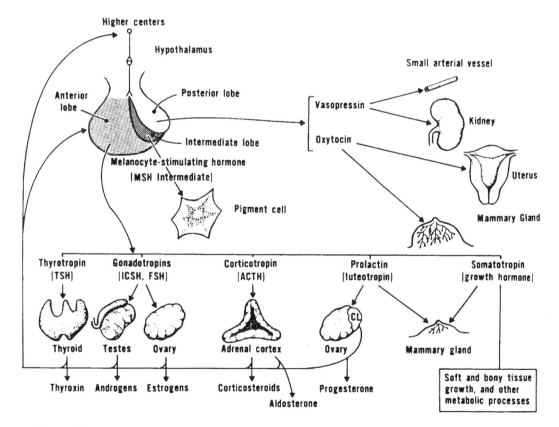

Figure 3.19 Cybernetic relations of the pituitary gland (anterior, intermediate, posterior lobes) with the hypothalamus, other endocrine organs, and tissues of the organism. (After Furth, 1975, reproduced with the permission of the author and publisher.)

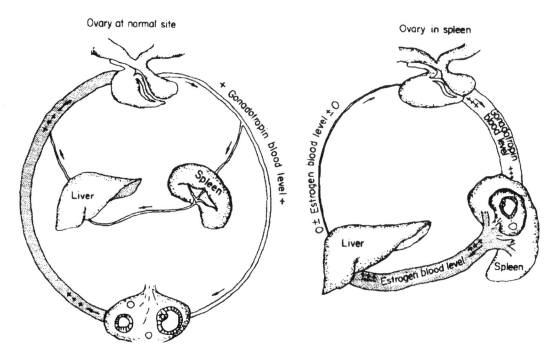

Figure 3.20 Scheme of the physiologic regulation of gonadotropin secretion of the pituitary by estrogen in the blood.(From Furth, 1969, with permission of publisher.)

A similar mechanism is likely to be involved in the production of thyroid neoplasms either by the administration of goitrogens (chemicals that inhibit the synthesis and/or secretion of normal thyroid hormone) or by a marked increase in the circulating levels of thyrotropin secreted by transplanted thyrotropin-secreting pituitary neoplasms (Chapter 18). In the former instance, there is a break in the feedback loop, and the pituitary gland produces high levels of thyrotropin in the absence of the normal feedback regulation by the thyroid hormone (cf. Furth, 1975). In fact, in the human there is substantial evidence that this mechanism may play an important role in the development of many thyroid cancers (Williams, 1989). In the latter case, high levels of circulating thyrotropin result from the unregulated production of this hormone by the transplanted neoplasm (Ueda and Furth, 1967). Thyroidectomy and neonatal gonadectomy result in the development of neoplasms of the pituitary, presumably because of the lack of inhibition by the hormone from the target end organ (cf. Furth, 1975). Chronic administration of pituitary growth hormone also induces a variety of neoplasms in the rat (Moon et al., 1950a,b). Theoretically, then, neoplasms of any of the end organs seen in Figure 3.17 may be produced by some manipulation that breaks the feedback loop between the pituitary and the end organ.

Some examples of carcinogenesis resulting from the interruption of the cybernetics of hormonal relationships seen in Figure 3.19 are listed in Table 3.7. In addition to effecting carcinogenesis in the ovary (Biskind and Biskind, 1944), endogenous gonadotropins are also involved in the development of adrenocortical and interstitial (Leydig) cell neoplasms in mice and rats respectively (Table 3.7). Unleaded gasoline acts like an antiestrogen, thus removing the estrogen protection usually provided against the development of liver neoplasms in the mouse (Standeven et al., 1994), leading to an increased number of hepatic neoplasms in the female. Phenobarbital acts to decrease serum levels of thyroid hormone (T_3) by stimulating enzymes that metabolize

Table 3.7 Interrupted Cybernetics of Hormonal Carcinogenesis in Rodents

Species/Tissue	Inducing Agent	Hormonal Carcinogen	Interrupted Pathway	Reference
Mouse/ovary	Ovary transplant to spleen	Gonadotropin	Estrogen → hypo-thalamus	Biskind and Biskind, 1944
Rat/thyroid	Goitrogen or thyrotropin-secreting tumor	Thyrotropin	$T_3 \rightarrow$ hypothalamus	cf. Furth, 1975
Mouse/adrenal cortex	Ovariectomy	Gonadotropins	Estrogen → hypo-thalamus	Kawashima et al., 1980
Female mouse/liver	Unleaded gasoline	Androgens	Estrogen synthesis	Standeven et al., 1994
Rat/thyroid	Phenobarbital	Thyrotropin?	$T_3 \rightarrow$ hypothalamus	McClain, 1989
Rat/pituitary	Estrogens		Dopamine → pituitary	cf. Neumann, 1991
Rat/Leydig cells	Antiantrogens	Gonadotropins	Androgens → hypo-thalamus	cf. Neumann, 1991
Rat/mammary gland	Estrogens	Prolactin	Dopamine → pituitary	cf. Neumann, 1991

and eliminate the hormone before it can be recycled to the hypothalamus. This mechanism (McClain, 1989) is very similar to the effects of goitrogens, which prevent T_3 formation and release from the thyroid. The induction of pituitary adenomas, which themselves produce large amounts of prolactin, is due to an inhibition of the formation of dopamine in the hypothalamus. Dopamine acts like an inhibitor of prolactin synthesis and release by the pituitary. When this inhibition is eliminated by estrogen inhibition of dopamine formation, prolactin-producing pituitary cells replicate at a very high rate. Furthermore, they produce extensive amounts of prolactin, which, in turn, in the presence of estrogens, leads to mammary neoplasia (Neumann, 1991).

Figure 3.21 shows some representative structures of naturally occurring hormones for which there is substantial evidence of carcinogenicity in lower animals and/or humans. In addition to the structure of growth hormone, two other growth factors expressed in adult tissues—transforming growth factor a (TGFα) expressed in the small intestine (Barnard et al., 1991), the major salivary glands (Wu et al., 1993), and other tissues (Lee et al., 1993), and insulin growth factor II (IGF-II), which is expressed in forebrain, uterus, kidney, heart, skeletal muscle, and to a very small degree in liver (Murphy et al., 1987)—may be considered as chemical carcinogens. The carcinogenic action of these latter two growth factor hormones in vivo has been demonstrated by the use of transgenic mice, wherein animals overexpressing TGFα developed liver neoplasms in dramatic excess of controls (Lee et al., 1992), and animals expressing high levels of IGF-II developed hepatocellular carcinomas and lymphomas in excess (Rogler et al., 1994).

As noted above (Table 3.7), neoplasms of the pituitary and of the peripheral endocrine organs may be induced by the administration of steroid sex hormones. Although the kidney is not usually considered to be a peripheral endocrine organ, its cells produce erythropoietin. Administration of synthetic (Figure 3.22) or natural estrogen can induce renal cortical carcinomas in male hamsters (Li and Li, 1990), and estradiol induces Leydig cell tumors of the testes in the mouse (Huseby, 1980). However, a closely related structural analog, 2-fluoroestradiol, which exhibits significant estrogenic potency, did not induce renal carcinoma in the same sex and species (Liehr, 1983). Recently, the synthetic antiestrogen tamoxifen was found to induce carcinomas of

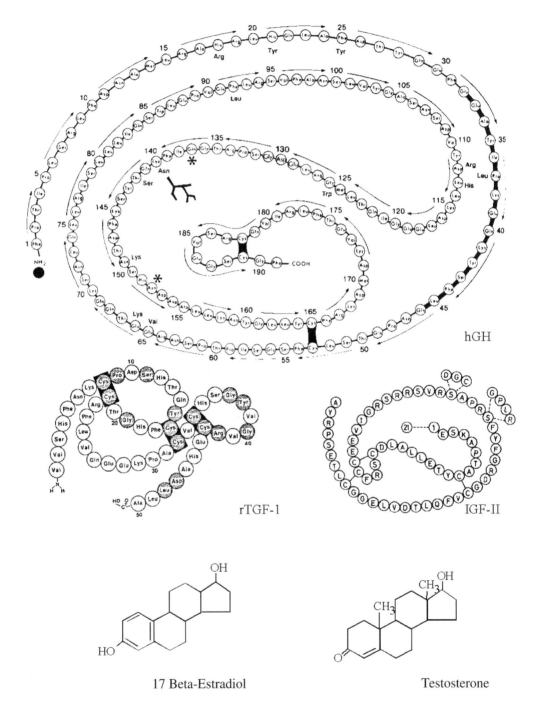

Figure 3.21 Structures of naturally occurring polypeptide hormones (hGH, human growth hormone; TGF-a, transforming growth factor alpha; IGF-II, insulin growth factor-II) and naturally occurring sex steroids (17 ß-estradiol and testosterone).

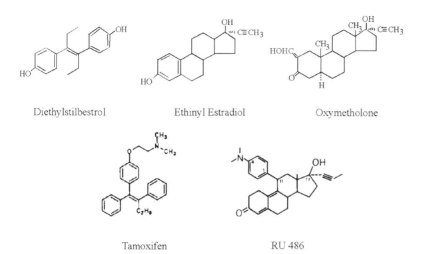

Figure 3.22   Structures of some synthetic sex steroid hormones and antihormones.

the liver in the rat as well (Williams et al., 1993). Evidence that male hormones, by themselves, are carcinogenic is not as strong as the data for the carcinogenicity of female hormones. The natural male hormone testosterone does exhibit a weak ability to "transform" hamster embryo cells in culture into a neoplastic phenotype (Lasne et al., 1990). The evidence that synthetic androgens are carcinogenic is somewhat greater, especially in the human. In addition, elevated serum testosterone levels are associated with an increased risk of hepatocellular carcinoma in the human (Yu and Chen, 1993). A number of reports (cf. Mays and Christopherson, 1984; Chandra et al., 1984) have indicated a causative relationship between the administration of synthetic androgens such as oxymetholone (Figure 3.22) for various clinical conditions and the appearance of hepatocellular neoplasms, predominantly benign.

In addition to the apparent direct induction of neoplasia by hormonal stimuli, hormones also act in concert with known carcinogenic agents to induce neoplasia. One of the better-studied examples of this phenomenon is the induction of mammary adenocarcinomas in rodents. Bittner (1956) demonstrated that three factors are essential for the production of mammary carcinoma in mice: genetic susceptibility, hormonal influence, and a virus transmitted through the milk. The importance of the first two factors has been repeatedly demonstrated in a variety of species including humans, but incontrovertible evidence for the participation of a virus in mammary carcinogenesis has been obtained only in mice. In the rat, high levels of endogenous prolactin enhance the induction of mammary carcinomas by dimethylbenz(a)anthracene (Ip et al., 1980). Chronic treatment with synthetic or natural estrogens alone may induce mammary carcinomas in rodents. Thus, mammary carcinogenesis in rodents is a complicated process, requiring several components that may differ from species to species.

Both male and female sex steroid hormones have also been shown to act in concert with known chemical carcinogens to increase the incidence of neoplasia. Various synthetic estrogens administered chronically to animals after dosing with a known carcinogen markedly enhance the development of hepatocellular carcinomas in the rat (Yager and Yager, 1980). Both testosterone and synthetic androgens given with or after chemical carcinogens enhance the induction of adenocarcinomas of the prostate and other accessory sex organs of the male (Hoover et al., 1990). A combination of testosterone and estradiol-17β after treatment with methylnitrosourea also resulted in the development of adenocarcinomas of the prostate (Bosland et al., 1991). In contrast,

Izbicki et al. (1990) reported evidence that androgens inhibit the development of colon cancer induced by azoxymethane.

Hormonal Relationships in the Development of Human Cancer

Although hints and reports of a role for hormones and the causation of human cancer had appeared over the past several centuries, the first practical application of hormones in oncology was their use in the therapy of specific human neoplasms. The first practical application to the human of what little knowledge existed at the time was the demonstration by Huggins and Hodges of the partial androgen dependence of many human prostatic cancers, as evidenced by the beneficial effects of orchiectomy or synthetic estrogens in many patients even with metastatic disease (Huggins and Hodges, 1941). Since then, significant evidence has developed to indicate a role for hormones in the development of several common human neoplasms. Miller (1978) pointed out such a relationship with breast, ovarian, endometrial, and prostate cancer in the human. More recently Henderson and colleagues (Henderson et al., 1988) have presented reasonable evidence to argue for a major role of estrogens in cancers of the breast and genital tissues in both males and females. However, as Kodama and Kodama (1987) have pointed out along with others, a variety of additional factors such as diet and other lifestyle components (Chapter 11) are involved in the hormonal interactions with tissues that lead ultimately to neoplasia.

To date there is little evidence for the carcinogenicity of polypeptide hormones in the human, such as with the animal systems indicated above. The best evidence is for a role of thyrotropin in the genesis of human thyroid cancer, as referred to above. In Williams' review (1989), several epidemiological studies indicated that risk factors such as iodide deficiency, "dyshormonogenesis," and ionizing radiation were all associated with elevated thyrotropin levels in the serum of these individuals. Furthermore, patients with neoplasms of the pituitary that secrete high levels of growth hormone (Chapter 18) do have an increased risk of several types of malignant neoplasms (Barzilay et al., 1991). Thus, based on animal experimentation together with these few epidemiological studies, the data are suggestive of a carcinogenic effect of endogenous polypeptide pituitary hormones in the human analogous to experimental investigations in the animal.

That estrogens are carcinogenic in the human, either by direct or indirect mechanisms, was first exemplified by the report of the development of primary vaginal adenocarcinoma in young women whose mothers had taken diethylstilbestrol (DES) during the first trimester of the relevant pregnancy (Herbst and Scully, 1970). A registry for such exposed women was developed, and in 1987 Melnick and associates (1987) reviewed 519 cases of clear-cell adenocarcinoma of the vagina and cervix in which the majority of the patients' mothers had received DES or a related hormone during pregnancy. The risk that such a neoplasm will develop in an exposed female from birth through age 34 was found to be approximately 1 in 1000. On the other hand, the incidence of a nonneoplastic condition resulting from the retention of embryonic glands in the vagina and cervix, termed vaginal adenosis, was much higher, approaching 70% of females exposed to DES in utero (Johnson et al., 1979). As further support for the causative relationship of DES and this vaginal pathology, Newbold and McLachlan (1982) reported that mice exposed prenatally or neonatally to DES developed both vaginal adenosis and adenocarcinoma.

For more than three decades, preparations of synthetic estrogens and progestogens, singly or combined, have been used as oral contraceptives by women in the United States (Huggins and Zucker, 1987). After the first decade of their widespread use, reports (Edmondson et al., 1976; Goldfarb, 1976) of a significant increase in the incidence of liver adenomas in women using such oral contraceptive preparations appeared. The increased risk of such lesions directly paralleled the duration of use; after 8 years, there was a 500-fold increase in the risk of the development of hepatocellular adenomas in women using oral contraceptives continuously for this period (cf. Huggins and Zucker, 1987). The use of sequential oral contraceptives, in which estrogen was given for 2 weeks followed by an estrogen-progestogen combination for 1 week, resulted in the occurrence of endometrial carcinoma in young women on this regimen (cf. Huggins and Zucker, 1987). Following the first reports of such occurrences (Silverberg and Makowski, 1975; Lyon, 1975), manufacturers voluntarily removed such preparations from the market. As further documentation of the carcinogenicity of estrogens in the human, the administration of synthetic or natural estrogens as hormone replacement therapy to postmenopausal women has revealed a strong association between estrogen use and cancer risk. The risk is in proportion to dose and duration of use, with a three- to sixfold increase in risk after 3 to 10 years of use and a more than tenfold increment in risk after more than 10 years of using unopposed estrogen (Barrett-Connor, 1992). Strikingly, when exogenous estrogens given to postmenopausal women are supplemented with progestogens, the risk of endometrial cancer is dramatically reduced (cf. Voigt et al., 1991). Thus, these findings with the use of exogenous estrogens further support the concepts of Henderson, Miller, and others of the importance of endogenous hormones, especially estrogens, in the development of human cancers of a variety of tissues, most of which are recognized as end organs for estrogen effects.

MECHANISTIC CONSIDERATIONS IN HORMONAL CARCINOGENESIS

Since all hormones are chemicals, their induction of neoplasia might be considered in the same light as chemical carcinogens discussed earlier (Figures 3.1, 3.3, 3.21, and 3.22). However, there is substantial evidence that, with few exceptions, the carcinogenic action of hormones is intimately associated with their hormonal activity. Thus, in determining the mechanism of carcinogenesis by hormones, it is important to consider the mechanisms by which these chemicals induce their hormonal effects on cells and tissues.

Unlike most chemical carcinogens, hormones in general need not be metabolized to exert their hormonal effects on cells. Rather, in all known instances, hormonal effects on cells are mediated through direct interaction of the hormone with a specific receptor molecule. A simplified diagram of the location of such receptors in cells is seen in Figure 3.23. In general, hormone receptors may occur either as soluble proteins dissolved in the internal milieu of the individual cell or as complex, membrane-associated glycoproteins whose initial action is primarily at the external plasma membrane. Low-molecular-weight hormones such as steroids and the thyroid hormone interact with intracellular receptors, producing a complex that, when transported into the nucleus by itself or complexed with other proteins, alters in a specific manner the transcription of certain genes. The soluble intracellular receptors for these molecules share a common set of structural motifs. A diagram of the structure of a number of these receptors can be seen in Figure 3.24 (cf. Vedeckis, 1992). The commonality of these receptors involves a modulating domain that is relatively unconserved among these various different receptors and is probably involved in the transcriptional regulation of gene expression. The "DNA-binding domain" interacts specifically with DNA response elements having specific sequences. This is the most highly conserved region of all of this superfamily of receptors. The carboxyl terminal region is designated the *ligand-binding domain*, which interacts specifically with the appropriate ligand (hormone) with high affinity and specificity. This domain also has a high degree of conservation within the superfamily, although not as exact as the DNA-binding domain. Thus, the ligand or hormone reacts with the receptor and in so doing causes an "activation" of the receptor, enabling it to interact with the specific DNA sequences (promoter) within DNA. This activation involves

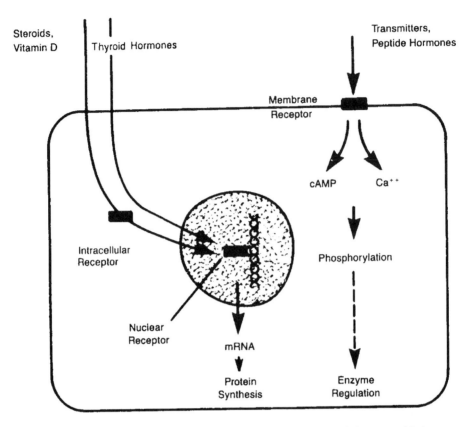

Figure 3.23   Location of receptors in cells. Receptor locations are as follows: peptide hormones such as insulin, growth hormone, gonadotropins, thyrotropin, parathyroid hormone, and corticotropin in plasma membrane; steroid hormones such as aldosterone, cortisol, estradiol, progesterone, testosterone, and dihydroxyvitamin D_3 in cytoplasm; and thyroid hormone in nucleus. cAMP indicates cyclic adenosine monophosphate; Ca^{++}, calcium ion; and mRNA, messenger RNA. (Adapted from Kaplan, 1984, with permission of the author and publisher.)

a conformational change in the receptor that not only allows for the interaction with DNA of the complex but also separates the receptor, steroid hormone receptors in particular, from proteins termed *heat-shock proteins*, which may maintain the receptor in its native form in the absence of the ligand (hormone); however, retinoic acid and thyroid hormone receptors are not associated with heat shock proteins (cf. Reichel and Jacob, 1993).

The structure of membrane-bound receptors is much more complex than the intracellular receptors described above. Receptors for neurotransmitters and glycoprotein hormones usually have a number of transmembrane segments as well as an extracellular and cytoplasmic domain. Receptors for a variety of growth factors—including growth hormone and prolactin, both hormones of the anterior pituitary—exhibit a single transmembrane domain with an extracellular and cytoplasmic domain as well. Examples of these two general types of receptors are indicated diagrammatically in Figure 3.25A and B. In all cases the ligand (hormone, neurotransmitter, growth factor)-binding domain is the extracellular component of the structure. The cytoplasmic domain in the case of the glycoprotein hormone-neurotransmitter type of receptor interacts directly with a transducing G protein (Reichert et al., 1991; Premont et al., 1995). A functionally

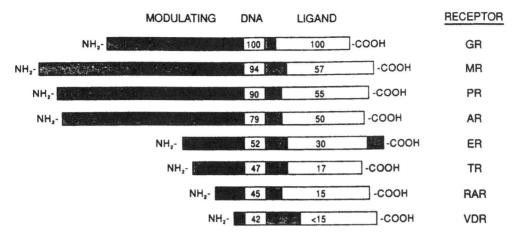

Figure 3.24 Structure of nuclear receptors. Nuclear receptors comprise three domains. The amino terminal region, called the "modulating domain," is not conserved among the superfamily of nuclear receptors, is of varying length, and may contain sequences that are involved in the transcriptional regulation of gene expression (transactivation). The second region is the "DNA-binding domain" that interacts specifically with DNA response element via two cysteine zinc fingers. It is the most highly conserved region of the nuclear receptors. The carboxyl terminal region is the "ligand-binding domain" that binds the appropriate ligand with high affinity and specificity. It is also quite conserved among nuclear receptors, although less so than the DNA-binding domain. The numbers in the DNA- and ligand-binding domains represent the percentage of amino acid identity in these regions, compared to those in the glucocorticoid receptor (GR). Other receptors diagrammed are the mineralocorticoid (aldosterone) receptor (MR), progesterone receptor (PR), androgen receptor (AR), estrogen receptor (ER), thyroid hormone receptor (TR), retinoic acid receptor (RAR), and vitamin D receptor (VDR). (From Vedeckis, 1992, with permission of the author and publisher.)

similar pathway occurs with the hormone and growth factor receptors exhibiting a single transmembrane domain but differs in that the cytoplasmic domain either possesses inherent protein tyrosine kinase activity, which is activated by interaction of the receptor with its ligand, or interacts with a cytoplasmic protein kinase upon interaction with ligand. For those monomeric receptors in Figure 3.25B, interaction with the ligand results in dimerization or trimerization (Heldin, 1995) of the single molecules, facilitating activation of the protein kinase either inherent or present in the cytoplasm. Dimeric receptors such as the structure seen in the center also occur—e.g., insulin or insulin growth factor-1 receptors, wherein activation of the inherent kinase only requires interaction with the ligand. Activation of these protein kinases results in further protein phosphorylations mediated through transducing G proteins (Chapter 7), thus allowing a "signal" to pass from membrane to the nucleus (Chapter 7) (Linder and Gilman, 1992). Hormone receptors with single transmembrane domains whose ligands include growth hormone, prolactin, and a number of peptide hormones and growth factors for lymphoid and hematopoietic tissues initiate signal transduction by association with specific cytoplasmic kinases that are not an integral part of the receptor molecule (cf. Kelly et al., 1994; Carter-Su et al., 1994).

The ultimate effect of the hormonal signal is the regulation of gene expression, probably by the interaction of proteins activated through the signal transduction pathway, and these in turn interact directly with specific sequences in the DNA. This has been shown for a cyclic AMP response element-binding protein (CREB) that interacts directly with a sequence in DNA known as CRE (cyclic AMP response element) (Lu et al., 1992). The initial signal between the growth factor and/or hormone and its receptor is limited by endocytosis of the complex into the cytoplasm, where the ligand is separated and destroyed while the receptor is recycled to the cell sur-

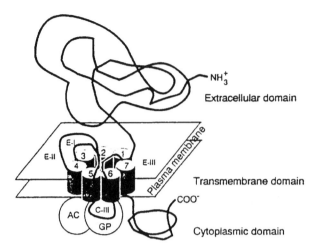

Figure 3.25A Model of glycoprotein hormone receptors. Schematic view of the membrane insertion and the coupling to the signaling complex. The receptors consist of a single polypeptide chain with a large extracellular amino terminal domain. The transmembrane domain is made up of 7 transmembrane helices with extracellular connecting loops E-I, E-II, and E-III (between helices 2 + 3, 4 + 5, 6 + 7) and cytoplasmic connecting loops C-I, C-I, and C-III (between helices 1 + 2, 3 + 4, 5 + 6). The carboxy terminus extends into the cytoplasm (cytoplasmic domain). The connecting loop C-III was proposed to achieve the coupling of the receptors to a stimulating G-protein (GP) of the signaling complex (AC, adenylyl cyclase). (From Merz, 1992, with permission of the author and publisher.)

face (cf. Dautry-Varsat and Lodish, 1984). However, for the initial signal from the interaction of the receptor with its ligand to occur, a highly specific interaction is necessary, comparable to the specific interaction of a steroid or thyroid hormone with its intracellular receptor. Thus, hormones in their native state induce changes in the expression of DNA within cells; in many instances this results in an increased proliferation of the target cell. Growth factors may be considered as polypeptide hormones with a more general target population than specific endo-

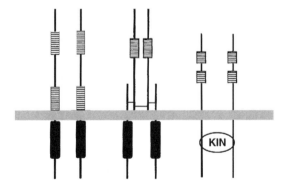

Figure 3.25B General structural features of receptors exhibiting a single transmembrane domain. The horizontal gray line represents the plasma membrane, and structures below this line are cytoplasmic. Hatched regions represent cysteine-rich repeat domains and closed boxes demarcate the protein tyrosine kinase domains. Horizontal lines connecting vertical structural components of the receptor represent disulfide bridges. KIN = protein kinase distinct from the receptor.

crine tissues targeted by polypeptide pituitary hormones. Growth factors, G proteins, signal transduction, and their role in neoplasia are discussed later in the text (Chapter 7).

Binding of Hormones to DNA

Although the mechanism of action of hormones involves few if any structural alterations in these chemical agents, in analogy to chemical carcinogenesis one might expect that some hormones, or more likely their metabolites, can interact directly with macromolecules, especially DNA, as has been described for nonhormonal chemical carcinogens (see above). One of the earliest studies demonstrating a low level of covalent interaction of hormones with proteins was that reported by Riegel and Mueller (1954), who demonstrated the formation of a protein-bound metabolite of estradiol in liver homogenates of female rats. Kappus and Remmer (1975) also described the irreversible binding of a synthetic estrogen to proteins of liver microsomes, possibly through an intermediate epoxide form. More recently Epe et al. (1990) have described the covalent binding of quinoid metabolites of diethylstilbestrol to microtubular protein in vitro and have proposed a role for such binding in the development of aneuploidy and the development of neoplasia induced by this synthetic estrogen.

The binding of both synthetic estrogens and their natural forms to DNA or the induction of DNA adducts revealed by ^{32}P-postlabeling (see above) has also been reported. Lutz and co-workers (1982) reported the covalent binding of diethylstilbestrol to DNA of rat and hamster liver and kidney, albeit at extremely low doses compared with the binding of nonhormonal chemical carcinogens. These workers (Jaggi et al., 1978) had earlier described the covalent binding of ethinylestradiol and estrone to liver DNA at levels four orders of magnitude lower than that of dimethylnitrosamine. Since these reports, Liehr and his associates (1986, 1987) have reported the appearance of new ^{32}P-postlabeling spots (DNA adducts) in hamster kidney, in which such hormones induce malignant neoplasms. Although it is not clear that the new adducts are formed from the hormones in most instances, Gladek and Liehr (1989) presented evidence that ^{32}P-postlabeled spots (adducts) appearing after diethylstilbesterol treatment of animals were likely to be generated from the reaction of the 4′,4″-quinone metabolite of diethylstilbesterol with DNA. Since steroid estrogens are metabolized to catechol estrogens, which are capable of forming quinones, Liehr (1990) has postulated a major role for such metabolites in estrogen-induced carcinogenesis. Interestingly, administration of the antiestrogen tamoxifen inhibited the development of renal neoplasms after 17β-estradiol administration but did not alter the DNA adduct levels (Liehr et al., 1988). Further support of a role for metabolic activation of synthetic and natural estrogens in their carcinogenic action is seen from the generation of unscheduled DNA synthesis (DNA damage) in cultured hamster cells by diethylstilbestrol and related compounds (Tsutsui et al., 1984) and the induction of sister chromatid exchanges both in vivo and in vitro by diethylstilbestrol (Mehnert et al., 1985). A similar increase in sister chromatid exchanges in human lymphocytes induced in vitro by diethylstilbestrol was not accompanied by a detectable change in ^{32}P-postlabeling patterns (Lundgren et al., 1988). That estrogens may induce neoplasia by other pathways that may be important for chemical carcinogenesis has been shown by Roy et al. (1991), who presented evidence for a role of active oxygen in DNA damage resulting from diethylstilbesterol treatment of hamsters in vivo. In addition, Lu et al. (1988) reported the hypomethylation of DNA in estrogen-induced hamster renal neoplasms. Thus, at least for synthetic and in one system natural estrogens, there is some evidence that metabolic activation may play a role in their carcinogenic activity, exemplified predominantly in the hamster. There is no evidence, however, that polypeptide hormones such as thyrotropin or gonadotropins, which exert their action at the cell surface and in all likelihood never reach the cell nucleus in an undegraded form, would exert their carcinogenic action by covalent adduction to DNA.

Furth suggested that the effect of hormones is to increase the rate of cell replication and that the rapidly dividing cell thus becomes more susceptible to "endogenous" carcinogenesis from genetic "mistakes" or mutations; the chance of such formations is increased by the more rapid rate of DNA synthesis. On this basis one should expect that carcinoma of the small intestine would be a very common neoplasm because of the extremely rapid rate of replication of intestinal epithelial cells. This is not the case either in humans or in animals. An earlier report by Málková and associates (1977) reported that the chronic administration of estrogen, as estradiol benzoate, induced hyperplasia in the cells of the pituitary of rats. For the first 2 months of the administration, hyperplastic cells exhibited normal karyotypes, but after that time the number of aneuploid cells increased, followed by neoplasms. In contrast, in the bone marrow, a rapidly replicating tissue, no detectable changes were seen in chromosomal morphology, although the mitotic index was lowered, as also occurred with the pituitary after four weeks of estrogen administration. Thus, rapid cell replication by itself does not appear to directly induce the neoplastic change, since rapidly replicating normal cells such as intestinal epithelial cells do not show an inordinate tendency to develop neoplasia. As discussed further on (Chapter 7), it seems likely that hormones may not act directly on cells to induce the neoplastic transformation; rather, they may act to enhance the replication and progression of a few cells already potentially neoplastic as a result of ambient environmental factors such as dietary contaminants, background radiation, and so on.

PHYSICAL CARCINOGENESIS

Radiation Carcinogenesis

Perhaps the first documented example of the induction of neoplasia by ionizing radiation was that of atypical epithelial hyperplasias and malignant epitheliomas observed on the hands of radiologists and scientists using x-ray devices and radium within a few years after their discovery near the turn of this century. In these cases, the human being was the experimental victim of radiation carcinogenesis. Fortunately, scientists rapidly became aware of the dangers of ionizing radiation and took precautions to prevent its effects in humans.

Radiant energy in our universe comes in a variety of general types, all related to the wavelength and frequency of the waves. A diagram of the electromagnetic spectrum is seen in Figure 3.26. With our present-day knowledge, there is no solid evidence that radiant energy of wavelengths greater than 5×10^{-5} cm is carcinogenic. However, ultraviolet, Roentgen or x-rays, and gamma rays have carcinogenic effects. In addition, high-energy particles such as electrons, neutrons, and alpha particles may also exhibit carcinogenic action. A major discussion of the physics of ionizing radiation, radiant or particulate, is beyond the scope of this text, and the reader is referred to more extensive reviews such as those by Upton (1975) and others or to the report of the United Nations Scientific Committee on the Effects of Atomic Radiation (Sources and Effects of Ionizing Radiation, 1977). Although in recent years substantial publicity has been given to the possible carcinogenic effect of electromagnetic field radiation of wavelengths greater than that of visible light, there has been little if any substantial evidence that such radiation is carcinogenic in experimental systems. However, some reports have suggested that low frequency electromagnetic fields may serve to enhance the development of neoplasia by mechanisms that are discussed later in the text (Chapter 12) (Goodman and Shirley-Henderson, 1990).

Since ultraviolet and ionizing radiations are known to have specific mutagenic effects, it has long been assumed that the mechanism of carcinogenesis by such radiation is related to its effects on the genome (cf. Strauss, 1977). A variety of specific radiation-induced lesions in DNA are now known; a number of examples are seen in Figure 3.15. Ultraviolet radiation induces pyrimidine dimers in DNA of two different types (Haseltine, 1983). The cyclobutane type of

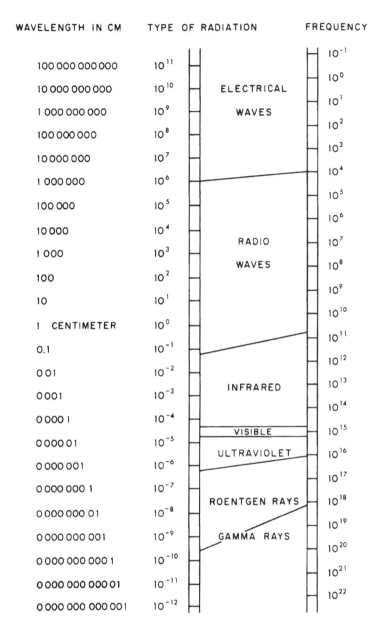

Figure 3.26 The electromagnetic spectrum showing the wavelength and frequency of the different classes of radiant energy. (Adapted from Glasser, 1944, with permission of the author and publisher.)

dimer is schematically noted in Figure 3.15, but there also occurs a 4,6 dimer which has significant mutagenic properties. Ultraviolet radiation also induces single-strand breaks in DNA and potentially protein-DNA crosslinks. Ionizing radiation, as indicated earlier (see above), has the greater propensity to produce DNA strand breaks, both single and double as well as protein-DNA crosslinks and hydroxylation of thymine, guanine, and other bases. In addition, ionizing radiation may cause a decrease in DNA methylation, possibly owing to the hydroxylation of 5-methylcytosine with subsequent repair (Kalinich et al., 1989).

The measurement of ionizing radiation has been of significant interest to physicists as well as physicians ever since the discovery of ionizing radiation and its biological effects. In Table 3.8 are listed many of the units of measurement employed for ionizing radiation. Within the last quarter century, terminology has altered from the original used in the earlier part of this century. Thus, the table indicates both the "old" and "new" units of measurement.

Some of the effects seen in Figure 3.15 may be termed the direct effects of radiation on DNA, such as DNA strand breaks and base elimination. However, there is substantial evidence that ionizing radiation has significant indirect effects that lead to base hydroxylation and other changes, not only of the genome, but also of other cellular structures (cf. Biaglow, 1981). Such indirect effects emanate largely from the formation of highly reactive species of other molecules in the biologic system. The predominant molecule in all biologic systems is water. High-energy irradiation of water leads to the formation of a variety of active molecules including the free radicals $\cdot OH$ and $\cdot H$, as well as other molecules such as the perhydroxyl radical ($HO_2 \cdot$) and singlet oxygen, $\cdot O_2$ (Piette, 1991). Such free radicals may react with cellular molecules in ways analogous to those of the "ultimate" forms of chemical carcinogens. Unsaturated fatty acids are converted to free radicals and to lipid peroxides by reaction with these products of the radiolysis of water. Proteins and nucleic acids may also be oxidized and/or converted to free radical forms, which in turn are highly reactive. This may cause the cross-linking of DNA and protein, as indicated in Figure 3.15. In addition, the perhydroxyl radical may combine with itself to form hydrogen peroxide or may ionize to form the superoxide ion ($O_2 \cdot^-$). Tissues irradiated at higher oxygen tension show greater effects of ionizing radiation than those irradiated at lower oxygen tensions. Although the exact mechanism of this "oxygen effect" is not yet fully understood, it is quite likely that the formation of oxygen radicals is a critical factor.

Other factors more directly related to the nature of the ionizing radiation itself are also important in the genesis of cancer by radiation. It is clear that the likelihood of carcinogenesis depends on the rate of energy loss of charged particles, either as incident radiation or induced by the radiation. This rate of loss is termed the *linear energy transfer* (LET). Higher LET radiation

Table 3.8 Units of Measurement for Ionizing Radiations

A. Field intensity (ionizations in air):
      1 Roentgen (R) (old) = 2.58×10^{-4} coulomb/kg
B. Absorbed energy:
      1 rad (old) = 100 ergs/g
      1 Gray (Gy) (new) = 100 rad = 1 joule/kg (J/kg)
C. Biological effect equivalent
      1 rem (*rad-equivalent-mammal*) (old) = dose of test radiation that produces the
      same biological effect as 1 rad of a standard (250 kVp x-rays or ^{60}Co gamma
      rays)
      1 Sievert (Sv) (new) = dose of test radiation that produces the same biological
      effect as 1 Gy of a standard radiation
D. Radioactivity
      1 Curie (Ci) (old) = that amount of radionuclide that yields 3.7×10^{10} disinte-
      grations per second
      1 Becquerel (Bq) (new) = nuclide amount that yields 1 disintegration per second
          1 petabecquerel (PBq) = 10^{15} Bq
             1 exabecquerel (EBq) = 10^{18} Bq
      energy per photon or accelerated particle
          1 electron volt (eV) = 1.602×10^{-19} joule (J)

is usually more carcinogenic than radiation with a low LET (Wiley et al., 1973). One may also characterize the dose of radiation by its relative biological effectiveness (RBE). Thus, the same doses of neutrons and gamma rays expressed in terms of roentgens have different carcinogenic potencies, the neutrons being more effective and thus having a greater RBE. The importance of these considerations has been documented in a number of studies (cf. Broerse et al., 1989, 1991) in that both LET and RBE are very important for the formation of neoplasms in relation to the radiation dose. The efficiency with which various forms of ionizing radiation induce cellular damage is quite variable and depends, as noted above, on the average density of energy loss along the path of the particle in the biological environment. Some examples of this LET for various sources of radiation are given in Table 3.9 (Tannock and Hill, 1992). The energy loss of a photon or particle as it traverses the biological system is dependent on its velocity, its charge, and the electron density of the target. Thus, as a particle loses energy and slows in its rate, its effective LET increases. Furthermore, the larger the LET of the photon or particle of a given energy, the shorter the distance traveled by the particle in the tissue. As the particle or photon travels through the tissue and interacts with structures within the cell, the energy loss is a summation of these interactive events along the particle track. Such events increase with increasing LET. Obviously, not all structures within the biological system will interact with a particle or photon track so that some will be altered or destroyed where interaction occurs, and others will not be affected in that no interaction with the particle or photon occurs. Such interactions become important in consideration of the carcinogenic effectiveness of ionizing radiation in relation to both LET and dose rate, as noted below.

Experimental Radiation Carcinogenesis

Although humans were the first "experimental animals" in which radiation-induced cancer was demonstrated, there are now many examples of the experimental induction of cancer by radiation. The experimental induction of skin cancer in mice by Findlay (1928) and later by Rusch

Table 3.9 Linear Energy Transfer (LET)
of Various Radiations

Radiation	LET (keV/μm)
Photons	
^{60}Co (~1.2 MeV)	0.3
200-keV X-ray	2.5
Electrons	
1 MeV	0.2
100 keV	0.5
10 keV	2
1 keV	10
Charged particles	
proton 2 MeV	17
alpha 5 MeV	90
carbon 100 MeV	160
Neutrons	
2.5 MeV	15–80
14.1 MeV	3–30

The units of LET are given in terms of energy
lost (keV) per unit path length (μm).

and colleagues (1941) paved the way for a better understanding of the ultraviolet light–induced cancer in patients with xeroderma pigmentosum and in the human population in general (Chapter 12).

DOSE-RESPONSE RELATIONSHIPS IN CHEMICAL AND PHYSICAL CARCINOGENESIS

The effectiveness of a chemical or physical carcinogen in inducing neoplasia is not only dependent on its structural and energetic properties, but also on the administered dose and the potency of the agent itself. The latter characteristic for chemicals will be considered in a later chapter (Chapter 13) and to some extent has already been spoken to for radiation carcinogenesis in relation to LET and RBE (see above). Both practical and theoretical considerations of quantitative aspects of chemical and radiation carcinogenesis must be taken into account in considering the effect of a specific dose of such agents in producing neoplasia. Theoretical dose-response curves are given in Figure 3.27, in which the dose in arbitrary units produces an effect, in this case cancer. The numbers on each of the curves indicate the number of "hits" that were required to produce that specific effect. Thus, if only a single hit is required for the production of cancer by radiation or by the ultimate form of a chemical carcinogen, an exponential curve beginning at the origin would be produced, and no "threshold" (dose below which there is no effect) would be seen. On the other hand, when a larger number of hits is required to produce an effect, a distinct threshold is noted. Biological data from both humans and experimental animals have demonstrated both types of responses, although the "no threshold" response is generally assumed for radiation and chemical carcinogenesis. Undoubtedly, a number of factors are involved in these differences, including hormonal relations within the organism, DNA repair capabilities of the

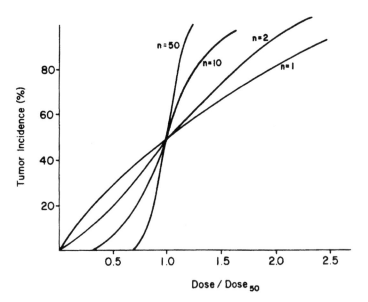

Figure 3.27   A family of dose-response curves relating tumor incidence to the dose of radiation in arbitrary units. For the sake of convenience, the actual dose is related to that dose producing 50% of the maximal effect or maximal tumor response. The numbers n = 1, 2, 10, 50 indicate the number of "hits" that were required to produce that specific response.

radiated cells, position in the cell cycle at the time of carcinogen administration, and the rate of cell proliferation in the target tissue. In particular, Swenberg et al. (1987) have pointed out that increased cell proliferation is a common phenomenon during chemical carcinogenesis associated with exposures to relatively high doses of carcinogenic chemicals.

Some of the more extensive and earlier studies on dose-response relationships of chemical carcinogens were carried out by Druckrey and associates (cf. Port et al., 1976). These studies were carried out by the chronic administration of chemicals at daily or weekly intervals by different dosage regimens. By investigating the median tumor induction times (the time at which half of the animals had developed neoplasms), as in Figure 3.27, they found this parameter to be directly related to the daily dose of the carcinogen administered plus a constant. When animals receiving a daily dose of a chemical carcinogen, 4-dimethylaminostilbene, were compared with animals receiving twice the daily dose but only every other week, the cumulative incidences of neoplasms in both groups were still the same. The target organ of a carcinogen may also depend on the dose; e.g., when a relatively few high doses of diethylnitrosamine are given, primarily kidney cancer resulted, whereas at much lower daily doses, liver cancer was the principal neoplasm induced. Although Druckrey's studies did seem to suggest that threshold doses of chemical carcinogens may occur, more recent investigations with extremely large numbers of rats (Peto et al., 1991) or mice (Brown and Hoel, 1983) dosed chronically with chemical carcinogens showed no evidence of threshold (no effect) doses.

In the case of radiation carcinogenesis, the relationship of dose to carcinoma incidence has been assumed to lack a threshold (National Academy of Sciences, 1990). However, both from animal studies as well as those in humans, evidence for thresholds does exist. Figure 3.28 is a schematic diagram of the induction of a specific neoplasm in mice exposed to various dose formats of ionizing radiation (Tannock and Hill, 1992). Neoplasms induced by intraperitoneal fractionated doses, given at a specific dose/time (day, week, etc.), exhibited distinct thresholds or no-effect levels (Tannock and Hill, 1992). Kohn and Fry (1984) have reported that in specific human situations, relatively small doses of radiation produce relatively greater carcinogenic effects than do high doses, such as those used to treat cancer. This phenomenon may reflect a saturation point for radiation-induced carcinogenesis—i.e., a dose of radiation above which no further cancers are induced and cancer production decreases, possibly owing to cytotoxicity. Apparent thresholds have also been seen for leukemias resulting from exposure to atomic bomb radiation at Nagasaki, Japan (Kondo, 1990).

One of the principal reasons for the continued emphasis on the presence or absence of a threshold is the need to estimate the risk to humans of carcinogens at very low doses. In general, as seen later (Chapter 11), exposure of humans to carcinogens occurs primarily at low doses. The extrapolation of high-dose data to very low doses may underestimate (Stenbäck et al., 1981) or overestimate (Figures 3.26 and 3.27) (Kondo, 1990) risks of neoplasia. Although safety considerations may direct evaluations of human risk strictly from the standpoint of the lack of threshold levels of chemical and physical carcinogens, practical consideration as well as expanding scientific knowledge makes such a blanket interpretation of dose-response relationships more and more untenable (Chapter 13).

In the case of neoplasms induced by ionizing radiation, it has become apparent that several factors may be involved. Lieberman and Kaplan (1959) demonstrated that the induction of leukemia by ionizing radiation in mice may be completely prevented by the removal of the thymus gland shortly after birth. Later, Kaplan and associates (Declève et al., 1976) demonstrated that radiation-induced leukemia in these animals occurred by the "activation" of a leukemogenic virus that normally occurs in the specific strain of animals used and that was activated by the ionizing radiation. However, Loutit and Ash (1978) question the direct causative effect of the virus in radiation-induced leukemia, suggesting that these infectious agents were passengers rather

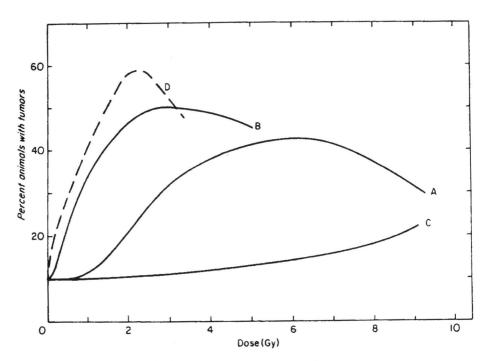

Figure 3.28 Schematic diagram of induction of a specific tumor type in mice exposed to various doses of ionizing radiation given to the whole body based on a review of a number of different in vivo results. Curve A: Tumors induced by single acute doses of low-LET ionizing radiation. Curve B: Tumors induced by single acute doses of high-LET radiation. Curve C: Tumors induced by fractionated doses (e.g., 1 Gy/day), of low-LET radiation. Curve D: Tumors induced by fractionated doses (e.g., 0.5 Gy/day), of high-LET radiation. (From Tannock and Hill, 1992, with permission of the authors and publisher.)

than causative in this condition. Later studies (cf. Janowski et al., 1990) indicated that the viruses involved in radiation-induced lymphomagenesis in mice played a role in the development of neoplasia rather than in its initiation (Chapter 8). Oncogenic viruses have also been isolated from radiation-induced osteosarcomas of rodents, although their relationship to the causation of these neoplasms is unclear (cf. Janowski et al., 1990). In male mice of the CBA/H strain, a single dose of ionizing radiation can induce acute myeloid leukemia. Months before the appearance of the leukemia, bone marrow cells exhibiting a specific deletion/rearrangement of chromosome 2 (Chapter 6) can be observed. However, other factors appear to be involved in the development of overt leukemia in these animals (cf. Janowski et al., 1990).

Major sites of radiogenic neoplasia in humans as well as in rodents include the mammary gland, bone marrow, skin, lung, and GI tract and a variety of other sites in nonhuman primates (Broerse et al., 1989). Earlier studies by Cole and Nowell (1965) demonstrated the interesting phenomenon of the potentiation of carcinogenesis by high-energy radiation when a mitotic stimulus was simultaneously administered to the animal. One of the best examples of this is the induction of radiation-induced hepatomas in rodents; partial hepatectomy or the administration of sublethal doses of a hepatotoxic chemical, such as carbon tetrachloride, markedly increases the incidence of hepatomas when radiation is given at specific times in relation to the operation or the administration of the chemical (Wiley et al., 1973). In addition, unlike most examples of the chemical induction of neoplasia, acute x-irradiation of mice of certain strains leads to a dramatic increase in the incidence of acute leukemias not only in exposed animals but also in their off-spring, persisting for several generations (cf. Nomura, 1991). This effect argues strongly for a direct action of ionizing radiation on germ cells, resulting in a genetic propensity for neoplastic development in later generations.

CHRONIC IRRITATION AND TRAUMA AS FACTORS IN CARCINOGENESIS

Although the general concept that chronic irritation is a carcinogenic stimulus is no longer accepted, in certain conditions chronic inflammation in humans may predispose to neoplasia. One of the best examples is the chronic draining sinus, usually resulting from chronic infections such as osteomyelitis. Such chronic infections are relatively rare today; however, in the past, when bone infections were rather common, epidermoid carcinomas occasionally arose in the skin near chronic draining sinuses. The histology of these lesions before the production of the neoplasm demonstrated a peculiar type of hyperplasia of the squamous epithelium known as pseudo-epitheliomatous hyperplasia (Sommerville, 1953). Other sites of chronic inflammation considered to be associated with higher incidences of neoplasia are the lower lips of pipe smokers and nevi or moles in locations on the body subject to chronic irritation, such as the belt region or the back of the neck. As has already been suggested and will be more thoroughly elaborated in subsequent chapters, chronic inflammation and, to a lesser degree, trauma stimulate cellular proliferation, which may increase the potential for the development of neoplasia (Chapter 9). In Chapter 7, we consider how trauma may enhance the production of certain experimental cancers of the skin. There is also significant evidence that metastatic spread of malignant neoplasms can be facilitated by trauma. However, there is no unequivocal evidence that either chronic irritation or trauma is *directly* causative of neoplastic transformation in the living animal (Monkman et al., 1974).

REFERENCES

Abell, C. W., and Heidelberger, C. Interaction of carcinogenic hydrocarbons with tissues. VIII. Binding of tritium-labeled hydrocarbons to the soluble proteins of mouse skin. Cancer Res., 22:931–946, 1962.

Ames, B. N., Durston, W. E., Yamasaki, E., and Lee, F. D. Carcinogens are mutagens: a simple test system combining liver homogenates for activation and bacteria for detection. Proc. Natl. Acad. Sci. U.S.A., 70:2281–2285, 1973.

Ames, B. N., Shigenaga, M. K., and Gold, L. S. DNA lesions, inducible DNA repair, and cell division: three key factors in mutagenesis and carcinogenesis. Environ. Health Perspect., 93:35–44, 1993.

Argetsinger, L. S., Campbell, G. S., Yang, X., Witthuhn, B. A., Silvennoinen, O., Ihle, J. N., and Carter-Su, C. Identification of JAK2 as a growth hormone receptor-associated tyrosine kinase. Cell, 74:237–244, 1993.

Ashby, J., and Paton, D. The influence of chemical structure on the extent and sites of carcinogenesis for 522 rodent carcinogens and 55 different human carcinogen exposures. Mutat. Res., 286:3–74, 1993.

Ashby, J., Tennant, R. W., Zeiger, E., and Stasiewicz, S. Classification according to chemical structure, mutagenicity to *Salmonella* and level of carcinogenicity of a further 42 chemicals tested for carcinogenicity by the U.S. National Toxicology Program. Mutat. Res., 223:73–103, 1989.

Barlow, D. P. Methylation and imprinting: from host defense to gene regulation? Science, 260:309–310, 1993.

Barrett, J. C., Wong, A., and McLachlan, J. A. Diethylstilbestrol induces neoplastic transformation without measurable gene mutation at two loci. Science, 212:1402–1404, 1981.

Barrett-Connor, E. Hormone replacement and cancer. Br. Med. Bull., 48:345–355, 1992.

Bartsch, H., Hietanen, E., and Malaveille, C. Carcinogenic nitrosamines: free radical aspects of their action. Free Rad. Biol. Med., 7:637–644, 1989.

Bartsch, H., Ohshima, H., Shuker, D. E. G., Pignatelli, B., and Calmels, S. Exposure of humans to endogenous N-nitroso compounds: implications in cancer etiology. Mutat. Res., 238:255–267, 1990.

Barzilay, J., Heatley, G. J., and Cushing, G. W. Benign and malignant tumors in patients with acromegaly. Arch. Intern. Med., 151:1629–1632, 1991.

Bast, A., and Goris, R. J. A. Oxidative stress. Biochemistry and human disease. Pharm. Weekbl., 11:199–206, 1989.

Bast, A., Haenen, G. R. M. M., and Doelman, C. J. A. Oxidants and antioxidants: State of the art. Am. J. Med., 91:3C-2S–3C-13S, 1991.

Beach, A. C., and Gupta, R. C. Human biomonitoring and the ^{32}P-postlabeling assay. Carcinogenesis, 13:1053–1074, 1992.

Beatson, G. T. On the treatment of inoperable cases of carcinoma of the mamma: suggestions for a new method of treatment, with illustrative cases. Lancet, 2:104–107, 1896.

Becker, R. A., and Shank, R. C. Kinetics of formation and persistence of ethylguanines in DNA of rats and hamsters treated with diethylnitrosamine. Cancer Res., 45:2076–2084, 1985.

Berger, M. R., Schmähl, D., and Zerban, H. Combination experiments with very low doses of three genotoxic N-nitrosamines with similar organotropic carcinogenicity in rats. Carcinogenesis, 8:1635–1643, 1987.

Bernard, C. Leçons sur les Phénomènes de la Vie. Paris: Baillière, 1878, 1879.

Bessho, T., Roy, R., Yamamoto, K., Kasai, H., Nishimura, S., Tano, K., and Mitra, S. Repair of 8-hydroxyguanine in DNA by mammalian N-methylpurine-DNA glycosylase. Proc. Natl. Acad. Sci. U.S.A., 90:8901–8904, 1993.

Biaglow, J. E. The effects of ionizing radiation on mammalian cells. J. Chem. Ed., 58:144–156, 1981.

Bichara, M., and Fuchs, R. P. P. DNA binding and mutation spectra of the carcinogen N-2-aminofluorene in Escherichia coli. A correlation between the conformation of the premutagenic lesion and the mutation specificity. J. Mol. Biol., 183:341–351, 1985.

Bischoff, F., and Bryson, G. Inert foreign-body implants in the mouse CNS. Res. Commun. Psychol. Psych. Behavior, 1:187–190, 1976.

Biskind, M. S., and Biskind, G. R. Development of tumors in the rat ovary after transplantation into the spleen. Proc. Soc. Exp. Biol. Med., 55:176–179, 1944.

Bittner, J. J. Mammary cancer in C3H mice of different sublines and their hybrids. J. Natl. Cancer Inst., 16:1263–1286, 1956.

Bohr, V. A., Phillips, D. H., and Hanawalt, P. C. Heterogeneous DNA damage and repair in the mammalian genome. Cancer Res., 47:6426–6436, 1987.

Bolt, H. M. Roles of etheno-DNA adducts in tumorigenicity of olefins. CRC Crit. Rev. Toxicol., 18:299–309, 1988.

Bolt, H. M., Peter, H., and Föst, U. Analysis of macromolecular ethylene oxide adducts. Int. Arch. Occup. Environ. Health, 60:141–144, 1988.

Bors, W., Michel, C., Dalke, C., Stettmaier, K., Saran, M., and Andrae, U. Radical intermediates during the oxidation of nitropropanes. The formation of NO_2 from 2-nitropropane, its reactivity with nucleosides, and implications for the genotoxicity of 2-nitropropane. Chem. Res. Toxicol., 6:302–309, 1993.

Bosland, M. C., Dreef-Van Der Meulen, H. C., Sukumar, S., Ofner, P., Leav, I., Han, X., and Liehr, J. G. Multistage prostate carcinogenesis: the role of hormones. Int. Symp. Princess Takamatsu Cancer Res. Fund, 22:109–123, 1991.

Boyland, E. The biological significance of metabolism of polycyclic compounds. Biochem. Soc. Symp., 5:40–54, 1950.

Brambilla, G., Carlo, P., Finollo, R., Bignone, F. A., Ledda, A., and Cajelli, E. Viscometric detection of liver DNA fragmentation in rats treated with minimal doses of chemical carcinogens. Cancer Res., 43:202–209, 1983.

Brand, K. G., Buoen, L. C., Johnson, K. H., and Brand, I. Etiological factors, stages, and the role of the foreign body in foreign body tumorigenesis: a review. Cancer Res., 35:279–286, 1975.

Brash, D. E., and Hart, R. W. DNA damage and repair in vivo. J. Environ. Pathol. Toxicol., 2:79–114, 1978.

Bresnick, E., and Eastman, A. Alkylation of mammalian cell DNA, persistence of adducts, and relationship to carcinogenesis. Drug Metab. Rev., 13:189–205, 1982.

Broerse, J. J., van Bekkum, D. W., and Zurcher, C. Radiation carcinogenesis in experimental animals. Experientia, 45:60–69, 1989.

Broerse, J. J., van Bekkum, D. W., Zoetelief, J., and Zurcher, C. Relative biological effectiveness for neutron carcinogenesis in monkeys and rats. Radiat. Res., 128:S128–S135, 1991.

Brooks, A. L., Benjamin, S. A., Jones, R. K., and McClellan, R. O. Interaction of ^{144}Ce and partial hepatectomy in the production of liver neoplasms in the Chinese hamster. Radiat. Res., 91:573–588, 1982.

Brown, K. G., and Hoel, D. G. Multistage prediction of cancer in serially dosed animals with application to the ED_{01} study. Fundam. Appl. Toxicol., 3:470–477, 1983.

Bryant, M. S., Skipper, P. L., Tannenbaum, S. R., and Maclure, M. Hemoglobin adducts of 4-aminobiphenyl in smokers and nonsmokers. Cancer Res., 47:602–608, 1987.

Butlin, H. J. Three lectures on cancer of the scrotum in chimney-sweeps and others. I. Secondary cancer without primary cancer. II. Why foreign sweeps do not suffer from scrotal cancer. III. Tar and paraffin cancer. Br. Med. J., 1:1341–1346, 1892; 2:1–6, 66–71, 1892.

Butterworth, B. E. Chemically induced cell proliferation as a predictive assay for potential carcinogenicity. In: Chemically Induced Cell Proliferation: Implications for Risk Assessment, pp. 457–467. New York: Wiley-Liss, 1991.

Carter-Su, C., Argetsinger, L. S., Campbell, G. S., Wang, X., Ihle, J., and Witthuhn, B. The identification of JAK2 tyrosine kinase as a signaling molecule for growth hormone. Proc. Soc. Exp. Biol. Med., 206:210–215, 1994.

Cavalieri, E. L., and Rogan, E. G. The approach to understanding aromatic hydrocarbon carcinogenesis: the central role of radical cations in metabolic activation. Pharmacol. Ther., 55:183–199, 1992.

Chandra, R. S., Kapur, S. P., Kelleher, J., Luban, N., and Patterson, K. Benign hepatocellular tumors in the young. Arch. Pathol. Lab. Med., 108:168–171, 1984.

Chang, L. W., Hsia, S. M. T., Chan, P.-C., and Hsieh, L.-L. Macromolecular adducts: biomarkers for toxicity and carcinogenesis. Annu. Rev. Pharmacol. Toxicol., 34:41–67, 1994.

Chung, F.-L., Chen, H.-J. C., Guttenplan, J. B., Nishikawa, A., and Hard, G. C. 2,3-Epoxy-4-hydroxynonanal as a potential tumor-initiating agent of lipid peroxidation. Carcinogenesis, 14:2073–2077, 1993.

Chung, F.-L., Chen, H.-J. C., and Nath, R. G. Lipid peroxidation as a potential endogenous source for the formation of exocyclic DNA adducts. Carcinogenesis, 17:2105–2111, 1996.

Clifton, K. H., and Sridharan, B. N. Endocrine factors and tumor growth. In: F. F. Becker (ed.), Cancer—A Comprehensive Treatise, Vol. 3, pp. 249–285. New York: Plenum, 1975.

Cohen, S. M., and Ellwein, L. B. Genetic errors, cell proliferation, and carcinogenesis. Cancer Res., 51:6493–6505, 1991.

Cole, L. J., and Nowell, P. C. Radiation carcinogenesis. The sequence of events. Science, 150:1782–1786, 1965.

Conaway, C. C., Nie, G., Hussain, N. S., and Fiala, E. S. Comparison of oxidative damage to rat liver DNA and RNA by primary nitroalkanes, secondary nitroalkanes, cyclopentanone oxime, and related compounds. Cancer Res., 51:3143–3147, 1991.

Conney, A. H. Induction of microsomal enzymes by foreign chemicals and carcinogenesis by polycyclic aromatic hydrocarbons: G. H. A. Clowes Memorial Lecture. Cancer Res., 42:4875–4917, 1982.

Costa, M. Molecular mechanisms of nickel carcinogenesis. Annu. Rev. Pharmacol. Toxicol., 31:321–337, 1991.

Costa, M. DNA-protein complexes induced by chromate and other carcinogens. Environ. Health Perspect., 92:45–52, 1991.

Dautry-Varsat, A., and Lodish, H. F. How receptors bring proteins and particles into cells. Sci. Am., 250:52–58, 1984.

Declève, A., Lieberman, M., Ihle, J. N., and Kaplan, H. S. Biological and serological characterization of radiation leukemia virus. Proc. Natl. Acad. Sci. U.S.A., 73:4675–4679, 1976.

Demple, B., and Harrison, L. Repair of oxidative damage to DNA: enzymology and biology. Annu. Rev. Biochem., 63:915–948, 1994.

Dipple, A., Michejda, C. J., and Weisburger, E. K. Metabolism of chemical carcinogens. Pharmacol. Ther., 27:265–296, 1985.

Dorgan, J. F., and Schatzkin, A. Antioxidant micronutrients in cancer prevention. Nutr. Cancer, 5:43–68, 1991.

Eastman, A., and Barry, M. A. The origins of DNA breaks: a consequence of DNA damage, DNA repair, or apoptosis? Cancer Invest., 10:229–240, 1992.

Edmondson, H. A., Henderson, B., and Benton, B. Liver-cell adenomas associated with use of oral contraceptives. N. Engl. J. Med., 294:470–472, 1976.

Emerit, I., Khan, S. H., and Esterbauer, H. Hydroxynonenal, a component of clastogenic factors? Free Radic. Biol. Med., 10:371–377, 1991.

Engelbergs, J., Thomale, J., Galhoff, A., and Rajewsky, M. F. Fast repair of O^6-ethylguanine, but not O^6-methylguanine, in transcribed genes prevents mutation of H-*ras* in rat mammary tumorigenesis induced by ethylnitrosourea in place of methylnitrosourea. Proc. Natl. Acad. Sci. U.S.A., 95:1635–1640, 1998.

Enslein, K., Gombar, V. K., and Blake, B. W. Use of SAR in computer-assisted prediction of carcinogenicity and mutagenicity of chemicals by the *TOPKAT* program. Mutat. Res., 305:47–61, 1994.

Epe, B., Harttig, U., Stopper, H., and Metzler, M. Covalent binding of reactive estrogen metabolites to microtubular protein as a possible mechanism of aneuploidy induction and neoplastic cell transformation. Environ. Health Perspect., 88:123–127, 1990.

Essigmann, J. M., and Wood, M. L. The relationship between the chemical structures and mutagenic specificities of the DNA lesions formed by chemical and physical mutagens. Toxicol. Lett., 67:29–39, 1993.

Farber, E. Ethionine carcinogenesis. Adv. Cancer Res., 7:383–474, 1963.

Featherstone, C., and Jackson, S. P. Ku. A DNA repair protein with multiple cellular functions? Mutat. Res., 434:3–15, 1999.

Ferguson, D. J. Cellular attachment to implanted foreign bodies in relation to tumorigenesis. Cancer Res., 37:4367–4371, 1977.

Findlay, G. M. Ultra-violet light and skin cancer. Lancet, 106:1070–1073, 1928.

Fishel, R., and Kolodner, R. D. Identification of mismatch repair genes and their role in the development of cancer. Curr. Opin. Genet. Dev., 5:382–395, 1995.

Fishel, R., and Wilson, T. MutS homologs in mammalian cells. Curr. Opin. Genet. Dev., 7:105–113, 1997.

Floyd, R. A. Role of oxygen free radicals in carcinogenesis and brain ischemia. FASEB J., 4:2587–2597, 1990.

Friedberg, E. C. DNA repair: looking back and peering forward. Bioessays, 16:645–649, 1994.

Fry, R. J. M., Ley, R. D., Grube, D., and Staffeldt, E. Studies on the multistage nature of radiation carcinogenesis. *In*: E. Hecker, N. E. Fusenig, W. Kunz, F. Marks, and H. W. Thielmann (Eds.). Carcinogenesis—A Comprehensive Survey, Vol. 7, Cocarcinogenesis and Biological Effects of Tumor Promoters, pp. 155–165. New York: Raven Press, 1982.

Furth, J. Pituitary cybernetics and neoplasia. Harvey Lect., 63:47, 1969.

Furth, J. Hormones as etiological agents in neoplasia. *In*: F. F. Becker (Ed.), Cancer—A Comprehensive Treatise, Vol. 1, Chap. 4, pp. 75–120. New York: Plenum, 1975.

Ghoshal, A. K., and Farber, E. The induction of liver cancer by dietary deficiency of choline and methionine without added carcinogens. Carcinogenesis, 5:1367–1370, 1984.

Gladek, A., and Liehr, J. G. Mechanism of genotoxicity of diethylstilbestrol *in vivo*. J. Biol. Chem., 264:16847–16852, 1989.

Glasser, O. Radiation spectrum. *In*: O. Glasser (Ed.), Medical Physics, p. 1969. Chicago: Yearbook Publishers, 1944.

Goldfarb, S. Sex hormones and hepatic neoplasia. Cancer Res., 36:2584–2588, 1976.

Goldstein, J. A., and Faletto, M. B. Advances in mechanisms of activation and deactivation of environmental chemicals. Environ. Health Perspect., 100:169–176, 1993.

Goodman, R., and Shirley-Henderson, A. Exposure of cells to extremely low-frequency electromagnetic fields: relationship to malignancy? Cancer Cells, 2:355–359, 1990.

Gorchev, H. G., and Jelinek, C. F. A review of the dietary intakes of chemical contaminants. Bull. World Health Organ., *63*:945–962, 1985.

Goth, R., and Rajewsky, M. F. Persistence of O^6-ethylguanine in rat-brain DNA: correlation with nervous system–specific carcinogenesis by ethylnitrosourea. Proc. Natl. Acad. Sci. U.S.A., *71*:639–643, 1974.

Guengerich, F. P. Reactions and significance of cytochrome P-450 enzymes. J. Biol. Chem., *266*:10019–10022, 1991.

Guengerich, F. P. Metabolic activation of carcinogens. Pharmacol. Ther., *54*:17–61, 1992.

Guenther, T. M., and Oesch, F. Metabolic activation and inactivation of chemical mutagens and carcinogens. Trends Pharmacol. Sci., *2*:129–132, 1981.

Gupta, R. C., Reddy, M. V., and Randerath, K. ^{32}P-postlabeling analysis of non-radioactive aromatic carcinogen-DNA adducts. Carcinogenesis, *3*:1081–1092, 1982.

Habs, M., and Schmähl, D. Diet and cancer. J. Cancer Res. Clin. Oncol., *96*:1–10, 1980.

Hanawalt, P. C. Transcription-coupled repair and human disease. Science, *266*:1957–1958, 1994.

Hansen, C., Asmussen, I., and Autrup, H. Detection of carcinogen-DNA adducts in human fetal tissues by the ^{32}P-postlabeling procedure. Environ. Health Perspect., *99*:229–231, 1993.

Harvey, R. G. Activated metabolites of carcinogenic hydrocarbons. Acc. Chem. Res., *14*:218–226, 1981.

Haseltine, W. A. Ultraviolet light repair and mutagenesis revisited. Cell, *33*:13–17, 1983.

Hathway, D. E., and Kolar, G. F. Mechanisms of reaction between ultimate chemical carcinogens and nucleic acid. Chem. Soc. Rev., *9*:241–253, 1980.

Hecht, S. S. Chemical carcinogenesis: an overview. Clin. Physiol. Biochem., *3*:89–97, 1985.

Heidelberger, C. Chemical carcinogenesis, chemotherapy: cancer's continuing core challenges. G. H. A. Clowes Memorial Lecture. Cancer Res., *30*:1549–1569, 1970.

Heldin, C.-H. Dimerization of cell surface receptors in signal transduction. Cell, *80*:213–223, 1995.

Henderson, B. E., Ross, R. K., Pike, M. C., and Casagrande, J. T. Endogenous hormones as a major factor in human cancer. Cancer Res., *42*:3232–3239, 1982.

Henderson, B. E., Ross, R., and Bernstein, L. Estrogens as a cause of human cancer: The Richard and Hinda Rosenthal Foundation Award Lecture. Cancer Res., *48*:246–253, 1988.

Herbst, A. L., and Scully, R. E. Adenocarcinoma of the vagina in adolescence. Cancer, *25*:745–757, 1970.

Herbst, A. L., Ulfelder, H., and Poskanzer, D. C. Adenocarcinoma of the vagina. Association of maternal stilbestrol therapy with tumor appearance in young women. N. Engl. J. Med., *284*:878–881, 1971.

Hirono, I., Kuhara, K., Yamaji, T., Hosaka, S., and Golberg, L. Carcinogenicity of dextran sulfate sodium in relation to its molecular weight. Cancer Lett., *18*:29–34, 1983.

Holland, J. H. Genetic algorithms. Sci. Am., *267*:66–72, July 1992.

Holliday, R. A different kind of inheritance. Sci. Am., *260*:60–73, 1989.

Hoover, D. M., Best, K. L., McKenney, B. K., Tamura, R. N., and Neubauer, B. L. Experimental induction of neoplasia in the accessory sex organs of male Lobund-Wistar rats. Cancer Res., *50*:142–146, 1990.

Horsfall, M. J., Gordon, A. J. E., Burns, P. A., Zielenska, M., van der Vliet, G. M. E., and Glickman, B. W. Mutational specificity of alkylating agents and the influence of DNA repair. Environ. Mol. Mutagen. *15*:107–122, 1990.

Hsieh, L.-L., and Hsieh, T.-T. Detection of aflatoxin B_1-DNA adducts in human placenta and cord blood. Cancer Res., *53*:1278–1280, 1993.

Huggins, G. R., and Zucker, P. K. Oral contraceptives and neoplasia: 1987 update. Fertil. Steril., *47*:733–761, 1987.

Huggins, C., and Hodges, C. L. Studies on prostatic cancer. I. The effect of castration, of estrogen and of androgen injection on serum phosphatase in metastatic carcinoma of the prostrate. Cancer Res., *1*:293, 1941.

Huh, N.-h., Satoh, M. S., Shiga, J., Rajewsky, M. F., and Kuroki, T. Immunoanalytical detection of O^4-ethylthymine in liver DNA of individuals with or without malignant tumors. Cancer Res., *49*:93–97, 1989.

Huseby, R. A. Demonstration of a direct carcinogenic effect of estradiol on Leydig cells of the mouse. Cancer Res., *40*:1006–1013, 1980.

IARC Monographs on the Evaluation of Carcinogenic Risks to Humans: Alcohol Drinking. Lyon, France: International Agency for Research on Cancer, *44*:101–105, 1987.

IARC Monographs on the Evaluation of the Carcinogenic Risk of Chemicals to Man: Some Inorganic and Organometallic Compounds, Vol. 2. Lyon, France: International Agency for Research on Cancer, 1973.

Ip, C., Yip, P., and Bernardis, L. L. Role of prolactin in the promotion of dimethylbenz[*a*]anthracene-induced mammary tumors by dietary fat. Cancer Res., *40*:374–378, 1980.

Ishak, K. G. Hepatic lesions caused by anabolic and contraceptive steroids. Semin. Liver Dis., *1*:116–128, 1981.

Ito, N., Hasegawa, R., Imaida, K., Kurata, Y., Hagiwara, A., and Shirai, T. Ingestion of 20 pesticides in combination at acceptable daily intake levels exerts no effects on rat liver carcinogenesis. Food Chem. Toxicol., *33*:159–163, 1995.

Ito, N., and Hirose, M. The role of antioxidants in chemical carcinogenesis. Jpn. J. Cancer Res. (Gann), *78*:1011–1026, 1987.

Izbicki, J. R., Hamilton, S. R., Wambach, G., Harnisch, E., Wilker, D. K., Dornschneider, G., Eibl-Eibesfeldt, B., and Schweiberer, L. Effects of androgen manipulations on chemically induced colonic tumours and on macroscopically normal colonic mucosa in male Sprague-Dawley rats. Br. J. Cancer, *61*:235–240, 1990.

Jaggi, W., Lutz, W. K., and Schlatter, C. Covalent binding of ethinylestradiol and estrone to rat liver DNA in vivo. Chem. Biol. Interact., *23*:13–18, 1978.

Janowski, M., Cox, R., and Strauss, P. G. The molecular biology of radiation-induced carcinogenesis: thymic lymphoma, myeloid leukaemia and osteosarcoma. Int. J. Radiat. Biol., *57*:677–691, 1990.

Jensen, H., and Madsen, J. L. Diet and cancer. Acta Med. Scand., *223*:293–304, 1988.

Jerina, D. M., Daly, J. W., Witkop, B. Zaltzman-Nirenberg, P., and Udenfriend, S. 1,2-Naphthalene oxide as an intermediate in the microsomal hydroxylation of naphthalene. Biochemistry, *9*:147–156, 1970.

Jerina, D. M., Sayer, J. M., Yagi, H., Croisy-Delcey, M., Ittah, Y., Thakker, D. R., Wood, A. W., Chang, R. L., Levin, W., and Conney, A. H. *In*: R. Snyder, D. V. Parke, J. J. Kocsis, D. J. Jollow, C. G. Gibson, C. M. Witmer (Eds.), Advances in Experimental Medicine and Biology: Biological Reactive Intermediates IIA, pp. 501–523. New York: Plenum, 1982.

Jiricny, J. Replication errors: cha(lle)nging the genome. EMBO J., *17*:6427–6436, 1998.

Johnson, K. H., Buoen, L. C., Brand, I., and Brand, K. G. Polymer tumorigenesis: clonal determination of histopathological characteristics during early preneoplasia: relationships to karyotype, mouse strain, and sex. J. Natl. Cancer Inst., *44*:785–793, 1970.

Johnson, L. D., Driscoll, S. G., Hertig, A. T., Cole, P. T., and Nickerson, R. J. Vaginal adenosis in stillborns and neonates exposed to diethylstilbestrol and steroidal estrogens and progestins. Obstet. Gynecol., *53*:671–679, 1979.

Kadlubar, F. F., Anson, J. F., Dooley, K. L., and Beland, F. A. Formation of urothelial and hepatic DNA adducts from the carcinogen 2-naphthylamine. Carcinogenesis, *2*:467–470, 1981.

Kalinich, J. F., Catravas, G. N., and Snyder, S. L. The effect of g radiation on DNA methylation. Radiat. Res., *117*:185–197, 1989.

Kaplan, S. A. Cell receptors. Am. J. Dis. Child., *138*:1140–1145, 1984.

Kappus, H., and Remmer, H. Metabolic activation of norethisterone (norethindrone) to an irreversibly protein-bound derivative by rat liver microsomes. Drug. Metab. Dispos., *3*:338–344, 1975.

Kaufmann, W. K. Pathways of human cell post-replication repair. Carcinogenesis, *10*:1–11, 1989.

Kawashima, S., Wakabayashi, K., Nishizuka, Y. Low incidence of nodular hyperplasia of the adrenal cortex after ovariectomy in neonatally estrogenized mice than in the controls. Proc. Jpn. Acad., *56*:350–354, 1980.

Kelly, P. A., Djiane, J., Postel-Vinay, M.-C., and Edery, M. The prolactin/growth hormone receptor family. Endocr. Rev., *12*:235–251, 1991.

Kelly, P. A., Edery, M., Finidori, J., Postel-Vinay, M.-C., Gougon, L., Ali, S., Dinerstein, H., Sotiropoulos, A., Lochnan, H., Ferrag, F., Lebrun, J.-J., Ormandy, C., Buteau, H., Esposito, N., Vincent, V., and Möldrup, A. Receptor domains involved in signal transduction of prolactin and growth hormone. Proc. Soc. Exp. Biol. Med., *206*:280–283, 1994.

Kennaway, E. The identification of a carcinogenic compound in coal-tar. Br. Med. J., 2:749–752, 1955.

Kinosita, R. Researches on the cancerogenesis of the various chemical substances. Gann, 30:423–426, 1936.

Kirkpatrick, C. J., Alves, A., Köhler, H., Kriegsmann, J., Bittinger, F., Otto, M., Williams, D. F., and Eloy, R. Biomaterial-induced sarcoma. A novel model to study preneoplastic change. Am. J. Pathol., 156:1455–1467, 2000.

Kodama, M., and Kodama, T. How valid is the concept of hormonal carcinogenesis in human neoplasias? Anticancer Res., 7:559–572, 1987.

Koga, N., Inskeep, P. B., Harris, T. M., and Guengerich, F. P. S-[2-N^7-Guanyl)ethyl]glutathione, the major DNA adduct formed from 1,2-dibromoethane. Biochemistry, 25:2192–2198, 1986.

Kohn, H. I., and Fry, R. J. M. Radiation carcinogenesis. N. Engl. J. Med., 310:504–511, 1984.

Kondo, S. Rational risk estimation in relation to atomic bomb radiation. J. Radiat. Res., 31:174–188, 1990.

Kritchevsky, D. Dietary effects in experimental carcinogenesis: Animal models. In: A. C. Beynen and C. E. West (Eds.), Use of Animal Models for Research in Human Nutrition. Comp. Anim. Nutr., Vol. 6, pp. 174–185. Basel, Switzerland: Karger, 1988.

Kuschner, M. The carcinogenicity of beryllium. Environ. Health Perspect., 40:101–105, 1981.

Landrigan, P. J. Arsenic—State of the art. Am. J. Ind. Med., 2:5–14, 1981.

Lasne, C., Lu, Y. P., Orfila, L., Ventura, L., and Chouroulinkov, I. Study of various transforming effects of the anabolic agents trenbolone and testosterone on Syrian hamster embryo cells. Carcinogenesis, 11:541–547, 1990.

Lawley, P. D. Historical origins of current concepts of carcinogenesis. Adv. Cancer Res., 64:17–111, 1994.

Levin, W., Thakker, D. R., Wood, A. W., Chang, R. L., Lehr, R. E., Jerina, D. M., and Conney, A. H. Evidence that benzo[a]anthracene 3,4-diol-1,2-epoxide is an ultimate carcinogen on mouse skin. Cancer Res., 38:1705–1710, 1978.

Li, A. P., Aaron, C. S., Auletta, A. E., Dearfield, K. L., Riddle, J. C., Slesinski, R. S., and Stankowski, L. F., Jr. An evaluation of the roles of mammalian cell mutation assays in the testing of chemical genotoxicity. Regul. Toxicol. Pharmacol., 14:24–40, 1991.

Li, D., and Randerath, K. Modulation of DNA modification (I-compound) levels in rat liver and kidney by dietary carbohydrate, protein, fat, vitamin, and mineral content. Mutat. Res., 275:47–56, 1992.

Li, D., Xu, D., and Randerath, K. Species and tissue specificities of I-compounds as contrasted with carcinogen adducts in liver, kidney and skin DNA of Sprague-Dawley rats, ICR mice and Syrian hamsters. Carcinogenesis, 11:2227–2232, 1990.

Li, G.-M., Wang, H., and Romano, L. J. Human MutSa specifically binds to DNA containing aminofluorene and acetylaminofluorene adducts. J. Biol. Chem., 271:24084–24088, 1996.

Li, J. J., and Li, S. A. Estrogen carcinogenesis in hamster tissues: a critical review. Endocr. Rev., 11:524–531, 1990.

Li, J. J., Li, S. A., Klicka, J. K., Parsons, J. A., and Lam, L. K. T. Relative carcinogenic activity of various synthetic and natural estrogens in the Syrian hamster kidney. Cancer Res., 43:5200–5204, 1983.

Lieber, M. R. Pathological and physiological double-strand breaks. Am. J. Pathol., 153:1323–1332, 1998.

Lieberman, M. W., and Forbes, P. D. Demonstration of DNA repair in normal and neoplastic tissues after treatment with proximate chemical carcinogens and ultraviolet radiation. Nature New Biol., 241:199–201, 1973.

Lieberman, M., and Kaplan, H. S. Leukemogenic activity of filtrates from radiation-induced lymphoid tumors of mice. Science, 130:387–388, 1959.

Liehr, J. G. 2-Fluoroestradiol. Separation of estrogenicity from carcinogenicity. Mol. Pharmacol., 23:278–281, 1983.

Liehr, J. G. Genotoxic effects of estrogens. Mutat. Res., 238:269–276, 1990.

Liehr, J. G., Avitts, T. A., Randerath, E., and Randerath, K. Estrogen-induced endogenous DNA adduction: possible mechanism of hormonal cancer. Proc. Natl. Acad. Sci., U.S.A., 83:5301–5305, 1986.

Liehr, J. G., Hall, E. R., Avitts, T. A., Randerath, E., and Randerath, K. Localization of estrogen-induced DNA adducts and cytochrome P-450 activity at the site of renal carcinogenesis in the hamster kidney. Cancer Res., 47:2156–2159, 1987.

Liehr, J. G., Sirbasku, D. A., Jurka, E., Randerath, K., and Randerath, E. Inhibition of estrogen-induced renal carcinogenesis in male Syrian hamsters by tamoxifen without decrease in DNA adduct levels. Cancer Res., *48*:779–783, 1988.

Lijinsky, W. Nitrosamines and nitrosamides in the etiology of gastrointestinal cancer. Cancer, *40*:2446–2449, 1977.

Lijinsky, W., Reuber, M. D., and Riggs, C. W. Carcinogenesis by combinations of *N*-nitroso compounds in rats. Food Chem. Toxicol., *21*:601–605, 1983.

Linder, M. E., and Gilman, A. G. G proteins. Sci. Am., *267*:56–65, 1992.

Loechler, E. L. Adduct-induced base-shifts: a mechanism by which the adducts of bulky carcinogens might induce mutations. Biopolymers, *28*:909–927, 1989.

Loutit, J. F., and Ash, P. J. N. D. Radiation leukaemogenesis: is virus really necessary? Br. J. Cancer, *38*:24–33, 1978.

Lowe, J. P., and Silverman, B. D. Predicting carcinogenicity of polycyclic aromatic hydrocarbons. Chem. Res., *17*:332–338, 1984.

Lu, G., Schlichter, D., and Wicks, W. D. Characterization of rat liver nuclear proteins which recognize the cAMP responsive element. Int. J. Biochem., *24*:1763–1771, 1992.

Lu, L.-J. W., Liehr, J. G., Sirbasku, D. A., Randerath, E., and Randerath, K. Hypomethylation of DNA in estrogen-induced and -dependent hamster kidney tumors. Carcinogenesis, 9:925–929, 1988.

Lundgren, K., Randerath, K., and Everson, R. B. Role of metabolism and DNA adduct formation in the induction of sister chromatid exchanges in human lymphocytes by diethylstilbestrol. Cancer Res., *48*:335–338, 1988.

Lutz, W. K., Jaggi, W., and Schlatter, C. Covalent binding of diethylstilbestrol to DNA in rat and hamster liver and kidney. Chem.-Biol. Interact., *42*:251–257, 1982.

Lutz, W. K., and Schlatter, J. The relative importance of mutagens and carcinogens in the diet. Pharmacol. Toxicol., *72*:s104–s107, 1993.

Lyon, F. A. The development of the endometrium in young women receiving long-term sequential oral contraception: report of four cases. Am. J. Obstet. Gynecol., *123*:299, 1975.

Magee, P. N., and Swann, P. F. Nitroso compounds. Br. Med. Bull., *25*:240–244, 1969.

Maher, V. M., Miller, E. C., Miller, J. A., and Szybalski, W. Mutations and decreases in density of transforming DNA produced by derivatives of the carcinogens 2-acetylaminofluorene and *N*-methyl-4-aminoazobenzene. Mol. Pharmacol., *4*:411–426, 1968.

Málková, J., Michalová, K., Pribyl, T., and Schreiber, V. Chromosomal changes in rat pituitary and bone marrow induced by long-term estrogen administration. Neoplasma, *24*:277–284, 1977.

Marnett, L. J. Polycyclic aromatic hydrocarbon oxidation during prostaglandin biosynthesis. Life Sci., *29*:531–546, 1981.

Marnett, L. J., and Burcham, P. C. Endogenous DNA adducts: potential and paradox. Chem. Res. Toxicol., *6*:771–785, 1993.

Martell, A. E. Chemistry of carcinogenic metals. Environ. Health Perspect., *40*:207–226, 1981.

Mauderly, J. L. Toxicological approaches to complex mixtures. Environ. Health Perspect., *101*:155–165, 1993.

Mays, E. T., and Christopherson, W. Hepatic tumors induced by sex steroids. Semin. Liver Dis., *4*:147–157, 1984.

McClain, R. M. The significance of hepatic microsomal enzyme induction and altered thyroid function in rats: implications for thyroid gland neoplasia. Toxicol. Pathol., *17*:294–306, 1989.

McCormick, J. J., and Maher, V. M. Mammalian cell mutagenesis as a biological consequence of DNA damage. DNA Repair Mech. 739, 1978.

Mehnert, K., Speit, G., and Vogel, W. Effect of diethylstilbestrol on the frequencies of sister chromatid exchange *in vitro* and *in vivo*. Cancer Res., *45*:3626–3630, 1985.

Melnick, S., Cole, P., Anderson, D., and Herbst, A. Rates and risks of diethylstilbestrol-related clear-cell adenocarcinoma of the vagina and cervix. N. Engl. J. Med., *316*:514–516, 1987.

Memoli, V. A., Urban, R. M., Alroy, J., and Galante, J. O. Malignant neoplasms associated with orthopedic implant materials in rats. J. Orthop. Res., *4*:346–355, 1986.

Merz, W. E. Properties of glycoprotein hormone receptors and post-receptor mechanisms. Exp. Clin. Endocrinol., *100*:4–8, 1992.

Michalopoulos, G., Strom, S. C., Kligerman, A. D., Irons, G. P., and Novicki, D. L. Mutagenesis induced by procarcinogens at the hypoxanthine-guanine phosphoribosyl transferase locus of human fibroblasts cocultured with rat hepatocytes. Cancer Res., *41*:1873–1878, 1981.

Michalowsky, L. A., and Jones, P. A. DNA methylation and differentiation. Environ. Health Perspect., *80*:189–197, 1989.

Mikol, Y. B., Hoover, K. L., Creasia, D., and Poirier, L. A. Hepatocarcinogenesis in rats fed methyl-deficient, amino acid-defined diets. Carcinogenesis, *4*:1619–1629, 1983.

Miller, A. B. An overview of hormone-associated cancers. Cancer Res., *38*:3985–3990, 1978.

Miller, A. B., Berrino, F., Hill, M., Pietinen, P., Riboli, E., and Wahrendorf, J. Diet in the aetiology of cancer: a review. Eur. J. Cancer, *30A*:207–220, 1994.

Miller, E. C. Studies on the formation of protein-bound derivatives of 3,4-benzopyrene in the epidermal fraction of mouse skin. Cancer Res., *11*:100–108, 1951.

Miller, E. C. Some current perspectives on chemical carcinogenesis in humans and experimental animals: Presidential address. Cancer Res., *38*:1479–1496, 1978.

Miller, E. C., and Miller, J. A. The presence and significance of bound aminoazo dyes in the livers of rats fed p-dimethylaminoazobenzene. Cancer Res., *7*:468–480, 1947.

Miller, J. A. Carcinogenesis by chemicals: an overview—G.H.A. Clowes Memorial Lecture. Cancer Res., *30*:559–576, 1970.

Miller, J. A. The need for epidemiological studies of the medical exposures of Japanese patients to the carcinogen ethyl carbamate (urethane) from 1950 to 1975. Jpn. J. Cancer Res., *82*:1323–1324, 1991.

Miller, J. A., Cramer, J. W., and Miller, E. C. The *N*- and ring-hydroxylation of 2-acetylaminofluorene during carcinogenesis in the rat. Cancer Res., *20*:950–962, 1960.

Mirsalis, J. C. Genotoxicity, toxicity, and carcinogenicity of the antihistamine methapyrilene. Mutat. Res., *185*:309–317, 1987.

Mirvish, S. S., Salmasi, S., Cohen, S. M., Patil, K., and Mahboubi, E. Liver and forestomach tumors and other forestomach lesions in rats treated with morpholine and sodium nitrite, with and without sodium ascorbate. J. Natl. Cancer Inst., *71*:81–85, 1983.

Modrich, P. Mismatch repair, genetic stability, and cancer. Science, *266*:1959–1960, 1994.

Modrich, P. Strand-specific mismatch repair in mammalian cells. J. Biol. Chem., *272*:24727–24730, 1997.

Monkman, G. R., Orwoll, G., and Ivins, J. C. Trauma and oncogenesis. Mayo Clin. Proc., *49*:157–163, 1974.

Monks, T. J., Anders, M. W., Dekant, W., Stevens, J. L., Lau, S. S., and van Bladeren, P. J. Contemporary issues in toxicology. Glutathione conjugate–mediated toxicities. Toxicol. Appl. Pharmacol., *106*:1–19, 1990.

Montesano, R., Brésil, H., Planche-Martel, G., Margison, G. P., and Pegg, A. E. Effect of chronic treatment of rats with dimethylnitrosamine on the removal of O^6-methylguanine from DNA. Cancer Res., *40*:452–458, 1980.

Müller, R., and Rajewsky, M. F. Enzymatic removal of O^6-ethylguanine *versus* stability of O^4-ethylthymine in the DNA of rat tissues exposed to the carcinogen ethylnitrosourea: possible interference of guanine-O^6 alkylation with 5-cytosine methylation in the DNA of replicating target cells. Z. Naturforsch., *38*:1023–1029, 1983.

Mumtaz, M. M., Sipes, I. G., Clewell, H. J., and Yang, R. S. H. Risk assessment of chemical mixtures: biologic and toxicologic issues. Fundam. Appl. Toxicol., *21*:258–269, 1993.

Myles G. M., and Sancar, A. DNA repair. Chem. Res. Toxicol., *2*:197–226, 1989.

Naegeli, H. Roadblocks and detours during DNA replication: mechanisms of mutagenesis in mammalian cells. Bioessays, *16*:557–564, 1994.

Nagata, C., Kodama, M., Ioki, Y., and Kimura, T. Free radicals produced from chemical carcinogens and their significance in carcinogenesis. *In*: R. A. Floyd (Ed.), Free Radicals and Cancer, pp. 1–62. New York: Marcel Dekker, 1982.

Nakagawa, T., Datta, A., and Kolodner, R. D. Multiple functions of MutS- and MutL-related heterocomplexes. Proc. Natl. Acad. Sci. U.S.A., *96*:14186–14188, 1999.

National Academy of Sciences: Health effects of exposure to low levels of ionizing radiation. BEIR V report. National Academy of Sciences. Washington D.C.: National Academy Press, 1990.

National Academy of Sciences: Biological significance of DNA adducts and protein adducts. *In*: Drinking Water and Health, Vol. 9, pp. 6–37. Washington D.C.: National Academy Press, 1989.

Neish, W. J. P., Parry, E. W., and Ghadially, F. N. Tumour induction in the rat by a mixture of two non-carcinogenic aminoazo dyes. Oncology, *21*:229–240, 1967.

Neumann, F. Early indicators for carcinogenesis in sex-hormone-sensitive organs. Mutat. Res., *248*:341–356, 1991.

Neumann, H.-G. Role of extent and persistence of DNA modifications in chemical carcinogenesis by aromatic amines. Recent Results Cancer Res., *84*:77–89, 1983.

Newbold, R. R., and McLachlan, J. A. Vaginal adenosis and adenocarcinoma in mice exposed prenatally or neonatally to diethylstilbestrol. Cancer Res., *42*:2003–2011, 1982.

Nomura, T. Multigeneration carcinogenesis. Radiat. Environ. Biophys., *30*:201–203, 1991.

Nordén, B., Edlund, U., and Wold, S. Carcinogenicity of polycyclic aromatic hydrocarbons studied by SIMCA pattern recognition. Acta Chem. Scand. B, *32*:602–608, 1978.

Ochi, T., and Kaneko, M. Active oxygen contributes to the major part of chromosomal aberrations in V79 Chinese hamster cells exposed to N-hydroxy-2-naphthylamine. Free Radic. Res. Commun., *5*:351–358, 1989.

Osler, M. Obesity and cancer. Danish Med. Bull., *34*:267–274, 1987.

Pariza, M. W. A perspective on diet, nutrition, and cancer. J.A.M.A., *251*:1455–1458, 1984.

Pastink, A., and Lohman, P. H. M. Repair and consequences of double-strand breaks in DNA. Mutat. Res., *428*:141–156, 1999.

Paulini, K., Beneke, G., Körner, B., and Enders, R. The relationship between the latent period and animal age in the development of foreign body sarcomas. Beitr. Pathol., *154*:161–169, 1975.

Pegg, A. E. Methylation of the O^6 position of guanine in DNA is the most likely initiating event in carcinogenesis by methylating agents. Cancer Invest., *2*:223–231, 1984.

Pegg, A. E., and Byers, T. L. Repair of DNA containing O^6-alkylguanine. FASEB J., *6*:2302–2310, 1992.

Pelkonen, O., and Nebert, D. W. Metabolism of polycyclic aromatic hydrocarbons: etiologic role in carcinogenesis. Pharmacol. Rev., *34*:189–222, 1982.

Perera, F., Mayer, J., Santella, R. M., Brenner, D., Jeffrey, A., Latriano, L., Smith, S., Warburton, D., Young, T. L., Tsai, W. Y., Hemminki, K., and Brandt-Rauf, P. Biologic markers in risk assessment for environmental carcinogens. Environ. Health Perspect., *90*:247–254, 1991.

Perera, F. P., and Weinstein, I. B. Molecular epidemiology and carcinogen-DNA adduct detection: new approaches to studies of human cancer causation. J. Chronic Dis., *35*:581–600, 1982.

Perera, F. P., Poirier, M. C., Yuspa, S. H., Nakayama, J., Jaretzki, A., Curnen, M. M., Knowles, D. M., and Weinstein, I. B. A pilot project in molecular cancer epidemiology: determination of benzo[a]pyrene–DNA adducts in animal and human tissues by immunoassays. Carcinogenesis, *3*:1405–1410, 1982.

Perrino, F. W., and Loeb, L. A. Animal cell DNA polymerases in DNA repair. Mutat. Res., *236*:289–300, 1990.

Peters, R. A. Mechanism of the toxicity of the active constituent of *Dichapetalum cymosum* and related compounds. Adv. Enzymol., *18*:113–159, 1957.

Petit, C., and Sancar, A. Nucleotide excision repair: from *E. coli* to man. Biochimie, *81*:15–25, 1999.

Peto, R., Gray, R., Brantom, P., and Grasso, P. Effects on 4080 rats of chronic ingestion of *N*-nitrosodiethylamine or *N*-nitrosodimethylamine: a detailed dose-response study. Cancer Res., *51*:6415–6451, 1991.

Piette, J. Biological consequences associated with DNA oxidation mediated by singlet oxygen. J. Photochem. Photobiol. B: Biol., *11*:241–260, 1991.

Port, R., Schmähl, D., and Wahrendorf, J. Some examples of dose-response studies in chemical carcinogenesis. Oncology, *33*:66–71, 1976.

Porter, T. D., and Coon, M. J. Cytochrome P-450: multiplicity of isoforms, substrates, and catalytic and regulatory mechanisms. J. Biol. Chem., *266*:13469–13472, 1991.

Pott, P. The Chirurgical Works of Percivall Pott, Vol. 5, Chirurgical observations relative to the cataract, the polypus of the nose, the cancer of the scrotum, the different kinds of ruptures, and the mortification of the toes and feet. London: L. Hawes, W. Clarke and R. Collins, 1775.

Premont, R. T., Inglese, J., and Lefkowitz, R. J. Protein kinases that phosphorylate activated G protein-coupled receptors. FASEB J., 9:175–182, 1995.

Pullman, A., and Pullman, B. Electronic structure and carcinogenic activity of aromatic molecules. New developments. Adv. Cancer Res., 3:117–169, 1955.

Randerath, E., Hart, R. W., Turturro, A., Danna, T. F., Reddy, R., and Randerath, K. Effects of aging and caloric restriction on I-compounds in liver, kidney and white blood cell DNA of male Brown-Norway rats. Mech. Ageing Dev., 58:279–296, 1991.

Randerath, K., van Golen, K. L., Dragan, Y. P., and Pitot, H. C. Effects of phenobarbital on I-compounds in liver DNA as a function of age in male rats fed two different diets. Carcinogenesis, 13:125–130, 1992.

Reddy, M. V., and Randerath, K. ^{32}P-Postlabeling assay for carcinogen-DNA adducts: nuclease P_1–mediated enhancement of its sensitivity and applications. Environ. Health Perspect., 76:41–47, 1987.

Regan, J. D., and Setlow, R. B. Two forms of repair in the DNA of human cells damaged by chemical carcinogens and mutagens. Cancer Res., 34:3318–3325, 1974.

Reichel, R. R., and Jacob, S. T. Control of gene expression by lipophilic hormones. FASEB J., 7:427–436, 1993.

Reichert, L. E. Jr., Dattatreyamurty, B., Grasso, P., and Santa-Coloma, T. A. Structure-function relationships of the glycoprotein hormones and their receptors. Trends Pharmacol. Sci., 12:199–203, 1991.

Richard, A. M., and Woo, Y.-t. A CASE-SAR analysis of polycyclic aromatic hydrocarbon carcinogenicity. Mutat. Res., 242:285–303, 1990.

Riegel, I. L., and Mueller, G. C. Formation of a protein-bound metabolite of estradiol-16-C^{14} by rat liver homogenates. J. Biol. Chem., 210:249–257, 1954.

Riggs, A. D., and Jones, P. A. 5-Methylcytosine, gene regulation, and cancer. Adv. Cancer Res., 40:1–30, 1983.

Roe, F. J. C., Dukes, C. E., and Mitchley, B. C. V. Sarcomas at the site of implantation of a polyvinyl plastic sponge: incidence reduced by use of thin implants. Biochem. Pharmacol., 16:647–650, 1967.

Rogers, A. E., Zeisel, S. H., and Groopman, J. Diet and carcinogenesis. Carcinogenesis, 14:2205–2217, 1993.

Rosenkranz, H. S., and Klopman, G. Structural implications of the ICPEMC method for quantifying geno-toxicity data. Mutat. Res., 305:99–116, 1994.

Ross, D. Mechanistic toxicology: a radical perspective. J. Pharm. Pharmacol., 41:505–511, 1989.

Roy, D., Floyd, R. A., and Liehr, J. G. Elevated 8-hydroxydeoxyguanosine levels in DNA of diethylstil-bestrol-treated Syrian hamsters: covalent DNA damage by free radicals generated by redox cycling of diethylstilbestrol. Cancer Res., 51:3882–3885, 1991.

Rusch, H. P., Kline, B. E., and Baumann, C. A. Carcinogenesis by ultraviolet rays with reference to wave-length and energy. Arch. Pathol., 31:135–146, 1941.

Sancar, A. Mechanisms of DNA excision repair . Science, 266:1954–1956, 1994.

Sancar, A., and Tang, M.-S. Nucleotide excision repair. Photochem. Photobiol. 57:905–921, 1993.

Sarasin, A., Bourre, F., and Benoit, A. Error-prone replication of ultraviolet-irradiated simian virus 40 in carcinogen-treated monkey kidney cells. Biochimie, 64:815–821, 1982.

Sasaki, T., and Yoshida, T. Experimentelle Erzeugung des Lebercarcinoms durch Fütterung mit o-Amido-azotoluol. Virchows Arch. Abt. A. Pathol. Anat., 295:175–200, 1935.

Satoh, M. S., and Lindahl, T. Enzymatic repair of oxidative DNA damage. Cancer Res., 54:1899s–1901s, 1994.

Schmidt, A. M., Whitehorn, W. V., and Martin, E. W. Estrogens and endometrial cancer. FDA Drug Bull., 6:18, 1976.

Scicchitano, D. A., and Hanawalt, P. C. Intragenomic repair heterogeneity of DNA damage. Environ. Health Perspect., 98:45–51, 1992.

Shamberger, R. J., Andreone, T. L., and Willis, C. E. Antioxidants and cancer. IV. Initiating activity of malonaldehyde as a carcinogen. J. Natl. Cancer Inst., 53:1771–1773, 1974.

Shapiro, R. Damage to DNA caused by hydrolysis. *In*: E. Seeberg and K. Kleppe (eds.), Chromosome Damage and Repair, pp. 3–18. New York: Plenum, New York, 1981.

Shearman, C. W. and Loeb, L. A. Effects of dupurination on the fidelity of DNA synthesis. J. Mol. Biol., *128*:197–218, 1979.

Shields, P. G., and Harris, C. C. Molecular epidemiology and the genetics of environmental cancer. J.A.M.A., *266*:681–687, 1991.

Siegfried, J. M. Strategies for identification of peptide growth factors. Pharmacol. Ther., *56*:233–245, 1992.

Silverberg, S. G., and Makowski, E. L. Endometrial carcinoma in young women taking oral contraceptives. Obstet. Gynecol., *46*:503, 1975.

Simic, M. G. Mechanisms of inhibition of free-radical processes in mutagenesis and carcinogenesis. Mutat. Res., *202*:377–386, 1988.

Sims, P., Grover, P. L., Swaisland, A., Pal, K., and Hewer, A. Metabolic activation of benzo[a]pyrene proceeds by a diol-epoxide. Nature, *252*:326–328, 1974.

Singer, B. N-nitroso alkylating agents: formation and persistence of alkylating agents: formation and persistence of alkyl derivatives in mammalian nucleic acids as contributing factors in carcinogenesis. J. Natl. Cancer Inst., *62*:1329–1339, 1979.

Singer, B. *O*-Alkyl pyrimidines in mutagenesis and carcinogenesis: occurrence and significance. Cancer Res., *46*:4879–4885, 1986.

Sirover, M. A., and Loeb, L. A. Infidelity of DNA synthesis in vitro: screening for potential metal mutagens or carcinogens. Science, *194*:1434–1436, 1976.

Smith, P. J. Carcinogenesis: molecular defences against carcinogens. Br. Med. Bull., *47*:3–20, 1991.

Sodum, R. S., Nie, G., and Fiala, E. S. 8-Aminoguanine: a base modification produced in rat liver nucleic acids by the hepatocarcinogen 2-nitropropane. Chem. Res. Toxicol., *6*:269–276, 1993.

Sommerville, J. Pseudo-epitheliomatous hyperplasia. Acta Derm. Venereol. (Stockh), *33*:236–251, 1953.

Sorof, S., Young, E. M., and Ott, M. G. Soluble liver h proteins during hepatocarcinogenesis by aminoazo dyes and 2-acetylaminofluorene in the rat. Cancer Res., *18*:33–46, 1958.

Sorof, S., Young, E. M., Coffey, C. B., and Morris, H. P. On protein binding of fluorenyl carcinogens by minimal deviation hepatomas. Cancer Res., *26*:81–88, 1966.

Soucek, P., and Gut, I. Cytochromes P-450 in rats: structures, functions, properties and relevant human forms. Xenobiotica, *22*:83–103, 1992.

Sources and Effects of Ionizing Radiation. United Nations Scientific Committee on the Effects of Atomic Radiation Report. New York: United Nations, 1977.

Srinivasan, S., and Glauert, H. P. Formation of 5-hydroxymethyl-2'-deoxyuridine in hepatic DNA of rats treated with g-irradiation, diethylnitrosamine, 2-acetylaminofluorene or the peroxisome proliferator ciprofibrate. Carcinogenesis, *11*:2021–2024, 1990.

Stafl, A., and Mattingly, R. F. Vaginal adenosis: a precancerous lesion? Am. J. Obstet. Gynecol., *120*:666–677, 1974.

Standeven, A. M., Wolf, D. C., and Goldsworthy, T. L. Investigation of antiestrogenicity as a mechanism of female mouse liver tumor induction by unleaded gasoline. Chem. Indust. Inst. Toxicol., *14*:1–5, 1994.

Stenbäck, F., Peto, R., and Shubik, P. Initiation and promotion at different ages and doses in 2200 mice. III. Linear extrapolation from high doses may underestimate low-dose tumour risks. Br. J. Cancer, *44*:24–34, 1981.

Stewart, B. W. Generation and persistence of carcinogen-induced repair intermediates in rat liver DNA *in vivo*. Cancer Res., *41*:3238–3243, 1981.

Stinson, N. E. The tissue reaction induced in rats and guinea-pigs by polymethylmethacrylate (acrylic) and stainless steel (18/8/Mo). Br. J. Exp. Pathol. *45*:21–29, 1964.

Stout, D. L., and Becker, F. F. Progressive DNA damage in hepatic nodules during 2-acetylaminofluorene carcinogenesis. Cancer Res., *40*:1269–1273, 1980.

Stowers, S. J., and Anderson, M. W. Formation and persistence of benzo(a)pyrene metabolite-DNA adducts. Environ. Health Perspect., *62*:31–39, 1985.

Strauss, B. S. Molecular biology of the response of cells to radiation and to radiomimetic chemicals. Cancer, *40*:471–480, 1977.

Sunderman, F. W., Jr. Carcinogenicity of metal alloys in orthopedic prostheses: clinical and experimental studies. Fund. Appl. Toxicol., *13*:205–216, 1989.

Sunderman, F. W., Jr. Mechanisms of nickel carcinogenesis. Scand. J. Work Environ. Health, *15*:1–12, 1989.

Swenberg, J. A., Dyroff, M. C., Bedell, M. A., Popp, J. A., Huh, N., Kirstein, U., and Rajewsky, M. F. O^4-Ethyldeoxythymidine, but not O^6-ethyldeoxyguanosine, accumulates in hepatocyte DNA of rats exposed continuously to diethylnitrosamine. Proc. Natl. Acad. Sci. U.S.A., *81*:1692–1695, 1984.

Swenberg, J. A., Richardson, F. C., Boucheron, J. A., and Dyroff, M. C. Relationships between DNA adduct formation and carcinogenesis. Environ. Health Perspect., *62*:177–183, 1985.

Swenberg, J. A., Richardson, F. C., Boucheron, J. A., Deal, F. H., Belinsky, S. A., Charbonneau, M., and Short, B. G. High- to low-dose extrapolation: critical determinants involved in the dose response of carcinogenic substances. Environ. Health Perspect., *76*:57–63, 1987.

Takayama, S., Hasegawa, H., and Ohgaki, H. Combination effects of forty carcinogens administered at low doses to male rats. Jpn. J. Cancer Res., *80*:732–736, 1989.

Tannock, I. F., and Hill, R. P. The Basic Science of Oncology, 2nd ed. New York: McGraw-Hill, 1992.

Teebor, G. W., and Frenkel, K. The initiation of DNA excision-repair. Adv. Cancer Res., *38*:23–59, 1983.

Thomassen, M. J., Buoen, L. C., Brand, I., and Brand, K. G. Foreign-body tumorigenesis in mice: DNA synthesis in surface-attached cells during preneoplasia. J. Natl. Cancer Inst., *61*:359–363, 1978.

Toyokuni, S. Reactive oxygen species–induced molecular damage and its application in pathology. Pathol. Int., *49*:91–102, 1999.

Tsapakos, M. J., Hampton, T. H., and Wetterhahn Jennette, K. The carcinogen chromate induces DNA cross-links in rat liver and kidney. J. Biol. Chem., *256*:3623–3626, 1981.

Tsurimoto, T. PCNA, a multifunctional ring on DNA. Biochim. Biophys. Acta, *1443*:23–39, 1998.

Tsutsui, T., Degen, G. H., Schiffmann, D., Wong, A., Maizumi, H., McLachlan, J. A., and Barrett, J. C. Dependence on exogenous metabolic activation for induction of unscheduled DNA synthesis in Syrian hamster embryo cells by diethylstilbestrol and related compounds. Cancer Res., *44*:184–189, 1984.

Tucker, G. T. Drug metabolism. Br. J. Anaesth., *51*:603–618, 1979.

Ueda, G., and Furth, J. Sacromatoid transformation of transplanted thyroid carcinoma. Arch. Pathol., *83*:3, 1967.

Umar, A., Boyer, J. C., Thomas, D. C., Nguyen, D. C., Risinger, J. I., Boyd, J., Ionov, Y., Perucho, M., and Kunkel, T. A. Defective mismatch repair in extracts of colorectal and endometrial cancer cell lines exhibiting microsatellite instability. J. Biol. Chem., *269*:14367–14370, 1994.

Upton, A. C. Physical carcinogenesis: radiation—history and sources. *In*: F. F. Becker (Ed.), Cancer—A Comprehensive Treatise, Vol. 1, Chap. 13, pp. 387–403. New York: Plenum, 1975.

Van Dyck, E., Stasiak, A. Z., Stasiak, A., and West, S. C. Binding of double-strand breaks in DNA by human Rad52 protein. Nature, *398*:728–731, 1999.

Vedeckis, W. V. Nuclear receptors, transcriptional regulation, and oncogenesis. Proc. Soc. Exp. Biol. Med., *199*:1–12, 1992.

Verschaeve, L., Driesen, M., Kirsch-Volders, M., Hens, L., and Susanne, C. Chromosome distribution studies after inorganic lead exposure. Hum. Genet., *49*:147–158 1979.

Voigt, L. F., Weiss, N. S., Chu, J., Daling, J. R., McKnight, B., and van Belle, G. Progestagen supplementation of exogenous oestrogens and risk of endometrial cancer. Lancet, *338*:274–276, 1991.

Warshawsky, D., Barkley, W., and Bingham, E. Factors affecting carcinogenic potential of mixtures. Fundam. Appl. Toxicol., *20*:376–382, 1993.

Weinstein, I. B., Jeffrey, A. M., Jennette, K. W., Blobstein, S. H., Harvey, R. G., Harris, C., Autrup, H., Kasai, H., and Nakanishi, K. Benzo[a]pyrene diol epoxides as intermediates in nucleic acid binding in vitro and in vivo. Science, *193*:592–595, 1976.

Weisburger, E. K., and Weisburger, J. H. Chemistry, carcinogenicity and metabolism of 2-fluorenamine and related compounds. Adv. Cancer Res., *5*:331–431, 1958.

Weisburger, J. H., and Williams, G. H. Metabolism of chemical carcinogens. *In*: F. F. Becker, (Ed), Cancer: A Comprehensive Treatise, Vol. 1, pp. 241–333. New York: Plenum, 1982.

Westra, J. G., Kriek, E., and Hittenhausen, H. Identification of the persistently bound form of the carcinogen *N*-acetyl-2-aminofluorene to rat liver DNA in vivo. Chem. Biol. Interact., *15*:149–164, 1976.

Wiley, A. L., Jr., Vogel, H. H., Jr., and Clifton, K. H. The effect of variations in LET and cell cycle on radiation hepatocarcinogenesis. Radiat. Res., *54*:284–293, 1973.

Willett, W. C., and MacMahon, B. Diet and cancer—an overview. N. Engl. J. Med., *310*:633–638 and 697–701, 1984.

Williams, E. D. TSH and thyroid cancer. *In*: E. F. Pfeiffer, and G. M. Reaven (Eds.), Hormone and Metabolic Research, Suppl. Series Vol. 23, pp. 72–75. New York: Theime, 1989.

Williams, G. M., Iatropoulos, M. J., Djordjevic, M. V., and Kaltenberg, O. P. The triphenylethylene drug tamoxifen is a strong liver carcinogen in the rat. Carcinogenesis, *14*:315–317, 1993.

Wilson, M. J., Shivapurkar, N., and Poirier, L. A. Hypomethylation of hepatic nuclear DNA in rats fed with a carcinogenic methyl-deficient diet. Biochem. J., *218*:987–990, 1984.

Wintersberger, U. Chemical carcinogenesis—the price for DNA-repair? Naturwissenschaften, *69*:107–113, 1982.

Wise, R. W., Zenser, T. V., Kadlubar, F. F., and Davis B. B. Metabolic activation of carcinogenic aromatic amines by dog bladder and kidney prostaglandin H synthase. Cancer Res. *44*:1893–1897, 1984.

Yager, J. D., and Yager, R. Oral contraceptive steroids as promoters of hepatocarcinogenesis in female Sprague-Dawley rats. Cancer Res., *40*:3680–3685, 1980.

Yamagawa, K., and Ichikawa, K. Experimentelle Studie über die Pathogenese der Epithelialgeschwülste. Mitteilungen Med. Fakultät Kaiserl. Univ. Tokyo, *15*:295–344, 1915.

Yang, S. K., McCourt, D. W., Roller, P. P., and Gelboin, H. V. Enzymatic conversion of benzo[*a*]pyrene leading predominantly to the diol-epoxide *r*-7,*t*-8-dihydroxy-*t*-9,10-oxy-7,8,9,10-tetrahydrobenzo[*a*]pyrene through a single enantiomer of *r*-7, *t*-8-dihydroxy-7,8-dihydrobenzo[*a*]pyrene. Proc. Natl. Acad. Sci. U.S.A., *73*:2594–2598, 1976.

Yu, M.-W., and Chen, C.-J. Elevated serum testosterone levels and risk of hepatocellular carcinoma. Cancer Res., *53*:790–794, 1993.

Zedeck, M. S. Polycyclic aromatic hydrocarbons. A review. J. Environ. Pathol. Toxicol., *3*:537–567, 1980.

4

The Etiology of Cancer as an Infectious Disease

INFECTIOUS AGENTS AS CAUSES OF CANCER

In 1913, Johannes Fibiger (cf. Clemmesen, 1978) reported the occurrence of papillomas of the stomach in rats infected with Spiroptera, a small parasitic worm. The intermediate host of the parasite was the cockroach. By feeding either cockroaches infested with the worm or the worm itself to rats, Fibiger was able to produce lesions that were interpreted as papillomatous growths of the stomach. In 1927, Fibiger was awarded the Nobel Prize for this work, the first such award for cancer research. Unfortunately, later studies did not bear out Fibiger's thesis that the stomach lesions were neoplasms but rather indicated that the tumors resulted from the combination of a deficiency of vitamin A in his experimental animals and the infestation by the parasite.

Despite this setback, over the years many investigators have reported that certain biological factors are important in the causation of cancer. The parasitic worm *Spirocerca lupi* is associated with esophageal sarcomas in the dog (Thrasher et al., 1963). Studies have demonstrated that the worms encyst in the wall of the esophagus, and a sarcoma may arise around this cyst. Shortly after Fibiger's discovery, Bullock and associates demonstrated genetic factors involved in the induction of sarcomas in rats by infection with *Cysticercus fasciolaris*, the common tapeworm of the cat (Curtis et al., 1933). Later studies demonstrated that sarcomas could be induced by the intraperitoneal injection of washed, ground larvae of the parasite in rats (Dunning and Curtis, 1953). The frequent association of *Schistosoma haematobium* infection with bladder cancer in various parts of the world, such as Egypt and other regions of Africa, has clearly indicated the association of the parasitic with the neoplastic disease (cf. Shimkin, 1977). Bladder cell hyperplasia and occasionally bladder carcinoma can be induced with some regularity in monkeys by infection with *S. haematobium*, and infection of mice with *Schistosoma mansoni* enhances the hepatocarcinogenicity of various chemicals (cf. Cheever, 1978). Chronic infection with the latter organism has also been associated with hepatic and colon cancer in the human (Chapter 12).

Infectious Agents in Plant Neoplasia

The first reported example of a biological agent inducing a neoplasm in plants was that of Smith and Townsend (1907), who reported that a bacterial infection in the region of wounds in a plant resulted in growths called crown galls. Since those classic experiments, investigations have demonstrated repeatedly that under suitable experimental conditions the crown gall plant tumor can be induced in practically all wounds in a large number of dicotyledonous plants inoculated with *Agrobacter tumefaciens* (cf. Braun, 1975; Kupila-Ahvenniemi and Therman, 1968). These authors pointed out that crown gall tumors cannot be induced in monocotyledonous plants, which show little or no reaction to wounding, whereas wounds in dicotyledonous plants stimulate a marked reaction in the plants, accompanied by DNA synthesis, mitosis, and increased ploidy of adjacent cells. Once infection by the bacterium has occurred and the crown gall tumor has formed, the bacterium is no longer necessary to maintain the existence and growth of the tumor.

Within the last three decades, rapid advances have been made in our understanding of the mechanism of tumor induction by *A. tumefaciens*. Only those bacteria containing a large extra-chromosomal plasmid are capable of inducing tumors (Watson et al., 1975). This plasmid, termed the Ti-plasmid, consists of a single circular molecule of DNA of molecular weight 90 to 150 million. That the plasmid is important in the transformation of normal to neoplastic cells was indicated by the fact that genes of the plasmid coded for the formation of enzymes synthesizing "opines," amino acids not found in normal plants but synthesized in crown gall tumors that resulted from the bacterial infection (cf. Schell, 1982). Chilton et al. (1977) and others showed the incorporation of Ti-plasmid DNA from the bacteria into the nuclear DNA of plant cells; these cells ultimately develop into the crown gall tumors. This incorporated DNA thus becomes part of the host cell genome and codes for enzymes involved in opine synthesis. This transfer of genetic information from the bacteria to the plant cell is a natural example of "genetic engineering." The soil bacterium forces plants, through the transfer of specific genes, to produce substrates, or opines, which are used solely by the soil bacterium containing the Ti-plasmids; this equips them to metabolize the opines for survival (Schell, 1982).

Thomashow et al. (1980) demonstrated that each line of crown gall tumor contained a "core" segment of Ti-plasmid DNA, which was postulated to be responsible for maintaining the transformed state. The infection of the plant by *A. tumefaciens* induces both chemical signaling from the plant cells by the production of phenolic compounds and the direct binding of the bacterium to the plant cell itself (Stachel and Zambryski, 1986; Winans, 1992). Roughly 25 Ti plasmid–encoded genes, termed *vir* genes, may be required for the development of tumors within the plants (cf. Winans, 1992). Many of these *vir* genes are involved in the processing of the T-DNA of the Ti plasmid. The gene products of the *vir* region facilitate the T-DNA transfer from the bacterium to the plant cell by a process very similar to bacterial conjugation (Beijersbergen et al., 1992). Furthermore, Hadley and Szalay (1982) and White et al. (1983) have presented evidence that the genome of the untransformed host plant cell contains sequences in its DNA that are homologous to sequences in or near the core region of the Ti plasmid. That DNA from the Ti plasmid is required for the maintenance of the neoplastic state in the plant cell is demonstrated by the fact that the neoplastic phenotype was lost concomitant with the loss of foreign DNA in the plant cell (Yang et al., 1980). Such loss of tumorigenicity always involved the loss of the *vir* region incorporated into all neoplasms studied (Yang and Simpson, 1981; Winans, 1992). This loss likely occurs during meiosis of the plant cell (Turgeon et al., 1976).

These findings are of considerable interest, especially in view of the findings of the infectious nature of some neoplasms in higher vertebrate animals. Some of the characteristics of crown gall tumor induction by *A. tumefaciens* are listed in Table 4.1. The reader should remember these characteristics and refer back to them after considering the later discussions in this chapter. This comparison will underline the similarity of the mechanisms involved in the induction of crown gall tumors in plants and the induction of malignant neoplasms in animals by oncogenic viruses.

Bacteria as Causal Agents of Neoplasia

As noted in Chapter 1, during the latter part of the nineteenth century, when bacteria were shown to be the causal agents of many infectious diseases, it was natural for scientists to consider neoplasia as the result of a similar cause. The studies by Doven and the claim that *Micrococcus*

Table 4.1 Characteristics of Crown Gall Tumor Induction by Infection
with *Agrobacter tumefaciens*

1. Tissue regeneration, mitosis, DNA synthesis of host cells of infected
   wound
2. Infection of plant with plasmid-containing bacterium
3. Incorporation of plasmid DNA into host plant cell genome
4. Presence of DNA sequences common to all plasmid-transformed host
   cells; these sequences are apparently necessary for maintenance of
   the neoplastic state
5. Presence of sequences in untransformed plant cells that are homologous to DNA sequences in plasmids of *A. tumefaciens*

neoformans was causative for many if not all human neoplasms are certainly examples of this. However, bacteria have actually only recently been clearly demonstrated to be causative agents in specific human neoplasms. In 1983, Warren reported the presence of an unidentified curved bacillus closely associated with the gastric epithelium in humans exhibiting active chronic gastritis. Subsequently, the organism was classified as *Campylobacter pylori* and shown by many others to be associated with gastritis and ulceration of the upper gastrointestinal tract (cf. Dooley and Cohen, 1988). Today this organism is known as *Helicobacter pylori* (DeCross and Marshall, 1993). Chronic infection with this bacterium in the human has now been associated, probably causally, not only with the development of chronic gastritis and ulceration of the gastric and upper intestinal mucosa, but also with the development of intestinal metaplasia of the gastric mucosa (Rugge et al., 1996), gastric carcinoma (Parsonnet et al., 1991; Hansson et al., 1993), and gastric lymphoma (Parsonnet et al., 1994) (Chapter 12). There is no evidence that the bacterium induces neoplasia by mechanisms seen with *Agrobacter* induction of crown gall tumors in plants. Mechanisms whereby this bacterium may induce neoplasia in the human are further considered in Chapter 12.

Following investigations in the human, it is now clear that species of *Helicobacter* occur in other mammals as well. *Helicobacter mustelae* has been associated with gastric carcinoma in the ferret (Fox et al., 1997) as well as with a gastric lymphoma (Erdman et al., 1997). Similar gastric lymphomas have been induced in mice with another member of this bacterial family, *Helicobacter felis* (Enno et al., 1995). A somewhat more practial problem is the demonstration that *Helicobacter hepaticus* is capable of inducing chronic hepatitis in specific strains of mice with the subsequent development of hepatocellular neoplasms (Ward et al., 1994). Infection causes a chronic stimulus to hepatocyte proliferation which increases the risk for the development of hepatocellular neoplasia (Nyska et al., 1997). Thus, with the discovery of this bacterial class, it is clear that such organisms may induce neoplasia both in humans and in experimental animals. The exact mechanisms for such induction will be considered later. The remainder of this chapter considers the primary infectious causative agents of neoplasia—viruses.

Intracellular parasites have long been implicated as the cause of certain types of neoplasms in vertebrate animals. In 1909, Ellerman and Bang demonstrated a viral causation for avian leukosis. In 1911, Rous reported that cell-free extracts of a sarcoma in chickens would in some instances produce sarcomas when injected into other chickens. In 1932, Shope described the Shope papillomavirus of rabbits, and in the 1930s the Bittner mouse mammary tumor virus was discovered (see below; Bittner, 1936). However, the general significance and potential importance of viruses in the causation of cancer was not generally appreciated until after the discovery of lysogeny in bacteria and the importance of latency in viral infections. In 1951, Gross reported that injection of cell-free filtrates from AKR mice with leukemia into newborn AKR mice resulted in a high percentage of leukemia in the inoculated animals at a later period. Since Gross's experiments, numerous individuals have extended these studies, and considerable biological knowledge is now available on the viral causation of neoplasms.

VIRUSES AS CAUSES OF CANCER

Viruses are ubiquitous obligate intracellular parasites. Because viruses replicate in and are dependent upon their host cells, they use the rules, signals, and regulatory pathways of the host cell. Viruses subvert and perturb normal cellular mechanisms and pathways as a means of replicating. These perturbations can have dire consequences for the host cell. It is not an uncommon consequence of a viral infection for the host cell to die. Though less common, viral infection can change or transform a normal cell into a neoplastic one, ultimately leading to a cancer. In fact, there is compelling evidence that several different human cancers are caused by viral infection (Chapter 12). Clearly, appreciation of this relationship can be critical in the epidemiological control of cancer. Prevention or cure of a viral infection may lower the incidence of the cancer induced by a given viral agent. Knowledge of cancer-causing viruses has served a second very important function. These viruses cause cancer by perturbing normal cellular processes or pathways. Understanding specifically how different viruses do this has led to an appreciation and understanding of various molecular pathways in the host cell that can contribute to the development of cancer. Moreover, these studies have led to an appreciation and understanding of the normal functions of these same processes and pathways. Many insights into cancer cell biology and normal cell biology have resulted from the study of viruses that either cause cancer in experimental animals or transform cells in culture. Viruses with oncogenic potential in humans, animals, or cell culture are known collectively as tumor viruses (for a review, see Vogt and Nevins, 1996).

Animal viruses can be divided into two broad groups: those with DNA genomes and those with RNA genomes. The DNA viruses with oncogenic potential are from six distinct virus groups: hepadnaviruses, papillomaviruses, polyomaviruses, herpesviruses, adenoviruses, and poxviruses. Two different families of RNA viruses have been found to have oncogenic potential: retroviruses and a flavivirus, hepatitis C virus (Figure 4.1, Table 4.2). Some viruses can act as carcinogens when infecting their natural host, either human or animal. Others, such as adenoviruses or SV40 (a polyomavirus), show their oncogenic potential only in experimental settings, such as infection of cell cultures (Chapter 14). The time it takes different tumor viruses to cause neoplasms can vary widely (Flint et al., 2000). Some induce tumors rapidly, within days or weeks (e.g., the transducing retroviruses), while others take months if not years for cancer development (e.g., human hepatitis B virus). Some tumor viruses, such as adenovirus or SV40 (polyomavirus), do not lead to neoplasms in cells in which they replicate, but only in cells that do not support their replication.

Retroviruses

Reports in the early 1900s described the induction of neoplasms in chickens inoculated with a "cell-free filtrate" (Ellerman and Bang, 1908; Rous, 1911). In retrospect, these early reports were describing the induction of cancer via infection with avian retroviruses. Later in the twentieth century, with the advent of cell culture methods, it became possible to induce oncogenic transformation of individual cells in culture via retroviral infection. The retrovirus, Rous sarcoma virus (RSV), was the first reported to transform cells in culture (Temin and Rubin, 1958). The study of retroviruses has a rich and long history that has yielded many seminal discoveries.

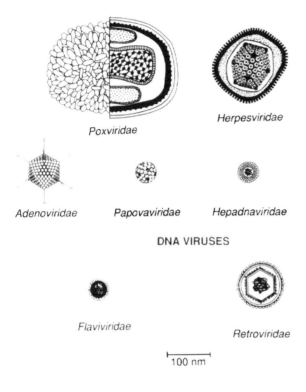

DNA VIRUSES

RNA VIRUSES

Figure 4.1   Artist's conception of shapes and sizes of viruses from different families that cause neo-plasms in vertebrates. On top are representations of five different DNA virus families that can cause neo-plasia. Below are the two RNA viruses families associated with cancer. Polyomaviruses and papillomavirus belong to the same family, the Papovaviridae. (Adapted from White and Fenner, 1994, with permission of authors and publisher.)

Table 4.2   Oncogenic Viruses and Cancer

Families	Associated Cancers
RNA viruses	
Flaviviridae	
Hepatitis C virus	Hepatocellular carcinoma
Retroviridae	Hematopoietic cancers, sarcomas, and carcinomas
DNA viruses	
Hepadnaviridae	Hepatocellular carcinoma
Papovaviridae	
Papillomaviruses	Papillomas and carcinomas
Polyomaviruses	Various solid tumors
Adenoviridae	Various solid tumors
Herpesviridae	Lymphomas, carcinomas, and sarcomas
Poxviridae	Myxomas and fibromas

For example, the discovery of oncogenes (see below) came from the study of retroviruses. Retroviruses are a large and diverse family of viruses, and not all family members are tumor viruses. The virion contains two identical copies of a single-stranded RNA. Depending on the family member, the RNA is 7 to 12 kb (Coffin et al., 1997). Retroviruses are enveloped (Figure 4.2). Their exterior is comprised of a lipid bilayer derived from the host cell. Embedded within this lipid bilayer are virally encoded proteins called envelope or env proteins. The envelope protein plays a major role in entry of the virus into a susceptible cell. Removal of the lipid bilayer reveals the nucleocapsid, a proteinaceous structure that contains the genomic RNA. The viral *gag* gene encodes the proteins comprising the nucleocapsid. Inside the nucleocapsid is found not only the genomic RNA, but two virally encoded proteins, reverse transcriptase and integrase, which are encoded by the *pol* gene. Entry into a susceptible cell is dependent not only on the virion envelope protein, but also on a cell surface receptor (Figure 4.3). Upon entry into the cell, the nucleocapsid is uncoated and released into the cytoplasm. At this time, reverse transcription takes place, the process in which the single-stranded RNA is converted into double-strand DNA by the action of reverse transcriptase. Next, the linear double-stranded DNA is transported into the nucleus of the cell and is integrated into the host DNA via the enzymatic action of the viral integrase protein. At this point the viral DNA, referred to as a provirus, has

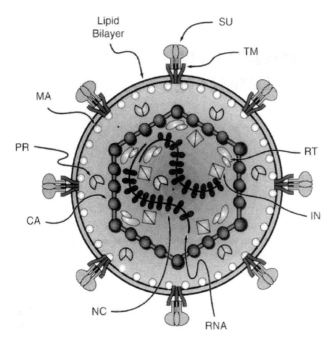

Figure 4.2 Generalized structure and organization of retroviral particle. The exterior of the virus is a cell-derived lipid bilayer or membrane. Embedded within the membrane are two viral proteins, SU and TM, which are encoded by the *env* gene. Env precursor polypeptide is proteolytically processed to give rise to SU and TM. Underneath the lipid envelope are viral structural proteins which are encoded by the *gag* gene. They are the matrix (MA), capsid (CA), and nucleocapsid (NC) proteins. CA is the subunit of the capsid, which is represented by a hexagon. Inside the capsid are two identical copies of RNA genome (which are coated with NC protein), the reverse transcriptase, RT, and the integrase, IN. The viral protease, PR, is responsible for processing the gag and gag-pol precursor polypeptides to yield mature proteins. (Adapted from Coffin et al., 1997, with permission of authors and publisher.)

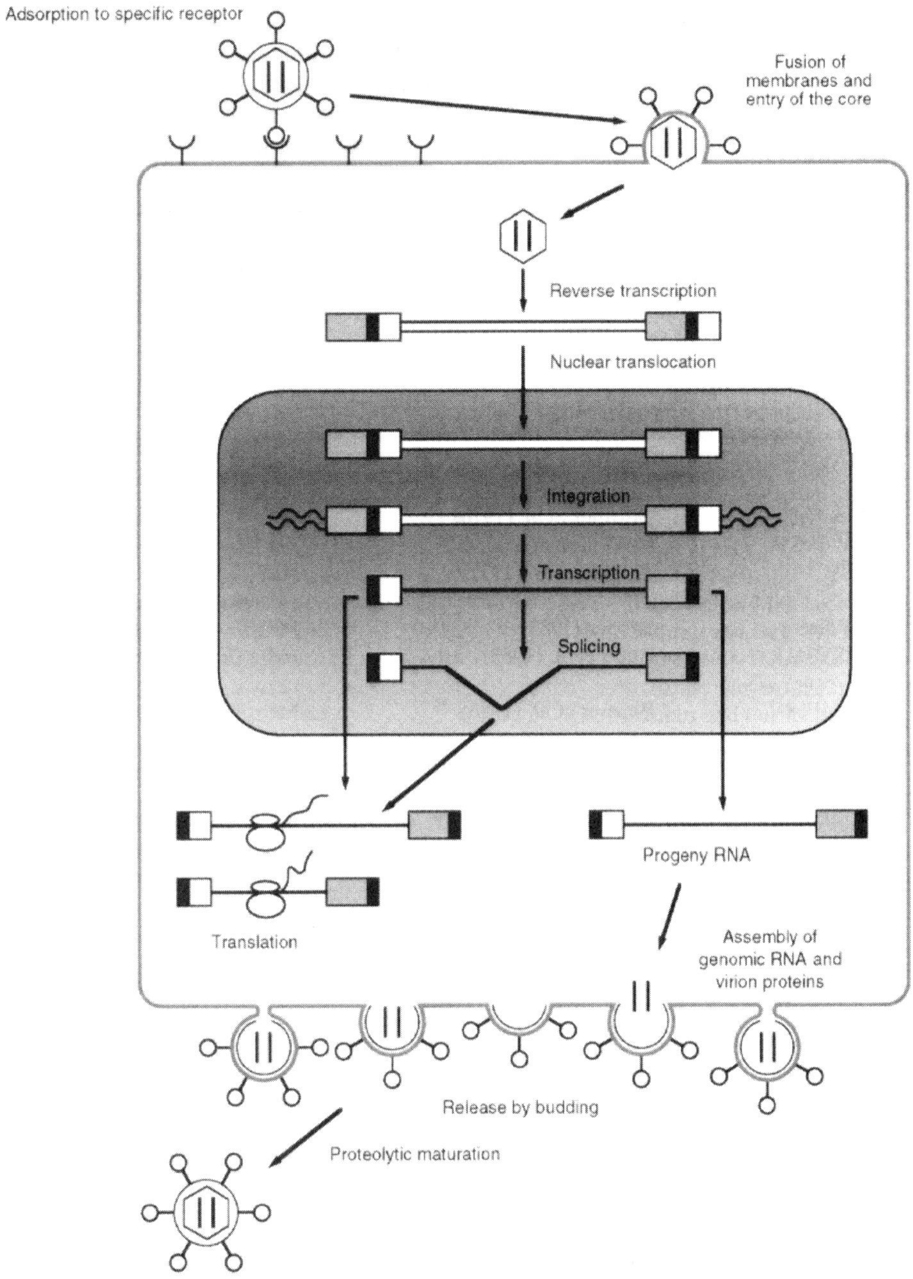

Figure 4.3 Retroviral replication cycle. The virus, via the SU portion of the viral Env protein, binds to a specific receptor on the surface of the susceptible cell. This interaction initiates a series of steps resulting in entry of the virus into the cell. Fusion of viral and cellular membranes is an example of one mechanism by which the viral capsid is uncoated and deposited into the cytoplasm. The process of reverse transcription generates a double-stranded DNA copy, called proviral DNA, of the RNA genome. Long terminal repeats, called LTRs, are at the 5′ and 3′ end of the proviral DNA. Proviral DNA is transported to the nucleus and integrated into chromosomal DNA. The integrated provirus is transcribed by cellular RNA polymerase. RNA transcription begins within the 5′ LTR and ends, via polyadenylation, within the 3′ LTR. Viral RNAs can be either full-length or spliced, and are mRNAs for translation of viral proteins. The full-length RNA is also the genomic RNA and becomes encapsidated into progeny virions. Viral proteins and two copies of the genomic RNA assemble and progeny virus bud from the plasma membrane of the cell, followed by proteolytic maturation of the virus. (Adapted from Coffin et. al., 1997, with permission of authors and publisher.)

become a stable component of the host chromosome and will be inherited by daughter cells. The proviral DNA contains long terminal repeats (LTRs), which are repeated sequences (up to several hundred nucleotides), found at the 5′ and 3′ ends of the proviral DNA, and generated during reverse transcription (Goff and Skalka, 1993; Varmus and Brown, 1989). The genomic organization of all retroviruses has general, common features (Figure 4.4). Between the 5′ and 3′ LTRs are the viral genes. All retroviruses capable of replicating have three genes in common: *gag*, *pol*, and *env*. Each of these genes gives rise to multiple polypeptides as a consequence of posttranslational processing. *gag* encodes the structural proteins that compose the caspid; *pol* encodes the reverse transcriptase and integrase, enzymes that function in the synthesis and integration of the provirus; *env* encodes the envelope glycoproteins that interact with cell surface receptors to mediate virus entry. The viral genome contains a number of *cis*-acting sequences that are important for viral replication. The LTRs contain regulatory sequences for the synthesis of the viral mRNAs. The 5′ LTR contains enhancer and promoter sequences that are used by the host RNA transcription machinery. The 3′ LTR contains sequences necessary for polyadenylation of the mRNA transcript.

Other *cis*-acting sequences include signals for packaging RNA into virus particles, sites of initiation of DNA synthesis, and specific sequences for correct integration of the proviral DNA. Once the proviral state is established, the cell can produce progeny virus. First, RNA transcrip-

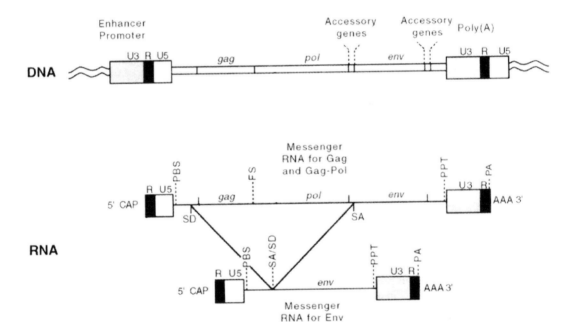

Figure 4.4 Generalized genetic organization of retrovirus. The proviral DNA has integrated into chromosomal DNA. LTRs are comprised of three domains, U3, R, and U5. The viral genes, *gag*, *pol*, and *env*, are between the LTRs. All replication-competent retroviruses have the above-mentioned genes. A subset of retroviruses (e.g., HIV-1) have additional genes, termed accessory genes, which are found in the 3′ half of the genome. The 5′ LTR contain enhancers and promoter elements, while the 3′ LTR contains the polyadenylation signal. Translation of genomic RNA gives rise to gag and gag-pol polyproteins, while the spliced RNA is translated to yield the env precursor polypeptide. PBS and PPT are the sites of initiation of the first and second strands of DNA, respectively. SA and SD are splice donor and acceptor sequences. (Adapted from Coffin et al., 1997, with permission of authors and publisher.)

tion, mediated by the host machinery, begins in the 5' LTR and terminates in the 3' LTR to produce a primary transcript that is essentially the genomic viral RNA. This will be the mRNA for the gag- and pol-encoded proteins as well as genomic RNA for progeny virus. A spliced version of the genomic RNA is synthesized and will be translated for the synthesis of env glycoprotein. Upon synthesis and accumulation of all of the necessary viral proteins, a new virus particle will assemble at the plasma membrane and bud from the cell, yielding a new progeny virus.

Oncogenic retroviruses can be isolated from neoplasms and, upon introduction into the appropriate host, cause malignant and benign tumors. They can be divided into two general groups on the basis of the time after infection at which the cancer phenotype appears: rapid (1 to a few weeks) or slow (6 months to 1 year) (Coffin, 1996). Members of the rapid group will efficiently transform cells in culture. This group of oncogenic retroviruses are also called the transducing retroviruses. The significance of this name is discussed below. A well-studied member of the transducing retroviruses is RSV. Within 1 to 2 weeks of infection with RSV, a chicken will develop several large sarcomas. In addition, infection of chicken embryo fibroblast cells in culture with RSV will result in nearly all cells becoming transformed. The second group of oncogenic retroviruses take a longer time to induce cancer in animals and are not transforming in cell culture. Members of this group are called the nontransducing retroviruses. The prototype member of this class is the avian leukosis virus (ALV). As can be inferred from their different cancer phenotypes, the two groups of oncogenic retroviruses induce cancer via different mechanisms.

Molecular analysis of the RSV genome reveals, in addition to the *gag*, *pol*, and *env* genes, the presence of a fourth gene (Figure 4.5) (Schwartz et al., 1983). This gene is located between the *env* gene and the 3' LTR. Mutants of RSV that have this gene deleted are not transforming but can still replicate, indicating that the new gene is not required for viral replication. But the fourth gene, called v-*src*, is required and is sufficient for the development of cancer. v-*src* was the first example of what is now called a viral oncogene or v-*onc*. Introduction and expression of the v-*src* gene in cells in culture can lead to their transformation. It was found that normal chicken cells contained a gene similar to v-*src* (Stehelin et al., 1976). In fact, sequences related to v-*src* are present in other vertebrate species, including humans. The cellular gene that is a homologue of v-*src* is called c-*src* (short for cellular-*src*) or proto-*src,* a proto-oncogene, and contains introns, unlike its viral counterpart (Figure 4.6). The protein encoded by c-*src* can be found in cells, and its expression does not lead to cell transformation in culture (Collet et al., 1978; Iba et al., 1984). The c-*src* gene has biological and biochemical properties different from v-*src*. Both c-*src* and v-*src* encode plasma membrane-associated proteins with tyrosine kinase activity. Comparison of the amino acid sequence of v-*src* and c-*src* proteins reveals several changes or mutations within v-*src* that are responsible for its transforming activities (Takeya and Hanafusa, 1983). We now know that the v-*src* gene in RSV was captured or derived from its cellular counterpart. The capture of an oncogene such as v-*src* is believed to happen during reverse transcription at a relatively low frequency. But because the selection and amplification of these infrequent events is very powerful (i.e., clonal expansion of the neoplasm), capture of a proto-oncogene by a retrovirus has been detected many times.

In addition to RSV, more than 60 other examples of transducing retroviruses that encode over 30 different oncogenes have been isolated from a variety of birds and mammals (but not from humans) (for a review, see Coffin et al., 1997) (Table 4.3). Each of these viruses has at least one oncogene that is not required for viral replication but that is responsible for the virus's cancer phenotype. For each example of a v-*onc*, a corresponding c-*onc* has been identified. The existence of multiple v-*onc* genes and their corresponding c-*onc* genes suggested that there are multiple ways to cause a cell to become cancerous. Proto-oncogenes have roles in the normal functioning of a variety of cellular processes such as proliferation, differentiation, and development. The v-*onc* gene almost always has changes or mutations that are responsible for the vi-

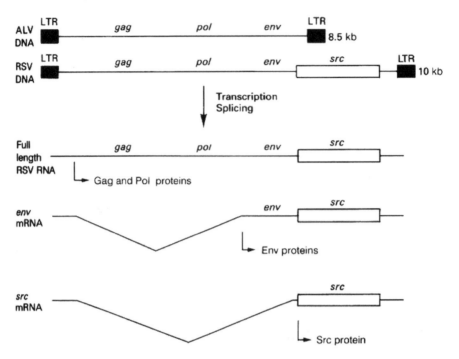

Figure 4.5 Rous sarcoma virus (RSV) contains an additional gene, *src*, not present in other retroviruses. The *src* gene is located between the *env* gene and the 3′ LTR. In comparison, avian leukosis virus (ALV), a closely related retrovirus, contains only the normal complement of genes, *gag*, *pol*, and *env*. RSV expresses Src protein from a spliced mRNA. (Adapted from Cooper, 1995, with permission of author and publisher.)

rus's ability to cause cancer. The role of oncogenes in cancer is further underscored by the fact that some nonviral cancers are due to mutation of proto-oncogenes and formation of cellular oncogenes (Table 6.2; Parada et al., 1982).

Other transducing retroviruses differ from RSV in one key respect (Figure 4.7). Whereas RSV can replicate on its own, all other examples of transducing retroviruses are replication defective (for a review, see Coffin et al., 1997). They are incapable of replicating on their own.

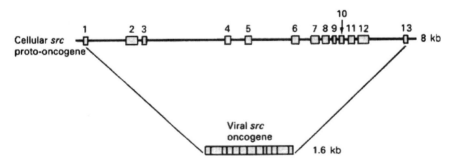

Figure 4.6 Comparison of the chicken *src* proto-oncogene and the RSV *src* oncogene. The cellular *src* proto-oncogene is comprised of 10 exons (filled boxes) that are separated by introns and spans 8 kb of chicken chromosomal DNA. The viral *src* oncogene does not contain introns, as a consequence of splicing and reverse transcription of a *src* mRNA. (Adapted from Cooper, 1995, with permission of author and publisher.)

They require coinfection with a replication-competent or helper retrovirus to be propagated. These viruses are replication defective because one or more of the viral replication genes (*gag*, *pol*, or *env*) are missing. In their place is the viral oncogene. As a consequence of replacing part of the viral genome, it is not uncommon for the v-*onc* to be expressed as a fusion with one of the viral replication proteins such as gag. In some cases, the fusion partner of the v-*onc* gene contributes to its oncogenic potential. There are two general mechanisms by which a v-*onc* of the transducing retroviruses contributes to the cancer phenotype. As mentioned above, v-*onc* genes contain mutations that confer an altered biochemical activity that in turn leads to an altered biological activity. In addition, in general, v-*onc* genes are expressed at levels higher than their c-*onc* counterparts as a consequence of being under the transcriptional control of the viral LTR (for a review, see Cooper, 1995). Higher levels of the v-*onc* mRNA can lead to higher levels of the v-onc protein, which can contribute to the cancer phenotype.

The group of retroviruses that take longer (6 months to 1 year) to induce cancer do not possess an oncogene. This group of oncogenic retroviruses induces neoplasms by integrating near a proto-oncogene. This phenomenon is termed proviral insertional mutagenesis or *cis*-activation (Figure 4.8). The presence of the provirus next to the proto-oncogene leads to its dysregulated expression, which plays a central role in induction of neoplasia (for a review, see Kung and Vogt, 1991). The prototypic member of *cis*-activating retroviruses is ALV, which causes lymphomas in chickens. Within a given ALV-induced lymphoma, all the cells contain an ALV provirus at the same chromosomal site, indicating that the neoplasm was clonal. When different independent lymphomas were examined, the ALV proviruses were found integrated into the same region of cellular DNA, adjacent to the c-*myc* locus (Hayward et al., 1981). c-*myc* is the cellular counterpart of a viral oncogene initially isolated from the transducing retrovirus, MC29. Insertion of the ALV provirus results in overexpression of the c-*myc* gene. RNA transcription from the ALV LTR, which is now next to the c-*myc* gene, leads to upregulation of its expression, which in turn leads to neoplastic transformation. ALV can upregulate expression of other proto-oncogenes, such as *erbB*, *fos*, and H-*ras*, by insertional activation to contribute to the induction of cancer (Cooper, 1995). A second example of a non-transducing oncogenic retrovirus is mouse mammary tumor virus (MMTV). MMTV has several preferred integration sites close to cellular genes, *Int-1*, *Int-2*, and *Int-3* (for a review, see Nusse, 1991; see Chapter 8). These three genes are located on different chromosomes and are not related to one another. In mammary tumors the MMTV provirus increases expression of the adjacent *int* locus, which likely contributes to tumor development. *Int-1*, now called *Wnt-1*, belongs to a family of genes that play a role in pattern formation during embryo development in organisms as diverse as Drosophila and mammals. *Int-2* gene encodes a member of the fibroblast growth factor family. The *Int-3* gene codes for a protein believed to have developmental function and is a member of the notch family of developmental regulators.

In summary, both transducing and nontransducing retroviruses contribute to the cancer phenotype via oncogenes. Proto-oncogenes are cellular genes that are important for a variety of cellular processes such as proliferation, differentiation, and development. There are two general mechanisms by which these oncogenic retroviruses contribute to the cancer phenotype: (1) by capture, delivery, and expression of a variant version (v-*onc*) of a proto-oncogene and (2) by integrating next to a proto-oncogene and causing its overexpression via the viral LTR. The study of oncogenic retroviruses has been revolutionary in that it led to the discovery of the oncogene. To date, no example of a transducing or a *cis*-activating oncogenic retrovirus has been identified in humans.

DNA Tumor Viruses

DNA tumor viruses have been isolated from six different virus families (Table 4.2). These represent a diverse set of viruses with differing structures, cell tropisms, genome organizations, and

Table 4.3 Functional Groups of Transduced Retroviral Oncogenes

Oncogene	Retrovirus	Viral Oncoprotein[a]	Function of Cellular Homolog
Growth factors			
sis	Simian sarcoma virus (SSV)	p28$^{env\text{-}sis}$	PDGF
Tyrosine kinase growth-factor receptors			
erbB	Avian erythroblastosis virus (AEV)-ES4,[b] AEV-R,[b] AEV-H	gp65^{erbB}	EGF receptor
fms	McDonough feline sarcoma virus (FeSV)	gp180gag-fms	CSF-1 receptor
sea	S13 avian erythroblastosis virus	gp160$^{env\text{-}sea}$	Receptor; ligand unknown
kit	Hardy-Zuckerman-4 FeSV	gp80$^{gag\text{-}kit}$	Hematopoietic receptor; product of the mouse W locus
ros	UR2 avian sarcoma virus (ASV)	p68$^{gag\text{-}ros}$	Receptor; ligand unknown
mpl	Mouse myeloproliferative leukemia virus	p31$^{env\text{-}mpl}$	Member of the hematopoietin receptor family
eyk	Avian retrovirus RPL30	gp37^{eyk}	Receptor; ligand unknown
Hormone receptors			
erbA	AEV-ES4,[b] AEV-R[b]	p75$^{gag\text{-}erbA}$	Thyroid hormone receptor
G proteins			
H-*ras*	Harvey murine sarcoma virus (MSV)	p21^{ras}	GTPase
K-*ras*	Kirsten MSV	p21^{ras}	GTPase
Adaptor protein			
crk	CT10, ASV-1	p47$^{gag\text{-}crk}$	Signal transduction
Nonreceptor tyrosine kinases			
src	Rous sarcoma virus (RSV)	pp60^{src}	Signal transduction
abl	Abelson murine leukemia virus (MuLV)	p460$^{gag\text{-}abl}$	Signal transduction
fps[c]	Fujinami ASV	p130$^{gag\text{-}fps}$	Signal transduction
	PRC 11 ASV	p105$^{gag\text{-}fps}$	
fes[c]	Snyder-Theilen FeSV	p85$^{gag\text{-}fes}$	Signal transduction

Oncogene	Virus	Oncoprotein	Function
	Gardner-Amstein FeSV	$p110^{gag\text{-}fes}$	
fgr	Gardner-Rasheed FeSV	$p70^{gag\text{-}actin\text{-}fgr}$	Signal transduction
yes	Y73 ASV	$p90^{gag\text{-}yes}$	Signal transduction
	Esh ASV	$p80^{gag\text{-}yes}$	
Serine-threonine kinases			
mos	Moloney MSV	$p37^{env\text{-}mos}$	Required for germ-cell maturation
raf[d]	3611-MSV	$p75^{gag\text{-}raf}$	Signal transduction
mil[d]	MH2 avian myelocytoma virus[b]	$p100^{gag\text{-}mil}$	Signal transduction
Nuclear proteins			
jun	ASV17	$p65^{gag\text{-}jun}$	Transcription factor (AP-1 complex)
fos	Finkel-Biskis-Jenkins MSV	$p55^{fos}$	Transcription factor (AP-1 complex)
myc	MC29 avian myelocytoma virus	$p100^{gag\text{-}myc}$	Transcription factor
	CM II avian myelocytoma virus	$p90^{gag\text{-}myc}$	
	OK10 avian leukemia virus	$p200^{gag\text{-}pol\text{-}myc}$	
	MH2 avian myelocytoma virus[b]	$p59^{gag\text{-}myc}$	
myb	Avian myeloblastosis virus (AMV) BAI/A, AMV-E26[b]	$p45^{myb}$	Transcription factor
$p135^{gag\text{-}myb\text{-}ets}$	Transcription factor		
ets	AMV-E26[b]	$p135^{gag\text{-}myb\text{-}ets}$	Transcription factor
rel	Avian reticuloendotheliosis virus T	$p64^{rel}$	Transcription factor
maf	Avian retrovirus AS42	$p100^{gag\text{-}maf}$	Transcription factor
ski	SKV ASV	$p110^{gag\text{-}ski\text{-}pol}$	Transcription factor
qin	Avian retrovirus ASV31	$p90^{gag\text{-}qin}$	Transcription factor of the forkhead/HNF-3 family

[a]These cumbersome but still widely used designations of viral oncoproteins contain basic structural data. p stands for protein, gp stands for glycoprotein, and pp stands for phosphoprotein; the latter is not applied consistently but, instead, is used mainly in conjunction with the *src* product. The numbers stand for estimated molecular weight in kilodaltons, and the superscript lists the genes from which the coding information is derived in 5′ to 3′ direction. In this chapter, we simply use the abbreviation of the oncogene; however, we use roman letters, with the first letter capitalized, to indicate the oncoprotein. Relevant contributions of viral genes to the oncoprotein are mentioned in the text.

[b]Transducing retrovirus with two oncogenes.

[c]*fps* and *fes* are the same oncogene derived from the avian and feline genomes, respectively.

[d]*raf* and *mil* are the same oncogene derived from the murine and avian genomes, respectively.

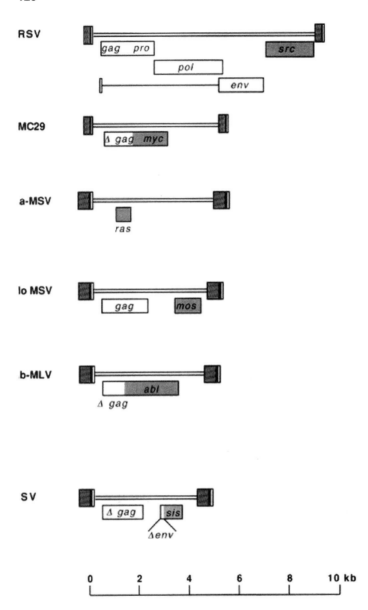

Figure 4.7 Examples of transducing retroviruses that are replication defective. Oncogenes are shaded. Top line represents RSV, which is replication competent and carries an intact *gag*, *pol*, and *env* gene. In contrast, each of the other retroviruses is missing at least some portion of the three essential replication genes. In their place is the oncogene. (MC29) avian myelocytomatosis virus (*myc* oncogene); (Ha-MSV) Harvey murine sarcoma virus (*ras* oncogene); (Mo-MSV) Moloney murine sarcoma virus (*mos* oncogene); (Ab-MLV) Abelson murine leukemia virus (*abl* oncogene); (SSV) simian sarcoma virus (*sis* oncogene). (Adapted from Coffin et al., 1997, with permission of authors and publisher.)

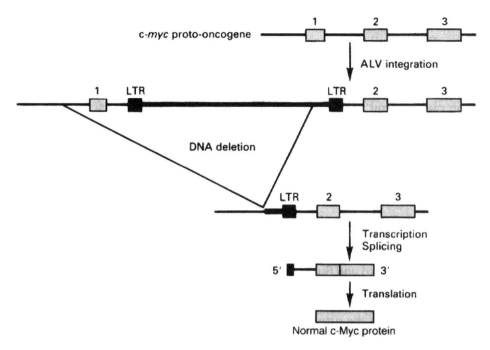

Figure 4.8   Example of proviral insertional mutagenesis or *cis*-activation. Activation of the c-*myc* proto-oncogene by ALV integration. The c-*myc* proto-oncogene has three exons. Exon 1 does not encode protein. In lymphomas, the most common integration site for ALV is in the first intron of the c-*myc* gene. Subsequently a deletion occurs that removes the first exon of c-*myc* and the 5' portion of the provirus. Transcription from the 3' LTR then leads to higher than normal levels of c-*myc* protein expression. (Adapted from Cooper, 1995, with permission of author and publisher.)

replication strategies. There is compelling evidence that some DNA tumor viruses can cause cancer in humans (Chapter 12). Others do not pose a cancer threat to humans, but cause cancer in animal hosts or transform cells in culture. Some important if not revolutionary insights have come from the study of DNA tumor viruses, such as adenovirus and SV40, which cause cancer only in experimental settings. The discovery of tumor suppressor genes (Chapter 5) was greatly facilitated by the study of the two aforementioned viruses in a manner similar to the way the study of retroviruses led to our understanding of cellular oncogenes and their functions. Tumor suppressor proteins function to prevent the cell from becoming cancerous, in that inactivation of all copies of a tumor suppressor gene or protein places a cell at an increased risk for cancer development. In this case, loss of gene function means increased cancer risk. This is in contrast to the oncogenes. Proto-oncogenes carry out a role in the normal functioning of a cell. Mutations within proto-oncogenes that result in gain of function can lead to the development of cancer (Chapter 5).

Adenoviruses

Adenoviruses are a large group of viruses that have been isolated from a wide range mammals and birds (for a review, see Schenk, 1996). Adenoviruses that infect humans can cause mild respiratory distress, conjunctivitis, or gastroenteritis. In general, adenovirus infection is relatively innocuous in humans. It does not lead to cancer. Adenoviruses have double-stranded linear DNA genomes of approximately 36 kb. Human cell cultures are permissive for human adenovirus replication. Productive infection results in virus multiplication, the death of the host cell, and spread of the virus. Rodent cells are not permissive for human adenovirus replication; instead, human adenovirus infection of rodent cells can result in cell transformation, albeit at a low frequency, one in 10^5 cells. Also, infection of newborn hamsters with some human adenoviruses leads to the development of tumors (Trentin et al., 1962). The study of the mechanism of adenovirus-induced cell transformation has helped to uncover the action of the class of cellular genes called tumor suppressor genes (see above and Chapter 5). In the transformed rodent cell, a piece of adenovirus DNA is always found integrated into the host DNA (Figure 4.9). In contrast to retroviruses, adenoviruses do not have a required integration step in their replication cycle. In a cell that is not permissive for adenovirus replication, the viral DNA can be integrated into one of the host chromosomes. This process is carried out by host enzymes and occurs infrequently. The integration is haphazard; usually incomplete copies of the viral DNA are present. Common to all transformed cells is the presence and expression of two adenovirus genes, *E1A* and *E1B* (Doerfler, 1968; Gallimore et al., 1974; Sharp et al., 1974). Expression of the *E1A* and *E1B* genes is required and is sufficient to transform rodent cells (Graham et al., 1975). Conversely, adenoviruses with certain mutations within *E1A* or *E1B* are not transforming. Each gene encodes several polypeptides. In a productive infection, E1A and E1B proteins are required for viral replication. E1A encodes two related proteins of 289 and 243 amino acids, while E1B codes for a 19- and 55-kDa protein. The 289-amino acid E1A protein is required for transformation and binds to several cellular proteins, including the retinoblastoma gene product (Rb). The ability of E1A to bind to Rb coincides with the transforming activity of adenoviruses (Whyte et al., 1988). In binding to Rb, E1A inactivates its function. Rb is an example of a protein with tumor suppressor activity. (Tumor suppressor proteins function to prevent the cell from growing out of control and becoming cancerous.) Two of the ways that tumor suppressors work are (1) by regulating progression through the cell cycle and (2) by regulating induction of programmed cell death or apoptosis. By inactivating Rb function, E1A contributes to the cancer phenotype. Similarly, the 55-kDa E1B protein inactivates a second tumor suppressor gene product, the p53 protein (Sar-

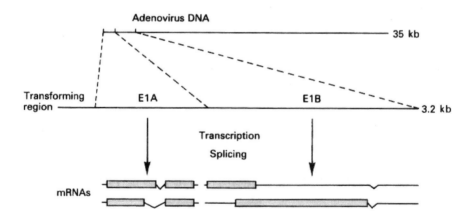

Figure 4.9 In adenovirus-transformed rodent cells, a common piece of viral genome is found integrated into cellular DNA. The adenovirus genome is a linear double-stranded DNA of approximately 35 kb. When a rodent cell is transformed by adenovirus, a portion of the viral DNA is found integrated into the cellular DNA. The exact boundaries of the fragment that is integrated in each transformed clone differ, but contain a common set of adenovirus sequences. The integrated DNA contains the adenovirus E1A and E1B genes, which each express two mRNAs and two proteins. Transformation of the cell is dependent on expression of the E1A and E1B polypeptides. (Adapted from Cooper, 1995, with permission of author and publisher.)

now et al., 1982). In lytically infected human cells, E1A proteins function to cause quiescent cells to enter S phase of the cell cycle, and E1B proteins block apoptosis. These changes make the cell a better host for adenovirus replication, which culminates in death of the cell. In the nonpermissive rodent cell, these same activities of E1A and E1B contribute to oncogenic transformation. *E1A* and *E1B* can be considered oncogenes. In addition to their role in virally induced cancers, tumor suppressor genes, such as *Rb* and *p53*, can play a crucial role in other nonviral human cancers (Chapter 5). In contrast to oncogenes of transducing retroviruses, the oncogenes of adenoviruses are not derived from cellular proto-oncogenes. In addition, adenoviral oncogenes are required for viral replication, whereas retroviral oncogenes are not. These themes in adenovirus-induced transformation are also seen in other DNA tumor viruses, namely, the SV40 virus and papillomaviruses.

Simian Virus 40 (SV40)

SV40, initially isolated from monkey kidney cells, has a covalently closed circular, double-stranded DNA genome of 5243 bp (for a review, see Cole, 1996). SV40 has five genes, three of which encode structural components of the virion (Figure 4.10). The other two genes encode the large and small T antigens. In permissive cells, the large T antigen is required for viral replication, and in nonpermissive cells it contributes to transformation. SV40 does not induce tumors in its natural host. Instead it replicates, killing the host cell with release of progeny virus. In a productive infection, SV40 DNA is replicated in the nucleus as an extrachromosomal plasmid. Rodent cells are not permissive for SV40 replication. Infection of rodent cells with SV40 can lead to their transformation, albeit at a low frequency (similar to adenovirus). The way SV40 transforms cells has a number of similarities to adenovirus transformation. In the transformed cell one finds SV40 DNA integrated into the host DNA. Integration of the SV40 genome is not a requisite step in its life cycle. Like adenoviruses (and unlike retroviruses), integration of SV40 DNA is not precise. Different integrants of SV40 are missing various and different portion of the genome. But common to all transformed cells is the presence and expression of the large T antigen gene (Sambrook et al., 1968; Botchan et al., 1976; Ketner and Kelly, 1976). The large T antigen is a 708–amino acid protein that is multifunctional and is required for viral DNA replication (for a review, see Pipas, 1992). During a productive infection, it binds to the viral DNA origin of replication and, in conjunction with host cellular DNA synthesis machinery, affects viral DNA synthesis. In addition, it causes the cell to enter the S phase, making the cell a more conducive host for viral DNA synthesis. Large T antigen accomplishes this by interfering with the functions of the tumor suppressor proteins Rb and p53 (Lane and Crawford, 1979; Linzer and Levine, 1979; DeCaprio et al., 1988). In a productive infection, these cells will ultimately die and release progeny virions. In the nonpermissive cell, in which SV40 DNA has integrated, expression of large T antigen ablates the tumor suppressor functions of Rb and p53, which leads to transformation of the cell. In this respect, SV40 and adenovirus employ a similar strategy except that SV40 uses one protein, large T antigen, instead of two. Large T antigen is a viral oncoprotein that does not have a cellular counterpart.

Papillomaviruses

The papillomaviruses are a family of DNA viruses that induce cutaneous papillomas or warts in a variety of mammals, including humans (for a review, see Howley, 1996). The Shope papillomavirus was an early if not the first example of a DNA tumor virus (Shope, 1932). This virus normally causes warts in its natural host, the cottontail rabbit. Domestic rabbits infected with the Shope papillomavirus will also develop warts, which develop to carcinomas in many instances. The bovine papillomaviruses (BPV) and human papillomaviruses (HPV) are the best experimen-

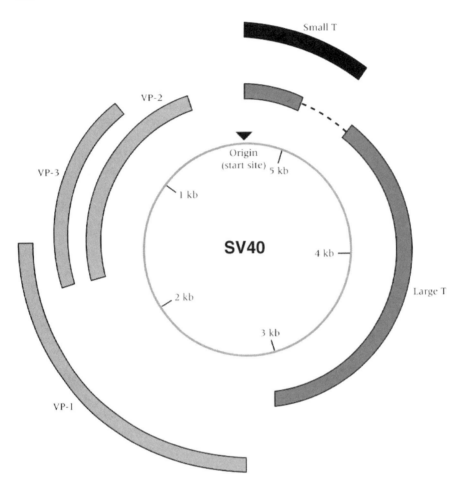

Figure 4.10 Genetic organization of SV40 genome. The genome of SV40 is a circular, double-stranded DNA of 5243 bp. The VP-1, 2, and 3 genes encode virion structural proteins. The small T and large T genes encode viral regulatory proteins. The protein encoded by the large T gene is named large T antigen. Rodent cells are not permissive for SV40 replication. At a low frequency, SV40 will transform rodent cells. All transformed cell clones contain an integrated, partial copy of the SV40 genome that expresses large T antigen. Large T antigen is necessary and sufficient for the transformation of rodent cells. (Adapted from Levine, 1992, with permission of author and publisher.)

tally studied members of this virus family. To date over 70 different HPVs and six BPVs have been described. In humans, some of the HPVs cause benign neoplasms, such as warts. Other human papillomaviruses are believed to be the causative agent of anogenital carcinomas, such as cervical cancer. Most anogenital cancers in humans have an integrated copy of HPV, primarily of the HPV-16 and HPV-18 subtypes. BPV-1 is the best-studied bovine family member. BPV causes benign warts in cattle. Both BPV-1 and HPV-16 and -18 cause transformation of cells in culture (Dvoretzky et al., 1980). The study of the ability of these viruses to transform cells has led to the identification of the genes that contribute to this phenotype.

The papillomavirus genome is covalently closed circular DNA of approximately 8 kb (Figure 4.11). The genetic organization of BPV and HPV is very similar, with some minor differences. BPV-1 has 10 genes, while the HPVs have nine, which are located in a clockwise ori-

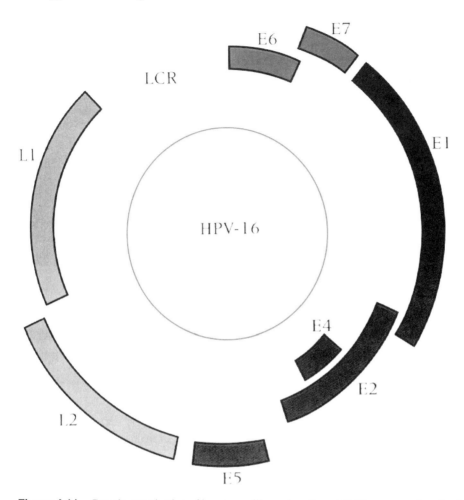

Figure 4.11   Genetic organization of human papillomavirus (type 16). The genome is a circular, double-stranded DNA molecule of 7,904 bp. The genes are E1 to E7, L1 and L2. The viral long control region (LCR) contains transcriptional and replication regulatory elements. Genetic organization of BPV-1 is similar, with the presence of an additional gene, E8. With HPV-16, E6 and E7 are the major transforming genes. The E3 gene, which is not indicated above, is not a consistent feature of all HPV isolates. (Adapted from Levine, 1992, with permission of author and publisher.)

entation. Two of the genes, *L1* and *L2*, code for subunits of the virion capsid. The remaining genes are named *E1* through *E8*. These code for non-structural proteins required for the viral life cycle. In terms of transformation of cells in culture, BPV and HPV share common features but also have some key differences. BPV-1 will transform the two mouse cell lines, C127 and NIH 3T3, in culture. In the transformed cell, BPV-1 DNA is commonly found as a multicopy plasmid, and integration is not required for the transformed state (Law et al., 1981). Three BPV-1 proteins, E5, E6, and E7 that contribute to the transforming potential of BPV-1 (Yang et al., 1985). BPV-1 E5 is believed to make the most significant contribution to the transformed state, with E6 and E7 playing ancillary roles (Schiller et al., 1986; Neary and DiMaio, 1989). BPV-1 E5 is a membrane protein that influences signaling of the platelet-derived growth factor (PDGF) receptor to mediate transformation (Schlegel et al., 1986; Petti et al., 1991). In contrast, transformation by the oncogenic HPVs is mediated by the E6 and E7 genes (Bedell et al., 1987; Phelps et al., 1988). E5 does not appear to play a role. The E6 and E7 proteins of the high risk HPVs act in a fashion similar to SV40 large T antigen and adenovirus E1A and E1B proteins. E6 leads to the degradation of the p53 tumor suppressor protein, while E7 binds to Rb to interfere with its tumor suppressor functions (Dyson et al., 1989; Scheffner et al., 1990; Werness et al., 1990).

Herpesviruses

Herpesviruses are a large (nearly 100 members) and diverse group of viruses found widely throughout vertebrates (for a review, see Roizman, 1996). Eight herpesviruses have been isolated so far from humans: herpes simplex virus 1 (HSV-1), herpes simplex virus 2 (HSV-2), human cytomegalovirus (hCMV), varicella zoster virus (VZV), Epstein-Barr virus (EBV), human herpesviruses 6 and 7 (HHV6 and HHV 7), and Kaposi sarcoma-associated herpes virus (KSHV). EBV and KSHV are believed to contribute to two different human cancers (see Chapter 12). Herpesviruses are enveloped viruses with very large DNA genomes ranging in size from 120 to 230 kb. Herpesviruses can establish two types of infections, lytic and latent. Lytic infections result in death of the host cell with production of virus. In a latent infection, the virus becomes dormant. The viral DNA is maintained in the host cell nucleus, as a circular plasmid, but few if any viral genes are expressed. Latent infections can become reactivated leading to the production of virus and sometimes pathological consequences for the host. Several animal herpesviruses are associated with tumor formation. These include the Ranid herpesvirus 1 (RaHV-1), which can cause renal adenocarcinomas in leopard frogs (Davison et al., 1999), and Marek's disease herpesvirus (MDV), which causes a T-cell lymphoma in chickens (for a review, see Ross, 1999). The mechanism by which these viruses cause cancer is not well understood.

Hepadnaviruses

Hepadnaviruses are a family of DNA viruses that infect the liver of their host. This family has five well-characterized members that infect different birds and mammals (for reviews, see Ganem, 1996; Seeger and Mason, 2000). Human hepatitis B virus (HBV) is the prototype member of this family. Other members include woodchuck hepatitis virus (WHV), ground squirrel hepatitis virus (GSHV), duck hepatitis B virus (DHBV), and heron hepatitis B virus (HHBV). The hepadnaviruses can cause either transient or persistent infections. In humans, transient infections are cleared within several months, while persistent infections are generally lifelong. The host immune response is a key determinant in the ultimate fate of the hepadnavirus infection. Chronic infections with HBV, WHV, and GSHV are associated with increased incidences of hepatocellular carcinoma (HCC). In fact, HBV is the leading cause of liver cancer worldwide (Beasley, 1988; also see Chapter 12).

The DNA genome of hepadnaviruses is only ~3 kb. Within the virus particle the DNA is in a relaxed circular conformation. Although they contain DNA, hepadnaviruses replicate via reverse transcription of an RNA intermediate (Summers and Mason, 1982). Even though retroviruses also replicate via reverse transcription, there are fundamental differences between the pathways employed by the two virus families. One difference is that hepadnaviruses do not have an integration step in their life cycle. Instead, hepadnaviruses maintain their genomes as a covalently closed, circular DNA in the nucleus.

As mentioned above, infection with the mammalian hepadnaviruses can lead to the development of HCC. In these liver tumors, it is common to find integrated pieces of hepadnaviral DNA even though hepadnaviruses do not have an obligate integration step in their life cycle. These findings raise the question whether DNA integration plays a role in the development of liver cancer. The answer is yes and no. Infection of woodchucks with WHV results in the development of hepatocellular carcinoma, with frequencies approaching 100% after 2 years. In a large percentage of liver tumors from infected animals, WHV DNA is found integrated near a member of the *myc* oncogene family, N-*myc* (Fourel et al., 1990, 1994). The integrated WHV DNA is thought to result in increased expression of the neighboring *myc* locus. This insertional activation of the *myc* oncogene locus contributes to the development of the cancer. As illuminating as the WHV story has been, HBV-induced tumors do not seem to result from insertional activation of a common oncogene. For HBV-induced liver cancers, a popular explanation is the "indirect model" (Ganem, 1996), which states that HBV, its genes, and their products make no direct contribution to transformation. Instead, HBV-induced liver injury, which is mediated by the host immune response, ultimately leads to liver cancer. During chronic infection, a persistent low level of liver damage is continuously occurring via the immune response. This immune response, which is not vigorous enough to clear the infection, is responsible for the hepatitis. In these individuals, the immune response leads to killing of infected cells. To replace the cells that die, the rate of hepatocyte proliferation increases, with a concomitant increase in the frequency of mutations. In humans, liver cancer develops after 20 to 40 years of chronic infection (Chapter 12). During this long latency period, the appropriate constellation of mutations accumulates, resulting in the development of HCC. In spite of the popularity of the above model, it should be emphasized that it is currently not well understood how HBV infection leads to the development of HCC. It is possible that HBV contributes to HCC by multiple mechanisms, both direct and indirect.

THE SIGNIFICANCE OF INFECTIOUS AGENTS IN THE CAUSATION OF NEOPLASIA

As noted in Chapter 1, the possibility that infectious agents are a significant cause of neoplasia was quite popular in the latter part of the nineteenth century. However, the popularity of this concept decreased during the twentieth century until about four decades ago, when several of the oncogenic viruses became known and subsequently were characterized both biologically and in a molecular sense. It is difficult to ascertain the importance of infectious agents as causes of neoplasia in lower forms of animals in their natural habitat, but it is apparent, as can be seen from many of the discussions in this chapter, that infectious agents can be a significant causative factor for neoplasia, either induced or spontaneous, in domestic and laboratory animals. As discussed in Chapter 12, infectious agents as causative of human cancer may represent as much as 15% of the total cancer problem. While this may seem alarming, it also presents the possibility that various preventive measures such as vaccination, better personal hygiene, and public health measures can potentially control if not eliminate a number of infectious causes of human neoplasia.

REFERENCES

Beasley, R. Hepatitis B virus: The major etiology of hepatocellular carcinoma. Cancer, *61*:1942–1956, 1988.

Bedell, M. A., Jones, K. H., and Laimins, L. A. The E6-E7 region of human papillomavirus type 18 is sufficient for transformation of NIH 3T3 and rat-1 cells. J Virol., *61*:3635–3640, 1987.

Beijersbergen, A., Dulk-Ras, A. D., Schilperoort, R. A., and Hooykaas, P. J. J. Conjugative transfer by the virulence system of *Agrobacterium tumefaciens*. Science, *256*:1324–1327, 1992.

Bittner, J. J. Some possible effects of nursing on the mammary gland tumor incidence in mice. Science, *84*:162, 1936.

Botchan, M., Topp, W., and Sambrook, J. The arrangement of simian virus 40 sequences in the DNA of transformed cells. Cell, *9*:269–287, 1976.

Braun, A. C. Plant tumors. *In*: F. F. Becker (Ed.), Cancer—A Comprehensive Treatise, Vol. 4, pp. 411–427. New York: Plenum, 1975.

Cheever, A. W. Schistosomiasis and neoplasia. J. Natl. Cancer Inst., *61*:13–18, 1978.

Chilton, M.-D., Drummond, M. H., Merlo, D. J., Sciaky, D., Montoya, A. L., Gordon, M. P., and Nester, E. W. Stable incorporation of plasmic DNA into higher plant cells: the molecular basis of crown gall tumorigenesis. Cell, *11*:263–271, 1977.

Clemmesen, J. Joannes Fibiger: Gonglyomena and vitamin A in carcinogenesis. Acta Pathol. Microbiol. Scand. A Suppl., *270*:1–13, 1978.

Coffin, J. M. Retroviridae: the viruses and their replication. *In*: B. N. Fields, D. M. Knipe, P. M. Howley, et al. (Eds.), Virology, 3rd ed., pp. 1767–1847. Philadelphia: Lippincott-Raven Publishers, 1996.

Coffin, J. M., Hughes, S. H., and Varmus, H. E. Retroviruses. Cold Spring Harbor, NY: Cold Spring Harbor Laboratory Press, 1997.

Cole, C. N. Polyomavirinae: the viruses and their replication. *In*: B. N. Fields, D. M. Knipe, P. M. Howley, et al. (Eds.), Virology, 3rd ed., pp. 1997–2025. Philadelphia: Lippincott-Raven Publishers, 1996.

Collet, M. S., Brugge, J. S., and Erikson, R. L. Characterization of a normal avian cell protein related to the avian sarcoma virus transforming gene product. Cell, *15*:1363–1369, 1978.

Cooper, G. M. Oncogenes, 2nd ed. Boston: Jones and Barlett Publishers, 1995.

Curtis, M. R., Dunning, W. F., and Bullock, F. D. Genetic factors in relation to the etiology of malignant tumors. Am. J. Cancer, *17*:894–923, 1933.

Davison, A. J., Sauerbier, W., Dolan, A., Addison, C., and McKinnell, R. G. Genomic studies of the Lucke tumor herpesvirus (RaHV-1). J. Cancer Res. Clin. Oncol., *125*:232–238, 1999.

DeCaprio, J. A., Ludlow, J. W., Figge, J., Shew, J. Y., Huang, C. M., Lee, W. H., Marsilio, E., Paucha, E., and Livingston, D. M. SV40 large tumor antigen forms a specific complex with the product of the retinoblastoma susceptibility. Cell, *54*:275–283, 1988.

DeCross, A. J., and Marshall, B. J. The role of *Helicobacter pylori* in acid-peptic disease. Am. J. Med. Sci., *306*:381–392, 1993.

Doerfler, W. The fate of the DNA of adenovirus type 12 in baby hamster kidney cells. Proc. Natl. Acad. Sci. USA *60*:636–643, 1968.

Dooley, C. P., and Cohen, H. The clinical significance of *Campylobacter pylori*. Ann. Int. Med., *108*:70–79, 1988.

Dunning, W. F., and Curtis, M. R. Attempts to isolate the active agent in *Cysticercus fasciolaris*. Cancer Res., *13*:838–842, 1953.

Dvoretzky, I., Shober, R., Chattopadhyay, S. K., and Lowy, D. R. A quantitative in vitro focus assay for bovine papilloma virus. Virology, *103*:369–375, 1980.

Dyson, N., Howley, P. M., Munger, K., and Harlow, E. The human papilloma virus-16 E7 oncoprotein is able to bind to the retinoblastoma gene product. Science, *243*:934–937, 1989.

Ellermann, V., and Bang, O. Experimentelle Leukamie bei Hühnern. Zentrbl. Bakteriol., *46*:595–609, 1908.

Ellerman, V., and Bang, O. Experimentelle Leukämie bei Hühnern. Z. Hyg. Infekt., *62*:231, 1909.

Enno, A., O'Rourke, J. L., Howlett, C. R., Jack, A., Dixon, M. F., and Lee, A. MALToma-like lesions in the murine gastric mucosa after long-term infection with *Helicobacter felis*. A mouse model of *Helicobacter pylori*–induced gastric lymphoma. Am. J. Pathol., *147*:217–222, 1995.

Erdman, S. E., Correa, P., Coleman, L. A., Schrenzel, M. D., Li, X., and Fox, J. G. *Helicobacter mustelae*–associated gastric MALT lymphoma in ferrets. Am. J. Pathol., *151*:273–280, 1997.

Flint, S. J., Enquist, L. W., Krug, R. M, Racaniello, V. R., and Skalka, A. M. Principles of Virology; Molecular Biology, Pathogenesis, and Control, pp. 553–593. Washington, D.C.: ASM Press, 2000.

Fourel, G., Trepo, C., Bougueleret, L., Henglein, B., Ponzetto, A., Tiollais, P., and Buendia, M. A. Frequent activation of N-*myc* genes by hepadnavirus insertion in woodchuck liver. Nature, *347*:294–298, 1990.

Fourel, G., Couturier, J., Wei, Y., Apiou, F., Tiollais, P., and Buendia, M. A. Evidence for long-range onco-gene activation by hepadnavirus insertion. EMBO J., *13*:2526–2534, 1994.

Fox, J. G. *Helicobacter* species and in vivo models of gastrointestinal cancer. Aliment. Pharmacol. Ther., *12*:37–60, 1998.

Fox, J. G., Dangler, C. A., Sager, W., Borkowski, R., and Gliatto, J. M. *Helicobacter mustelae*–associated gastric adenocarcinoma in ferrets (*Mustela putorius furo*). Vet. Pathol., *34*:225–229, 1997.

Gallimore, P. H., Sharp, P. A., and Sambrook, J. Viral DNA in transformed cells. II. A study of the se-quences of adenovirus 2 DNA in nine lines of transformed rat cells using specific fragments of the viral genome. J. Mol. Biol., *89*:49–72, 1974.

Ganem, D. Hepadnaviridae and their replication. *In*: B. N. Fields, D. M. Knipe, P. M. Howley, et al. (Eds.), Virology, 3rd ed., pp. 2703–2737. Philadelphia: Lippincott-Raven Publishers, 1996.

Goff, S. J., and Skalka, A. M. (Eds.). *Reverse Transcriptase*. Cold Spring Harbor, NY: Cold Spring Harbor Laboratory Press, 1993.

Graham, F. L., Abrahams, P. J., Mulder, C., Heijneker, H. L., Warnaar, S. O., De Vries, F. A., Fiers, W., and Van Der Eb, A. J. Studies on in vitro transformation by DNA and DNA fragments of human aden-oviruses and simian virus 40. Cold Spring Harbor Symp. Quant. Biol., *39* (*Pt 1*):637–650, 1975.

Gross, L. "Spontaneous" leukemia developing in C3H mice following inoculation, in infancy, with AK-leukemic extracts, or AK-embryos. Proc. Soc. Exp. Biol. Med., *76*:27–32, 1951.

Hadley, R. G., and Szalay, A. A. DNA sequences homologous to the T DNA region of *Agrobacterium tumefaciens* are present in diverse *Rhizobium* species. Mol. Gen. Genet., *188*:361–369, 1982.

Hansson, L. E., Engstrand, L., Nyrén, O., Evans, D. J., Jr., Lindgren, A., Bergstrom, R., Andersson, B., Athlin, L., Bendtsen, O., and Tracz, P. *Helicobacter pylori* infection: independent risk indicator of gastric adenocarcinoma. Gastroenterology, *105*:1098–1103, 1993.

Hayward, W. S., Neel, B. G., and Astrin, S. M. Activation of a cellular onc gene by promoter insertion in ALV-induced lymphoid leukosis. Nature, *290*:475–480, 1981.

Howley, P. M. Papillomavirinae: the viruses and their replication. *In*: B. N. Fields, D. M. Knipe, P. M. Howley, et al. (Eds.), Virology, 3rd ed., pp. 2045–2076. Philadelphia: Lippincott-Raven Publishers, 1996.

Iba, H., Takeya, T., Cross, F. R., Hanafusa, T., and Hanafusa, H. Rous sarcoma virus variants that carry the cellular *src* gene instead of the viral *src* gene cannot transform chicken embryo fibroblasts. Proc. Natl. Acad. Sci. USA, *81*:4424–4428, 1984.

Ketner, G., and Kelly, T. J. Integrated simian virus 40 sequences in transformed cell DNA: Analysis using restriction endonucleases. Proc. Natl. Acad. Sci. USA, *73*:1102–1106, 1976.

Kung, H. J., Boerkoel, C., and Carter, T. H. Retroviral mutagenesis of cellular oncogenes: a review with insights into the mechanisms of insertional activation. Curr. Top. Microbial. Immunol., *171*:1–25, 1991.

Kupila-Ahvenniemi, S., and Therman, E. Morphogenesis of crown gall. Adv. Morphogenesis, *7*:45–78, 1968.

Lane, D. P., and Crawford, L. V. T antigen is bound to a host protein in SV40-transformed. Nature, *278*:261–263, 1979.

Law, M. F., Lowy, D. R., Dvoretzky, I., and Howley, P. M. Mouse cells transformed by bovine papilloma-virus contain only extrachromosomal viral DNA sequences. Proc. Natl. Acad. Sci. U.S.A., *78*:2727–2731, 1981.

Levine, A. J. Viruses. New York: Scientific American Library, 1992.

Linzer, D. I., and Levine, A. J. Characterization of a 54-Kdalton cellular SV40 tumor antigen present in SV40-transformed cells and uninfected embryonal carcinoma. Cell, *17*:43–52, 1979.

Neary, K., and DiMaio, D. Open reading frames E6 and E7 of bovine papillomavirus type 1 are both re-quired for full transformation of mouse C127 cells. J. Virol., *63*:259–266, 1989.

Nusse, R. Insertional mutagenesis in mouse mammary tumorigenesis. *In*: H. J. Kung and P. Vogt (Eds.), Retroviral insertion and oncogene activation. Curr. Top. Microbiol. Immunol., *171*:43–65, 1991.

Nyska, A., Maronpot, R. R., Eldridge, S. R., Haseman, J. K., and Hailey, J. R. Alteration in cell kinetics in control B6C3F$_1$ mice infected with *Helicobacter hepaticus*. Toxicol. Pathol., *25*:591–596, 1997.

Parada, L. F., Tabin, C. J., Shih, C., and Weinberg, R. A. Human EJ bladder carcinoma oncogene is homologue of Harvey sarcoma virus *ras* gene. Nature, *297*:474–478, 1982.

Parsonnet, J., Friedman, G. D., Vandersteen, D. P., Chang, Y., Vogelman, J. H., Orentreich, N., and Sibley, R. K. *Helicobacter pylori* infection and the risk of gastric carcinoma. N. Engl. J. Med., *325*:1127–1131, 1991.

Parsonnet, J., Hansen, S., Rodriguez, L., Gelb, A. B., Warnke, R. A., Jellum, E., Orentreich, N., Vogelman, J. H., and Friedman, G. D. *Helicobacter pylori* infection and gastric lymphoma. N. Engl. J. Med., *330*:1267–1271, 1994.

Petti, L., Nilson, L. A., and DiMaio, D. Activation of the platelet-derived growth factor receptor by the bovine papillomavirus E5 transforming protein. EMBO J., *10*:845–855, 1991.

Phelps, W. C., Yee, C. L., Munger, K., and Howley, P. M. The human papillomavirus type 16 E7 gene encodes transactivation and transformation functions similar to those of adenovirus E1A. Cell, *53*:539–547, 1988.

Pipas, J. M. Common and unique features of T antigens encoded by the polyomavirus. J. Virol., *66*:3979–3985, 1992.

Roizman, B. Herpesviridae. *In*: B. N. Fields, D. M. Knipe, P. M. Howley, et al. (Eds.), Virology, 3rd ed., pp. 2221–2230. Philadelphia: Lippincott-Raven Publishers, 1996.

Ross, N. L. T-cell transformation by Marek's disease virus. Trends Microbiol., *7*:22–29, 1999.

Rous, P. A transmissible avian neoplasm: sarcoma of the common fowl. J. Exp. Med., *12*:696–705, 1911.

Rous, P. Transmission of a malignant new growth by means of a cell-free filtrate. JAMA, *56*:198, 1911.

Rugge, M., Cassaro, M., Leandro, G., Baffa, R., Avellini, C., Bufo, P., Stracca, V., Battaglia, G., Fabiano, A., Guerini, A., and di Mario, F. *Helicobacter pylori* in promotion of gastric carcinogenesis. Digest. Dis. Sci., *41*:950–955, 1996.

Sambrook, J., Westphal, H., Srinivasan, P. R., and Dulbecco, R. The integrated state of viral DNA in SV40-transformed cells. Proc. Natl. Acad. Sci. U.S.A., *60*:1288–1295, 1968.

Sarnow, P., Ho, Y. S., Williams, J., and Levine, A. J. Adenovirus E1b-58kd tumor antigen and SV40 large tumor antigen are physically associated with the same 54 kd cellular protein in transformed cells. Cell, *28*:387–394, 1982.

Scheffner, M., Werness, B. A., Huibregtse, J. M., Levine, A. J., and Howley, P. M. The E6 oncoprotein encoded by human papillomavirus types 16 and 18 promotes the degradation of p53. Cell, *63*:1129–1136, 1990.

Schell, J. Crown gall: tumor as a result of oncogenic DNA transfer. Natl. Cancer Inst. Monogr., *60*:229–233, 1982.

Schenk, T. Adenoviridae: the viruses and their replication. *In*: B. N. Fields, D. M. Knipe, P. M. Howley, et al. (Eds.), Virology, 3rd ed., pp. 2111–2148. Philadelphia: Lippincott-Raven Publishers, 1996.

Schiller, J. T., Vass, W. C., Vousden, K. H., and Lowy, D. R. E5 open reading frame of bovine papillomavirus type 1 encodes a transforming gene. J. Virol., *57*:1–6, 1986.

Schlegel, R., Wade-Glass, M., Rabson, M. S., and Yang, Y. C. The E5 transforming gene of bovine papillomavirus encodes a small, hydrophobic polypeptide. Science, *233*:464–467, 1986.

Schwartz, D. E., Tizard, R., and Gilbert, W. Nucleotide sequence of Rous sarcoma virus. Cell, *32*:853–869, 1983.

Seeger, C., and Mason, W. S. Hepatitis B virus biology. Microbiol. Mol. Biol. Rev., *64*:51–68, 2000.

Sharp, P. A., Pettersson, U., and Sambrook, J. Viral DNA in transformed cells. I. A study of the sequences of adenovirus 2 DNA in a line of transformed rat cells using specific fragments of the viral genome. J. Mol. Biol., *86*:709–726, 1974.

Shimkin, M. B. Contrary to Nature. Washington, D.C.: United States Government Printing Office, 1977.

Shope, R. E. A transmissible tumor-like condition in rabbits. J. Exp. Med., *56*:793–802, 1932.

Smith, E. F., and Townsend, C. O. A plant-tumor of bacterial origin. Science, *25*:671, 1907.

Stachel, S. E., and Zambryski, P. C. Agrobacterium tumefaciens and the susceptible plant cell: a novel adaptation of extracellular recognition and DNA conjugation. Cell, *47*:155–157, 1986.

Stehelin, D., Varmus, H. E., Bishop, J. M., and Vogt, P. K. DNA related to the transforming gene(s) of avian sarcoma viruses is present in normal avian DNA. Nature, *260*:170–173, 1976.

Summers, J., and Mason, W. S. Replication of the genome of a hepatitis B-like virus by reverse transcription of an RNA intermediate. Cell, *29*:403–415, 1982.

Takeya, T., and Hanafusa, H. Structure and sequence of the cellular gene homologous to the RSV *src* gene and the mechanism for generating the transforming virus. Cell, *32*:881–890, 1983.

Temin, H. M., and Rubin, H. Characteristics of an assay for Rous sarcoma virus and Rous sarcoma cells in tissue culture. Virology, *6*:669–688, 1958

Thomashow, M. F., Nutter, R., Montoya, A. L., Gordon, M. P., and Nester, E. W. Integration and organization of Ti plasmid sequences in crown gall tumors. Cell, *19*:729–739, 1980.

Thrasher, J. P., Ichinose, H., and Pitot, H. C. Osteogenic sarcoma of the canine esophagus associated with *Spirocerca lupi* infection. Am. J. Vet. Res., *24*:808, 1963.

Trentin, J. J., Yabe, Y., and Taylor, G. The quest for human cancer viruses. Science, *137*:835–849, 1962.

Turgeon, R., Wood, H. N., and Braun, A. C. Studies on the recovery of crown gall tumor cells. Proc. Natl. Acad. Sci. USA, *73*:3562–3564, 1976.

Varmus, H., and Brown, P. Retroviruses. *In*: M. Howe and D. Berg (Eds.), Mobile DNA, pp. 53–108. Washington, D.C.: ASM Press, 1989.

Vogt, P. K., and Nevins, J. R. Cell transformation by viruses. *In*: B. N. Fields, D. M. Knipe, P. M. Howley et al. (Eds.), Virology, 3rd ed., pp. 301–343. Philadelphia: Lippincott-Raven Publishers, 1996.

Ward, J. M., Fox, J. G., Anver, M. R., Haines, D. C., George, C. V., Collins, Jr., M. J., Gorelick, P. L., Nagashima, K., Gonda, M. A., Gilden, R. V., Tully, J. R., Russell, R. J., Benveniste, R. E., Paster, B. J., Dewhirst, F. E., Donovan, J. C., Anderson, L. M., and Rice, J. M. Chronic active hepatitis and associated liver tumors in mice caused by a persistent bacterial infection with a novel *Helicobacter* species. J. Natl. Cancer Inst., *86*:1222–1227, 1994.

Warren, J. R. Unidentified curved bacillus on gastric epithelium in active chronic gastritis. Lancet, *1*:1273, 1983.

Watson, B., Currier, T. C., Gordon, M. P., Chilton, M. D., and Nester, E. W. Plasmid required for virulence of *Agrobacterium tumefaciens*. J. Bacteriol., *123*:255–264, 1975.

Werness, B. A., Levine, A. J., and Howley, P. M. Association of human papillomavirus types 16 and 18 E6 proteins with p53. Science, *248*:76–79, 1990.

White, D. O., and Fenner, F. J. Medical Virology, 4th ed., San Diego, CA: Academic Press, 1994.

White, F. F., Garfinkel, D. J., Huffman, G. A., Gordon, M. P., and Nester, E. W. Sequences homologous to *Agrobacterium rhizogenes* T-DNA in the genomes of uninfected plants. Nature, *301*:348–350, 1983.

Whyte, P., Buchkovich, K. J., Horowitz, J. M., Friend, S. H., Raybuck, M., Weinberg, R. A., and Harlow, E. Association between an oncogene and an anti-oncogene: The adenovirus E1A proteins bind to the retinoblastoma gene product. Nature, *334*:124–129, 1988.

Winans, S. C. Two-way chemical signaling in *Agrobacterium*-plant interactions. Microbiol. Rev., *56*:12–31, 1992.

Yang, F., and Simpson, R. B. Revertant seedlings from crown gall tumors retain a portion of the bacterial Ti plasmid DNA sequences. Proc. Natl. Acad. Sci. USA, *78*:4151–4155, 1981.

Yang, F., Montoya, A. L., Merlo, D. J., Drummond, M. H., Chilton, M.-D., Nester, E. W., and Gordon, M. P. Foreign DNA sequences in crown gall teratomas and their fate during the loss of the tumorous traits. Mol. Gen. Genet., *177*:707–714, 1980.

Yang, Y. C., Okayama, H., and Howley, P. M. Bovine papillomavirus contains multiple transforming genes. Proc. Natl. Acad. Sci. U.S.A., *82*:1030–1034, 1985.

5
The Etiology of Cancer:
Germline Genetic Factors

The predominant environmental factors in the causation of cancer include chemicals, ionizing and ultraviolet radiation, as well as specific infectious agents, predominantly viruses. Although the majority of these agents may have as a principal component of their etiological mechanism some interaction with and/or alteration of the cellular genome, neoplastic disease resulting from the action of such agents is not generally thought of as hereditary or genetic disease. The term *hereditary* or *genetic disease* usually connotes an abnormality transmitted through the germline from parent to offspring. In this sense it is reasonable to state that, in considering all cases of human neoplasia, most cancers are not the direct result of heredity but are acquired through an interaction of the host with the environment. However, the interaction of the environment with the genetic composition of the host, either directly or indirectly through the regulation of the expression of the host genome, is important in the development of all human and animal neoplasms. Therefore, although relatively few human neoplasms exhibit a clearly defined Mendelian pattern of heredity, polygenic and multifactorial inheritance may play a significant role in increasing the risk of cancer for a large number of humans. This discussion centers largely on hereditary factors in human cancer, because there is a larger body of knowledge on this subject in this species; however, germline genetic factors in the development of cancer in lower animals are also considered.

DOMINANT AND RECESSIVE DISORDERS ASSOCIATED WITH A HIGH INCIDENCE OF HUMAN CANCER

Although the total number of cases of human cancer with a distinct Mendelian genetic mode of inheritance is small relative to the incidence of neoplasia in general, a variety of autosomal and sex-linked disorders, both dominant and recessive, are associated with or clearly causative of specific neoplasms both in humans and in animals. For obvious reasons, the largest number of examples of such conditions have been described and studied in humans. Some of these are listed in Table 5.1, with the associated neoplasm(s) and the mode of inheritance of the specific condition.

In the majority of autosomal recessive disorders, the principal biochemical defect concerns some aspects of DNA metabolism or chromosomal structure, especially DNA repair. The lack of capacity of cells from patients with xeroderma pigmentosum to repair ultraviolet damage to their DNA is well known (cf. Cleaver, 1990). Studies of mutations in this disease have led to the finding and characterization of 14 or more genes (Hoeijmakers, 1994) involved in nucleotide

Table 5.1 Cancers and Precancerous Diseases Exhibiting a Distinct Mendelian Mode of Inheritance

Disease	Associated Neoplasm(s)	Mode of Inheritance
Clastogenic and multiple syndromes		
Bloom syndrome	Leukemia, intestinal cancer (chromosomal breaks)	AR
Fanconi anemia	Acute monomyelogenous leukemia, squamous cell carcinoma of mucocutaneous junctions, hepatocarcinoma, adenoma (chromosomal breaks)	AR
Dyskeratosis congenita (Zinsser-Colde-Engman syndrome)	Leukoplakia with squamous cell carcinoma, including that of cervix	XR AD
Incontinentia pigmenti	Wilms tumor, acute leukemia retinoblastoma (all in infancy)	XD
Noonan syndrome	Schwannoma	AD
Beckwith-Wiedemann syndrome	Visceromegaly, cytomegaly, macroglossia, adrenal cortical neoplasia, Wilms tumor, hepatocarcinoma	AD
Hereditary nonpolyposis colorectal cancer	Colorectal cancer and adenomas Endometrial, gastric, and ovarian cancers	AD
Genodermatoses		
Neurocutaneous melanosis	Malignant melanoma of skin and meninges	AR
Xeroderma pigmentosum	Skin cancer	AR
Xerodermoid pigmentosum (including De Sanctis-Cacchione syndrome)		AD
Multiple sebaceous gland tumors and visceral carcinoma (Torre syndrome)	Diverse gastrointestinal and urogenital cancers	AR
Acrokeratosis verruciformis, van den Bosch syndrome	Warty hyperkeratosis	AD XR
Nevoid basal cell carcinoma syndrome	Basal cell carcinomas, jaw cysts, and skeletal deformities	AD
Pachyonychia congenita	Hyperkeratosis, cutaneous horns, leukoplakia	AD
Multiple trichoepithelioma (Spiegler-Brooke tumors; cylindromatosis)	Basal and squamous cell carcinomas, carcinomas, adenocarcinoma of salivary gland	AD XD
Dysplastic nevus syndrome	Dysplastic nevi, malignant melanomas, pancreatic cancer (?)	AD
Hidrotic ectodermal dysplasia	Squamous cell carcinoma of palms and soles	AD
Maffucci syndrome	Hemangiomata, chondrosarcoma	AD
Porokeratosis of Mibelli	Squamous cell carcinoma within the lesion	AD
Breast cancer in females	Mammary carcinoma	AD
Endocrine system		
Multiple endocrine neoplasia 1 (Werner syndrome, MEN 1)	Adenomas of islet cells, parathyroid, pituitary and adrenal glands, malignant schwannoma, nonappendiceal carcinoid, thyroid adenomas)	AD
Zollinger-Ellison syndrome	Alpha cell nesidioblastoma and lymphatic metastases	AD
Multiple endocrine neoplasia II (Sipple syndrome, MEN 11a)	Medullary carcinoma of thyroid, parathyroid adenoma, pheochromocytoma	AD

Table 5.1   (continued)

Disease	Associated Neoplasm(s)	Mode of Inheritance
Endocrine system (continued)		
Mucosal neuromas and endocrine adenomatosis MEN (11b)	Pheochromocytoma, medullary carcinoma of the thyroid, neurofibroma, submucosa' neuromas of tongue, lips, eyelids; intestinal ganglioneuromatosis	AD
Nervous system		
Retinoblastoma, bilateral	Sarcoma	AD
Neurofibromatosis type 2	Acoustic neuromas, bilateral, gliomas, meningiomas	AD
Neuroblastoma	Ganglioneurofibroma, pheochromocytoma	AR AD
Megalencephaly	Ganglioneuroblastoma, glioblastoma	AD
Gastrointestinal system		
Familial polyposis coli	Intestinal polyps, carcinoma of colon, hepato-blastoma, medullablastoma, desmoids	AD
Gardner syndrome	Intestinal polyps, osteomas, fibromas, seba-ceous cysts, carcinoma of colon, ampulla of Vater, pancreas, thyroid and adrenal	AD
Peutz-Jeghers syndrome	Intestinal polyps, ovarian (granulosa cell) tumors in 5% of females	AD
Tylosis with esophageal cancer	Carcinoma of esophagus	AD
Pulmonary and vascular systems		
Fibrocystic pulmonary dysplasia	Bronchial adenocarcinoma	AD
Hereditary hemorrhagic telangiectasia of Rendu-Osler-Weber	Angioma	AD
Lymphedema with distichiasis	Lymphangiosarcoma of edematous limb	AD
Urogenital system		
Gonadal dysgenesis, hermaphroditism, Reifenstein syndrome	Gonadoblastoma, dysgerminoma	AR
Stein-Leventhal syndrome	Endometrial carcinoma	AD
Wilms tumor	Wilms tumor (nephroblastoma)	AD
Hydronephrosis, familial	Congenital sarcoma of kidney	AD
Hypernephroma (renal cell carcinoma)	Renal cell carcinoma	AD
Denys-Drash syndrome	Wilms tumor	AD
Phakomatosis		
von Recklinghausen neurofibroma-tosis (type 1)	Fibrosarcoma, neuroma, schwannoma, meningi-oma, polyps, optic glioma, pheochromocy-toma, myelogenous leukemia, neurosarcoma in children	AD
Tuberous sclerosis	Adenoma sebaceum, periungual fibroma, glial tumors, rhabdomyoma of heart, renal tumor, lung cysts	AD

(table continues)

Table 5.1   (continued)

Disease	Associated Neoplasm(s)	Mode of Inheritance
Phakomatosis (continued)		
von Hippel–Lindau syndrome, hemangiomatosis	Retinal angioma, cerebellar hemangioblastoma, other hemangiomas, pheochromocytoma, hypernephroma, cysts	AD
Sturge-Weber syndrome	Angioma of numerous organs	AD
Mesodermal and skeletal systems		
Nevoid basal cell carcinoma syndrome	Basal cell carcinoma, medulloblastoma, jaw cysts, ovarian fibroma, and carcinoma	AD
Multiple hamartoma syndrome (Cowden disease)	Papillomatosis of lip and mouth, hypertrophic and cystic breast with early cancer, thyroid adenoma and carcinoma, bone and liver cysts, lipoma, polyps, meningioma	AD
Multiple lipomatosis, sometimes site specific, neck or conjunctiva, cervical	Skin cancer	AD
Multiple exostosis	Osteosarcoma, chondrosarcoma	AD
Fibro-osseous dysplasia	Osteosarcoma, medullary fibrosarcoma	AD
Hematopoietic malignancies		
Kostmann infantile genetic agranulocytosis	Acute monocytic leukemia (chromosomal breakage)	AR
Family cancer syndrome	Breast, colon, endometrium, lung carcinomas, lymphoma, or leukemia	AD
Ataxia telangiectasia	Lymphocytic leukemia and lymphomas, carcinoma of stomach, brain tumors (chromosomal breakage)	AR
DiGeorge syndrome	Squamous cell carcinoma of upper respiratory tract	AD
X-linked agammaglobulinemia	Leukemia, lymphoma	XR
Wiskott-Aldrich syndrome	Lymphoma	XR
Severe combined immunodeficiency	Lymphoma, leukemia, sarcoma	XR
X-linked recessive lymphoproliferative syndrome	B-cell lymphomas, fatal infectious mononucleosis, agammaglobulinemia	XR
Miscellaneous (multiple systems)		
Family cancer syndromes (Li-Fraumeni syndrome)	Colon, endometrium, ovary, breast, stomach carcinomas, lymphoma, sarcomas	AD

Key: AR, autosomal recessive; XR, X-linked recessive; AD, autosomal dominant.
Excerpted from a listing by Purtilo et al., 1978, as in Pitot, 1986.

excision repair (Chapter 3). Other autosomal recessive diseases with associated increased incidences of neoplasia may exhibit genetic abnormalities related to defects in the maintenance or repair of the structure of the genome. These include Bloom syndrome, Fanconi anemia, and ataxia telangiectasia (cf. Hanawalt and Sarasin, 1986). Several diseases in this category, such as Bloom syndrome, although manifest in all tissues, do not result in cancer of a wide variety of tissues, but the malignant lesions in such diseases are limited to specific and often uncommon organ sites (German, 1993). Individuals heterozygous for these diseases show little if any clinical abnormalities (Heim et al., 1992) with the exception of patients heterozygous for the gene of ataxia telangiectasia. A number of sites for cancer development have been reported in such heterozygous individuals (Swift et al., 1990), but a significant excess cancer risk occurs only for the breast in female relatives of ataxia telangiectasia patients (Easton, 1994). From an estimate of 1.4% incidence of ataxia telangiectasia heterozygotes in the U.S. population, Swift et al. (1990) have suggested that 9% to 18% of all cases of breast cancer in this country may occur in women heterozygous for mutation(s) in the ataxia telangiectasia gene, which has recently been cloned (Savitsky et al., 1995).

In addition to the specific disease entities mentioned above and listed in the table, it is now apparent that some individuals exhibit higher spontaneous mutation rates, as monitored by chromosome breakage rates, than other individuals (see below). Furthermore, it has been reported (Pero et al., 1989) that individuals with a family history of cancer exhibit a significant reduction in unscheduled DNA synthesis resulting from DNA repair, as evidenced in mononuclear leukocytes, compared with individuals with no family history of any major cancer. These factors, together with the evidence that certain nonneoplastic diseases that may be associated with an increased incidence of malignancy can also exhibit chromosomal instability—e.g., sarcoidosis (Okabe et al., 1986), Down's syndrome (Countryman et al., 1977), celiac disease (Fundia et al., 1994), and ulcerative colitis (Emerit et al., 1972)—suggest that a significant segment of the population may be at increased genetic risk for the development of neoplasia because of abnormalities in chromosomal stability. Several aspects of this phenomenon are considered later in this chapter.

Almost all of the neoplasms resulting from the diseases listed in Table 5.1 show the following characteristics: (1) a relatively early age of the clinical onset of the neoplasm, the same histogenetic type of neoplasm often occurring 20 or more years earlier than its occurrence in the general population in the absence of a specific genetic background; (2) an unusual excess of neoplasms occurring bilaterally in paired organs such as breast, adrenal, thyroid, kidney, acoustic nerve; (3) the appearance of multiple primary or multicentric cancers in nonpaired organs at a much higher frequency than seen in comparable histogenetic neoplasms not having a genetic basis; and (4) a predominance of autosomal dominant inheritance (Lynch et al., 1979).

Autosomal dominant disorders associated with an increased incidence of neoplasia usually exhibit an increase in one or a few specific types of neoplasms. One such disorder is familial polyposis of the colon, which is primarily associated with numerous polyps and ultimately carcinomas of the large bowel. A related and probably identical condition is Gardner syndrome, which was originally felt to involve primarily adenomas of the small bowel as well as other neoplasms, including those of the thyroid gland and the ampulla of Vater. However, recent investigations (Iida et al., 1989) strongly argue that these two conditions are the same disease, because both exhibit tumors in the tissues mentioned above as well as osteomas, benign tumors of soft tissue (desmoids), medulloblastomas of the cerebellum (Jagelman, 1991), and hepatoblastomas (cf. Bülow, 1989). Chromosomes of cells, both intestinal and others, have been found by a number of investigators to exhibit both numerical and structural aberrations (Gardner et al., 1982; Takai et al., 1986), and the morphology of skin fibroblasts grown in cell culture from patients with familial polyposis/Gardner syndrome exhibits changes indicating that such cells are abnormal and more closely resemble cells in the process of the neoplastic transformation in vitro (Antecol, 1988). Thus, alterations in a single gene, the APC gene (discussed below), can lead to the development of neoplasms in a variety of tissues as well as the cellular changes noted above.

Clinically, a closely related disease is hereditary nonpolyposis colorectal cancer (HNPCC), which was initially described by Warthin but studied most extensively by Lynch and his associates (1995). This disease differs from hereditary polyposis, discussed above, in that very few adenomas or polyps are present in affected individuals, their incidence not being increased relative to the general population (cf. Smyrk, 1994). The adenomas that are present are more often villous than polypoid, with a flat, spreading pattern that has a much greater tendency to progress to malignancy. As in familial polyposis, patients develop colon cancer at a young age and exhibit multiple cancers of the colon, with almost three-fourths occurring proximal to the splenic flexure (cf. Smyrk, 1994). Originally this disease was termed the "cancer family syndrome," because several other sites where neoplasia commonly developed in these patients had been noted. These included the endometrium, small intestine, stomach, ovary, and genitourinary tract (Watson and Lynch, 1993). HNPCC is decidedly more prevalent than familial polyposis, its occurrence being estimated at from 2% to 6% of all colorectal cancers (Kee and Collins, 1991; Lynch et al., 1991). If one considers individuals less than 35 years of age, the percentage exhibiting this genetic abnormality increases dramatically (Liu et al., 1995).

Another autosomal dominant condition in which neoplasms, primarily of mesenchymal origin, have been reported is that of von Recklinghausen neurofibromatosis. This condition is a relatively common trait, with a frequency of about 1 in 3000. Although the heterogeneous nature of the disease was recognized by von Recklinghausen himself, only recently has the disease been separated into at least two distinct clinical pictures, termed neurofibromatosis 1 and 2. The latter has also been termed bilateral acoustic neurofibromatosis (Martuza and Eldridge, 1988). Neurofibromatosis 1 affects approximately 100,000 people in the United States and is characterized by multiple brown skin macules (café au lait spots), intertriginous freckling, iris hamartomas (Lisch nodules), and multiple skin neurofibromas. Other benign mesenchymal tumors, neurological impairment, and bone abnormalities may also be seen. The hallmark of neurofibromatosis 2 is bilateral acoustic neuromas. Patients with mutations in the neurofibromatosis 2 gene are usually severely affected, and offspring show that the gene is almost completely penetrant. As with adenomas in familial polyposis, the neurofibromas may degenerate into neurofibrosarcomas and malignant schwannomas. In addition, other neoplasms—such as rhabdomyosarcoma, leukemia, pheochromocytoma, and Wilms tumor—may also be found in these patients (Riccardi, 1981). Another autosomal dominant disease affecting the skin is the dysplastic nevus syndrome, which is associated with a marked increase in atypical (dysplastic) nevi of the skin, which exhibit a propensity to develop into malignant melanomas, especially in younger affected individuals (Greene, 1984; Goldstein et al., 1994). Although there have been examples of the dysplastic nevus syndrome in patients with neurofibromatosis (Stokkel et al., 1993), a more extensive study revealed no significant excess of cancers other than malignant melanoma in patients with the dysplastic nevus syndrome (Tucker et al., 1993). Interestingly, at least two studies (Lynch et al., 1993; Caporaso et al., 1987) reported that nonneoplastic cells of patients with the dysplastic nevus syndrome exhibited significant chromosomal instability.

In various tissues with symmetrical distribution within the human body—including the retina, kidney, breast, and thyroid—the bilateral occurrence of neoplasia at a relatively early age usually indicates an autosomal dominant form of disease. Perhaps best known of these conditions is bilateral retinoblastoma, which is also clinically inherited as an autosomal dominant condition. The hereditary form of the disease represents about 40% of all cases of retinoblastoma; of these, 15% are unilateral and 25% bilateral. The remaining 60% are nonhereditary and unilateral (cf. Newsham et al., 1995). With respect to the hereditary form, there is nearly a 50%

risk that a child of an affected parent will receive the gene for the retinoblastoma, with a 90% chance (penetrance) of manifesting the neoplasm. Complete penetrance (50% incidence) resulted in offspring from parents with bilateral hereditary retinoblastoma, while only 42% of offspring of parents with hereditary unilateral retinoblastoma exhibited the disease (cf. Newsham et al., 1995). The vast majority of cases becine manifest during the first few years of life, and many patients may be treated successfully for this disease. However, such individuals have a dramatically increased risk of developing other neoplasms later in life, especially sarcomas of bone and connective tissue, malignant melanoma, neoplasms of the brain, and a variety of other cancers (Eng et al., 1993). Mortality from a second neoplasm is dramatically greater in patients with bilateral retinoblastoma than in those with unilateral disease. In addition, while somewhat controversial in the past, the study by Eng and his associates clearly indicates that patients with bilateral hereditary retinoblastoma receiving radiotherapy have a significantly greater risk of developing second primary neoplasms. This finding conforms to the results of a number of other studies indicating that cells of patients with hereditary retinoblastoma exhibit a hypersensitivity to DNA-damaging agents, including ionizing radiation (Heras and Larripa, 1988).

Another example of a bilateral neoplasm exhibiting an autosomal dominant mode of inheritance is Wilms tumor of the kidney. The incidence of synchronous bilateral Wilms tumor varies between 4.4% and 9% of all cases (Mesrobian, 1988); Knudson and Strong (1972) have presented evidence that all bilateral cases and a substantial number of unilateral cases of Wilms tumor are the result of a germinal mutation. On this basis, although the exact incidence of the hereditary form of Wilms tumor is not as clear as that of retinoblastoma, more than 10% of all cases of Wilms tumor exhibit a Mendelian type of inheritance. Furthermore, most cases of the hereditary form arise in multiple sites in both kidneys, at times producing a condition known as nephroblastomatosis, a phenomenon related to the normal method of growth of the renal blastema (Mesrobian, 1988). Of patients with bilateral Wilms tumor, 60% also exhibit various congenital abnormalities, the most common of which is aniridia. In this latter instance, the combination of Wilms tumor with aniridia (lack of ocular irises), genitourinary malformations, and mental retardation forms a syndrome known as the WAGR syndrome. Two other syndromes in which Wilms tumor occurs are the Denys-Drash syndrome, in which many patients exhibit intersexual disorders along with the Wilms tumor, and the Beckwith-Wiedemann syndrome, in which patients sometimes exhibit Wilms tumor in association with enlargement of a number of organs. Genes for each of these conditions occur near that for Wilms tumor on the short arm of chromosome 11 (cf. Coppes et al., 1994). Patients with hereditary Wilms tumor show little if any evidence of an increased risk for the development of other neoplasms; however, another autosomal dominant condition, von Hippel-Lindau disease (vHL), is manifest by the development of renal adenocarcinoma and, in addition, exhibits complex manifestations in multiple organ systems with tumors, both benign and malignant, in the brain, pancreas, and adrenals (Lamiell et al., 1989). Renal malignancy is seen in about 25% of vHL patients, and about 60% of these exhibit bilateral incidence of neoplasms. Evidence of neoplasia in vHL patients occurs prior to age 40; by careful screening, the diagnosis may be made much earlier. Unlike the histology of Wilms tumor, which exhibits an embryonic pattern, tumors in vHL are renal cell (clear cell) carcinomas or hypernephromas (Linenan et al., 1995). In addition, at least two other forms of hereditary renal cell cancer, one exhibiting a pattern similar to that of vHL and the other exhibiting a papillary pattern, have been described (Maher and Yates, 1991; Linenan et al., 1995). Interestingly, several investigators (Foster et al., 1994; Shuin et al., 1994; Whaley et al., 1994) have reported that from one-third to more than one-half of sporadic renal cell carcinomas exhibit mutations in the vHL gene.

The endocrine system is another organ system exhibiting bilaterality of hereditary neoplasia. As noted in Table 5.1, there are two general types of multiple endocrine neoplasia (MEN)—

types I and II. Type II is separated into A and B subtypes, since the clinical picture in these cases differs somewhat, resulting from different mutations within the affected gene. The bilateral neoplasms seen in MEN I are those of the parathyroids, small glands associated with the lateral aspects of the thyroid gland, usually occurring in pairs on each side of the neck. Patients exhibit abnormalities in calcium metabolism resulting from the hyperfunctioning of both hyperplasias and neoplasms of the parathyroid. In addition, neoplasms of the pancreatic islet cells as well as the pituitary are found (Bone, 1990). The age of onset of this disease is variable but is rare in childhood and uncommonly seen after age 60. Years may elapse between the discovery of one neoplasm and the appearance of the next (Schimke, 1984). In MEN II, the predominant neoplasms seen in both the A and B subtypes are medullary thyroid carcinoma and pheochromocytoma. The A form of this condition also exhibits parathyroid neoplasia, whereas the B form does not. Conversely, the B form exhibits striking facial features, such as enlargement of the lips, and abnormalities of the peripheral nervous system, including neuromatous nodules in and around the mouth, as well as mucosal neuromas in the gastrointestinal tract and other abnormalities of the nerves in the digestive tract, especially the colon. In the A form, the parafollicular C cell of the thyroid becomes focally hyperplastic at an early age; from it, multifocal, bilateral medullary thyroid cancers may develop (Schimke, 1984; Gagel, 1994). Medullary thyroid cancers in the B form develop at an even earlier age and are usually more malignant than those in the A form (Schimke, 1984).

One of the more obvious bilateral organs exhibiting a high incidence of neoplasia is the female breast. The environmental risks associated with the development of breast cancer are the subject of a later chapter (Chapter 10). The genetic risks to relatives of patients with breast cancer have been a topic of considerable study for the past several decades. In general, the risk of developing breast cancer in immediate relatives of cases diagnosed prior to age 40 is fivefold greater than that in individuals with no family history and twofold greater for relatives of cases diagnosed over age 50 (cf. Easton et al., 1993). The risk of breast cancer is much greater in women with two or more affected first-degree relatives than in women with only one affected relative. The risk of developing breast cancer is also significantly greater in the relatives of metachronous bilateral cases of breast cancer than in those relatives of patients with unilateral breast cancer (Bernstein et al., 1992). These findings, which have developed during the past decade, led to the suggestion that a small proportion of breast cancer cases are likely due to the inheritance of a highly penetrant gene, the proportion of genetic cases being highest at younger ages, especially in those under age 30 (Easton et al., 1993). In the last few years, several candidate genes for dominant breast cancer susceptibility have been discovered and/or proposed (Eeles et al., 1994). In a recent estimation, Friedman et al. (1994) suggested that as many as 1 in 200 women will develop breast cancer over the normal life span as a result of a germline inherited susceptibility in the United States. It is likely that more than a single gene is involved in this inherited susceptibility, and breast cancer is still one of the most common genetic diseases in the world. To date the most frequent single gene associated with hereditary breast cancer is the *BRCA1* gene, first localized by Hall et al. (1990b) through linkage studies and recently isolated and characterized by Miki and his colleagues (1994). The frequency of significant mutations in the *BRCA1* gene contributing to breast and also ovarian cancer has been estimated to be 7 in 10,000 individuals or roughly 0.1% of the population (Easton et al., 1993). For patients bearing a mutated copy of the *BRCA1* gene, the cumulative risk of developing breast and ovarian cancer is seen in Figure 5.1. The data in this figure, developed from a study of human patients, are drawn for two different susceptibility alleles or mutations conferring high or moderate risk of ovarian cancer, whereas the same two alleles show little difference in the risk of breast cancer. In contrast, if one considers the proportion of breast cancer cases that result from dominant gene mutations as a function of age at diagnosis, the curves are the reverse of that seen in Figure 5.1

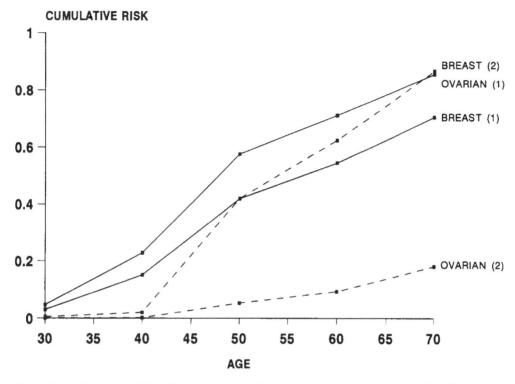

Figure 5.1 Cumulative risks of breast cancer (continuous lines) and ovarian cancer (dashed lines) in carriers of the *BRCA1* mutation. These risk estimates assume allelic heterogeneity in which there are two susceptibility alleles, one of which is associated with a high ovarian cancer risk (1) and the other with moderate to low ovarian cancer risk (2). (Reproduced from Easton et al., 1993, with permission of authors and publisher.)

(Figure 5.2). Interestingly, Tulinius et al. (1994) have presented evidence that the risk of cancer at all sites in relatives of breast cancer patients is increased over that of the general, unrelated population. While this latter study was carried out in Iceland, it still further emphasizes that the genetics of breast cancer development is complex and in many instances, where there is some genetic predisposition, is likely to be multifactorial.

The onset of breast cancer at a relatively early age is also a characteristic of the Li-Fraumeni syndrome, which is a clinically dominant disease in which gene carriers exhibit a high risk of childhood sarcomas, early onset of breast cancer, brain tumors, leukemia, and adrenocortical carcinoma (Li et al., 1988; Malkin, 1994). However, this is a relatively rare disease and is causative in far less than 1% of all breast cancers (Eeles et al., 1994). In cultured fibroblasts from these patients, spontaneous aneuploidy and relative resistance to the killing effect of ionizing radiation are noted (Bischoff et al., 1990; Chang et al., 1987). The gene whose mutations are the basis for most patients with the Li-Fraumeni syndrome, the *p53* gene, has been well characterized and is discussed later.

Although Mendelian inheritance suggests that the genetic constitution of the host is the prime causative factor in the development of benign and malignant neoplasms listed in Table 5.1, it should be obvious that the environment also plays a significant role. This becomes even more important in consideration of the multigenic inheritance of a predisposition to cancer.

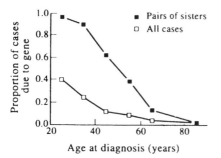

Figure 5.2 The proportion of breast cancer cases resulting from dominant mutations in autosomal genes as a function of the age of the patient. (Reproduced from Eeles et al., 1994, with permission of authors and publisher.)

A MUTATIONAL THEORY OF INHERITED AND SPONTANEOUS (SPORADIC) CANCER

While the diseases listed in Table 5.1 presumably develop as a result of mutations within a single gene, mostly unique to that disease, this knowledge tells us little about how the disease actually develops. In fact, if the mutation is in the germline, then every cell of the organism possesses a copy of that mutated gene within its nucleus. If such a mutational change were truly dominant in all cells, the host would be expected to develop neoplasms of numerous if not all tissues. This does not occur, although in many diseases listed in Table 5.1, both dominant and recessive, neoplasia of several tissues may develop. Thus, the expression of the abnormal gene that leads to the neoplastic change must require a number of other accompanying changes that may be genetic, environmental, or both.

A reasonable solution to this dilemma was first proposed by Knudson (1971), who hypothesized a two-mutational (two-hit) theory of carcinogenesis. His theory was developed primarily to explain the epidemiological findings seen in hereditary retinoblastoma, in which nearly two-thirds of the hereditary cases were bilateral but all of the sporadic cases were unilateral. The former cases occurred in very young patients (mean age, 18 months), whereas the sporadic unilateral cases developed at an average of 30 months or more. On the assumption that mutational events occur at random and a relatively fixed rate, Knudson reasoned that at least two mutational events, now understood to be frequently in each allele of the same gene, were necessary to convert a normal cell into a neoplastic cell. If the first mutation or hit were postzygotic (spontaneous or sporadic), the progeny of this mutated cell would then be at an increased risk of developing into a neoplasm when one or more cells received a second hit involving the normal allele. However, since spontaneous mutagenic events are of the order of 1 in 10^5 per genetic locus (Bridges et al., 1994; Glickman et al., 1994) the chance of a spontaneous two-mutational event would be 1 in 10^{10}, which is highly unlikely and conforms, at the cellular level, to a very rare occurrence, as is generally true of spontaneous cancer. If, however, the first hit were present in the germline (prezygotic), with all cells in the organism having a mutation in one allele of the disease gene, then a second hit would be 10^5 times more common. Thus, in such individuals, neoplasms would be expected to develop much earlier, more frequently, and bilaterally in tissues in which neoplasia commonly developed. Furthermore, in this model, the neoplastic susceptibility would be transmitted as an autosomal dominant trait, as noted clinically (Bolande and Vekemans, 1983). A diagram of the two-hit theory of Knudson is seen in Figure 5.3.

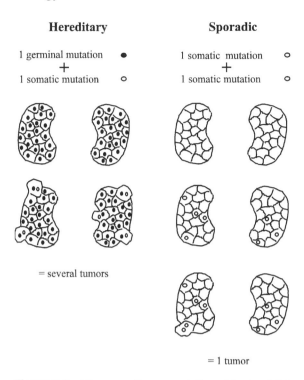

Hereditary   **Sporadic**

1 germinal mutation   ●   1 somatic mutation   ○
        +   +
1 somatic mutation   ○   1 somatic mutation   ○

= several tumors

= 1 tumor

Figure 5.3   Diagrammatic representation of the two-hit theory of Knudson and associates. (Reproduced from Junien, 1989, with permission of author and publisher.)

When first proposed, this theory or model was felt to be potentially applicable to certain germline-dominant diseases associated with a high incidence of neoplasia. Today, Knudson's theory is regarded as a major basis for our understanding of the process of carcinogenesis, the pathogenesis of neoplasia. Furthermore, the theory set the stage for a more complete understanding of many of the genetic and environmental factors in neoplastic development. Thus, while almost all of the evidence points to a genetic basis for the conversion of a normal to a neoplastic cell, Knudson's theory made a clear distinction between germline genetic changes and somatic (nongermline) genetic changes. In the clinically autosomal dominant conditions leading to neoplasia, the germline mutation put all cells of the organism at some degree of risk for a somatic mutation that would result in a neoplastic cell. In the development of nonhereditary cancer, both mutations or hits must have occurred in both alleles in individual somatic cells. If the two hits occur, one in each allele of the gene whose abnormal function leads to the development of neoplasia, then the normal or wild-type gene must give rise to a product that protects the cell from undergoing the neoplastic transformation. Expression of only one normal copy of the gene is sufficient to prevent the appearance of the neoplastic phenotype. The genotypes of normal and neoplastic cells in wild-type, heterozygous, and homozygous abnormal cells may be seen in Table 5.2. This table shows the number of somatic events required before neoplasia develops, along with the genotypes of the host cell and the neoplastic cell. Because of their function in preventing or suppressing the neoplastic transformation of somatic cells, such genes have been termed *tumor suppressor genes*. A more complete discussion of these genes appears later in this chapter.

Table 5.2 Tumors Caused by Recessive Tumor Suppressor Genes in Hosts of Different Genotypes

Germline Genotype	Normal Host Cell	Neoplastic Cell	Number of Somatic Events	Probability of Neoplasms
Normal	+/+	–/–	2	Rare
Heterozygote	+/–	–/–	1	≈1
Homozygous abnormal	–/–	–/–	0	Many? (lethal)

Key: +, wild-type or normal gene; –, defective or deleted allele.
Based on Knudson, 1985.

Genetic Evidence Supporting the "Two-Hit" Development of Neoplasia

As noted above, Knudson's original proposal of the two-mutational concept of neoplastic development was based primarily on epidemiological data and appropriate models to explain the data. It was not until a number of years after the proposal was first enunciated that cytogenetic and molecular genetic evidence developed in its support. Both of these technologies are considered here, as well as much of the evidence that has developed in support of Knudson's thesis.

The Cytogenetics of Germline, Dominantly Inherited Cancer

Each species of living organism has evolved in such a way that its genome is packaged into a number of structures termed *chromosomes*. Both the number and the structure of chromosomes are characteristic of the species, so that, for example, the human exhibits a haploid (one copy of each chromosome only) number of 23 chromosomes in its karyotype. However, most vertebrates exhibit two copies of the chromosome within each somatic cell in the female, while the male has one copy of the X and one copy of the Y chromosome. These last two are termed *sex chromosomes*, while all others in the karyotype are termed *autosomes*. Thus, the human karyotype for all cells except certain germ cells and cells of some glandular organs is 46 chromosomes. This number differs for other species; e.g., the rat karyotype is 42 chromosomes, that of the mouse 40 chromosomes, the hamster 44, etc.

Appropriate methods have been developed to allow the microscopic examination of chromosomes and karyotypes of cells. In 1970, Caspersson and associates were among the first to develop techniques that allowed studies of the substructure of chromosomes with the light microscope and assured definitive identification of individual autosomes. These techniques, which have now been modified and extended by a variety of workers, have allowed the identification of "bands" or regions of differential staining of the arms of individual chromatids in a variety of species. Specific patterns of banding, characteristic of the species as well as of each of the chromosomes within any one species, have now been described. Furthermore, the localization of individual genes on specific chromosomes and in relation to specific bands has been described in a number of mammalian species as well as other species, both vertebrate and invertebrate. Figure 5.4 shows a diagram of chromosome 13 of the human karyotype, including its banding patterns and indicating the position of a number of genes in the two arms of the chromosome. As noted in the figure, the short arm is designated as the *p* arm, while the long arm is the *q* arm. The two are separated by the centromere. In chromosome 13 the short arm (*p*) is polymorphic in nature, and variations in size may occur in the heterochromatic satellite region (*p*13), the nucleolar organizer or secondary constriction (*p*12), and the short arm proper (*p*11) (Yunis et al., 1979). One should

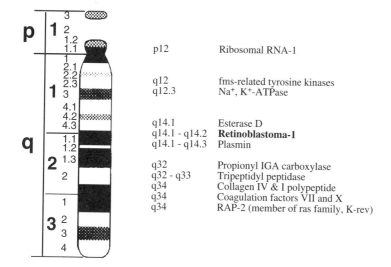

p12   Ribosomal RNA-1

q12   fms-related tyrosine kinases
q12.3   Na⁺, K⁺-ATPase

q14.1   Esterase D
q14.1 - q14.2   **Retinoblastoma-1**
q14.1 - q14.3   Plasmin

q32   Propionyl IGA carboxylase
q32 - q33   Tripeptidyl peptidase
q34   Collagen IV & I polypeptide
q34   Coagulation factors VII and X
q34   RAP-2 (member of ras family, K-rev)

Figure 5.4 Diagrammatic representation of human chromosome 13 in early metaphase, showing major and minor bands, with the designation of the band positions of a number of genes shown on the right. (Modified from Yunis et al., 1979; McKusick and Amberger, 1995.)

also note that each arm is separated into regions designated by the large numbers within the blocked spaces and bands designated by the smaller numbers adjacent to individual bands of the chromatid in the figure. This nomenclature was first standardized at an international conference held in Paris in 1971 (Paris Conference, 1972). Later refinements have been undertaken in this country for international use (ISCN, 1985). Thus, it is now possible to designate specific regions of the chromosome according to the specific banding pattern as standardized by this nomenclature. Although aberrations in karyotypes are not only characteristic of but perhaps ubiquitously associated with malignant neoplasia (see below), it is only in the last two decades that specific chromosomal alterations have been associated with neoplasms resulting from specific inheritance patterns.

As indicated earlier, the recessive conditions of Bloom syndrome, Fanconi anemia, and ataxia telangiectasia are associated with chromosomal instability, but no specific chromosomal alterations have been demonstrated in these and other conditions that exhibit a more generalized instability of karyotypes. However, in cancer-prone syndromes of a dominant type of inheritance, in a number of instances either specific chromosomal alterations or specific structural gene alterations have been demonstrated during the past 15 years, as evidenced by techniques of cytogenetics or molecular biology, respectively. These findings have, in turn, led to the localization of specific gene(s) that appear to be responsible for the defect and the resulting neoplasm.

Table 5.3 lists some specific chromosomal changes associated with autosomal dominant inherited cancers. Best known is the association of hereditary retinoblastoma with a small deletion in the long arm of chromosome 13 (Francke and Kung, 1976; Wilson et al., 1973). Less than 5% of patients with retinoblastoma show such deletions (Horsthemke, 1992), but recent evidence indicates that even those patients with normal chromosomal karyotype express molecular biological and biochemical evidence of genetic abnormalities in this chromosomal structure. Benedict et al. (1983) reported that patients with the characteristic chromosomal deletion exhibit only half the normal activity of esterase D, the gene for which appears to be closely linked to the area of deletion. In one patient with bilateral retinoblastoma and a normal karyotype, only 50%

Table 5.3   Specific Chromosomal Changes Associated with Cancer-Prone Autosomal
Dominant Conditions

Neoplasm	Chromosomal Abnormality	References
Familial polyposis coli	5p21 deletion	Hockey et al., 1989; Herrera et al., 1986
Familial renal cell carcinoma	3p;8q (p14.2; q24.1) translocation	Drabkin et al., 1985; LaFargia et al., 1993
von Hippel–Lindau disease	3p13-pter deletion	Kovacs, 1991
Retinoblastoma	13(q14.1 q14.3) deletion	Sparkes, 1984
von Recklinghausen neurofibromatosis 1	17q;22q translocation	Ledbetter et al., 1989
neurofibromatosis 2	4q; 22q (q12; q12.2) translocation	Arai et al., 1992
Wilms tumor	11p13 deletion	cf. Housman, 1992

of the normal esterase D activity was found in the patient's normal cells. Interestingly, in cells isolated from the neoplasm of this patient and exhibiting abnormalities of chromosome 13, no detectable esterase D activity was found. More recent studies have demonstrated that the esterase D gene is closely linked to that coding for retinoblastoma (van der Heiden et al., 1988; Table 5.3). In further support of the two-hit theory, the second retinoblastoma allele frequently is lost by chromosomal mechanisms (Cavenee et al., 1983).

Another example of chromosomal abnormalities in hereditary neoplasms is the demonstration of a constitutional deletion on the short arm of chromosome 11 in some patients with Wilms tumor, specifically those with the WAGR syndrome, which includes a predisposition to Wilms tumor (W), aniridia (A), genitourinary abnormalities (G), and mental retardation (R). There is much variation in the size of these deletions, but chromosome band 11p13 is invariably involved in the WAGR syndrome (Riccardi et al., 1978). Other phenotypic features frequently associated with these deletions include congenital absence of the irises (aniridia), gonadal dysplasia, and mental retardation. However, only 50% of patients with the congenital defects actually develop Wilms tumor, indicative of the incomplete penetrance of the mutation predisposing to the neoplasm or linked genes with different functions being deleted. More recently, several authors have also demonstrated that hereditary renal cell carcinoma, an autosomal dominant condition, is associated with translocations between the short arm of chromosome 3 and other chromosomes, especially 11 and 8 (cf. Table 5.3). Although this condition is quite rare, when the translocation involves chromosome 8, it has also been reported to involve the c-*myc* proto-oncogene, reminiscent of similar translocations seen in Burkitt's lymphoma, resulting from somatic changes in the karyotype (Drabkin et al., 1985). However, no rearrangement or abnormality in the structure of the translocated proto-oncogene has yet been described. Finally, the balanced translocation between chromosomes 17 and 22 seen in a female patient with von Recklinghausen neurofibromatosis 1 was actually an unusual manifestation, but, as shown below, it offered a clue to the localization of the gene for this condition. Not shown in the table is the fact that hereditary medullary carcinoma of the thyroid has also been found to be associated with a preponderance of chromosomal structural abnormalities, as noted in karyotype preparations (Hsu et al., 1991).

Obviously, chromosomal deletions visible in the light microscope represent major alterations in the genome, reflecting thousands of kilobases of DNA lost from that chromosome. Localization of the gene involved (usually 15 to 40 kilobases in size) requires more refined technology, which has now been employed not only in the localization of genes for neoplasms exhibiting a Mendelian type of heredity but also for numerous other genetic diseases as well.

The Molecular Genetics of Germline, Dominantly Inherited Cancer

The constitutional chromosomal deletions in several dominant neoplastic diseases supported the two-hit hypothesis, but such examples (Table 5.3) were relatively unusual, and the biochemical evidence, like that exemplified by the esterase D changes noted in hereditary retinoblastoma, was exceptional. More recent techniques have allowed more detailed analysis of genetic material to the point of and including the isolation and structural characterization of the genes involved in many dominantly inherited diseases with high incidences of neoplasia (Table 5.4).

As we have already noted (Table 5.2), by the two-hit theory, both alleles of the gene involved in a specific neoplasm, whether of hereditary or spontaneous origin, will have lost the function of the gene in question. In the case of a germline inherited neoplastic condition, all cells of the organism will exhibit heterozygosity of the gene locus, one allele being functional and the other not. Thus, the neoplasm will have lost this heterozygous state to become homozygous for the defective gene. Below it is shown that loss of heterozygosity can also be determined in diseases of somatic cell origin since, by the two-hit theory, they would also be expected to exhibit a homozygous genotype, as noted in Table 5.2.

The mutated gene in dominantly inherited neoplastic disease may be the result of point mutations, small or larger deletions, or nonsense mutations leading to a truncation of the protein. Mutation in the second allele, especially in dominantly inherited neoplasms, will be the result of chromosomal abnormalities such as translocations, major deletions, recombination, etc. (Lasko et al., 1991). It is also possible, however, that loss of function of the second allele may be far more subtle, such as point mutations or minor deletions. When such changes occur, examination of the karyotype may not be informative, since no chromosomal aberration can be detected. However, one may use a molecular analysis, termed restriction fragment length polymorphism (RFLP) analysis, which involves the use of restriction enzymes that cleave DNA strands at spe-

Table 5.4 Structure and Function of Genes of Dominantly Inherited Neoplastic Diseases

Gene	Disease	Gene Product	Subcellular Location	Function
RB1	Retinoblastoma	pRB	Nucleus	Transcription factor
NF1	Neurofibromatosis type 1	Neurofibromin	Cytoplasm	GTPase activating protein (GAP)
p53	Li-Fraumeni syndrome	p53	Nucleus	Transcription factor
NF2	Neurofibromatosis type 2	Merlin	Cytoskeleton	Integration of cytoskeleton with plasma membrane
ret	MEN II	*ret* kinase	Plasma membrane	Receptor tyrosine kinase
WT1	Wilms tumor syndrome	WT1	Nucleus	Transcription factor
DCC	Familial colon cancer	DCC	Plasma membrane	Cell adhesion
APC	Familial polyposis	APC	Cytoplasm	β-catenin binding
MTS1	Familial melanoma	p16	Nucleus	Kinase inhibitor
VHL	von Hippel–Lindau syndrome	VHL	Unknown	Unknown
MSH2	Hereditary nonpolyposis colorectal cancer	MSH2	Nucleus	DNA repair
MLH1	Hereditary nonpolyposis colorectal cancer	MLH1	Nucleus	DNA repair

Modified from Skuse and Ludlow, 1995.

cific base sequences. Since numerous such restriction enzymes, each acting on a specific sequence of DNA extending from four to seven or more bases, are known (Roberts and Macelis, 1992), one may survey a variety of sequences in the DNA for changes. Such an RFLP analysis is diagrammed in Figure 5.5 between normal and tumor DNA, using two examples of DNA structure. In one case the normal DNA of a gene is cleaved in three places by a single restriction enzyme. This leads to three possible fragments of different sizes. In the second instance the diagram involves a segment of DNA containing numerous repeated sequences. In each instance shown, each horizontal line represents a segment of one allele of the gene investigated. In the case where tandem repeats are present and the restriction enzyme cuts adjacent to the repeats as well as somewhere else in the genome, only two fragments are obtained. If there is a deletion of one of the copies or of the segment with a restriction sequence or if there is a mutation of the restriction sequence, then digestion of the DNA in each case results in only a single band. Electrophoresis of the bands and their reaction with the probe, a complementary sequence to a portion of the DNA, as shown in the figure, results in a pattern shown in the lower portion of the

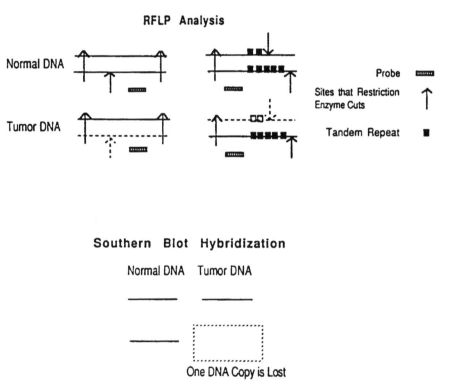

Figure 5.5 Restriction fragment length polymorphism (RFLP) method for the detection of allelic loss in somatic cells. Minor variation in base sequences or repetitive sequences may occur without alteration of the proteins encoded. Such alterations induce variations in recognition sites for restriction enzymes which cleave DNA at specific sequences. Following cleavage the DNA is electrophoresed, bands (molecules) separated, blotted to a filter and hybridized with a radiolabeled DNA probe which recognizes a sequence involved in the restriction reaction. In the Southern blot hybridization depicted, the normal genomic DNA on the left contains a polymorphism recognized by the probe as two bands of different molecular sizes, each of which corresponds to one of the two allelic copies. If one of the alleles has been deleted as a result of restriction digestion, then one band will be missing allowing molecular confirmation of the deletion event. (Modified from Viallet and Minna, 1990, with permission of the authors and publisher.)

figure. The small band expected in the digestion of normal DNA without repeats would have migrated off the gel and not be seen. As noted, in both instances one copy of the DNA is lost in the neoplasm as a result of genetic alteration, thus demonstrating the loss of heterozygosity in the tumor DNA. Table 5.5 lists dominantly inherited neoplastic diseases in which a loss of heterozygosity has been demonstrated. Examination of the table reveals that a number of regions of loss of heterozygosity do not necessarily indicate the chromosomal localization of the gene for the disease (Table 5.6), and in some instances several different chromosomal sites with loss of heterozygosity may be noted in the same genetic condition—e.g., MEN II, familial breast cancer. Furthermore, in this example, the chromosomal localization of the gene primarily affected in MEN II does not exhibit loss of heterozygosity (Table 5.6). This conforms to the nature of the gene involved, the *ret* proto-oncogene, which was first isolated from DNA originating from a human T-cell lymphoma (Takahashi et al., 1985). As discussed previously (Chapter 4), alterations in proto-oncogenes are dominant in their effects, and thus mutation in a single allele of the *ret* gene might be expected to result in neoplastic disease. In Table 5.5, there are also several instances in which the loss of heterozygosity has been used to aid in the localization and ultimate isolation and characterization of the gene affected in the disease under study—e.g., von Hippel–Lindau syndrome, familial melanoma, tuberous sclerosis.

Through the use of the two techniques described above, cytogenetic analysis and RFLP analysis, the chromosomal localization of a number of autosomal dominant conditions predisposing to specific neoplastic disease has been elucidated (Table 5.6). With localization of the genes to specific chromosomal regions coupled with a knowledge of other genes and genetic markers in the region of the locus being investigated (Figure 5.4), several of these genes have been isolated and characterized through the use of a variety of molecular biological and molecular genetic techniques. A reasonably up-to-date listing of genes that are mutated in specific dominantly inherited neoplastic disease and whose sequence structure has been elucidated are listed

Table 5.5 Loss of Heterozygosity in Dominantly Inherited Neoplasms

Chromosome region	Neoplasm	Reference
1p	Familial breast carcinoma	Lindblom et al., 1993b
1p	MEN IIA	Mathew et al., 1987
1q	Familial breast carcinoma	Lindblom et al., 1993b
3p25-p26	von Hippel–Lindau syndrome	Richards et al., 1993
3p	Familial renal cell carcinoma	Zbar et al., 1987
3q	MEN IIA	Mulligan et al., 1993
5	Familial polyposis	Sasaki et al., 1989
9p13-p22	Familial melanoma	Walker et al., 1994
9q23.1-q31	Nevoid basal cell carcinoma syndrome	Chenevix-Trench et al., 1993
11p	Wilms tumor	Wadey et al., 1990
11p13-pter	MEN II	Mulligan et al., 1993
11q13	MEN I	Radford et al., 1990
16p13	Tuberous sclerosis	Nellist et al., 1993
16q	Wilms tumor	Maw et al., 1992
16q	Familial breast cancer	Lindblom et al., 1993a
17p	Neurofibromatosis 1	Menon et al., 1990
17p	Familial breast cancer	Lindblom et al., 1993b
17q12-q21	Familial breast cancer	Lalle et al., 1994
22q	Neurofibromatosis 2	Couturier et al., 1990

Table 5.6 Chromosomal Localization of Genes for Dominantly Inherited Neoplastic Disease

Disease	Chromosomal Locus	Reference
Beckwith-Wiedemann syndrome	11p15	Koufos et al., 1989
Familial glomus tumors	11q23-qter	Heutink et al., 1992
Familial melanoma	9p21	Hussussian et al., 1994
Familial breast cancer	17q21 (BRCA1)	Hall et al., 1990b
	13q12-13 (BRCA2)	Wooster et al., 1994
Familial polyposis	5q21-22	Bodmer et al., 1987
Hereditary nonpolyposis colon cancer	3p21.3-23	Bronner et al., 1994
	2p21-22	Fishel et al., 1993
Li-Fraumeni syndrome	17p13	McBride et al., 1986
Multiple endocrine neoplasia		
Type I	11q12-13	Larsson et al., 1988
Type IIA,B	10q11-12	Mathew et al., 1987
Neurofibromatosis		
Type 1	17q12-22	Seizinger et al., 1987
Type 2	22q11.1-13.1	Wertelecki et al., 1988
Retinoblastoma	13q14.1-14.3	Sparkes, 1984
Tuberous sclerosis	16p13.3	Nellist et al., 1993
von Hippel–Lindau disease	3p25	Seizinger et al., 1991
Wilms tumor (WAGR and Denys-Drash syndrome)	11p13 (WT1)	cf. Gerald, 1994

in Table 5.6. While it is beyond the scope of this text to depict the structure and sequences of the genes listed in Tables 5.4 and 5.6, examples of a single, relatively large gene, that for retinoblastoma (over 200 kb pairs), and a relatively small gene (about 50 kb pairs), that for the von Hippel–Lindau syndrome, are depicted in Figure 5.6. Thus, the degree of complexity of the genes is not a factor in whether they served as the basis for dominantly inherited neoplastic disease. All of the genes listed in Table 5.6 with the exception of that for MEN IIA and B conform to the two-hit theory of Knudson, in that both alleles of the gene must be mutated in order that one or more neoplasms arise. As noted earlier, the principal exception to this to date is MEN IIA and B, in which only one of the two alleles need be mutated for neoplasia to arise.

At this point the student should appreciate that the evidence in support of the two-hit theory is quite substantial for a number of dominantly inherited neoplastic conditions. However, other mechanisms have been described in which the neoplastic phenotype may result from mutations in only one of the alleles of the gene in question. Dominant negative mutations of some genes noted in Table 5.6 have been described and are the result of specific alterations in the tumor suppressor gene such that the mutant protein may disrupt the function of the products of the normal allele through the formation of protein complexes between mutant and normal proteins or through abnormal interactions with DNA sequences that are the target of the normal gene. This phenomenon has now been described for the WT1 (Reddy et al., 1995) and the *p53* genes (Srivastava et al., 1993).

Another mechanism resulting in the loss of function of both alleles in neoplastic tissues may be seen when the gene in question is imprinted in one or the other parent (Rainier and Feinberg, 1994). Gene imprinting occurs when the allele of a gene inherited from one parent is repressed and not expressed in cells of the offspring. A diagram of such a phenomenon is seen in Figure 5.7 in relation to the imprinting of a tumor suppressor gene. Imprinting of the gene is presumed to involve methylation of the DNA bases, resulting in repression and nonexpression of

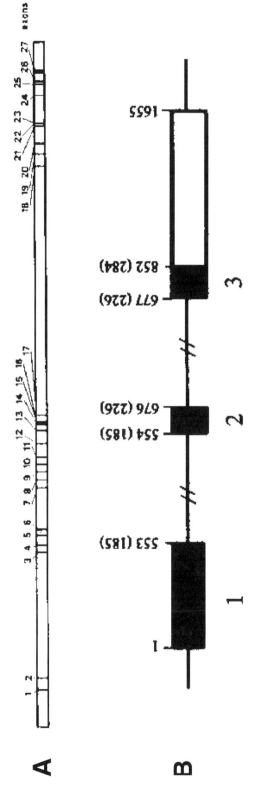

Figure 5.6 A. Diagram of the *RB-1* gene, which consists of 27 exons spread over a length of 200 kb. (From Kloss et al., 1991, with permission of the authors and publisher.) B. Structure of the VHL tumor suppressor gene. The boxes show the exons with the coding region dark and the 3′ untranslated region unshaded. The numbers correspond to the nucleotide numbers in the cDNA, and the codon numbers are in parenthesis. (Reproduced from Foster et al., 1994, with permission of the authors and publisher.)

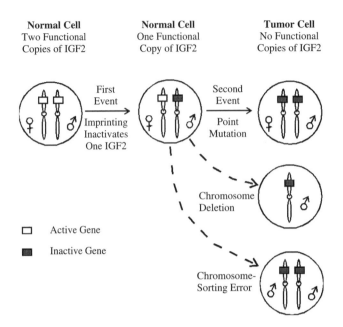

Figure 5.7 Parental imprinting of the insulin growth factor-2 (IGF2) gene, which is potentially involved in Wilms tumor development. With imprinting of one gene, only mutation or loss of the other gene is required to eliminate its function. (Reproduced from Sapienza, 1990, with permission of the author and publisher.)

the gene from that parent (Razin and Cedar, 1994). The methylation is inherited epigenetically from one or the other parent, thus resulting in the expression of only a single, nonmethylated gene from the other parent. While as yet there is no clear and distinct example that has been proven to follow the scheme seen in Figure 5.7, there is evidence of the imprinting of tumor suppressor genes or other related genes affecting or affected by the expression of a tumor suppressor gene. In Table 5.7 are listed some examples of dominantly inherited neoplasia for which there is some evidence for the imprinting (repression) of genes, both known and un-known. New mutations giving rise to bilateral retinoblastoma exhibit a marked preference for the paternal allele of the RB gene, suggesting as one mechanism that imprinting early in embryonic life affects chromosomal susceptibility to mutation (Zhu et al., 1989). Similarly, in MEN II, all new mutations were of paternal origin (Carlson et al., 1994). Alleles in the neoplasms of familial and sporadic cases of embryonal rhabdomyosarcoma are of paternal origin (Scrable et al., 1989). In contrast, in familial glomus tumors it is the maternal allele that appears to be imprinted (repressed), although the exact nature of the gene is as yet unknown (van der Mey et al., 1989).

A potential role for genomic imprinting in carcinogenesis is best exhibited by findings of the Beckwith-Wiedemann syndrome. In addition to various somatic manifestations including organomegaly (kidney, liver, and adrenal), hemihypertrophy, and gigantism, neoplasms arise in these individuals, including Wilms tumor and embryonal rhabdomyosarcoma (cf. Tycko, 1994). Although there is not substantial evidence for imprinting of the WT1 gene, two genes found very close to WT1, H19 and IGF2, are imprinted from different parents. H19 is expressed from the maternal allele and IGF2 from the paternal allele. Rainier demonstrated that more than two-thirds of Wilms tumors exhibiting no loss of heterozygosity in the region of the WT1 gene ex-

Table 5.7 Gene Imprinting and Dominantly Inherited Neoplasia

Neoplasm	Imprinted Gene (parental)	Reference
Bilateral retinoblastoma	RB (P)	Dryja et al., 1989
	RB (?)	Zhu et al., 1989
		Naumova and Sapienza, 1994
MEN II	*ret* (?)	Carlson et al., 1994
Rhabdomyosarcoma	? (P)	Scrable et al., 1989
Familial glomus tumors	? (M)	van der Mey et al., 1989
Beckwith-Wiedemann syndrome	H19 (P)	Rainier et al., 1993
	IGF2 (M)	Rainier et al., 1993

Key: P, paternal imprint; M, maternal imprint

hibited biallelic expression of one or both of these genes. Since IGF2 codes for a growth factor, one possible mechanism contributing to the development of this neoplasm is the loss of the regulation of imprinting of this growth factor gene as well as H19, a function for which is as yet unknown.

The two-hit theory of Knudson has gained substantial evidence in favor of its functioning as a major mechanism in carcinogenesis. However, it is clear from this brief discussion that other genetic and epigenetic mechanisms are involved in the development of malignant neoplasia. A number of these mechanisms are the subject of later chapters in the text.

SPONTANEOUS AND INDUCED DOMINANT AND RECESSIVE GENETIC DISORDERS ASSOCIATED WITH HIGH CANCER INCIDENCE IN LOWER ANIMALS

Until relatively recently, the germline genetics of cancer in lower animals was far less well studied than that in the human with a few specific exceptions—in particular, strains of mice where genetic factors could be well controlled. However, specific dominant or recessive genes predisposing to a high incidence of neoplasia have not as yet been frequently seen in animal systems. On the other hand, with the advent of molecular genetic techniques, it has become possible to program genetic factors leading directly to the incidence of specific neoplasms.

Spontaneously Occurring, Dominantly Inherited Neoplasia in Lower Animals

Although our knowledge of dominantly inherited neoplasia in lower animals has not developed rapidly, several excellent systems have been studied rather extensively. In the rodent these include the Eker rat (Eker et al., 1981) and the *Min* mouse (Moser et al., 1990). In the former example, renal cell carcinomas develop in virtually all rats bearing the dominant mutation by the age of 1 year. In addition, later in the life of these animals, pituitary adenomas, splenic sarcomas, leiomyomas, and leiomyosarcomas of the female genital tract can be seen (Hino et al., 1994; Everitt et al., 1995). The gene responsible for this condition is the rat equivalent of the tuberous sclerosis gene (Table 5.6), which is found in the rat on chromosome 10q (Kobayashi et al., 1995; Yeung et al., 1994). Allelic loss at the 10q locus of this gene has been reported in both spontaneous and chemically induced renal cell carcinomas in the Eker rat (Kubo et al., 1994). However, the phenotype of tuberous sclerosis in humans (see above) differs from that seen in the Eker rat except for the occurrence of renal neoplasms (Kobayashi et al., 1995).

Another well-studied, dominantly inherited neoplasm is that of intestinal adenomas in *Min* mice. In these animals, at a young age, multiple adenomas develop throughout the intestine, and the mice are prone to develop mammary neoplasms (Moser et al., 1993). In this condition the gene involved is completely homologous to the APC gene responsible for the development of familial polyposis in the human (Table 5.4). In the original *Min* mouse, the mutation in the APC gene is a nonsense mutation occurring as the result of a conversion of a leucine (TTG) to a stop (TAG) codon by the transversion from T to A at nucleotide 2549 (Su et al., 1992). Studies on allelic loss of the APC locus indicated that the gene was on mouse chromosome 18 (Luongo et al., 1994). Other genes have been linked to the development of papillomas and squamous cell carcinomas in the mouse (Lutzner et al., 1985) and thymomas in certain strains of rats (Matsuyama et al., 1986; Murakumo et al., 1993).

Another well-studied model occurs in fish of the genus *Xiphophorus*, in which a dominant tumor formation gene (*Tu*) is under the control of a repressor gene (R). If the R gene is absent, these animals develop fatal melanomas (cf. Anders et al., 1984). The *Tu* gene appears to encode a membrane receptor tyrosine kinase (cf. Friend, 1993), but the function of the product of the R gene is not known to date. A variety of malignant neoplasms of genetic origin have also been described in the fruit fly, *Drosophila melanogaster* (Gateff, 1978). More recently, Watson et al. (1994) have reviewed the more than 50 identified genes in which loss-of-function mutations may lead to a variety of abnormalities in cell proliferation, including neoplasia in both the developing and adult *Drosophila*. Mutations in several genes termed *lethal* result in neoplastic overgrowth of tissues during development, including that of the brain. Abnormalities in several other genes result in tumors of gonadal origin. Several of these genes involved in the development of neoplasms appear to regulate differentiation under normal conditions; but when they are mutated, they cause the appearance of benign and malignant neoplasms in the insect.

Transgenic and Gene-targeting Carcinogenesis

Although there are very few examples of dominantly inherited neoplastic disease in lower animals, as indicated above, the ability to manipulate the genome of mammalian organisms has made enormous technological advances during the last decade. This has led to the production of transgenic animals bearing oncogene or related constructs as a component of their genome (Jaenisch, 1988) and the production of animals with specific gene alterations resulting from gene targeting (knockout) methods (Bronson and Smithies, 1994). Figure 5.8 presents a diagram of the method used in producing transgenic animals. In this technique it is necessary to introduce a specific genetic construct by means of microinjection into the fertilized egg. This is then implanted in the uterus of a pseudopregnant female, allowing embryonic development to proceed through the birth of the fetus (cf. Camper, 1995). Pups are tested for the presence of the transgene by securing samples of their DNA and analyzing it for the introduced genetic material. Usually the transgene is expressed in a dominant manner. In contrast, when gene targeting is employed, blastocysts (Chapter 2) are isolated from pregnant females, and the inner cell mass is cultured to produce embryonic stem (ES) cells (Chapter 14). The gene construct used to target the gene of interest is then transfected into the ES cells. Those cells exhibiting the altered gene structure are isolated and injected directly into blastocysts, which are implanted into a foster mother as with the microinjected fertilized eggs above. From this is produced a chimera which, if the targeted ES cell has populated the germline, will be heterozygous for the gene alteration. Subsequent breeding will produce homozygous progeny. This technique is outlined in Figure 5.9, along with a diagram depicting the results and mechanisms of the transfection step. Basically this step depends on homologous recombination of the transfected gene into the position of

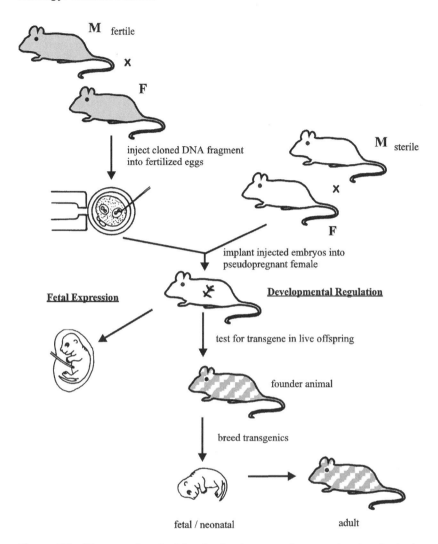

Figure 5.8   Diagram of method for the development of transgenic mice, beginning with injection of cloned DNA construct into the nucleus of a fertilized egg, implantation into pseudopregnant female, and monitoring of offspring for the presence of the transgene. With subsequent breeding of transgene-positive founder animals, inheritance of the transgene through the germline can be determined.

the normal gene, with subsequent recombination and replacement of one copy of the normal gene with the gene construct containing a selectable marker in place of one or more of the genetic components of the gene. Culture of ES cells having undergone this process of homologous recombination will allow enrichment and isolation of the ES cells. The selectable marker allows growth of cells containing such a gene in the presence of a drug which would be toxic to cells not having this selectable gene. Complications arise in that some random incorporation of the transfected gene occurs, and thus all clones must be tested to ensure that the one to be utilized contains the disrupted or "knocked out" gene.

By means of these two techniques, it thus becomes possible to develop animals having extra copies of a specific gene in their germline as well as animals missing one or both alleles of a critical gene, such as a tumor suppressor gene.

a.

b.

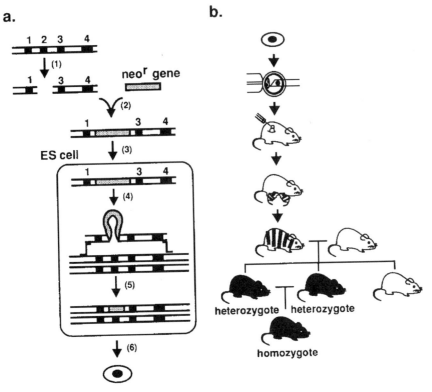

neo^r gene

ES cell

heterozygote   heterozygote

homozygote

Figure 5.9 Diagram of the procedure for homologous recombination (a) and the scheme for the development of animals with a homozygous loss of the targeted gene (b). In the homologous recombination procedure there is deletion of exon 2 (1) and its replacement by a selectable gene (the neo^r gene). This construct is transfected into ES cells (3) in which homologous recombination occurs with replacement of the normal gene by the gene containing the selectable sequence. In the scheme on the right, ES cells are cultured and those containing the selectable genes isolated and grown in the presence of the drug (neo). Surviving cells are implanted into a foster mother, and progeny in which the germ cells have been populated by the targeted ES cell are obtained by selective breeding. Such chimeras are then bred to produce homozygous offspring exhibiting complete loss of the targeted gene. (From Yamamura and Wakasugi, 1991, with permission of the authors and publisher.)

Gene targeting (knockout) has been used in mice to study the effects of complete elimination as well as heterozygosity of the RB and *p53* tumor suppressor genes. Mice in which one allele of the Rb gene is mutated do not exhibit retinoblastomas, but some of the animals have pituitary neoplasms that arise from cells in which the wild-type RB allele is absent (Jacks et al., 1992). The elimination of both alleles results in death prior to the 16th day of embryonic life. Such animals exhibit multiple defects with abnormalities in the hematopoietic system and central nervous system (Lee et al., 1992a). On the other hand, mice with mutations in one or both of the *p53* tumor suppressor genes appear normal during the first few months of life but then begin to develop a variety of mesenchymal and epithelial neoplasms (Donehower et al., 1992; Hooper, 1994).

In contrast, considerable work has been done with the transgenic approach, largely with viral and cellular oncogenes as the structural gene within the constructs. In addition, constructs in which growth factors, hormones, and even homeobox genes are the structural component of the construct have been utilized (Table 5.8). Table 5.8 shows some examples of transgenic car-

Table 5.8 Examples of Transgenic Carcinogenesis in the Mouse

Construct		Sites of Neoplasia	Latency Period	Reference
Promoter/Enhancer	Structural Gene			
A. Viral Transgene Constructs				
Bovine keratin 6	HPV-16 early region genes	Stomach	300 days	Searle et al., 1994
Insulin promoter	Polyoma early region genes	β-cell of isle of Langerhans	13 months	Bautch, 1989
HTLV-LTR	HTLV *tat* gene	Neurofibromas	3 months	Hinrichs et al., 1987
Human granzyme B promoter	HTLV *tax* gene	Leukemia	?	Grossman et al., 1995
Glucagon gene promoter/enhancer	SV40 large T antigen	Colon carcinoma	4 weeks	Lee et al., 1992c
Adipocyte P2 gene regulatory region	SV40 early genes	Hibernoma	1 month	Ross et al., 1992
Rabbit uteroglobin gene regulatory region	SV40 T antigen	Bronchioalveolar adenocarcinomas	5 months	Sandmöller et al., 1995
Prostate-specific probasin promoter	SV40 large T antigen	Prostatic carcinomas	10 weeks	Greenberg et al., 1995
MMTV enhancer/promoter	SV40 large T antigen	Lymphomas, adenocarcinomas of lung, kidney and mammary gland	?	cf. Muller, 1991
Albumin promoter	HBV sequences	Hepatocellular carcinoma	12 months	Dunsford et al., 1990
B. c- and v-Oncogene Constructs				
Immunoglobulin enhancer	c-*myc* proto-oncogene	Lymphoma	3 months	Adams et al., 1985
Prostate-specific antigen promoter	Ha-*ras* with codon 12 mutation	Salivary gland and GI carcinomas	10.5 months	Schaffner et al., 1995
Human β globin promoter	v-*gag-fps* oncogene	Lymphomas, fibrosarcomas, hemangiomas, angiosarcomas	2–12 months	Yee et al., 1989
Moloney virus LTR	c-*mos* protooncogene	Pheochromocytomas, medullary thyroid neoplasms	8 months	Schulz et al., 1992
C. Growth Factor, Hormonal and Homeobox Constructs				
Metallothionine I promoter	TGFα	Hepatocellular	13–15 months	Lee et al., 1992
Human keratin I gene	TGFα	Skin papillomas	2–5 months	Dominey et al., 1993
Major urinary protein promoter	IGF-II	Hepatocellular, squamous, and thyroid carcinoma, sarcoma	18 months	Rogler et al., 1994
Metallothionine I promoter	Bovine growth hormone	Hepatocellular carcinomas	43 weeks	Orian et al., 1990
Immunoglobulin heavy chain enhancer	E2A-PBX 1 homeobox	T-cell leukemia/lymphoma	2–3 months	Dedera et al., 1993

cinogenesis with various constructs following the technique depicted in Figure 5.8. The listing is only representative and by no means exhaustive. In addition, transgenic carcinogenesis has also been established in other rodent species including the rat (Hully et al., 1994) and the rabbit (Knight et al., 1988). One may assume that neoplasms resulting from transgenic carcinogenesis as exemplified in Table 5.8 are the result of dominant effects of the structural genes utilized to produce the animals, but some phenotypes resemble dominantly inherited neoplastic disease syndromes of the human. For example, mice made transgenic with the HTLV *tat* gene under the regulation of its LTR produce a syndrome very similar to neurofibromatosis I in the human (see above). In addition, mice made transgenic with the c-*mos* proto-oncogene under the regulation of the Moloney virus LTR develop a syndrome very similar to MEN II (Schalz et al., 1992). As shown in the table, in some instances the regulatory region (promoter/enhancer) of the gene construct targets the expression of the structural gene to specific tissues, with resultant neoplasms arising only in those tissues. An exception to this is the description by Schaffner et al. (1995) of the use of the promoter for prostate-specific antigen with a mutated Ha-*ras* gene in which no prostatic neoplasms developed, but rather carcinomas of the salivary gland and the gastrointestinal tract. Some regulatory components, especially the metallothionine promoter, have been utilized so that the expression of the structural gene may be regulated by external factors, in this instance zinc administration (Lee et al., 1992b; Dyer and Messing, 1989).

Although the induction of cancer by modern genetic techniques is, on the surface, quite different from carcinogenesis by chemical and physical agents, there are many similarities in the development of neoplasms from genetic, chemical, and physical carcinogens. Thus, the genetic changes that occur during the process of carcinogenesis initiated by any of these methods may have more similarities than differences, and both careful investigation and comparison of the development of neoplasia from several different carcinogenic mechanisms may prove to be extremely fruitful in ultimately elucidating the critical mechanisms of cancer development.

MULTIFACTORIAL GENETICS OF CANCER

As indicated above, genetic predisposition to neoplasia resulting from alteration in a single gene locus is a relatively rare cause of cancer in humans as well as in lower animals. A much greater contribution of genetics to the causation of neoplastic disease are those conditions having patterns of inheritance that conform to a polygenic or multifactorial mode of inheritance, recently termed *complex traits* (Lander and Schork, 1994). Many common chronic diseases of adults (including types of hypertension, coronary heart disease, diabetes mellitus, and schizophrenia) as well as certain developmental defects (including cleft lip and palate, spina bifida, and congenital heart disease) are known to be more frequent in those with family histories of such disorders. A number of these diseases may be due to single gene defects and others to chromosomal abnormalities, but most are the result of multiple genetic and environmental factors combined. In polygenic inheritance, multiple genes at independent loci interact in a cumulative fashion with environmental factors that move an individual beyond the "threshold of risk," so that the disease becomes of biological and clinical significance, with environmental influences determining whether and to what extent the individual is actually affected by the disease (Carter, 1970). Thus, the heritability for a threshold trait is a simple measure of the degree to which the liability is inherited. Figure 5.10 shows the distribution of such a disease liability in the general population and among relatives of affected individuals. The location of the threshold (T) is the same in both populations; however, the potential for disease is higher among relatives than in the general population, in part because of the genes shared by affected individuals and their relatives. Thus, the distribution of liability or potential for disease among the relatives of affected individuals is

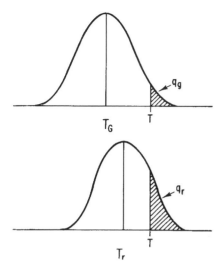

Figure 5.10   The distribution of the risk (liability or potential for disease) in the general population (upper curve) and that of a family exhibiting a threshold or multigenic trait (lower curve) in which there is a fixed threshold (T) that is identical in both populations. Individuals that are affected with the disease are those with risks or liabilities above (to the right of) the threshold, as shown by all individuals within the shaded areas of the curves. (Adapted from Duggleby et al., 1981, with permission of the authors and publisher.)

shifted to the right, that is, toward a greater risk, compared with the general population. For another individual in the same family to exhibit the disease syndrome, a similar combination of affected genes must be inherited. Since siblings share half their genes, the probability of a brother or sister inheriting the same combination of genes is $(1/2)^n$, where n is the number of genes required to express the disease trait, assuming that none of the genes are linked. In contrast disorders of single genes affect 25% or 50% of the first-degree relatives who are at genetic risk as based on mathematical inheritance patterns. On the other hand, multifactorial genetic disorders usually affect no more than 5% to 10% of first-degree relatives, and the recurrence risk of multifactorial disease varies from family to family. Risk estimation is significantly influenced by two factors: (1) the number of affected persons already present in the family and (2) the severity of the disorder in the index case. The greater the number of affected relatives and the more severe the clinical presentation of the disease, the higher the risk to remaining relatives (Beaudet et al., 1995). In general, just as with most monogenic neoplastic disease, a multifactorial genetic etiology for disease is less frequently seen with increasing age beyond adolescence.

Genes That Modify Cancer Predisposition

In the earlier part of this chapter we discussed specific genes, abnormalities of which lead to the development of specific neoplasms, usually in a fairly high percentage of affected individuals. However, in multifactorial genetic traits, as noted above, a number of genes may be involved in the expression of a predisposition to neoplastic disease. This may be the case even in those situations where cancer predisposition may result from mutations in a tumor suppressor or proto-oncogene. Obvious proof of this latter statement is the fact that germline inherited mutations in tumor suppressor genes do not result in neoplasms of all tissues, proliferating or not, but usually only in certain tissues of the organism. Presumably, genes expressed in some tissues prevent the neoplastic transformation seen in other tissues. Furthermore, it is well known that exposures to carcinogenic agents will result in only a proportion of the exposed individuals developing cancer. This may be due in part to a dose-response effect; but if the population is exposed to basically the same dose throughout, then the differential neoplastic response is probably the result of individual differences in susceptibility during the development of neoplasia.

It has been estimated that up to 20% of all cancers in humans exhibit some form of inherited predisposition (Müller and Scott, 1994). In many of these examples, it is likely that the basic stimulus for the development of neoplasia is genetic and that environmental factors acting on a variety of genes may alter the expression and neoplastic potential of the one or two critical genes involved. On the other hand, the major etiological factors for cancer development may be environmental, but the induction of neoplasia by environmental carcinogenic influences is modified by the expression of various genes within the organism. It is not always easy to distinguish these two "pathways," and in a number of instances one may make a cogent argument that modifying genes affect neoplastic development no matter what the inciting cause, genetic or environmental.

Genetic Modification of Germline Genetic Cancer Predisposition

As our knowledge of the specific genetic factors involved in the development of certain types of neoplasms increases, the characterization of subsets of specific neoplasms as "complex traits" is also enhanced. In some cases, such as retinoblastoma, where the penetrance of the gene exceeds 95%, it is unlikely that many cases can be attributed to a complex genetic trait, although other genetic factors such as imprinting may play a significant role in the expression of a few such neoplasms. On the other hand, with some of the more common neoplasms in which there is a known genetic predisposition, an understanding of the genetic foundations for the disease has become clarified. One such example is that of breast cancer, where (see above) two genes, the *BRCA1* and *BRCA2*, have been characterized as causally related, when mutated, to a significant number of inherited cases. But if one examines the genetics of mammary and ovarian cancer in general, one sees a spectrum of diseases ranging from Cowden's disease to postmenopausal breast cancer, in which it is likely that all women affected with this dominantly inherited predisposition to multiple neoplasms exhibit either frank malignancy of mammary tissue or mammary dysplasia (cf. Wolman and Dawson, 1991). Figure 5.11 shows a pie chart indicating the frequency of several inherited syndromes in which mammary cancer is predominant, these fading off into a larger group of polygenic diseases, with the majority of breast cancer resulting from unknown, presumably environmental causes and thus termed *sporadic* mammary cancer (Lynch et al., 1990). However, even in individuals bearing a mutated *BRCA1* gene, the risk of developing mammary cancer is not absolute and is partly age-dependent, being greater prior to age 50 and decreasing somewhat by age 65 or 70 (King et al., 1993). Interestingly, these workers describe families in which some members develop mammary cancer and others ovarian cancer, but the mutation in the *BRCA1* gene is identical. A variety of environmental factors can increase or decrease the risk of development of mammary cancer even in patients exhibiting genetic predisposition. These include diet, age at first pregnancy, parity, abortions, or artificially imposed menopause (Henderson, 1993; Andrieu et al., 1993). The age of onset of the disease is also related to the breast cancer incidence of immediate relatives, such that the risk is much greater among women whose mother or sibling was diagnosed with breast cancer prior to age 40, but the risk remains elevated even for those whose mothers were diagnosed with the disease at the age of 70 years or older (Colditz et al., 1993). An equally important example of genetic predisposition to a common human neoplasm is that seen in polygenic colon cancer. While the two major Mendelian genetic causes of colon cancer are shown, there are several others, as can be noted in

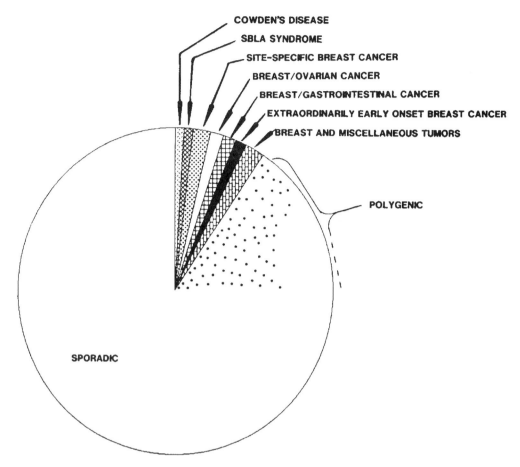

Figure 5.11   Schematic representation of the genetic heterogeneity seen in breast cancer in humans. (After Lynch et al., 1990, with permission of authors and publisher.)

Table 5.1, that contribute very small numbers to the chart. During the last decade there have been at least two studies suggesting that polyps and colorectal cancers occur primarily in genetically susceptible individuals in the human population, although the studies could not eliminate non-heritable causes of the disease (Cannon-Albright et al., 1988; Houlston et al., 1992). These studies suggested that perhaps as many as 80% of patients with this disease exhibit some sort of genetic predisposition in which one or a few genes may be the primary factors but multiple genes are probably involved in the ultimate expression of the disease. As with breast cancer, development of the disease at an earlier age increases the risk to siblings and close relatives (Fuchs et al., 1994; St. John et al., 1993).

On the other hand, although there is little if any evidence that human leukemia is inherited in a Mendelian fashion, there is good evidence to indicate that a number of patients with leukemia may have had a significant predisposition for the disease. The groups at greatest risk are listed in Table 5.9. One of the most interesting aspects of this listing is that, when one member of identical twins develops leukemia at a relatively early age, the risk is about 20% that the unaffected twin will also succumb to the disease; but this means that 80% do not appear to be at risk.

Table 5.9 Groups at Exceptionally High Risk of Leukemia

Group	Approximate Risk	Average Age at Onset
Identical twin of child with leukemia	1 in 5[a]	Weeks or months
Radiation-treated polycythemia vera	1 in 6	10–15 years
Bloom syndrome	1 in 8[b]	30 years
Hiroshima survivors who were within 1000 meters of the hypocenter	1 in 60	12 years
Down syndrome	1 in 95	10 years
Radiation-treated patients with anky-losing spondylitis	1 in 270	15 years
Sibs of leukemic children	1 in 720	10 years
U.S. Caucasian children 15 years of age	1 in 2880	10 years

[a]Of 22 sets of identical twins with one leukemic twin, the cotwin was affected in five instances.
[b]Three leukemics among 23 persons with Bloom syndrome.
From Miller, 1971, with permission of the author and publisher.

At least one extensive study (Gunz et al., 1975) indicated that polygenic mechanisms may be involved in the incidence of certain cases of chronic lymphocytic as well as acute leukemia but not of chronic myelogenous leukemia.

Of the examples given in Table 5.9, the majority are associated with radiation effects or genomic abnormalities. Several investigations of radiation-induced damage and DNA repair in individuals with and without a family history of cancer have indicated that abnormalities tend to occur, especially in patients with cancer or who are cancer-prone (Parshad et al., 1983; Pero et al., 1989; Kovacs and Langemann, 1991). Hsu and associates (1991) used a standardized test with the mutagen bleomycin to assay the mutagen sensitivity of the general population. These investigators demonstrated that moderately sensitive to hypersensitive individuals make up almost 23% of the total population. Recently Lipkowitz et al. (1992) demonstrated an increased frequency of abnormal rearrangements of immune receptor loci in peripheral blood lymphocytes of agricultural workers. This may relate to an observed increased risk for lymphoid malignancy in this occupational group. As noted earlier, patients who are heterozygous for the genetic disease ataxia-telangiectasia (see above), composing 0.7% to almost 8% of the population (Murnane and Kapp, 1993), exhibit a slight but significant increase in radiosensitivity to ionizing radiation. Since the genetics of DNA repair in response to chemical and physical insults is quite complex (Chapter 3), multiple genes are likely to be involved in the genesis of many complex trait neoplasms.

Other Genes Modifying Susceptibility to Inherited and Environmental Neoplastic Disease

The identification of specific genes involved in the multifactorial inheritance of neoplasia may be grouped into a number of different general categories. We have already discussed the involvement of genes involved in DNA repair. Three other areas involve gene products of the HLA locus coding for surface membrane antigens involved in immune mechanisms (Chapter 17), proto-oncogenes, and pharmacogenetics. In the former category there is substantial evidence that specific HLA haplotypes (genotypes) are associated with an increased incidence of specific human neoplasms, as reported in sporadic instances. As can be seen from Table 5.10, the greatest risks related to specific HLA antigen haplotypes are associated with leukemias and lymphomas, the

Table 5.10 HLA and Malignancy Associations and Linkages

Diseases	Unrelated Patients		Family Studies
	HLA Antigen	Relative Risk	
Leukemia			
A.L.L.	A2	1.39	Excess of shared HLA-A,B antigens and haplotypes in parents
A.M.L.			Excess of shared haplotype in sibs and in the proband
C.L.L.	DR5	8.08	
Cancer			
Nasopharynx (Chinese)	A2 Bw46	2.38	
(African)	A29	19.5	
Kidney	DR5	4.7	
Breast	Bw35	1.35	
Testicle	Dw7	8.12	
Uterus	B12	1.46	
Lymphoma			
Hodgkin	A1	1.38	Probable linkage with HLA
	B5	1.33	Excess of HLA identical pairs of affected sibs
	B8	1.23	
	B18	1.30	
Non-Hodgkin			
B Lymphoma (Negroid)	B37	37.59	
Kaposi sarcoma			
(Mediterranean)	DR5	12.7	
(Other Caucasoid)	DR2		
Familial malignant melanoma			Possible linkage with HLA

Main data from the International HLA and Disease Registry as reviewed by Hors et al., 1984.

notable exceptions being neoplasms of the kidney and testicle. Since many leukemias and lymphomas arise from cells of the immune system where HLA haplotypes play a major role in gene expression, the results seen in Table 5.10 might be expected, perhaps in relation to the immunobiology of the host-tumor relationship (Chapter 19). In another cell surface gene family, the ABO blood groups, a relationship between blood group A and cancer of the stomach was found among black and white patients in the southern United States (Newell et al., 1974).

Proto-Oncogenes in Multifactorial Cancer Susceptibility

On the basis of studies in animals with carcinogenic retroviruses, one might expect that mutations in proto-oncogenes would be a major cause of germline neoplasia in the human. We have already seen that this is generally not true, with the *ret* proto-oncogene being the only known example of a causative association with specific human neoplasms (Tables 5.4 and 5.6). Evidence that mutations in proto-oncogenes play any role in a genetic predisposition to neoplasia has been somewhat controversial. In 1987 Krontiris reported that rare alleles of the Ha-*ras* proto-oncogene were almost exclusively seen in the genomes of cancer patients (Krontiris et al., 1987). Since that time, other studies (Klingel et al., 1991; Ryberg et al., 1992) have shown a somewhat similar effect in German patients with colorectal cancer and in Norwegians with lung cancer, respectively. Krontiris and associates (1993) have also extended their investigations and proposed that 1 in 11 cancers of the breast, colon, and bladder possess such mutant alleles. On the other hand, Hall et al. (1990a) were unable to find such an association, and Peto et al. (1988) argued that there was no clear evidence of Ha-*ras* polymorphic alleles and cancer development. A number of other negative studies in leukemias and lymphomas have been reported (Trench et al., 1989; Knauf and Ho, 1991). A germline mutation in the *mos* proto-oncogene was uniquely detected in a small series of patients with breast cancer (Lidereau et al., 1988), while a specific allele of the *myc* proto-oncogene was significantly increased in males with bone and soft-tissue sarcomas (Kato et al., 1990). Thus, the role of germline mutations in proto-oncogenes in cancer susceptibility with the exception noted above has not yet been clarified. On the other hand, given the considerable experimental basis and the suggestion of positive effects noted above, it is likely that mutations in such genes may play a role in the multifactorial origin of neoplasia. In contrast, as noted further on (Chapter 6), somatic mutations in proto-oncogenes appear to play significant roles in cancer growth and development.

The Role of Pharmacogenetics in Multifactorial Neoplasia

As noted in Chapter 3, the metabolism of many chemical carcinogens is critical to their carcinogenic action. Thus, one might expect that the susceptibility to the development of neoplastic disease resulting from exposure to a chemical carcinogen will depend on the host's capability of "activating" the agent to its ultimate form through appropriate metabolic pathways. Genetic alteration in such pathways can lead to an enhanced or decreased susceptibility of the individual to neoplasia induced by the carcinogenic agent.

Phase I Genes

As discussed in Chapter 3, the principal components of the phase I xenobiotic metabolizing enzymes are those of the cytochrome P450 family. Table 5.11 lists the cytochrome P450 genes of the human, their chromosomal location where known, the number of amino acids in the gene product, the organs of major expression, and, where known, those carcinogens that are activated by the individual members of the family.

More than two decades ago, a report indicated that high inducibility of the aromatic hydrocarbon hydroxylation pathway was a significant risk factor for human lung cancer (Kellerman et al., 1973). These studies were performed with human lymphocytes, and it was assumed that changes seen in this peripheral tissue reflected changes in the lung, since a high level of inducibility of AHH in lymphocytes was more frequently observed in lung cancer patients than in patients with other diseases. These results became quite controversial, since others were unable to reproduce these data, but more recent studies in Japan have related a specific mutation in a codon of exon 7 in the cytochrome P-450IA1 gene exhibits a different genotypic distribution between controls and lung cancer patients, as noted in Table 5.12 (Hayashi et al., 1992).

The mutation in the gene is the result of a transition from an adenine residue to that of a guanine, resulting in a change from an isoleucine (Ile) to a valine (Val) residue, as depicted in Figure 5.12. Individuals with the homozygous mutation (Val/Val) tend to develop lung cancer at a greater frequency with lower consumption of cigarettes (Figure 5.13). A different polymorphism revealed by the restriction enzyme *Msp*I also demonstrated polymorphisms in the Japanese population that were related to increased risk of lung cancer, especially at low numbers of cigarettes smoked (Nakachi et al., 1991). Studies in other races, especially in Scandinavians, did

Table 5.11 Nomenclature of Human Cytochrome P450 Gene Family Together with Some Characteristics of the Gene, Its Product, Its Expression, and the Carcinogens Activated

P450 Gene Symbol	Trivial Name	Chromosomal Location	Amino Acid Residues	Organs	Carcinogens Activated
CYP1A1	P_1, c, form6	15q22-qter	512	Extrahepatic	B(a)P, 2-AAF etc.
1A2	P_3, d, form 4	15	516	Liver	2-AAF, 4-ABP, Glu-P-1, IQ, AFB_1, Trp-P-2, 2-AF etc.
CYP2A6	IIA3, P450(I)	19q13.1-13.2	494	Liver	AFB_1, NDEA etc.
2B6				Liver and extrahepatic	6-AC
2B7	IIB1	19q12-q13.2	491	Liver	AFB_1
2C8	form 1, IIC2		490	Liver	
2C9	IIC1, mp-4	10q24.1-24.3	490	Liver	
2C10	mp, mp-8		490	Liver	
2D6	dbl	22q11.2-qter	497	Liver	NNK
2E1	j	10	493	Liver	NDMA, NDEA etc.
2F1	IIF1	19q12-13.2	491	Lung	
CYP3A3	HLp		504	Liver	AFB_1
3A4	NF		503	Liver	AFB_1, B(a)P-7, 8-diol, 6-AC etc.
3A5	hPCN3, HLp2	7q21.3-q22	502	Liver	
3A7	HFL33		503	Liver	AFB_1, IQ
CYP4B1	IVB1, P450HP	1p12-p34	511	Placenta, lung	
CYP7	7α		504	Liver	
CYP11A1	SCC	15	521	Steroidogenic	
11B1	11β	8q21-22	503	Adrenal	
CYP17	17α	10	508	Steroidogenic	
CYP19	arom	15q21.1-21.3	503	Steroidogenic	
CYP21A2	C21B	6p21.3	494	Adrenal	
CYP27		2q33-qter	499	Liver	

Key: B(a)P, benzo(a)pyrene; 2-AAF, 2-acetylaminofluorene; 4-ABP, 4-aminobiphenyl; Glu-P-1, 2-amino-6-methyldipy-rido[1,2-a:3',2'-d]imidazole; IQ, 2-amino-3-methylimidazo[4,5-f]quinoline; AFB_1, aflatoxin B_1; Trp-P-2, 3-amino-1-methyl-5 H-pyrido[4,3-b]indole; 2-AF, 2-aminofluorene; NDEA, N-nitrosodiethylamine; NNK, 4-(methylnitrosamino)-1-(3-pyridyl)-1-butanone; 6-AC, 6-aminochrysene.
Adapted from Kawajiri and Fujii-Kuriyama, 1991, with permission of authors and publisher.

not give evidence of the relationship of such polymorphisms, as noted in the Japanese population to lung cancer or cigarette dose (Hirvonen et al., 1992; Alexandrie et al., 1994). On the other hand, homozygosity for the *Msp*I mutant genotype was positively associated with in situ colorectal cancer in Japanese and Hawaiians (Sivaraman et al., 1994).

Another phase I enzyme exhibiting significant genetic polymorphism and related to different cancer susceptibility is cytochrome P-4502D6. This cytochrome is responsible for the metabolism of a number of clinically used drugs, especially those involved in the treatment of hypertension, depression, cardiac arrhythmias, and some analgesics. In general, humans may be divided into "extensive metabolizers" (EM) and "poor metabolizers" (PM). About 8% of the Caucasian population are PM individuals (cf. Nebert, 1991). The structures of the best known variant alleles and the normal (*wt*) gene (EM) may be seen in Figure 5.14 (Nebert, 1991).

Table 5.12 Distribution of P450IA1 Genotypes in Healthy Controls and Lung
Cancer Patients

	Genotypes [# patients (% of total)]			
	Ile/Ile	Ile/Val	Val/Val	Total
Controls	233 (65.1)	108 (30.2)	17 (4.7)	358 (100)
Lung cancer	120 (56.6)	66 (31.1)	26 (12.3)	212 (100)
Kreyberg I	66 (56.9)	34 (29.3)	16 (13.8)	116 (100)
Squamous cell carcinoma	41 (61.2)	16 (23.9)	10 (14.9)	67 (100)
Kreyberg II adenocarcinoma	54 (56.3)	32 (33.3)	10 (10.4)	96 (100)
Stomach cancer	54 (56.8)	37 (39.6)	4 (4.2)	95 (100)
Colon cancer	59 (69.4)	21 (24.7)	5 (5.9)	85 (100)
Breast cancer	65 (66.5)	29 (29.6)	4 (4.1)	98 (100)

Modified from Hayashi et al. (1992).

Phase II Metabolism

Of the phase II genes, those studies most extensively are the N-acetyltransferases and glu-
tathione-S-transferases in relation to the pharmacogenetics of neoplasia. It is the former gene
family that have been studied in relation to human cancer for the longest period. In the human, at
least three N-acetyltransferase (NAT) gene loci exist. One of these is probably a pseudogene,
while the two expressed genes, NAT 1 and NAT 2, are both located on chromosome 8 but are
separated by at least 25 kb (Grant, 1993). It is the NAT 2 gene locus that is involved in human
acetylation polymorphism. A schematic diagram of most of the variant alleles is shown in Figure
5.15. In this diagram the wildtype alleles are designated as R, the mutant alleles as S. These

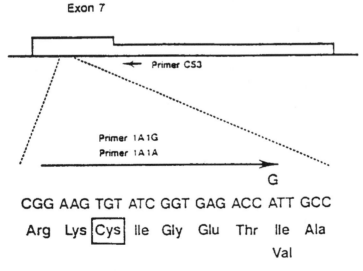

Figure 5.12 Structure of the polymorphic site in exon 7 of the P-450IA1 gene. The cysteine residue, a
heme-binding thiolate ligand, is noted as enclosed with a box. The mutant codon is indicated by the G over
the A reflecting the transition giving rise to the valine (Val) as noted below the normal amino acid
sequence. (Adapted from Hayashi et al., 1992, with permission of authors and publisher.)

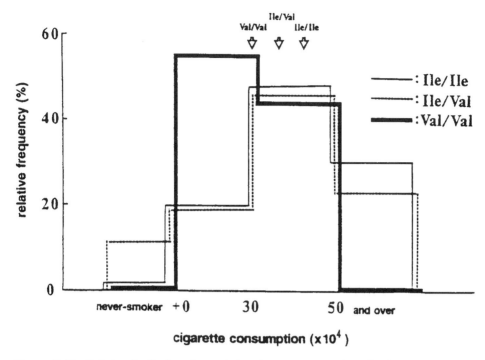

Figure 5.13   Relative distribution of cumulative cigarette consumption of patients in the Ile-Val genotypes, where the total number of patients with each of the genotypes is considered as 100%. Vertical arrowheads indicate mean cigarette consumption of patients with each genotype. (Adapted from Nakachi et al.,
1993, with permission of authors and publisher.)

designations also indicate the rate at which the transacetylation is catalyzed, R indicating rapid
and S slow acetylator phenotypes.

   Although the mechanism of the ineffective acetylation by the mutant slow acetylator phenotypes is not generally known, the M1 mutant appears to cause a decrease in the amount of
NAT 2 protein in the liver because of defective translation, whereas M2 translation results in an
unstable enzyme (Blum et al., 1991).

   Since N-acetyltransferases are involved in the formation of the ultimate forms of aromatic
amine carcinogens (Chapter 3), studies of the frequency of the rapid and slow acetylator phenotypes in workers exposed to such agents became an important project. Table 5.13 shows the relationship of bladder cancer incidence in industrial chemical workers classified as to whether each
individual was a slow or rapid acetylator. From these data, workers with the slow acetylator phenotype were at a far greater risk of developing bladder cancer than rapid acetylators (cf. Nebert,
1991). Fettman et al. (1991) have suggested that such slow acetylators appear to be predisposed
to bladder cancer as a result of the shift in metabolism of arylamines to oxidation and glucu-
ronidation with concentration of the metabolites in the urine, thus increasing the risk of bladder
cancer. In contrast, according to these investigators, the rapid acetylator phenotype may be identified in a disproportionately large number of colorectal cancer patients presumably through the
enhanced production of mutagenic arylamides and acetoxyarylamines initiated by the N-acetyltransferase pathway. However, not all investigations have supported this latter concept (Probst-
Hensch et al., 1995; Oda et al., 1994). A scheme of the metabolic pathway of an arylamine
showing the two alternative paths indicated above may be seen in Figure 5.16.

Allele

Phenotype

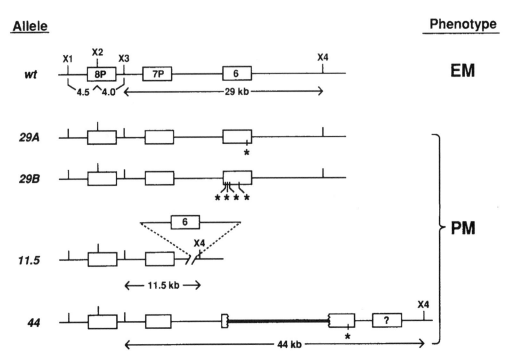

Figure 5.14 Diagram of the wild-type (*wt*) and variant alleles of the human CYP2D6 8P and 7P are pseudogenes, while 6 is the functional CYP2D6 gene. The box with a question mark may be an additional CYP2D gene or pseudogene. The mutations that have been characterized are denoted by asterisks. X1, X2, X3, and X4 are restriction sites (*Xba*I). In the 11.5 allele the functional gene is completely missing, while in the 44 allele a large insertion (heavy bar) is present in the 5' half of the functional CYP2D6 gene. Other alleles are also known (cf. Shields, 1994), and a particularly interesting allele is that exhibiting a 12-fold amplification of the functional gene resulting in an ultrarapid metabolism of the enzyme's normal substrates (Johansson et al., 1993). The major association with human cancer is the strong association of the EM phenotype with lung cancer as shown in several studies (Caporaso et al., 1992; Hirvonen et al., 1993). CYP2D6 polymorphism is not related to human colorectal cancer (Ladero et al., 1991a), but these individuals have presented some evidence suggesting an increased risk of breast cancer among women with the PM phenotype (Ladero et al., 1991b). (Adapted from Nebert, 1991, with permission of the author and publisher.)

Another metabolic phase II pathway is the inactivation of various chemical carcinogens by their conjugation with the tripeptide glutathione, catalyzed by glutathione S-transferase. One form of this enzyme, termed GST1, is dominant in the population with approximately 50% of individuals exhibiting the recessive characteristic resulting in little or no measurable GST1 activity (Seidegård and Pero, 1985). The distribution of GST1 in lung cancer patients and appropriate controls expressed as a fraction or percentage of patients expressing the gene (dominant expression) in relation to the total patients studied is seen in Table 5.14. Again, patients with lung cancer exhibit lower proportions of the dominant gene activity than do controls.

When the expression of both genes is studied in the same population, the relative risks of the patients bearing the mutant form of P450IA1 and the recessive expression of GST1 exhibit extremely high relative risks, demonstrating the complexity of the genetic background of individuals and their risk of developing cancer on exposure to chemical carcinogens (Table 5.15). As noted in Figure 5.13, the relative risks can increase to 40 or 50 when one takes into consideration the age and total cigarette consumption.

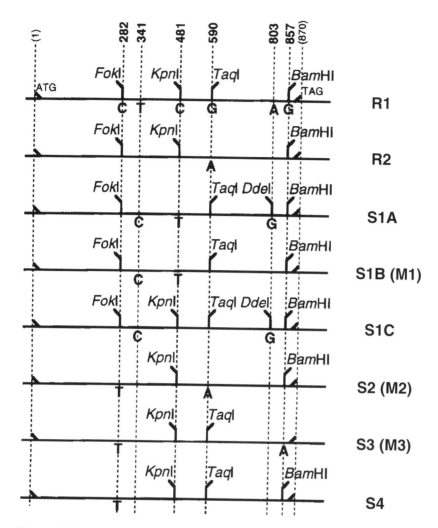

Figure 5.15 Schematic diagram of variant alleles at the NAT 2 gene locus. Identities of the nucleotides at the six variable regions of the 870-bp NAT 2 coding sequence are indicated for the allele, R1. Deviations from this are indicated as base changes (G, C, A, T) on each of the other alleles are as any gains and losses of recognition sites for the various restriction endonucleases indicated. (Adapted from Grant, 1993, with permission of author and publisher.)

Table 5.13 Acetylator Phenotypes and Industrial Bladder Cancer

Acetylator Type	Chemical Workers	Never Chemical Workers	Cancer Invasiveness	
			Low	High
Slow	22 (96%)	52 (59%)	59	14
Rapid	1	36	33	3
Total	23	88		

Data from Cartwright et al., 1982.

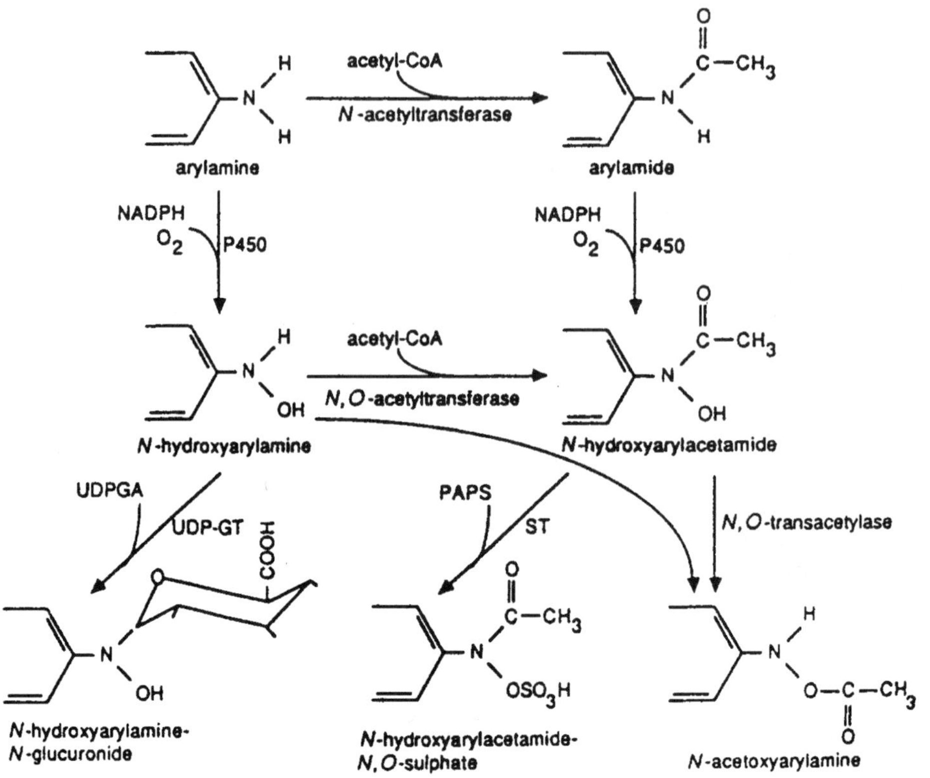

Figure 5.16 Potential pathways for the metabolism of arylamines. Abbreviations used: UDPGA, uridine diphosphoglucuronic acid; UDP-GT, UDP-glucuronosyltransferase; PAPS, phosphoadenosine phosphosulfate; ST, sulfotransferase. (From Fettman et al., 1991, with permission of the author and publisher.)

In addition to the above noted relationship of alterations in glutathione S-transferase I expression and lung cancer, the null or decreased expression of this gene has also been associated with increased risk for hepatocellular carcinoma (McGlynn et al., 1995), adenocarcinoma of the stomach and colon (Strange et al., 1991), bladder cancer (Bell et al., 1993), and mesothelioma (Hirvonen et al., 1995). In addition, the null phenotype of the glutathione-S-transferase I gene is associated with larger amounts of polycyclic aromatic hydrocarbon-dGMP adducts in the lungs of smokers.

Table 5.14 Distribution of Glutathione S-Transferase I in Smokers with Various Types of Lung Cancer and in Matched Controls

	Males (+/ratio of t/total)	Females (+/ratio of t/total)
Controls	70/127 (0.55)	42/65 (0.65)
Squamous cell carcinoma	21/45 (0.47)	6/17 (0.35)
Adenocarcinoma	19/61 (0.31)	9/32 (0.28)
All lung neoplasms	47/129 (0.36)	23/62 (0.37)

Data from Seidegård et al., 1990.

Table 5.15 Relative Risk Estimate of the Combined Genotypes of the
P450IA1 and GST1 Genes for Lung Cancer

	Genotypes					
P450IA1	Ile/Ile		Ile/Val		Val/Val	
GST1	+	−	+	−	+	−
Lung cancer	1.0		1.19		2.97	
	1.0	1.74	1.74	1.42	2.30	5.83
Kreyberg I	1.0		1.11		3.32	
	1.0	1.84	1.33	1.75	1.63	7.94
Squamous cell	1.0		0.84		3.34	
carcinoma	1.0	2.31	1.16	1.54	2.02	9.07
Kreyberg II	1.0		1.28		2.54	
(adenocarcinoma)	1.0	1.62	2.21	1.04	3.07	3.45

Adapted from Hayashi et al., 1992.

Multifactorial Carcinogenesis in Animal Systems

Surprisingly, given our relatively detailed knowledge of the genomes of several murine and insect species, fewer studies aimed at identifying genes whose expression modifies the development of neoplasia have been carried out in these lower species. Studies in the mouse are perhaps
the best documented. In Table 5.16 may be seen a listing of most of the known genes that have
been found to modify the development of neoplasia in animals treated with chemical carcino-

Table 5.16 Modifying Genes in Germline Genetic (GG) and Chemical (C) Carcinogenesis in Animals

Species	Neoplasm(s)	Carcinogen	Modifying gene, Locus, or Linkage	Reference
Mouse	Intestinal tumors	Mutated APC gene (GG)	*Mom 1*	Dietrich et al., 1993
Mouse	Hepatomas	Ethylnitrosourea (C)	*Hcs*	Drinkwater, 1989
Mouse	Lung adenomas	Urethan (C)	*pas* (K-*ras*)	Malkinson, 1991 Malkinson and You, 1994
Rat	Pituitary tumors	Estrogen (C)	Prl-linked	Shepel and Gorski, 1990
Mouse	Plasmacytomas	Tetramethyl-pentadecan (C)	Linkage near Gt10 on chromosome 4 and Frgr2 on chromosome 1	Mock et al., 1993
Mouse	Small intestinal cancer	Ethylnitroso-urea (C)	*ssic1*	Fijneman and Demant, 1995
Rat	Thymic lymphoma	N-propyl-N-nitroso-urea (C)	*Tls-1, -2, -3*	Ogiu et al., 1995
Rat	Hepatoma	Spontaneous	Atp7b	Wu et al., 1994
Rat	Mammary carcinoma	Dimethylbenz-anthracene	Mcs	Zhang et al., 1989

gens. In at least one instance, that of the *Min* mouse, a germline genetic mutation in the APC gene (see above) is the basis for neoplastic development. In this latter case, the modifying gene termed *Mom1* has been reported to be identical to the gene for secretory type II phospholipase A2 (Pla2s), as reported by MacPhee et al. (1995). These latter authors suggest that the modifying gene acts to alter the cellular microenvironment within the intestinal crypts, thereby modifying the number of polyps that develop.

A number of examples of genes, all of which have been only partially or very little characterized, have been shown to alter the tumor response to the administration of one or a few doses of a chemical carcinogen. The *Hcs* locus first described by Drinkwater modifies the development of hepatomas in the liver of the mouse after ethylnitrosourea administered during neonatal life or hepatomas that develop spontaneously. The action of the gene is to alter the rate of replication of preneoplastic hepatocytes. Manenti et al. (1994) have also reported at least five other *Hcs* loci in the mouse, but the functions of these are as yet unknown. Malkinson and his associates have reported the existence of multiple pulmonary adenoma susceptibility (*pas*) genes that affect the spontaneous or chemically induced numbers of pulmonary adenomas in appropriate mouse strains (Malkinson, 1991). In studies directed towards identifying such genes, they have presented evidence that different forms of *Ki-ras* proto-oncogene in which a 37-bp sequence within the first intron of the gene is present once in the DNA of sensitive strains and twice in that of resistant mice (Malkinson and You, 1994). The authors have considered several possible mechanisms for the modifying action of this mutation. Fijneman et al. (1994) have also shown that other loci within the major histocompatibility complex are likely to modify lung tumor susceptibility in the mouse as well. Susceptibility to estrogen-induced pituitary tumors in rats segregates with the prolactin (*Prl*) gene or in some closely linked gene (Shepel and Gorski, 1990).

There have also been reported instances of enhanced spontaneous and chemically induced neoplasia in both rats and mice exhibiting specific genotypes. One of the most extensively studied is the viable yellow gene (A^{vy}), the expression of which increases the incidence of spontaneous and induced tumors in mouse strains carrying the nude (nu/nu) mutation (Chapter 15; Stutman, 1979). In addition, mice of the C3H strain carrying the A^{vy} gene show an extremely high spontaneous incidence of mammary and liver neoplasms (Heston and Vlahakis, 1968). In rats, two separate mutations not obviously related to cancer development have been shown to act as modifiers in the development of specific neoplasms. Rats of the LEC strain bearing a deletion in the copper transporting ATPase gene homologous to that causing Wilson's disease (Wu et al., 1994) in the human exhibit a high spontaneous rate of both renal and liver cancer (Izumi et al., 1994; Ono et al., 1991). Whether this is related to the abnormality in copper metabolism must await further investigation. Another rat strain bearing a small deletion mutation in the albumin gene, in which homozygotes exhibit almost no measurable serum albumin, exhibit a higher incidence of neoplasms of the kidney (Nagase et al., 1983) after dimethylnitrosamine administration and of the brain after a single transplacental administration of ethylnitrosourea to homozygous rats (Usuki et al., 1992).

Pharmacogenetics as a Multifactorial Variable in Animal Cancer

The study of multiple forms of phase I and phase II genes in animals has, for some species, been almost as extensive as that in humans. However, the initial studies relating the metabolic activation of chemical carcinogens to specific genes was carried out in the mouse more than two decades ago, when the relationship between the induction of a phase I activity, aryl hydrocarbon hydroxylase (AHH) by the carcinogen methylcholanthrene was related to the "carcinogenic index" or susceptibility to chemical carcinogenesis of the skin in a series of inbred mouse strains. These data are depicted in Figure 5.17. These studies stimulated investigations mentioned above

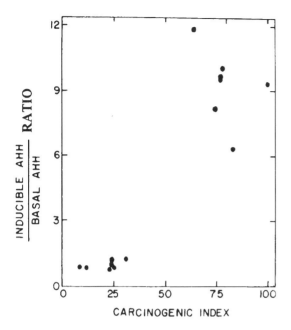

Figure 5.17 Relationship between the carcinogenic index (Iball index) for the induction of neoplasms in mice by subcutaneous administration of 3-methylcholanthrene as a function of the induction of aryl hydrocarbon hydroxylase (AHH) activity by 3-methylcholanthrene in the liver for each of 14 genetically distinct inbred strains of mice, each indicated by a separate solid circle. The Iball index is defined as:

$$I = \frac{\text{tumor yield (\%)}}{\text{latent period (days)}} \times 100$$

The carcinogenic potency (I) of a chemical is thus related to both the number (as %) of neoplasms induced and the time required (latent period) for neoplasms to appear (Chapter 13). By this reference potent carcinogens usually induce many neoplasms in a short time, whereas weak carcinogens induce fewer neoplasms only after a prolonged period. (After Thorgeirsson and Nebert et al., 1977, with permission of the authors and publisher.)

in relation to aryl hydrocarbon hydroxylase induction in human cells in patients with lung cancer. Interestingly, induction of sarcomas by the subcutaneous implantation of the same carcinogen gave various results in relation to the aryl hydrocarbon hydroxylase activity, depending on the dose of the carcinogen implanted (Prehn and Lawler, 1979). The genetic locus that is critical for the environmentally induced response in these phase I genes as well as a number of phase II genes has been termed the *Ah* locus. This locus codes for one member of a family of proteins that are ligand-activated transcription factors involved in the regulation of the expression of a number of genes. The molecular mechanisms of this regulatory process are being elucidated but are beyond the scope of this text. The interested reader is referred to recent reviews (Swanson and Bradfield, 1993; Okey et al., 1994).

A mutation in the cytochrome P450–metabolizing debrisoquine has been reported in the rat (Matsunaga et al., 1989) owing to an absence of expression of the gene. No carcinogenesis investigations have yet been carried out on this strain, but in another study (Aitio et al., 1991)—with outbred rats administered the carcinogen diethylnitrosamine for 20 weeks—a correlation of individual susceptibility to the development of liver cancer was related to the pattern of a number of cytochrome P450 gene products. This relationship was most accentuated at low dose levels and thus was felt to be a closer reflection of human exposure.

Several phase II genes have also been investigated in rodents, but most extensively investigated and compared with the human are the N-acetyltransferases. Polymorphic forms of slow and rapid acetylator phenotypes have been described in the hamster (Ferguson et al., 1994), mouse (Chung et al., 1993), rabbit (Sasaki et al., 1991), and rat (Hein et al., 1991). Mutations in the hamster are somewhat analogous to those seen in the human, but those in the rabbit appear to be quite different. McQueen et al. (1982) demonstrated that, in hepatocytes from rapid and slow acetylator rabbits maintained in culture and treated with hydralazine, DNA repair was present in cells from the slow acetylators but not in those from the rapid acetylators. This suggested a potential difference in the susceptibility to amine carcinogens as well. A similar result was seen in hepatocytes of rapid and slow acetylator strains of mice treated with aminofluorene (cf. Weber and Hein, 1985).

GENETIC CARCINOGENESIS: THE KEY TO UNLOCKING THE SECRETS OF CANCER?

From this overview, the student will hopefully appreciate that the explosion in our knowledge of genetic mechanisms is reflected in a dramatic increase in our understanding of neoplasia and its genesis. In the remainder of this text, there are numerous other examples verifying this statement. However, as indicated earlier in this chapter, germline genetic alterations do not constitute the major cause of neoplasia in the human, although especially the multifactorial, polygenic area may be involved in the causation of a great percentage of all human cancer. The next chapter views the genetics of neoplasia not from the germline but from the inheritance of somatic cells. This process, as we have noted from our definition of neoplasia (Chapter 2), is ubiquitous, and much of our knowledge of somatic cell genetics has now evolved from the genetic revolution of the latter part of this century.

REFERENCES

Adams, J. M., Harris, A. W., Pinkert, C. A., Corcoran, L. M., Alexander, W. S., Cory, S., Palmiter, R. D., and Brinster, R. L. The c-*myc* oncogene driven by immunoglobulin enhancers induces lymphoid malignancy in transgenic mice. Nature, *318*:533–538, 1985.

Aitio, A., Aitio, M-L., Camus, A-M., Cardis, E., and Bartsch, H. Cytochrome P-450 isozyme pattern is related to individual susceptibility to diethylnitrosamine-induced liver cancer in rats. Jpn. J. Cancer Res., *82*:146–156, 1991.

Alexandrie, A-K., Sundberg, M. I., Seidegård, J., Tornling, G., and Rannug, A. Genetic susceptibility to lung cancer with special emphasis on *CYP1A1* and *GSTM1*: A study on host factors in relation to age at onset, gender and histological cancer types. Carcinogenesis, *15*:1785–1790, 1994.

Anders, F., Schartl, M., Barnekow, A., and Anders, A. *Xiphophorus* as an *in vivo* model for studies on normal and defective control of oncogenes. Adv. Cancer Res., *42*:191–275, 1984.

Andrieu, N., Clavel, F., Auquier, A., Lê, M. G., Gairard, B., Piana, L., Brémond, A., Lansac, J., Flamant, R., and Renaud, R. Variations in the risk of breast cancer associated with a family history of breast cancer according to age at onset and reproductive factors. J. Clin. Epidemiol., *46*:973–980, 1993.

Antecol, M. H., and Mukherjee, B. B. Effects of 12-*O*-tetradecanoylphorbol-13-acetate on fibroblasts from individuals genetically predisposed to cancer. Cancer Res., *42*:3870–3879, 1982.

Arai, E., Ikeuchi, T., Karasawa, S., Tamura, A., Yamamoto, K., Kida, M., Ichimura, K., Yuasa, Y., and Tonomura, A. Constitutional translocation t(4;22) (q12;q12.2) associated with neurofibromatosis type 2. Am. J. Med. Genet., *44*:163–167, 1992.

Bautch, V. L. Effects of polyoma virus oncogenes in transgenic mice. Mol. Biol. Med., *6*:309–317, 1989.

Beaudet, A. L., Scriver, C. R., Sly, W. S., and Valle, D. Genetics, biochemistry, and molecular basis of variant human phenotypes. *In*: C. R. Scriver et al. (Eds.), The Metabolic Bases of Inherited Disease, 7th ed., pp. 53–118. New York: McGraw-Hill, 1995.

Bell, D. A., Taylor, J. A., Paulson, D. F., Robertson, C. N., Mohler, J. L., and Lucier, G. W. Genetic risk and carcinogen exposure: a common inherited defect of the carcinogen-metabolism gene glutathione *S*-transferase M1 (GSTM1) that increases susceptibility to bladder cancer. J. Natl. Cancer Inst., *85*:1159–1164, 1993.

Benedict, W. F., Murphree, A. L., Banerjee, A., Spina, C. A., Sparkes, M. C., and Sparkes, R. S. Patient with 13 chromosome deletion: evidence that the retinoblastoma gene is a recessive cancer gene. Science, *219*:973–975, 1983.

Bernstein, J. L., Thompson, W. D., Risch, N., and Holford, T. R. The genetic epidemiology of second primary breast cancer. Am. J. Epidemiol., *136*:937–948, 1992.

Bischoff, F. Z., Yim, S. O., Pathak, S., Grant, G., Siciliano, M. J., Giovanella, B. C., Strong, L. C., and Tainsky, M. A. Spontaneous abnormalities in normal fibroblasts from patients with Li-Fraumeni cancer syndrome: aneuploidy and immortalization. Cancer Res., *50*:7979–7984, 1990.

Blum, M., Demierre, A., Grant, D. M., Heim, M., and Meyer, U. A. Molecular mechanism of slow acetylation of drugs and carcinogens in humans. Proc. Natl. Acad. Sci. U.S.A., *88*:5237–5241, 1991.

Bodmer, W. F., Bailey, C. J., Bodmer, J., Bussey, H. J. R., Ellis, A., Gorman, P., Lucibellow, F. C., Murday, V. A., Rider, S. H., Scambler, P., Sheer, D., Solomon, E., and Spurr, N. K. Localization of the gene for familial adenomatous polyposis on chromosome 5. Nature, *328*:614–616, 1987.

Bolande, R. P., and Vekemans, M. J.-J. Genetic models of carcinogenesis. Hum. Pathol., *14*:658–662, 1983.

Bone, H. G. III. Diagnosis of the multiglandular endocrine neoplasias. Clin. Chem., *36*:711–718, 1990.

Bridges, B. A., Cole, J., Favor, J., Glickman, B. W., Mohrenweiser, H., Sankaranarayanan, K., and Skopek, T. R. Spontaneous mutation and its place in risk assessment for chemical mutagens. Mutat. Res., *304*:3–11, 1994.

Bronner, C. E., Baker, S. M., Morrison, P. T., Warren, G., Smith, L. G., Lescoe, M. K., Kane, M., Earabino, C., Lipford, J., Lindblom, A., Tannergård, P., Bollag, R. J., Godwin, A. R., Ward, D. C., Nordenskjøld, M., Fishel, R., Kolodner, R., and Liskay, R. M. Mutation in the DNA mismatch repair gene homologue *hMLH 1* is associated with hereditary non-polyposis colon cancer. Nature, *368*:258–261, 1994.

Bronson, S. K., and Smithies, O. Altering mice by homologous recombination using embryonic stem cells. J. Biol. Chem., *269*:27155–27158, 1994.

Bülow, S. Familial adenomatous polyposis. Ann. Med., *21*:299–307, 1989.

Camper, S. A., Saunders, T. L., Kendall, S. K., Keri, R. A., Seasholtz, A. F., Gordon, D. F., Birkmeier, T. S., Keegan, C. E., Karolyi, I. J., Roller, M. L., Burrows, H. L., and Samuelson, L. C. Implementing transgenic and embryonic stem cell technology to study gene expression, cell-cell interactions and gene function. Biol. Reprod., *52*:246–257, 1995.

Cannon-Albright, L. A., Skolnick, M. H., Bishop, T., Lee, R. G., and Burt, R. W. Common inheritance of susceptibility to colonic adenomatous polyps and associated colorectal cancers. N. Engl. J. Med., *319*:533–537, 1988.

Caporaso, N., Greene, M. H., Tsai, S., Pickle, L. W., and Mulvihill, J. J. Cytogenetics in hereditary malignant melanoma and dysplastic nevus syndrome: is dysplastic nevus syndrome a chromosome instability disorder? Cancer Genet. Cytogenet., *24*:299–314, 1987.

Caporaso, N. E., Shields, P. G., Landi, M. T., Shaw, G. L., Tucker, M. A., Hoover, R., Sugimura, H., Weston, A., and Harris, C. C. The debrisoquine metabolic phenotype and DNA-based assays: implications of misclassification for the association of lung cancer and the debrisoquine metabolic phenotype. Environ. Health Perspect., *98*:101–105, 1992.

Carlson, K. M., Bracamontes, J., Jackson, C. E., Clark, R., Lacroix, A., Wells, S. A., Jr., and Goodfellow, P. J. Parent-of-origin effects in multiple endocrine neoplasia type 2B. Am. J. Hum. Genet., *55*:1076–1082, 1994.

Carter, C. O. Multifactorial genetic disease. Hosp. Pract., pp. 45–59, May 1970.

Cartwright, R. A., Glashan, R. W., Rogers, H. J., Ahmad, R. A., Barham-Hall, D., Higgins, E., and Kahn, M. A. Role of N-acetyltransferase phenotypes in bladder carcinogenesis: a pharmacogenetic epidemilogical approach to bladder cancer. Lancet, October 16, 842–845, 1982.

Caspersson, T., Zech, L., Johansson, C., and Modest, E. J. Identification of human chromosomes by DNA-binding fluorescent agents. Chromosoma, *30*:215–227, 1970.

Cavenee, W. K., Dryja, T. P., Phillips, R. A., Benedict, W. F., Godbout, R., Gallie, B. L., Murphree, A. L., Strong, L. C., and White, R. L. Expression of recessive alleles by chromosomal mechanisms in retinoblastoma. Nature, *305*:779–784, 1983.

Chang, E. H., Pirollo, K. F., Zou, Z. Q., Cheung, H.-Y., Lawler, E. L., Garner, R., White, E., Bernstein, W. B., Fraumeni, J. W., Jr., and Blattner, W. A. Oncogenes in radioresistant, noncancerous skin fibroblasts from a cancer-prone family. Science, *237*:1036–1038, 1987.

Chenevix-Trench, G., Wicking, C., Berkman, J., Sharpe, H., Hockey, A., Haan, E., Oley, C., Ravine, D., Turner, A., Goldgar, D., Searle, J., and Wainwright, B. Further localization of the gene for nevoid basal cell carcinoma syndrome (NBCCS) in 15 Australasian families: linkage and loss of heterozygosity. Am. J. Hum. Genet., *53*:760–767, 1993.

Chung, J. G., Levy, G. N., and Weber, W. W. Distribution of 2-aminofluorene and *p*-aminobenzoic acid *N*-acetyltransferase activity in tissues of C57BL/6J rapid and B6.A-*Nat*^{s} slow acetylator congenic mice. Drug Metab. Dispos., *21*:1057–1062, 1993.

Cleaver, J. E. Do we know the cause of xeroderma pigmentosum? Carcinogenesis, *11*:875–882, 1990.

Colditz, G. A., Willett, W. C., Hunter, D. J., Stampfer, M. J., Manson, J. E., Hennekens, C. H., Rosner, B. A., and Speizer, F. E. Family history, age, and risk of breast cancer. J. Am. Med. Assoc., *270*:338–343, 1993.

Coppes, M. J., Haber, D. A., and Grundy, P. E. Genetic events in the development of Wilms' tumor. N. Engl. J. Med., *331*:586–590, 1994.

Countryman, P. I., Heddle, J. A., and Crawford, E. The repair of x-ray-induced chromosomal damage in trisomy 21 and normal diploid lymphocytes. Cancer Res., *37*:52–58, 1977.

Couturier, J., Delattre, O., Kujas, M., Philippon, J., Peter, M., et al. Assessment of chromosome 22 anomalies in neurinomas by combined karyotype and RFLP analyses. Cancer Genet. Cytogenet., *45*:55–62, 1990.

Dedera, D. A., Waller, E. K., LeBrun, D. P., Sen-Majumdar, A., Stevens, M. E., Barsh, G. S., and Cleary, M. L. Chimeric homeobox gene *E2A-PBX1* induces proliferation, apoptosis, and malignant lymphomas in transgenic mice. Cell, *74*:833–843, 1993.

Dietrich, W. F., Lander, E. S., Smith, J. S., Moser, A. R., Gould, K. A., Luongo, C., Borenstein, N., and Dove, W. Genetic identification of *Mom-1*, a major modifier locus affecting *Min*-induced intestinal neoplasia in the mouse. Cell, *75*:631–639, 1993.

Dominey, A. M., Wang, X.-J., King, L. E., Jr., Nanney, L. B., Gagne, T. A., Sellheyer, K., Bundman, D. S., Longley, M. A., Rothnagel, J. A., Greenhalgh, D. A., and Roop, D. R. Targeted overexpression of transforming growth factor α in the epidermis of transgenic mice elicits hyperplasia, hyperkeratosis, and spontaneous, squamous papillomas. Cell Growth Differ., *4*:1071–1082, 1993.

Donehower, L. A., Harvey, M., Slagle, B. L., McArthur, M. J., Montgomery, C. A., Jr., Butel, J. S., and Bradley, A. Mice deficient for p53 are developmentally normal but susceptible to spontaneous tumours. Nature, *356*:215–221, 1992.

Drabkin, H. A., Bradley, C., Hart, I., Bleskan, J., Li, F. P., and Patterson, D. Translocation of c-*myc* in the hereditary renal cell carcinoma associated with a t(3;8)(p14.2;q24.13) chromosomal translocation. Proc. Natl. Acad. Sci. U.S.A., *82*:6980–6984, 1985.

Drinkwater, N. R. Genetic control of hepatocarcinogenesis in inbred mice. *In*: N. Colburn (Ed.), Genes and Signal Transduction in Multistage Carcinogenesis, pp. 3–17. New York: Marcel Dekker, 1989.

Dryja, T. P., Mukai, S., Petersen, R., Rapaport, J. M., Walton, D., and Yandell, D. W. Parental origin of mutations of the retinoblastoma gene. Nature, *339*:556–558, 1989.

Duggleby, W. F., Stoll, H., Priore, R. L., Greenwald, P., and Graham, S. A genetic analysis of melanoma—polygenic inheritance as a threshold trait. Am. J. Epidemiol., *114*:63–72, 1981.

Dunsford, H. A., Sell, S., and Chisari, F. V. Hepatocarcinogenesis due to chronic liver cell injury in hepatitis B virus transgenic mice. Cancer Res., *50*:3400–3407, 1990.

Dyer, K. R., and Messing, A. Metal-inducible pathology in the liver, pancreas, and kidney of transgenic mice expressing SV40 early region genes. Am. J. Pathol., *135*:401–410, 1989.

Easton, D. F. Cancer risks in A-T heterozygotes. Int. J. Radiat. Biol., *66*:S177–S182, 1994.

Easton, D., Ford, D., and Peto, J. Inherited susceptibility to breast cancer. Cancer Surv., *18*:95–113, 1993.

Eeles, R. A., Stratton, M. R., Goldgar, D. E., and Easton, D. F. The genetics of familial breast cancer and their practical implications. Eur. J. Cancer, *30A*:1383–1390, 1994.

Eker, R., Mossige, J., Johannessen, J. V., and Aars, H. Hereditary renal adenomas and adenocarcinomas in rats. Diagn. Histopathol., *4*:99–110, 1981.

Emerit, I., Emerit, J., Tosoni-Pittoni, A., Bousquet, O., and Sarrazin, A. Chromosome studies in patients with ulcerative colitis. Humangenetik, *16*:313–322, 1972.

Eng, C., Li, F. P., Abramson, D. H., Ellsworth, R. M., Wong, F. L., Goldman, M. B., Seddon, J., Tarbell, N., and Boice, J. D., Jr. Mortality from second tumors among long-term survivors of retinoblastoma. J. Natl. Cancer Inst., *85*:1121–1128, 1993.

Everitt, J. I., Wolf, D. C., Howe, S. R., Goldsworthy, T. L., and Walker, C. Rodent model of reproductive tract leiomyomata. Am. J. Pathol., *146*:1556–1567, 1995.

Ferguson, R. J., Doll, M. A., Baumstark, B. R., and Hein, D. W. Polymorphism arylamine *N*-acetyltransferase encoding gene (*NAT2*) from homozygous rapid and slow acetylator congenic Syrian hamsters. Gene, *140*:247–249, 1994.

Fettman, M. J., Butler, R. N., McMichael, A. J., and Roberts-Thomson, I. C. Metabolic phenotypes and colorectal neoplasia. J. Gastroenterol. Hepatol., *6*:81–89, 1991.

Fijneman, R. J. A., and Demant, P. A gene for susceptibility to small intestinal cancer, *ssic1*, maps to the distal part of mouse chromosome 4. Cancer Res., *55*:3179–3182, 1995.

Fijneman, R. J. A., Ophoff, R. A., Hart, A. A. M., and Demant, P. *Kras-2* alleles, mutations, and lung tumor susceptibility in the mouse—an evaluation. Oncogene, *9*:1417–1421, 1994.

Fishel, R., Lescoe, M. K., Rao, M. R. S., Copeland, N. G., Jenkins, N. A., Garber, J., Kane, M., and Kolodner, R. The human mutator gene homolog *MSH2* and its association with hereditary nonpolyposis colon cancer. Cell, *75*:1027–1038, 1993.

Foster, K., Prowse, A., van den Berg, A., Fleming, S., Hulsbeek, M. M. F., Crossey, P. A., Richards, F. M., Cairns, P., Affara, N. A., Ferguson-Smith, M. A., Buys, C. H. C. M., and Maher, E. R. Somatic mutations of the von Hippel-Lindau disease tumour suppressor gene in non-familial clear cell renal carcinoma. Hum. Mol. Genet., *3*:2169–2173, 1994.

Francke, U., and Kung, F. Sporadic bilateral retinoblastoma and 13q–chromosomal deletion. Med. Pediatr. Oncol., *2*:379–385, 1976.

Friedman, L. S., Ostermeyer, E. A., Lynch, E. D., Szabo, C. I., Anderson, L. A., Dowd, P., Lee, M. K., Rowell, S. E., Boyd, J., and King, M.-C. The search for *BRCA1*. Cancer Res., *54*:6374–6382, 1994.

Friend, S. H. Genetic models for studying cancer susceptibility. Science, *259*:774–775, 1993.

Fuchs, C. S., Giovannucci, E. L., Colditz, G. A., Hunter, D. J., Speizer, F. E., and Willett, W. C. A prospective study of family history and the risk of colorectal cancer. N. Engl. J. Med., *331*:1669–1674, 1994.

Fundia, A. F., González Cid, M. B., Bai, J., Gómez, J. C., Mazure, R., Vazquez, H., Larripa, I. B., and Slavutsky, I. R. Chromosome instability in lymphocytes from patients with celiac disease. Clin. Genet., *45*:57–61, 1994.

Gagel, R. F. Multiple endocrine neoplasia type II. *In*: J. P. Bilezikian, M. A. Levine, and R. Marcus (Eds.), The Parathyroids, pp. 681–698. New York: Raven Press, 1994.

Gardner, E. J., Rogers, S. W., and Woodward, S. Numerical and structural chromosome aberrations in cultured lymphocytes and cutaneous fibroblasts of patients with multiple adenomas of the colorectum. Cancer, *49*:1413–1419, 1982.

Gateff, E. Malignant neoplasms of genetic origin in *Drosophila melanogaster*. Science, *200*:1448–1459, 1978.

Gerald, W. L. The molecular genetics of Wilms tumor: a paradigm of heterogeneity in tumor development. Cancer Invest., *12*:350–359, 1994.

German, J. Bloom syndrome: a Mendelian prototype of somatic mutational disease. Medicine, *72*:393–406, 1993.

Glickman, B. W., Saddi, V. A., and Curry, J. Spontaneous mutations in mammalian cells. Mutat. Res., *304*:19–32, 1994.

Goldstein, A. M., Fraser, M. C., Clark, W. H., Jr., and Tucker, M. A. Age at diagnosis and transmission of invasive melanoma in 23 families with cutaneous malignant melanoma/dysplastic nevi. J. Natl. Cancer Inst., *86*:1385–1390, 1994.

Grant, D. M. Molecular genetics of the N-acetyltransferases. Pharmacogenetics, *3*:45–50, 1993.

Greenberg, N. M., DeMayo, F., Finegold, M. J., Medina, D., Tilley, W. D., Aspinall, J. O., Cunha, G. R., Donjacour, A. A., Matusik, R. J., and Rosen, J. M. Prostate cancer in a transgenic mouse. Proc. Natl. Acad. Sci. U.S.A., *92*:3439–3443, 1995.

Greene, M. H. Dysplastic nevus syndrome. Hosp. Pract., pp. 91–108, January 1984.

Grossman, W. J., Kimata, J. T., Wong, F.-H., Zutter, M., Ley, T. J., and Ratner, L. Development of leukemia in mice transgenic for the *tax* gene of human T-cell leukemia virus type I. Proc. Natl. Acad. Sci. U.S.A., *92*:1057–1061, 1995.

Gunz, F. W., Gunz, J. P., Veale, A. M. O., Chapman, C. J., and Houston, I. B. Familial leukaemia: a study of 909 families. Scand. J. Haematol., *15*:117–131, 1975.

Hall, J. M., Huey, B., Morrow, J., Newman, B., Lee, M., Jones, E., Carter, C., Buehring, G. C., and King, M-C. Rare HRAS alleles and susceptibility to human breast cancer. Genomics, *6*:188–191, 1990a.

Hall, J. M., Lee, M. K., Newman, B., Morrow, J. E., Anderson, L. A., Huey, B., and King, M.-C. Linkage of early-onset familial breast cancer to chromosome 17q21. Science, *250*:1684–1689, 1990b.

Hanawalt, P. C., and Sarasin, A. Cancer-prone hereditary diseases with DNA processing abnormalities. Trends Genet., *2*:124–129, 1986.

Hayashi, S-i., Watanabe, J., and Kawajiri, K. High susceptibility to lung cancer analyzed in terms of combined genotypes of P450IA1 and Mu-class glutathione *S*-transferase genes. Jpn. J. Cancer Res., *83*:866–870, 1992.

Heim, R. A., Lench, N. J., and Swift, M. Heterozygous manifestations in four autosomal recessive human cancer-prone syndromes: ataxia telangiectasia, xeroderma pigmentosum, Fanconi anemia, and Bloom syndrome. Mutat. Res., *284*:25–36, 1992.

Hein, D. W., Rustan, T. D., Bucher, K. D., Martin, W. J., and Furman, E. J. Acetylator phenotype-dependent and -independent expression of arylamine *N*-acetyltransferase isozymes in rapid and slow acetylator inbred rat liver. Drug Metab. Dispos., *19*:933–937, 1991.

Henderson, I. C. Risk factors for breast cancer development. Cancer, *71*:2127–2140, 1993.

Heras, J. G., and Larripa, I. Radiation sensitivity in retinoblastoma: current perspectives for cancer research on this disease. Mutat. Res., *202*:1–8, 1988.

Herrera, L., Kakati, S., Gibas, L., Pietrzak, E., and Sandberg, A. A. Gardner syndrome in a man with an interstitial deletion of 5q. Am. J. Med. Genet., *25*:473–476, 1986.

Heston, W. E., and Vlahakis, G. C3H-A^{vy}—a high hepatoma and high mammary tumor strain of mice. J. Natl. Cancer Inst., *40*:1161–1166, 1968.

Heutink, P., van der Mey, A. G. L., Sandkuijl, L. A., van Gils, P. G., Bardoel, A., Breedveld, G. J., van Vliet, M., van Ommen, G.-J. B., Cornelisse, C. J., Oostra, B. A., Weber, J. L., and Devilee, P. A gene subject to genomic imprinting and responsible for hereditary paragangliomas maps to chromosome 11q23-qter. Hum. Mol. Genet., *1*:7–10, 1992.

Hino, O., Mitani, H., Katsuyama, H., and Kubo, Y. A novel cancer predisposition syndrome in the Eker rat model. Cancer Lett., *83*:117–121, 1994.

Hinrichs, S. H., Nerenberg, M., Reynolds, R. K., Khoury, G., and Jay, G. A transgenic mouse model for human neurofibromatosis. Science, *237*:1340–1343, 1987.

Hirvonen, A., Husgafvel-Pursiainen, K., Karjalainen, A., Anttila, S., and Vainio, H. Point-mutational *Msp*I and *Ile-Val* polymorphisms closely linked in the *CYP1A1* gene: lack of association with susceptibility to lung cancer in a Finnish study population. Cancer Epidemiol. Biomark. Prevent., *1*:485–489, 1992.

Hirvonen, A., Husgafvel-Pursiainen, K., Anttila, S., Karjalainen, A., Pelkonen, O., and Vainio, H. PCR-based *CYP2D6* genotyping for Finnish lung cancer patients. Pharmacogenetics, *3*:19–27, 1993.

Hirvonen, A., Pelin, K., Tammilehto, L., Karjalainen, A., Mattson, K., and Linnainmaa, K. Inherited *GSTM1* and *NAT2* defects as concurrent risk modifiers in asbestos-related human malignant mesothelioma. Cancer Res., *55*:2981–2983, 1995.

Hockey, K. A., Mulcahy, M. T., Montgomery, P., and Levitt, S. Deletion of chromosome 5q and familial adenomatous polyposis. J. Med. Genet., *26*:61–62, 1989.

Hoeijmakers, J. H. J. Human nucleotide excision repair syndromes: molecular clues to unexpected intricacies. Eur. J. Cancer, *30A*:1912–1921, 1994.

Hooper, M. L. The role of the *p53* and *Rb-1* genes in cancer, development and apoptosis. J. Cell Sci. Suppl., *18*:13–17, 1994.

Hors, J., Andrieu, J. M., and Gony, J. HLA and cancer. Transplant. Proc., *16*:455–457, 1984.

Horsthemke, B. Genetics and cytogenetics of retinoblastoma. Cancer Genet. Cytogenet., *63*:1–7, 1992.

Houlston, R. S., Collins, A., Slack, J., and Morton, N. E. Dominant genes for colorectal cancer are not rare. Ann. Hum. Genet., *56*:99–103, 1992.

Housman, D. E. Role of the Wilms' tumor 1 tumor-suppressor gene in the etiology of Wilms' tumor. *In*: Nuclear Processes and Oncogenes, pp. 147–160. New York: Academic Press, 1992.

Hsu, T. C., Spitz, M. R., and Schantz, S. P. Mutagen sensitivity: a biological marker of cancer susceptibility. Cancer Epidemiol. Biomarkers Prevention, *1*:83–89, 1991.

Hussussian, C. J., Struewing, J. P., Goldstein, A. M., Higgins, P. A. T., Ally, D. S., Sheahan, M. D., Clark, W. H., Jr., Tucker, M. A., and Dracopoli, N. C. Germline p16 mutations in familial melanoma. Nature Genet., *8*:15–21, 1994.

Iida, M., Yao, T., Itoh, H., Watanabe, H., Matsui, T., Iwashita, A., and Fujishima, M. Natural history of duodenal lesions in Japanese patients with familial adenomatosis coli (Gardner's syndrome). Gastroenterology, *96*:1301–1306, 1989.

ISCN. *In*: D. G. Harnden and H. P. Klinger (Eds.), An International System for Human Cytogenetic Nomenclature. Published in collaboration with Cytogenet. Cell Genet. Basel, Karger, 1985.

Izumi, K., Kitaura, K., Chone, Y., Tate, H., Nakagawa, T., Suzuki, Y., and Matsumoto, K. Spontaneous renal cell tumors in Long-Evans cinnamon rats. Jpn. J. Cancer Res., *85*:563–566, 1994.

Jacks, T., Fazeli, A., Schmitt, E. M., Bronson, R. T., Goodell, M. A., and Weinberg, R. A. Effects of an *Rb* mutation in the mouse. Nature, *359*:295–300, 1992.

Jaenisch, R. Transgenic animals. Science, *240*:1468–1474, 1988.

Jagelman, D. G. Extra-colonic manifestations of familial adenomatous polyposis. Oncology, *5*:23–33, 1991.

Johansson, I., Lundqvist, E., Bertilsson, L., Dahl, M-L., Sjöqvist, F., and Ingelman-Sundberg, M. Inherited amplification of an active gene in the cytochrome P450 *CYP2D* locus as a cause of ultrarapid metabolism of debrisoquine. Proc. Natl. Acad. Sci. U.S.A., *90*:11825–11829, 1993.

Junien, C. Genes of susceptibility to cancer. Horm. Res., *32*:30–33, 1989.

Kato, M., Toguchida, J., Honda, K., Sasaki, M. S., Ikenaga, M., Sugimoto, M., Yamaguchi, T., Kotoura, Y., Yamamuro, T., and Ishizaki, K. Elevated frequency of a specific allele of the L-*myc* gene in male patients with bone and soft-tissue sarcomas. Int. J. Cancer, *45*:47–49, 1990.

Kawajiri, K., and Fujii-Kuriyama, Y. P450 and human cancer. Jpn. J. Cancer Res., *82*:1325–1335, 1991.

Kee, F., and Collins, B. J. How prevalent is cancer family syndrome? Gut, *32*:509–512, 1991.

Kellermann, G., Shaw, C. R., and Luyten-Kellerman, M. Aryl hydrocarbon hydroxylase inducibility and bronchogenic carcinoma. N. Engl. J. Med., *289*:934–937, 1973.

King, M-C., Rowell, S., and Love, S. M. Inherited breast and ovarian cancer. What are the risks? What are the choices? J.A.M.A., *269*:1975–1980, 1993.

Klingel, R., Mittelstaedt, P., Dippold, W. G., and Meyer zum Büschenfelde, K-H. Distribution of Ha-ras alleles in patients with colorectal cancer and Crohn's disease. Gut, *32*:1508–1513, 1991.

Kloss, K., Währisch, P., Greger, V., Messmer, E., Fritze, H., Höpping, W., Passarge, E., and Horsthemke, B. Characterization of deletions at the retinoblastoma locus in patients with bilateral retinoblastoma. Am. J. Med. Genet., *39*:196–200, 1991.

Knauf, W. U., and Ho, A. D. Polymorphism of the human Ha-ras oncogene locus in chronic lymphocytic and chronic myelogenous leukemia. Hematol. Oncol., *9*:157–162, 1991.

Knight, K. L., Spieker-Polet, H., Kazdin, D. S., and Oi, V. T. Transgenic rabbits with lymphocytic leukemia induced by the c-*myc* oncogene fused with the immunoglobulin heavy chain enhancer. Proc. Natl. Acad. Sci. U.S.A., *85*:3130–3134, 1988.

Knudson, A. G. Mutation and cancer: statistical study of retinoblastoma. Proc. Natl. Acad. Sci. U.S.A., *60*:820, 1971.

Knudson, A. G., Jr., and Strong, L. C. Mutation and cancer: a model for Wilms' tumor of the kidney. J. Natl. Cancer Inst., *48*:313–324, 1972.

Knudson, A. G., Jr. Hereditary cancer, oncogenes, and antioncogenes. Cancer Res., *45*:1437–1443, 1985.

Kobayashi, T., Hirayama, Y., Kobayashi, E., Kubo, Y., and Hino, O. A germline insertion in the tuberous sclerosis (*Tsc2*) gene gives rise to the Eker rat model of dominantly inherited cancer. Nature Genet., 9:70–75, 1995.

Koufos, A., Grundy, P., Morgan, K., et al. Familial Wiedemann-Beckwith syndrome and a second Wilms' tumor locus map to 11p15.5. Am. J. Hum. Genet., 44:711–719, 1989.

Kovacs, G., Emanuel, A., Neumann, H. P. H., and Kung, H.-f. Cytogenetics of renal cell carcinomas associated with von Hippel-Lindau disease. Genes Chromosom. Cancer, 3:256–262, 1991.

Kovacs, E., and Langemann, H. Differences in the kinetics of DNA repair in cancer patients and healthy controls. Oncology, 48:312–316, 1991.

Krontiris, T. G., DiMartino, N. A., Mitcheson, H. D., Lonergan, J. A., Begg, C., and Parkinson, D. R. Human hypervariable sequences in risk assessment: rare Ha-*ras* alleles in cancer patients. Environ. Health Perspect., 76:147–153, 1987.

Krontiris, T. G., Devlin, B., Karp, D. D., Robert, N. J., and Risch, N. An association between the risk of cancer and mutations in the HRAS1 minisatellite locus. N. Engl. J. Med., 329:517–523, 1993.

Kubo, Y., Mitani, H., and Hino, O. Allelic loss at the predisposing gene locus in spontaneous and chemically induced renal cell carcinomas in the Eker rat. Cancer Res., 54:2633–2635, 1994.

Ladero, J. M., Benítez, J., González, J. F., Vargas, E., and Díaz-Rubio, M. Oxidative polymorphism of debrisoquine is not related to human colorectal cancer. Eur. J. Clin. Pharmacol., 40:525–527, 1991a.

Ladero, J. M., Benítez, J., Jara, C., Llerena, A., Valdivielso, M. J., Muñoz, J. J., and Vargas, E. Polymorphic oxidation of debrisoquine in women with breast cancer. Oncology, 48:107–110, 1991b.

LaForgia, S., Lasota, J., Latif, F., Boghosian-Sell, L., Kastury, K., Ohta, M., Druck, T., Atchison, L., Cannizzaro, L. A., Barnea, G., Schlessinger, J., Modi, W., Kuzmin, I., Tory, K., Zbar, B., Croce, C. M., Lerman, M., and Huebner, K. Detailed genetic and physical map of the 3p chromosome region surrounding the familial renal cell carcinoma chromosome translocation, t(3;8)(p14.2;q24.1). Cancer Res., 53:3118–3124, 1993.

Lalle, P., De Latour, M., Rio, P., and Bignon, Y.-J. Detection of allelic losses on 17q12-q21 chromosomal region in benign lesions and malignant tumors occurring in a familial context. Oncogene, 9:437–442, 1994.

Lamiell, J. M., Salazar, F. G., and Hsia, Y. E. von Hippel–Lindau disease affecting 43 members of a single kindred. Medicine, 68:1–29, 1989.

Lander, E. S., and Schork, N. J. Genetic dissection of complex traits. Science, 265:2037–2048, 1994.

Larsson, C., Skogseid, B., Öberg, K., Nakamura, Y., and Nordenskjöld, M. Multiple endocrine neoplasia type 1 gene maps to chromosome 11 and is lost in insulinoma. Nature, 332:85–86, 1988.

Lasko, D., Cavenee, W., and Nordenskjöld, M. Loss of constitutional heterozygosity in human cancer. Annu. Rev. Genet., 25:281–314, 1991.

Ledbetter, D. H., Rich, D. C., O'Connell, P., Leppert, M., and Carey, J. C. Precise localization of NF1 to 17q11.2 by balanced translocation. Am. J. Hum. Genet., 44:20–24, 1989.

Lee, E. Y.-H. P., Chang, C.-Y., Hu, N., Wang, Y.-C. J., Lai, C.-C., Herrup, K., Lee, W.-H., and Bradley, A. Mice deficient for Rb are nonviable and show defects in neurogenesis and haematopoiesis. Nature, 359:288–294, 1992a.

Lee, G.-H., Merlino, G., and Fausto, N. Development of liver tumors in transforming growth factor α transgenic mice. Cancer Res., 52:5162–5170, 1992b.

Lee, Y. C., Asa, S. L., and Drucker, D. J. Glucagon gene 5′-flanking sequences direct expression of Simian virus 40 large T antigen to the intestine, producing carcinoma of the large bowel in transgenic mice. J. Biol. Chem., 267:10705–10708, 1992c.

Li, F. P., Fraumeni, J. F., Jr., Mulvihill, J. J., Blattner, W. A., Dreyfus, M. G., Tucker, M. A., and Miller, R. W. A cancer family syndrome in twenty-four kindreds. Cancer Res., 48:5358–5362, 1988.

Lidereau, R., Mathieu-Mahul, D., Escot, C., Theillet, C., Champeme, M-H., Cole, S., Mauchauffe, M., Ali, I., Amione, J., Callahan, R., and Larsen, C-J. Genetic variability of proto-oncogenes for breast cancer risk and prognosis. Biochimie, 70:951–959, 1988.

Lindblom, A., Rotstein, S., Skoog, L., Nordenskjöld, M., and Larsson, C. Deletions on chromosome 16 in primary familial breast carcinomas are associated with development of distant metastases. Cancer Res., 53:3707–3711, 1993a.

Lindblom, A., Skoog, L., Andersen, T. I., Rotstein, S., Nordenskjöld, M., and Larsson, C. Four separate regions on chromosome 17 show loss of heterozygosity in familial breast carcinomas. Hum. Genet., *91*:6–12, 1993b.

Lindblom, A., Skoog, L., Rotstein, S., Werelius, B., Larsson, C., and Nordenskjöld, M. Loss of heterozygosity in familial breast carcinomas. Cancer Res., *53*:4356–4361, 1993c.

Linenan, W. M., Brenan, M., and Zbar, B. Identification of the von Hippel-Lindau (VHL) gene. Its role in renal cancer. J.A.M.A., *273*:564–570, 1995.

Lipkowitz, S., Garry, V. F., and Kirsch, I. R. Interlocus V-J recombination measures genomic instability in agriculture workers at risk for lymphoid malignancies. Proc. Natl. Acad. Sci. U.S.A., *89*:5301–5305, 1992.

Liu, B., Farrington, S. M., Petersen, G. M., Hamilton, S. R., Parsons, R., Papadopoulos, N., Fujiwara, T., Jen, J., Kinzler, K. W., Wyllie, A. H., Vogelstein, B., and Dunlop, M. G. Genetic instability occurs in the majority of young patients with colorectal cancer. Nature Med., *1*:348–352, 1995.

Luongo, C., Moser, A. R., Gledhill, S., and Dove, W. F. Loss of Apc^+ in intestinal adenomas from Min mice. Cancer Res., *54*:5947–5952, 1994.

Lutzner, M. A., Guenet, J.-L., and Breitburd, F. Multiple cutaneous papillomas and carcinomas that develop spontaneously in a mouse mutant, the repeated epilation heterozygote Er/+. J. Natl. Cancer Inst., *75*:161–166, 1985.

Lynch, H. T., and Lynch, J. Genetics, natural history, surveillance, management, and gene mapping in the Lynch syndrome. Pathol. Biol., *43*:151–158, 1995.

Lynch, H. T., Lynch, P. M., Albano, W. A., Edney, J., Organ, C. H., and Lynch, J. F. Hereditary cancer: ascertainment and management. CA, *29*:216–232, 1979.

Lynch, H. T., Fitzgibbons, R. J. Jr., and Lynch, J. F. Heterogeneity and natural history of hereditary breast cancer. Surg. Clin. North Am., *70*:753–774, 1990.

Lynch, H. T., Lanspa, S., Smyrk, T., et al. Hereditary nonpolyposis colorectal cancer (Lynch syndromes I & II). Genetics, pathology, natural history, and cancer control, part 1. Cancer Genet. Cytogenet., *53*:143–160, 1991.

Lynch, H. T., Fusaro, R. M., Sandberg, A. A., Bixenman, H. A., Johnsen, L. R., Lynch, J. F., Ramesh, K. H., and Leppert, M. Chromosome instability and the FAMMM syndrome. Cancer Genet. Cytogenet., *71*:27–39, 1993.

MacPhee, M., Chepenik, K. P., Liddell, R. A., Nelson, K. K., Siracusa, L. D., and Buchberg, A. M. The secretory phospholipase A2 gene is a candidate for the *Mom1* locus, a major modifier of Apc^{Min}-induced intestinal neoplasia. Cell, *81*:957–966, 1995.

Maher, E. R., and Yates, J. R. W. Familial renal cell carcinoma: clinical and molecular genetic aspects. Br. J. Cancer, *63*:176–179, 1991.

Malkin, D. *p53* and the Li-Fraumeni syndrome. Biochim. Biophys. Acta, *1198*:197–213, 1994.

Malkinson, A. M. Genetic studies on lung tumor susceptibility and histogenesis in mice. Environ. Health Perspect., *93*:149–159, 1991.

Malkinson, A. M., and You, M. The intronic structure of cancer-related genes regulates susceptibility to cancer. Mol. Carcinog., *10*:61–65, 1994.

Manenti, G., Binelli, G., Gariboldi, M., Canzian, F., de Gregorio, L., Falvella, F. S., Dragani, T. A., and Pierotti, M. A. Multiple loci affect genetic predisposition to hepatocarcinogenesis in mice. Genomics, *23*:118–124, 1994.

Martuza, R. L., and Eldridge, R. Neurofibromatosis 2. N. Engl. J. Med., *318*:684–688, 1988.

Mathew, C. G. P., Smith, B. A., Thorpe, K., Wong, Z., Royle, N. J., et al. Depletion of genes on chromosome 1 in endocrine neoplasia. Nature, *328*:524–527, 1987.

Matsunaga, E., Zanger, U. M., Hardwick, J. P., Gelboin, H. V., Meyer, U. A., and Gonzalez, F. J. The *CYP2D* gene subfamily: analysis of the molecular basis of the debrisoquine 4-hydroxylase deficiency in DA rats. Biochemistry, *28*:7349–7355, 1989.

Matsuyama, M., Yamada, C., and Hiai, H. A single dominant susceptible gene determines spontaneous development of thymoma in BUF/Mna rat. Jpn. J. Cancer Res., *77*:1066–1068, 1986.

Maw, M. A., Grundy, P. E., Millow, L. J., Eccles, M. R., Dunn, R. S., Smith, P. J., Feinberg, A. P., Law, D. J., Paterson, M. C., Telzerow, P. E., Callen, D. F., Thompson, A. D., Richards, R. I., and Reeve, A. E. A third Wilms tumor locus on chromosome 16q. Cancer Res., *52*:3094–3098, 1992.

McBride, O. W., Merry, D., and Givol, D. The gene for human p53 cellular tumor antigen is located on chromosome 17 short arm (17p13). Proc. Natl. Acad. Sci. U.S.A., *83*:130–134, 1986.

McGlynn, K. A., Rosvold, E. A., Lustbader, E. D., Hu, Y., Clapper, M. L., Zhou, T., Wild, C. P., Xia, X-L., Baffoe-Bonnie, A., Ofori-Adjei, D., Chen, G-C., London, W. T., Shen, F-M., and Buetow, K. H. Susceptibility to hepatocellular carcinoma is associated with genetic variation in the enzymatic detoxification of aflatoxin B$_1$. Proc. Natl. Acad. Sci. U.S.A., *92*:2384–2387, 1995.

McKusick, V. A., and Amberger, J. S. Genetic map of the human genome: the autosomes and X, Y, and mitochondrial chromosomes. *In*: C. R. Scriver et al. (Eds.), The Metabolic Bases of Inherited Disease, 7th ed., pp. 119–228. New York: McGraw-Hill, 1995.

McQueen, C. A., Maslansky, C. J., Glowinski, I. B., Crescenzi, S. B., Weber, W. W., and Williams, G. M. Relationship between the genetically determined acetylator phenotype and DNA damage induced by hydralazine and 2-aminofluorene in cultured rabbit hepatocytes. Proc. Natl. Acad. Sci. U.S.A., *79*:1269–1272, 1982.

Menon, A. G., Anderson, K. M., Riccardi, V. M., Chung, R. Y., Whaley, J. M., Yandell, D. W., Farmer, G. E., Freiman, R. N., Lee, J. K., Li, F. P., Barker, D. F., Ledbetter, D. H., Kleider, A., Martuza, R. L., Gusella, J. F., and Seizinger, B. R. Chromosome 17p deletions and p53 gene mutations associated with the formation of malignant neurofibrosarcomas in von Recklinghausen neurofibromatosis. Proc. Natl. Acad. Sci. U.S.A., *87*:5435–5439, 1990.

Mesrobian, H.-G. J. Wilms tumor: past, present, future. J. Urol., *140*:231–238, 1988.

Miki, Y., Swensen, J., Shattuck-Eidens, D., Futreal, P. A., Harshman, K., Tavtigian, S., Liu, Q., Cochran, C., Bennett, L. M., Ding, W., Bell, R., Rosenthal, J., Hussey, C., Tran, T., McClure, M., Frye, C., Hattier, T., Phelps, R., Haugen-Strano, A., Katcher, H., Yakumo, K., Gholami, Z., Shaffer, D., Stone, S., Bayer, S., Wray, C., Bodgen, R., Dayananth, P., Ward, J., Tonin, P., Narod, S., Bristow, P. K., Norris, F. H., Helvering, L., Morrison, P., Rosteck, P., Lai, M., Barrett, J. C., Lewis, C., Neuhausen, S., Cannon-Albright, L., Goldgar, D., Wiseman, R., Kamb, A., and Skolnick, M. H. A strong candidate for the breast and ovarian cancer susceptibility gene *BRCA1*. Science, *266*:66–71, 1994.

Miller, R. W. Transplacental chemical carcinogenesis in man. J. Natl. Cancer Inst., *47*:1169–1171, 1971.

Mock, B. A., Krall, M. M., and Dosik, J. K. Genetic mapping of tumor susceptibility genes involved in mouse plasmacytomagenesis. Proc. Natl. Acad. Sci. U.S.A., *90*:9499–9503, 1993.

Moser, A. R., Pitot, H. C., and Dove, W. F. A dominant mutation that predisposes to multiple intestinal neoplasia in the mouse. Science, *247*:322–324, 1990.

Moser, A. R., Mattes, E. M., Dove, W. F., Lindstrom, M. J., Haag, J. D., and Gould, M. N. *Apc^{Min}*, a mutation in the murine *Apc* gene, predisposes to mammary carcinomas and focal alveolar hyperplasias. Proc. Natl. Acad. Sci. U.S.A., *90*:8977–8981, 1993.

Müller, H., and Scott, R. J. How common is hereditary cancer? Ann. Med., *26*:173–175, 1994.

Muller, W. J. Expression of activated oncogenes in the murine mammary gland: transgenic models for human breast cancer. Cancer Metast. Rev., *10*:217–227, 1991.

Mulligan, L. M., Gardner, E., Smith, B. A., Mathew, C. G. P., and Ponder, B. A. J. Genetic events in tumour initiation and progression in multiple endocrine neoplasia type 2. Genes Chromosom. Cancer, *6*:166–177, 1993.

Murakumo, Y., Takahashi, M., Arakawa, A., Saito, M., Amo, H., Katoh, H., and Matsuyama, M. Chromosomal mapping of genetic locus associated with thymus-size enlargement in BUF/Mna rats. Jpn. J. Cancer Res., *84*:838–840, 1993.

Murnane, J. P., and Kapp, L. N. A critical look at the association of human genetic syndromes with sensitivity to ionizing radiation. Cancer Biol., *4*:93–104, 1993.

Nagase, S., Shumiya, S., Emori, T., and Tanaka, H. High incidence of renal tumors induced by N-dimethylnitrosamine in analbuminemic rats. Gann, *74*:317–318, 1983.

Nakachi, K., Imai, K., Hayashi, S-i., Watanabe, J., and Kawajiri, K. Genetic susceptibility to squamous cell carcinoma of the lung in relation to cigarette smoking dose. Cancer Res., *51*:5177–5180, 1991.

Nakachi, K., Imai, K., Hayashi, S-i., and Kawajiri, K. Polymorphisms of the *CYP1A1* and glutathione *S*-transferase genes associated with susceptibility to lung cancer in relation to cigarette dose in a Japanese population. Cancer Res., *53*:2994–2999, 1993.

Naumova, A., and Sapienza, C. The genetics of retinoblastoma, revisited. Am. J. Hum. Genet., *54*:264–273, 1994.

Nebert, D. W. Polymorphism of human *CYP2D* genes involved in drug metabolism: possible relationship to individual cancer risk. Cancer Cells, *3*:93–96, 1991.

Nellist, M., Janssen, B., Brook-Carter, P. T., Hesseling-Janssen, A. L. W., Maheshwar, M. M., Verhoef, S., Van den Ouweland, A. M. W., Lindhout, D., Eussen, B., Cordeiro, I., Santos, H., Halley, D. J. J., Sampson, J. R., Ward, C. J., Peral, B., Thomas, S., Hughes, J., Harris, P. C., Roelfsema, J. H., Saris, J. J., Spruit, L., Peters, D. J. M., Dauwerse, J. G., and Breuning, M. H. Identification and characterization of the tuberous sclerosis gene on chromosome 16. Cell, *75*:1305–1315, 1993.

Newell, G. R., Gordon, J. E., Monlezun, A. P., and Horwitz, J. S. ABO blood groups and cancer. J. Natl. Cancer Inst., *52*:1425–1430, 1974.

Newsham, I. F., Hadjistilianou, T., and Cavenee, W. K. Retinoblastoma. *In*: C. R. Scriver, A. L. Beaudet, W. S. Sly, and D. Valle (Eds.), The Metabolic and Molecular Bases of Inherited Disease, 7th ed., Vol. 1, Chapter 11, pp. 613–642. New York: McGraw-Hill, 1995.

Oda, Y., Tanaka, M., and Nakanishi, I. Relation between the occurrence of K-*ras* gene point mutations and genotypes of polymorphic *N*-acetyltransferase in human colorectal carcinomas. Carcinogenesis, *15*:1365–1369, 1994.

Ogiu, T., Fukami, H., Nishimura, M., and Matsuyama, M. Genetic regulation of development of thymic lymphomas induced by *N*-propyl-*N*-nitrosourea in the rat. Jpn. J. Cancer Res., *86*:638–644, 1995.

Okabe, T., Suzuki, A., Ishikawa, H., Watanabe, I., and Takaku, F. Chromosomal aneuploidy in sarcoid granuloma cells. Am. Rev. Respir. Dis., *134*:300–304, 1986.

Okey, A. B., Riddick, D. S., and Harper, P. A. Molecular biology of the aromatic hydrocarbon (dioxin) receptor. Trends Pharmacol. Sci., *15*:226–232, 1994.

Ono, T., Abe, S., and Yoshida, M. C. Hereditary low level of plasma ceruloplasmin in LEC rats associated with spontaneous development of hepatitis and liver cancer. Jpn. J. Cancer Res., *82*:486–489, 1991.

Orian, J. M., Tamakoshi, K., Mackay, I. R., and Brandon, M. R. New murine model for hepatocellular carcinoma: transgenic mice expressing metallothionein-ovine growth hormone fusion gene. J. Natl. Cancer Inst., *82*:393–398, 1990.

Paris Conference. Standardization in Human Cytogenetics. Birth Defects, Original Article Ser. 8, No. 7, 1972. New York: The National Foundation.

Parshad, R., Sanford, K. K., and Jones, G. M. Chromatid damage after G_2 phase x-irradiation of cells from cancer-prone individuals implicates deficiency in DNA repair. Proc. Natl. Acad. Sci. U.S.A., *80*:5612–5616, 1983.

Pero, R. W., Johnson, D. B., Markowitz, M., Doyle, G., Lund-Pero, M., Seidegard, J., Halper, M., and Miller, D. G. DNA repair synthesis in individuals with and without a family history of cancer. Carcinogenesis, *10*:693–697, 1989.

Peto, T. E. A., Thein, S. L., and Wainscoat, J. S. Statistical methodology in the analysis of relationships between DNA polymorphisms and disease: putative association of Ha-ras-I hypervariable alleles and cancer. Am. J. Hum. Genet., *42*:615–617, 1988.

Pitot, H. C. Fundamentals of Oncology, 3rd ed. New York: Marcel Dekker, 1986.

Prehn, L. M., and Lawler, E. M. Rank order of sarcoma susceptibility among mouse strains reverses with low concentrations of carcinogen. Science, *204*:309–310, 1979.

Probst-Hensch, N. M., Haile, R. W., Ingles, S. A., Longnecker, M. P., Han, C-Y., Lin, B. K., Lee, D. B., Sakamoto, G. T., Frankl, H. D., Lee, E. R., and Lin, H. J. Acetylation polymorphism and prevalence of colorectal adenomas. Cancer Res., *55*:2017–2020, 1995.

Purtilo, D. T., Paquin, L., and Gindhart, T. Genetics of neoplasia—impact of ecogenetics on oncogenesis. Am. J. Pathol., *91*:609–688, 1978.

Radford, D. M., Ashley, S. W., Wells, S. A., Jr., and Gerhard, D. S. Loss of heterozygosity of markers on chromosome 11 in tumors from patients with multiple endocrine neoplasia syndrome type 1. Cancer Res., *50*:6529–6533, 1990.

Radice, P., Pierotti, M. A., Borrello, M. G., Illeni, M. T., Rovini, D., and Della Porta, G. HRAS1 proto-oncogene polymorphisms in human malignant melanoma: TaqI defined alleles significantly associated with the disease. Oncogene, *2*:91–95, 1987.

Rainier, S., Johnson, L. A., Dobry, C. J., Ping, A. J., Grundy, P. E., and Feinberg, A. P. Relaxation of imprinted genes in human cancer. Nature, *362*:747–749, 1993.

Razin, A., and Cedar, H. DNA methylation and genomic imprinting. Cell, *77*:473–476, 1994.

Reddy, J. C., Morris, J. C., Wang, J., English, M. A., Haber, D. A., Shi, Y., and Licht, J. D. WT1-mediated transcriptional activation is inhibited by dominant negative mutant proteins. J. Biol. Chem., *270*:10878–10884, 1995.

Riccardi, V. M. von Recklinghausen neurofibromatosis. N. Engl. J. Med., *305*:1617–1627, 1981.

Riccardi, W. M., Sujansky, E., Smith, A. C., and Francke, U. Chromosomal imbalance in the aniridia-Wilms tumor association: 11p interstitial deletion. Pediatrics, *61*:604–610, 1978.

Richards, F. M., Maher, E. R., Latif, F., Phipps, M. E., Tory, K., Lush, M., Crossey, P. A., Oostra, B., Gustavson, K. H., Green, J., Turner, G., Yates, J. R. W., Linehan, W. M., Affara, N. A., Lerman, M., Zbar, B., and Ferguson-Smith, M. A. Detailed genetic mapping of the von Hippel-Lindau disease tumour suppressor gene. J. Med. Genet., *30*:104–107, 1993.

Roberts, R. J., and Macelis, D. Restriction enzymes and their isoschizomers. Nucleic Acids Res., *20*:2167–2180, 1992.

Rogler, C. E., Yang, D., Rossetti, L., Donohoe, J., Alt, E., Chang, C. J., Rosenfeld, R., Neely, K., and Hintz, R. Altered body composition and increased frequency of diverse malignancies in insulin-like growth factor-II transgenic mice. J. Biol. Chem., *269*:13779–13784, 1994.

Ross, S. R., Choy, L., Graves, R. A., Fox, N., Solevjeva, V., Klaus, S., Ricquier, D., and Spiegelman, B. M. Hibernoma formation in transgenic mice and isolation of a brown adipocyte cell line expressing the uncoupling protein gene. Proc. Natl. Acad. Sci. U.S.A., *89*:7561–7565, 1992.

Ryberg, D., Tefre, T., Skaug, V., Stangeland, L., Øvrebø, S., Naalsund, A., Børresen, A-L., and Haugen, A. Allele diversity of the H-*ras*-1 variable number of tandem repeats in Norwegian lung cancer patients. Environ. Health Perspect., *98*:187–189, 1992.

Sandmöller, A., Halter, R., Suske, G., Paul, D., and Beato, M. A transgenic mouse model for lung adenocarcinoma. Cell Growth Differ., *6*:97–103, 1995.

Sapienza, C. Parental imprinting of genes. Sci. Am., *263, October*:52–60, 1990.

Sasaki, M., Okamoto, M., Sato, C., Sugio, K., Soejima, J.-i., Iwama, T., Ikeuchi, T., Tonomura, A., Miyaki, M., and Sasazuki, T. Loss of constitutional heterozygosity in colorectal tumors from patients with familial polyposis coli and those with nonpolyposis colorectal carcinoma. Cancer Res., *49*:4402–4406, 1989.

Sasaki, Y., Ohsako, S., and Deguchi, T. Molecular and genetic analyses of arylamine *N*-acetyltransferase polymorphism of rabbit liver. J. Biol. Chem., *266*:13243–13250, 1991.

Savitsky, K., Bar-Shira, A., Gilad, S., Rotman, G., Ziv, Y., Vanagaite, L., Tagle, D. A., Smith, S., Uziel, T., Sfez, S., Ashkenazi, M., Pecker, I., Frydman, M., Harnik, R., Patanjali, S. R., Simmons, A., Clines, G. A., Sartiel, A., Gatti, R. A., Chessa, L., Sanal, O., Lavin, M. F., Jaspers, N. G. J., Taylor, A. M. R., Arlett, C. F., Miki, T., Weissman, S. M., Lovett, M., Collins, F. S., and Shiloh, Y. A single ataxia telangiectasia gene with a product similar to P1-3 kinase. Science, *268*:1749–1753, 1995.

Schaffner, D. L., Barrios, R., Shaker, M. R., Rajagopalan, S., Huang, S. L., Tindall, D. J., Young, C. Y. F., Overbeek, P. A., Lebovitz, R. M., and Lieberman, M. W. Transgenic mice carrying a PSA*ras*T24 hybrid gene develop salivary gland and gastrointestinal tract neoplasms. Lab. Invest., *72*:283–290, 1995.

Schimke, R. N. Genetic aspects of multiple endocrine neoplasia. Annu. Rev. Med., *35*:25–31, 1984.

Schulz, N., Propst, F., Rosenberg, M. P., Linnoila, R. I., Paules, R. S., Kovatch, R., Ogiso, Y., and Vande Woude, G. Pheochromocytomas and C-cell thyroid neoplasms in transgenic c-*mos* mice: a model for the human multiple endocrine neoplasia type 2 syndrome. Cancer Res., *52*:450–455, 1992.

Scrable, H., Cavenee, W., Ghavimi, F., Lovell, M., Morgan, K., and Sapienza, C. A model for embryonal rhabdomyosarcoma tumorigenesis that involves genome imprinting. Proc. Natl. Acad. Sci. U.S.A., *86*:7480–7484, 1989.

Searle, P. F., Thomas, D. P., Faulkner, K. B., and Tinsley, J. M. Stomach cancer in transgenic mice expressing human papillomavirus type 16 early region genes from a keratin promoter. J. Gen. Virol., *75*:1125–1137, 1994.

Seidegård, J., and Pero, R. W. The hereditary transmission of high glutathione transferase activity towards *trans*-stilbene oxide in human mononuclear leukocytes. Hum. Genet., *69*:66–68, 1985.

Seidegård, J., Pero, R. W., Markowitz, M. M., Roush, G., Miller, D. G., and Beattie, E. J. Isoenzyme(s) of glutathione transferase (class Mu) as a marker for the susceptibility to lung cancer: a follow up study. Carcinogenesis, *11*:33–36, 1990.

Seizinger, B. R., Rouleau, G. A., Ozelius, L. J., Lane, A. H., Faryniarz, A. G., Chao, M. V., Huson, S., Korf, B. R., Parry, D. M., Pericak-Vance, M. A., Collins, F. S., Hobbs, W. J., Falcone, B. G., Iannazzi, J. A., Roy, J. C., St. George-Hyslop, P. H., Tanzi, R. E., Bothwell, M. A., Upadhyaya, M., Harper, P., Goldstein, A. E., Hoover, D. L., Bader, J. L., Spence, M. A., Mulvihill, J. J., Aylsworth, A. S., Vance, J. M., Rossenwasser, G. O. D., Gaskell, P. C., Roses, A. D., Martuza, R. L., Breakefield, X. O., and Gusella, J. F. Genetic linkage of von Recklinghausen neurofibromatosis to the nerve growth factor receptor gene. Cell, *49*:589–594, 1987.

Seizinger, B. R., Smith, D. I., Filling-Katz, M. R., Neumann, H., Green, J. S., Choyke, P. L., Anderson, K. M., Freiman, R. N., Klauck, S. M., Whaley, J., Decker, H.-J. H., Hsia, Y. E., Collins, D., Halperin, J., Lamiell, J. M., Oostra, B., Waziri, M. H., Gorin, M. B., Scherer, G., Drabkin, H. A., Aronin, N., Schinzel, A., Martuza, R. L., Gusella, J. F., and Haines, J. L. Genetic flanking markers refine diagnostic criteria and provide insights into the genetics of von Hippel Lindau disease. Proc. Natl. Acad. Sci. U.S.A., *88*:2864–2868, 1991.

Shepel, L. A., and Gorski, J. Relationship of polymorphisms near the rat prolactin, N-*ras*, and retinoblastoma genes with susceptibility to estrogen-induced pituitary tumors. Cancer Res., *50*:7920–7925, 1990.

Shields, P. G. Pharmacogenetics: detecting sensitive populations. Environ. Health Perspect., *102*:81–87, 1994.

Shuin, T., Kondo, K., Torigoe, S., Kishida, T., Kubota, Y., Hosaka, M., Nagashima, Y., Kitamura, H., Latif, F., Zbar, B., Lerman, M. I., and Yao, M. Frequent somatic mutations and loss of heterozygosity of the von Hippel-Lindau tumor suppressor gene in primary human renal cell carcinomas. Cancer Res., *54*:2852–2855, 1994.

Sivaraman, L., Leatham, M. P., Yee, J., Wilkens, L. R., Lau, A. F., and Le Marchand, L. *CYP1A1* genetic polymorphisms and *in situ* colorectal cancer. Cancer Res., *54*:3692–3695, 1994.

Skuse, G. R., and Ludlow, J. W. Tumour suppressor genes in disease and therapy. Lancet, *345*:902–906, 1995.

Smyrk, T. C. Cancer syndrome meets molecular biology meets histopathology. Am. J. Pathol., *145*:1–6, 1994.

Sparkes, R. S. Cytogenetics of retinoblastoma. Cancer Surv., *3*:479–496, 1984.

Srivastava, S., Wang, S., Tong, Y. A., Hao, Z.-M., and Chang, E. H. Dominant negative effect of a germline mutant *p53*: a step fostering tumorigenesis. Cancer Res., *53*:4452–4455, 1993.

St. John, D. J., McDermott, F. T., Hopper, J. L., Debney, E. A., Johnson, W. R., and Hughes, E. S. R. Cancer risk in relatives of patients with common colorectal cancer. Ann. Intern. Med., *118*:785–790, 1993.

Stewart, T. A., and Mintz, B. Successive generations of mice produced from an established culture line of euploid teratocarcinoma cells. Proc. Natl. Acad. Sci. U.S.A., *78*:6314–6318, 1981.

Stokkel, M. P. M., Kroon, B. B. R., van der Sande, J. J., and Neering, H. Malignant cutaneous melanoma associated with neurofibromatosis in two sisters from a family with familial atypical multiple mole melanoma syndrome. Cancer, *72*:2370–2375, 1993.

Strange, R. C., Matharoo, B., Faulder, G. C., Jones, P., Cotton, W., Elder, J. B., and Deakin, M. The human glutathione S-transferases: a case-control study of the incidence of the GST1 0 phenotype in patients with adenocarcinoma. Carcinogenesis, *12*:25–28, 1991.

Stutman, O. Spontaneous tumors in nude mice: effect of the viable yellow gene. Exp. Cell Biol., *47*:129–135, 1979.

Su, L.-K., Kinzler, K. W., Vogelstein, B., Preisinger, A. C., Moser, A. R., Luongo, C., Gould, K. A., and Dove, W. F. Multiple intestinal neoplasia caused by a mutation in the murine homolog of the APC gene. Science, *256*:668–670, 1992.

Swanson, H. I., and Bradfield, C. A. The AH-receptor: genetics, structure and function. Pharmacogenetics, *3*:213–230, 1993.

Swift, M., Chase, C. L., and Morrell, D. Cancer predisposition of ataxia-telangiectasia heterozygotes. Cancer Genet. Cytogenet., *46*:21–27, 1990.

Takahashi, M., Ritz, M., and Cooper, G. M. Activation of a novel human transforming gene, *ret*, by DNA rearrangement. Cell, *42*:581–588, 1985.

Takai, S., Iwama, T., and Tonomura, A. Chromosome instability in cultured skin fibroblasts from patients with familial polyposis coli and Peutz-Jeghers' syndrome. Jpn. J. Cancer Res., *77*:759–766, 1986.

Thorgeirsson, S. S., and Nebert, D. W. The *Ah* locus and the metabolism of chemical carcinogens and other foreign compounds. Adv. Cancer Res., *25*:149–193, 1977.

Trench, G. C., Southall, M., Smith, P., and Kidson, C. Allelic variation of the c-*raf*-1 proto-oncogene in human lymphoma and leukemia. Oncogene, *4*:507–510, 1989.

Tucker, M. A., Fraser, M. C., Goldstein, A. M., Elder, D. E., Guerry IV, D., and Organic, S. M. Risk of melanoma and other cancers in melanoma-prone families. J. Invest. Dermatol., *100*:350S–355S, 1993.

Tulinius, H., Olafsdottir, G. H., Sigvaldason, H., Tryggvadottir, L., and Bjarnadottir, K. Neoplastic diseases in families of breast cancer patients. J. Med. Genet., *31*:618–621, 1994.

Tycko, B. Genomic imprinting: mechanism and role in human pathology. Am. J. Pathol., *144*:431–443, 1994.

Usuki, S., Maekawa, A., Kang, H-i., Shumiya, S., and Nagase, S. High susceptibility of analbuminemic rats to neurogenic tumor induction by transplacental administration of N-ethyl-N-nitrosourea. Jpn. J. Cancer Res., *83*:146–152, 1992.

van der Heiden, C., Geurtzen, A. F. M., Brink, W., de Klerk, J. B. C., and Beemer, F. A. Esterase D: evaluation of a potential derived gene marker for hereditary retinoblastoma. Clin. Chim. Acta, *173*:81–88, 1988.

van der Mey, A. G. L., Maaswinkel-Mooy, P. D., Cornelisse, C. J., Schmidt, P. H., and van de Kamp, J. J. P. Genomic imprinting in hereditary glomus tumours: evidence for new genetic theory. Lancet, 2:1291–1294, 1989.

Viallet, J., and Minna, J. D. Dominant oncogenes and tumor suppressor genes in the pathogenesis of lung cancer. Am. J. Respir. Cell Mol. Biol., *2*:225–232, 1990.

Wadey, R. B., Pal, N., Buckle, B., Yeomans, E., Pritchard, J., and Cowell, J. K. Loss of heterozygosity in Wilms tumour involves two distinct regions of chromosome 11. Oncogene, *5*:901–907, 1990.

Walker, G. J., Palmer, J. M., Walters, M. K., Nancarrow, D. J., Parsons, P. G., and Hayward, N. K. Refined localization of the melanoma (MLM) gene on chromosome 9p by analysis of allelic deletions. Oncogene, *9*:819–824, 1994.

Watson, K. L., Justice, R. W., and Bryant, P. J. *Drosophila* in cancer research: the first fifty tumor suppressor genes. J. Cell Sci., *18*:19–33, 1994.

Watson, P., and Lynch, H. T. Extracolonic cancer in hereditary nonpolyposis colorectal cancer. Cancer, *71*:677–685, 1993.

Weber, W. W., and Hein, D. W. N-Acetylation pharmacogenetics. Pharmacol. Rev., *37*:25–78, 1985.

Wertelecki, W., Rouleau, G. A., Superneau, D. W., Forehand, L. W., Williams, J. P., Haines, J. L., and Gusella, J. F. Neurofibromatosis 2: clinical and DNA linkage studies of a large kindred. N. Engl. J. Med., *319*:278–283, 1988.

Whaley, J. M., Naglich, J., Gelbert, L., Hsia, Y. E., Lamiell, J. M., Green, J. S., Collins, D., Neumann, H. P. H., Laidlaw, J., Li, F. P., Klein-Szanto, A. J. P., Seizinger, B. R., and Kley, N. Germ-line mutations in the von Hippel-Lindau tumor-suppressor gene are similar to somatic von Hippel-Lindau aberrations in sporadic renal cell carcinoma. Am. J. Hum. Genet., *55*:1092–1102, 1994.

Wilson, M. G., Towner, J. W., and Fujimoto, A. Retinoblastoma and D-chromosome deletions. Am. J. Human Genet., *25*:57–61, 1973.

Wolman, S. R., and Dawson, P. J. Genetic events in breast cancer and their clinical correlates. Crit. Rev. Oncog., *2*:277–291, 1991.

Wooster, R., Neuhausen, S. L., Mangion, J., Quirk, Y., Ford, D., Collins, N., Nguyen, K., Seal, S., Tran, T., Averill, D., Fields, P., Marshall, G., Narod, S., Lenoir, G., Lynch, H., Feunteun, J., Devilee, P.,

Cornelisse, C. J., Menko, F. H., Daly, P. A., Ormiston, W., McManus, R., Pye, C., Lewis, C. M., Cannon-Albright, L. A., Peto, J., Ponder, B. A. J., Skolnick, M. H., Easton, D. F., Goldgar, D., E., and Stratton, M. R. Localization of a breast cancer susceptibility gene, *BRCA2*, to chromosome 13q12-13. Science, *265*:2088–2090, 1994.

Wu, J., Forbes, J. R., Chen, H. S., and Cox, D. W. The LEC rat has a deletion in the copper transporting ATPase gene homologous to the Wilson disease gene. Nature Genet., *7*:541–545, 1994.

Yamamura, K-i., and Wakasugi, S. Manipulating the mouse genome: new approaches for the dissection of mouse development. Dev. Growth Differ., *33*:93–100, 1991.

Yee, S.-P., Mock, D., Greer, P., Maltby, V., Rossant, J., Bernstein, A., and Pawson, T. Lymphoid and mesenchymal tumors in transgenic mice expressing the v-*fps* protein-tyrosine kinase. Mol. Cell. Biol., *9*:5491–5499, 1989.

Yeung, R. S., Xiao, G.-H., Jin, F., Lee, W.-C., Testa, J. R., and Knudson, A. G. Predisposition to renal carcinoma in the Eker rat is determined by germ-line mutation of the tuberous sclerosis 2 (*TSC2*) gene. Proc. Natl. Acad. Sci. U.S.A., *91*:11413–11416, 1994.

Yunis, J. J., Ball, D. W., and Sawyer, J. R. G-banding patterns of high-resolution human chromosomes 6-22, X, and Y. Hum. Genet., *49*:291–306, 1979.

Zbar, B., Brauch, H., Talmadge, C., and Linehan, M. Loss of alleles of loci on the short arm of chromosome 3 in renal cell carcinoma. Nature, *327*:721–724, 1987.

Zhu, X., Dunn, J. M., Phillips, R. A., Goddard, A. D., Paton, K. E., Becker, A., and Gallie, B. L. Preferential germline mutation of the paternal allele in retinoblastoma. Nature, *340*:312–313, 1989.

6

The Etiology of Cancer: Somatic Cell Genetics

While germline genetic factors are likely to be involved as major causes in the genesis and development of 20% or more of human cancers, it is now evident that genetic alterations in somatic cells occur in virtually all neoplasms. A somatic mutation results in a hereditary alteration in the non-germ cells of the mature or maturing organism. Although this definition does not require that the heritably transmitted change necessarily be due to an alteration in the genome itself, epigenetic alterations that result in the neoplastic transformation are not usually considered as mutations.

Early in this century Theodore Boveri (1914), after extensive studies of the mitotic apparatus and chromosomes of both normal and neoplastic cells, proposed that cells of malignant neoplasms possess the uniform characteristic of abnormal karyotypic morphology. Such abnormalities might reside in the mitotic apparatus as well as in the structure and/or chromosomes themselves. While Boveri's thesis lay almost dormant until the revolution in molecular genetics during the last several decades, today it is apparent that his original thesis probably applies to virtually all known neoplasms. A number of studies over the years have reported normal karyotypes in both human (Tseng and Jones, 1969; Joensuu et al., 1986; Mitelman, 1981) and animal neoplasms (Mitelman, 1974; Nowell et al., 1967), but more recent studies have questioned the significance of "normal" karyotypes in malignant cells. While nearly one-third of more than 300 cases of acute lymphoblastic leukemia exhibited normal karyotypes, as evidenced in a workshop in 1980 (Mitelman, 1981), more recent advances have questioned the normalcy of earlier studies (Yunis, 1984; Misawa et al., 1988). In addition, more extensive investigation of "diploid" transplantable hepatomas in rats (Wolman et al., 1973) did not confirm earlier reports of normal karyotypes in these solid tumors. Thus, it is likely that with refinement of cytogenetic methods, virtually all malignant neoplasms will be found to exhibit abnormal karyotypes, as Boveri postulated.

TYPES OF STRUCTURAL MUTATIONS: SOMATIC AND GERMLINE GENETICS

We have already noted (Chapter 5) that a variety of different types of mutations including chromosomal deletions may result in germline inherited cancer predisposition. However, the variety of known genetic mutations that can be found in neoplastic cells is quite extensive and likely to be expanded as more detailed knowledge of structural alterations in DNA occurs. Table 6.1 lists structural mutations in genes that may result in the alteration of genetic expression, the hallmark of the "relative autonomy" of our original definition of neoplasia (Chapter 2). While "silent" mutations occur, even some of these may lead ultimately to alterations in expression and/or reg-

Table 6.1   Structural Mutations in Genes That Result in Altered Gene Expression

Event	Consequence	Examples
Base mutation or deletion in coding sequences	New gene product with altered activity	Hormone independence Activation of tyrosine kinase activity Dominant negative mutations
Base mutation or deletion in noncoding sequences	Altered regulation of expression and function of normal gene product	Transcriptional regulation Activation of proto-oncogene
Frameshift mutations	Altered or deleted gene product	Loss of gene product
Insertion or substitution with repetitive DNA elements ("transposons") or "external" DNA	Altered regulation of gene expression	Loss of gene product or altered transcription
Chromosomal translocation	Altered mRNA, new gene product, altered regulation of gene expression	*bcr-abl* gene fusion c-*myc* regulation
Dynamic mutations (increase in repeated sequences)	Blockage of transcription	Fragile X syndrome, Kennedy disease
Recombination Somatic crossing over Gene conversion	Change or block in transcription rate	Gene disruption Genetic instability
Gene amplification	Increased expression of normal gene	Human cancers Drug resistance
Hyper- or hypomethylation of regulatory sequences in genes	Altered regulation of gene expression, normal gene product	Developmental gene expression Genomic imprinting

ulation of genetic information (Shub and Goodrich-Blair, 1992). The events listed in Table 6.1 may potentially occur in most genes, but they are most relevant to the expression and function of genes that play a significant role in the neoplastic transformation, i.e., proto- and cellular oncogenes and tumor suppressor genes. Although we have discussed several of these genes already (Chapters 4 and 5), their characteristics are reviewed in Table 6.2. Point mutations in genes can lead to structural alterations in the gene product that change its function, as in the case of the *ras* proto- and cellular oncogenes that code for G proteins important in signal transduction (Chapter 7). Dominant negative mutations (Herskowitz, 1987) result in a new gene product that interferes with the function of the normal gene product, which is encoded by the remaining normal allele. Probably the most common somatic mutation in neoplasia involves structural alterations in genes that govern chromosomal alterations, insertional mutagenesis, and gene amplification (Table 6.1). In fact, the frequency of the latter type of mutations is significantly higher than that of point mutations in cells (Holliday, 1991). Dynamic mutations are the result of changes in the copy number of repeated sequences within genes. In the fragile X syndrome, there is more than a fourfold increase in the number of CGG repeats within the coding sequence of a specific X-linked gene, the FMR-1 gene (Fu et al., 1991). This syndrome is a leading cause of mental retardation worldwide (Nelson, 1995) and has been associated with a possible increase in neoplastic disease (Cunningham and Dickerman, 1988). On the other hand, fragile sites—i.e., regions of chromosomes exhibiting instability toward breakage in the presence of antifolates, ionizing radiation—and certain carcinogens have been related to chromosomal rearrangements commonly

Table 6.2   Characteristics of Proto-Oncogenes, Cellular Oncogenes, and Tumor Suppressor Genes

Proto-Oncogenes	Cellular Oncogenes	Tumor Suppressor Genes
Dominant	Dominant	Recessive
Broad tissue specificity for cancer development	Broad tissue specificity for cancer development	Considerable tissue specificity for cancer development
Germline inheritance rarely involved in cancer development	Germline inheritance rarely involved in cancer development	Germline inheritancy frequently involved in cancer development
Analogous to certain viral oncogenes	No known analogs in oncogenic viruses	No known analogs in oncogenic viruses
Somatic mutations are activated during all stages of neoplastic development	Somatic mutations activate during all stages of neoplastic development	Germline mutations may be initiated, but mutation to neoplasia occurs only during the stage of progression

From Pitot, 1993, with permission of publisher.

seen in a variety of different types of neoplasms (Yunis and Hoffman, 1989; De Braekeleer et al., 1985). These mutations are to be distinguished from those induced by "mutator" genes, which cause microsatellite instability resulting from a lack or alteration of "mismatch" DNA repair (Chapter 3). Although mutations in such genes have been linked to the germline inheritance of nonpolyposis colon cancer, somatic mutations in these "mutator" genes occur as somatic mutations in colon and other neoplasms (Rüschoff et al., 1995). Recombinatorial events are many times associated with chromosomal alterations but may occur within the individual chromosome, as evidenced by various rates of sister chromatid exchange in both normal (Elbling and Colot, 1986) and neoplastic (Slavutsky et al., 1984) cells.

Theoretically, somatic mutations may reflect any one or several of the mutations (Table 6.1) occurring within a single cell. Furthermore, spontaneous mutations occur in somatic cells quite frequently (Chapter 3; Bridges et al., 1994). In studying somatic mutations in neoplastic cells, until recently the principal evidence for the occurrence of somatic mutations in neoplasia was the presence of chromosomal abnormalities. The expansion of methods and increased knowledge of gene structure have now made it possible to identify point, frameshift, and small deletion mutations in individual genes involved in carcinogenesis, i.e., oncogenes and tumor suppressor genes. However, the major dilemma in the importance of somatic mutagenesis in neoplastic disease is whether such mutations are the result or the primary cause of the neoplastic process.

BASE, FRAMESHIFT, AMPLIFICATION, AND INSERTIONAL OR SUBSTITUTIONAL MUTATIONS IN SPECIFIC GENES IN SOMATIC CELLS AS FACTORS IN NEOPLASTIC DEVELOPMENT

Somatic Mutations in Proto- and Cellular Oncogenes

With the advent, during the last two decades, of a clearer understanding of primary target genes for the action of carcinogenic agents, the search for mutations within specific genes has advanced dramatically. Prior to the development of modern methods of DNA sequencing and the use of the polymerase chain reaction (PCR), analysis of specific mutations in oncogenes was determined by indirect methods followed by specific sequencing. This procedure was first exemplified by demonstrating that the *Ha-ras-1* proto-oncogene bearing a single base substitution in the 12th codon resulted in the substitution of valine for glycine in the mutated gene product. Initial evidence for this alteration came from studies of transfection of DNA from the human bladder carcinoma cell line, T24, transfected into mouse 3T3 cells, which resulted in their morphological transformation (Chapter 9; Tabin et al., 1982). The transfection assay became a method for the rapid screening of "activated" proto-oncogenes in neoplasms. When such activation was discovered, analysis of mutations in candidate proto- and cellular oncogenes could be determined by more detailed nucleic acid sequence methods.

It has now become apparent that the *Ha-ras-1* proto-oncogene is only one of a family of genes coding for G proteins whose function is involved in the mediation of signal transduction pathways (Chapter 7). Several other *ras* proto- and cellular oncogenes have been studied (Tables 6.3 and 6.4), but the most extensive investigations into the structure and effects of mutations on the protein function have been carried out on the *Ha-ras-1* proto-oncogene and its product. Figure 6.1 shows a ribbon drawing of the *Ha-ras-1* (p21) proto-oncogene product showing the loops (λ_{1-10}) and helices (shown as multilined bands). The positions of important amino acid residues are labeled for orientation, as noted in the figure. Most of the known mutations in the *ras* gene family occur in codons 12, 13, and 61 (Bos, 1989). While the details of how amino acid substitutions at these positions affect the function of the p21 molecule have not been completely clarified (Bokoch and Der, 1993), such mutations cause a loss of the ability of the p21 protein to become inactivated, thus resulting in a constant stimulation of the signal transduction pathway(s) resulting in cell growth, cell function, or cell differentiation on a constitutive basis (cf. Kiaris and Spandidos, 1995). Through such a mechanism, mutations at codons 12, 13, or 61 would thus confer a proliferative advantage to the cell bearing such mutations, allowing its selective overgrowth and overfunction in a general population of its normal peers.

Since the *ras* proto- and cellular oncogene family has been most extensively studied, most investigations have observed specific mutations in one member of this family. Table 6.3 lists examples of human and animal neoplasms in which 50% or more of the tumors exhibited a mutated oncogene. This is not meant to imply that other lesions exhibited no evidence of such mutations. Rather, one finds that in the majority of human neoplasms as well as many animal

Table 6.3 Somatic Mutations in Proto-Oncogenes in Neoplasms

Neoplasm	Oncogene Mutated	Percent	Reference
Human			
Colon carcinoma	c-*Ki-ras*	60% (37/61)	Burmer et al., 1991
Lung adenocarcinoma (in smokers)	c-*Ki-ras*	80% (8/10)	Reynolds et al., 1991
Pancreas adenocarcinoma	c-*Ki-ras*	92% (35/38)	Nagata et al., 1990
Cholangiocarcinoma	c-*Ki-ras*	50% (9/18)	Tada et al., 1992
Thyroid adenomas	N, c-*Ha*, c-*Ki-ras*	85% (25/25)	Shi et al., 1991
Thyroid follicular carcinomas	N, c-*Ha*, c-*Ki-ras*	50% (8/16)	Shi et al., 1991
Acute myelogenous leukemia	N-*ras*	19–70%	Bos, 1989
	c-*fms*	100% (28/28)	Dubreuil et al., 1988
Animal			
Hepatoma (mouse, B6C3F$_1$ strain) (spontaneous)	c-*Ha-ras*	65% (67/103)	Anderson et al., 1992
Mammary carcinoma (methylnitrosourea-induced)	c-*Ha-ras*	87% (61/70)	Anderson et al., 1992
Epidermal neoplasms (dimethylbenzanthracene-induced	c-*Ha-ras*	95% (58/61)	Anderson et al., 1992

Table 6.4 Activation of Human Proto- and Cellular Oncogenes

Gene	Activation as Oncogenes		Mechanism of activation
	Type of tumor	Frequency	
dbl	Diffuse B-cell lymphoma	Single case	Unknown
erbB-1/HER	Glial tumors, A431 cells	5–10%	Amplification
erbB-2/neu	Adenocarcinomas, several organs	5–10%	Amplification
mas	Activated during gene transfer	Single case	Rearrangement
mcf-3/ros	Activated during gene transfer	Single case	Rearrangement
mel	Melanoma	Single case	Unknown
met	MNNG-HOS cells	Single case	Translocation and rearrangement
myb	AML, COLO 201 cells	Isolated cases	Amplification
L-myc	Small cell lung carcinoma	20%[a]	Amplification
N-myc	Neuroblastomas stages III and IV	50%	Amplification
raf-1	Stomach cancer, glioblasts	Isolated cases	Rearrangement
H-ras	Several carcinomas	1–5%	Point mutation
K-ras	Most types of tumors	10–15%	Point mutation
	Lung and bladder carcinomas	1%	Amplification
N-ras	Leukemias, other types of tumors	5–25%	Point mutation
ret	Activated during gene transfer	Single case	Rearrangement
trk	Colon carcinoma	Single case	Rearrangement with tropomyosin
hst	Esophageal cancer	>50%	Amplification
ROS1	Glioblastoma cell line	Single case	Rearrangement
gsp	Pituitary adenoma	18%	Point mutation

Modified from Martin-Zanca et al., 1986. The last three genes, hst, ROS1, and gsp are from the reports by Terada et al., 1990; Birchmeier et al., 1987; and Lyons et al., 1990.

tumors similar mutations may be found. In humans an average of 5% to 10% of all neoplasms exhibit mutation(s) in at least one oncogene studied (Nishimura and Sekiya, 1987). However, several human neoplasms including some sarcomas (Castresana et al., 1993), adrenal neoplasms (Moul et al., 1993), and neuroendocrine neoplasms of the lung (Wagner et al., 1993) are not associated specifically with mutations in ras oncogenes. While spontaneous hepatomas arising in the B6C3F$_1$ strain exhibited a high incidence (65%) of mutations in the c-Ha-ras gene, other mouse strains having a lower incidence of spontaneous liver tumors, including the C57BL/6J and BALB/c strains, possess few if any such mutations in hepatomas arising spontaneously (Buchmann et al., 1991). Interestingly, Sugio et al. (1994) indicated that mutations in the c-Ki-ras gene occurred relatively late in the development of lung cancer, since early lesions did not exhibit these mutagenic changes. c-Ki-ras mutations may be found in normal colonic mucosa in the human (Ronai et al., 1994) as well as in very early lesions prior to the appearance of frank cancer (Smith et al., 1994).

Proto- and cellular oncogenes other than those of the ras family may also be found in a variety of human neoplasms, as exemplified in Table 6.4. While many of the changes noted in the table were reported only in single cases, the variety of mutation type and loci involved exemplify the extent of such changes in the human. A number of examples of amplification of proto-oncogenes have been described. Similarly, mutations in proto-and cellular oncogenes other than the ras gene family have also been reported in lower animals including c-myb (Shen-Ong and

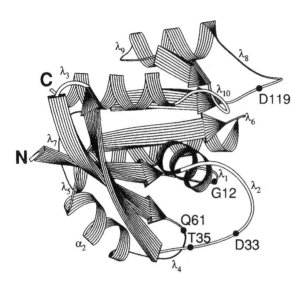

Figure 6.1 Schematic representation of the three-dimensional structure of the *ras* protein. In the figure, loops and several important amino acid residues are labeled, including glycine-12 and glutamine-61. (After Pai et al., 1989, with permission of the authors and publisher.)

Wolff, 1987), the *neu* activated in rat neoplasms of the central nervous system (Perantoni et al., 1994), and the *Spi-1* cellular oncogene in murine erythroleukemia (Moreau-Gachelin, 1994).

Somatic Mutations in Tumor Suppressor Genes

As indicated by our earlier discussions (see above), somatic mutations in tumor suppressor genes will effect the neoplastic transformation only if both alleles of the suppressor gene are affected. Because of the relative tissue specificity of neoplasms developing in patients with germline mutations in these genes, one might expect that a similar specificity would be found in somatic mutations. In part this is true, as noted earlier (Chapter 5) by somatic mutations seen in up to 56% of clear-cell renal carcinomas (Shuin et al., 1994; Foster et al., 1994); but no mutations were found in non-clear-cell renal carcinomas. In addition, about 20% of sporadic central nervous system hemangioblastomas, benign neoplasms often associated with the von Hippel–Lindau (VHL) syndrome, also exhibit somatic mutations in the VHL gene (Kanno et al., 1994). Similarly, mutations in the APC tumor suppressor gene of hereditary familial polyposis are seen in about 60% of esophageal and gastric cancers in the human (Tahara, 1995).

Somatic mutations in tumor suppressor genes have been most extensively investigated in the Rb (retinoblastoma) (Table 6.5) and *p53* tumor suppressor genes. A surprisingly high frequency of mutations has been noted in the Rb gene in a number of different neoplasms in the human. As noted in the table, several of these determinations have been made through the use of the Southern blot analyses in which allelic loss (loss of heterozygosity, or LOH) can be determined (Chapter 5). Specific point mutations have not been determined in most instances, and the majority of changes are seen in carcinomas rather than benign neoplasms as exemplified by the virtual absence of Rb mutations in parathyroid adenomas (Cryns et al., 1994). The presence of deletions within the promoter region of the Rb gene in prostatic carcinomas, as reported by Bookstein et al. (1990), was later not confirmed by Sarkar et al. (1992). Osteosarcomas are the most common second malignancy found in individuals with hereditary retinoblastoma. A loss of

Table 6.5   Somatic Mutations in the Rb Tumor Suppressor Gene

Type of Neoplasm	Species	Frequency	Mutation(s)	Reference
Colorectal carcinoma	Human	35%	LOH,* amplification	Meling et al., 1991
Esophageal				
Squamous cell carcinoma	Human	54%	LOH	Boynton et al., 1991
Adenocarcinoma	Human	36%		
Lung, small cell carcinoma	Human	30%	LOH, deletion	Hensel et al., 1990
Lymphomas	Human	5%	rearrangement	Ginsberg et al., 1991
Mammary carcinoma	Human	59%	LOH	Tamura et al., 1994
Osteosarcoma	Human	43%	structural changes in Rb gene	Toguchida et al., 1988
Parathyroid carcinoma	Human	100%	allelic loss	Cryns et al., 1994
Prostate carcinoma	Human	1 of 7	deletion within promoter region	Bookstein et al.,1990

*LOH = loss of heterozygosity

heterozygosity for chromosome 13 probes has been observed in individuals with osteosarcoma, whether or not these patients had a previous history of retinoblastoma (cf. Benedict et al., 1990). In a series of some 30 cases of primary osteosarcoma, 13 exhibited structural abnormalities in the Rb gene (Toguchida et al., 1988). Other sporadic soft-tissue sarcomas exhibited somatic mutations in the Rb gene (Weichselbaum et al., 1988) with the exception of childhood rhabdomyosarcomas (De Chiara et al., 1993). However, in osteosarcomas arising in mixed gonadal neoplasms, somatic mutations in Rb are unusual (Reuvekamp et al., 1992). Thus, somatic mutations in the Rb tumor suppressor gene have been reported in a number of nonocular neoplasms. This phenomenon is even more extensively seen in the *p53* tumor suppressor gene.

Somatic Mutations in the *p53* Tumor Suppressor Gene

Somatic mutations in the *p53* tumor suppressor gene in human cancer have been seen more commonly than somatic mutations in any other single gene. About half of all cases of human cancer studied exhibit somatic mutations in the *p53* gene (Harris, 1993), including nearly 70% of colorectal cancers, 50% of lung cancers, and 40% of breast cancers (Culotta and Koshland, 1993). As Harris (1993) has noted, mutations in the *p53* tumor suppressor gene are different from those seen in other tumor suppressor genes. Whereas Rb and APC are commonly inactivated by nonsense mutations, causing truncation or instability of the protein, more than 90% of the mutations in the *p53* tumor suppressor gene are missense mutations, transitions, or transversions that result in a change of an amino acid within the protein. Such changes may alter the conformation and increase the stability of the protein. This observation has led a number of authors to utilize immunohistochemistry of tissue slices with antibodies specific to a mutant *p53* protein to obtain evidence for presumed mutation in the *p53* gene (Bartek et al., 1991; Zusman, 1995). Guinee et al. (1995) extended these studies, demonstrating that enhanced immunohistochemical staining for *p53* correlated predominantly with the presence of missense mutations in specific exons (5–8) of the *p53* gene. The *p53* protein consists of 393 amino acids with functional and evolutionarily conserved domains (Harris, 1995). A diagram of the relative frequency of mutations at specific sites in the human *p53* tumor suppressor gene is seen in Figure 6.2. The majority of missense mutations occur in the conserved hydrophobic region, while nonmissense mutations are distributed throughout the protein. Direct mutagenesis of *p53* cDNA by benzo[a]pyrene di-

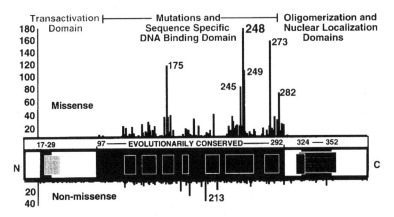

Figure 6.2 Schematic representation of the *p53* molecule. The protein extending from the amino terminus (N) on the left to the carboxy terminus (C) on the right is diagramed with its functional and evolutionarily conserved domains. The numbers indicate the codons where a very high incidence of mutation (mutational hot spots) occurs. (Adapted from Harris, 1995, with permission of the author and publisher.)

olepoxide and the epoxide of aflatoxin B_1 results in G:C-T:A transversions in a number of locations in the conserved region by the diolepoxide and a similar change with the ultimate form of aflatoxin. These mutations were localized to a considerable extent to codon 249 (Puisieux et al., 1991), but this codon was not a target for the benzo[a]pyrene diolepoxide. Interestingly, in hepatocellular carcinomas developing in individual regions of the world where aflatoxin B_1 exposure is endemic, a similar transversion in codon 249 was noted (Hsu et al., 1991). A diagram of the proportion and types of various mutations seen in a number of cancer types as well as the distribution of *p53* mutations in general is given in Figure 6.3. As noted in the figure, there are distinct, different distributions of the various types of mutations in each of the types of cancer depicted. This is particularly notable in colon cancer, which develops in adenomatous polyposis coli in patients exhibiting a germline mutation in APC, compared with sporadic colon cancer where only somatic mutation in this gene is presumably involved. The proportions of the transition mutations G:C to A:T at CpG dinucleotide positions where the C is presumably methylated are quite different in colon and lung cancer. Rideout et al. (1992) have suggested that this indicates a more important role for endogenous mutagens in colon cancer than in lung cancer, where presumably exogenous tobacco smoke is the primary carcinogenic factor.

In later chapters (Chapters 9 and 15) the molecular functions of *p53* and other tumor suppressor genes are considered. However, it is obvious that this gene in particular is the target for a variety of exogenous and endogenous mutagens. It is also clear that many other somatic mutations may occur in both oncogenes and tumor suppressor genes, and it is unlikely that any single mutation in any single gene is the ubiquitous lesion that leads directly to cancer.

Somatic Mutations of the *p53* Tumor Suppressor Gene in Experimental Neoplasia

Concurrent with the extensive work done on the somatic mutations in the *p53* tumor suppressor gene in humans, a number of animal systems have been investigated in a similar manner. Fortunately, the gene and protein structure of *p53* is conserved within the mammalian kingdom, and thus reagents can be used to some extent across species. Table 6.6 lists a number of studies in rats and mice in which mutations have been discovered and for the most part characterized as to

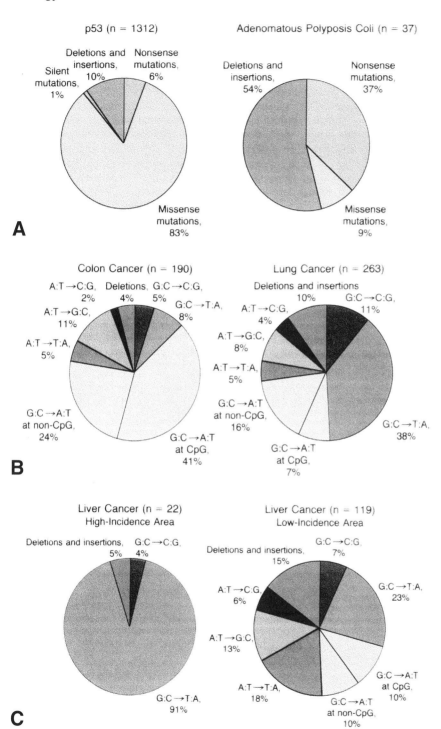

Figure 6.3 Proportions of various types of somatic mutations in the *p53* tumor suppressor gene in a large number of cancers [upper left, *p53* (n = 1312)] and in several types of neoplasms. The numbers in parentheses next to the type of cancer and *p53* indicate the numbers of mutations. (Adapted from Harris and Hollstein, 1993, with permission of the authors and publisher.)

Table 6.6 Somatic Mutations of the *p53* Tumor Suppressor Gene in Experimental Carcinogenesis

Organ/Species	Carcinogen	Mutation	Frequency	Reference
Bladder/rat	FANFT	Missense, non-sense frameshift	7.4%	Asamoto et al., 1994
Epidermis/mouse	Benzo[a]pyrene	G to T transversion	60%	Ruggeri et al., 1993
Epidermis/mouse	UV radiation	C to T transition	20–30%	Kress et al., 1992b van Kranen et al., 1995
Epidermis/mouse	β radiation	Point, insertion, deletion	47%	Ootsuyama et al., 1994
Kidney/rat	Ethylnitrosourea (transplacental)	G to T transversion	75–100%	Ohgaki et al., 1992
Liver/rat	Choline-deficient diet	Point, deletion	73%	Smith et al., 1993b
Liver/rat	Acetylaminofluorene	Point	31%	Ho et al., 1995
Liver/rat	Aflatoxin B_1	?	20%	Lilleberg et al., 1992
Lung/mouse	Methylene chloride	?	8%	Hegi et al., 1993
Mammary HAN/mouse	Spontaneous	Point, deletion, insertion	3/5	Jerry et al., 1993
Thymic lymphomas/ mouse	Methylnitrosourea or γ radiation	Point	4/30	Brathwaite et al., 1992
Zymbal gland/rat	2-amino-3-methylimid-azo[4,5-*f*]quinoline	Point, deletion	4/15	Makino et al., 1992

specific codons and base changes. Numerous other studies have examined the immunohistochemical staining of *p53* in tissue sections, but since this is not an absolute method for identifying somatic mutations in the gene, these are not included here.

As can be noted from the table, the frequency of mutations in the various systems shown ranges from very high to less than 10% of the neoplasms examined. Since almost all of these examples are from neoplasms resulting from chemical carcinogenesis, the sequence alterations are of significance. Interestingly, aflatoxin B1 administered to rats does not induce mutations at codon 249 (Hulla et al., 1993) such as seen in *p53* from humans exposed to this carcinogen (Figure 6.3). Furthermore, *p53* mutations are virtually absent from mouse liver tumors, either spontaneous or chemically induced (Kress et al., 1992a; Goodrow et al., 1992; Rumsby et al., 1994), as well as from neoplasms induced in rat liver by a peroxisome proliferator that has no known direct covalent interaction with DNA (Smith et al., 1993a). In addition, administration of nickel subsulfide and iron, a mixture carcinogenic for the rat kidney, resulted in neoplasms that did not exhibit mutations in the *p53* gene (Weghorst et al., 1994). Thus, for a number of chemical carcinogens, the *p53* tumor suppressor gene is either not a target or one that is hit only in frequently, although it is possible that the *p53* gene is mutated often but not selected for in these tumors.

SOMATIC MUTATIONS AS REFLECTED BY CHROMOSOMAL ABERRATIONS

Quantitatively, neoplasia is a disease more commonly seen in older individuals (Chapter 9), and there is ample evidence to indicate that both point mutations (Lee et al., 1994) and chromosomal aberrations increase with age (Nisitani et al., 1990; Liu et al., 1994). Despite this correlation, the genome of most species is reasonably stable throughout their lifetime, and there is little if any evidence that the aging process is itself carcinogenic (Chapter 8). Even so, the search for somatic mutations that are characteristic of neoplasia amidst the apparent randomness of background mutations has been the goal of many investigators since the time of Boveri. This search was initially rewarded by the demonstration of a specific chromosomal change associated with a specific neoplasm, chronic myeloid leukemia in humans, by Nowell and Hungerford (1960). This condition is a neoplasm of polymorphonuclear leukocytes, is chronic in that the neoplastic cells are reasonably well differentiated, and the disease has a relatively protracted course. The original observation of an abnormally small G group (chromosomes 21 and 22) led to later studies that confirmed it to be chromosome 22 with an abnormal shortening of the long arm of the chromosome. The resultant chromosome has been termed the "Philadelphia" chromosome (Ph[1]) after the city where it was first described. The Ph[1] chromosome occurs in over 90% of patients with chronic myeloid leukemia (CML). It has also been reported in about 20% of adults with acute lymphoblastic leukemia (ALL), 5% of children with ALL, and about 2% of adults with acute myeloid leukemia (AML) (Barton and Westbrook, 1994).

In 1973 Rowley reported that the "shortening" of the long arm of chromosome 22, resulting in the Ph[1] chromosome, was actually the result of a translocation of this chromosomal segment to the long arm of chromosome 9. In Figure 6.4 may be seen an artist's representation of this translocation. Later studies by Geraedts and Van der Ploeg (1980) showed that the translocation is not

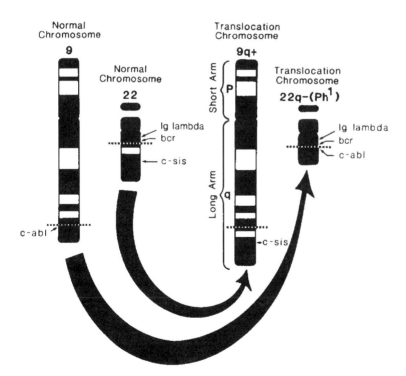

Figure 6.4   Diagram of chromosome translocation in chronic myeloid leukemia. The break occurs in chromosomes 9 and 22 in the area of the dotted lines. The translocation chromosome 9 is labeled 9q+ because of the additional genetic information on the long arm (q), extending it to a greater length than normal. Conversely, the translocation chromosome 22q-(Ph1) exhibits a shortening of the long arm because the translocated segment of chromosome 9 is smaller than that translocated from chromosome 22 to chromosome 9. (Adapted from Rowley, 1990b, with permission of the author and publisher.)

accompanied by any measurable loss in the DNA of the two chromosomes involved. Studies after Rowley's initial observation indicated that, while a majority of translocations resulting in the Ph[1] chromosome are to chromosome 9q, translocations to other chromosomes have been seen, including 12q, 17q, and 19q as well as more complex rearrangements (Sandberg, 1980).

In 1982 the Abelson (*abl*) proto-oncogene was localized to chromosome 9 by DeKlein and his associates. In 1984 Groffen and his associates cloned the translocation breakpoint. In these studies it was demonstrated that the *abl* gene translocated from chromosome 9 to 22, and the region of the breakpoint on chromosome 22 was limited to a small 5.8-kb region termed *bcr* (breakpoint cluster region). Thus, the gene on chromosome 22 in which this breakage occurs bears the terminology, *bcr*. As a result of the translocation, there is produced a chimeric *bcr-abl* fusion gene. A diagram of the genes at the breakpoints and on the translocated chromosomes is seen in Figure 6.5, which shows two translocation schemes. In A, the resultant protein has a molecular weight of 210,000, while in B the resultant protein is smaller, 190,000 Da (Rowley, 1990a; Barton and Westbrook, 1994). As noted, the breakpoints involve the 5′ region of the *abl* proto-oncogene, but the *bcr* gene is cleaved nearer the middle of the gene in the small p210 fusion gene. In the smaller p190 fusion gene, the *bcr* breakpoint is in the first intron of the *bcr* gene (Barton and Westbrook, 1994). Although the normal *abl* protein has relatively weak tyrosine kinase activity, the protein product of the fused gene exhibits a much stronger tyrosine kinase activity (cf. Barton and Westbrook, 1994). Nearly 98% of CML cases exhibit the breakpoint patterns seen in Figure 6.5. In the remaining 2%, other aberrant transcripts have been reported (cf. Barton and Westbrook, 1994). None of the different CML fusion genes examined to date have a breakpoint in the c-*abl* gene of chromosome 9 at exactly the same location. The breakpoints appear to be distributed more or less at random within the 5′ region of the c-*abl* gene (cf. Groffen and Heisterkamp, 1989).

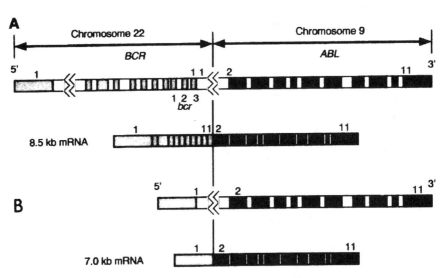

Figure 6.5   A. Map of the BCR/ABL fusion gene seen in CML and some adult patients with ALL. The breakpoint has occurred between the third and fourth exons included in the BCR region. These are equivalent to exons 11 and 12 in the *bcr* gene. The chimeric mRNA is diagramed below the gene. B. Map of the fusion gene in some ALL patients showing the breakpoint in the first intron of the *bcr* gene. The breakpoint in the *abl* gene is identical with that seen in CML in this example. The mRNA is much smaller than that seen in CML. (Adapted from Rowley, 1990b, with permission of the author and publisher.)

The importance of the presence of the BCR/ABL fusion gene in CML is exemplified by the finding that even in patients lacking an identifiable Ph[1] chromosome, a number do exhibit the fusion gene probably representing an interstitial insertion or *bcr* rearrangement (cf. Dobrovic et al., 1991). Patients not exhibiting the fusion gene in the absence of a Ph[1] chromosome usually exhibit atypical disease features and a more rapid and progressive course (cf. Dobrovic et al., 1991; Barton and Westbrook, 1994). The exact mechanism by which the BCR/ABL fusion gene is related to the neoplastic transformation in CML is not clear. Recently, the function of the *bcr* gene was reportedly to encode a GTPase-activating protein whose function is involved with that of several proto-oncogenes, especially the *ras* gene family (Diekmann et al., 1991). Thus, the BCR/ABL protein may function to form a complex of an intrinsic GTPase-activating signal transduction pathway with an activated protein tyrosine kinase, both of which functions have been implicated in carcinogenesis (Chapter 16).

KARYOTYPIC CHANGES IN NEOPLASIA: RANDOM AND NONRANDOM

Prior to the discovery of the Philadelphia chromosome, no specific pattern of chromosomal abnormalities in neoplasia had been observed. This is the likely reason that Boveri's initial proposal was generally disregarded. However, following Rowley's observation of the translocation resulting in the formation of the Philadelphia chromosome in CML, investigators employed newer techniques to determine whether any karyotypic changes were specific to one or more histogenetic types of neoplasms.

Figure 6.6 portrays the chromosomes of the human karyotype, indicating positions of certain proto- and cellular oncogenes and tumor suppressor genes as well as sites of translocations, deletions, trisomies, and inversions. The banding pattern seen is that of a single chromatid of each of the chromosomes from the human karyotype. All of the chromosomes, including those which as yet have not been involved in the genesis of any specific histogenetic neoplasm, are represented in the figure. As noted in the figure, most of the neoplasms associated with translocations, inversions, or deletions are leukemias. The reason for this is technical, in that examination of the karyotypes of leukemic cells is much easier than of the karyotypes of solid neoplasms. However, the figure also shows chromosomal alterations characteristically seen in several sarcomas as well as epithelial neoplasms. In most of the examples, the percentage of patients exhibiting the specific chromosomal abnormality is less than 50%. However, in a number of neoplasms the chromosomal abnormality is characteristically greater than 50%, as noted in Table 6.7.

Since it is the leukemias and lymphomas that have revealed the most consistent and easily studied chromosomal aberrations, detailed investigations of a number of chromosomal translocations analogous to the Ph[1] chromosome have been carried out and in turn have served as models for similar chromosomal aberrations in neoplasms of diverse types (Figure 6.6 and Table 6.7). Here three examples of structural aberrations occurring in a high percentage in specific neoplasms are considered in more detail.

The 8:14 Translocation in Burkitt Lymphoma

Burkitt lymphoma is endemic in certain parts of the continent of Africa (Chapter 11). A variant form of this disease is seen in the North American continent and other parts of the world. As noted from Table 6.7, an extremely high proportion of individuals with this disease exhibit a specific chromosomal translocation. A diagram of the translocation is seen in Figure 6.7; the translocation involves a disruption of two genes involved in the breakpoint. These are c-*myc*

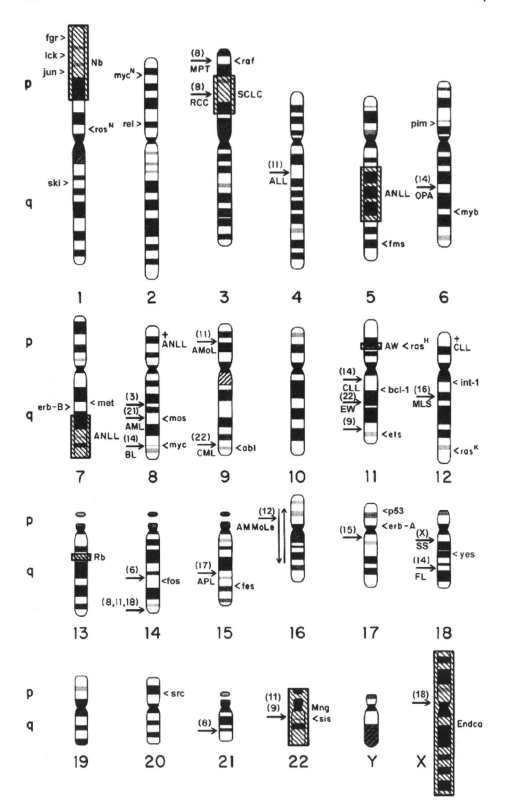

Table 6.7 Nonrandom Chromosome Abnormalities in Malignant Diseases

Disease	Chromosome Abnormality	Percent of Patients
Leukemias		
CML	t(9;22)(q34;q11)	~100
CML blast phase	t(9;22)(q34;q11) with +8, +Ph[1], +19, or I(17q)	~70
APL-M3, M3V	t(15;17)(q22;q11-12)	60–100
AMMoL-M4Eo	inv(16)(p13q22) or t(16;16)(p13;q22)	100 (25% of M4)
Therapy-related AML	–7 or del(7q) and/or –5 or del(5q)	90
Solid tumors		
Small-cell lung carcinoma	del(3p14-23)	~90% Mitelman and Heim (1990)
Meningioma	del(22)	~64% Dumanski et al. (1990)
Synovial sarcoma	t(X;18)(p11.2;q11.2)	~80% Turc-Carel et al. (1987)
Myxoid liposarcoma	t(12;16)(q13;p11)	~90% Panagopoulos et al. (1994)
Ewing sarcoma	t(11;22)(q24;q12)	88% Turc-Carel et al. (1988)
Burkitt lymphoma	t(8;14)(q24;q32)	~90% Manolov and Manolova, 1972
Follicular lymphoma	t(14;18)(q32;q21)	~90% Weiss et al., 1987

Key: AML, acute myeloblastic leukemia; AMMoL-M4Eo, acute myelomonocytic leukemia with abnormal eosinophils; APL-M3, M3V, hypergranular (M3) and microgranular (M3V) acute promyelocytic leukemia; CML, chronic myelogenous leukemia.
The references for the solid tumors are noted in the table. The findings in leukemias are taken from Rowley, 1990.

Figure 6.6 Human chromosome map showing position of oncogenes (< lowercase), translocation and breakage sites (arrow with number in parentheses designating other chromosome involved in the translocation), deletions (boxes with diagonal lines), trisomies (+), inversions (two-way arrows), and the notation of the specific neoplasm associated with the designated chromosomal abnormality (uppercase or combination of upper- and lowercase letters). The karyotype represents Giemsa bands at the 400 band stage. The nomenclature for the cellular oncogenes is identical with that in Table 4.4, Chapter 4. The key to the abbreviations of the neoplastic conditions designated in the figure is as follows, in alphabetical order: ALL, acute lymphocytic leukemia with t(4;11); AML, acute myelogenous leukemia with t(8;21); AMoL, acute monocytic leukemia with t(9;11); AMMoLe, acute myelomonocytic leukemia with inversion of chromosome 16 (double reversed arrows); ANLL, acute nonlymphocytic leukemia with deletion in chromosome 5; APL, acute promyelocytic leukemia with t(15;17); AW, aniridia "Wilms" tumor syndrome with small deletion of short arm of chromosome 11; BL, Burkitt's lymphoma and B-cell lymphoma with t(8;14); CLL, chronic lymphocytic leukemia with t(11;14) and trisomy of chromosome 12; CML, chronic myelogenous leukemia with t(9;22); Endca, endometrial carcinoma with deletion of the X chromosome; EW, Ewing sarcoma with t(11;22)(q24;q12); FL, follicular lymphoma with t(14;18); MLS, myxoid liposarcoma t(12;16)(q13;p11); Mng, meningioma with deletion of chromosome 22; MPT, mixed parotid gland tumor with t(3;8); Nb, neuroblastoma with deletion of portion of long arm of chromosome 1; OPA, ovarian papillary adenocarcinoma with t(6;14); Rb, retinoblastoma with deletion of segment of short arm of chromosome 13; RCC, renal cell carcinoma with t(3;8); SCLC, small-cell lung cancer with deletion of short arm of chromosome 3; SS, synovial sarcoma t(X:18)(p11;q11). For further details of this map, the reader is referred to the text and the review by Yunis (1983) as well as Rowley (1990) and Mitelman and Heim (1990).

present on chromosome 8 and the heavy chain of the immunoglobulin gene family (Chapter 15). The figure indicates two different genes resulting from the translocation, one seen predominantly in African Burkitt lymphoma and the other seen more commonly in North American Burkitt lymphoma (Haluska et al., 1987). Other variants have also been reported involving chromosome 8 with translocations to chromosome 2 or chromosome 22 (Aisenberg, 1984). In many B-cell lymphomas with translocations that involve immunoglobulin genes (Chapter 16), a significant rearrangement of the immunoglobulin genes may be found in the lymphoma cell genomes (Cleary et al., 1984; Haluska et al., 1986). Because of the nature of the normal somatic recombination seen in immunoglobulin genes (Chapter 16), it is possible that the formation of the translocation may be related to this normal process seen in B cells. A similar finding of the relationship of chromosomal abnormalities to the T-cell receptor genes (Chapter 19) has led to similar proposals of the mechanisms of chromosomal abnormalities in T-cell neoplasms (Boehm and Rabbitts, 1989).

Despite extensive knowledge of the detailed structure of the fusion of the c-*myc* and immunoglobulin genes at the breakpoint, the molecular mechanism of the dysregulation of the c-*myc* proto-oncogene that occurs in this condition remains unclear (Aisenberg, 1993). As seen in Figure 6.7, the sites of disruption of the two genes involved may differ slightly between different neoplasms, especially in different parts of the world. Croce and Nowell (1985) suggested that enhancer elements within the immunoglobulin gene that had been translocated may serve to increase transcription of the c-*myc* proto-oncogene, but as yet this concept remains theoretical.

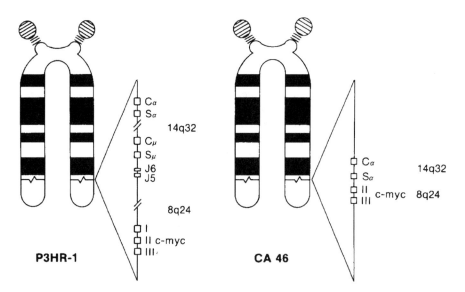

Figure 6.7 Differences in the t(8:14) chromosome translocation of the African Burkitt lymphoma (P3HR-1) and sporadic Burkitt lymphoma (CA 46) with only the 14q+ chromosome illustrated in each case. In the case of African Burkitt lymphoma, the breakpoint lies upstream of the joining (J5) region of the heavy immunoglobulin chain on chromosome 14 and more than 50 kb 5′ of the intact c-*myc* on chromosome 8. In contrast, in sporadic Burkitt lymphoma, this example demonstrates a breakpoint much farther 3′ into the immunoglobulin heavy chain gene region and the elimination of the first exon of c-*myc*. (From Haluska et al., 1987, with permission of the authors and publisher.)

The 14:18 Translocation in Follicular Lymphomas

In general, it has been stated that translocation between chromosomes 14 and 18 is the most common cytogenetic abnormality observed in malignant lymphomas (Rowley, 1988). As noted in Table 6.7, as many as 90% of follicular lymphomas may exhibit this abnormality. The translocation places the IgM heavy chain gene on chromosome 14 in juxtaposition to the *bcl-2* cellular oncogene on chromosome 18 (Figure 6.8). The *bcl-2* gene, designation for *B-cell lymphoma/leukemia*, has been shown to play an important role in apoptosis, programmed cell death (cf. Bagg and Cossman, 1993). The *bcl-2* gene product appears to inhibit the process of apoptosis in both normal and neoplastic cells. In the translocation, the coding region of the *bcl-2* gene is left intact, and there is a marked deregulation of the gene following translocation. This in turn leads to an inhibition of programmed cell death of B lymphocytes with continued expansion and potential for other secondary genetic events that are seen in lymphomas.

The 15:17 Translocation in Acute Promyelocytic Leukemia

Acute promyelocytic leukemia is a distinct subtype of acute nonlymphocytic leukemias in which a translocation occurs between chromosomes 15 and 17 with the breakpoints noted in Table 6.7. Larson et al. (1984) have argued that every patient with this condition exhibits the 15:17 translocation. A more detailed scheme of the translocation may be seen in Figure 6.9. As noted, the genes involved are the retinoic acid receptor-α (RAR-α) and a gene termed PML (abbreviation for *pro*myelocytic *l*eukemia). The gene resulting from the translocation involves the amino terminal two-thirds of the coding region of the PML gene. A large portion but not all of the RAR-a receptor comprises the other portion of the fused gene (de Thé et al., 1991). While there have been several suggested mechanisms by which the fused gene product interferes with the normal function of the receptor that plays a role in promyelocytic differentiation, the important clinical characteristic of this disease is that more than 85% of patients respond to the administration of retinoids by an induced differentiation in vivo of the leukemic cells, resulting in a remission of the disease.

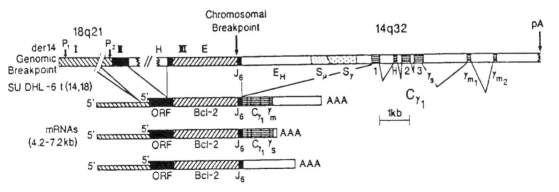

Figure 6.8 Schematic presentation of the *bcl-2/Ig* fusion gene and multiple chimeric mRNA products. In the figure P$_1$ and P$_2$ denote separate promoter regions for the *bcl-2* gene. (From Seto et al., 1988, with permission of the authors and publisher.)

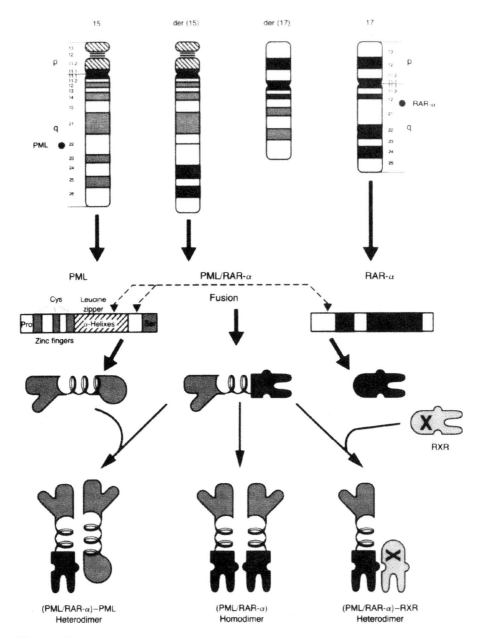

Figure 6.9 Diagram of the genesis and dimerization of the PML/RAR-α fusion protein. At the upper part of the figure the reciprocal translocations between the long arms of chromosomes 15 and 17 in APL are shown with the derived (der) chromosomes in the center. In the middle of the figure are shown the protein sequences for the PML and RAR-α genes with the upper single arrowheads associated with the dashed line indicating the most common breakpoints involved in the translocations in APL. At the bottom of the figure are shown possible mechanisms by which the fusion of the two genes may lead to leukemogenesis, including heterodimerization with wild-type PML and inactivation of the latter, inactivation of other retinoid receptors (RXR), and inactivation of these as well as homodimerization of the fusion proteins with subsequent binding to PML and/or RAR-α target genes. (From Warrell et al., 1993, with permission of the authors and publisher.)

The Significance of Fusion Genes Resulting from Chromosomal Somatic Mutations in Neoplasia

The original observation of the Ph[1] chromosome by Nowell and Hungerford (1960), a seemingly isolated fact when first reported, has given rise to a major increase in our understanding of the ramifications of somatic mutations in the neoplastic cells. The four examples discussed thus far of the detailed analysis of the translocation-derived chromosomes seen in various lymphomas and leukemias are in fact only the beginning of what promises to be an enormous increase in our understanding not only of the ramification of genetic changes in neoplasia, but also in the structure of the human genome and the potential for genetic alterations residing therein. In Table 6.8 is a reasonably complete listing through 1994 of the known fusion genes and the proteins resulting from specific translocations not only in lymphomas and leukemias, but also in a number of other solid neoplasms. A number of generalizations resulting from these investigations are slowly developing. As one views the functions of the various genes involved, one is struck by the large numbers of transcription factors and DNA-binding proteins involved in the translocations and ultimately in the fusion proteins. In addition, although thus far a minority, genes involved in signal transduction, including protein kinases and receptors make up most of the remaining functions of the known fusion proteins. There is also the question of the de- or dysregulation of the production of the active component of the fusion protein in which the genes are usually activated either by an increase in their transcription or by an enhanced functional efficiency of the fusion protein itself. Translocations involving immunoglobulin genes or T-cell receptor (TCR) genes (Chapter 19) might be considered a special case since these genes are naturally rearranged in their normal cells for the generation of active immunoglobulins or antigen-receptor genes. As noted from the table, fusion genes may involve tumor suppressor genes (EWS/WT1) or proto-oncogenes as in myc/IgH, TPR/MET, and RET/D10S170. In addition, an interesting fusion of the FUS (also termed the TLS, translocated in liposarcoma) gene fused to the chop gene is seen in myxoid liposarcoma. In this instance the FUS gene codes a nuclear RNA-binding protein, while the chop gene codes a growth arrest gene. Fusion of the two seems to eliminate the RNA-binding domain of FUS with subsequent potential inappropriate targeting of the fusion gene product to regulatory elements normally interacting with FUS alone (Crozat et al., 1993). Interestingly, approximately 50% of benign lipomas are characterized by cytogenetic rearrangements involving 12q14-15 in a presumably balanced translocation with a variety of other autosomes as well as the X chromosome (Sreekantaiah et al., 1991). One of the partners in the fusion is the gene, HMGI-C, belonging to the high-mobility group (HMG) family of DNA-binding proteins, possibly playing a role in adipogenesis and mesenchyme differentiation (Ashar et al., 1995). For further information on some of the fusion genes listed in Table 6.8, the references cited should be examined more closely.

NONRANDOM CHROMOSOMAL ABNORMALITIES CHARACTERISTIC OF SPECIFIC ANIMAL NEOPLASMS

While there have been numerous investigations of the karyotypes of many neoplasms in experimental and domestic animals (cf. Sasaki, 1982; Kerler and Rabes, 1994), relatively few constant karyotypic changes occurring in specific histogenetic types of neoplasms have been noted. Table 6.9 shows some examples of known chromosomal abnormalities characteristic of certain neoplasms in the mouse and the rat. One of the earliest and most frequently studied is the trisomy of chromosome 15 in the mouse, which is found in the vast majority of T-cell lymphomas and leukemias regardless of the inducing agent (Sasaki, 1982; Spira, 1983). This change occurs both in

Table 6.8 Fusion Genes in Neoplasia

Type	Affected Gene	Protein Domain	Fusion Protein	Disease	Reference
Hematopoietic tumors					
inv14 (q11; q32)	TCR-α (14q11) / VH (14q32)	TCR-Cα / Ig VH	VH-TCR-Cα	T/B-cell lymphoma	Rabbitts, 1994
t(9; 22)(q34; q11)	CABL (9q34) / BCR (22q11)	Tyrosine kinase / Serine kinase	serine + tyrosine kinase	CML/ALL	Rabbitts, 1994
t(1; 19)(q23; p13.3)	PBX1 (1q23) / E2A (19p13.3)	HD / AD-b-HLH	AD + HD	pre-B-ALL	Rabbitts, 1994
t(17; 19)(q22; p13)	HLF (17q22) / E2A (19p13)	bZIP / AD-b-HLH	AD + bZIP	pro-B-ALL	Rabbitts, 1994
t(15; 17)(q21-q11-22)	PML (15q21) / RARA (17q21)	Zinc-finger / Retinoic acid receptor-α	Zinc-finger + RAR DNA and ligand binding	APL	Rabbitts, 1994
t(11; 17)(q23; q21.1)	PLZF (11q23) / RARA (17q21)	Zinc-finger / Retinoic acid receptor-α	Zn-finger + RAR DNA and ligand binding	APL	Rabbitts, 1994
t(4; 11)(q21; q23)	MLL (11q23) / AF4 (4q21)	A-T hook/Zn-finger, Ser-Pro rich	A-T hook + Ser-Pro	ALL/preB-ALL/ANLL	Rabbitts, 1994
t(9; 11)(q21; q23)	MLL (11q23) / AF9/MLLT3 (9p22)	A-T hook/Zn-finger, Ser-Pro rich	A-T hook + Ser-Pro	ALL/preB-ALL/ANLL	Rabbitts, 1994
t(11; 19)(q23; p13)	MLL (11q23) / ENL (19p13)	A-T hook/Zn-finger, Ser-Pro rich	A-T hook + Ser-Pro	pre-B-ALL/T-ALL/ANLL	Rabbitts, 1994
t(X; 11)(q13; q23)	MLL (11q23) / AFX1 (Xq13)	A-T hook/Zn-finger, Ser-Pro rich	A-T hook + Ser-Pro	T-ALL	Rabbitts, 1994
t(1; 11)(p32; q23)	MLL (11q23) / AF1P (1p32)	A-T hook/Zn-finger Eps-15 homolog	A-T hook + ?	ALL	Rabbitts, 1994
t(6; 11)(q27; q23)	MLL (11q23) / AF6 (6q27)	A-T hook/Zn-finger Myosin homolog	A-T hook + ?	ALL	Rabbitts, 1994
t(11; 17)(q23; q21)	MLL (11q23) / AF17 (17q21)	A-T hook/Zn-finger Cys-rich/leucine zipper	A-T hook + leucine zipper	AML	Rabbitts, 1994
t(8; 21)(q22; q22)	AML1/CBFα (21q22) / ETO/MTG8 (8q22)	DNA binding/runt homology Zn-finger	DNA binding + Zn-fingers	AML	Rabbitts, 1994

(table continues)

Translocation	Gene (location)	Function	Fusion product	Disease	Reference
t(3; 21)(q26; q22)	AML1 (21q22)	DNA binding	DNA binding + Zn-fingers	CML	Rabbitts, 1994
	EVI-1 (3q26)	Zn-finger			
t(3; 21)(q26; q22)	AML1 (21q22)	DNA binding	DNA binding + out-of-frame EAP	Myelodysplasia	Rabbitts, 1994
	EAP (3q26)	Sn protein			
t(16; 21)(p11; q22)	FUS (16p11)	Gln-Ser-Tyr/Gly-rich/RNA binding	Gln-Ser-Tyr + DNA binding	Myeloid	Rabbitts, 1994
	ERG (21q22)	Ets-like DNA binding			
t(6; 9)(p23; q34)	DEK (6p23)	?	? + ZIP	AML	Rabbitts, 1994
	CAN (9q34)	ZIP			
t(6; 9)(p23; q34)	SET (9q34)	?	? + ZIP	AUL	Rabbitts, 1994
	CAN (9p34)	ZIP			
t(4; 46)(q26; p13)	IL-2 (4q26)	IL2	IL-2/TM	T-lymphoma	Rabbitts, 1994
	BCM (16p13.1)	?/TM domain			
inv(2; 2)(p13; p11.2-14)	REL (2p13)	DNA binding-activator	DNA binding + ?	NHL	Rabbitts, 1994
	NRG (2p11.2-14)	Not known			
inv(16)(p13q22)	Myosin MYH11 (16p13)		DNA binding ?	AML	Rabbitts, 1994
	CBF-β (16q22)				
t(5; 12)(q33; p13)	PDGF-β (5q33)	Receptor kinase	Kinase + DNA binding	CMML	Rabbitts, 1994
	TEL (12p13)	Ets-like DNA binding			
t(2; 5)(2p23; q35)	NPM (5q35)	Nucleolar phospho-protein	N terminus NPM + kinase	NHL	Rabbitts, 1994
	ALK (2p23)	Tyrosine kinase			
t(7; 19)(q35; p13)	Lyl-1	HLH, DNA binding	Lyl-1/TCR-Cβ	T-cell leukemia	Mellentin et al., 1989
	TCR-Cβ	TCR-Cβ			
t(12; 21)(p13; q22)	TEL	ETS-like transcription factor	TEL/AML1	ALL	Golub et al., 1995
	AML1	DNA binding (HLH)			
Solid tumors					
inv10(q11.2; q21)	RET (10q11.2)	Tyrosine kinase	Unk + tyrosine kinase	Papillary thyroid carcinoma	Rabbitts, 1994
	D10S170 (q21)	Uncharacterized			
t(11; 22)(q24; q12)	FLI1 (11q24)	Ets-like DNA binding	Gln-Ser-Tyr + DNA binding	Ewing sarcoma	Rabbitts, 1994
	EWS (22q12)	Gln-Ser-Tyr/Gly-rich/RNA binding			

(table continues)

Table 6.8 (continued)

Solid tumors (continued)

Type	Affected Gene	Protein Domain	Fusion Protein	Disease	Reference
t(21; 22)(?; q12)	ERG (21q22) EWS (22q12)	Ets-like DNA binding Gln-Ser-Tyr/Gly-rich/RNA binding	Gln-Ser-Tyr + DNA binding	Ewing sarcoma	Rabbitts, 1994
t(12; 22)(q13; q12)	ATF1 (12q13) EWS (22q12)	bZIP Gln-Ser-Tyr/Gly-rich/RNA binding	Gln-Ser-Tyr + bZIP	Melanoma of soft parts	Rabbitts, 1994
t(12; 16)(q13; p11)	CHOP (12q13) FUS (16p11)	(DNA binding?)/ZIP Gln-Ser-Tyr/Gly-rich/RNA binding	Gln-Ser-Tyr + (DNA binding?)/ZIP	Liposarcoma	Rabbitts, 1994
t(2; 13)(q35; q14)	PAX3 (2q35) FKHR (13q14)	Paired box/homeo-domain Forkhead domain	PB/HD + DNA binding	Rhabdomyosarcoma	Rabbitts, 1994
t(X; 18)(p11.2; q11.2)	SYT (18q11.2) SSX (Xp11.2)	None identified None identified	Synovial sarcoma	Rabbitts, 1994	
t(1; 7)	TPR MET	Translated promoter region Growth factor receptor	TPR/MET	Gastric carcinoma	Sornan et al., 1991
t(11; 22)(p13; q12)	EWS WT1	Gln-Ser-Tyr/Gly-rich/RNA binding Transcription factor	EWS/WT1	Desmoplastic small round Cell tumor	Gerald et al., 1995

The motifs indicated in the putative fusion proteins are those likely to be the important molecule in tumor pathogenesis. In most cases this is an assumption that is not yet confirmed by functional data.

Key: Known and putative DNA binding and/or protein dimerization motifs—PB, paired box; HD, homeodomain; bZIP, basic region leucine zipper; b-HLH, basic helix-loop-helix motif; ZIP, leucine zipper motif; LIM, cysteine-rich motif. Disease nomenclature: BL, Burkitt lymphoma; FL, follicular lymphoma; AL, acute leukemia; CL, chronic leukemia; ALL, acute lymphocytic leukemia (T- or B-cell); CLL, chronic lymphocytic leukemia (T- or B-cell); PLL, prolymphocytic leukemia; CML, chronic myelogenous leukemia; AML, acute myelogenous leukemia; APL, acute promyelocytic leukemia; AUL, acute undifferentiated leukemia; NHL, non–Hodgkin lymphoma; CMML, chronic myelomonocytic leukemia; DLCL, diffuse large-cell lymphoma; AD, transcriptional activation domain; TM, TM sequence; RARA, retinoic acid receptor-α receptor; IL, interleukin; Ph, Philadelphia chromosome; Unk, unknown. Further details and specific references may be obtained from the primary source of this table.

From Rabbitts, 1994, with permission of the author and publisher.

Table 6.9 Neoplasms in Mice and Rats Exhibiting Consistent Chromosomal Abnormalities

Species	Disease	Chromosome (Abnormality)	Incidence	Reference
Mouse	Myeloid leukemia	2 (partial deletion)	93%	Blatt & Sachs, 1988
Mouse	Plasmacytoma (Pristane-induced)	6;15 or 12;15 (trans- location)	100%	Ohno et al., 1979
Mouse	Plasmacytoma (Pristane/Abelson virus)	15;16 translocation	100%	Wiener et al., 1990
		11 (trisomy)	52%	Wiener et al., 1995
Mouse	T-cell leukemia/lymphoma	15 (trisomy)	65–95%	cf. Sasaki, 1982
Mouse	Skin carcinoma			
	(DMBA/TPA induced)	7 (trisomy)	95+%	Bremner et al., 1994
	(v-*Ha-ras* transgene + TPA)	15 (trisomy)	33%	French et al., 1994
Rat	Erythroblastic leukemia (DMBA-induced)	2 (trisomy)	24%	Sugiyama et al., 1978
	"Neurogenic" neoplasms (ENU-induced)	4 (trisomy)	92%	Au et al., 1977

spontaneous and chemically and physically induced T-cell neoplasms as well as some B-cell tumors in mice (Spira, 1983). In a related neoplasm, the plasmacytoma induced by pristane in the mouse, regularly translocations involving chromosome 15 are noted in virtually all such neoplasms including those infected with the oncogenic Abelson virus, wherein a somewhat different characteristic translocation and a trisomy of chromosome 11 is noted in contrast to those neoplasms induced by pristane alone (Table 6.9). The (12;15) chromosome translocation causes a juxtaposition of the c-*myc* proto-oncogene to one of the heavy chain immunoglobulin genes in a head-to-head orientation very much like that seen in the Burkitt lymphoma (8;14) translocation (Wirschubsky et al., 1985; Figure 6.7). The high incidence of the trisomy of chromosome 7 seen in mouse skin carcinomas had earlier been seen to a large extent in premalignant skin lesions in the mouse induced by a similar protocol (Aldaz et al., 1989). Interestingly, the virtual absence of trisomy 7 in skin carcinomas induced in mice transgenic for the v-*Ha-ras* oncogene may be related to the fact that the c-*Ha-ras* proto-oncogene occurs on that chromosome (French et al., 1994).

Kerler and Rabes (1994) have reviewed much of the literature on the cytogenetics of rat neoplasms. By combining a number of studies they concluded that the majority (about two-thirds) of the studies exhibited abnormalities in chromosome 2, either numerical or structural. The reference in the table is to a specific study (Sugiyama et al., 1978) which showed that about one quarter of erythroblastic leukemias induced by DMBA exhibited a trisomy of this chromosome. A trisomy of chromosome 4 was noted in almost all of ENU-induced "neurogenic" neoplasms in the rat (Au et al., 1977). The most commonly affected chromosome in rat neoplasms is chromosome 1 (Kerler and Rabas, 1994). This is also true in hepatic neoplasms, although abnormalities in chromosomes 2, 3, 4, 6, 7, 10, and 11 exhibit substantial abnormalities. A major portion of the alterations in chromosome 1 are noted in the distal portion of the long arm (Kerler and Rabas, 1994).

Thus, consistent chromosomal abnormalities characteristic of specific histogenetic neoplasms can be noted in lower animals as well as in humans. Despite these consistencies in both animals and the human, we are still faced with the dilemma of the extensive, apparently random nature of the majority of chromosome abnormalities seen in malignant neoplasms, as well as the question of the primacy of the more specific chromosomal abnormalities in the causation of such neoplasms.

NEOPLASIA AS A DISEASE OF CELL DIFFERENTIATION

In the past, the term *somatic mutation* has been used broadly to encompass cell differentiation. However, it is likely that most processes of cell differentiation occurring in the development of multicellular organisms do not involve a series of directed genetic mutations with the possible exception of the hypermutation seen in the development of immunoglobulins and related molecules (Neuberger and Milstein, 1995). Rather, the heritable phenotypes that occur during differentiation are associated with alterations in the regulation of genetic expression of a genome identical in most cells of the organism. The mechanisms of cell differentiation are for the most part still relatively obscure, but despite rapid advances in our understanding of the molecular biology of both germline and somatic mutations, significant efforts have been directed toward understanding neoplasia in the light of developmental biology.

Many experimental and histopathological investigations in oncology during the past century have pointed to a loss of the capacity of neoplastic cells to differentiate. However, during the last several decades, investigators have pointed out examples in plants (Braun and Wood, 1976), lower animals (Pierce and Wallace, 1971; Pierce, 1974), and humans (Rangecroft et al., 1978) in which neoplastic cells have exhibited the capability of specific differentiation. As we shall see in Chapter 9, continued differentiation of malignant neoplasms may lead to regression and conversion to a benign or nonneoplastic condition. In addition, studies beginning with those of Friend and her associates (1971) have demonstrated that experimental and even human neoplasms can be induced to differentiate in vitro by the addition of a variety of chemicals (cf. Freshney, 1985). Furthermore, Sachs (1993) and colleagues have demonstrated that both normal and leukemic hepatopoietic cells can be induced to differentiate by a variety of endogenous growth factors and hormones. These studies and others (cf. Lynch, 1995) have led to the concept that endogenous factors may be capable of regulating the development and differentiation of neoplastic cells.

That such endogenous factors are important in the regulation and suppression of neoplasia was best exemplified by the studies of Mintz and Illmensee (1975), Papaioannou et al. (1975), and others. These experiments, which were the actual forerunners of the embryonic stem cell technology discussed in Chapter 5, were carried out by the inoculation of malignant teratoma cells that had originated from a genetically distinct line of mice, the line 129 inoculated into blastocysts of normal mice of another line (Figure 6.10). The resultant animals exhibited cells of the genotype of the 129 line but no neoplasms. Later studies by Stewart and Mintz (1981) demonstrated that cells from the malignant teratoma line had populated the germline of the chimeric animal. It was found, however, that this phenomenon was not always reproducible with the teratoma cells, and thus for controlled experiments embryonic stem cells were preferable.

As extensions of these investigations, attempts have been made to suppress the neoplastic phenotype by inoculation of neoplastic cells at later stages of embryonic development and even in the adult. Gootwine and his associates (1982) inoculated myeloid leukemia cells into mouse embryos in utero at 10 days of gestation with the result that healthy adult mice were obtained, although the cells contained a genetic marker derived from the leukemic cells, implying the suppression of their neoplastic phenotype. Somewhat similar experiments were carried out with neuroblastoma cells, with a different end point (Pierce et al., 1982). More recently, Coleman and his associates (1993) have demonstrated that malignant liver epithelial cells in culture, when inoculated directly into the liver or the spleen of an adult rat, resulted in the suppression of their

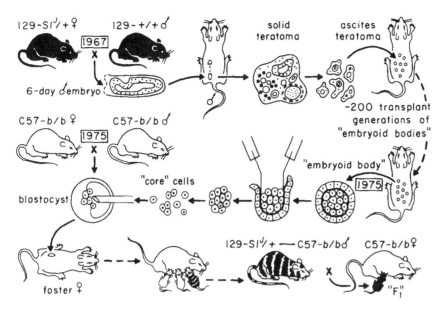

Figure 6.10 Experimental demonstration of the normal development of malignant teratoma cells originating from strain 129 mice inoculated into the normal blastocyst of strain C57 mice with subsequent production of chimeric offspring (seen as striped 129/C57 progeny). Details of the experiment may be obtained from the original reference (Mintz and Illmensee, 1975). (From Mintz and Illmensee, 1975, with permission of the authors and publisher.)

malignancy and their incorporation into hepatic plates in a differentiated state. In sum, these experiments suggest that, under appropriate environmental conditions, malignant cells can be induced to revert to a normal phenotype and lose all obvious characteristics of the neoplastic transformation for the apparent lifetime of the host.

REFERENCES

Aisenberg, A. C. New genetics of Burkitt's lymphoma and other non-Hodgkin's lymphomas. Am. J. Med., 77:1083–1090, 1984.

Aisenberg, A. C. Utility of gene rearrangements in lymphoid malignancies. Annu. Rev. Med., 44:75–84, 1993.

Aldaz, C. M., Trono, D., Larcher, F., Slaga, T. J., and Conti, C. J. Sequential trisomization of chromosomes 6 and 7 in mouse skin premalignant lesions. Mol. Carcinog., 2:22–26, 1989.

Anderson, M. W., Reynolds, S. H., You, M., and Maronpot, R. M. Role of proto-oncogene activation in carcinogenesis. Environ. Health Perspect., 98:13–24, 1992.

Asamoto, M., Mann, A. M., and Cohen, S. M. *p53* mutation is infrequent and might not give a growth advantage in rat bladder carcinogenesis *in vivo*. Carcinogenesis, 15:455–458, 1994.

Ashar, H. R., Schoenberg Fejzo, M., Tkachenko, A., Zhou, X., Fletcher, J. A., Weremowicz, S., Morton, C. C., and Chada, K. Disruption of the architectural factor HMGI-C: DNA-binding AT hook motifs fused in lipomas to distinct transcriptional regulatory domains. Cell, 82:57–65, 1995.

Au, W., Soukup, S. W., and Mandybur, T. I. Excess chromosome #4 in ethylnitrosourea-induced neurogenic tumor lines of the rat. J. Natl. Cancer Inst., 59:1709–1716, 1977.

Bagg, A., and Cossman, J. BCL-2: physiology and role in neoplasia. *In*: C. C. Benz and E. T. Liu (Eds.), Oncogenes and Tumor Suppressor Genes in Human Malignancies, pp. 141–166. Boston: Kluwer Academic Publishers, 1993.

Bártek, J., Bártková, J., Vojtesek, B., Stasková, Z., Lukás, J., Rejthar, A., Kovarík, J., Midgley, C. A., Gannon, J. V., and Lane, D. P. Aberrant expression of the *p53* oncoprotein is a common feature of a wide spectrum of human malignancies. Oncogene, *6*:1699–1703, 1991.

Barton, K., and Westbrook, C. A. Chronic myelogenous leukemia: a model for the genetic and biochemical basis of neoplasia. *In*: Biochemical and Molecular Aspects of Selected Cancers, Vol. 2, pp. 1–17. New York: Academic Press, 1994.

Benedict, W. F., Xu, H.-J., and Takahashi, R. The retinoblastoma gene: its role in human malignancies. Cancer Invest., *8*:535–540, 1990.

Birchmeier, C., Sharma, S., and Wigler, M. Expression and rearrangement of the *ROS1* gene in human glioblastoma cells. Proc. Natl. Acad. Sci. U.S.A., *84*:9270–9274, 1987.

Blatt, C., and Sachs, L. Deletion of a homeobox gene in myeloid leukemias with a deletion in chromosome 2. Biochem. Biophys. Res. Commun., *156*:1265–1270, 1988.

Boehm, T., and Rabbitts, T. H. The human T cell receptor genes are targets for chromosomal abnormalities in T cell tumors. FASEB J., *3*:2344–2359, 1989.

Bokoch, G. M., and Der, C. J. Emerging concepts in the *Ras* superfamily of GTP-binding proteins. FASEB J., *7*:750–759, 1993.

Bookstein, R., Rio, P., Madreperla, S. A., Hong, F., Allred, C., Grizzle, W. E., and Lee, W-H. Promoter deletion and loss of retinoblastoma gene expression in human prostate carcinoma. Proc. Natl. Acad. Sci. U.S.A., *87*:7762–7766, 1990.

Bos, J. L. *ras* oncogenes in human cancer: a review. Cancer Res., *49*:4682–4689, 1989.

Boveri, T. Zur Frage der Entstehung maligner Tumoren. Jena: Gustav Fischer, 1914.

Boynton, R. F., Huang, Y., Blount, P. L., Reid, B. J., Raskind, W. H., Haggitt, R. C., Newkirk, C., Resau, J. H., Yin, J., McDaniel, T., and Meltzer, S. J. Frequent loss of heterozygosity at the retinoblastoma locus in human esophageal cancers. Cancer Res., *51*:5766–5769, 1991.

Brathwaite, O., Bayona, W., and Newcomb, E. W. *p53* mutations in C57BL/6J murine thymic lymphomas induced by γ-irradiation and *N*-methylnitrosourea. Cancer Res., *52*:3791–3795, 1992.

Braun, A. C., and Wood, H. N. Suppression of the neoplastic state with the acquisition of specialized functions in cells, tissues, and organs of crown gall teratomas of tobacco. Proc. Natl. Acad. Sci. U.S.A., *73*:496–500, 1976.

Bremner, R., Kemp, C. J., and Balmain, A. Induction of different genetic changes by different classes of chemical carcinogens during progression of mouse skin tumors. Mol. Carcinog., *11*:90–97, 1994.

Bridges, B. A., Cole, J., Favor, J., Glickman, B. W., Mohrenweiser, H., Sankaranarayanan, K., and Skopek, T. R. Spontaneous mutation and its place in risk assessment for chemical mutagens. Mutat. Res., *304*:3–11, 1994.

Buchmann, A., Bauer-Hofmann, R., Mahr, J., Drinkwater, N. R., Luz, A., and Schwarz, M. Mutational activation of the c-Ha-*ras* gene in liver tumors of different rodent strains: correlation with susceptibility to hepatocarcinogenesis. Proc. Natl. Acad. Sci. U.S.A., *88*:911–915, 1991.

Burmer, G. C., Rabinovitch, P. S., and Loeb, L. A. Frequency and spectrum of c-Ki-*ras* mutations in human sporadic colon carcinoma, carcinomas arising in ulcerative colitis, and pancreatic adenocarcinoma. Environ. Health Perspect., *93*:27–31, 1991.

Castresana, J. S., Rubio, M-P., Kunimi, K., Barrios, C., and Kreicbergs, A. Lack of mutation at codon 12 of the c-H-*ras* oncogene in 51 human sarcomas assessed by PCR-RFLP. Int. J. Oncol., *2*:823–825, 1993.

Cleary, M. L., Chao, J., Warnke, R., and Sklar, J. Immunoglobulin gene rearrangement as a diagnostic criterion of B-cell lymphoma. Proc. Natl. Acad. Sci. U.S.A., *81*:593–597, 1984.

Coleman, W. B., Wennerberg, A. E., Smith, G. J., and Grisham, J. W. Regulation of the differentiation of diploid and some aneuploid rat liver epithelial (stemlike) cells by the hepatic microenvironment. Am. J. Pathol., *142*:1373–1382, 1993.

Croce, C. M., and Nowell, P. C. Molecular basis of human B cell neoplasia. J. Am. Soc. Hematol., *65*:1–7, 1985.

Crozat, A., Åman, P., Mandahl, N., and Ron, D. Fusion of CHOP to a novel RNA-binding protein in human myxoid liposarcoma. Nature, *363*:640–644, 1993.

Cryns, V. L., Thor, A., Xu, H-J., Hu, S-X., Wierman, M. E., Vickery, A. L., Jr., Benedict, W. F., and Arnold, A. Loss of the retinoblastoma tumor-suppressor gene in parathyroid carcinoma. N. Engl. J. Med., *330*:757–761, 1994.

Culotta, E., and Koshland, D. E., Jr. *p53* sweeps through cancer research. Science, *262*:1958–1961, 1993.

Cunningham, M., and Dickerman, J. D. Fragile X syndrome and acute lymphoblastic leukemia. Cancer, *62*:2383–2386, 1988.

De Braekeleer, M., Smith, B., and Lin, C. C. Fragile sites and structural rearrangements in cancer. Hum. Genet., *69*:112–116, 1985.

De Chiara, A., T'Ang, A., and Triche, T. J. Expression of the retinoblastoma susceptibility gene in childhood rhabdomyosarcomas. J. Natl. Cancer Inst., *85*:152–157, 1993.

DeKlein, A., Geurts van Kessel, A., Grosveld, G., Bartram, C. R., Hagemeijer, A., Bootsma, D., Spurr, N. K., Heisterkamp, N., Groffen, J., and Stephenson, J. R. A cellular oncogene is translocated to the Philadelphia chromosome in chronic myelocytic leukemia. Nature, *300*:765–767, 1982.

de Thé, H., Lavau, C., Marchio, A., Chomienne, C., Degos, L., and Dejean, A. The PML-RARα fusion mRNA generated by the t(15;17) translocation in acute promyelocytic leukemia encodes a functionally altered RAR. Cell, *66*:675–684, 1991.

Diekmann, D., Brill, S., Garrett, M. D., Totty, N., Hsuan, J., Monfries, C., Hall, C., Lim, L., and Hall, A. *Bcr* encodes a GTPase-activating protein for p21^{rac}. Nature, *351*:400–402, 1991.

Dobrovic, A., Peters, G. B., and Ford, J. H. Molecular analysis of the Philadelphia chromosome. Chromosoma, *100*:479–486, 1991.

Dubreuil, P., Torrès, H., Courcoul, M-A., Birg, F., and Mannoni, P. c-*fms* expression is a molecular marker of human acute myeloid leukemias. Blood, *72*:1081–1085, 1988.

Dumanski, J. P., Rouleau, G. A., Nordenskjöld, M., and Collins, V. P. Molecular genetic analysis of chromosome 22 in 81 cases of meningioma. Cancer Res., *50*:5863–5867, 1990.

Elbling, L., and Colot, M. In vitro SCE discrepancy between embryonic and extraembryonic mouse tissues. Mutat. Res., *163*:175–180, 1986.

Foster, K., Prowse, A., van den Berg, A., Fleming, S., Hulsbeek, M. M. F., Crossey, P. A., Richards, F. M., Cairns, P., Affara, N. A., Ferguson-Smith, M. A., Buys, C. H. C. M., and Maher, E. R. Somatic mutations of the von Hippel-Lindau disease tumour suppressor gene in non-familial clear cell renal carcinoma. Hum. Mol. Genet., *3*:2169–2173, 1994.

French, J. E., Libbus, B. L., Hansen, L., Spalding, J., Tice, R. R., Mahler, J., and Tennant, R. W. Cytogenetic analysis of malignant skin tumors induced in chemically treated TG·AC transgenic mice. Mol. Carcinog., *11*:215–226, 1994.

Freshney, R. I. Induction of differentiation in neoplastic cells. Anticancer Res., *5*:111–130, 1985.

Friend, C., Scher, W., Holland, J. G., and Sato, T. Hemoglobin synthesis in murine virus-induced leukemic cells *in vitro*: stimulation of erythroid differentiation by dimethyl sulfoxide. Proc. Natl. Acad. Sci. U.S.A., *68*:378–382, 1971.

Fu, Y-H., Kuhl, D. P. A., Pizzuti, A., Pieretti, M., Sutcliffe, J. S., Richards, S., Verkerk, A. J. M. H., Holden, J. J. A., Fenwick, R. G., Jr., Warren, S. T., Oostra, B. A., Nelson, D. L., and Caskey, C. T. Variation of the CGG repeat at the fragile X site results in genetic instability: resolution of the Sherman paradox. Cell, *67*:1047–1058, 1991.

Geraedts, J. P. M., and Van der Ploeg, M. DNA measurements of chromosomes 9 and 22 of six patients with t(9;22) and chronic myeloid leukemia. Cytometry, *1*:152–156, 1980.

Gerald, W. L., Rosai, J., and Ladanyi, M. Characterization of the genomic breakpoint and chimeric transcripts in the *EWS-WT1* gene fusion of desmoplastic small round cell tumor. Proc. Natl. Acad. Sci. U.S.A., *92*:1028–1032, 1995.

Ginsberg, A. M., Raffeld, M., and Cossman, J. Inactivation of the retinoblastoma gene in human lymphoid neoplasms. Blood, *77*:833–840, 1991.

Golub, T. R., Barker, G. F., Bohlander, S. K., Hiebert, S. W., Ward, D. C., Bray-Ward, P., Morgan, E., Raimondi, S. C., Rowley, J. D., and Gilliland, D. G. Fusion of the *TEL* gene on 12p13 to the *AML1* gene on 21q22 in acute lymphoblastic leukemia. Proc. Natl. Acad. Sci. U.S.A., *92*:4917–4921, 1995.

Goodrow, T. L., Storer, R. D., Leander, K. R., Prahalada, S. R., van Zwieten, M. J., and Bradley, M. O. Murine *p53* intron sequences 5-8 and their use in polymerase chain reaction/direct sequencing analysis of *p53* mutations in CD-1 mouse liver and lung tumors. Mol. Carcinog., *5*:9–15, 1992.

Gootwine, E., Webb, C. G., and Sachs, L. Participation of myeloid leukaemic cells injected into embryos in haematopoietic differentiation in adult mice. Nature, *299*:63–65, 1982.

Groffen, J., and Heisterkamp, N. C. Philadelphia chromosome translocation. Crit. Rev. Oncogen., *1*:53–64, 1989.

Groffen, J., Stephenson, J. R., Heisterkamp, N., DeKlein, A., Bartram, C. R., and Grosveld, G. Philadelphia chromosome breakpoints are clustered within a limited region, *bcr*, on chromosome 22. Cell, *36*:93–99, 1984.

Guinee, D. G., Jr., Travis, W. D., Trivers, G. E., De Benedetti, V. M. G., Cawley, H., Welsh, J. A., Bennett, W. P., Jett, J., Colby, T. V., Tazelaar, H., Abbondanzo, S. L., Pairolero, P., Trastek, V., Caporaso, N. E., Liotta, L. A., and Harris, C. C. Gender comparisons in human lung cancer: analysis of *p53* mutations, anti-*p53* serum antibodies and C-*erb*B-2 expression. Carcinogenesis, *16*:993–1002, 1995.

Haluska, F. G., Finver, S., Tsujimoto, Y., and Croce, C. M. The t(8;14) chromosomal translocation occurring in B-cell malignancies results from mistakes in V-D-J joining. Nature, *324*:158–161, 1986.

Haluska, F. G., Tsujimoto Y., and Croce, C. M. Mechanisms of chromosome translocation in B- and T-cell neoplasia. Trends Genet., *3*:11–15, 1987.

Harris, C. C. *p53*: at the crossroads of molecular carcinogenesis and risk assessment. Science, *262*:1980–1981, 1993.

Harris, C. C. *p53*: at the crossroads of molecular carcinogenesis and risk assessment. CIIT Activities, *15*:1–6, 1995.

Harris, C. C., and Hollstein, M. Clinical implications of the *p53* tumor-suppressor gene. N. Engl. J. Med., *329*:1318–1327, 1993.

Hegi, M. E., Söderkvist, P., Foley, J. F., Schoonhoven, R., Swenberg, J. A., Kari, F., Maronpot, R., Anderson, M. W., and Wiseman, R. W. Characterization of *p53* mutations in methylene chloride-induced lung tumors from B6C3F1 mice. Carcinogenesis, *14*:803–810, 1993.

Hensel, C. H., Hsieh, C-L., Gazdar, A. F., Johnson, B. E., Sakaguchi, A. Y., Naylor, S. L., Lee, W-H., and Lee, E. Y-H. P. Altered structure and expression of the human retinoblastoma susceptibility gene in small cell lung cancer. Cancer Res., *50*:3067–3072, 1990.

Herskowitz, I. Functional inactivation of genes by dominant negative mutations. Nature, *329*:219–222, 1987.

Ho, Y-S., Cheng, H-T., Wang, Y-J., and Lin, J-K. *p53* gene mutational spectra in hepatocellular carcinomas induced by 2-acetylaminofluorene and *N*-nitroso-2-acetylaminofluorene in rats. Mol. Carcinog., *13*:182–190, 1995.

Holliday, R. Mutations and epimutations in mammalian cells. Mutat. Res., *250*:351–363, 1991.

Hsu, I. C., Metcalf, R. A., Sun, T., Welsh, J. A., Wang, N. J., and Harris, C. C. Mutational hotspot in the *p53* gene in human hepatocellular carcinomas. Nature, *350*:427–428, 1991.

Hulla, J. E., Chen, Z. Y., and Eaton, D. L. Aflatoxin B₁-induced rat hepatic hyperplastic nodules do not exhibit a site-specific mutation within the *p53* gene. Cancer Res., *53*:9–11, 1993.

Jerry, D. J., Ozbun, M. A., Kittrell, F. S., Lane, D. P., Medina, D., and Butel, J. S. Mutations in *p53* are frequent in the preneoplastic stage of mouse mammary tumor development. Cancer Res., *53*:3374–3381, 1993.

Joensuu, H., Klemi, P., and Eerola, E. DNA aneuploidy in follicular adenomas of the thyroid gland. Am. J. Pathol., *124*:373–376, 1986.

Kanno, H., Kondo, K., Ito, S., Yamamoto, I., Fujii, S., Torigoe, S., Sakai, N., Hosaka, M., Shuin, T., and Yao, M. Somatic mutations of the Von Hippel-Lindau tumor suppressor gene in sporadic central nervous system hemangioblastomas. Cancer Res., *54*:4845–4847, 1994.

Kerler, R., and Rabes, H. M. Rat tumor cytogenetics: a critical evaluation of the literature. Crit. Rev. Oncogen., *5*:271–295, 1994.

Kiaris, H., and Spandidos, D. A. Mutations of *ras* genes in human tumours. Int. J. Oncol., *7*:43–421, 1995.

Kress, S., König, J., Schweizer, J., Löhrke, H., Bauer-Hofmann, R., and Schwarz, M. *p53* mutations are absent from carcinogen-induced mouse liver tumors but occur in cell lines established from these tumors. Mol. Carcinog., *6*:148–158, 1992a.

Kress, S., Sutter, C., Strickland, P. T., Mukhtar, H., Schweizer, J., and Schwarz, M. Carcinogen-specific mutational pattern in the *p53* gene in ultraviolet B radiation-induced squamous cell carcinomas of mouse skin. Cancer Res., *52*:6400–6403, 1992b.

Larson, R. A., Kondo, K., Vardiman, J. W., Butler, A. E., Golomb, H. M., and Rowley, J. D. Evidence for a 15;17 translocation in every patient with acute promyelocytic leukemia. Am. J. Med., *76*:827–840, 1984.

Lee, A. T., DeSimone, C., Cerami, A., and Bucala, R. Comparative analysis of DNA mutations in *lacI* transgenic mice with age. FASEB J., *8*:545–550, 1994.

Lilleberg, S. L., Cabonce, M. A., Raju, N. R., Wagner, L. M., and Kier, L. D. Alterations in the structural gene and the expression of *p53* in rat liver tumors induced by aflatoxin B$_1$. Mol. Carcinog., *6*:159–172, 1992.

Liu, Y., Hernandez, A. M., Shibata, D., and Cortopassi, G. A. *BCL2* translocation frequency rises with age in humans. Proc. Natl. Acad. Sci. U.S.A., *91*:8910–8914, 1994.

Lynch, R. G. Differentiation and cancer: the conditional autonomy of phenotype. Proc. Natl. Acad. Sci. U.S.A., *92*:647–648, 1995.

Lyons, J., Landis, C. A., Harsh, G., Vallar, L., Grünewald, K., Feichtinger, H., Duh, Q-Y., Clark, O. H., Kawasaki, E., Bourne, H. R., and McCormick, F. Two G protein oncogenes in human endocrine tumors. Science, *249*:655–658, 1990.

Makino, H., Ishizaka, Y., Tsujimoto, A., Nakamura, T., Onda, M., Sugimura, T., and Nagao, M. Rat *p53* gene mutations in primary Zymbal gland tumors induced by 2-amino-3-methylimidazo[4,5-*f*]quinoline, a food mutagen. Proc. Natl. Acad. Sci. U.S.A., *89*:4850–4854, 1992.

Manolov, G., and Manolova, Y. Marker band in one chromosome 14 from Burkitt lymphoma. Nature, *237*:33–34, 1972.

Martin-Zanca, D., Mitra, G., Long, L. K., and Barbacid, M. Molecular characterization of the human *trk* oncogene. Cold Spring Harbor Symp. Quant. Biol., *51*:983–990, 1986.

Meling, G. I., Lothe, R. A., Børresen, A.-L., Hauge, S., Graue, C., Clausen, O. P. F., and Rognum, T. O. Genetic alterations within the retinoblastoma locus in colorectal carcinomas. Relation to DNA ploidy pattern studied by flow cytometric analysis. Br. J. Cancer, *64*:475–480, 1991.

Mellentin, J. D., Smith, S. D., and Cleary, M. L. *Iyl*-1, a novel gene altered by chromosomal translocation in T cell leukemia, codes for a protein with a helix-loop-helix DNA binding motif. Cell, *58*:77–83, 1989.

Mintz, B., and Illmensee, K. Normal genetically mosaic mice produced from malignant teratocarcinoma cells. Proc. Natl. Acad. Sci. U.S.A., *72*:3585–3589, 1975.

Misawa, S., Yashige, H., Horiike, S., Taniwaki, M., Nishigaki, H., Okuda, T., Yokota, S., Tsuda, S., Edagawa, J., Imanishi, H., Takino, T., Inazawa, J., Abe, T., Nakanishi, S., Nakagawa, M., Kobayashi, H., Maekawa, T., Fujii, H., Akaogi, T., Hayashi, H., Fujiyama, Y., and Kohsaki, M. Detection of karyotypic abnormalities in most patients with acute nonlymphocytic leukemia by adding ethidium bromide to short-term cultures. Leuk. Res., *12*:719–729, 1988.

Mitelman, F. Different chromosome morphology of diploid and aneuploid malignant cells. J. Natl. Cancer Inst., *52*:561–564, 1974.

Mitelman, F. The Third International Workshop on Chromosomes in Leukemia, Lund, Sweden, July 21–25, 1980. Cancer Genet. Cytogenet., *4*:95–142, 1981.

Mitelman, F., and Heim, S. Chromosome abnormalities in cancer. Cancer Detect. Prev., *14*:527–537, 1990.

Moreau-Gachelin, F. Spi-1/PU.1: an oncogene of the Ets family. Biochim. Biophys. Acta, *1198*:149–163, 1994.

Moul, J. W., Bishoff, J. T., Theune, S. M., and Chang, E. H. Absent *ras* gene mutations in human adrenal cortical neoplasms and pheochromocytomas. J. Urol., *149*:1389–1394, 1993.

Nagata, Y., Abe, M., Motoshima, K., Nakayama, E., and Shiku, H. Frequent glycine-to-aspartic acid mutations at codon 12 of c-Ki-*ras* gene in human pancreatic cancer in Japanese. Jpn. J. Cancer Res., *81*:135–140, 1990.

Nelson, D. L. The fragile X syndromes. Cell Biol., *6*:5–11, 1995.

Neuberger, M. S., and Milstein, C. Somatic hypermutation. Curr. Opin. Immunol., *7*:248–254, 1995.

Nishimura, S., and Sekiya, T. Human cancer and cellular oncogenes. Biochem. J., *243*:313–327, 1987.

Nisitani, S., Hosokawa, M., Sasaki, M. S., Yasuoka, K., Naiki, H., Matsushita, T., and Takeda, T. Acceleration of chromosome aberrations in senescence-accelerated strains of mice. Mutat. Res., *237*:221–228, 1990.

Nowell, P. C., and Hungerford, D. A. A minute chromosome in human chronic granulocytic leukemia. Science, *132*:1497, 1960.

Nowell, P. C., Morris, H. P., and Potter, V. R. Chromosomes of "minimal deviation" hepatomas and some other transplantable rat tumors. Cancer Res., *27*:1565–1579, 1967.

Ohgaki, H., Hard, G. C., Hirota, N., Maekawa, A., Takahashi, M., and Kleihues, P. Selective mutation of codons 204 and 213 of the *p53* gene in rat tumors induced by alkylating *N*-nitroso compounds. Cancer Res., *52*:2995–2998, 1992.

Ohno, S., Babonits, M., Wiener, F., Spira, J., and Klein, G. Nonrandom chromosome changes involving the Ig gene-carrying chromosomes 12 and 6 in pristane-induced mouse plasmacytomas. Cell, *18*:1001–1007, 1979.

Ootsuyama, A., Makino, H., Nagao, M., Ochiai, A., Yamauchi, Y., and Tanooka, H. Frequent *p53* mutation in mouse tumors induced by repeated β-irradiation. Mol. Carcinog., *11*:236–242, 1994.

Pai, E. F., Kabsch, W., Krengel, U., Holmes, K. C., John, J., and Wittinghofer, A. Structure of the guanine-nucleotide-binding domain of the Ha-*ras* oncogene product p21 in the triphosphate conformation. Nature, *341*:209–214, 1989.

Panagopoulos, I., Mandahl, N., Ron, D., Höglund, M., Nilbert, M., Mertens, F., Mitelman, F., and Åman, P. Characterization of the *CHOP* breakpoints and fusion transcripts in myxoid liposarcomas with the 12;16 translocation. Cancer Res., *54*:6500–6503, 1994.

Papaioannou, V. E., McBurney, M. W., and Gardner, R. L. Fate of teratocarcinoma cells injected into early mouse embryos. Nature, *258*:70–73, 1975.

Perantoni, A. O., Turusov, V. S., Buzard, G. S., and Rice, J. M. Infrequent transforming mutations in the transmembrane domain of the *neu* oncogene in spontaneous rat schwannomas. Mol. Carcinog., *9*:230–235, 1994.

Pierce, G. B. Neoplasms, differentiations and mutations. Am. J. Pathol., *77*:103–118, 1974.

Pierce, G. B., and Wallace, C. Differentiation of malignant to benign cells. Cancer Res., *31*:127–134, 1971.

Pierce, G. B., Pantazis, C. G., Caldwell, J. E., and Wells, R. S. Specificity of the control of tumor formation by the blastocyst. Cancer Res., *42*:1082–1087, 1982.

Pitot, H. C. The molecular biology of carcinogenesis. Cancer, *72*:962–970, 1993.

Puisieux, A., Lim, S., Groopman, J., and Ozturk, M. Selective targeting of *p53* gene mutational hotspots in human cancers by etiologically defined carcinogens. Cancer Res., *51*:6185–6189, 1991.

Rabbits, T. H. Chromosomal translocations in human cancer. Nature, *372*:143–149, 1994.

Rangecroft, L., Lander, I., and Wagget, J. Spontaneous maturation of stage IV-S neuroblastoma. Arch. Dis. Child., *52*:815–817, 1978.

Reuvekamp, P. T. W., Stulp, R. P., Schraffordt Koops, H., Wolter Oosterhuis, J., Scheffer, H., and Buys, C. H. C. M. Analysis of a metastasizing testicular mixed gonadal stromal tumor with osteosarcoma components suggests that a malignant tumor with the histology of osteosarcoma may develop without primary involvement of *RB1* and *TP53*. Cancer Res., *52*:6705–6707, 1992.

Reynolds, S. H., Anna, C. K., Brown, K. C., Wiest, J. S., Beattie, E. J., Pero, R. W., Iglehart, J. D., and Anderson, M. W. Activated protooncogenes in human lung tumors from smokers. Proc. Natl. Acad. Sci. U.S.A., *88*:1085–1089, 1991.

Rideout, W. M., III, Coetzee, G. A., Olumi, A. F., Spruck, C. H., and Jones, P. A. 5-methylcytosine as an endogenous mutagen in the *p53* tumor suppressor gene. *In*: C. C. Harris et al. (Eds.), Multistage Carcinogenesis, pp. 207–219. Tokyo: Japan Scientific Societies Press; Boca Raton, FL: CRC Press, 1992.

Ronai, Z., Luo, F. C., Gradia, S., Hart, W. J., and Butler, R. Detection of K-*ras* mutation in normal and malignant colonic tissues by an enriched PCR method. Int. J. Oncol., *4*:391–396, 1994.

Rowley, J. D. A new consistent chromosomal abnormality in chronic myelogenous leukaemia identified by quinacrine fluorescence and Giemsa staining. Nature, *243*:290–293, 1973.

Rowley, J. D. Chromosome studies in the non-Hodgkin's lymphomas: the role of the 14;18 translocation. J. Clin. Oncol., *6*:919–925, 1988.

Rowley, J. D. Molecular cytogenetics: rosetta stone for understanding cancer—twenty-ninth G.H.A. Clowes memorial award lecture. Cancer Res., *50*:3816–3825, 1990a.

Rowley, J. D. The Philadelphia chromosome translocation. A paradigm for understanding leukemia. Cancer, *65*:2178–2184, 1990b.

Ruggeri, B., DiRado, M., Zhang,. S. Y., Bauer, B., Goodrow, T., and Klein-Szanto, A. J. P. Benzo[*a*]pyrene-induced murine skin tumors exhibit frequent and characteristic G to T mutations in the *p53* gene. Proc. Natl. Acad. Sci. U.S.A., *90*:1013–1017, 1993.

Rumsby, P. C., Davies, M. J., and Evans, J. G. Screening for *p53* mutations in C3H/He mouse liver tumors derived spontaneously or induced with diethylnitrosamine or phenobarbitone. Mol. Carcinog., *9*:71–75, 1994.

Rüschoff, J., Bocker, T., Schlegel, J., Stumm, G., and Hofstaedter, F. Microsatellite instability: new aspects in the carcinogenesis of colorectal carcinoma. Virchows Arch., *426*:215–222, 1995.

Sachs, L. Regulators of normal development and tumor suppression. Int. J. Dev. Biol., *37*:51–59, 1993.

Sandberg, A. A. Chromosomes and causation of human cancer and leukemia: XL. The Ph[1] and other translocations in CML. Cancer, *46*:2221–2226, 1980.

Sarkar, F. H., Sakr, W., Li, Y-W., Macoska, J., Ball, D. E., and Crissman, J. D. Analysis of retinoblastoma (RB) gene deletion in human prostatic carcinomas. Prostate, *21*:145–152, 1992.

Sasaki, M. Current status of cytogenetic studies in animal tumors with special reference to nonrandom chromosome changes. Cancer Genet. Cytogenet., *5*:153–172, 1982.

Seto, M., Jaeger, U., Hockett, R. D., Graninger, W., Bennett, S., Goldman, P., and Korsmeyer, S. J. Alternative promoters and exons, somatic mutation and deregulation of the *Bcl-2-Ig* fusion gene in lymphoma. EMBO J., *7*:123–131, 1988.

Shen-Ong, G. L. C., and Wolff, L. Moloney murine leukemia virus-induced myeloid tumors in adult BALB/c mice: requirement of c-*myb* activation but lack of v-*abl* involvement. J. Virol., *61*:3721–3725, 1987.

Shi, Y., Zou, M., Schmidt, H., Juhasz, F., Stensky, V., Robb, D., and Farid, N. R. High rates of *ras* codon 61 mutation in thyroid tumors in an iodide-deficient area. Cancer Res., *51*:2690–2693, 1991.

Shub, D. A., and Goodrich-Blair, H. Protein introns: a new home for endonucleases. Cell, *71*:183–186, 1992.

Shuin, T., Kondo, K., Torigoe, S., Kishida, T., Kubota, Y., Hosaka, M., Nagashima, Y., Kitamura, H., Latif, F., Zbar, B., Lerman, M. I., and Yao, M. Frequent somatic mutations and loss of heterozygosity of the von Hippel-Lindau tumor suppressor gene in primary human renal cell carcinomas. Cancer Res., *54*:2852–2855, 1994.

Slavutsky, I., Labal de Vinuesa, M., Larripa, I., Mudry de Pargament, M., and Brieux de Salum, S. Sister chromatid exchange in malignant lymphomas. Cancer Genet. Cytogenet., *13*:153–158, 1984.

Smith, A. J., Stern, H. S., Penner, M., Hay, K., Mitri, A., Bapat, B. V., and Gallinger, S. Somatic *APC* and K-*ras* codon 12 mutations in aberrant crypt foci from human colons. Cancer Res., *54*:5527–5530, 1994.

Smith, M. L., Yeleswarapu, L., Lombardi, B., and Shinozuka, H. Lack of mutations of the *p53* tumor suppressor gene in hepatocellular carcinomas induced in rats by a peroxisome proliferator. Mol. Carcinog., *7*:89–93, 1993a.

Smith, M. L., Yeleswarapu, L., Scalamogna, P., Locker, J., and Lombardi, B. *p53* mutations in hepatocellular carcinomas induced by a choline-devoid diet in male Fischer 344 rats. Carcinogenesis, *14*:503–510, 1993b.

Soman, N. R., Correa, P., Ruiz, B. A., and Wogan, G. N. The *TPR-MET* oncogenic rearrangement is present and expressed in human gastric carcinoma and precursor lesions. Proc. Natl. Acad. Sci. U.S.A., *88*:4892–4896, 1991.

Spira, J. Similar translocation pattern in B cell derived tumors of human, mouse, and rat origin. *In* Chromosomes and Cancer, pp. 85–97. New York: Academic Press, 1983.

Sreekantaiah, C., Leong, S. P. L., Karakousis, C. P., McGee, D. L., Rappaport, W. D., Villar, H. V., Neal, D., Fleming, S., Wankel, A., Herrington, P. N., Carmona, R., and Sandberg, A. A. Cytogenetic profile of 109 lipomas. Cancer Res., *51*:422–433, 1991.

Stewart, T. A., and Mintz, B. Successive generations of mice produced from an established culture line of euploid teratocarcinoma cells. Proc. Natl. Acad. Sci. U.S.A., *78*:6314–6318, 1981.

Sugio, K., Kishimoto, Y., Virmani, A. K., Hung, J. Y., and Gazdar, A. F. K-*ras* mutations are a relatively late event in the pathogenesis of lung carcinomas. Cancer Res., *54*:5811–5815, 1994.

Sugiyama, T., Uenaka, H., Ueda, N., Fukuhara, S., and Maeda, S. Reproducible chromosome changes of polycyclic hydrocarbon-induced rat leukemia: incidence and chromosome banding pattern. J. Natl. Cancer Inst., *60*:153–160, 1978.

Tabin, C. J., Bradley, S. M., Bargmann, C. I., Weinberg, R. A., Papageorge, A. G., Scolnick, E. M., Dhar, R., Lowy, D. R., and Chang, E. H. Mechanism of activation of a human oncogene. Nature, *300*:143–149, 1982.

Tada, M., Omata, M., and Ohto, M. High incidence of *ras* gene mutation in intrahepatic cholangiocarcinoma. Cancer, *69*:1115–1118, 1992.

Tahara, E. Genetic alterations in human gastrointestinal cancers. Cancer, *75*:1410–1417, 1995.

Tamura, G., Maesawa, C., Suzuki, Y., Kashiwaba, M., Ishida, M., Saito, K., and Satodate, R. Improved detection of loss of heterozygosity at retinoblastoma gene locus in human breast carcinoma. Pathol. Int., *44*:34–38, 1994.

Terada, M., Yoshida, T., Sakamoto, H., Miyagawa, K., Katoh, O., Hattori, Y., and Sugimura, T. Biological significance of the *hst-1* gene. *In*: A. G. Knudson, Jr., et al. (Eds.), Genetic Basis for Carcinogenesis: Tumor Suppressor Genes and Oncogenes, pp. 71–80. Tokyo: Japan Scientific Societies Press; Bristol: Taylor & Francis, 1990.

Toguchida, J., Ishizaki, K., Sasaki, M. S., et al. Chromosomal reorganization for the expression of recessive mutation of retinoblastoma susceptibility gene in the development of osteosarcoma. Cancer Res., *48*:3939–3943, 1988.

Tseng, P-Y., and Jones, H. W., Jr. Chromosome constitution of carcinoma of the endometrium. Obstet. Gynecol., *33*:741–752, 1969.

Turc-Carel, C., Dal Cin, P., Limon, J., Rao, U., Li, F. P., Corson, J. M., Zimmerman, R., Parry, D. M., Cowan, J. M., and Sandberg, A. A. Involvement of chromosome X in primary cytogenetic change in human neoplasia: nonrandom translocation in synovial sarcoma. Proc. Natl. Acad. Sci. U.S.A., *84*:1981–1985, 1987.

Turc-Carel, C., Aurias, A., Mugneret, F., Lizard, S., Sidaner, I., Volk, C., Thiery, J. P., Olschwang, S., Philip, I., and Berger, M. P. Chromosomes in Ewing's sarcoma. I. An evaluation of 85 cases of remarkable consistency of t(11;22)(q24;q12). Cancer Genet. Cytogenet., *32*:229–238, 1988.

van Kranen, H. J., de Gruijl, F. R., de Vries, A., Sontag, Y., Wester, P. W., Senden, H. C. M., Rozemuller, E., and van Kreijl, C. F. Frequent *p53* alterations but low incidence of *ras* mutations in UV-B-induced skin tumors of hairless mice. Carcinogenesis, *16*:1141–1147, 1995.

Wagner, S. N., Müller, R., Boehm, J., Pütz, B., Wünsch, P. H., and Höfler, H. Neuroendocrine neoplasms of the lung are not associated with point mutations at codon 12 of the Ki-*ras* gene. Virchows Arch. B Cell Pathol., *63*:325–329, 1993.

Warrell, R. P., Jr., de Thé, H., Wang, Z-Y., and Degos, L. Acute promyelocytic leukemia. N. Engl. J. Med., *329*:177–189, 1993.

Weghorst, C. M., Dragnev, K. H., Buzard, G. S. Thorne, K. L., Vandeborne, G. F., Vincent, K. A., and Rice, J. M. Low incidence of point mutations detected in the *p53* tumor suppressor gene from chemically induced rat renal mesenchymal tumors. Cancer Res., *54*:215–219, 1994.

Weichselbaum, R. R., Beckett, M., and Diamond, A. Some retinoblastomas, osteosarcomas, and soft tissue sarcomas may share a common etiology. Proc. Natl. Acad. Sci. U.S.A., *85*:2106–2109, 1988.

Weiss, L. M., Warnke, R. A., Sklar, J., and Cleary, M. L. Molecular analysis of the t(14;18) chromosomal translocation in malignant lymphomas. N. Engl. J. Med., *317*:1185–1189, 1987.

Wiener, F., Coleman, A., Mock, B. A., and Potter, M. Nonrandom chromosomal change (trisomy 11) in murine plasmacytomas induced by an ABL-MYC retrovirus. Cancer Res., *55*:1181–1188, 1995.

Wiener, F., Silva, S., Sugiyama, H., Babonits, M., and Klein, G. The "missing" mouse plasmacytoma (MPC) associated translocation T(15;16) occurs repeatedly in new MPC induction systems. Genes Chromosome Cancer, *2*:36–43, 1990.

Wirschubsky, Z., Ingvarsson, S., Carstenssen, A., Wiener, F., Klein, G., and Sümegi, J. Gene localization on sorted chromosomes: definitive evidence on the relative positioning of genes participating in the mouse plasmacytoma-associated typical translocation. Proc. Natl. Acad. Sci. U.S.A., *82*:6975–6979, 1985.

Wolman, S. R., Horland, A. A., and Becker, F. F. Altered karyotypes of transplantable "diploid" tumors. J. Natl. Cancer Inst., *51*:1909–1914, 1973.

Yunis, J. J. The chromosomal basis of human neoplasia. Science, *221*:227–236, 1983.

Yunis, J. J. Recurrent chromosomal defects are found in most patients with acute nonlymphocytic leukemia. Cancer Genet. Cytogenet., *11*:125–137, 1984.

Yunis, J. J., and Hoffman, W. R. Nuclear enzymes, fragile sites, and cancer. J. Gerontol., *44*:37–44, 1989.

Zusman, I. The clinical relevance of *p53* oncoprotein determination in cancer diagnosis and prognosis. Oncol. Rep., *2*:143–150, 1995.

7
The Natural History of Neoplastic Development: Initiation and Promotion

The nature of disease can be fully understood only in light of its pathogenesis or natural development within the organism. An understanding of the pathogenesis of disease is the basis for rational medical management and therapy. The pathogenesis of most infectious diseases was elucidated prior to the discovery of antibiotics, thus permitting the use of these drugs in the rational management and therapy of these diseases. Similarly, a better understanding of the pathogenesis of arteriosclerosis has led to the rational use of diet in the control and management of this disease, which ultimately kills more individuals in our society than does cancer. Thus, it is reasonable to predict that enlarging our understanding of the pathogenesis of neoplastic disease will be equally useful.

THE LATENCY OF NEOPLASIA

One of the ubiquitous characteristics of the natural history of the development of a neoplasm in vivo is the extended period of time between the initial application of a carcinogen—be it physical, chemical, or biological—and the appearance of a neoplasm. This latency phenomenon or tumor induction time, which can be demonstrated most readily following treatment with chemical carcinogens, has been shown to occur even when the carcinogen is administered continuously to an experimental animal. There is no obvious evidence of neoplastic growth or clinical neoplasia during the latency period. For example, when the carcinogen diethylstilbestrol is administered to a pregnant animal, neoplasms appear only much later in the offspring. This latency phenomenon may also be seen after infection by some oncogenic viruses, ionizing radiation, or in the enigmatic production of sarcomas by the subcutaneous implantation of plastic or metal disks. Thus, the latency period of the carcinogenic process may be considered as a general feature of the natural history of neoplasia. The period of latency varies with the type of agent, its dosage, and certain characteristics of the target cells as well as of the host.

Although morphological changes occurring during the early stages of neoplasia were described during the early decades of this century, it was in the 1940s that a better understanding of the biological changes that occur after exposure to a carcinogen was obtained. The beginnings of our understanding for the basis for the latency phenomenon in carcinogenesis was pioneered by Rous and Kidd (1941). Rous and his associates coined the term *initiate* in reference to the application of tar to the ear of a rabbit; subsequent wounding of the treated area *promoted* the appearance of neoplasms growing along the edge of the wound. In 1944 Mottram reported that treatment of mice with the irritant croton oil after a brief treatment with a small amount of

223

benz[a]pyrene resulted in a much higher incidence of skin tumors in the treated area than when the carcinogen was given alone. In 1947, Berenblum and Shubik's extension of the work of Mottram clearly demonstrated that skin carcinogenesis in the mouse could be divided into a stage of *initiation*, which resulted from the direct administration of a single dose of a known chemical carcinogen such as benz[a]pyrene or another carcinogenic polycyclic hydrocarbon, followed by a stage of *promotion*, which did not require the application of a carcinogenic agent but rather the repeated application of a second agent that by itself was incapable of inducing the neoplastic transformation. These latter authors employed the irritant croton oil as the agent given repeatedly, as had Mottram (1944), to complete the second stage, *promotion*.

The basic experimental protocol used by these investigators to demonstrate initiation and promotion in the development of skin cancer in the mouse, extended and refined by Boutwell (1964), is depicted in Figure 7.1. The experiment was designed so that administration of the "initiating agent" induced no tumors. When initiation was followed by chronic administration of croton oil, the promoting agent, in multiple doses, tumors developed whether the administration of croton oil was begun immediately after initiation or delayed for even as much as a year (Loehrke et al., 1983; Van Duuren et al., 1975), although the aging of the animal might decrease the efficiency of promotion (Chapter 8). Administration of croton oil prior to initiation or with-

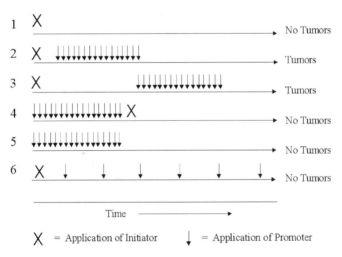

Figure 7.1 Outline of the format of experiments demonstrating initiation and promotion as developed from studies of carcinogenesis of mouse skin. Each line represents an experimental condition in which there is either no application or a single application (x) of the initiating agent, usually a carcinogenic polycyclic hydrocarbon. The multiple vertical arrows represent multiple applications of the promoting agent (phorbol ester, phenobarbital, or other known promoters for mouse skin). The time span may extend from 15 to more than 70 weeks, depending on the dosages of the initiator and promoter used, the mouse species and strain employed in the experiment, or the format of the experiment such as line 3, in which the delay between initiation and promotion may be more than a year. In line 6 the time intervals between applications of the promoting agent may be 4 weeks or more, whereas in the other experiments the promoting agent is administered twice weekly. The term *tumors* refers to papillomas or carcinomas, the latter occurring when the experiment is extended for a sufficiently long time.

out initiation resulted in no tumors. Interestingly, when the frequency of administration of the promoting agent was decreased to a tenth or less of the carcinogenic format, no tumors resulted (Boutwell, 1964). This last experiment suggested that the effects of the promoting agent were not very long lasting, in contrast to the effects of the initiating agent (line 3). Boutwell and others have maintained that the effects of promoting agents are reversible (see below).

THE STAGES OF INITIATION AND PROMOTION AS GENERAL CHARACTERISTICS OF CARCINOGENESIS

As indicated above, the initial studies of the basis for the latency of neoplastic development were carried out primarily in the mouse epidermis. Later studies by Foulds and others (Foulds, 1949; Medina, 1976) on the intermediate lesions occurring during the development of mammary adenocarcinomas in the mouse represented another system for the study of neoplastic development, but the initial emphasis was on the fate of early lesions rather than on the entire process. Within the last two decades, the development of a number of different histogenetic neoplasms in a variety of species has been investigated and found to have characteristics very similar to those originally described in the mouse epidermis model. Table 7.1 lists many of the animal systems in

Table 7.1 Animal Systems Exhibiting the Stages of Initiation and Promotion during Carcinogenesis

Tissue	End-Point Lesion	Species	Initiator	Promoter
Bladder	Papilloma, carcinoma	Dog	2-Naphthylamine	D,L-Tryptophan
Bladder	Papilloma,	Rat	MNU, FANFT	Saccharin
	Carcinoma	Rat	BBN	BHA, Urolithiasis
Colon	Adenoma	Rat	MNNG	Lithocholate
	Adenocarcinoma	Rat	DMH	Na barbiturate
Dermis	Fibrosarcoma	Mouse	3-MC	TPA
Embryo cells (in vitro)	Foci of altered morphology	Hamster	BP, MNNG	TPA, 1,25-$(OH)_2D_3$
Epidermis	Papilloma, carcinoma	Mouse, rat, hamster	BP, DMBA, 3-MC, 7-BrMeBA, TEM, Trp-P-2	TPA, skin abrasion, Telcocidin B, Aplysiatoxin, Okadiac acid, Pristane, Chrysartoxin, Dioctanoylglycerol
Epidermis	Melanoma	Hamster, mouse	DMBA	TPA Croton oil
Esophagus	Carcinoma	Rat	AMN	TPA
	Carcinoma	Rat	NNP	NaCl
Forestomach	Papilloma, carcinoma	Rat	MNNG	BHA
	Carcinoma	Rat	MNNG	Histamine

(table continues)

Table 7.1 (continued)

Tissue	End-Point Lesion	Species	Initiator	Promoter
Liver	Neoplastic nodule, adenoma, hepato-cellular carcinoma	Rat	AAF, DMH, DEN, DMN, DAB, or NNM	PB αHCH, CPA, Nafenopin PenCDF Wy-14,643 Choline deficiency Dietary tryptophan TCDD DDT BHT Ethinyl estradiol Mestranol Orotic acid $CHCl_3$ Deoxycholic acid Polyhalogenated biphenyls Dibromoethane
Liver	Hepatocellular carcinoma	Hamster	BHP	PB
	Cholangiocarcinoma			DCA
	Adenomas		DMN	CCl_4
Liver	Hepatocellular adenoma	Mouse	DEN	PB, BHA, DEHP
	Hepatocellular carcinoma	(C3H, DBA, CD-1, B6C3F1 strains)		Polychlorinated biphenyls TCPOBOP
Liver	Hepatoma	Trout	Aflatoxin	Me-sterculate
Lung	Pulmonary adenomas	Mouse	Urethan	BHT
			4NQO	Glycerol
Mammary gland	Adenoma/carcinoma	Rat	DMBA	Prolactin, dietary fat, caloric content, and energy utilization
			NMU	Dietary fat
Pancreas	Adenoma, acinar	Rat	Azaserine	Unsaturated fat
	Adenocarcinoma, acinar	Rat	Rat	Rat
	Ductular carcinoma	Rat	HAQO	Testosterone
Prostate	Adenocarcinoma	Rat	NMU	Testosterone
Stomach, glandular	Adenomas and carcinomas	Rat	MNNG	Nataurocholate
	Adenocarcinoma	Rat	MNNG	Formaldehyde
	Adenocarcinoma	Rat	MNNG	P-methylcatechol

(table continues)

Table 7.1 (continued)

Tissue	End-Point Lesion	Species	Initiator	Promoter
Stomach, glandular (continued)	Adenocarcinoma	Rat	MNNG	Somatostatin
	Adenocarcinoma	Rat	MNNG	Meth and Leu Enkephalins
Thyroid	Adenomas	Rat	DHPN	PB, AT
			DEN	PB, EPH
			NMU	I_2-deficient diet
Vagina	Stromal polyp	Rat	NMU	Estradiol
	Papilloma, carcinoma	Mouse	DMBA	TPA

Key: Abbreviations used in this table are as follows: MNU, N-methyl-N-nitrosourea; FANFT, N[4-(5-Nitro-2-furyl)-2-thiazolyl]formamide; BBN, N-butyl-N-(4-hydroxybutyl)nitrosamine; BHA, butylated hydroxyanisole; MNNG, N-methyl-N1-nitro-N-nitrosoguanidine; 1,2-DMH, dimethylhydrazine; TPA, tetradecanoyl phorbol acetate; 3-MC, 3-methylcholanthrene; BP, benzo[a]pyrene; 1,25-(OH)$_2$-D$_2$, 1α,25-dihydroxycholecalciferol; DMBA, 7,12-dimethyl-benzanthracene; 7-BrMeBA, 7-bromomethyl benzanthracene; TEM, triethylene melamine; Trp-P-2, 3-Amino-1-methyl-5H-pyrido[4,3-b]-indole; AMN, N-amyl-N-methylnitrosamine; AAF, 2-acetylaminofluorene; DEN, diethylnitrosamine; DMN, dimethylnitrosamine; DAB, dimethylaminoazobenzene; NNM, N-nitrosomorpholine; αHCH, αhexachloro-cyclohexane; PenCDF, 2,3,4,7,8-pentachlorodibenzofuran; CPA, cyproterone acetate; PB, phenobarbital; TCDD, 2,3,7,8-tetrachlorodibenzo-p-dioxin; DDT, dichlorodiphenyltrichloroethane; BHT, butylated hydroxytoluene; DCA, deoxycholic acid; DEHP, di(2-ethylhexyl)-phthalate; TCPOBOP, 1,4-bis[2-(3,5-dichloropyridyloxy)]benzene; 4NQO, 4-nitroquinoline-1-oxide; NMU, N-nitrosomethylurea; HAQO, 4-hydroxyaminoquinoline 1-oxide; DHPN, N-bis(2-hydroxypropyl)nitrosamine; AT, 3-amino-1,2,4-triazole; EPH, 5-ethyl-5-phenylhydantoins; AOM, azoxymethane; PB, phenobarbital.
Modified from Pitot, 1996, with permission of the publisher.

which the stages of initiation and promotion may be identified. The exact characteristics of the stages in different tissues may vary somewhat with the experimental conditions and as a result of the biology of the system itself. There is also substantial evidence for the existence of the stages of initiation and promotion in the development of a number of human neoplasms, considered later (Chapter 11).

In Table 7.1, most of the end-point lesions induced are malignant neoplasms. However, the development of malignancy implies that the final stage, progression, in which cancer develops (Chapter 9) has also occurred. Thus, strictly speaking, a study of the stages of initiation and promotion should be restricted to the development of *preneoplastic* lesions that have distinct characteristics (see below) distinguishing them from malignant neoplasms. *Preneoplasia* thus may be defined as lesions in the stage of initiation and/or promotion, while *neoplastic* lesions are restricted to those in the stage of progression (Chapters 9 and 10). Although it has not been possible to identify preneoplastic lesions in the genesis of all neoplasms listed in Table 7.1, a large number of putative preneoplastic lesions have been described in animal carcinogenesis. A number of these are listed in Table 7.2. Most of the examples in Table 7.2 may be found in Table 7.1 as examples of two-stage carcinogenesis. As discussed in Chapter 10, many of these preneo-plastic lesions in rodents have their counterparts in the development of neoplasia in the human.

Table 7.2 Preneoplastic Lesions in Rodent Carcinogenesis

Tissue	Species	Preneoplastic Lesion	Reference
Adrenal	Rat	Altered proliferative foci	Furuya and Williams, 1985
Bladder	Rat	NADH:menadione oxidoreductase-positive foci	Vanderlaan et al., 1982
Bladder	Dog	Alkaline phosphatase-negative foci	Radomski et al., 1978
Brain	Rat	Focal oligodendroglial hyperplasia	Lantos and Pilkington, 1979 Galloway et al., 1990
Cholangioles (bile ducts)	Rat	Cholangiofibrosis	Bannasch, 1986
Colon	Rat	Aberrant crypts	Pretlow, 1994 Bird, 1995
Fibrous tissue	Rat	Atypical proliferative foci	Nikitin et al., 1993
Esophagus	Mouse	Epithelial dysplasia papilloma	Rubio, 1983
Kidney	Mouse	Succinic dehydrogenase-negative foci of tubules	Ahn et al., 1994
Kidney	Rat	"Proliferative tubules"	Bannasch, 1986
Liver	Rat	Altered hepatic foci	Pitot, 1990
Mammary gland	Rat	Hyperplastic terminal end buds	Russo et al., 1983
Pancreas	Rat	Acidophilic foci	Murata et al., 1987
Stomach	Rat	Intestinal metaplasia	Sasajima et al., 1979
		Dysplastic mucin-positive foci	Tsiftsis et al., 1980
Thyroid	Rat	γ-Glutamyltranspeptidase-positive foci	Moriyama et al., 1983
Tracheobronchial epithelium	Rat	Atypical metaplasia	Nettesheim et al., 1981

THE STAGE OF INITIATION

As noted in Figure 7.1, the application of a single appropriate low dose of a carcinogenic poly-cyclic hydrocarbon does not of itself result in the development of any tumors. However, the po-tential for preneoplastic development may be realized by addition of the promoting agent, strongly arguing for the presence of cells altered or "initiated" in the carcinogen-treated skin.

Until recently, characterization and quantification of the stage of initiation could be ac-complished well only after the process of carcinogenesis had begun. Thus, the presence of pre-neoplastic and/or neoplastic lesions implied that initiation had occurred. Many preneoplastic and neoplastic lesions appear to be derived from single cells (cf. Tanooka, 1988). It is on this basis, then, that some of the characteristics of the stage of initiation have been delineated. To date, it has not been possible to identify in an unequivocal manner single initiated cells, although single cells having some of the characteristics of initiated cells have been described in several experi-mental systems (Moore et al., 1987; Nakano et al., 1994; Solt et al., 1985). Therefore most of the discussion on the cellular and molecular biology of initiation has been deduced from experi-ments in which the implication is that the characteristics of the stage of initiation are being investigated.

Morphologic and Biological Characteristics of the Stage of Initiation

One of the striking characteristics of the stage of initiation, deduced from the experiments outlined in Figure 7.1, was the irreversibility of its effects. An extensive delay of administration of the promoting agent after initiation still led to the development of tumors. Other biological characteristics of initiation could also be concluded from the experiments of Figure 7.1. Application of the promoting agent must follow initiation, although in some investigations in the skin, Fürstenberger et al. (1985) suggested that a partial inversion of this sequence could induce mouse skin carcinogenesis. Other biological characteristics of the stage of initiation are given in Table 7.3. The effectiveness of initiation by chemicals is sensitive to alterations in xenobiotic metabolism (Talalay et al., 1988) and in trophic hormones (Liao et al., 1993). As discussed in Chapter 3, the ability of a carcinogenic agent to initiate cells may depend on the ability of the cell to metabolize the agent to its ultimate carcinogenic form. The process of initiation appears to be most effective when the agent is administered during the DNA synthesis phase of the cell cycle, as noted both in vivo (Rabes et al., 1986) and in cell culture (Grisham et al., 1980). Several studies (Borek and Sachs, 1968; Columbano et al., 1981; Kakunaga, 1975) have indicated the critical importance of one or several rounds of cell division that must occur in the presence of the initiating agent for a cell to become initiated.

An important characteristic of the stage of initiation is the fact that spontaneous (endogenous or fortuitous) initiation occurs in living organisms, probably rather frequently. The existence of spontaneously initiated cells can be deduced from the occurrence of spontaneous neoplasms in both the human and in experimental animals. Single putatively initiated cells have been described in the rat liver (Moore et al., 1987), and their spontaneous clonal progeny have been identified by several investigators (Schulte-Hermann et al., 1983; Xu et al., 1990). Other spontaneous preneoplastic lesions have been described in experimental systems (Maekawa and Mitsumori, 1990; Pretlow, 1994) as well as in the human (Dunham, 1972; Pretlow, 1994). Therefore it would appear that the spontaneous or fortuitous initiation of cells in a variety of tissues is a very common occurrence. It follows, then, that the development of neoplasia may be a function solely of the action of agents at the stages of promotion and/or progression.

The absence of either a readily measurable threshold or no-effect dose level and of a maximal response of the formation of initiated cells short of lethal cellular toxicity to the tissue and/or animal are major characteristics of the process of initiation. Such a dose-response curve is seen in Figure 7.2. As noted in the figure, extrapolation of the data points of those animals administered the carcinogen will extend the curve to the ordinate where some tumors are seen to

Table 7.3 Morphological and Biological Characteristics of the Stage of Initiation

---

Irreversible in viable cells
Initiated "stem cell" usually not morphologically identified
Efficiency sensitive to metabolic and other cellular factors and the cell cycle
Spontaneous (endogenous) occurrence of initiated cells
Requires cell division for "fixation"
Dose-response does not exhibit a readily measurable threshold
Relative potency of initiators depends on quantitation of the *numbers* of preneo-
    plastic lesions after defined period of promotion

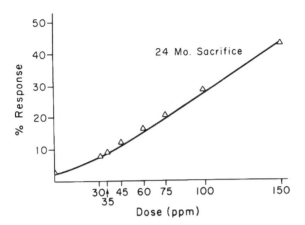

Figure 7.2 Liver tumor incidence expressed as percentage response in mice given various daily doses of 2-acetylaminofluorene for 24 months. These data were taken from the review by Fishbein (1980). A small percentage of animals not receiving any of the carcinogen developed liver neoplasms within the 24-month period, as evidenced by the symbol slightly above the origin on the y axis. However, extrapolation of the data points through the origin of animals given 2-acetylaminofluorene can be accomplished.

occur in the absence of any administered carcinogen. As the curve is drawn, however, even at the lowest theoretical doses, one must presume an ever-so-slight increase in tumor incidence over that seen in the absence of the carcinogen. While the potential pitfalls in the extrapolation of data points have been considered by a number of individuals (Preussmann, 1980; Aldridge, 1986), at present there is insufficient evidence for the existence of measurable thresholds of the effects of initiation. Further support for this concept may be seen in Figure 7.3, which depicts a dose-response curve of the appearance of single putative initiated hepatocytes as a function of the amount of a single dose of the chemical carcinogen diethylnitrosamine. Although this curve

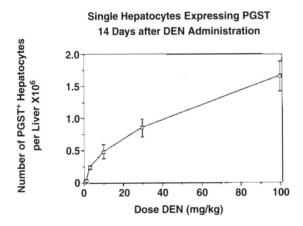

Figure 7.3 The effect of varying the dose of diethylnitrosamine administered to rats 24 hours after a 70% partial hepatectomy on the number of single hepatocytes expressing the placental form of glutathione S-transferase (PGST[+]) per liver 14 days after carcinogen administration.

appears to exhibit a threshold, the data points may readily be extrapolated through the origin. Other studies in which DNA adducts of a specific carcinogenic agent are measured as a function of dose similarly result in a linear relationship extrapolatable through the origin (cf. Zeise et al., 1987). While the determination of the initiating potency of chemical agents has generally not been done in rat liver, a measure of the relative potency of several initiating agents has been made on the basis of the quantitation of numbers of preneoplastic focal lesions (Pitot et al., 1987).

THE BIOLOGY OF THE STAGE OF PROMOTION

A variety of chemicals have been shown to induce and/or influence the stage of promotion. However, unlike chemicals inducing the stage of initiation, there is no evidence that promoting agents or their metabolites directly interact with DNA or that metabolism is required at all for their effectiveness (Chapter 3). Figure 7.4 shows some representative structures of various promoting agents. Tetradecanoyl phorbol acetate (TPA) is a naturally occurring alicyclic chemical that is the active ingredient of croton oil, a promoting agent used for mouse skin tumor promotion. Saccharin is an effective promoting agent for the bladder, and phenobarbital is an effective promoting agent for hepatocarcinogenesis. 2,3,7,8-Tetrachlorodibenzo-*p*-dioxin (TCDD) is probably the most effective promoting agent known for rat liver carcinogenesis, but is also effective in the lung and skin. Butylated hydroxytoluene (BHT) is an antioxidant chemical that has been added to foodstuffs to prevent oxidation and spoiling. Estradiol is shown as a representative of endogenous hormones that are effective promoting agents. Both androgens and estrogens, natural and synthetic, are effective promoting agents in their target end organ as well as in liver (Taper, 1978; Sumi et al., 1980; Kemp et al., 1989). Cholic acid enhances preneoplastic and neoplastic lesions in the rat colon (Magnuson et al., 1993), whereas 2,2,4-trimethylpentane and unleaded gasoline effectively promote renal tubular cell tumors in rats (Short et al., 1989). The final two structures noted, Wy-14,643 and nafenopin, are two members of the large class of carcinogenic peroxisome proliferators that induce the synthesis of peroxisomes in liver, are effective promoting agents, and, with long-term administration at high doses, induce hepatic neoplasms (Reddy and Lalwani, 1983). Multiple other agents—including polypeptide hormones (see above), dietary factors including total calories, many halogenated hydrocarbons, and numerous other chemicals—have been found to enhance the development of preneoplastic and neoplastic lesions in one or more systems of carcinogenesis including the human.

The distinctive characteristic of promotion, as contrasted with the stage of initiation, is the reversible nature of this stage (cf. Pitot and Dragan, 1996 and Table 7.4). Boutwell (1964) first demonstrated that, by decreasing the frequency of application of the promoting agent after initiation in mouse skin with a carcinogenic aromatic polycyclic hydrocarbon, a lower yield of papillomas was obtained in comparison with that obtained by a more frequent application of the promoting agent. Other investigators (Andrews, 1971; Burns et al., 1978) later demonstrated that papillomas developing during the stage of promotion in mouse epidermal carcinogenesis regress in large numbers on removal of the promoting agent. The regression of preneoplastic lesions upon withdrawal of the promoting agents may be owing to apoptosis (Schulte-Herrmann et al., 1990). This proposed mechanism is supported by the demonstration that many promoting agents inhibit apoptosis in preneoplastic lesions (Schulte-Herrmann et al., 1993; Wright et al., 1994). Another potential pathway of this operational reversibility is "redifferentiation" or remodeling (Tatematsu et al., 1983). This remodeling process is said to occur in hepatocarcinogenesis in the rodent when focal or nodular lesions appear to change to adult, normal-appearing liver. Thus, cells in the stage of promotion are dependent for their continued existence on continued admin-

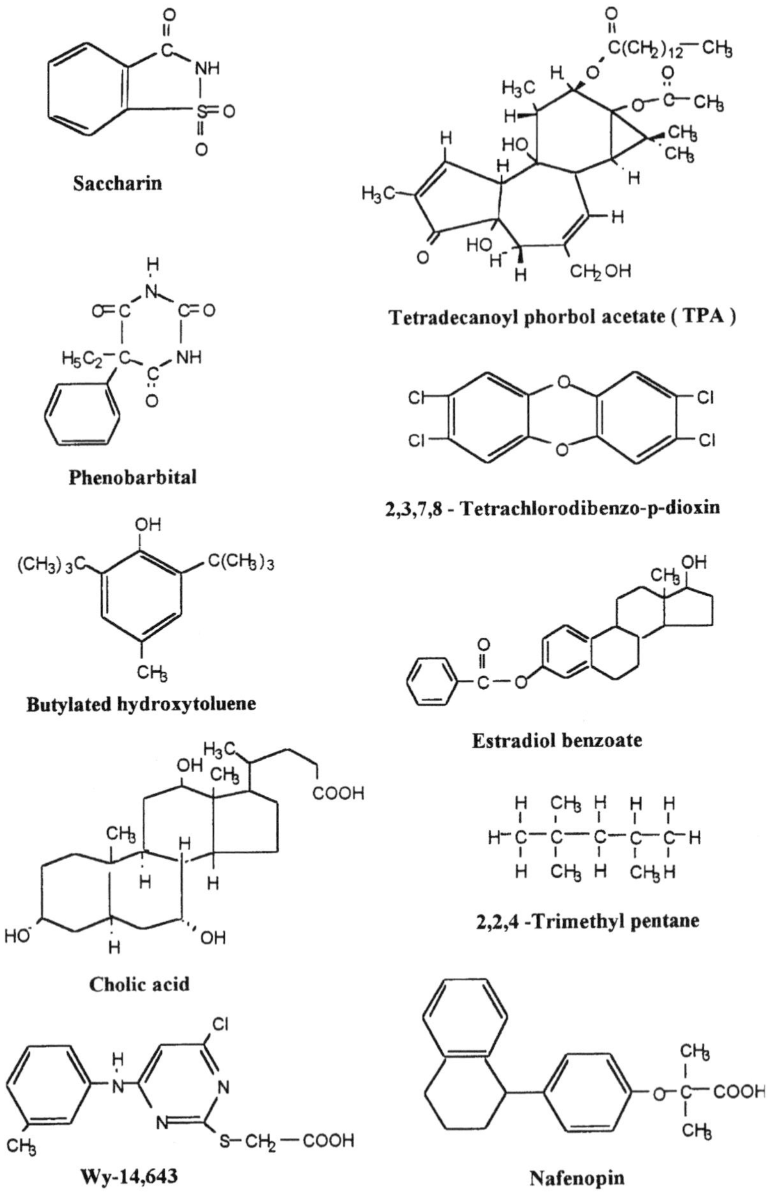

Figure 7.4 Structures of representative promoting agents. (From Pitot and Dragan, 1996, with permission of publisher.)

istration of the promoting agent (Hanigan and Pitot, 1985), as implied by the early studies of Furth (1959) on hormonally dependent neoplasia.

Another characteristic of the stage of promotion is its susceptibility to modulation by physiological factors. The stage of promotion may be modulated by the aging process (Van Duuren et al., 1975), as well as by dietary and hormonal factors (Sivak, 1979). Glauert et al. (1986) demonstrated that promotion of hepatocarcinogenesis was less effective in rats fed a relatively defined, semisynthetic diet than in those fed a crude, undefined, cereal-based diet. The

Table 7.4 Morphological and Biological Characteristics of the Stage of Promotion

Operationally reversible both at the level of gene expression and at the cell level

Promoted cell population existence dependent on continued administration of the promoting agent

Efficiency sensitive to aging and dietary and hormonal factors

Endogenous promoting agents may affect "spontaneous" promotion

Dose-response exhibits measurable threshold and maximal effect

Relative potency of promoters is measured by their effectiveness to cause an expansion of the progeny of the initiated cell population

promotion stage of chemically induced rat mammary cancer is also modulated by dietary (Cohen et al., 1991) and hormonal (Carter et al., 1988) factors. Many of these topics will be considered more extensively in Chapter 8. Many such modulating factors are themselves promoting agents. Several hormones are carcinogenic. Such hormones are effective promoting agents and thus may serve as an exogenous or endogenous source for modulation of cell proliferation during carcinogenesis (Pitot, 1991). Thus, endogenously produced, potentially carcinogenic promoting agents may cause the endogenous promotion of initiated cells.

The dose-response relationships of promoting agents exhibit sigmoid-like curves with an observable threshold and maximal effect. Such relationships are depicted in Figure 7.5, in which the dose-response curve for binding of TPA with its receptor is compared with the dose-response curve for the TPA promotion of dimethylbenzanthracene-initiated papillomas in mouse skin (Ashendel, 1985; Verma and Boutwell, 1980). The threshold effects of promoting agents may be

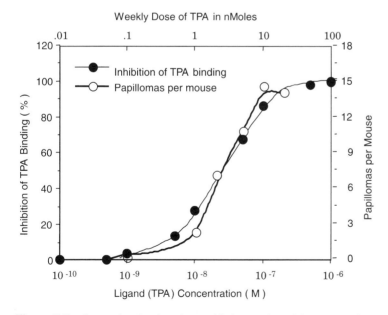

Figure 7.5 Composite showing the specific interaction of the receptor for phorbol esters with its ligand determined as the inhibition of radioactive TPA binding (closed circles). The tumor response expressed as papillomas per mouse on mice initiated with dimethylbenzanthracene and promoted with various weekly doses of TPA is noted in the open circles.

considered a consequence of the reversible nature of their effects at the cellular level (see above). The maximal effect is due to a saturation of ligand binding in the former case and to the promotion of all initiated cells in the latter (Figure 7.5). Although one may not directly equate the variables in the two processes, the similarity in the shapes of the curves is striking (Figure 7.5). The relative potency of promoting agents may be determined as a function of their ability to induce the clonal growth of initiated cells. Thus, the net rate of growth of preneoplastic lesions can be employed to determine relative potencies for promoting agents (Pitot et al., 1987). The end point analyzed in studies of the stage of promotion is a preneoplastic lesion that develops clonally from initiated cells in the tissue under study. While the listing of such lesions as noted in Table 7.2 would in many cases be the appropriate end point, a number of studies still utilize malignant lesions as the end point for the studies of the stage of promotion (Table 7.1). The reader should be aware of this discrepancy in reading the literature and interpret the results appropriately.

There is also a controversy surrounding the question of thresholds for initiating agents and promoting agents. In essence, it is statistically impossible to prove or disprove the presence or absence of thresholds in either case by experimental means. Since extrapolation is necessary to state that no threshold exists for initiating agents, one can never be certain that the extrapolation faithfully reflects the actual situation at extremely low dose levels. Furthermore, if the single altered hepatocytes expressing glutathione S-transferase aberrantly are initiated cells, then, from Figure 7.3, it might be possible to argue the existence of a threshold. On the other hand, it is virtually impossible to prove the existence of a threshold either in this case or that of promoting agents despite data such as seen in Figures 7.3, 7.4, and 7.5. The reason for this is again statistical in that, if sufficient numbers of animals were used in the experiment, it is possible that an occasional one might exhibit a neoplastic response. Since statistics cannot answer this question, we are faced with interpreting the experimental data in light of the best experimental evidence available combined with our knowledge of the most probable mechanisms involved in the action of initiators and promoters. Since most, if not all, initiating agents act through a mutagenic mechanism permanently altering the structure of DNA in an irreversible manner (Chapter 3), no threshold of effect would theoretically be possible, since even a single molecule of the active, mutagenic form of the initiating agent could induce a single mutation. Promoting agents exert their effects by a reversible mechanism at the level of either gene expression or cell replication, whereby a single molecule would have essentially no effect in inducing changes characteristic of promoting agents (see below). Therefore, at the present time, one may conclude that initiation exhibits no practical threshold, whereas promoting agents do exhibit threshold or no-effect levels that will vary dramatically from agent to agent. Further discussion of the practical aspects of this problem may be found in Chapter 13.

Cell and Molecular Mechanisms of the Stages of Initiation and Promotion

Although the descriptive and morphological characteristics of the stages of carcinogenesis are critical to our initial understanding of the pathogenesis of neoplasia, a complete knowledge of the molecular mechanisms of carcinogenesis may be necessary to control the disease through rational therapy, earlier diagnosis, and reasonable methods of prevention. However, our understanding of the molecular mechanisms of carcinogenesis is incomplete. On the other hand, there has been an explosion of knowledge in this area during the past decade. From some of this knowledge, it has now become possible to establish some reasonably valid mechanisms for the stages of initiation and promotion. Some of these mechanisms for these two stages are given in Table 7.5.

Table 7.5 Some Cell and Molecular Mechanisms in the Stages of Initiation and Promotion

Initiation	Promotion
Mutational microlesions (transitions, transversions, frameshift, base-pair substitutions) involving the cellular genome	Reversible enhancement or repression of gene expression mediated directly via receptors specific for the individual promoting agent and/or indirectly through the formation of reactive oxygen intermediates and their reversible effect on gene expression
In some species and tissues, point mutations occur in proto-oncogenes and/or potential cellular oncogenes	Inhibition of apoptosis by promoting agents
Mutations in genes of signal transduction pathways may result in altered phenotype	No direct structural alteration in DNA results from action or metabolism of promoting agent

Initiation

While the morphological and biological characterization of the stage of initiation has been somewhat limited, mechanistic studies of this stage have been more extensive, especially in relation to the metabolic activation of chemical carcinogens and the structure of their DNA adducts. As indicated earlier, however, the molecular mechanisms of this stage must conform to the observable biological characteristics of this stage. At least three processes are important in initiation, including metabolism, DNA repair, and cell proliferation. Perturbation of any of these pathways has an impact on initiation. Just as initiated cells are difficult to distinguish morphologically and phenotypically from their normal counterparts, the molecular alterations responsible for initiation may be equally subtle. As already indicated, initiating agents or their metabolites are mutagenic to DNA (see above). Thus, carcinogenic agents that are capable of initiating cells when administered at doses that do not induce neoplasia (incomplete carcinogenesis) initiate cells in experimental models of multistage carcinogenesis (Boutwell, 1964; Dragan et al., 1994a). Furthermore, such subcarcinogenic doses of initiating agents may induce substantial DNA alkylation (Pegg and Perry, 1981; Brambilla et al., 1983; Ward, 1987) but do not appear to induce karyotypic alterations.

More than three decades ago, mutational lesions were classified into two general groups, microlesions and macrolesions. While our knowledge of mutational events has increased since then, the classification is still generally applicable (Table 7.6). The stage of initiation appears to result from the formation of microlesions in DNA, while macrolesions are characteristic of the

Table 7.6 Classification of Mutations

Microlesions	Base-pair substitutions (transitions, transversions)
	Frameshifts
Macrolesions	Deletions
	Gene amplification (duplications)
	Chromosomal rearrangement, clastogenesis

Modified from Banks, 1971.

stage of progression. By definition (Chapter 9), direct induction of major chromosomal alterations in a cell can immediately induce the stage of progression directly, thereby bypassing the stages of initiation and promotion, provided that the altered cell remains viable and capable of replication. Sargent et al. (1989) demonstrated normal karyotypes of cells from altered hepatic foci in the stage of promotion in the rat, and Aldaz et al. (1987) showed that epidermal papillomas in the mouse that occurred early during promotion were diploid in character. A number of investigations have demonstrated specific point mutations in genes that are compatible with those induced in vitro by the adducts resulting from treatment with carcinogenic chemicals (cf. Anderson et al., 1992). The potential genetic targets for initiating agents have now been elucidated to some extent (Chapter 6). Individual variability, species differences, and organotropism of the stage of initiation are a balance of carcinogen metabolism, cell proliferation, and DNA repair.

The activation of proto-oncogenes and cellular oncogenes by specific base mutations, small deletions, and frameshift mutations results from DNA synthesis in the presence of DNA damage, including the presence of adducts. Methods for determining such alterations in specimens consisting of only a few hundred or a thousand cells have been available only during the last decade (cf. Komminoth and Long, 1993; Alard et al., 1993), permitting the analysis of mutations in specific genes potentially involved in the neoplastic transformation of DNA from very small samples.

The *ras* genes code for guanosine triphosphatases, which function as molecular switches for signal transduction pathways involved in the control of growth, differentiation, and other cellular functions (Hall, 1994). Table 7.7 lists a number of examples in rodent tissues of specific mutations in two of the *ras* genes, the Ha-*ras* proto-oncogene and the Ki-*ras* cellular oncogene. With the exception of mouse skin, the frequency of such mutations in preneoplastic lesions in experimental animals in the stage of promotion is about 20% to 60%. In multistage carcinogenesis in mouse skin, the frequency increases to nearly 100% (Bailleul et al., 1989). In general, the mutations noted are those which theoretically could result from DNA adducts formed by the particular carcinogen.

Interestingly, spontaneously occurring neoplasms in mice also exhibit a significant incidence of point mutations in the *ras* proto- and cellular oncogenes (Rumsby et al., 1991; Candrian et al., 1991), but neoplasms in corresponding tissues in other species do not necessarily exhibit activating mutations in proto- or cellular oncogenes (Tokusashi et al., 1994; Kakiuchi et al., 1993; Schaeffer et al., 1990). In addition, mutated *ras* genes have been described in normal-appearing mouse skin after DMBA or urethane application (Nelson et al., 1992). On the other hand, Cha et al. (1994) have reported that a very high percentage of untreated rats contained detectable levels of Ha-*ras* mutations in normal mammary tissue. Thus, mutations seen in neoplasms in untreated animals may result from the selective proliferation of cells containing preexisting mutations.

While several classes of genes appear appropriate as targets for DNA-damaging carcinogens, the actual role of proto- and cellular oncogene mutations in establishing carcinogenesis is not entirely clear. In the earliest preneoplastic lesions studied (Table 7.7), only about one-third exhibit mutations in the *ras* gene family, but it is quite possible that other proto- and cellular oncogenes may be targets. Evidence that tumor suppressor genes may be targets for the initiation of early malignant development comes largely from studies of genetically inherited neoplasia. In these rare hereditary cancers, one of the alleles of a tumor suppressor gene contains a germline mutation in all cells of the organism (Paraskeva and Williams, 1992; Knudson, 1993), thus, in theory, initiating all cells in the organism. However, the exact gene(s) critical for the initiation of a specific cell type after administration of a specific carcinogen has not yet been defined in any instance. Furthermore, as noted from Chapter 5, other genes may be involved in the stage of

Table 7.7 Mutational Activation of *ras* Oncogenes during the Stage of Initiation

Species/Tissue	Carcinogen	Lesion	Gene/Mutation[a]	Frequency[b]	Reference
Rat/colon	Azoxymethane	Aberrant crypt foci	K-*ras*/G→A/12	5/16	Shivapurkar et al., 1994
Mouse/liver	Diethylnitrosamine	G6Pase⁻ foci	Ha-*ras*/C→A/61 A→G61	12/127	Bauer-Hofmann et al., 1992
Mouse/lung	Urethane	Small adenomas	Ki-*ras*/A→G/61 A→T61	32/100	Nuzum et al., 1990
Rat/mammary gland	N-methyl-N-nitrosourea	Initiated cell clones	H-*ras*/G→A/12	17%	Zhang et al., 1991
Hamster/pancreas	N-nitroso-bis(2-oxopropyl)-amine	Papillary hyperplasia	K-*ras*/G→A/12	12/26	Cerny et al., 1992
Mouse/skin	DMBA/TPA	Papilloma	Ha-*ras*/A→T/61	12/14	Quintanilla et al., 1986

[a]The numbers in this column refer to the codon position in the cDNA (mRNA) of the gene product.
[b]The numerator indicates the number of animals exhibiting the mutation; the denominator refers to the total number of animals studied.

initiation, although it is likely that alterations in one or a very few genes constitute the "rate-limiting step" in the initiation of any individual cell.

Promotion

Boutwell (1974) was the first to propose that promoting agents induce their effects through their ability to alter gene expression. During the past decade, our understanding of mechanisms involving the alteration of gene expression by environmental agents has increased exponentially (Morley and Thomas, 1991; Rosenthal, 1994). The regulation of genetic information is mediated through recognition of the environmental effector—hormone, promoting agent, drug, etc.—and its specific molecular interaction with either a surface or a cytosolic receptor. Several types of receptors exist in cells (Mayer, 1994; Pawson, 1993; Strader et al., 1994) and are depicted in Figure 7.6. Plasma membrane receptors may or may not possess a tyrosine protein kinase domain on their intracellular region (Figure 3.25B), while others have multiple transmembrane domains with the intracellular signal transduced through G proteins and cyclic nucleotides (Figure 3.25A) (Mayer, 1994; Collins et al., 1992). The other general type of receptor mechanism involves a cytosolic receptor that interacts with the ligand (usually lipid-soluble) that has diffused through the plasma membrane (Figure 3.24). The ligand-receptor complex then travels to the nucleus before interacting directly with specific DNA sequences known as response elements (Figure 7.6).

The figure shows in a highly simplified manner the cascade effect of receptor-ligand and protein kinase interactions, resulting in changes in transcription as well as cell replication within the nucleus. As shown in the figure, interaction of transmembrane receptors containing a tyrosine protein kinase domain involves initially their dimerization, induced by ligand interaction. This activates the protein kinase domain of the receptor, causing autophosphorylation. This, in turn, attracts a cytoplasmic complex, Grb2-Sos, to the plasma membrane (Aronheim et al., 1994; Egan et al., 1993). Sos is a member of a family of regulatory proteins termed guanine-nucleotide exchange factors (GEFs) (Feig, 1994). Sos association with the G protein Ras stimulates, along with other protein interactions, the exchange of GDP with GTP on the Ras α subunit. The GTP-Ras, in turn, interacts with B-raf, a cytoplasmic serine-threonine protein kinase, with subsequent activation of its catalytic activity and initiation of a kinase cascade, ultimately resulting in the phosphorylation and activation of transcription factors including Jun, Fos, Myc, CREB, and ultimately E2F and Rb, the tumor suppressor gene (Lewis et al., 1998; Janknecht et al., 1995; Roussel, 1998). A number of other transcription factors are also activated by other pathways involving phospholipase C, phosphatidylinositol kinase, and protein kinase C (Vojtek and Der, 1998; Takuwa and Takuwa, 1996).

As indicated in Figure 7.5, the critical, rate-limiting step in this process is the mediation of the signal through the G-protein family. The G proteins are targeted to the plasma membrane through lipid moieties, both isoprenoid and fatty acyl, covalently linked to the carboxyl terminal region of the protein (Yamane and Fung, 1993). In this way, the initiation of the signal by the ligand-receptor interaction can be physically related to the rate-limiting G-protein activation step. The activation cycle of the G-protein family is seen in Figure 7.7. As seen from the figure, activation is accompanied by GTP binding to the α subunit of the G protein, such binding being dramatically stimulated by GEF proteins such as Sos. Activation also involves dissociation of the α from the β and γ subunits, allowing the α subunit to interact with and activate downstream members of the pathway, a protein kinase in the case of the growth factor-related pathway (Figure 7.6) or with other membrane molecules such as adenyl cyclase in the case of multiple transmembrane domain receptors (Figure 7.6). The activated G protein has an extremely short half-life because of the action of RGS (regulator of G-protein signaling) proteins, which stimulate

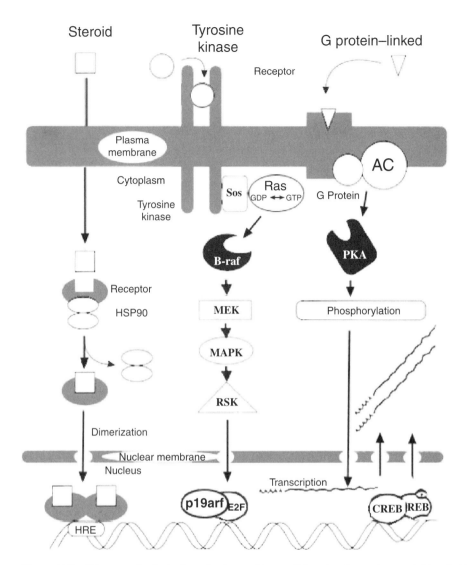

Figure 7.6 Diagram of principal mechanisms of intracellular signal transduction initiated either within the cytosol or at the plasma membrane. Lipid-soluble molecules such as steroid hormones interact directly with a cytoplasmic receptor after passing through the plasma membrane, this receptor being in association with heat shock protein 90 (HSP 90). Following association and dissociation with different protein species, the ligand receptor complex enters the nucleus and interacts with DNA in association with specific DNA sequences known as hormone response elements (HRE). Receptors for many polypeptides hormones (Chapter 3) and growth factors (Chapter 16) have a single transmembrane domain and associate or dimerize after interaction with its ligand. This association activates the tyrosine kinase activity of the cytoplasmic component of the receptor, phosphorylating both itself and other proteins. In the figure, an intermediate protein, Sos, complexes with the G protein, Ras, which interacts with a protein kinase, B-*raf*, activating its kinase activity and initiating the kinase cascade shown in the figure, ultimately ending up with activation of transcription factors, in this case the E2F class. The G protein–linked receptors have multiple transmembrane domains, and interaction with the ligand results in the activation of a membrane-associated G protein, which in turn activates adenylcyclase (AC) to produce increased levels of cyclic AMP. This small molecule, termed a second messenger, activates the cyclic AMP–dependent protein kinase (PKA), which in turn phosphorylates several other substrates, ultimately including the cyclic AMP response element (CRE)–binding protein (CREB). This protein interacts with its DNA response element, CRE, resulting in enhanced transcription. MAPK, mitogen activated protein kinase; MEK, MAPK kinase; RSK, ribosomal S6 kinase. p91[ARF] and E2F are specific transcription factors.

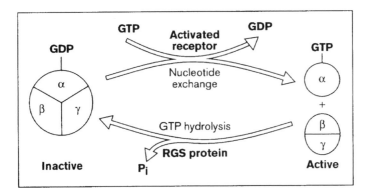

Figure 7.7 The guanine nucleotide cycle for heterotrimeric G proteins. The inactive G protein on the left is a GDP-bound heterotrimer. Ligand-bound activated receptors, either directly or indirectly, catalyze the exchange of GDP for GTP, leading to association of the α subunit from the βγ dimer (right). The separated G-protein subunits are thus activated for signaling. The G protein becomes an inactive heterotrimer again following action of the intrinsic GTPase activity of the α subunit returning it to the GDP bound form. RGS proteins can bind to activated G-protein α subunits and greatly accelerate the GTP-hydrolysis reaction. P_i, phosphate. (Adapted from Koelle, 1997, with permission of author and publisher.)

GTP hydrolysis to GDP with subsequent reassociation of the G protein in its inactive state (Koelle, 1997). Some receptors having a single transmembrane domain do not possess tyrosine protein kinase activity but require interaction with a cytoplasmic protein kinase. The exact mechanism of this interaction, which does not involve protein phosphorylation, is not clear at the present (Silvennoinen et al., 1997). The kinases involved have a direct interaction with the cytoplasmic domain of the receptor and are termed Jak or janus (two-faced) kinases. These in turn may cause phosphorylation of the tyrosines in the cytoplasmic region of the receptor with subsequent activation via the pathway seen in Figure 7.6. In some cells, especially those of the immune system, the Jak kinases may cause phosphorylation of specific transcription factors known as STATs (Chapter 19; Silvennoinen et al., 1997).

The multiple transmembrane domain receptors are in direct association with G proteins and, on activation of the receptor by interaction with a ligand, may activate a kinase termed a G-protein receptor kinase (GRK) or another effector such as adenyl cyclase (AC, Figure 7.6) (Böhm et al., 1997; Rasenick et al., 1995). While the α subunits of G proteins are major factors in this signaling pathway, the β and γ subunits also appear to be involved (Pitcher et al., 1992).

In addition to the plasma membrane receptors, gene expression can be regulated through the interaction of cytoplasmic receptors with their ligands as previously discussed in Chapter 3 (Figures 3.23 and 3.24). Just as with membrane receptors, the pathways of the cytoplasmic receptors involve multiple interactions with proteins, phosphorylation, and ultimate alteration of transcription through factor interaction with DNA (Weigel, 1996; Pratt and Toft, 1997). In all of these pathways, in addition to alteration of transcription and gene expression, enhancement or inhibition of cell replication may also be an end point achieved through transcriptional modulation of the cell cycle (Chapter 9).

Many promoting agents exert their effects on gene expression through perturbation of one of the signal transduction pathways, as indicated in Figure 7.6. One may, in general, classify receptor mechanisms into three broad classes—steroid, tyrosine kinase, and G protein–linked. The majority of the more commonly studied promoting agents exert their actions by mediation of one or more of the receptor pathways indicated in Figure 7.6. In Table 7.8 are listed some of

Table 7.8   Some Promoter-Receptor Interactions in Target Tissues

Promoting Agent	Target Tissue(s)	Receptor Status	Type
Tetradecanoylphorbol acetate (TPA)	Skin	Defined (protein kinase C)	Tyrosine kinase/ G protein–linked
2,3,7,8-Tetrachlorodibenzo-*p*-dioxin (TCDD); planar PCBs	Skin, liver	Defined (Ah receptor)	Steroid
Sex steroids (androgens and estrogens	Liver, mammary tissue, kidney	Defined (estrogen and androgen receptors	Steroid
Synthetic antioxidants (butylated hydroxytoluene, BHT; butylated hydroxyanisole, BHA)	Liver, lung, fore-stomach	Postulated	Steroid (?)
Phenobarbital	Liver	Postulated	Unknown
Peroxisome proliferators (WY-14,643, nafenopin, clofibrate)	Liver	Defined [peroxisome proliferator-activated receptor (PPAR)]	Steroid
Polypeptide trophic hormones and growth factors (prolactin, EGF, glucagon)	Liver, skin, mammary gland	Defined or partially characterized (Chapters 3 and 11)	G protein–linked/ tyrosine kinase
Okadaic acid	Skin	Defined (?) (protein phosphatase-2A)	Unknown
Cyclosporine	Liver, lymphoid tissue	Defined (cyclophilin)	Tyrosine kinase/ G protein–linked

Adapted from Pitot and Dragan, 1996, with permission of the publisher. Further references may be found in the text. Cyclosporine as a promoter of murine lymphoid neoplasms has been described by Hattori et al. (1988).

the most studied promoting agents known or postulated to be effectors in signal transduction pathways. While protein kinase C (PKC) is not itself one of the three types of receptors noted in Figure 7.6, it is a mediator of the signal transduction pathways of both the tyrosine kinase and G protein–linked transduction pathways. TPA interacts directly with membrane-bound PKC, displacing the normal activator, diacylglycerol, and serving to maintain the kinase in its active and soluble form (Ashendel, 1985). The continual activation of this kinase then stimulates further transduction pathways by phosphorylation of specific proteins (Stabel and Parker, 1991). TCDD acts in the steroid pathway via a specific receptor, the Ah receptor, the ligand-receptor complex together with other proteins, ultimately altering the transcriptional rate of genes possessing specific regulatory sequences (HRE). In a similar manner, sex steroids, some synthetic antioxidants, and peroxisome proliferators interact with specific soluble receptors and altered gene expression by presumed mechanisms similar to that of TCDD (Chapter 3, Figures 3.23 and 3.24). While in some instances the actual receptor is still not defined, those for polypeptide hormones and growth factors consist of either the tyrosine kinase or G protein–linked types depending on the structure of the polypeptide. The "receptors" for okadaic acid and cyclosporine have been reported to be protein phosphatase 2A and cyclophilin-A respectively (Fujiki and Suganuma, 1993). These proteins, like PKC, are involved in phosphorylation mechanisms of the tyrosine kinase and G protein–linked pathways, although specific sites and mechanisms have not been completely clarified at this time. Thus, the action of promoting agents in altering gene expression may be mediated through specific receptors. This hypothesis provides a reasonable explanation for the tissue specificity demonstrated by many promoting agents. The receptor-ligand concept of promoting agent action is based on the dose-response relationships involving pharmacological agents. The basic assumptions of such interactions argue that the effect of the agent is directly proportional to the number of receptors occupied by the ligand. The intrinsic activities of the chemical and the signal transduction pathways available in the tissue are important factors in the type and degree of response observed (Saltiel, 1995).

Indirect Pathways of Tumor Promotion. In addition to the specific action of tumor promoters on gene expression mediated directly via specific ligand (promoting agent)-receptor interactions, another mechanism of tumor promotion has been identified that involves the indirect action of promoting agents in inducing the formation of reactive oxygen radicals (Chapter 3), which in turn involve signal transduction pathways specifically activated by such "oxidative stress." Cells may also be subjected to other types of stress involving changes in temperature, pressure, substrate availability, etc., but the roles of these mechanisms in tumor promotion, if any, have not been clarified. On the other hand, reactive oxygen radicals, whether developing internally within the cell from the indirect action of chemical agents or directly from the action of chemical and physical agents, alter a number of signal transduction pathways. One mechanism for such alteration appears to be a change in the redox state of several of the protein species themselves (Cimino et al., 1997). Cerutti and colleagues (Cerutti, 1985) were among the first to argue that reactive oxygen species played a major role in tumor promotion. Since that time, it has become apparent that many extracellular ligands generate and/or require reactive oxygen radicals and their derived species in the transmission of some of their signals to the nucleus (Lander, 1997). Such pathways include those involving growth factors and hormones, ion transport, transcription factors, and apoptosis (Lander, 1997). In particular, the oxidation state of transcription factors is of paramount importance in the effects of free radicals, especially of oxygen metabolism, and redox potential in governing signal transduction pathways. In Figure 7.8 may be seen several examples of the effect of reactive oxygen species (ROS) in regulating the function of several transcription factors (cf. Cimino et al., 1997). Notable in the figure are zinc-finger transcription factors such as the AP-1 family of transcription factors, which are involved in a variety of signal transduction pathways including that from TPA, ultraviolet-A, TCDD, and ionizing radiation (cf. Dalton et al., 1999). Another transcription factor noted in the figure (B) is NF-κB, which plays a central role in the regulation of many genes involved in cellular defense mechanisms, pathogen defenses, immunological responses, and expression of cytokines and cell adhesion molecules (Dalton et al., 1999). As shown in the figure, NF-κB consists of two subunits, p50 and p65, which are restricted to the cytoplasm because of their association with an inhibitory subunit, I-κB. NF-κB translocates to the nucleus following phosphorylation of I-κB which frees NF-κB from the complex. This allows NF-κB to interact with specific sequences in DNA (cf. Cimino et al., 1997). Such interaction with DNA is markedly altered by oxidation of the proteins, as is the phosphorylation of I-κB. As noted in C of the figure, heat-shock proteins (HSF) may also be altered in their function as chaperones and in the ability of the cell to cope with external stress by alteration in the ROS (cf. Cimeno et al., 1997). There is also substantial evidence that ROS may alter the function of a variety of kinases involved in signal transduction including protein kinase C (Konishi et al., 1997) and the mitogen-activated protein kinase (MAPK) family (Guyton et al., 1996). Even G proteins themselves, such as members of the *ras* family, play a significant role in the signal transduction effects resulting from ROS, sometimes themselves being important targets for redox changes (cf. Finkel, 1998).

Promoting agents, which themselves are responsible for the direct induction of reactive oxygen molecules (e.g., growth factors, phorbol esters), induce the production of ROS in a variety of cell types. Some examples of this are seen in Table 7.9. The table was restricted to nonphagocytic cells and is modified from a similar table by Gamaley and Klyubin (1999). Thus, the specific signal transduction pathway resulting from the specific interaction of ligand with receptor is complemented by the mostly indirect production of ROS, which, in turn, may enhance the

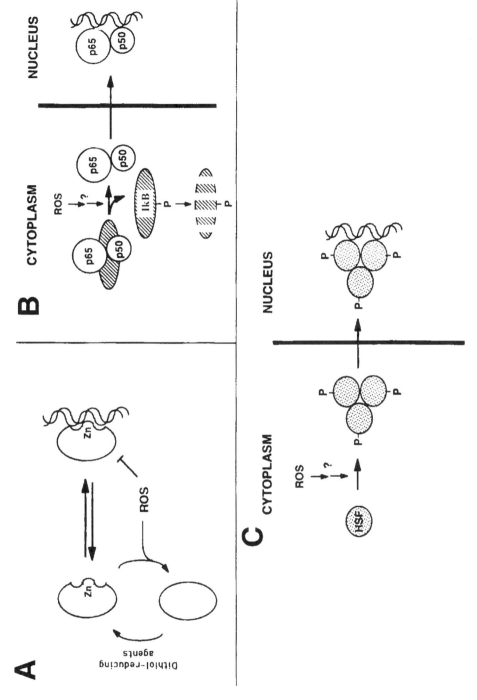

Figure 7.8 Models of the mediation by ROS in the regulation of transcription factors. A. A zinc-finger transcription factor (Zn) and its alteration by ROS preventing its interaction with DNA in the oxidized state. B. NF-κB (p65-p50) and I-κB association in the cytoplasm indicating areas of change induced by ROS prior to entrance into the nucleus. C. Heat-shock proteins (HSF) and their interaction with each other and other proteins as chaperones (not shown) indicating the potential action of ROS. (Adapted from Cimino et al., 1997, with permission of the authors and publisher.)

Table 7.9 Some Promoting Agents That Induce ROS Production in Various Cells

Agonist	Cell Type
Epidermal growth factor	A431, fibroblasts, keratinocytes
Fibroblast growth factor	3T3 L1 cells, chondrocytes
Insulin	3T3 L1 cells, fat cells
Phorbol esters	B lymphocytes, fibroblasts, platelets
Platelet-derived growth factor	3T3 L1 cells, fibroblasts, smooth muscle cells
Thyrotropin	Thyroid cells
Transforming growth factor	Endothelial cells, fibroblasts, osteoblasts
Tumor necrosis factor	B lymphocytes, endothelial cells, fat cells, fibroblasts, mesangial cells, smooth muscle cells

induced alteration of genetic expression by the promoting agent. The importance of the induction of ROS by promoting agents is perhaps best noted by the effect of antioxidants and related chemical species capable of significantly inhibiting the promoting action of many promoting agents (Chapter 8). In addition, since ROS are capable of altering the structure of DNA in a variety of ways (Chapter 3), this effect may also play a role in the action of promoting agents. However, that such is unlikely is seen by the reversible nature of the action of promoting agents (see above), in contrast to the irreversibility of the induction of mutations by ROS. Furthermore, as the student may recall from Table 3.6, extensive endogenous DNA damage resulting from ROS and other factors is occurring all of the time. Repair of such damage is largely the function of the mismatch repair system also discussed in Chapter 3. Although theoretically ROS may initiate cells, there has been little if any evidence that such occurs (Glauert and Clark, 1989; Denda et al., 1991; Takaba et al., 1997). It is more likely that structural alterations induced by ROS during the action of promoting agents may play a major role in the transition of cells from the stage of promotion to that of progression (Chapter 9).

Cell Cycle Regulation

Although the exact mechanism(s) by which promoting agents selectively enhance cell replication in preneoplastic cells is unknown, our understanding of the interaction of ligand-receptor signaling with the cell cycle and its regulation has dramatically increased in recent years. Figure 7.9 diagrams an integration of the cell cycle and apoptosis with the signal transduction pathways (Figure 7.6). Phosphorylation of the mitogen-activated protein kinase (MAPK) via the signal transduction pathway activates this kinase (Figure 7.9), which then activates various transcription factors, the proto-oncogene products, c-*myc*, c-*jun*, and c-*fos* (Seger and Krebs, 1995). Rb, the retinoblastoma tumor suppressor gene, is made throughout the cell cycle. It becomes highly phosphorylated at the beginning of DNA synthesis (G1,S). This releases a transcription factor, E2F, which is complexed with the highly phosphorylated but not the hypophosphorylated Rb protein. E2F then is available to stimulate the transcription of a variety of genes needed for the transition from G1 and the initiation of DNA synthesis. As noted above, ligand-receptor interactions can result in the activation of E2F and thus the transcription of genes needed for continuation of the cell cycle. This continuation involves a variety of protein kinases and proteins known as cyclins (cf. Oratta, 1994) that are discussed more exhaustively in Chapters 9 and 15. Another tumor suppressor gene, the p53 gene, also plays a role as a transcription factor, preventing continuance of the cell cycle on the occasion of DNA damage (Wu and Levine, 1994). Such a pause allows the cells to repair such damage or, if the damage is excessive, to undergo apoptosis (Figure 7.9). If

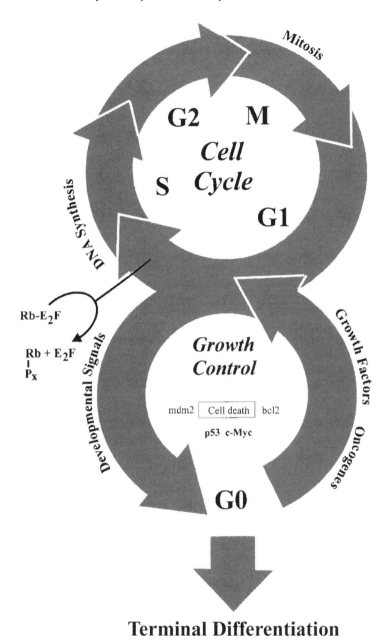

Figure 7.9 Diagram of the cell cycle and its associated cycle to apoptosis or terminal differentiation with potential to return to the active cycle under the influence of growth factors and related components. Signal transduction may regulate the cell cycle through kinase activation involving the E_2F-Rb interaction or other kinases and related molecules involved in the cell cycle (Chapter 9). (From Laird and Shalloway, 1997; Müller et al., 1993.)

the p53 gene is mutated or absent, such a pause does not occur and the cell cycle continues replicating despite the presence of damage, resulting in mutations and clastogenesis (Lane, 1992; Sander et al., 1993; Dulic et al., 1994). Obviously, the missing mechanistic link is a clear understanding of the selective enhancement of the cell cycle in preneoplastic cells by promoting agents (Jacobs, 1992). A variety of possibilities exist, including increased concentrations of receptors or any one or more of the components of the signal transduction pathway, as well as mutations in transcription factors, cyclins, cdks, or other components of the cell cycle. As yet, however, definitive studies to pinpoint such mechanisms have not been performed.

Role of Cell Division in Tumor Promotion

In recent years there has been an increased appreciation of the role of promoting agents in enhancing cell replication in the entire carcinogenic process. In some models, cell replication during this and the final stage of carcinogenesis has been postulated to be the key to the entire developmental process of neoplasia (Cohen and Ellwein, 1990). The significance of the enhancement of proliferation of cells already possessing a mutated genome on their advancement into the final stage of progression and malignant neoplasia is considered in Chapter 9.

It is now clear that many tumor-promoting agents are mitogenic, at least for certain cell populations. TPA when applied to mouse skin results in a rapid increase in DNA synthesis in most basal skin cells (Frankfurt and Raitcheva, 1972). From studies in liver, Cayama et al. (1978) and others have argued strongly that the initiation of chemical carcinogenesis requires cell proliferation. The role of cell proliferation in "fixing" the initiated change is discussed further in Chapter 14. However, numerous studies have shown that, although cell replication may be necessary for the "fixation" of tumor initiation, it is not sufficient in itself to assure the continuance of the process of promotion and ultimate tumor formation by the initiated cell(s) or their progeny (Boutwell, 1974).

Studies with cultured cells have demonstrated that several of the phorbol esters are capable of increasing the frequency of amplification of specific genes within these cells in culture (Barsoum and Varshavsky, 1983; Hayashi et al., 1983). Such direct effects of tumor promoters on the genome of the cell have not in the past been considered a significant factor in tumor promotion. On the other hand, studies by several authors (Emerit and Cerutti, 1982; Birnboim, 1982) have demonstrated that TPA, added to leukocytes in vitro, induces the formation of chromosomal breaks and other abnormalities. Such changes may be the result of the action of oxygen metabolites, especially superoxide radicals (Chapter 3), since the enzyme superoxide dismutase strongly inhibits the clastogenic activity of this tumor promoter in such a system. Earlier studies in support of these findings included the demonstration of the induction of sister chromatid exchanges by TPA in cultured cells, a process clearly involving DNA strand breakage (Nagasawa and Little, 1979). Although other investigators had some difficulty in reproducing these results (Thompson et al., 1980), Nagasawa and Little (1981) indicated that the effect is markedly dependent on the medium in which the cells are maintained during the experiment. That such effects are active in vivo is supported by the findings of Kozumbo and associates (1983), who demonstrated the inhibition of ornithine decarboxylase induction and tumor promotion by antioxidants that eliminate the accumulation of oxygen metabolites, such as the superoxide radical. In addition, several studies (cf. Verma et al., 1977) have shown that inhibitors of prostaglandin synthesis also prevent tumor promotion. Since the synthesis of prostaglandins involves oxygen radical formation, these effects further support a possible role of oxygen metabolites in the process of tumor promotion.

Early studies by Boutwell (1964) suggested that the process of tumor promotion could be divided into at least two stages. Boutwell used limited treatments with croton oil that were insufficient to produce skin papillomas. This was followed by repeated treatments with turpentine, which then allowed the development of papillomas (cf. DiGiovanni, 1992). Slaga et al. (1980) and Fürstenberger et al. (1981) confirmed these studies and extended them into the use of other agents, some of which were effective only during the "second stage" of promotion, such as mezerein or derivatives of TPA (Marks and Fürstenberger, 1986). The "first stage" of promotion was termed *conversion*, which could be effected by several applications of TPA. This resulted in no tumors when no further treatment was given. Repeated application of a second-stage promoter such as mezerein would then lead to the development of papillomas, although mezerein given alone after initiation did not result in a significant number of skin lesions (cf. Perchellet and Perchellet, 1988). Fürstenberger et al. (1983) have also shown that the effects of a single dose of TPA may last for at least 8 weeks; this suggests that the "reversibility" of tumor promotion is largely related to the second stage of this process. The exact nature of each of the stages of tumor promotion in the skin is not clear, but it is quite possible that the first stage of tumor promotion is closely related to the process of fixation (see above), whereas the second stage involves a more direct effect on the subsequent cellular population. By this concept, most known promoting agents for liver carcinogenesis are second-stage promoters.

The selective induction of proliferation of initiated cell populations was first intimated by the work of Solt and Farber (1976), who used 2-acetylaminofluorene administration as a "selection agent" for the enhancement of proliferation of altered hepatic foci in a modified initiation-promotion protocol. A similar "selection" of certain initiated clones by TPA promotion has also been postulated as occurring during multistage carcinogenesis in mouse skin (cf. DiGiovanni, 1992). Later studies demonstrated that 2-acetylaminofluorene was acting as a promoting agent in this protocol (Saeter et al., 1988). Farber and his colleagues (Roomi et al., 1985) espoused the concept that the lowered xenobiotic metabolism of preneoplastic cell populations gave such cells a competitive advantage in toxic environments such as those provided by the chronic administration of carcinogens. Schulte-Hermann and associates (1981) demonstrated that several hepatic promoting agents—including phenobarbital, certain steroids, and peroxisome proliferators—selectively enhanced the proliferation of cells within preneoplastic lesions in rat liver. A similar effect was reported by Klaunig in preneoplastic and neoplastic hepatic lesions in mice responding to promotion by phenobarbital (Klaunig, 1993). The response of preneoplastic hepatocytes in the rat to partial hepatectomy is also greater than that of normal hepatocytes (Laconi et al., 1994). Preneoplastic hepatocytes in culture exhibit an inherently higher level of replicative DNA synthesis than normal hepatocytes (Xu et al., 1988). Thus, the characteristic of promoting agents at the cell and molecular level to increase cell proliferation of preneoplastic cell populations selectively more than that of their normal counterparts may be the result of altered mechanisms of cell cycle control within the preneoplastic cell.

Mechanisms of Action of Three Promoting Agents

Although the signal transduction pathways for promoting agents discussed above are generally applicable, it is useful to consider the more specific molecular mechanisms and pathways of the most commonly employed promoting agents in experimental systems. These are tetradecanoylphorbolacetate (TPA) and 2,3,7,8-tetrachlorodibenzo-*p*-dioxin (TCDD), promoting agents effective in a variety of tissues, and phenobarbital (PB), a promoting agent effective in only a few tissues.

Tetradecanoylphorbolacetate

The receptor for TPA was shown to be a cytosolic serine/threonine protein kinase termed protein kinase C (Leach et al., 1983; Ashendel et al., 1983). Pathways activated by the TPA interaction with protein kinase C in its membrane-bound form are outlined in Figure 7.10 (Kazanietz and Blumberg, 1996). Diacylglycerol, the normal endogenous activator of protein kinase C, may be produced by the action of phospholipases after being activated either from a transmembrane growth factor receptor or a multiple transmembrane protein receptor (Figure 7.6). TPA is a more effective ligand activator than the endogenous diacylglycerol, thus causing the enhancement of the various pathways noted that involve the activation of another protein kinase, Raf-1 (B-raf), and the subsequent cascade of various events ending with the phosphorylation. This ultimately results in the changes in phosphorylation levels of a dimeric transcription factor, AP-1, usually consisting of a heterodimer comprising one molecule each of the proto-oncogenes c-*jun* and c-*fos*. This heterodimer interacts with a DNA sequence, termed the TPA-responsive element (TRE), whose sequence is TGA(G/C)TCA (Kazanietz and Blumberg, 1996). The regulatory regions of many genes possess AP-1 sites thus resulting in the numerous effects of TPA on cells (Chapter 14, Table 14.9).

The other signal transduction pathway activated by TPA is that involving the nuclear transcription factor NFκB. This protein is normally maintained in the cytoplasm in a complex with another protein, IkB, which prevents its entrance into the nucleus by formation of the complex. Phosphorylation of IFκB by specific protein kinases (cf. Karin, 1999) that themselves may be phosphorylated by protein kinase C causes the degradation of IFκB by the ubiquitin pathway, freeing the NFκB protein for entrance into the nucleus and interaction at its specific sequence motif, GGG(A/G)NNYYCC (Miyamoto and Verma, 1995). NFκB may also be activated by alteration in intracellular thiols, presumably involving oxidative stress (cf. Keyse, 1997). Just as with AP-1, which is also affected by oxidative stress, the target genes for NFκB comprise an extensive list, a number of which are concerned with the immune system (Schreck et al., 1997).

It is of interest that although TPA activates protein kinase C, chronic administration of the promoting agent causes a downregulation of this gene in mouse epidermis and in preneoplastic papillomas (Hansen et al., 1990). The activation of protein kinase C appears also to phosphorylate the epidermal growth factor receptor at serine residues (Davis and Czech, 1984), which may be related to the demonstration that the epidermal growth factor receptor binding to EGF is dramatically inhibited by TPA. This inhibition is reversed in the absence of the promoting agent (Magun et al., 1980). While these seemingly discordant results may be explained by a variety of mechanisms, it is clear that TPA induces cell replication in the epidermis, the overriding factor in its promoting action.

2,3,7,8-Tetrachlorodibenzo-*p*-dioxin

Another model promoting agent to be considered is 2,3,7,8-tetrachlorodibenzo-*p*-dioxin (TCDD), an effective promoter in a variety of tissues but primarily in liver and skin in the rodent (Pitot et al., 1980; Poland et al., 1982). TCDD is an environmental contaminant that is both a by-product of a variety of chemical syntheses and a product of various types of combustion (Hites, 1990; Bumb et al., 1980). TCDD is extremely toxic (cf. Lilienfeld and Gallo, 1989; Pohjanvirta and Tuomisto, 1994) and is likely the most effective promoting agent on a per-molecule basis that has been described (Pitot et al., 1980). Virtually all of the toxicities of TCDD (Pohjanvirta and Tuomisto, 1994) are mediated through the interaction of TCDD with the Ah receptor as first described by Poland (cf. Poland and Knutson, 1982). The signal transduction pathway effecting the toxicity and promoting activity of TCDD has now been established to some degree

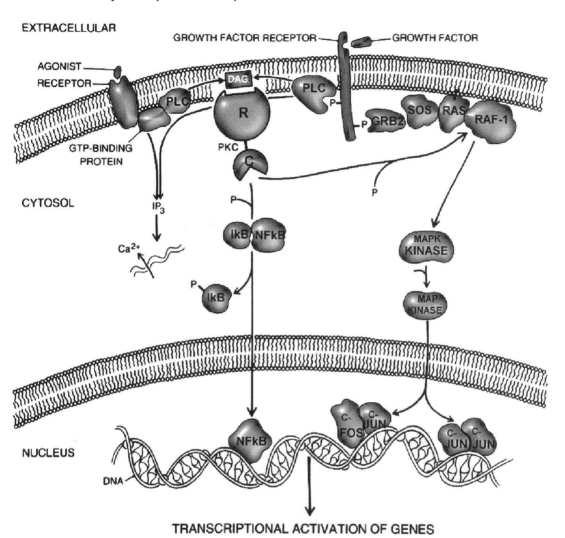

Figure 7.10 Pathways of protein kinase C–activated signal transduction. Interaction of TPA with the membrane-associated protein kinase C leads to an enhancement of its catalytic domain (C), which in turn may phosphorylate several different substrates as noted in the figure. This leads to a phosphorylation cascade with ultimate transcriptional activation of phorbol ester-inducible genes. Transcriptional activation is mediated by two independent routes, the *ras/raf-1* and the IkB/NF-κB pathways. Abbreviations: R, regulatory domain of PKC; C, catalytic domain of PKC; PLC, phospholipase C; GRB-2, growth receptor–bound protein 2 (an adapter between the growth receptor tyrosine kinase and SOS through its SH2 domain; SOS (son of sevenless), a guanine-nucleotide dissociation protein that releases GDP from RAS and allows GTP to bind and activate RAS; MAP kinase, mitogen-activated protein kinase; NF-κB, nuclear factor κB; IκB, inhibitory subunit of nuclear factor κB. (Adapted from Kazanietz and Blumberg, 1996, with permission of the authors and publisher.)

(Figure 7.11). As shown in the figure, TCDD interacts with the Ah receptor in the cytoplasm, the receptor being maintained in a native form through interaction with heat-shock proteins or chaperones (Henry and Gasiewicz, 1993; Whitlock, 1993). Interaction of the receptor with the ligand (TCDD) in the cytoplasm leads to a dissociation of the chaperone-Ah receptor complex and its binding to another somewhat related protein, the Ah receptor nuclear translocator protein (Arnt) (Reyes et al., 1992). This complex is then translocated into the nucleus, where it interacts with a specific core nucleotide sequence, T_GCGTG (Whitlock, 1993). Just as with TPA, this complex transcriptionally activates a large number of different genes, including many of the phase I xenobiotic metabolizing genes such as members of the cytochrome P450 family and a variety of others (DeVito and Birnbaum, 1994; Grassman et al., 1998). Like TPA, TCDD administration in vivo, albeit at doses considerably in excess of those used for tumor promotion, downregulated both the epidermal growth factor receptor (Sewall et al., 1995) and protein kinase C (Bombick et al., 1985). In addition, in cell culture, TCDD inhibited intercellular communication, like many other tumor promoting agents (Chapter 14) (De Haan et al., 1994). Like TPA, TCDD induces DNA synthesis and cell replication in preneoplastic foci but has very little if any effect on the nonfocal hepatocytes in such livers (Buchmann et al., 1994). This finding is in concert with that of its similar selective effect in inhibiting apoptosis of cells of altered hepatic foci without significantly altering the apoptotic index of the nonfocal liver (Stinchcombe et al., 1995). A potential mechanistic explanation of this latter finding is the demonstration that TCDD also suppresses apoptosis in rat hepatocytes treated in vitro with an apoptogenic dose of ultraviolet light. TCDD administration resulted in a dose-dependent increase in the phosphorylation of the p53 tumor suppressor protein (Wörner and Schrenk, 1998). This suggests that phosphorylation of key sites on the p53 protein prevents its action as a mediator of apoptosis (Bates and Vousden, 1999).

Phenobarbital

Phenobarbital (PB), the more classic tumor promoter of rodent hepatocarcinogenesis, appears to have a somewhat more complex mechanism of signal transduction than either TPA or TCDD. TPA inhibited the PB induction of phase I genes (Steele and Virgo, 1988), while PB inhibited the translocation of protein kinase C from the soluble to the particulate or membrane fraction of the cell (Brockenbrough et al., 1991), which is the normal pathway by which TPA activates protein kinase C to initiate signal transduction pathways. Like that of TPA, chronic administration of PB caused a decrease in epidermal growth factor receptor protein levels (Orton et al., 1996). PB also increased expression of the transcription factor c-*fos*, which is important in the enhancement of gene expression by TPA through the AP-1 regulatory site on DNA (see above) as well as in enhancing the expression of glutathione S-transferase in preneoplastic foci in rodent liver (Bitsch et al., 1999). However, the exact signal transduction pathway of phenobarbital has not been as readily elucidated as those of TPA and TCDD. In 1991, He and Fulco reported on a sequence in DNA which had some of the characteristics of a PB-responsive element. Later studies from this laboratory (Liang et al., 1995) defined the wild-type sequence, termed a Barbie box, as AT(A/C)AAAAGCTGGTG. Such sequences were found in the regulatory regions of several PB-responsive genes (Fournier et al., 1994). More recently, Negishi and associates defined another regulatory DNA element involved in the phenobarbital induction of cytochrome P450 CYP2B genes (cf. Honkakoski and Negishi, 1998). This sequence, termed the PB-responsive enhancer module (PBREM), did not contain any sequences of the Barbie box but usually occurred distal in the 5′ region of genes containing Barbie boxes. The sequence of the PBREM 51 base-pair enhancer element is seen in Figure 7.12.

These same workers have now demonstrated that several regulatory factors including a constitutively active receptor (CAR) are capable of transactivating the PBREM (Kawamoto et

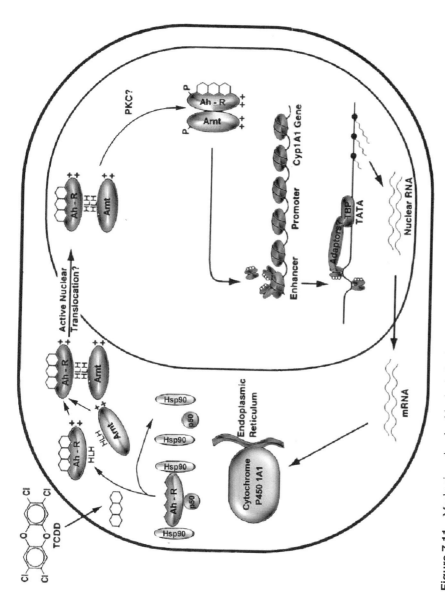

Figure 7.11 Mechanisms involved in the induction of cytochrome P450 1A1 gene transcription by TCDD. The figure demonstrates the various steps occurring from interaction of TCDD with the Ah receptor (Ah-R), the complex being an association with heat shock proteins and chaperones, Hsp90 and p50. This complex dissociates with an interaction of the ligand, TCDD, with the Ah-R, the complex then interacting with the Ah receptor nuclear translocator, Arnt, through helix-loop-helix (HLH) domains in the two proteins. This complex is translocated into the nucleus, where it may be phosphorylated by kinases such as protein kinase C, then interacting with specific regions of DNA and other proteins of the RNA polymerase complex. This complex is shown associating with adapter proteins and the TATA-box binding protein (TBP), ultimately resulting in transcription of the specific gene. (Modified from Whitlock, 1993, and DeVito and Birnbaum, 1994.)

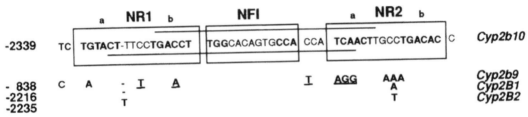

Figure 7.12 The 51-bp enhancer element (PBREM) as delineated by transfection in mammalian cells. The two putative nuclear receptor binding motifs are within the boxes as well as an NFI binding sequence. Variations in other cytochrome P450IIB genes are noted below the primary sequence with the differences indicated. (Adapted from Honkakoski et al., 1998, with permission of the authors and publisher.)

al., 1999). Phenobarbital appears to have an active function in this process, since it is capable of altering protein binding to this unit in native chromatin (Kim and Kemper, 1997). Thus, the phenobarbital signal transduction pathway appears to be quite analogous to that seen with TCDD in relation to the CAR receptor, but this does not explain the function of the Barbie box. Other studies (Stolz et al., 1998) indicate that phenobarbital induction of the PB-responsive cytochrome P450s requires interactions among multiple regulatory proteins and multiple *cis*-acting elements in the regulatory regions of these genes.

The mechanisms described for the action of these three promoting agents—TPA, TCDD, and PB—are responsible for the phenotypes noted in preneoplastic lesions, which differ significantly from those of their normal cellular counterparts. However, based on studies up to the present time, these mechanisms involved in both preneoplastic and normal cells appear to be the same. How these mechanisms result in selective cell replication and gene expression within preneoplastic tissues, giving them a growth advantage over their normal counterparts but being totally dependent on a continued presence of the promoting agent, is not clear at the present time.

The Molecular Basis of the Reversibility of the Stage of Tumor Promotion

The theoretical and practical aspects of ligand-receptor interactions have been previously reviewed (cf. Pitot, 1995). Herein such relationships are considered as they concern the action of tumor promoters. The basic assumption of the ligand-receptor interaction is that the effect of the agent is directly proportional to the number of receptors occupied by that chemical ligand and that a maximum response of the target is obtained only when all receptors are occupied. As seen in Figure 7.13, a simple bimolecular interaction between the ligand and receptor can be utilized to determine a dissociation constant, K_L, of the receptor-ligand complex. Although a variety of mathematical relationships may be derived from this simple equation (cf. Ruffolo, 1992), only the dose-response relationship is considered here. The dose-response of the receptor-ligand interaction takes the shape of a sigmoidal curve identical to that seen with the inhibition of TPA binding depicted in Figure 7.5. The figure denotes a threshold response at very low doses and a maximal effect above a specific dose. Theoretically, the linear conversion of the sigmoidal curves, such as seen in Figure 7.5, may indicate effects at even lower doses than those usually studied, but this depends on the association constant of the ligand-receptor complex and the subsequent fate of the complex (Aldridge, 1986). Withdrawal of the ligand reverts the system to its original state. Thus, the regulation of genetic expression that occurs by the ligand-receptor mechanism predicts a threshold and reversible effect unlike that of genotoxic carcinogenic agents, in which an irreversible nonthreshold response is assumed on theoretical grounds and can be demonstrated in a variety of instances (Druckrey, 1967; Zeise et al., 1987). Furthermore,

**Ligand (L) – Receptor (R)
Interactions**

$$R + L \rightleftharpoons RL \text{ (complex)}$$

$$K_L = \frac{[R] \cdot [L]}{[RL]}$$

where K_L = the dissociation constant of RL complex

Figure 7.13 Representation of receptor–ligand interaction and dissociation with derivation of the K_L, dissociation constant of the receptor–ligand complex.

at very low doses of some carcinogenic agents, an apparent reversal or "protective" effect of the agent can actually be demonstrated. This phenomenon has been termed *hormesis* (Teeguarden et al., 1998). Regardless of whether this latter effect can be more generalized, it is apparent that both the measured dose response and the receptor mechanisms of tumor promotion imply a no-effect or threshold level for the action of these agents during carcinogenesis. Thus, the stage of tumor promotion, unlike that of initiation and progression, does not involve mutational or structural events in the genome but rather is concerned with the reversible alteration of the expression of genetic information.

Role of Apoptosis in Tumor Promotion

As noted from Figure 7.9, there occurs a period during the cell cycle when the cell may enter into a differentiated, usually G_0 state and remain so for hours, days, or years. In some instances such a decision to enter G_0 also culminates in terminal differentiation and apoptosis or programmed cell death (Chapter 2). Although Figure 7.9 indicates that such decisions are made at the G_0/G_1 switchpoint or checkpoint, deviation of the cell cycle to apoptosis may occur during any of the stages of the cycle (cf. King and Cidlowski, 1995).

We have already considered (Chapter 2) some of the biological characteristics of apoptosis, and during the last few years a considerable body of knowledge has accumulated related to molecular characteristics and controls of this process. Figure 7.14 is an extension of Figure 2.5 and shows a hypothetical diagram of the sequence of events leading to apoptosis. It indicates the genes and gene products involved during the various phases noted—induction, mediation, modulation (effector stage in Figure 2.5), and degradation. DNA strand breakage by ionizing radiation induces an increase in the amount of p53 tumor suppressor gene by a posttranscriptional mechanism (cf. Canman and Kastan, 1995). In turn, the p53 protein acts as a transcriptional activator of several genes that serve to inhibit the cell cycle, thus presumably allowing time for the cell to repair the DNA damage. If the damage is excessive or repair mechanisms fail, the presence of excessive amounts of p53 protein appear to enhance cellular apoptosis. The Rb-1 gene normally suppresses cell proliferation in its underphosphorylated form, in which it binds to the transcription factor E2F-1. A deficiency of the Rb-1 protein results in activation of E2F-1 responsive genes and an inappropriate entry of cells into the S phase, leading ultimately to apoptosis or division of a cell with a mutated genome (Almasan et al., 1995).

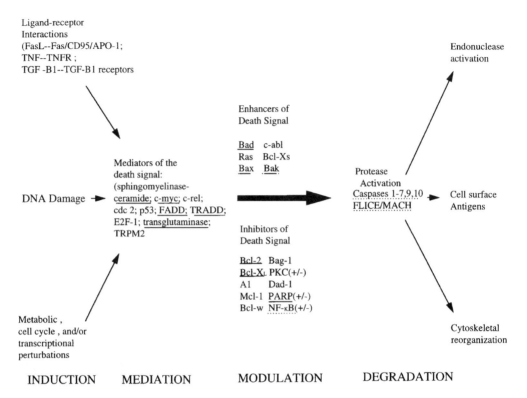

Figure 7.14 A theoretical scheme showing the general classes of perturbations which can initiate the "death signal" mediated by a variety of intracellular effectors. The intracellular effectors are then modulated by both enhancers and inhibitors, resulting ultimately in the activation of proteases, leading to alterations in cellular structure as well as the activation of nucleases causing DNA fragmentation. Descriptions of the various genes noted in the figure may be found in the text and/or the references. Those genes whose actions have been shown to be involved in apoptosis in hepatocytes are *underlined with solid lines*. The genes whose action is assumed to occur during hepatocyte apoptosis are *underlined with dotted lines*. (From Pitot, 1998. Reproduced with permission of the publisher.)

Another pathway leading to apoptosis is that of ligand-receptor interactions, including the interaction of TGFβ-1 (see above) with its receptor, and the Fas ligand interaction with its receptor (Nagata and Golstein, 1995). In addition, the deprivation of growth factors from cells may also lead to apoptosis (Thompson, 1995). Mechanisms involved in such ligand-receptor–mediated apoptosis may be similar to those involved in ligand-receptor enhancement of cell proliferation. Some of the effector molecules, as noted in the figure, include the *ras* G protein and protein kinase C (PKC).

Metabolic or cell cycle perturbations that induce apoptosis include the effect of ceramide, a product of sphingomyelin hydrolysis (Bose et al., 1995) and a variety of drugs capable of inhibiting or altering the cell cycle (Smets, 1994). Ceramide-induced apoptosis may involve signal transduction pathways, which involve ligand-receptor mechanisms as well (Obeid and Hannun, 1995). The effects of many chemotherapeutic drugs may involve mechanisms causing a mitotic catastrophe, which occurs when cell cycle (Spruck et al., 1999) or mitotic (Pihan and Doxsey, 1999) components are themselves overexpressed or defective. This latter phenomenon has a number of characteristics similar to those of apoptosis, and many cells showing such changes ultimately undergo apoptosis (King and Cidlowski, 1995).

Effector genes may modify the development of apoptosis either in a positive enhancing or negative inhibitory manner. Predominant among gene products that prevent the development of apoptosis is the *Bcl-2* gene, which codes for a protein in the mitochondrial membrane (Hockenbery et al., 1990). The *Bcl-2* gene has a variety of demonstrated functions involving mitochondrial permeability, especially to proteins such as cytochrome c, ions, and protective actions against reactive oxygen species produced by the mitochondrion (cf. Mignotte and Vayssiere, 1998). Cells expressing high levels of this protein are resistant to apoptosis induced by several different mechanisms (cf. Hoffman and Liebermann, 1994). In contrast, *Bax*, a gene whose transcription is enhanced by the p53 protein, results in an acceleration of apoptosis. Just as in mitosis, checkpoints (Chapter 9) have been proposed, first during the modulation stage, when enhancers and inhibitors of the death signal are opposed, and second at the initiation of the degradation stage, by activation of the protease caspases (Oltvai and Korsmeyer, 1994) in a cascade of activation of the 10 or more known caspases (cf. Cohen, 1997).

The exact role of poly(ADP-ribosyl)ation catalyzed by poly ADP-ribose polymerase (PARP) is not clear. This enzyme is activated by DNA strand breaks and is somehow involved in the more efficient repair of DNA. In some cell types, inhibition of PARP inhibits apoptosis (Tanaka et al., 1995); in other cell types, it either has no effect or causes a questionable enhancement of the process of programmed cell death (cf. Binder and Hiddemann, 1994). The common pathway of the degradation phase of apoptosis is protease activation, which may occur directly, as by the action of cytotoxic T cells, or by other mechanisms possibly involving signal transduction (Martin and Green, 1995). The first protease that was identified as an effector during apoptosis in several cell types was the interleukin-1β-converting enzyme (ICE) (Kumar, 1995). A number of similar proteases have been implicated in apoptosis in lower forms of life, and proteolysis itself is necessary for the activation of ICE-like proteases (Kumar, 1995, 1999). While the relationship between the various genes apparently acting earlier in the effector phase and ICE-like proteases is not entirely clear, evidence has indicated that ICE-like proteases do cleave PARP, thus eliminating it as an effective factor (Gu et al., 1995). A number of other proteins including kinases, the retinoblastoma, and APC tumor suppressor genes are cleaved by the caspases (cf. Thornberry et al., 1997). Caspases activate, by proteolysis, a DNase that is capable of degrading chromosomal DNA (Enari et al., 1998).

A number of promoting agents, including growth factors, are effective inhibitors of apoptosis in preneoplastic cells (Table 7.10). Although the mechanisms underlying the inhibition of apoptosis by promoting agents are not clear, it would appear from the list that growth factor inhibition of apoptosis may be largely the result of maintaining cells within the cell cycle, not allowing ready exit to the apoptotic pathway (Figure 7.9). Other hormones may act through signal transduction pathways involving nuclear receptors such as the sex hormones, TCDD, and nafenopin, a peroxisome proliferator.

The inhibition of apoptosis by TPA may well be mediated by the protein kinase C pathway, which is the principal method by which this promoting agent effects its action as a tumor promoter (cf. Evans, 1993). Just as cell replication is enhanced selectively in preneoplastic cells by the action of promoting agents (see above), apoptosis appears to be more selectively inhibited by promoting agents in preneoplastic lesions as compared with normal tissues (Stinchcombe et al., 1995; Schulte-Hermann et al., 1993). Inhibition of the apoptosis of single initiated cells may also occur in the presence of tumor promotion (Dragan et al., 1994a,b). Dietary restriction appears to eliminate initiated cells, probably through apoptosis (Grasl-Kraupp et al., 1994). Thus, programmed cell death plays a major role in both the stages of initiation and promotion. In particular, the reversibility of the stage of promotion, shown at the molecular level in a diagrammatic manner in Figure 7.13, at the cellular level involves the relief of the inhibition of apoptosis by removal or inhibition of action (Chapter 8) of the promoting agent. Withdrawal of the pro-

Table 7.10 Promoting Agents as Inhibitors of Apoptosis in Vivo

	Reference
Growth Factors	
Nerve growth factor	Binder and Hiddemann, 1994
Fibroblast growth factor	Binder and Hiddemann, 1994
Platelet-derived growth factor	Binder and Hiddemann, 1994
Colony-stimulating growth factors	Binder and Hiddemann, 1994
Hormones	
Estrogens, progesterone, androgens	Binder and Hiddemann, 1994
Adrenocorticotrophic hormone	Schulte-Hermann et al., 1993
Pharmacological Agents	
α Hexachlorocyclohexane	Schulte-Hermann et al., 1993
Phenobarbital	Schulte-Hermann et al., 1993
TPA	Schulte-Hermann et al., 1993
Nafenopin	Schulte-Hermann et al., 1993
TCDD	Stinchcombe et al., 1995
Metabolites	
Cholic acid	Magnuson et al., 1994

moting agent results in loss of all or almost all of the preneoplastic cells in the stage of promotion through apoptosis stimulated by both humoral and cellular mechanisms which are inactive as long as the promoting agent is present. Apoptosis also plays significant roles in the stage of progression and the therapy of neoplasia, as discussed further on (Chapter 20).

DEFINITIONS OF INITIATING AND PROMOTING AGENTS

Some of the characteristics of initiation and promotion, stages in the natural history of the development of neoplasia, have already been noted (Tables 7.1 and 7.3). On the basis of these characteristics as well as our knowledge of carcinogenic agents, it is possible to formulate working definitions of the two types of agents.

Initiating Agent

An initiating agent is a chemical, physical, or biological agent that is capable of directly altering the genetic component (DNA) of the cell irreversibly. Such alteration(s) may be the result of a covalent reaction of DNA with the initiating agent itself or with one of its metabolites, but this alteration may, at least theoretically, also include a distortion of the structure of DNA without covalent binding to its components. Alternatively or in addition, the agent may cause DNA strand breaks, an elimination of one of its component parts (e.g., bases or sugars), or errors in DNA repair. Many initiating agents at high doses may produce more extensive genetic abnormalities characteristic of the stage of progression.

Promoting Agent

A promoting agent is an agent capable of altering the expression of genetic information of the cell as well as, in many cases, inhibiting programmed cell death or apoptosis of the cell. While promoting agents may be metabolized by the cell, most or all of their promoting effects are the result of interaction of the native agent with specific cellular components, especially receptors, thereby resulting in an alteration of gene expression and altered mitosis and apoptosis. *In essence, promoting agents <u>selectively</u> enhance cell replication of preneoplastic cells and <u>selectively</u> inhibit apoptosis of neoplastic cells.*

The above definitions have the advantage over other terminology of being applicable to almost all examples of initiating and promoting agents. Oncogenic viruses and radiation have the properties of initiating agents, since they alter the basic structure of the DNA of the cell. Inasmuch as neoplasms result from the action of a number of viruses and types of radiation, many of these also possess promoting activity and thus may be considered *complete carcinogens*, i.e., having both initiating and promoting activity. Many agents that have been shown to be carcinogenic—such as polycyclic hydrocarbons, carcinogenic aromatic amines, nitrosamines (Chapter 3), oncogenic RNA and DNA viruses (Chapter 4), and ionizing and ultraviolet irradiation—may be considered complete carcinogens. As discussed earlier in this chapter, *incomplete carcinogens* (agents capable of initiation but not promotion) have been shown to exist, but as yet only rarely. The classic experiments of Berenblum and Haran-Ghera (1957a,b), demonstrating incomplete carcinogenesis by urethane in mouse skin, indicated the existence of such chemicals, but since urethane is a complete carcinogen for several other tissues, its action as a "pure" initiator was quite restricted. Furthermore, studies by Deringer (1962) with specific strains of mice indicated that, under certain circumstances, urethane may act as a complete carcinogen in the skin as well. Scribner and Scribner (1980) demonstrated that dibenzo[a,c]anthracene does have the characteristics of an incomplete carcinogen for mouse skin, although its carcinogenicity for other tissues has not been adequately tested.

The diversity of promoting agents may be seen from the structures depicted in Figure 7.4. Several of these compounds act as promoting agents in various tissues with a relatively high degree of specificity. For example, saccharin is an effective promoting agent in bladder carcinogenesis but not in hepatocarcinogenesis (Nakanishi et al., 1982). These authors also demonstrated that phenobarbital, although an effective promoting agent in the liver, was totally ineffective as a promoter for bladder carcinogenesis. Not only estrogens, but a variety of hormones have been shown to serve as effective promoting agents in vivo (Berenblum, 1978). Berenblum proposed that hormones should be considered as a class of promoting agents that effectively promote initiated cells, whether initiated specifically by known environmental intervention or by background environmental factors. Not shown in Figure 7.4 is the "foreign body" or "plastic film" carcinogenesis discussed in Chapter 3. Several experimental studies (Ryan et al., 1981; Brand et al., 1975) have indicated that such foreign bodies can act as promoting agents. Furthermore, Topping and Nettesheim (1980) presented evidence that asbestos acts like a promoting agent in experimental tracheal carcinogenesis. This finding correlates well with the known epidemiological phenomenon of the marked enhancement of bronchogenic carcinoma in humans exposed to asbestos who are smokers as compared with those smokers not exposed to asbestos (Chapter 11).

THE STAGES OF INITIATION AND PROMOTION IN HUMAN CARCINOGENESIS

Evidence for the existence of the stages of initiation and promotion in the human have come largely from clinicopathological and epidemiological studies. That initiation occurs in the human is evidenced by the spontaneous incidence of cancer in the human population, implying initiation as an essential component for the development of such neoplasms. Evidence for the existence of the stage of promotion in human neoplasia is not so definitive as that seen in the animal, but since the pathogenesis of cancer development in the human may be recapitulated in the animal, one may use such model systems to potentially identify the stage of promotion in the development of human neoplasia.

Morphological evidence for the clonal expansion of initiated cells during tumor promotion is based on the description of preneoplastic lesions and attempts to relate such lesions to the development of specific malignancies (cf. Henson and Albores-Saavedra, 1986; Dunham, 1972). Table 7.11 lists some preneoplastic lesions of the human and their related or analogous lesions in the rodent. The preneoplastic nature of the human lesions has been inferred from both histopathological and epidemiological studies. The similarity of putative human preneoplastic lesions to comparable lesions known to be preneoplastic that develop in experimental animal models further supports the preneoplastic nature of the human alterations. For example, nodular hyperplasia of the adrenal cortex is quite commonly seen in the rodent, and the preneoplastic potential of the lesions has been implied for many years in the animal (Dunn, 1970). The lesions observed in mammary carcinogenesis are also quite analogous in animals and humans (van Bogaert, 1984). In addition, the lesions observed in the liver and colon of animals are strikingly similar to their human counterparts. Although examples exist where the congruence of the preneoplastic counterpart in the human is not distinct during pathogenesis of the developing neoplasm in animals (e.g., the dysplastic nevus to malignant melanoma), in general the similarities of preneoplastic lesions in the human and experimental animal strongly argue that the stages of the carcinogenic process in mammals are very similar across species.

Table 7.11 Preneoplastic Lesions in the Human and Their Counterparts in Rodents

Tissue	Human	Rodent
Skin	Keratoacanthoma	Papilloma
Tracheobronchial epithelium	Atypical metaplasia (Trump et al., 1978)	Atypical metaplasia
Esophagus	Moderate to severe dysplasia (Kuwano et al., 1993)	Moderate to severe dysplasia
Stomach	Intestinal metaplasia (Correa, 1983) Gastric dysplasia (Saraga et al., 1987)	Glandular dysplasia
Colon	Aberrant crypts (Pretlow et al., 1992a,b)	Aberrant crypts
Pancreas	Focal acinar cell dysplasia	Atypical acinar cell foci
Liver	Liver cell dysplasia Focal nodular hyperplasia	Altered hepatic foci "Neoplastic" nodules
Bladder	Moderate to severe dysplasia (Coon et al., 1983)	Papillary hyperplasia
Adrenal	Adrenocortical nodules (Cohen, 1966)	Adrenocortical hyperplasia
Mammary gland	Atypical lobule type A (Jensen et al., 1976)	Hyperplastic terminal end buds

Adapted from Pitot and Dragan, 1995, with permission of the publisher.

Reversal of Human Preneoplasia

As noted above, the primary characteristic of the promotion stage seen in models of cancer development is its operational reversibility (Williams and Watanabe, 1978; Iversen, 1982; Moore et al., 1983; Hill et al., 1989). Several examples of the reversibility of human preneoplasia are provided in Table 7.12. Lung cancer risk has been reported to decrease exponentially with the time after cessation of smoking. After 15 to 20 years of nonsmoking, the risk of lung cancer in the smokers that stopped smoking was essentially equivalent to that for nonsmokers (cf. Reif, 1981). In addition, Zatonski et al. (1990) demonstrated a dramatic decrease in the risk of laryngeal cancers in smokers who had stopped smoking, as well as in those who stopped smoking for 1 to 4 years but then resumed the habit. This last finding is very similar to the lessened effect of intermittent compared with continual exposure to a promoting agent on the subsequent yield of preneoplastic lesions (Boutwell, 1964; Xu et al., 1991). In addition, atypical epithelial hyperplasia of the oral cavity seen in tobacco users disappears upon cessation of tobacco product use (Table 7.12). Furthermore, the administration of retinoids can also lead to the reversible disappearance of oral leukoplakia (Hong et al., 1986).

Several other organ systems also exhibit preneoplastic lesions that regress under some conditions. For example, preneoplastic lesions of the stomach and colon display an instability based on their regression with or without intervention (Table 7.12). In addition, chemopreventive trials with nonsteroidal anti-inflammatory agents have demonstrated a regression of the polyps that are believed to be precursors to colonic adenocarcinomas (Giardiello et al., 1993). Perhaps the clearest example of regression of a human preneoplastic lesion is that of regression of nodular hyperplasia and adenomas of the liver induced by administration of some synthetic estrogen preparations to premenopausal women (Edmondson et al., 1977; Steinbrecher et al., 1981; Bühler et al., 1982). Most of these lesions disappeared upon cessation of use of these contraceptive preparations (Table 7.12).

Table 7.12 Reversibility of Carcinogenesis at the Stage of Tumor Promotion (Preneoplasia) in Humans

Lesion	Promoting Agent	Reversal Effect	Reference
Gastric epithelial dysplasia	Dietary factors	Regression and disappearance of dysplasia	Rugge et al., 1991
Lung cancer	Cigarette smoke	Decrease in risk as function of time after cessation	Reif, 1981
Laryngeal cancer	Cigarette smoke	Decrease in risk after complete and interval cessation	Zatonski et al., 1990
Hepatic nodular hyperplasia (adenomas?)	Synthetic estrogens	Loss of lesion after cessation of use	Bühler et al., 1982 Steinbrecher et al., 1981 Edmondson et al., 1977
Leukoplakia	Chewing tobacco and/or tobacco smoke	Disappearance of lesion after cessation of tobacco abuse	Eveson, 1983 Larsson et al., 1991
Rectal and colonic polyps	Dietary factors (?) in patients with familial polyposis	Regression of polyps after anti-inflammatory therapy or dietary change	Giardiello et al., 1993 DeCosse et al., 1989

Adapted from Pitot and Dragan, 1995, with permission of the publisher.

Thus, it is apparent that the stages of initiation and promotion, including the major characteristic of the latter, operational reversibility, can be demonstrated in the human. Thus, it is likely that the genesis of many if not the majority of human neoplasms may involve the stages of initiation and promotion, accounting not only for the extensive known latent period in the development of human neoplasia (Chapter 11) but also the effects of a variety of chemopreventive (Chapter 8) agents acting during the stage of promotion to prevent further development of the neoplastic process.

REFERENCES

Ahn, Y. S., Chemeris, G. Y., Turusov, V. S., and Bannasch, P. Enzymic pattern of preneoplastic and neoplastic lesions induced in the kidney of CBA mice by 1,2-dimethylhydrazine. Toxicol. Pathol., *22*:415–422, 1994.

Alard, P., Lantz, O., Sebagh, M., Calvo, C. F., Weill, D., Chavanel, G., Senik, A., and Charpentier, B. A versatile ELISA-PCR assay for mRNA quantitation from a few cells. Biotechniques, *15*:730–737, 1993.

Aldaz, C. M., Conti, C. J., Klein-Szanto, A. J. P., and Slaga, T. J. Progressive dysplasia and aneuploidy are hallmarks of mouse skin papillomas: relevance to malignancy. Proc. Natl. Acad. Sci. U.S.A., *84*:2029–2032, 1987.

Aldridge, W. N. The biological basis and measurement of thresholds. Annu. Rev. Pharmacol. Toxicol., *26*:39–58, 1986.

Almasan, A., Yin, Y., Kelly, R. E., Lee, E. Y.-H. P., Bradley, A., Li, W., Bertino, J. R., and Wahl, G. M. Deficiency of retinoblastoma protein leads to inappropriate S-phase entry, activation of E2F-responsive genes, and apoptosis. Proc. Natl. Acad. Sci. U.S.A., *92*:5436–5440, 1995.

Anderson, M. W., Reynolds, S. H., You, M., and Maronpot, R. M. Role of proto-oncogene activation in carcinogenesis. Environ. Health Perspect., *98*:13–24, 1992.

Andrews, E. J. Evidence of the nonimmune regression of chemically induced papillomas in mouse skin. J. Natl. Cancer Inst., *47*:653–665, 1971.

Aronheim, A., Engelberg, D., Li, N., Al-Alawi, N., Schlessinger, J., and Karin, M. Membrane targeting of the nucleotide exchange factor Sos is sufficient for activating the Ras signaling pathway. Cell, *78*:949–961, 1994.

Ashendel, C. L. The phorbol ester receptor: a phospholipid-regulated protein kinase. Biochim. Biophys. Acta, *822*:219–242, 1985.

Ashendel, C. L., Staller, J. M., and Boutwell, R. K. Protein kinase activity associated with a phorbol ester receptor purified from mouse brain. Cancer Res., *43*:4333–4337, 1983.

Bailleul, B., Brown, K., Ramsden, M., Akhurst, R. J., Fee, F., and Balmain, A. Chemical induction of oncogene mutations and growth factor activity in mouse skin carcinogenesis. Environ. Health Perspect., *81*:23–27, 1989.

Banks, G. R. Mutagenesis: a review of some molecular aspects. Sci. Prog., Oxf., *59*:475–503, 1971.

Bannasch, P. Preoplastic lesions as end points in carcinogenicity testing. II. Preneoplasia in various nonhepatic tissues. Carcinogenesis, *7*:849–852, 1986.

Barsoum, J., and Varshavsky, A. Mitogenic hormones and tumor promoters greatly increase the incidence of colony-forming cells bearing amplified dihydrofolate reductase genes. Proc. Natl. Acad. Sci. U.S.A., *80*:5330–5334, 1983.

Bates, S., and Vousden, K. H. Mechanisms of p53-mediated apoptosis. Cell. Mol. Life Sci., *55*:28–37, 1999.

Bauer-Hofmann, R., Klimek, F., Buchmann, A., Müller, O., Bannasch, P., and Schwarz, M. Role of mutations at codon 61 of the c-Ha-*ras* gene during diethylnitrosamine-induced hepatocarcinogenesis in C3H/He mice. Mol. Carcinog., *6*:60–67, 1992.

Berenblum, I. Guest editorial. Established principles and unresolved problems in carcinogenesis. J. Natl. Cancer Inst., *60*:723–726, 1978.

Berenblum, I., and Haran-Ghera, N. A quantitative study of the systemic initiating action of urethane (ethyl carbamate) in mouse skin carcinogenesis. Br. J. Cancer, *11*:77–84, 1957a.

Berenblum, I., and Haran-Ghera, N. The induction of the initiating phase of skin carcinogenesis in the mouse by oral administration of 9:10-dimethyl-1:2-benzanthracene, 20-methylcholanthrene, 3:4-benzpyrene, and 1:2:5:6-dibenzanthracene. Br. J. Cancer, *11*:85–87, 1957b.

Berenblum, I., and Shubik, P. The role of croton oil applications, associated with a single painting of a carcinogen, in tumour induction of the mouse's skin. Br. J. Cancer, *1*:379–382, 1947.

Binder, C., and Hiddemann, W. Programmed cell death—many questions still to be answered. Ann. Hematol., *69*:45–55, 1994.

Bird, R. P. Role of aberrant crypt foci in understanding the pathogenesis of colon cancer. Cancer Lett., *93*:55–71, 1995.

Birnboim, H. C. DNA strand breakage in human leukocytes exposed to a tumor promoter, phorbol myristate acetate. Science, *215*:1247–1249, 1982.

Bitsch, A., Deubelbeiss, C., and Greiner, A. c-fos Gene expression in rat liver is induced by phenobarbital. Cancer Lett., *135*:215–222, 1999.

Böhm, S. K., Grady, E. F., and Bunnett, N. W. Regulatory mechanisms that modulate signalling by G-protein-coupled receptors. Biochem. J., *322*:1–18, 1997.

Bombick, D. W., Madhukar, B. V., Brewster, D. W., and Matsumura, F. TCDD (2,3,7,8-tetrachlorodibenzo-p-dioxin) causes increases in protein kinases particularly protein kinase C in the hepatic plasma membrane of the rat and the guinea pig. Biochem. Biophys. Res. Commun., *127*:296–302, 1985.

Borek, C., and Sachs, L. The number of cell generations required to fix the transformed state in x-ray–induced transformation. Proc. Natl. Acad. Sci. U.S.A., *59*:83–85, 1968.

Bose, R., Verheij, M., Haimovitz-Friedman, A., Scotto, K., Fuks, Z., and Kolesnick, R. Ceramide synthase mediates daunorubicin-induced apoptosis: an alternative mechanism for generating death signals. Cell, *82*:405–414, 1995.

Boutwell, R. K. Some biological aspects of skin carcinogenesis. Prog. Exp. Tumor Res., *4*:207–250, 1964.

Boutwell, R. K. Function and mechanism of promoters of carcinogenesis. CRC Crit. Rev. Toxicol., *2*:419–443, 1974.

Brambilla, G., Carlo, P., Finollo, R., Bignone, F. A., Ledda, A., and Cajelli, E. Viscometric detection of liver DNA fragmentation in rats treated with minimal doses of chemical carcinogens. Cancer Res., *43*:202–209, 1983.

Brand, K. G., Buoen, L. C., Johnson, K. H., and Brand, I. Etiological factors, stages, and the role of the foreign body in foreign body tumorigenesis: a review. Cancer Res., *35*:279–286, 1975.

Brockenbrough, J. S., Meyer, S. A., Li, C., and Jirtle, R. L. Reversible and phorbol ester-specific defect of protein kinase C translocation in hepatocytes isolated from phenobarbital-treated rats. Cancer Res., *51*:130–136, 1991.

Buchmann, A., Stinchcombe, S., Körner, W., Hagenmaier, H., and Bock, K. W. Effects of 2,3,7,8-tetrachloro- and 1,2,3,4,6,7,8-heptachlorodibenzo-p-dioxin on the proliferation of preneoplastic liver cells in the rat. Carcinogenesis, *15*:1143–1150, 1994.

Bühler, H., Pirovino, M., Akovbiantz A., et al. Regression of liver cell adenomas. A follow-up study of three consecutive patients after discontinuation of oral contraceptive use. Gastroenterology, *82*:775–782, 1982.

Bumb, R. R., Crummett, W. B., Cutie, S. S., Gledhill, J. R., Hummel, R. H., Kagel, R. O., Lamparski, L. L., Luoma, E. V., Miller, D. L., Nestrick, T. J., Shadoff, L. A., Stehl, R. H., and Woods, J. S. Trace chemistries of fire: a source of chlorinated dioxins. Science, *210*:385–390, 1980.

Burns, F. J., Vanderlaan, M., Snyder, E., and Albert, R. E. Induction and progression kinetics of mouse skin papillomas. *In*: T. J. Slaga, A. Sivak, and R. K. Boutwell (Eds.), Carcinogenesis, Vol. 2, Mechanism of Tumor Promotion and Cocarcinogenesis, pp. 91–96. New York: Raven Press, 1978.

Candrian, U., You, M., Goodrow, T., Maronpot, R. R., Reynolds, S. H., and Anderson, M. W. Activation of protooncogenes in spontaneously occurring non-liver tumors from C57BL/6 x C3H F_1 mice. Cancer Res., *51*:1148–1153, 1991.

Canman, C. E., and Kastan, M. B. Induction of apoptosis by tumor suppressor genes and oncogenes. Cancer Biol., *6*:17–25, 1995.

Carter, J. H., Carter, H. W., and Meade, J. Adrenal regulation of mammary tumorigenesis in female Sprague-Dawley rats: incidence, latency, and yield of mammary tumors. Cancer Res., 48:3801–3807, 1988.

Cayama, E., Tsuda, H., Sarma, D. S. R., and Farber, E. Initiation of chemical carcinogenesis requires cell proliferation. Nature, 275:60–62, 1978.

Cerny, W. L., Mangold, K. A., and Scarpelli, D. G. K-ras mutation is an early event in pancreatic duct carcinogenesis in the Syrian golden hamster. Cancer Res., 52:4507–4513, 1992.

Cerutti, P. A. Prooxidant states and tumor production. Science, 227:375–381, 1985.

Cerutti, P. A. Oxidant stress and carcinogenesis. Eur. J. Clin. Invest., 21:1–5, 1991.

Cha, R. S., Thilly, W. G., and Zarbl, H. N-Nitroso-N-methylurea-induced rat mammary tumors arise from cells with preexisting oncogenic Hras1 gene mutations. Proc. Natl. Acad. Sci. U.S.A., 91:3749–3753, 1994.

Cimino, F., Esposito, F., Ammendola, R., and Russo, T. Gene regulation by reactive oxygen species. Curr. Top. Cell. Regul., 35:123–148, 1997.

Cohen, G. M. Caspases: the executioners of apoptosis. Biochem. J., 326:1–16, 1997.

Cohen, L. A., Kendall, M. E., Zang, E., Meschter, C., and Rose, D. P. Modulation of N-nitrosomethylurea-induced mammary tumor promotion by dietary fiber and fat. J. Natl. Cancer Inst., 83:496–501, 1991.

Cohen, R. B. Observations on cortical nodules in human adrenal glands. Cancer, 19:552–556, 1966.

Cohen, S. M., and Ellwein, L. B. Cell proliferation in carcinogenesis. Science, 249:1007–1011, 1990.

Collins, S., Caron, M. G., and Lefkowitz, R. J. From ligand binding to gene expression: new insights into the regulation of G-protein-coupled receptors. Trends Biochem. Sci., 17:37–40, 1992.

Columbano, A., Rajalakshmi, S., and Sarma, D. S. R. Requirement of cell proliferation for the initiation of liver carcinogenesis as assayed by three different procedures. Cancer Res., 41:2079–2083, 1981.

Coon, J. S., Pauli, B. U., and Weinstein, R. S. Precancer of the urinary bladder. Cancer Surv., 2:479–494, 1983.

Correa, P. The gastric precancerous process. Cancer Surv., 2:437–450, 1983.

Dalton, T. P., Shertzer, H. G., and Puga, A. Regulation of gene expression by reactive oxygen. Annu. Rev. Pharmacol. Toxicol., 39:67–101, 1999.

Davis, R. J., and Czech, M. P. Tumor-promoting phorbol diesters mediate phosphorylation of the epidermal growth factor receptor. J. Biol. Chem., 259:8545–8549, 1984.

DeCosse, J. J., Miller, H. H., and Lesser, M. L. Effect of wheat fiber and vitamins C and E on rectal polyps in patients with familial adenomatous polyposis. J. Natl. Cancer Inst., 81:1290–1297, 1989.

De Haan, L. H. J., Simons, J.-W. F. A., Bos, A. T., Aarts, J. M. M. J. G., Denison, M. S., and Brouwer, A. Inhibition of intercellular communication by 2,3,7,8-tetrachlorodibenzo-p-dioxin and dioxin-like PCBs in mouse hepatoma cells (Hepa1c1c7): involvement of the Ah receptor. Toxicol. Appl. Pharmacol., 129:283–293, 1994.

Denda, A., Sai, K., Tang, Q., Tsujiuchi, T., Tsutsumi, M., Amanuma, T., Murata, Y., Nakae, D., Maruyama, H., Kurokawa, Y., and Konishi, Y. Induction of 8-hydroxydeoxyguanosine but not initiation of carcinogenesis by redox enzyme modulations with or without menadione in rat liver. Carcinogenesis, 12:719–726, 1991.

Deringer, M. K. Response of strain HR/De mice to painting with urethan. J. Natl. Cancer Inst., 29:1107–1121, 1962.

DeVito, M. J., and Birnbaum, L. S. Toxicology of dioxins and related chemicals. In: A. Schecter (Ed.), Dioxins and Health, Chapter 5, pp. 139–162. New York: Plenum Press, 1994.

DiGiovanni, J. Multistage carcinogenesis in mouse skin. Pharmac. Ther., 54:63–128, 1992.

Draetta, G. F. Mammalian G_1 cyclins. Curr. Opin. Cell Biol., 6:842–846, 1994.

Dragan, Y. P., Campbell, H. A., Baker, K., Vaughan, J., Mass, M., and Pitot, H. C. Focal and nonfocal hepatic expression of placental glutathione S-transferase in carcinogen-treated rats. Carcinogenesis, 15:2587–2591, 1994a.

Dragan, Y. P., Hully, J. R., Nakamura, J., Mass, M. J., Swenberg, J. A., and Pitot, H. C. Biochemical events during initiation of rat hepatocarcinogenesis. Carcinogenesis, 15:1451–1458, 1994b.

Druckrey, H. Quantitative aspects in chemical carcinogenesis. In: R. Truhant (ed.), Potential Carcinogenic Hazards from Drugs. Evaluation of Risks, UICC Monograph Series, Vol. 7, pp. 60–77. Berlin: Springer-Verlag, 1967.

Dulic, V., Kaufmann, W. K., Wilson, S. J., Tlsty, T. D., Lees, E., Harper, J. W., Elledge, S. J., and Reed, S. I. p53-Dependent inhibition of cyclin-dependent kinase activities in human fibroblasts during radiation-induced G1 arrest. Cell, 76:1013–1023, 1994.

Dunham, L. J. Cancer in man at site of prior benign lesion of skin or mucous membrane: a review. Cancer Res., 32:1359–1374, 1972.

Dunn, T. B. Normal and pathologic anatomy of the adrenal gland of the mouse, including neoplasms. J. Natl. Cancer Inst., 44:1323–1389, 1970.

Edmondson, H., Reynolds, T., Henderson, B., and Benton, B. Regression of liver cell adenomas associated with oral contraceptives. Ann. Intern. Med., 86:180–182, 1977.

Egan, S. E., Giddings, B. W., Brooks, M. W., Buday, L., Sizeland, A. M., and Weinberg, R. A. Association of Sos Ras exchange protein with Grb2 is implicated in tyrosine kinase signal transduction and transformation. Nature, 363:45–50, 1993.

Emerit, I., and Cerutti, P. A. Tumor promoter phorbol 12-myristate 13-acetate induces a clastogenic factor in human lymphocytes. Proc. Natl. Acad. Sci. U.S.A., 79:7509–7513, 1982.

Enari, M., Sakahira, H., Yokoyama, H., Okawa, K., Iwamatsu, A., and Nagata, S. A caspase-activated DNase that degrades DNA during apoptosis, and its inhibitor ICAD. Nature, 391:43–50, 1998.

Evans, V. G. Multiple pathways to apoptosis. Cell Biol. Int., 17:461–476, 1993.

Eveson, J. W. Oral premalignancy. Cancer Surv., 2:403–424, 1983.

Feig, L. A. Guanine-nucleotide exchange factors: a family of positive regulators of Ras and related GT-Pases. Curr. Opin. Cell Biol., 6:204–211, 1994.

Finkel, T. Oxygen radicals and signaling. Curr. Opin. Cell Biol., 10:248–253, 1998.

Fishbein, L. New concepts of design and utility of large-scale carcinogenicity studies. J. Toxicol. Environ. Health, 6:1081–1100, 1980.

Foulds, L. Mammary tumours in hybrid mice: growth and progression of spontaneous tumours. Br. J. Cancer, 3:345–375, 1949.

Fournier, T., Mejdoubi, N., Lapoumeroulie, C., Hamelin, J., Elion, J., Durand, G., and Porquet, D. Transcriptional regulation of rat α_1-acid glycoprotein gene by phenobarbital. J. Biol. Chem., 269:27175–27178, 1994.

Frankfurt, O., and Raitcheva, E. Effect of tumor promoters on cell kinetics in mouse epidermis. J. Natl. Cancer Inst., 49:131–137, 1972.

Fujiki, H., and Suganuma, M. Tumor promotion by inhibitors of protein phosphatases 1 and 2A: the okadaic acid class of compounds. Adv. Cancer Res., 61:143–194, 1993.

Fürstenberger, G., Berry, D. L., Sorg, B., and Marks, F. Skin tumor promotion by phorbol esters is a two-stage process. Proc. Natl. Acad. Sci. U.S.A., 78:7722–7726, 1981.

Fürstenberger, G., Sorg, B., and Marks, F. Tumor promotion by phorbol esters in skin: evidence for a memory effect. Science, 220:89–91, 1983.

Fürstenberger, G., Kinzel, V., Schwarz, M., and Marks, F. Partial inversion of the initiation-promotion sequence of multistage tumorigenesis in the skin of NMRI mice. Science, 230:767–778, 1985.

Furth, J. A meeting of ways in cancer research: thoughts on the evolution and nature of neoplasms. Cancer Res., 19:241–256, 1959.

Furuya, K., and Williams. G. M. Iron exclusion by proliferative foci and neoplastic lesions induced by 7,12-dimethylbenz(a)anthracene in the rat adrenal cortex. Histochem. J., 17:213–221, 1985.

Galloway, P. G., Likavec, M. J., and Perry, G. Immunohistochemical recognition of ethylnitrosourea induced rat brain microtumors by anti-Leu 7 monoclonal antibody. Cancer Lett., 49:243–248, 1990.

Gamaley, I. A., and Klyubin, I. V. Roles of reactive oxygen species: signaling and regulation of cellular functions. Int. Rev. Cytol., 188:203–255, 1999.

Giardiello, F. M., Hamilton, S. R., Krush, A. J., et al. Treatment of colonic and rectal adenomas with sulindac in familial adenomatous polyposis. N. Engl. J. Med., 328:1313–1316, 1993.

Glauert, H. P., and Clark, T. D. Lack of initiating activity of the peroxisome proliferator ciprofibrate in two-stage hepatocarcinogenesis. Cancer Lett., 43:95–100, 1989.

Glauert, H. P., Schwarz, M., and Pitot, H. C. The phenotypic stability of altered hepatic foci: effect of the short-term withdrawal of phenobarbital and of the long-term feeding of purified diets after the withdrawal of phenobarbital. Carcinogenesis, 7:117–121, 1986.

Grasl-Kraupp, B., Bursch, W., Ruttkay-Nedecky, B., Wagner, A., Lauer, B., and Schulte-Hermann, S. Food restriction eliminates preneoplastic cells through apoptosis and antagonizes carcinogenesis in rat liver. Proc. Natl. Acad. Sci. U.S.A., *91*:9995–9999, 1994.

Grassman, J. A., Masten, S. A., Walker, N. J., and Lucier, G. W. Animal models of human response to dioxins. Environ. Health Perspect., *106*:761–775, 1998.

Grisham, J. W., Greenberg, D. S., Kaufman, D. G., and Smith, G. J. Cycle-related toxicity and transformation in 10T1/2 cells treated with *N*-methyl-*N'*-nitro-*N*-nitrosoguanidine. Proc. Natl. Acad. Sci. U.S.A., *77*:4813–4817, 1980.

Gu, Y., Sarnecki, C., Aldape, R. A., Livingston, D. J., and Su, M. S.-S. Cleavage of poly(ADP-ribose) polymerase by interleukin-1β converting enzyme and its homologs TX and Nedd-2. J. Biol. Chem., *270*:18715–18718, 1995.

Guyton, K. Z., Liu, Y., Gorospe, M., Xu, Q., and Holbrook, N. J. Activation of mitogen-activated protein kinase by H_2O_2. Role in cell survival following oxidant injury. J. Biol. Chem., *271*:4138–4142, 1996.

Hall, A. A biochemical function for ras—at last. Science, *264*:1413–1414, 1994.

Hanigan, M. H., and Pitot, H. C. Growth of carcinogen-altered rat hepatocytes in the liver of syngeneic recipients promoted with phenobarbital. Cancer Res., *45*:6063–6070, 1985.

Hansen, L. A., Monteiro-Riviere, N. A., and Smart, R. C. Differential down-regulation of epidermal protein kinase C by 12-*O*-tetradecanoylphorbol-13-acetate and diacylglycerol: association with epidermal hyperplasia and tumor promotion. Cancer Res., *50*:5740–5745, 1990.

Hattori, A., Kunz, H. W., Gill, T. J. III, Pan, S. F., and Shinozuka, H. Diversity of the promoting action of cyclosporine on the induction of murine lymphoid tumors. Carcinogenesis, *9*:1091–1094, 1988.

Hayashi, K., Fujiki, H., and Sugimura, T. Effects of tumor promoters on the frequency of metallothionein I gene amplification in cells exposed to cadmium. Cancer Res., *43*:5433–5436, 1983.

He, J.-S., and Fulco, A. J. A barbiturate-regulated protein binding to a common sequence in the cytochrome P450 genes of rodents and bacteria. J. Biol. Chem., *266*:7864–7869, 1991.

Henry, E. C., and Gasiewicz, T. A. Transformation of the aryl hydrocarbon receptor to a DNA-binding form is accompanied by release of the 90 kDa heat-shock protein and increased affinity for 2,3,7,8-tetrachlorodibenzo-*p*-dioxin. Biochem. J., *294*:95–101, 1993.

Henson, D. E., and Albores-Saavedra, J. The Pathology of Incipient Neoplasia. Philadelphia: Saunders, 1986.

Hill, R. N., Erdreich, L. S., Paynter, O. E., Roberts, P. A., Rosenthal, S. L., and Wilkinson, C. F. Thyroid follicular cell carcinogenesis. Fundam. Appl. Toxicol., *12*:629–697, 1989.

Hites, R. A. Environmental behavior of chlorinated dioxins and furans. Accounts Chem. Res., *23*:194–201, 1990.

Hockenbery, D., Nuñez, G., Milliman, C., Schreiber, R. D., and Korsmeyer, S. J. Bcl-2 is an inner mitochondrial membrane protein that blocks programmed cell death. Nature, *348*:334–336, 1990.

Hoffman, B., and Liebermann, D. A. Molecular controls of apoptosis: differentiation/growth arrest primary response genes, proto-oncogenes, and tumor suppressor genes as positive and negative modulators. Oncogene, *9*:1807–1812, 1994.

Hong, W. K., Endicott, J., Itri, L. M., Doos, W., Batsakis, J. G., Bell, R., Fofonoff, S., Byers, R., Atkinson, E. N., Vaughan, C., Toth, B. B., Kramer, A., Dimery, I. W., Skipper, P., and Strong, S. 13-cis-retinoic acid in the treatment of oral leukoplakia. N. Engl. J. Med., *315*:1501–1505, 1986.

Honkakoski, P., and Negishi, M. Regulatory DNA elements of phenobarbital-responsive cytochrome P450 CYP2B genes. J. Biochem. Mol. Toxicol., *12*:3–9, 1998.

Honkakoski, P., Moore, R., Washburn, K. A., and Negishi, M. Activation by diverse xenochemicals of the 51-base pair phenobarbital-responsive enhancer module in the *CYP2B10* gene. Mol. Pharmacol., *53*:597–601, 1998.

Iversen, O. H. Hairless mouse skin in two-stage chemical carcinogenesis. An experimental study with special reference to cell kinetics, papilloma regression and the possible development of increased cellular resistance. Virchows Arch. (Cell. Pathol.), *38*:263–272, 1982.

Jacobs, T. Control of the cell cycle. Dev. Biol., *153*:1–15, 1992.

Janknecht, R., Cahill, M. A., and Nordheim, A. Signal integration at the c-*fos* promoter. Carcinogenesis, *16*:443–450, 1995.

Jensen, H. M., Rice, J. R., and Wellings, S. R. Preneoplastic lesions in the human breast. Science, *191*:295–297, 1976.

Kakiuchi, H., Ushijima, T., Ochiai, M., Imai, K., Ito, N., Yachi, A., Sugimura, T., and Nagao, M. Rare frequency of activation of the Ki-*ras* gene in rat colon tumors induced by heterocyclic amines: possible alternative mechanisms of human colon carcinogenesis. Mol. Carcinog., *8*:44–48, 1993.

Kakunaga, T. The role of cell division in the malignant transformation of mouse cells treated with 3-methylcholanthrene. Cancer Res., *35*:1637–1642, 1975.

Karin, M. The beginning of the end: IκB kinase (IKK) and NF-κB activation. J. Biol. Chem., *274*:27339–27342, 1999.

Kawamoto, T., Sueyoshi, T., Zelko, I., Moore, R., Washburn, K., and Negishi, M. Phenobarbital-responsive nuclear translocation of the receptor CAR in induction of the *CYP2B* gene. Mol. Cell. Biol., *19*:6318–6322, 1999.

Kazanietz, M. G., and Blumberg, P. M. Protein kinase C and signal transduction in normal and neoplastic cells. *In*: A. E. Sirica (Ed.), Cellular and Molecular Pathogenesis, pp. 389–402. Philadelphia: Lippincott-Raven Publishers, 1996.

Kemp, C. J., Leary, C. N., and Drinkwater, N. R. Promotion of murine hepatocarcinogenesis by testosterone is androgen receptor-dependent but not cell autonomous. Proc. Natl. Acad. Sci. U.S.A., *86*:7505–7509, 1989.

Keyse, S. M. Oxidative stress responses in mammalian cells. *In*: J. D. Hayes and C. R. Wolf (Eds.), Molecular Genetics of Drug Resistance, pp. 335–372. Reading, UK: Harwood Academic Publishers, 1997.

Kim, J., and Kemper, B. Phenobarbital alters protein binding to the *CYP2B1/2* phenobarbital-responsive unit in native chromatin. J. Biol. Chem., *272*:29423–29425, 1997.

King, K. L., and Cidlowski, J. A. Cell cycle and apoptosis: common pathways to life and death. J. Cell. Biochem., *58*:175–180, 1995.

Klaunig, J. E. Selection induction of DNA synthesis in mouse preneoplastic and neoplastic hepatic lesions after exposure to phenobarbital. Environ. Health Perspect., *101*:235–240, 1993.

Knudson, A. G. Antioncogenes and human cancer. Proc. Natl. Acad. Sci. U.S.A., *90*:10914–10921, 1993.

Koelle, M. R. A new family of G-protein regulators—the RGS proteins. Curr. Opin. Cell Biol., *9*:143–147, 1997.

Komminoth, P., and Long, A. A. In-situ polymerase chain reaction. Virchows Archiv. B Cell Pathol., *64*:67–73, 1993.

Konishi, H., Tanaka, M., Takemura, Y., Matsuzaki, H., Ono, Y., Kikkawa, U., and Nishizuka, Y. Activation of protein kinase C by tyrosine phosphorylation in response to H_2O_2. Proc. Natl. Acad. Sci. U.S.A., *94*:11233–11237, 1997.

Kozumbo, W. J., Seed, J. L., and Kensler, T. W. Inhibition by 2(3)-*tert*–butyl-4-hydroxyanisole and other antioxidants of epidermal ornithine decarboxylase activity induced by 12-*O*-tetradecanoylphorbol-13-acetate. Cancer Res., *43*:2555–2559, 1983.

Kumar, S. ICE-like proteases in apoptosis. TIBS, *20*:198–202, 1995.

Kumar, S. Mechanisms mediating caspase activation in cell death. Cell Death Differ., *6*:1060–1066, 1999.

Kuwano, H., Watanabe, M., Sadanaga, N., et al. Squamous epithelial dysplasia associated with squamous cell carcinoma of the esophagus. Cancer Lett., *72*:141–147, 1993.

Laconi, E., Vasudevan, S., Rao, P. M., Rajalakshmi, S., Pani, P., and Sarma, D. S. R. An earlier proliferative response of hepatocytes in γ-glutamyl transferase positive foci to partial hepatectomy. Cancer Lett., *81*:229–235, 1994.

Laird, A. D., and Shalloway, D. Oncoprotein signaling and mitosis. Cell. Signal., *9*:249–255, 1997.

Lander, H. M. An essential role for free radicals and derived species in signal transduction. FASEB J., *11*:118–124, 1997.

Lane, D. P. p53, guardian of the genome. Cancer, *358*:15–16, 1992.

Lantos, P. L., and Pilkington, G. J. The development of experimental brain tumours. A sequential light and electron microscope study of the subependymal plate. Acta Neuropathol., *45*:167–175, 1979.

Larsson, A., Axéll, T., and Andersson, G. Reversibility of snuff dippers' lesion in Swedish moist snuff users: a clinical and histologic follow-up study. J. Oral Pathol. Med., *20*:258–264, 1991.

Leach, K. L., James, M. L., and Blumberg, P. M. Characterization of a specific phorbol ester aporeceptor in mouse brain cytosol. Proc. Natl. Acad. Sci. U.S.A., *80*:4208–4212, 1983.

Lewis, T. S., Shapiro, P. S., and Ahn, N. G. Signal transduction through MAP kinase cascades. Adv. Cancer Res., *74*:49–139, 1998.

Liang, Q., He, J.-S., and Fulco, A. J. The role of Barbie box sequences as *cis*-acting elements involved in the barbiturate-mediated induction of cytochromes $P450_{BM-1}$ and $P450_{BM-3}$ in *Bacillus megaterium*. J. Biol. Chem., *270*:4438–4450, 1995.

Liao, D., Porsch-Hällström, I., Gustafsson, J.-Å., and Blanck, A. Sex differences at the initiation stage of rat liver carcinogenesis—influence of growth hormone. Carcinogenesis, *14*:2045–2049, 1993.

Lilienfeld, D. E., and Gallo, M. A. 2,4-D, 2,4,5-T, and 2,3,7,8-TCDD: an overview. Epidemiol. Rev., *11*:28–58, 1989.

Loehrke, H., Schweizer, J., Dederer, E., Hesse, B., Rosenkranz, G., and Goerttler, K. On the persistence of tumor initiation in two-stage carcinogenesis on mouse skin. Carcinogenesis, *4*:771–775, 1983.

Maekawa, A., and Mitsumori, K. Spontaneous occurrence and chemical induction of neurogenic tumors in rats—influence of host factors and specificity of chemical structure. Crit. Rev. Toxicol., *20*:287–310, 1990.

Magnuson, B. A., Carr, I., and Bird, R. P. Ability of aberrant crypt foci characteristics to predict colonic tumor incidence in rats fed cholic acid. Cancer Res., *53*:4499–4504, 1993.

Magnuson, B. A., Shirtliff, N., and Bird, R. P. Resistance of aberrant crypt foci to apoptosis induced by azoxymethane in rats chronically fed cholic acid. Carcinogenesis, *15*:1459–1462, 1994.

Magun, B. E., Matrisian, L. M., and Bowden, G. T. Epidermal growth factor. Ability of tumor promoter to alters its degradation, receptor affinity and receptor number. J. Biol. Chem., *255*:6373–6381, 1980.

Marks, F., and Fürstenberger, G. Experimental evidence that skin carcinogenesis is a multistep phenomenon. Br. J. Dermatol., *115*:1–8, 1986.

Martin, S. J., and Green, D. R. Protease activation during apoptosis: death by a thousand cuts? Cell, *82*:349–352, 1995.

Mayer, E. A. Signal transduction and intercellular communication. *In*: J. H. Walsh and G. J. Dockray (Eds.), Gut Peptides: Biochemistry and Physiology, pp. 33–73. New York: Raven Press, 1994.

Medina, D. Preneoplastic lesions in murine mammary cancer. Cancer Res., *36*:2589–2595, 1976.

Mignotte, B., and Vayssiere, J.-L. Mitochondria and apoptosis. Eur. J. Biochem., *252*:1–15, 1998.

Miyamoto, S., and Verma, I. M. REL/NF-κB/IκB story. Adv. Cancer Res., *66*:255–292, 1995.

Moore, M. A., Hacker, H.-J., and Bannasch, P. Phenotypic instability in focal and nodular lesions induced in a short term system in the rat liver. Carcinogenesis, *4*:595–603, 1983.

Moore, M. A., Nakagawa, K., Satoh, K., Ishikawa, T., and Sato, K. Single GST-P positive liver cells—putative initiated hepatocytes. Carcinogenesis, *8*:483–486, 1987.

Moriyama, S., Kawaoi, A., Hirota, N. Localization and significance of gamma-glutamyl transpeptidase during experimental thyroid carcinogenesis in rats. Acta Histochem. Cytochem., *16*:567–576, 1983.

Morley, S. J., and Thomas, G. Intracellular messengers and the control of protein synthesis. Pharmacol. Ther., *50*:291–319, 1991.

Mottram, J. C. A developing factor in experimental blastogenesis. J. Pathol. Bacteriol., *56*:181–187, 1944.

Müller, R., Mumberg, D., and Lucibello, F. C. Signals and genes in the control of cell-cycle progression. Biochim. Biophys. Acta, *1155*:151–179, 1993.

Murata, Y., Denda, A., Obara, T., Yokose, Y., and Konishi, Y. Histochemical studies on γ-glutamyltranspeptidase activity of pancreatic acinar cell lesions induced by 4-hydroxyaminoquinoline 1-oxide and/or azaserine in rats. Exp. Pathol., *32*:41–53, 1987.

Nagasawa, H., and Little, J. B. Effect of tumor promoters, protease inhibitors, and repair processes on x-ray-induced sister chromatid exchanges in mouse cells. Proc. Natl. Acad. Sci. U.S.A., *76*:1943–1947, 1979.

Nagasawa, H., and Little, J. B. Factors influencing the induction of sister chromatid exchanges in mammalian cells by 12-O-tetradecanoyl-phorbol-13-acetate. Carcinogenesis, *2*:601–607, 1981.

Nagata, S., and Golstein, P. The Fas death factor. Science, *267*:1449–1456, 1995.

Nakanishi, K., Fukushima, S., Hagiwara, A., Tamano, S., and Ito, N. Organ-specific promoting effects of phenobarbital sodium and sodium saccharin in the induction of liver and urinary bladder tumors in male F344 rats. J. Natl. Cancer Inst., *68*:497–500, 1982.

Nakano, H., Hatayama, I., Satoh, K., Suzuki, S., Sato, K., and Tsuchida, S. c-Jun expression in single cells and preneoplastic foci induced by diethylnitrosamine in B6C3F1 mice: comparison with the expression of pi-class glutathione *S*-transferase. Carcinogenesis, *15*:1853–1857, 1994.

Nelson, M. A., Futscher, B. W., Kinsella, T., Wymer, J., and Bowden, G. T. Detection of mutant Ha-*ras* genes in chemically initiated mouse skin epidermis before the development of benign tumors. Proc. Natl. Acad. Sci. U.S.A., *89*:6398–6402, 1992.

Nettesheim, P., Klein-Szanto, A. J. P., Marchok, A. C., Steele, V. E., Terzaghi, M., and Topping, D. C. Studies of neoplastic development in respiratory tract epithelium. Arch. Pathol. Lab. Med., *105*:1–10, 1981.

Nikitin, A. Y., Rajewsky, M. F., and Pozharisski, K. M. Development of malignant fibrous histiocytoma induced by 7,12-dimethylbenz[a]anthracene in the rat: characterization of early atypical cells. Virchows Archiv B Cell Pathol., *64*:151–159, 1993.

Nuzum, E. O., Malkinson, A. M., and Beer, D. G. Specific Ki-*ras* codon 61 mutations may determine the development of urethan-induced mouse lung adenomas or adenocarcinomas. Mol. Carcinog., *3*:287–295, 1990.

Obeid, L. M., and Hannun, Y. A. Ceramide: a stress signal and mediator of growth suppression and apoptosis. J. Cell. Biochem., *58*:191–198, 1995.

Oltvai, Z. N., and Korsmeyer, S. J. Checkpoints of dueling dimers foil death wishes. Cell, *79*:189–192, 1994.

Orton, T. C., Doughty, S. E., Kalinowski, A. E., Lord, P. G., and Wadsworth, P. F. Expression of growth factors and growth factor receptors in the liver of C57BL/10J mice following administration of phenobarbitone. Carcinogenesis, *17*:973–981, 1996.

Paraskeva, C., and Williams, A. C. Promotability and tissue specificity of hereditary cancer genes: do hereditary cancer patients have a reduced requirement for tumor promotion because all their somatic cells are heterozygous at the predisposing locus? Mol. Carcinog., *5*:4–8, 1992.

Pawson, T. Signal transduction—a conserved pathway from the membrane to the nucleus. Dev. Genet., *14*:333–338, 1993.

Pegg, A. E., and Perry, W. Alkylation of nucleic acids and metabolism of small doses of dimethylnitrosamine in the rat. Cancer Res., *41*:3128–3132, 1981.

Perchellet, J.-P., and Perchellet, E. M. Phorbol ester tumor promoters and multistage skin carcinogenesis. *In* ISI Atlas of Science: Pharmacology, pp. 325–332, 1988.

Pihan, G. A., and Doxsey, S. J. The mitotic machinery as a source of genetic instability in cancer. Semin. Cancer Biol., *9*:289–302, 1999.

Pitcher, J. A., Inglese, J., Higgins, J. B., Arriza, J. L., Casey, P. J., Kim, C., Benovic, J. L., Kwatra, M. M., Caron, M.G., and Lefkowitz, R. J. Role of βγ subunits of G proteins in targeting the β-adrenergic receptor kinase to membrane-bound receptors. Science, *257*:1264–1267, 1992.

Pitot, H. C. Altered hepatic foci: their role in murine hepatocarcinogenesis. Annu. Rev. Pharmacol. Toxicol., *30*:465–500, 1990.

Pitot, H. C. Endogenous carcinogenesis: the role of tumor promotion. Proc. Soc. Exp. Biol. Med., *198*:661–666, 1991.

Pitot, H. C. The role of receptors in multistage carcinogenesis. Mutat. Res., *333*:3–14, 1995.

Pitot, H. C. The stages in neoplastic development. *In*: D. Schottenfeld and J. Fraumeni (Eds.), Cancer Epidemiology and Prevention, pp. 65–79. New York: Oxford University Press, 1996.

Pitot, H. C. Hepatocyte death in hepatocarcinogenesis. Hepatology, *28*:1–5, 1998.

Pitot, H. C., and Dragan, Y. P. The instability of tumor promotion in relation to human cancer risk. *In*: R. M. McClain, T. J. Slaga, R. LeBoeuf, and H. Pitot (Eds.), Growth Factors and Tumor Promotion: Implications for Risk Assessment, pp. 21–38. New York: Wiley-Liss, Inc., 1995.

Pitot H. C. III, and Dragan, Y. P. Chemical carcinogenesis. *In*: C. D. Klaasen (Ed.), Casarett and Doull's Toxicology—The Basic Science of Poisons. pp. 201–267. New York: McGraw-Hill 1996.

Pitot, H. C., Goldsworthy, T., Campbell, H. A., and Poland, A. Quantitative evaluation of the promotion by 2,3,7,8-tetrachlorodibenzo-*p*-dioxin of hepatocarcinogenesis from diethylnitrosamine. Cancer Res., *40*:3616–3620, 1980.

Pitot, H. C., Goldsworthy, T. L., Moran, S., Kennan, W., Glauert, H. P., Maronpot, R. R., and Campbell, H. A. A method to quantitate the relative initiating and promoting potencies of hepatocarcinogenic agents in their dose-response relationships to altered hepatic foci. Carcinogenesis, *8*:1491–1499, 1987.

Pohjanvirta, R., and Tuomisto, J. Short-term toxicity of 2,3,7,8-tetrachlorodibenzo-*p*-dioxin in laboratory animals: effects, mechanisms, and animal models. Pharmacol. Rev., *46*:483–549, 1994.

Poland, A., and Knutson, J. C. 2,3,7,8-Tetrachlorodibenzo-*p*-dioxin and related halogenated aromatic hydrocarbons: examination of the mechanism of toxicity. Annu. Rev. Pharmacol. Toxicol., *22*:517–554, 1982.

Poland, A., Palen, D., and Glover, E. Tumour promotion by TCDD in skin of HRS/J hairless mice. Nature, *300*:271–273, 1982.

Pratt, W. B., and Toft, D. O. Steroid receptor interactions with heat shock protein and immunophilin chaperones. Endocr. Rev., *18*:306–360, 1997.

Pretlow, T. P. Alterations associated with early neoplasia in the colon. *In*: T. G. Pretlow and T. P. Pretlow (Eds.), Biochemical and Molecular Aspects of Selected Cancers, Vol. 2, pp. 93–141. San Diego, CA: Academic Press, 1994.

Pretlow, T. P., O'Riordan, M. A., Somich, G. A., et al. Aberrant crypts correlate with tumor incidence in F344 rats treated with azoxymethane and phytate. Carcinogenesis, *13*:1509–1512, 1992a.

Pretlow, T. P., O'Riordan, M. A., Pretlow, T. G., and Stellato, T. A. Aberrant crypts in human colonic mucosa: putative preneoplastic lesions. J. Cell. Biochem., *16G*:55–62, 1992b.

Preussmann, R. The problem of thresholds in chemical carcinogenesis. Some views on theoretical and practical aspects. J. Cancer Res. Clin. Oncol., *97*:1–14, 1980.

Quintanilla, M., Brown, K., Ramsden, M., and Balmain, A. Carcinogen-specific mutation and amplification of Ha-*ras* during mouse skin carcinogenesis. Nature, *322*:78–80, 1986.

Rabes, H. M., Müller, L., Hartmann, A., Kerler, R., and Schuster, C. Cell cycle-dependent initiation of adenosine triphosphatase-deficient populations in adult rat liver by a single dose of *N*-methyl-*N*-nitrosourea. Cancer Res., *46*:645–650, 1986.

Radomski, J. L., Krischer, C., and Krischer, K. N. Histologic and histochemical preneoplastic changes in the bladder mucosae of dogs given 2-naphthylamine. J. Natl. Cancer Inst., *60*:327–333, 1978.

Rasenick, M. M., Caron, M. G., Dolphin, A. C., Kobilka, B. K., and Schultz, G. Receptor-G protein-effector coupling: coding and regulation of the signal transduction process. *In*: A. C. Cuello and B. Collier (Eds.), Pharmacological Sciences: Perspectives for Research and Therapy in the Late 1990s, pp. 91–102. Basel, Switzerland: Birkhäuser Verlag, 1995.

Reddy, J. K., and Lalwani, N. D. Carcinogenesis by hepatic peroxisome proliferators: evaluation of the risk of hypolipidemic drugs and industrial plasticizers to humans. CRC Crit. Rev. Toxicol., *12*:1–58, 1983.

Reif, A. E. Effect of cigarette smoking on susceptibility to lung cancer. Oncology, *38*:76–85, 1981.

Reyes, H., Reisz-Porszasz, S., and Hankinson, O. Identification of the Ah receptor nuclear translocator protein (Arnt) as a component of the DNA binding form of the Ah receptor. Science, *256*:1193–1195, 1992.

Roomi, M. W., Ho, R. K., Sarma, D. S. R., and Farber, E. A common biochemical pattern in preneoplastic hepatocyte nodules generated in four different models in the rat. Cancer Res., *45*:564–571, 1985.

Rosenthal, N. Molecular medicine. Regulation of gene expression. N. Engl. J. Med., *331*:931–933, 1994.

Rous, P., and Kidd, J. G. Conditional neoplasms and subthreshold neoplastic states. J. Exp. Med., *73*:365–390, 1941.

Roussel, M. F. Key effectors of signal transduction and G1 progression. Adv. Cancer Res., *74*:1–24, 1998.

Rubio, C. A. Epithelial lesions antedating oesophageal carcinoma. Pathol. Res. Pract., *176*:269–275, 1983.

Ruffolo, R. R., Jr. Fundamentals of receptor theory: basics for shock research. Circ. Shock, *37*:176–184, 1992.

Rugge, M., Farinati, F., Di Mario, F., et al. Gastric epithelial dysplasia: a prospective multicenter follow-up study from the interdisciplinary group on gastric epithelial dysplasia. Hum. Pathol., *22*:1002–1008, 1991.

Rumsby, P. C., Barrass, N. C., Phillimore, H. E., and Evans, J. G. Analysis of the Ha-*ras* oncogene in C3H/He mouse liver tumors derived spontaneously or induced with diethylnitrosamine or phenobarbitone. Carcinogenesis, *12*:2331–2336, 1991.

Russo, J., Tait, L., and Russo, I. H. Susceptibility of the mammary gland to carcinogenesis. III. The cell of origin of rat mammary carcinoma. Am. J. Pathol., *113*:50–66, 1983.

Ryan, W. L., Stenback, F., and Curtis, G. L. Tumor promotion by foreign bodies (IUD). Cancer Lett., *13*:299–302, 1981.

Saeter, G., Schwarze, P. E., Nesland, J. M., and Seglen, P. O. 2-Acetylaminofluorene promotion of liver carcinogenesis by a non-cytotoxic mechanism. Carcinogenesis, 9:581–587, 1988.

Saltiel, A. R. Signal transduction pathways as drug targets. Sci. Am. Sci. Med., *2*, Nov./Dec., pp. 58–67, 1995.

Sander, C. A., Yano, T., Clark, H. M., Harris, C., Longo, D. L., Jaffe, E. S., and Raffeld, M. p53 Mutation is associated with progression in follicular lymphomas. Blood, *82*:1994–2004, 1993.

Saraga, E.-P., Gardiol, D., and Costa, J. Gastric dysplasia. A histological follow-up study. Am. J. Surg. Pathol., *11*:788–796, 1987.

Sargent, L., Xu, Y.-h., Sattler, G. L., Meisner, L., and Pitot, H. C. Ploidy and karyotype of hepatocytes isolated from enzyme-altered foci in two different protocols of multistage hepatocarcinogenesis in the rat. Carcinogenesis, *10*:387–391, 1989.

Sasajima, K., Kawachi, T., Matsukura, N., Sano, T., and Sugimura, T. Intestinal metaplasia and adenocarcinoma induced in the stomach of rats by N-propyl-N'-nitro-N-nitrosoguanidine. J. Cancer Res. Clin. Oncol., *94*:201–206, 1979.

Schaeffer, B. K., Zurlo, J., and Longnecker, D. S. Activation of c-Ki-*ras* not detectable in adenomas or adenocarcinomas arising in rat pancreas. Mol. Carcinog., *3*:165–170, 1990.

Schreck, R., Kistler, B., and Wirth, T. The NF-κB/Rel system of transcriptional activators. *In*: A. G. Papayassiliou (Ed.), Transcription Factors in Eukaryotes, pp. 154–188. Landes Bioscience, 1997.

Schulte-Hermann, R., Ohde, G., Schuppler, J., and Timmermann-Trosiener, I. Enhanced proliferation of putative preneoplastic cells in rat liver following treatment with the tumor promoters phenobarbital, hexachlorocyclohexane, steroid compounds, and nafenopin. Cancer Res., *41*:2556–2562, 1981.

Schulte-Hermann, R., Timmermann-Trosiener, I., and Schuppler, J. Promotion of spontaneous preneoplastic cells in rat liver as a possible explanation of tumor production by nonmutagenic compounds. Cancer Res., *43*:839–844, 1983.

Schulte-Hermann, R., Timmermann-Trosiener, I., Barthel, G., and Bursch, W. DNA synthesis, apoptosis, and phenotypic expression as determinants of growth of altered foci in rat liver during phenobarbital promotion. Cancer Res., *50*:5127–5135, 1990.

Schulte-Hermann, R., Bursch, W., Kraupp-Grasl, B., Oberhammer, F., Wagner, A., and Jirtle, R. Cell proliferation and apoptosis in normal liver and preneoplastic foci. Environ. Health Perspect., *101*:87–90, 1993.

Scribner, N. K., and Scribner, J. D. Separation of initiating and promoting effects of the skin carcinogen 7-bromomethylbenz(a)anthracene. Carcinogenesis, *1*:97–100, 1980.

Seger, R., and Krebs, E. G. The MAPK signaling cascade. FASEB J., *9*:726–735, 1995.

Sewall, C. H., Clark, G. C., and Lucier, G. W. TCDD reduces rat hepatic epidermal growth factor receptor: comparison of binding, immunodetection, and autophosphorylation. Toxicol. Appl. Pharmacol., *132*:263–272, 1995.

Shivapurkar, N., Tang, Z., Ferreira, A., Nasim, S., Garett, C., and Alabaster, O. Sequential analysis of K-*ras* mutations in aberrant crypt foci and colonic tumors induced by azoxymethane in Fischer-344 rats on high-risk diet. Carcinogenesis, *15*:775–778, 1994.

Short, B. G., Steinhagen, W. H., and Swenberg, J. A. Promoting effects of unleaded gasoline and 2,2,4-trimethylpentane on the development of atypical cell foci and renal tubular cell tumors in rats exposed to N-ethyl-N-hydroxyethylnitrosamine. Cancer Res., *49*:6369–6378, 1989.

Silvennoinen, O., Saharinen, P., Paukku, K., Takaluoma, K., and Kovanen, P. Cytokine receptor signal transduction through Jak tyrosine kinases and Stat transcription factors. APMIS, *105*:497–509, 1997.

Sivak, A. Cocarcinogenesis. Biochim. Biophys. Acta, *560*:67–89, 1979.

Slaga, T. J., Fischer, S. M., Nelson, K., and Gleason, G. L. Studies on the mechanism of skin tumor promotion: evidence for several stages in promotion. Proc. Natl. Acad. Sci. U.S.A., *77*:3659–3663, 1980.

Smets, L. A. Programmed cell death (apoptosis) and response to anti-cancer drugs. Anticancer Drugs, *5*:3–9, 1994.

Solt, D., and Farber, E. New principle for the analysis of chemical carcinogenesis. Nature, *263*:701–703, 1976.

Solt, D. B., Calderon-Solt, L., and Odajima, T. Rapid induction of carcinomas and γ-glutamyl transpeptidase-rich clones in *N*-methyl-*N*-benzylnitrosamine-treated hamster buccal pouch. J. Natl. Cancer Inst., *74*:437–445, 1985.

Spruck, C. H., Won, K.-A., and Reed, S. I. Deregulated cyclin E induces chromosome instability. Nature, *401*:297–300, 1999.

Stabel, S., and Parker, P. J. Protein kinase C. Pharmacol. Ther., *51*:71–95, 1991.

Steele, D. F., and Virgo, B. B. Cytochrome P450 induction by phenobarbital (PB) is inhibited by 12-O-tetradecanoylphorbol-13-acetate (TPA): evidence that protein kinase C regulates induction. Biochem. Biophys. Res. Commun., *153*:728–733, 1988.

Steinbrecher, U. P., Lisbona, R., Huang, S. N., and Mishkin, S. Complete regression of hepatocellular adenomas after withdrawal of oral contraceptives. Digest. Dis. Sci., *26*:1045–1050, 1981.

Stinchcombe, S., Buchmann, A., Bock, K. W., and Schwarz, M. Inhibition of apoptosis during 2,3,7,8-tetrachlorodibenzo-*p*-dioxin-mediated tumour promotion in rat liver. Carcinogenesis, *16*:1271–1275, 1995.

Stolz, C., Vachon, M.-H., Trottier, E., Dubois, S., Paquet, Y., and Anderson, A. The *CYP2B2* phenobarbital response unit contains an accessory factor element and a putative glucocorticoid response element essential for conferring maximal phenobarbital responsiveness. J. Biol. Chem., *273*:8528–8536, 1998.

Strader, C. D., Fong, T. M., Tota, M. R., and Underwood, D. Structure and function of G protein-coupled receptors. Annu. Rev. Biochem., *63*:101–132, 1994.

Sumi, C., Yokoro, K., Kajitani, T., and Ito, A. Synergism of diethylstilbestrol and other carcinogens in concurrent development of hepatic, mammary, and pituitary tumors in castrated male rats. J. Natl. Cancer Inst., *65*:169–175, 1980.

Takaba, K., Hirose, M., Yoshida, Y., Kimura, J., Ito, N., and Shirai, T. Effects of *n*-tritriacontane-16,18-dione, curcumin, chlorophyllin, dihydroguaiaretic acid, tannic acid and phytic acid on the initiation stage in a rat multi-organ carcinogenesis model. Cancer Lett., *113*:39–46, 1997.

Takuwa, N., and Takuwa, Y. Signal transduction of cell-cycle regulation: its temporo-spacial architecture. Jpn. J. Physiol., *46*:431–449, 1996.

Talalay, P., De Long, M. J., and Prochaska, H. J. Identification of a common chemical signal regulating the induction of enzymes that protect against chemical carcinogens. Proc. Natl. Acad. Sci. U.S.A., *85*:8261–8265, 1988.

Tanaka, Y., Yoshihara, K., Tohno, Y., Kojima, K., Kameoka, M., and Kamiya, T. Inhibition and down-regulation of poly(ADP-ribose) polymerase results in a marked resistance of HL-60 cells to various apoptosis-inducers. Cell. Mol. Biol., *41*:771–781, 1995.

Tanooka, H. Monoclonal growth of cancer cells: experimental evidence. Jpn. J. Cancer Res., *79*:657–665, 1988.

Taper, H. S. The effect of estradiol-17-phenylpropionate and estradiol benzoate on N-nitrosomorpholine-induced liver carcinogenesis in ovariectomized female rats. Cancer, *42*:462–467, 1978.

Tatematsu, M., Nagamine, Y., and Farber, E. Redifferentiation as a basis for remodeling of carcinogen-induced hepatocyte nodules to normal appearing liver. Cancer Res., *43*:5049–5058, 1983.

Teeguarden, J. G., Dragan, Y. P., and Pitot, H. C. Implications of hormesis on the bioassay and hazard assessment of chemical carcinogens. Human Exp. Toxicol., *17*:254–258, 1998.

Thompson, C. B. Apoptosis in the pathogenesis and treatment of disease. Science, *267*:1456–1462, 1995.

Thompson, L. H., Baker, R. M., Carrano, A. V., and Brookman, K. W. Failure of the phorbol ester 12-O-tetradecanoylphorbol-13-acetate to enhance sister chromatid exchange, mitotic segregation, or expression of mutations in Chinese hamster cells. Cancer Res., *40*:3245–3251, 1980.

Thornberry, N. A., Rosen, A., and Nicholson, D. W. Control of apoptosis by proteases. Adv. Pharmacol., *41*:155–177, 1997.

Tokusashi, Y., Fukuda, I., and Ogawa, K. Absence of *p53* mutations and various frequencies of Ki-*ras* exon 1 mutations in rat hepatic tumors induced by different carcinogens. Mol. Carcinog., *10*:45–51, 1994.

Topping, D. C., and Nettesheim, R. Two-stage carcinogenesis studies with asbestos in Fischer 344 rats. J. Natl. Cancer Inst., *65*:627–630, 1980.

Trump, B. F., McDowell, E. M., Glavin, F., et al. The respiratory epithelium. III. Histogenesis of epidermoid metaplasia and carcinoma in situ in the human. J. Natl. Cancer Inst., *61*:563–575, 1978.

Tsiftsis, D., Jass, J. R., Filipe, M. I., and Wastell, C. Altered patterns of mucin secretion in precancerous lesions induced in the glandular part of the rat stomach by the carcinogen *N*-methyl-*N'*-nitro-*N*-nitrosoguanidine. Invest. Cell Pathol., *3*:399–408, 1980.

van Bogaert, L.-J. Mammary hyperplastic and preneoplastic changes: taxonomy and grading. Breast Cancer Res. Treat., *4*:315–322, 1984.

Vanderlaan, M., Fong, S., and King, E. B. Histochemistry of NADH diaphorase and γ-glutamyltranspeptidase in rat bladder tumors. Carcinogenesis, *3*:397–402, 1982.

Van Duuren, B. L., Sivak, A., Katz, C., Seidman, I., and Melchionne, S. The effect of aging and interval between primary and secondary treatment in two-stage carcinogenesis on mouse skin. Cancer Res., *35*:502–505, 1975.

Verma, A. K., and Boutwell, R. K. Effects of dose and duration of treatment with the tumor-promoting agent, 12-O-tetradecanoylphorbol-13-acetate on mouse skin carcinogenesis. Carcinogenesis, *1*:271–276, 1980.

Verma, A. K., Rice, H. M., and Boutwell, R. K. Prostaglandins and skin tumor promotion: inhibition of tumor promoter-induced ornithine decarboxylase activity in epidermis by inhibitors of prostaglandin synthesis. Biochem. Biophys. Res. Commun., *79*:1160–1166, 1977.

Vojtek, A. B., and Der, C. J. Increasing complexity of the Ras signaling pathway. J. Biol. Chem., *273*:19925–19928, 1998.

Ward, E. J. Persistent and heritable structural damage induced in heterochromatic DNA from rat liver by *N*-nitrosodimethylamine. Biochemistry, *26*:1709–1717, 1987.

Weigel, N. L. Steroid hormone receptors and their regulation by phosphorylation. Biochem. J., *319*:657–667, 1996.

Whitlock, J. P., Jr. Mechanistic aspects of dioxin action. Chem. Res. Toxicol., *6*:754–763, 1993.

Williams, G. M., and Watanabe, K. Quantitative kinetics of development of *N*-2-fluorenylacetamide-induced, altered (hyperplastic) hepatocellular foci resistant to iron accumulation and of their reversion or persistence following removal of carcinogen. J. Natl. Cancer Inst., *61*:113–121, 1978.

Wörner, W., and Schrenk, D. 2,3,7,8-Tetrachlorodibenzo-*p*-dioxin suppresses apoptosis and leads to hyperphosphorylation of p53 in rat hepatocytes. Environ. Toxicol. Pharmacol., *6*:239–247, 1998.

Wright, S. C., Zhong, J., and Larrick, J. W. Inhibition of apoptosis as a mechanism of tumor promotion. FASEB J., *8*:654–660, 1994.

Wu, X., and Levine, A. J. p53 and E2F-1 cooperate to mediate apoptosis. Proc. Natl. Acad. Sci. U.S.A., *91*:3602–3606, 1994.

Xu, Y.-D., Dragan, Y., Young, T., and Pitot, H. The effect of the format of administration and the total dose of phenobarbital on altered hepatic foci following initiation in female rats with diethylnitrosamine. Carcinogenesis, *12*:1009–1016, 1991.

Xu, Y.-H., Sattler, G. L., and Pitot, H. C. A method for the comparative study of replicative DNA synthesis in GGT-positive and GGT-negative hepatocytes in primary culture isolated from carcinogen-treated rats. In Vitro Cell. Dev. Biol., *24*:995–1000, 1988.

Xu, Y.-h., Campbell, H. A., Sattler, G. L., Hendrich, S., Maronpot, R., Sato, K., and Pitot, H. C. Quantitative stereological analysis of the effects of age and sex on multistage hepatocarcinogenesis in the rat by use of four cytochemical markers. Cancer Res., *50*:472–479, 1990.

Yamane, H. K., and Fung, B. K.-K. Covalent modifications of G-proteins. Annu. Rev. Pharmacol. Toxicol., *32*:201–241, 1993.

Zatonski, W., Becher, H., and Lissowska, J. Smoking cessation: intermediate nonsmoking periods and reduction of laryngeal cancer risk. J. Natl. Cancer Inst., *82*:1427–1428, 1990.

Zeise, L., Wilson, R., and Crouch, E. A. C. Dose-response relationships for carcinogens: a review. Environ. Health Perspect., *73*:259–308, 1987.

Zhang, R., Haag, J. D., and Gould, M. N. Quantitating the frequency of initiation and cH-ras mutation in *in situ* N-methyl-N-nitrosourea-exposed rat mammary gland. Cell Growth Differ., *2*:1–6, 1991.

8

The Natural History of Neoplastic Development: Host Effects During Carcinogenesis

In the last chapter, characteristics and mechanisms of the early stages of neoplastic development—initiation and promotion—were presented as being the result of cellular and molecular changes induced by specific carcinogenic agents. However, one must not forget that a neoplasm, by definition, develops within a complete, viable, multicellular organism. In a later chapter (Chapter 14) the "transformation" of normal cells to cells having distinctive characteristics while cultured in vitro is considered. However, in order to relate such transformation in vitro to the neoplastic process in vivo, the whole animal must be utilized as a testing arena in order to determine the neoplastic potential of cells that have been altered in culture.

The host plays a variety of modifying roles in carcinogenesis as the result of its interaction with exogenous modifying factors, factors present within the organism (termed endogenous modifiers), or both. For all general categories of carcinogenic agents—chemicals, viruses, radiation, and genetics—the interplay of exogenous and endogenous modifiers with the host as defined both phenotypically and genotypically is a major factor in the development of neoplasia.

The stage of neoplastic development that appears most susceptible to the action of exogenous and endogenous modifiers is promotion. On the other hand, genetic factors, which may be less susceptible to modification, may play a role at more than one stage in neoplastic development. Just as the host-tumor relationship (Chapters 17, 18, and 19) is critical to our ultimate understanding of the control and therapy of established neoplastic disease, a complete comprehension of host effects during carcinogenesis may be vital for the practical prevention of neoplasia or termination of its natural history prior to significant clinical effects in the host.

ENDOGENOUS MODIFIERS

Within the organism, a variety of substances can affect the development of neoplasia. Some of these are products of specific genes within the organism, some of which have already been discussed (Chapter 5). Others are factors inherent in the development of the organism, as well as hormones and related endogenous components that under normal circumstances maintain the "internal milieu" of the organism. As has been pointed out, several of these latter factors are carcinogenic in their own right and thus might be important in the development of spontaneous neoplasia (Pitot, 1993).

Genetic Modifiers in Spontaneous and Chemically Induced Carcinogenesis

The most basic of the endogenous factors that may modify the process of carcinogenesis is the genetic constitution of the host and the resultant gene products produced by the expression of a number of "modifier" genes, many of which were discussed in Chapter 5. However, it is important to distinguish between such "modifying" genes and those genes, tumor suppressor genes and proto-oncogenes, that are directly involved in the origin of the stages of initiation and progression (see Chapters 5 and 9). Modifying genes, discussed in Chapter 5, can generally be grouped as those involved in xenobiotic metabolism and the major histocompatibility complex (MHC) in both humans and animals. In animals, a number of modifying genes do not appear to be involved in either xenobiotic metabolism or in the MHC system (Drinkwater, 1995; Table 5.16). The functions of the products of several of these genes are known, whereas others are only speculative. A genetic alteration in the MHC in the rat has been associated with a marked increase in the development of liver cancer in males and breast cancer in females (Melhem et al., 1991). Similarly, in several mouse strains differing genetically in the MHC (termed H-2 in the mouse), substantial differences in the incidence of neoplasms of the liver, lung, mammae, ovary, and uterus were seen and correlated with different alleles of the H-2 locus (cf. Smith and Walford, 1978). These situations may be analogous to that seen with the relationship of specific MHC alleles and an enhanced incidence of specific neoplasms in humans (Chapter 5). On the other hand, modifying genes in the development of neoplasia other than genes of xenobiotic metabolism and the MHC region in the human have not been extensively characterized. Table 8.1 shows several examples of such modifying genes that fall into a number of categories, including receptors or mutations in the G-CSF receptor gene, that are involved in the pathogenesis of severe congenital neutropenia with progression to acute myeloid leukemia in many cases (Dong et al., 1995). Enhanced susceptibility to prostate cancer has been seen with genetic polymorphisms in the vitamin D receptor and the androgen receptor (Ingles et al., 1997), while an increase in pulmonary cancer and a number of other cancers, especially in the black population, appears to be related to a deletion in the poly(ADP-ribose) polymerase gene (Bhatia et al., 1990). Interestingly, hereditary pancreatitis resulting from a mutation in the cationic trypsinogen gene increases the risk of pancreatic cancer dramatically (Lowenfels et al., 1997). Thus, it is likely from this and animal studies that there are numerous genes whose products exhibit a variety of different functions that may modify, in a positive or negative manner, the development of neoplasia.

Table 8.1 Modifying Genes in the Development of Cancer in the Human

Neoplasm	Modifying Gene, Locus, or Linkage	Function of Gene Product	Reference
Breast	Aromatase	Converts C19 androgens to estrogens	Kristensen et al., 2000
Acute myeloid leukemia	G-CSF receptor gene	Receptor for granulocyte colony-stimulating factor	Dong et al., 1995
Pancreas	Cationic trypsinogen gene	Precursor of proteolytic enzyme	Lowenfels et al., 1997
Prostate	AR	Androgen receptor	Ingles et al., 1997
	VDR	Vitamin D receptor	Ingles et al., 1997
Pulmonary cancer	PADPRP gene	Poly(ADP-ribose) polymerase	Bhatia et al., 1990

This is not unexpected in view of the discussion presented on polygenic inheritance of neoplasia in Chapter 5.

Genetic Factors in Viral Carcinogenesis

Host genes that regulate the expression of virus-induced leukemia in animals have been studied to a much greater extent than host genes involved in chemical and physical carcinogenesis (cf. Meruelo and Bach, 1983; Kozak et al., 1989). The susceptibility of mice to the Friend virus (FV), a typical oncogenic RNA virus, has been shown to be the result of a multiple-gene trait (cf. Steeves and Lilly, 1977). In particular, a locus in the host's genome termed the *Fv-1* locus on chromosome 4 significantly affects the susceptibility of the host to the virus. The function of the gene product of the *Fv-1* locus is not entirely clear. Recently, Best et al. (1996) have cloned the *Fv-1* gene and demonstrated that it appears to be derived from the *gag* region of an endogenous retrovirus unrelated to murine leukemia viruses. Since genetic restriction at the *Fv-1* locus results in failure of the Friend murine leukemia virus DNA to integrate into the host genome (cf. Axelrad, 1989), Goff (1996) has pointed out that the *Fv-1* gene product is able to block virus development during the early phase of the viral life cycle after reverse transcription but before establishment of the integrated provirus in the host genome. The site within the cell where the *Fv-1* gene product acts is uncertain. At least two alleles of this locus occur, and one may separate mouse strains into two types (N type and B type) depending on which of the two alleles is present in their genome. It is possible to characterize viruses as N-tropic or B-tropic—that is, whether the virus replicates in NIH (*N*-type) mice or in BALB/c (*B*-type) mice. Thus, the gene is quite important for the susceptibility of specific mouse strains to certain RNA oncogenic viruses.

Another genetic locus, the *Fv-2* gene, has a major effect on the response of mice to the Friend and to the Rauscher murine retroviruses. Mice recessive for this gene are completely resistant to these viruses, whereas heterozygotes and homozygotes for the normal gene product are susceptible. Risser (1979) suggested that the *Fv-2* locus codes for a specific hematopoietic differentiation antigen. More recently, Hoatlin et al. (1990) have presented evidence that the *Fv-2* protein controls the response to a leukemogenic membrane glycoprotein (gp55) encoded by the Friend spleen focus-forming virus and the hormone erythropoietin. Through such regulatory effects, the *Fv-2* gene product can modulate infection by the virus in hematopoietic tissue.

As shown in Table 8.2, at least three other *Fv* genes have been described, each of which regulates different aspects of the expression of the Friend virus. A large number of other genetic loci associated with expression of viruses or viral products have also been described in various strains of mice. In strain AKR mice and their hybrids, loci coding for the endogenous form of the virus have been found within their genomes—that is, the *Akv* locus localized to chromosome 7. The nomenclature for the latter locus has been changed to *Emr-11* (Bedigian et al., 1983). Other examples of such structural genes for endogenous viruses within the genome of the host have been described in the BALB/c strain of mouse (Kozak and Rowe, 1979), as well as another locus on chromosome 1 in at least five different mouse strains (Kozak and Rowe, 1980).

Although these genes have been most carefully studied in the mouse, similar genes have also been described in other species including the *Bvr-1* locus in the cat, which restricts the expression of a type-C RNA virus (O'Brien, 1976) and the *Bevi* locus on human chromosome 6, which controls the replication of baboon type-C virus in human cells (Lemons et al., 1977).

Hormones as Endogenous Modifiers of Carcinogenesis

In Chapter 3 the carcinogenic effects of a variety of hormones within the organism were presented. In Chapter 7 it was noted that in general the carcinogenic action of such endogenous

Table 8.2 Loci Affecting Leukemogenesis by Type C RNA Viruses in Mice

Genetic locus	Function	Chromosome Location	Dominance
Akv-1	Controls initial expression of virus in AKR mice and hybrids containing an AKR background	7	Susceptibility
Akv-2	Controls initial expression of virus in AKR mice and hybrids containing an AKR background	?	Susceptibility
Akvr-1	Resistance to viremia of AKR endogenous retrovirus and of virus-mediated lymphoma	?	Resistance[a]
Fv-1	Controls efficiency of initial virus infection	4	Resistance
Fv-2	Determines the response of mice to the spleen focus-forming virus component of FV preparations	9	Susceptibility
Fv-3	Controls the in vitro susceptibility of lymphocytes to the suppressive action of Friend murine leukemia virus	?	Resistance[b]
Fv-4	Controls resistance to NB-tropic Friend murine leukemia virus in wild mice	12	Resistance[c]
Fv-5	Controls the types of erythropoiesis induced by Friend erythroleukemia virus	?	Expression is codominant[d]
Rfv-1	Resistance to FV associated with *H-2G* or *H-2D* region	17	Resistance
Rfv-2	Resistance to FV associated with the *H-2K* or *H-2L* region	17	Resistance
f	Flexed—involved in hereditary anemia—confers resistance to Friend virus by reducing available erythroid precursors	?	Resistance
Gv-1	Controls expression of G_{IX} antigen	17 or 4 (?)	Expression is semidominant
Gv-2	Controls expression of G_{IX} antigen	7	Expression is dominant
Rgv-1	Confers resistance to Gross virus-induced leukemia and is linked to *H-2*	17	Resistance
Rgv-2	Confers resistance to Gross virus-induced leukemia; remains a statistical construct and may turn out to be *Fv-1*	?	Resistance
Rrv-1	Influences resistance to the A-RadLV strain	17	?
S1	Steel—a mutation involved in hereditary anemia, which reduces susceptibility to FV by decreasing available erythroid targets for infection	?	Resistance
W	Dominant spotting—involved in hereditary anemia, causes reduction of erythroid precursors for FV	?	Resistance
Rec-1	Required for binding of Rauscher murine leukemia virus envelope protein, gp70	5	Susceptibility[e]
Fhe	Controls susceptibility to Friend helper virus erythroplastosis	?	Resistance[f]
Rmcf	Restricts the replication of MCF viruses	5	Resistance[g]
Ram-1	Required for binding of amphotropic murine leukemia virus to cell	8	Susceptibility[h]

Modified from Meruelo and McDevitt, 1978, with the following additions: [a]Gardner et al., 1980; [b]Odaka, 1973; [c]Odaka et al., 1981; [d]Shibuya et al., 1982; [e]Hilkens et al., 1979; [f]Silver and Fredrickson, 1983; [g]Hartley et al., 1983; [h]Gazdar et al., 1977.

hormones is their effectiveness as promoting agents. Thus, it would be expected that hormones play a significant role as endogenous modifiers within a multicellular organism.

As noted in Chapter 3, particularly Figures 3.19 and 3.20 as well as Table 3.7, dramatic changes in circulating levels of specific hormones maintained for long periods of time can result in the development of neoplasms, especially in endocrine tissues. In a similar manner, alteration of internal levels of several different hormones can affect the development of neoplasia induced by chemicals and viruses. One of the earlier studies on the effects of alterations in the endocrine status of rats on their susceptibility to chemical hepatocarcinogens was carried out by Bielschowsky (1961). Dramatic inhibition of the development of hepatic neoplasms by thyroidectomy and adrenalectomy was noted. Administration of growth hormone or cortisone to thyroidectomized animals reversed this inhibition to a very great degree (Figure 8.1). Since these original studies, a number of similar investigations have been carried out. Most of these studies involve carcinogenesis of the liver or mammary gland (Table 8.3). In rat liver, the effects described by Bielschowsky have been extended by use of a number of different chemical carcinogens. The predominant effect noted has been an inhibition of carcinogenesis—with the exception of ovariectomy in both the mouse and the rat, which has been reported to enhance carcinogenesis by 2-AAF and urethane respectively (Table 8.3). Hypophysectomy inhibited or eliminated carcinogenesis in rat liver and mammary gland by several different chemical carcinogens with a notable exception of dimethylnitrosamine (Yamamoto and Weisburger, 1977). Orchiectomy inhibits carcinogenesis in rat and mouse liver by several different chemical carcinogens, as it did also in one study in rat kidney (Takizawa and Hirose, 1978). Ovariectomy inhibits carcinogenesis in rat mammary glands by both ionizing radiation and DMBA (Table

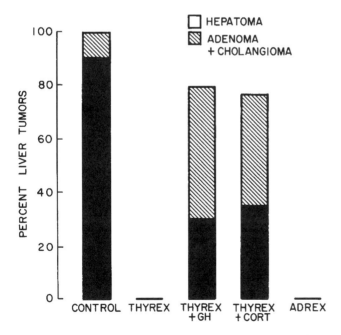

Figure 8.1   The effect of the endocrine status of male rats given 2-acetylaminofluorene on the induction of liver neoplasms. THYREX, thyroidectomized; ADREX, adrenalectomized; GH, growth hormone; CORT, cortisone. (After Bielschowsky, 1961.)

Table 8.3 The Effect of Endocrine Ablations on Carcinogenesis in Animals

Procedure	Tissue	Carcinogen	Effect	Reference
Adrenalectomy	Rat liver	2-AAF	No effect	Reuber, 1969
	Rat mammary gland	DMBA	Enhancement	Carter et al., 1988
Hypophysectomy	Rat liver	2-AAF	Inhibition	Reuber, 1969
	Rat liver	Aflatoxin B_1	Inhibition	Goodall & Butler, 1969
	Rat liver	3′Me-DAB	Inhibition	Griffin et al., 1953
	Rat liver	DMN	No effect	Lee & Goodall, 1968
	Rat mammary gland	DMBA	Inhibition	Carter et al., 1988
Orchiectomy	Rat liver	DEN/AAF	Inhibition	Matsuura et al., 1994
	Rat liver	2-AAF	Inhibition	Tokumo et al., 1993
	Mouse liver	Urethan	Inhibition	Vesselinovitch & Mihailovich, 1967
	Rat kidney	N-nitrosobutylurea	Inhibition	Takizawa & Hirose, 1978
	Rat liver	Aflatoxin/CQ_4	Inhibition	Cardeilhac & Nair, 1973
	Rat colon	azoxymethane	Enhancement	Izbicki et al., 1990
Ovariectomy	Rat liver	2-AAF	Enhancement	Mulay & O'Gara, 1962
			No effect	Katayama et al., 1984
	Mouse liver	Urethane	Enhancement	Vesselinovitch & Mihailovich, 1967
	Mouse kidney and partial hepatectomy	Ethylnitrosourea	Enhancement	Vesselinovitch et al., 1973
	Rat mammary gland	Ionizing radiation	Inhibition	Solleveld et al., 1986
	Rat mammary gland	DMBA	Inhibition	cf. Russo and Russo, 1996
Sialoadenectomy	Mouse mammary gland (C3H/HeN strain)	None	Inhibition	Kurachi et al., 1985
Thyroidectomy	Rat liver	2-AAF	Inhibition	Reuber, 1969

8.3). In both rats and mice, ovariectomy appeared to enhance chemical carcinogenesis in liver and in mouse kidney when a partial hepatectomy was performed simultaneously (Vesselinovitch et al., 1973). Interestingly, sialoadenectomy (removal of the submandibular salivary gland) inhibited spontaneous mouse mammary carcinogenesis (Kurachi et al., 1985). In addition, the number of colonic tumors induced by azoxymethane in rats was increased by surgical orchiectomy, but most efficiently by chemical orchiectomy plus the antiandrogen cyproterone acetate (Izbicki et al., 1990).

Sex Hormones as Endogenous Modifiers of Carcinogenesis

As noted in Table 8.3, removal of the primary sources of male and female hormones in mammals can have significant effects on chemical and radiation carcinogenesis. Thus, one must conclude that sex hormones can play a significant role as endogenous modifiers in carcinogenesis. This should already be obvious from the statistical information presented in Chapter 1 and becomes even more so from the epidemiological studies of human cancer (Chapter 11). In experimental animals, a highly significant effect of sex on chemical carcinogenesis is seen in the liver. With several aromatic amine carcinogens, especially 2-AAF, hepatoma incidence is much higher in the male than in the female, as is the incidence of preneoplastic lesions after 2-AAF administration (Tokumo et al., 1993). Interestingly, N-hydroxy-AAF is equally carcinogenic for both sexes in several strains of rats. In mice, there is a significant effect of the sex of the animal on spontaneous mouse hepatoma incidence (Table 8.4). The incidence of hepatomas in female mice is slightly to markedly lower than the incidence of such lesions in males (Grasso and Hardy, 1975). Induced alterations in the endogenous sex hormone concentrations also affect the incidence of mouse hepatomas. Breeding enhanced the incidence of hepatomas in males but inhibited the incidence in females (Burns and Schenken, 1943a,b). Castration of male C3H mice reduced the incidence of hepatomas in these animals by one-third but had little influence in CBA mice (Andervont, 1950). The incidence of hepatic neoplasms was increased in female C3H mice treated with testosterone (Agnew and Gardner, 1952). Thus, with few exceptions, one may conclude that in the mouse, androgens promote hepatocarcinogenesis while estrogenic hormones tend to inhibit this process (Poole and Drinkwater, 1996).

The mechanism for this differential effect of sex on hepatocarcinogenesis is not entirely clear, but to some extent it is a function of the control of xenobiotic metabolism of endogenous and exogenous carcinogenic agents. Early studies by Lotlikar (1970) demonstrated that the enzymic esterification of 2-N-hydroxy-AAF was significantly higher in the male than in the female rat, while earlier studies by this investigator (Lotlikar et al., 1964) demonstrated that hypophysectomy decreased the urinary excretion of N-hydroxy-AAF. Weisburger et al. (1964) had earlier reported a difference in the excretion of hydroxylated forms of 2-AAF by males and females. Male rats are also more sensitive than females to the toxic actions of aflatoxin B_1 (Kamdem et al., 1982).

A more subtle mechanism of hormonal modification of carcinogenesis may be seen in the effects of gonadectomy and sex hormone administration during the neonatal period. This "imprinting" of the expression of genes of xenobiotic and steroid metabolism by hormones and xenobiotics, as distinguished from genetic imprinting (Chapter 5), is a more general phenomenon, the molecular basis of which is unclear (Skett and Gustafsson, 1979). Such "imprinting" may result from the exposure of newborn rats to a number of drugs including phenobarbital (Haake and Safe, 1988), thus effecting a more or less permanent increase in specific xenobiotic enzymes that can alter the metabolism of carcinogens in later life (Faris and Campbell, 1981). In addition, carcinogens themselves may imprint genes of xenobiotic metabolism when administered during the neonatal period (Herd and Greene, 1980; Soyka, 1980). However, with reference to sex hormones, testosterone administered in the neonatal period causes a subsequent enhancement of specific cytochrome P450 forms (Chang and Bellward, 1996; Shimada et al., 1987) as well as enzymes of steroid metabolism (Chang and Bellward, 1996; cf. Skett and Gustafsson, 1979). Administration of diethylstilbesterol, a potent synthetic estrogen, during the neonatal period alters the capacity of adult female rats to form and/or dispose of DNA adducts of aflatoxin B_1 metabolites after a single dose of the carcinogen to the adult (Lamartiniere, 1990).

Table 8.4 Incidence of Hepatomas in Various Strains of Mice

Strain	Substrain	Number		Incidence, %	
		Male	Female	Male	Female
C3H					
		20	10	20	0
		320	–	26	–
		19	–	18	–
		102	85	–	
	f	96	–	71	–
	e	79	–	78	–
	f	108	–	57	–
	Y/AYA	63	–	100	–
	Y/A$_a$	94	–	88	–
	eB/Fe	←——134——→		←——7——→	
	AHe	10		30 (20 m^a)	
	eB/De			90	59
	f/He			–	17
	HeO	323		32	
BALB/c					
		49	51		Nil
		30	–	Nil	–
		–	131	–	<1
Charles River					
		137	144	2	1.5
		4	4	Nil	Nil
A					
		←——400——→		←——1.5——→	
		←——?——→		←——1——→	
		5	5	0	0
		–	20	–	Nil
	AHe	39	36	7	Nil
CF					
	CF-W	107	119	Nil	Nil
	CF-W	23	30	Nil	Nil
	CF-1	125	117	15	Nil
	CF-1	288	297	20 (0.7m^a)	13
C57					
	BL	?10	?10	1	1
	BL	143	171	<1	<1
	IF	19	31	0	3
	BL/6/C3H	79	87	10	Nil
	BL/6/AKR	90	82	5	1.0
Y		←——129——→		←——1.6——→	
C		–	150	–	Nil
STS		–	18	–	Nil
DBA/2eBDE				–	5
HR/De				12	6

(table continues)

Table 8.4   (continued)

Strain	Substrain	Number		Incidence, %	
		Male	Female	Male	Female
Wild Mice				9	3
CBA/Cb/Se		37	47	11	4
ICR		28	–	Nil	–
RF		262	–	3	–
ASH CS1		429	420	5	Nil
				(0.2m)[a]	
TF1		107	91	13 (2m)[a]	5
CF-LP		240	24	16 (2m)[a]	6
BDH-SPF		106	112	2	0

[a]malignant tumors.
From Grasso and Hardy, 1975, with permission of the authors and publisher. The reader is referred to the original publication for references to the individual substrains.

Inhibition of Carcinogenesis by Hormones

Although a number of hormones may act as endogenous carcinogens, presumably through their promoting action (Pitot, 1993), in several examples treatment with exogenous hormones actually inhibited the development of neoplasia. Chedid et al. (1980) demonstrated that the administration of corticosteroids as well as adrenocorticotrophic hormone (ACTH) inhibited the development of hepatocellular carcinomas after administration of aflatoxin B_1. Similarly, administration of the neural hormone neurotensin inhibited the induction of pancreatic carcinomas by azaserine in rats (Tatsuta et al., 1991). This latter finding was somewhat surprising, since chronic administration of this hormone had previously been shown to induce growth of the pancreas as well as to enhance exocrine pancreatic secretion. The mechanism of this effect was not clear; but in another observation by Russo et al. (1990), a biological mechanism for the effect of an exogenous hormone was proposed. These investigators had observed that mammary carcinogenesis is inhibited in rats that had completed a pregnancy prior to exposure to the carcinogenic polycyclic hydrocarbon DMBA. As a mechanism, they proposed that the placental hormone, chorionic gonadotropin (hCG), was the mediator of these effects. They demonstrated that administration of hCG simulated mammary gland differentiation, depressing the labeling indices of the terminal structures in the glands of hCG-treated animals. This induction of terminal differentiation thus prevented the "fixation" of DMBA initiation (Chapter 7) and inhibited carcinogenesis by this agent. The potential for the use of hCG in the human as a chemopreventative agent for mammary cancer has never been adequately studied or exploited.

Endogenous Hormones as Modifiers of Viral Carcinogenesis

Since genetic factors of the host are important in the expression of oncogenic viruses in vivo, one might suspect that hormones and growth factors, as products of specific genes in the host, might affect the expression of viruses within the host. A prime example of such an effect is the induction of transcription of the mouse mammary tumor virus (MMTV) genome by glucocorticoids (cf. Beato, 1991). Treatment of cells with one or more integrated copies of the MMTV genome with glucocorticoids leads to an accumulation of MMTV particles (cf. Beato, 1991). The mechanism of this hormonal stimulation involves the interaction of glucocorticoid and progestin receptors with a specific hormone-responsive element (HRE) present in a proximal region of the U3 portion of the long terminal repeat (LTR) (see Chapter 4). This HRE contains four overlapping recognition sites to which the activated receptors bind (cf. Günzburg and Salmons, 1992). In many cells the levels of glucocorticoid and progestin receptors appear to be the limiting factor in MMTV transcription (cf. Beato, 1991). However, other hormones and growth factors, including prolactin and transforming growth factor β, also appear to modulate expression of MMTV (cf. Beato, 1991; Munoz and Bolander, 1989). In these latter instances, the exact mechanism by which these factors enhance or inhibit MMTV transcription is not clear at present. Other oncogenic viruses, including the SV40 DNA papovavirus (Chapter 4), contain hormone-responsive elements in their genomes that may, in turn, alter the expression of the virus in the host (e.g., Zuo et al., 1997). From these few examples, then, one may appreciate the dramatic effects of hormones as endogenous modifiers in virtually all types of carcinogenesis.

Aging as an Endogenous Modifier of Carcinogenesis

Cancer is a disease that increases with age both in the human and in animal populations that have been studied thus far. Persons 65 years of age and older bear the greatest burden of cancer, with 55% of all neoplasms occurring in this age group (Yancik and Ries, 1991). In the human, however, this increase is not continuous from birth in that, from shortly after birth until the age of puberty, in the United States and many other Western countries, cancer is the second most common cause of death from disease (Chapter 1). The high incidence of cancer at an early stage appears to reflect genetic as well as intrauterine and neonatal environmental influences. However, the number of individuals with cancer at this early age is an extremely small fraction of the total, as can be seen in Figure 8.2. The curve in Figure 8.2 is actually a composite of a number of curves, each for a specific histogenetic type of neoplasm. Examples of the general types of curves are shown in Figure 8.3A and B. In this instance, a number of the major cancers seen in older age groups—i.e., prostate, rectum, pancreas, etc.—increase exponentially after midlife (Figure 8.3A). However, in several neoplasms more commonly seen in the younger age groups, the curves are quite different, as noted in Figure 8.3B. Neoplasms of the bone as well as acute lymphoblastic leukemia show a biphasic curve, with a significant increase in the younger age groups, a low plateau during middle age, and then a continuing increase in the older age groups above age 55. Cancer of the testis may be considered a cancer of young adults, with its peak incidence at about 30 years of age, decreasing then almost exponentially for most of the remainder of the life span, with a small increase between ages 70 and 80. A somewhat different pattern of breast cancer incidence in the human is noted, with a relatively rapid increase between ages 20 and 40 and a flattening out of the curve after age 40, most dramatically seen in the 40- to 50-year-old range, with increases as age increases after that (Kessler, 1992). Interestingly, there is a gradual decline in breast cancer incidence after age 55 in Japanese women (Kodama et al., 1992).

Spontaneous carcinogenesis in rodents is also age-related, with relatively few neoplasms appearing within the first 12 months in most but not all strains (Tamano et al., 1988; Yamate et al., 1990; Chandra and Frith, 1992a,b). Interestingly, in a comparison of cancer mortality in the Beagle dog and humans, Albert et al. (1994) demonstrated that the age dependence and total cancer mortality was the same in both sexes in both species, although the total cancer mortality was somewhat greater in female Beagles owing primarily to an increase in the incidence of

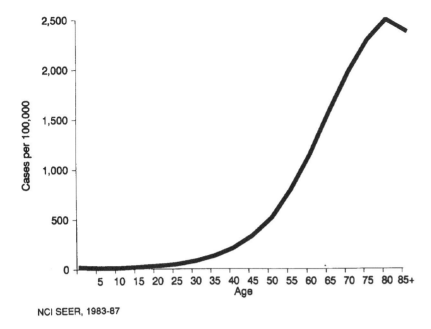

NCI SEER, 1983-87

Figure 8.2 Cancer incidence rates by 5-year age groups including all races and both sexes. The data for this figure are taken from the National Cancer Institute SEER program from 1983 to 1987. (Adapted from Yancik and Ries, 1991, with permission of authors and publisher.)

breast cancer. Thus, it is likely that, in general, there is little if any difference in the effect of aging on spontaneous carcinogenesis in humans and domesticated and experimental animals.

The reason for the dramatic increase in both the incidence and death rate from cancer as a function of increasing age in these mammalian species is not entirely clear. The two major theories to explain this phenomenon are the following: (1) the aging process itself is responsible for this high incidence of neoplasia; (2) the increasing cancer incidence is due to a continuous effect of environmental influences as organisms age; or (3) both (1) and (2). It is unlikely that specific genetic mechanisms, such as those that may play a role in prepubertal cancer incidence, are involved. Peto et al. (1975) attempted to distinguish experimentally between environmental and intrinsic aging as mechanisms for the increased incidence of neoplasms seen with advancing age, using skin tumor induction in mice by multiple applications of benzo[a]pyrene as a model system.

These authors predicted results from such an experiment on the basis of the two theories stated above. These predictions are seen in Figure 8.4. In hypothesis I, the incidence rate of neoplasia depends wholly on age and not at all on the duration of the treatment (exposure). In hypothesis II, the incidence rate depends wholly on the duration of the treatment (exposure) but not at all on age. These are the two extreme predictions, but the data obtained experimentally (Peto et al., 1975) agree very closely with hypothesis II. These authors concluded that skin carcinogenesis by this agent in this model system was independent of any intrinsic effects of aging, such as failing immunosurveillance (Chapter 19) or age-related hormonal alterations.

When a protocol of epidermal carcinogenesis, which distinguishes the stages of initiation and promotion, is employed in the mouse, an intrinsic effect of the aging animal, especially on the latter process, may be discerned. Van Duuren et al. (1975) were the first to show a general decrease in tumor production when promotion by TPA was carried out at later ages. Later studies by Stenbäck et al. (1981) confirmed this finding and indicated a significant decrease in the

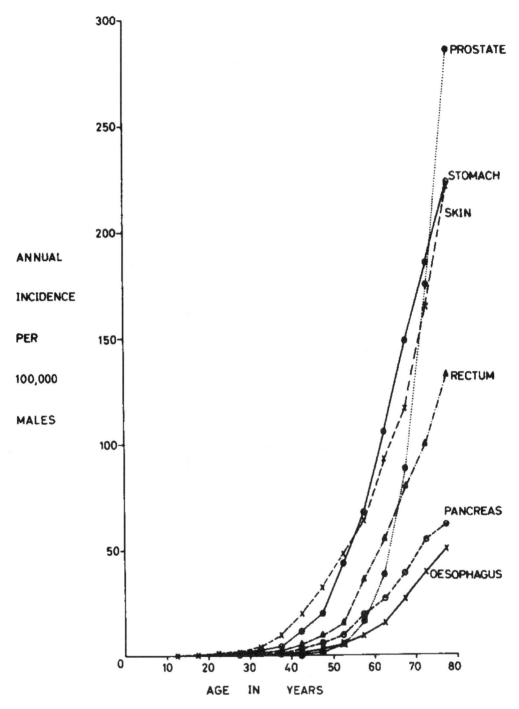

Figure 8.3A The pattern of continued increase of incidence in several different types of cancer from adolescence to old age.

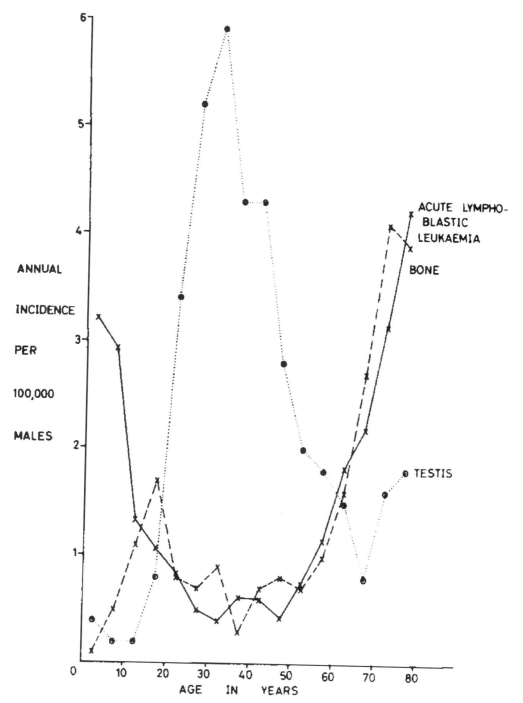

Figure 8.3B   The pattern of the peak incidence of cancer in the young followed by a decline and in some cases a secondary rise in the elderly. (Adapted from Miller, 1980, with permission of author and publisher.)

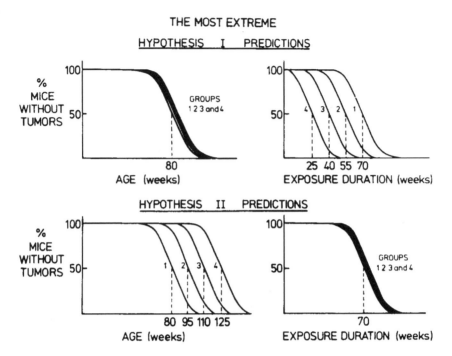

THE MOST EXTREME
HYPOTHESIS   I   PREDICTIONS

HYPOTHESIS   II   PREDICTIONS

Figure 8.4   Life tables depicting percentages of mice without tumors against age and duration of exposure to benzo[a]pyrene under hypotheses I and II. Details of the hypotheses are given in the text. (From Peto et al., 1975, with permission of the authors and publisher.)

promotional efficacy of TPA in aging mice, as evidenced by epidermal carcinogenesis initiated with DMBA on the skin. On the other hand, Loehrke et al. (1983) saw no such effect when initiation was carried out systemically by intragastric administration of DMBA. Other data indicate that phenobarbital may be somewhat more effective in promoting the growth and appearance of hepatocellular foci (Chapter 7) in aged as compared with young rats (Ward, 1983).

Mechanisms of the Effect of Aging on Carcinogenesis

In view of Peto's finding that carcinogenesis was dependent on the presence of the carcinogen rather than the age of the animal, one possible mechanism for the effect of aging is a differential effect of chemical carcinogens in inducing neoplasia as a function of age. Anisimov has reviewed much of the data on organ-specific carcinogenesis by a variety of chemicals and radiation and found no distinct pattern of modification of the carcinogenic effect by the aging process (Anisimov, 1989). Somewhat similar discrepancies have been seen in a few examples of chemical carcinogenesis in aging humans (Leutzinger and Richie, 1995). An interesting effect of aging was noted in the development of sarcomas from foreign-body implantation in rats (Paulini et al., 1975). In this study, young animals were seen to first develop malignant mesenchymal neoplasms after a mean of 17.2 months, whereas old rats had developed similar lesions after only 6.3 months. Furthermore, Lijinsky et al. (1993) demonstrated that, with rare exceptions, the administration of chemical carcinogens to rats did not alter the incidence of spontaneous neoplasms occurring with age.

Another potential mechanism of the increased incidence of neoplasia with age is that the immune system fails to suppress spontaneous and induced neoplasms. In a later chapter (Chapter 19) there is a more extensive discussion of the immune system in relation to carcinogenesis and neoplasia. In old animals, the thymus, an important organ of the immune system, is atrophic. This is accompanied by excessive apoptosis of mature lymphocytes from the thymus (T lymphocytes) in humans (Phelouzat et al., 1996). There is also an increase in the proportion of committed or memory-type T (thymic) lymphocytes as compared with naïve T cells and a decline in the response of naïve T cells to activation and their capacity to enter the cell cycle (Globerson, 1995). In part, this may be due to a decline in the production of interleukin-2, a growth factor for T lymphocytes (Pahlavani and Richardson, 1996). Natural killer (NK) cell functions in humans and mice are somewhat discrepant. In the mouse, there is a profound loss of NK cell function in spleen and lymph nodes in older animals, while in the human, blood-derived NK cells show little if any age effect (Miller, 1996). Both T cell–mediated immunity and NK-cell cytotoxicity have been implicated in the host immune response to some neoplasms (Chapter 19). Thus, the aging process, in modifying this immune response, may allow the growth of neoplasms that would otherwise be suppressed by the immune response.

Just as aging of the immune response is a theoretical mechanism for the increased incidence of cancer seen in the aged, our increasing understanding of genes involved in cellular senescence and apoptosis may also offer a genetic or inherent mechanism for the effect of aging resulting in an increased incidence of neoplasia (Barrett et al., 1994; Benson et al., 1996). Such a hypothesis, however, is not in line with the experiment of Peto (1975; Figure 8.4), which argues that the aging process itself is not a major factor in the increased incidence of neoplasia noted in older organisms. A better understanding of the interrelated mechanisms of the process of aging and of neoplasia offers promise of potential applications of this area to the control of neoplastic disease.

EXOGENOUS MODIFIERS

In a general sense, all carcinogenic agents may be considered exogenous modifiers of carcinogenesis. However, below are discussed the effects of specific agents and processes not usually considered to be carcinogenic as exogenous modifiers of the various stages of carcinogenesis. Here it becomes obvious that, because of the characteristics of the stage of tumor promotion in its responsiveness to environmental factors, both endogenous and exogenous, most exogenous agents affecting carcinogenesis appear to act at the stage of tumor promotion. Furthermore, agents exhibiting promoting activity may also inhibit the effect of some carcinogens when given prior to or concomitant with a complete carcinogen or an initiating agent (Chapter 7).

Effects of Drugs and Other Agents and Procedures on the Stages of Carcinogenesis

Earlier in this chapter, it was already noted that changes in hormones can alter the process of carcinogenesis, probably through their effects on the stage of promotion. However, in view of the requirement for the metabolism of many complete carcinogenic agents to a reactive form, which is probably the actual initiating agent, modifications of the metabolic activation by exogenous agents may lead to alterations in the efficiency and/or repair of the initiation process. In Chapter 3, the effect of the administration of mixtures of carcinogenic agents was briefly considered. The discussion here focuses on the effect of combining carcinogenic agents, which can result in an enhancement or synergistic effect or, conversely, an inhibitory or antagonistic effect.

In a recent review, Berger (1995) used the term *synergism* when a combination of carcinogens exerts an effect exceeding the arithmetic sum of the effects of the chemicals individually. In the extreme, combinations of chemicals each at a specific dose may be carcinogenic while each chemical administered individually at the same dose is noncarcinogenic. *Antagonism* is defined as the combination of carcinogens exerting an effect less than additive or even lower than the effect of one of the carcinogens singly. Berger (1995) has reviewed a number of the synergistic and antagonistic effects of binary and ternary mixtures of chemical carcinogens. The variables associated with the carcinogenic effect of combinations of chemicals are multiple, including the sequence of the administration of the individual chemicals, the toxicity of one or more of the members of the mixture at the doses employed, and the organ specificity of the individual agents. In some instances, combinations of carcinogens led to the development of neoplasms of tissues that are not usually induced by either of the agents employed (cf. Newberne and Connor, 1980). In an earlier study, Berger et al. (1987) administered to rats a mixture of three different carcinogenic nitrosamines, each at doses that were not carcinogenic when given alone. The mixture was carcinogenic. In a series of studies by Ito and colleagues (Takayama et al., 1989; Fukushima et al., 1991; Uwagawa et al., 1991), the administration of up to 40 carcinogenic agents or multiple mixtures of carcinogenic with noncarcinogenic agents resulted, as expected, in a variety of effects, both synergistic and additive, but no attempt at determining mechanisms was undertaken with these extremely complex experiments. In some instances, a change in the solvent in which the carcinogenic agent is applied to tissues such as skin may enhance the carcinogenic action of such an agent, e.g., specific polycyclic hydrocarbons (Warshawsky et al., 1993). While the toxicity of one or more components of the mixture may tend to inhibit the carcinogenic effect of the mixture, in other instances, especially in hepatocarcinogenesis, toxicity results in an enhancement of the proliferative activity of hepatocytes, thereby enhancing the carcinogenic action of carcinogenic agents even at low doses (Taylor et al., 1974; Pitot et al., 1978). Enhancing effects of the hepatoproliferative agent α-hexachlorocyclohexane have been demonstrated with several hepatocarcinogens (Schulte-Hermann and Parzefall, 1981).

Chemical inhibition of carcinogenesis has been most extensively studied during hepatocarcinogenesis. The carcinogenic action of some nitrosamines and azo dyes is inhibited by the prior or simultaneous administration of carcinogenic polycyclic hydrocarbons, the latter not usually considered as complete carcinogens for the liver (cf. Venkatesan et al., 1970). The inhibition of azo dye hepatocarcinogenesis by benzimidazole derivatives such as chloramphenicol and diethylstilbesterol (Akao and Kuroda, 1978; Blunck et al., 1971/1972) gives further examples of this inhibition. A most likely mechanism for the inhibition of carcinogenesis of the liver by these agents is their effect on altering the metabolism of the carcinogen and inhibiting the formation of reactive metabolites (Berger, 1995). Both β-naphthoflavone and pregnenolone-16α-carbonitrile are inducers of xenobiotic metabolism and inhibitors of hepatocarcinogenesis induced by dimethylnitrosamine (Argus et al., 1978). In other tissues, chloroform administration inhibits 1,2-dimethylhydrazine-induced gastrointestinal tract neoplasms in rats (Daniel et al., 1989), while some polycyclic hydrocarbons that are noncarcinogenic or weakly carcinogenic inhibit initiation of epidermal carcinogenesis by DMBA or benzo[a]pyrene (cf. Berger, 1995). Inhibition of hepatocarcinogenesis by azo dyes can also be accomplished by surgical alteration of the blood supply of the liver to produce a portacaval anastomosis, that is, diversion of the portal blood supply from the liver to the systemic circulation via the vena cava (Ricco et al., 1977). Thus, one can appreciate that the addition of agents or procedures to simple carcinogenic experiments may produce a variety of alterations in the process of carcinogenesis, especially experimental hepatocarcinogenesis. While many of these agents act to alter the stage of initiation, others may affect the stages of promotion and/or progression. The next section shows a similar complexity of dietary effects on carcinogenesis.

Dietary Factors Influencing Stages of Carcinogenesis

One of the major exogenous modifiers of carcinogenesis is diet (cf. Rogers et al., 1993). Effectors of such modification include the caloric content of the diet; its major constituents, such as protein, lipid, and carbohydrate; and trace factors in the diet such as various vitamins, minerals, and contaminants. Dietary contaminants, where their identity is known, may exert direct carcinogenic effects. Examples of such are aflatoxin B_1, lipid peroxides, and toxic metals. Since these are covered in other sections, the composition of the diet in relation to normal constituents is considered here.

Caloric Restriction

One of the earliest observations on the dietary modification of carcinogenesis was the effect of caloric restriction on tumor incidence. This relatively simple modification significantly decreased tumor incidence, both experimentally induced by chemicals and spontaneously induced in animals and possibly in humans. An early example of this effect was the reduction of the incidence of skin tumors induced by dibenz[a,h]anthracene by more than one-half by stringent caloric restriction (cf. Tannenbaum, 1947). In addition, caloric restriction to about 50% of ad libitum markedly reduced the incidence of spontaneous mammary tumors (Sarkar et al., 1982) as well as of pulmonary neoplasms, hepatomas, and leukemias in mice. Tucker (1979) demonstrated that, under the conditions of caloric restriction described by Tannenbaum, mice lived longer and exhibited fewer hepatic neoplasms than mice fed ad libitum. The effect was much more marked in the males than in the females. Caloric restriction of 25% reduced both lung and lymphoid tumors, but the most dramatic decrease was seen in the incidence of hepatic neoplasms (Conybeare, 1980). On the other hand, caloric restriction had no effect on the progression of hyperplastic nodules to hepatocellular carcinoma (M.S. Rao et al., 1983); this suggested that both the development and the stage of tumor progression are not sensitive to this dietary effect.

Concomitant with the decrease in spontaneous tumor incidence with caloric restriction is an extension of the life span of the animal (Weindruch, 1992; Masoro, 1996) as well as a greater maintenance of immune function (Fernandes et al., 1997), amelioration of chronic renal disease (Gumprecht et al., 1993), and age-related changes in the small intestine of the rat (Heller et al., 1990). In Figure 8.5 may be seen the relation of survival to age as well as tumor incidence in female mice (Weindruch, 1992). There was an increase of approximately 35% in life span in the group that ate about 60% of the calories of the normal group. Overall tumor incidence for the control group was 78%, and for the restricted group 38%. The caloric effect on neoplastic development, induced or spontaneous, is not limited to one organ system but rather can be noted in the development of a number of different histogenetic types of neoplasms (Albanes, 1987; Birt, 1987). Furthermore, as expected, in both hepatocarcinogenesis in mice (Lagopoulos and Stalder, 1987; Kolaja et al., 1996) and in pancreatic carcinogenesis in the rat (Roebuck et al., 1993), preneoplastic lesions also decreased in number and in size in calorically restricted animals. This indicates that caloric restriction exerts its effect very early in the stage of promotion, inhibiting this stage during its development. Keenan et al. (1996) showed that the incidence of spontaneous tumors in restricted and ad libitum fed rats was similar, indicating that caloric restriction does not affect the initiation stage. Furthermore, in concert with the earlier findings of M.S. Rao et al.

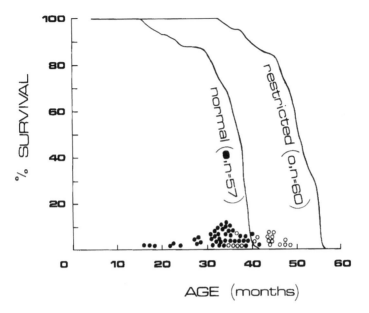

Figure 8.5 Influence of caloric restriction initiated at 3 weeks of age on the life span and tumor incidence of female mice of the long-lived C3B10RF$_1$ hybrid strain. The circles depict the age at death for tumor-bearing mice on normal (closed circles) and restricted (open circles). (Adapted from Weindruch, 1992, with permission of author and publisher.)

(1983), Keenan et al. (1995) demonstrated that moderate dietary restriction does not affect the stage of progression in spontaneous neoplastic development.

In the diet, the most concentrated source of calories is from fat. Thus, there has been considerable discussion of the role of dietary fat vis-à-vis total dietary calories in effecting the alterations of caloric restriction and ad libitum feeding. Several studies have now indicated that it is total caloric intake rather than fat intake that governs the ultimate yield of neoplasms both in mouse skin carcinogenesis and rat mammary carcinogenesis (cf. Boutwell, 1992). This effect is noted in Table 8.5. However, Birt et al. (1992) demonstrated that restriction of fat calories resulted in a greater inhibition of papillomas than when carbohydrate was restricted in the diet.

Table 8.5 Restriction of Caloric Intake Modulates the Enhancing Effect of Fat on Mouse Skin Carcinogenesis and Rat Mammary Carcinogenesis

Mouse Skin Carcinogenesis			
Caloric intake (% of ad libitum)	Fat level (% of diet)	Fat intake (grams per mouse per day)	Skin carcinomas (%)
100	5	0.06	54
66	15	0.24	28
Rat Mammary Carcinogenesis			
Caloric intake (% of ad libitum)	Fat level (% of diet)	Fat intake (grams per rat per day)	Mammary neoplasms (%)
100	5	0.6	43
81	30	2.2	7

Adapted from Boutwell, 1992, with permission of the author and publisher.

Still, the majority of experimental evidence argues that the caloric content of the diet is paramount in importance in producing the effects of caloric restriction. However, later in this chapter, we note that the composition of the fat can actually make significant differences in modifying the effects of carcinogenesis.

In addition to the dramatic effects of caloric restriction on spontaneous and chemically induced carcinogenesis, caloric restriction also alters carcinogenesis by radiation and viruses. Gross and Dreyfuss (1990), in a study with female rats, found that 89% of animals fed ad libitum developed neoplasms, predominantly leukemias and mammary carcinomas. When fed a restricted diet (about 50% of control calories), only 23% of irradiated animals developed neoplasms. Of the controls, 48% of the ad libitum unirradiated females developed similar neoplastic lesions, while none of the unirradiated females on a restricted diet developed neoplasms. Males showed a similar effect but at lower incidences. In another study with mice bearing the MMTV/v-Ha-*ras* transgene, Fernandes et al. (1995) examined the effect of caloric restriction on the expression of the transgene in mammary tissue of transgenic mice. Using a diet containing 60% of the calories of the ad libitum control group, they found that, whereas the tumor incidence was 83% in the ad libitum animals, it was 27% in the calorie-restricted animals. Since the transgene construct utilized the MMTV long terminal repeat as a promoter of the v-Ha-*ras* oncogene, this study suggests that both virus-induced and transgene-induced carcinogenesis are subject to the inhibitory effect of caloric restriction. In contrast, while caloric restriction inhibited the induction of intestinal neoplasms in rats by methylazoxymethanol acetate, which requires metabolic activation to exert its carcinogenic effect, caloric restriction had no effect on the induction of these neoplasms in rats administered the direct-acting carcinogen N-methylnitrosourea (Pollard and Luckert, 1985). In this latter study the restricted animals were fed at 75% of the caloric level of the ad libitum animals. Thus, whether carcinogenesis by direct-acting carcinogens is not affected by caloric restriction or requires a higher degree of caloric restriction to show the effect has yet to be determined.

Unlike chronic caloric restriction, acute complete caloric restriction by fasting has not been intensively studied. Initiation by diethylnitrosamine in rats is quantitatively unaffected by a 48-hour fast (Schmitt et al., 1993). When the fasting period is followed by refeeding, a significant enhancement of the initiation of preneoplastic focal lesions occurred (Tessitore et al., 1996) as well as an enhancing effect on the growth of nodules after a selection protocol of hepatocarcinogenesis (Laconi et al., 1995). It is likely that the enhancement of initiation is the result of an enhancement of DNA synthesis on refeeding, as was shown later by Hikita et al. (1997), with simultaneous enhancement of "fixation" of initiation. These last authors fasted animals for two 5-day periods interspersed by a 2-day feeding respite. At the end of the fasting periods, preneoplastic lesions had essentially disappeared, but reappeared quantitatively within 1 week of refeeding at levels identical to those of nonfasted animals. These authors demonstrated that the loss of preneoplastic cells was due to apoptosis with sparing of a stem cell(s) to allow rapid regrowth of preneoplastic lesions on refeeding. Thus, acute fasting and refeeding can modulate the stage of promotion in hepatocarcinogenesis and may enhance the efficiency of initiation through increased cell replication upon refeeding.

Mechanisms of the Effect of Dietary Restriction on Carcinogenesis

A number of potential mechanisms have been proposed to explain the inhibitory effect of caloric restriction on normal aging (Masoro, 1996). While some of these theories, including a retardation of "growth" and the decrease in endogenous formation of reactive oxygen molecules, can be applied to the effect of caloric restriction on carcinogenesis, other mechanistic factors undoubtedly play a role (Hocman, 1988b).

Paramount among the mechanisms of the effect of caloric restriction on aging and neo-plastic development are endogenous hormones. A striking effect is that described by Schwartz and Pashko (1994) in the demonstration that adrenalectomy could reverse the inhibition of skin papilloma development by food restriction in a two-stage carcinogenesis experiment involving DMBA initiation and TPA promotion. Furthermore, these authors demonstrated that adrenalec-tomy 2 weeks before initiating food restriction abolished the effect of the latter on the induction of pulmonary adenomas in A/J mice by DMBA (Pashko and Schwartz, 1996). The inhibition of mammary carcinogenesis by caloric restriction is also accompanied by a reduction in serum con-centrations of prolactin and estrogens in rats (Sylvester, 1986) and decreases in serum insulin-like growth factor I and insulin (Ruggeri et al., 1989).

A major potential mechanism for both the antiaging and anticarcinogenic effects of dietary restriction is the latter's effect on intracellular oxidative stress (Yu, 1996). Caloric restriction inhibits the oxidative damage to DNA that occurs normally (Djuric et al., 1992; Gao and Chou, 1992). The significance of this finding is emphasized by the demonstration that caloric restric-tion enhances activities of enzymes involved in antioxidant processes including superoxide dis-mutase, catalase, and glutathione peroxidase (G. Rao et al., 1990). However, these authors demonstrated that the effects on antioxidant enzymes did not occur in all tissues—e.g., intestinal mucosa—and in other tissues varied quite significantly (Xia et al., 1995). On the other hand, mitochondria in general and the electron transport system in particular are probably the most significant sources of active oxygen radicals (Feuers et al., 1993). Xenobiotic metabolism is sig-nificantly affected by caloric restriction. In Table 8.6 may be seen the effect of caloric restriction on some phase I and phase II enzyme levels in ad libitum and calorie-restricted animals (cf. Hart et al., 1992). Similarly, the formation of aflatoxin B_1-DNA adducts in liver of calorie-restricted animals is decreased (Chou and Chen, 1997) and increased with dimethylnitrosamine (Prasanna et al., 1989). In the skin, food restriction inhibits the formation of DMBA-DNA adducts

Table 8.6   Effect of Caloric Restriction on Selected Hepatic Drug-Metabolizing Enzymes

Enzyme	*Ad libitum*	Restricted	% Change
Phase I enzymes			
Testosterone-6β-hydroxylase	0.12	0.09	−25
Testosterone-16α-hydroxylase	2.67	1.71	−36
Lauric acid 12-hydroxylase	3.45	12.21	+253
4-Nitrophenol hydroxylase	0.43	0.91	+111
7-Ethoxyresorufin-*O*-deethylase	0.037	0.045	N.S.
Aminopyrene-*N*-demethylase	3.54	3.24	N.S.
7-Ethoxycoumarin-*O*-deethylase	0.43	0.68	+58
Testosterone-17-oxidase	0.87	1.79	+105
Phase II enzymes			
Glutathione *S*-transferase			
1,2-Dichloro-4-nitrobenzene	27.6	39.2	+42
1-Chloro-2,4-dinitrobenzene	1130	1050	N.S.
N-Acetyltransferase	2.09	4.60	+123
UDP-glucuronyltransferase			
2-Aminophenol	3.33	5.43	+63
Bilirubin	2.09	3.49	+67

N.S. = not studied.
Adapted from Hart et al., 1992, with permission of authors and publisher.

(Schwartz and Pashko, 1986) after DMBA application but increases the formation of benzo[a]pyrene-DNA adducts in the lung of the mouse, with a concomitant increase in cytochrome P4501A1, which metabolizes benzo[a]pyrene en route to its active form (Chen et al., 1996). Furthermore, caloric restriction increases the formation of endogenous I compounds (Chapter 3), spontaneous DNA adducts of largely unknown structure (Randerath et al., 1993). Thus, the role(s) of oxidative stress, xenobiotic metabolism, and DNA adduct formation in the mechanism of the antiaging and anticarcinogenic effect of caloric restriction are not entirely clear, but a lowering of intracellular oxidant reactions is a universal effect of caloric restriction.

Cell Replication and Apoptosis during Caloric Restriction

Generally, as one might expect, caloric restriction tends to decrease cell replication, DNA and RNA synthesis in various tissues of both the rat (Merry and Holehan, 1985) and the mouse (Lok et al., 1990). Interesting exceptions to this generalization have been noted, however. Klurfeld et al. (1987) found, in concert with earlier studies, that caloric restriction inhibited by almost 50% the formation of colon neoplasms in rats administered 1,2-dimethylhydrazine. However, caloric restriction induced a significant increase in the DNA labeling index of normal colonic mucosal cells. Similarly, Keenan and associates (1994) noted that both male and female rats fed for a year at a level of 65% of the ad libitum caloric intake exhibited a dramatic increase in the labeling index of hepatocytes. The mechanism of this effect may be related to a compensatory hyperplasia of the liver, resulting from the increased rate of apoptosis of hepatocytes that occurs with caloric restriction (James and Muskhelishvili, 1994; Grasl-Kraupp et al., 1994) in both mice and rats. Both of these groups suggested that the enhanced apoptotic rate occurring in the liver during caloric restriction might also explain the effect of caloric restriction in inhibiting the development of spontaneous neoplasms. Muskhelishvili et al. (1996) presented evidence for this in demonstrating that dietary restriction induced apoptosis in approximately 70% of putatively initiated glutathione S-transferase-π-positive hepatocytes, occurring after only 1 week of dietary restriction to 2-year-old ad libitum–fed mice. Grasl-Kraupp et al. (1994) and associates reported a similar experiment in rats, utilizing a 95-day period of caloric restriction with subsequent administration of nafenopin, a promoting agent and peroxisome proliferator (Chapter 7). These authors continued their study to 900 days, examining both preneoplastic and neoplastic lesions, and demonstrated a dramatic decrease in the growth of preneoplastic lesions as well as the number of neoplastic lesions (Figure 8.6). These studies, taken together, offer substantial evidence for a major role in the altered regulation of cell turnover in the calorically restricted animal by the elimination of initiated cells as well as the inhibition of proliferation and enhancement of apoptosis of cells in the stage of promotion, leading to lower rates of development of preneoplastic lesions (Wachsman, 1996).

Dietary Constituents and Carcinogenesis

The caloric content of the diet is made up of the caloric values of its various constituents. The constituents of the diet consist of protein, fat, and carbohydrate as the major components and vitamins, minerals, and related factors as the minor components. As shown above in relation to the overall carcinogenic process, the caloric content of the diet plays a major role. However, individual constituents of the diet also modify the carcinogenic process.

Dietary Protein. Early studies with rats demonstrated that the incidences of certain spontaneous neoplasms are very dependent on the level of the protein in the diet (Ross and Bras, 1973). In these animals the spontaneous incidence of thymoma increased more than threefold in animals on a low-protein diet (10% casein), while increasing the dietary protein content by a factor of five decreased the incidence of thymoma by a factor of eight. In most other examples,

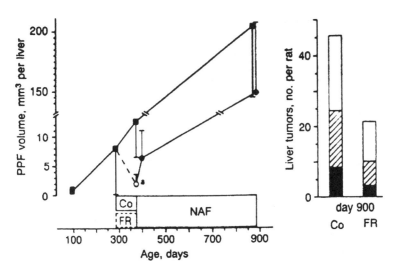

Figure 8.6 Effect of a 95-day period of caloric restriction on the volume of spontaneously occurring altered hepatic foci (PPF) and on the formation of liver tumors in animals administered nafenopin, a peroxisome proliferator and tumor promoting agent. Animals were fed ad libitum except for a group that were calorically-restricted to 60% of the calories of the control diet from day 285 to day 380 at the end of which time the volume of altered hepatic foci had decreased considerably (open circle, [a]). The insert at the right shows the number of liver tumors per rat in control (Co) and calorically restricted (FR) animals at the end of the experiment (day 900). The total column represents the number of grossly detectable lesions per liver, the hatched and solid part of the bar represents the numbers of adenomas and carcinomas. (Adapted from Grasl-Kraupp et al., 1994, with permission of authors and publisher.)

feeding either a 10% or a 50% casein diet lowered the spontaneous incidence of epithelial neoplasms compared with that of animals on a 22% casein diet. While total tumor risk was found to be correlated with caloric consumption, the diet containing a higher amount of protein for a given caloric intake resulted in a higher risk of malignancy. Furthermore, a high absolute protein consumption shortly after weaning and that relative to body weight during the early adult period were correlated with a higher probability of developing spontaneous neoplasms (cf. Mohr and Lewkowski, 1989).

The chemical induction of neoplasia in various rodent tissues is likewise affected by the protein content of the diet. Early studies in rats showed that when animals were fed a 5% (casein) protein diet, they exhibited significantly fewer aflatoxin-induced hepatomas than rats fed four to six times higher levels of casein (Madhaven and Gopalan, 1968; Wells et al., 1976). More recent investigations by Campbell and associates (O'Connor and Campbell, 1987; Schulsinger et al., 1989) demonstrated that lowering the dose of casein dramatically inhibits the growth of altered hepatic foci induced by aflatoxin B_1 in vivo. Furthermore, if the casein in the diet were replaced by wheat gluten, a low-quality protein, the development of altered hepatic foci was significantly inhibited compared with animals fed a casein diet at the same level for the same period. Lysine supplementation of the wheat gluten in the diet during the stage of promotion returned the growth of altered hepatic foci to normal (Schulsinger et al., 1989).

The protein content of the diet does not influence the growth of skin tumors, but a high-protein diet enhances DMBA-induced lung tumors in mice and DMH-induced neoplasms in rats (cf. Kritchevsky, 1988). In his discussion, the author points out that most studies have been carried out with casein as the protein source, emphasizing the significance of the study by Schulsinger et al. (1989). An increase in intake of protein prior to the administration of DMBA to induce mammary neoplasms decreased the number of tumors induced (Clinton et al., 1979). However, increasing the protein content of the diet after initiation, during the promotion phase, resulted in an increased incidence of mammary neoplasms. These results can be explained on the basis of an increased rate of metabolism of the carcinogen to noncarcinogenic metabolites in the liver of animals on a high-protein diet when DMBA is administered, resulting in a decreased level of potentially active metabolites of DMBA reaching the mammary gland (Hawrylewicz et al., 1982). The composition of the diet also appears to be important in determining the incidence of mouse hepatomas. In early studies, Tannenbaum and Silverstone (1949) showed that the incidence of mouse hepatomas increased with the rising content of casein in a partially purified diet until 26% of the diet consisted of protein. At a higher level of dietary casein, the incidence decreased significantly. Thus, the effect of the high protein content of the diet on carcinogenesis may occur at the stage of initiation by stimulating the metabolism of the chemical carcinogen to noncarcinogenic metabolites, with subsequent inhibition of this stage. The effect of high-protein diets on the stage of promotion may be either an enhancement or an inhibition, as noted above. Unfortunately, our knowledge of the mechanism of this effect is very limited.

Of the amino acid constituents of protein, tryptophan has been most widely studied for its effects on carcinogenesis in several different species in both bladder and liver (Sidransky, 1998). The initial studies in this area were described by Dunning et al. (1950), wherein Fischer female rats fed a purified diet, that had been supplemented with DL-tryptophan and contained 0.06% 2-AAF, exhibited a high incidence of bladder carcinomas, but no carcinomas developed when 2-AAF was administered in the absence of dietary tryptophan. Later Radomski and associates (1977) reported that female beagle dogs fed a diet containing 4-aminobiphenyl with supplemental DL-tryptophan developed a low incidence of bladder tumors, while animals receiving 4-aminobiphenyl in the absence of supplemental dietary tryptophan developed no such neoplasms. A number of studies on hepatocarcinogenesis in the rat gave variable results when tryptophan was added to the diet, in some cases an enhancing effect and in other cases no effect (cf. Sidransky, 1998). L-Tryptophan has many of the characteristics of a promoting agent, including an apparent interaction with a nuclear receptor (cf. Sidransky, 1998). Thus, some of the effects of increased dietary protein on carcinogenesis may be related to the tryptophan content of the diet causing a promoting action in the carcinogenic process.

Dietary Lipids and Carbohydrates. As suggested earlier in this chapter, the effect of lipids in the diet on carcinogenesis may be controversial in that the effects noted are the result primarily of the caloric content of the diet rather than specifically of the lipid content and of individual lipids themselves (see above). This is emphasized by the data depicted in Table 8.5. However, the fact still remains that dietary lipids do have significant effects, primarily in enhancing the development of a number of neoplasms induced by a variety of chemical and physical factors, as noted by the listing depicted in Table 8.7 from Birt (1987). Almost all of the effects of dietary fat listed in Table 8.7 are to enhance the development of neoplasms of a variety of tissues as a result of spontaneous and induced carcinogenesis.

Notably absent from the table is the effect of dietary lipids on mammary carcinogenesis, which has been the subject of considerable investigation, both experimentally (Pariza et al., 1986) and in the human (Prentice et al., 1989; Hunter et al., 1996). A variety of studies in experimental animals have indicated that the caloric and fat contents of the diet independently enhanced mammary tumor incidence in rats and mice (Freedman et al., 1990). However, Welsch et al. (1990) indicated that the increase in mammary neoplasia following DMBA administration in rats occurred only in animals fed ad libitum. Mammary carcinogenesis induced by the direct-acting carcinogen N-nitrosomethylurea (NMU) was primarily enhanced by the level of calories

Table 8.7 Effects of Dietary Fat on Carcinogenesis at Sites Other Than the Mammary Gland in Several Rodent Species

Site	Animal	Agent	Effect of High-Fat Diet
Skin	Mouse	None (spontaneous)	↑
		Polycyclic hydrocarbon	↑
		UV light	↑
Lung	Mouse	None	↑, NE
	Hamster	Benzo[a]pyrene (BP) on ferric oxide	↑
		N-nitrosobis(2-oxopropyl)-amine (BOP)	↑
Colon	Rat	1,2-dimethylhydrazine (DMH)	↑, NE
		Azoxymethane (AOM)	↑
		Methylazoxymethanol acetate (MAM)	↑, NE
		3,2′-Dimethyl-4-amino-biphenyl (DMAB)	↑
		Methylnitrosourea (MNU)	↑
Liver	Mouse	None	↑
	Rat	Aminoazo dyes	↑
	Hamster	Aflatoxin B_1 (AFB)	↑
		Acetylaminofluorene (AAF)	↑
		BOP	↑
Pancreas	Hamster	BOP	↑
	Rat	Azaserine (AZA)	↑
Prostate	Rat	None (promoted with testosterone)	↑
Brain	Mouse	None	↑
Ear duct	Rat	DMH	NE
Kidney	Rat	DMH	NE
	Hamster	BOP	↑

Key: NE, no effect; ↑, enhanced carcinogenesis.
Adapted from Birt, 1987, with permission of author and publisher.

in the diet (Beth et al., 1987) although the tumor-promoting effects of dietary fat manifested a threshold rather than a linear dose-response effect (Cohen et al., 1986). Furthermore, these effects of dietary fat were reportedly not related in a significant way to changes in endogenous levels of estrogen or prolactin (Clinton et al., 1995). However, early studies (Gammal et al., 1967) suggested that the type of dietary fat—i.e., corn oil versus coconut oil—significantly affected the development of mammary neoplasms in that animals receiving the corn oil diet developed a greater number of tumors. Subsequent studies demonstrated that fish oils rich in ω3 fatty acids, particularly eicosapentaenoic and docosahexaenoic acids, consistently inhibited mammary carcinogenesis in mice and rats when administered during the promotion stage (cf. Welsch, 1992). In contrast, safflower and corn oil, which contain predominantly ω6 fatty acids such as linoleic acid, exhibited a significant tumor-promoting effect in mouse mammary carcinogenesis induced by DMBA (Cameron et al., 1989). The structures of representative ω3 and ω6 fatty acids are depicted in Figure 8.7. The mechanism of this difference in effect on tumor promotion of ω3 and ω6 fatty acids is not known but may be related to their differential effect on the synthesis of prostaglandins, a series of hormones derived from these molecules (Lands, 1992).

As indicated from Table 8.7, increases in dietary fat enhance the development of neoplasms in a number of other tissues. The early studies of Miller and Rusch demonstrated the importance of the type of fatty acids in the diet on the incidence of azo dye–induced liver neoplasms (cf. Miller et al., 1944). When animals were fed unsaturated fat together with the carcin-

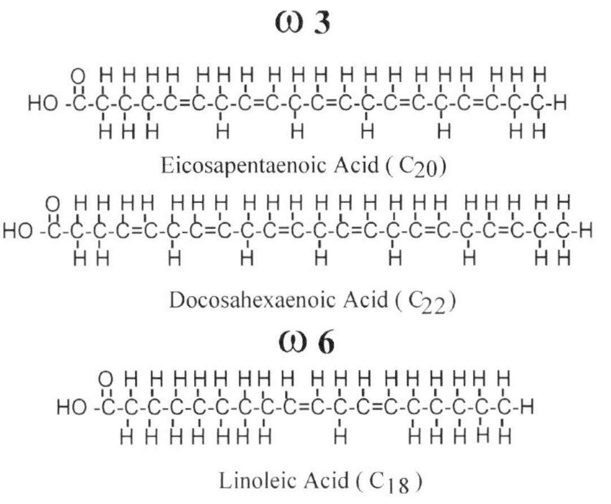

ω 3

Eicosapentaenoic Acid (C_{20})

Docosahexaenoic Acid (C_{22})

ω 6

Linoleic Acid (C_{18})

Figure 8.7   Structures of representative ω3 and ω6 polyunsaturated fatty acids.

ogen, the tumor incidence was much greater than when animals were fed an isocaloric amount of saturated lipids. Birt et al. (1989) reported that in Syrian hamsters initiated with N-nitrosobis-(2-oxopropyl)amine (BOP) at 8 weeks of age, a three- to fourfold enhancement of pancreatic carcinogenesis occurred in those hamsters fed high-fat diets ad libitum or fed equivalent caloric intakes. Rats initiated with azaserine, which induces acinar cell adenomas and carcinomas—in contrast to the BOP-induction of ductular carcinomas of the pancreas in hamsters—were studied during the promotion stage of carcinogenesis. Azaserine induces acinar foci of acidophilic and basophilic appearance. A diet containing 20% unsaturated fat induced an increase in the number of acidophilic foci as well as an increase in the thymidine labeling index of their nuclei compared with rats fed a 20% saturated fat diet or a control diet of 5% unsaturated fat (Roebuck, 1986). Later studies by O'Connor et al. (1989) demonstrated an inhibition of the development of these preneoplastic acinar cell foci and nodules by ω3 fatty acids in the diet, whereas ω6 fatty acids induced a significant increase in the growth of these preneoplastic lesions. Furthermore, dietary linoleic acid acts to promote pancreatic lesions in rats and hamsters (Appel et al., 1994). In the rat, an apparent threshold for this effect of linoleic acid is seen at concentrations between 4% and 8% in the diet, above which both the number and size of acidophilic foci increase (cf. Roebuck, 1992).

Dietary lipid content also enhances the development of preneoplasia and neoplasia in the intestine of mice and rats. In the mutant mouse strain *min*, which is genetically prone to develop polyps in the intestine, increasing the dietary fat content increased the number of polyps in the large and small bowel as well as increasing the size of the polyps in the small bowel (Wasan et al., 1997). In a review of some 14 studies of such experiments, a positive relationship was found between the incidence of colon carcinoma and fat intake (Zhao et al., 1991). This association was seen with the inbred Fischer 344 strain, but no such association was apparent for Sprague-Dawley rats. In contrast, while a high-fat diet enhanced the early development of colon neoplasms in rats after azoxymethane administration for 2 weeks, alteration in the fat content of the diet after neoplasms had developed did not change the neoplastic outcome, suggesting a lack of effect of dietary fat on the stage of progression in this tissue (Bird et al., 1996). As with mammary and pancreatic carcinogenesis, the type of lipid in the diet has significant effects on the carcinogenic process in the intestine. Dietary cholesterol enhances both the development of pre-neoplastic aberrant crypts and ultimately the number of colon neoplasms in mice and rats (Kendall et al., 1992; Hiramatsu et al., 1983). In mice administered 1,2-dimethylhydrazine (DMH), corn oil containing a large percentage of unsaturated fats markedly enhanced both the number and volume of neoplasms in the intestine as compared with mice fed an equivalent amount of beef tallow, which is composed primarily of saturated fats (Nutter et al., 1990). Also, as in the case of pancreatic and mammary carcinogenesis, dietary ω3 fatty acids inhibited while ω6 fatty acids enhanced the development of intestinal neoplasms induced by azoxymethane (Reddy and Sugie, 1988; Minoura et al., 1988).

The effect of carbohydrate administration on carcinogenesis seems to be of less importance and to exert less influence than protein and lipid components of the diet. A high-carbohydrate diet inhibited the development of hyperplastic nodules and neoplasms of the liver induced by 3′-methyl-4-dimethylaminoazobenzene (DEN) (Sato et al., 1984), whereas a high-sucrose diet—in comparison with an equivalent (65%) level of glucose—significantly enhanced the growth of preneoplastic hepatic foci initiated with DEN (Hei and Sudilovsky, 1985). Treatment of Sprague-Dawley rats with azoxymethane for 8 weeks resulted in a lower growth rate and less dysplasia of preneoplastic aberrant crypts when animals were administered cornstarch rather than sucrose in the diet (Caderni et al., 1994, 1997). In general, however, neither sucrose feeding nor systemic administration of sucrose enhanced spontaneous or induced carcinogenesis (cf. Kritchevsky, 1988).

Mechanisms of the Effects of Protein, Lipid, and Carbohydrate on Carcinogenesis. Mechanisms of the effects of the major dietary constituents on carcinogenesis differ where evidence for a mechanism exists. As indicated earlier (see above), inhibition of carcinogenesis by dietary protein may be related to its effect on xenobiotic metabolism to enhance the latter, causing the formation of noncarcinogenic metabolites of the agent involved (cf. Mohr and Lewkowski, 1989). It has also been suggested that enhanced dietary protein levels may produce effects on the immune system that could enhance or inhibit the development of carcinogenesis, although how this might directly relate to effects of dietary protein on carcinogenesis is not clear (Mohr and Lewkowski, 1989). The enhancement effect of dietary sucrose, especially in hepatocarcinogenesis, may be related to the fact that dietary fructose significantly enhanced the growth of altered hepatic foci in livers of rats initiated with N-nitrosomorpholine (Enzmann et al., 1989). Since fructose is one of the two sugars in the sucrose molecule and glucose does not appear to have a similar enhancing effect (Hei and Sudilovsky, 1985), the effects of sucrose may be that of the fructose resulting from hydrolysis in the intestine.

In contrast to our lack of knowledge of the mechanisms involved in the effects of protein and carbohydrate on carcinogenesis, there is significant information available on potential mechanisms of the effect of dietary lipids on carcinogenesis. The differential effect of ω3 and ω6 fatty acids on mammary carcinogenesis was not reflected in the number of mammary neoplasms induced by NMU in rats that exhibited an Ha-*ras* codon 12 mutation (Ronai et al., 1991). However, Lu et al. (1995) did find that a much larger proportion of mammary neoplasms in rats from this protocol exhibited a wild-type Ha-*ras* genotype when fed a high-fat diet in comparison with a low-fat diet. In colon carcinogenesis induced by azoxymethane, Singh et al. (1997) demonstrated that diets high in ω6 fatty acids exhibited an enhanced expression of the small *ras*-p21 proto-oncogene as well as an increased accumulation of the protein product in the cytoplasm in comparison with animals fed an ω3 fatty acid–rich diet. These studies suggest mechanism(s) by which high-fat diets of different composition may affect the process of initiation through altering the expression of wild-type and mutant *ras* proto-oncogenes. In this vein, dietary fat was also found to promote spontaneous carcinogenesis of the mammary gland in MMTV/v-Ha-*ras* transgenic mice (DeWille et al., 1993), and studies by others (Etkind et al., 1995) have indicated a more rapid development of mammary neoplasms in mice containing an endogenous MMTV proviral DNA in their genome. That ω6 fatty acids act as promoting agents in the development of colon neoplasia in rats was seen from the demonstration of a significantly lower number of apoptotic cells/crypts in the proximal colon of rats compared with those receiving ω3 fatty acids in the diet (Chang et al., 1997). This further indicates that the promoting action of ω6 fatty acids is in part to inhibit apoptosis, presumably selectively in altered cells within the colonic mucosa. The fact that dietary cholesterol may enhance the development of intestinal neoplasms is probably related to its metabolic conversion to bile salts, a number of which are known promoting agents for intestinal cancer in the rodent (Klurfeld et al., 1983). Corn oil diets, high in ω6 fatty acids, also enhance the metabolism of chemical carcinogens through a direct effect on xenobiotic metabolism, leading, in this case, to an increased production of the proximate and ultimate forms of such agents (Newberne et al., 1979; Wade et al., 1982). These studies on the mechanisms of the effects of dietary protein, lipid, and carbohydrate on the stages of carcinogenesis further substantiate their effectiveness in influencing the stages of initiation and promotion, primarily the latter.

Dietary Micronutrients in Carcinogenesis

While the bulk of the diet is made up of protein, carbohydrate, and lipid as well as significant nondigestible components in crude diets, a number of so-called micronutrients, vitamins, minerals, and related substituents are necessary for the survival and growth of the multicellular organism (Hunt and Groff, 1990). Table 8.8 lists most of the macro- and micronutrients that serve as exogenous modifiers in carcinogenesis in experimental animals. A number of these in relation to the human are discussed later in the text (Chapter 11). Since the macronutrients in relation to carcinogenesis have already been discussed, this section emphasizes the effect of micronutrients as exogenous modifiers of carcinogenesis.

In the strict sense, vitamins are micronutrients that are essential for the nutrition and viability of a multicellular organism and that cannot be synthesized in amounts sufficient for growth and/or normal function of the organism. The effects of the listed vitamins and minerals on the carcinogenic process are primarily to inhibit the process of carcinogenesis when present in sufficient or more than sufficient quantities. However, when the organism is deficient in one or more of these micronutrients, the carcinogenic process in one or more tissues is enhanced. It will also be noted that, as with macronutrients, the stages of carcinogenesis at which micronutrients exert their primary effects are, in most cases, initiation and/or promotion.

Retinoids. Over the past two decades, a remarkable effect of excess vitamin A and/or its derivatives on the development of epidermal, pulmonary, and other types of neoplasia has been demonstrated (cf. Lotan, 1980; Sporn and Roberts, 1983; Birt, 1986). In early studies in the hamster given carcinogenic hydrocarbons intranasally (a regimen that induces squamous cell carcinoma of the lung), carcinogenesis could be completely inhibited by the administration of high levels of vitamin A. The feeding of a diet containing high levels of vitamin A inhibited skin carcinogenesis by 7,12-dimethylbenz[a]anthracene in mice (Bollag, 1972). In addition, when vitamin A was applied directly to the skin after carcinogenesis was well under way, the morphological type of neoplasm produced was altered. This latter effect was inhibited by actinomycin D (Prutkin, 1971). These earlier studies have now been extended to a variety of other tissues and the development of neoplasms therein. Table 8.9 from Birt (1986) lists many of the more dramatic effects of retinoids on experimental carcinogenesis in several organs. Some of the most dramatic effects, as noted in this table, can be seen in the inhibition of carcinogenesis in the mouse skin by chemicals through the use of a variety of retinoids (Table 8.9; DeLuca et al., 1996). Retinoic acid was found to enhance or inhibit the development of papillomas in mouse epidermis during the two-stage process of carcinogenesis (Hennings et al., 1982; Verma et al., 1982). The differences in this effect are not clear, although Verma et al. (1982) demonstrated that

Table 8.8 Dietary Factors That Alter Cancer Incidence in Lower Animals

Dietary Component	Cancer Type	Change	Stage of Action
Macronutrients			
Calories	Breast, skin, liver, colon	+	Promotion
Carbohydrate	Liver, pancreas	–	Initiation
	Kidney	+	Initiation
Protein	Liver	–	Initiation
	Liver	+	Promotion
Fat	Breast, pancreas, skin	+	Promotion
Micronutrients			
Vitamins			
Vitamin A (retinoids)	Skin, bladder, lung, colon, breast	–	Promotion
Vitamin C	Breast, kidney	–	?
Vitamin D	Colon	–	Promotion
Vitamin E	Skin, breast	–	Promotion/?Progression
Folic acid	Colon, cervix, lung, brain	–	Initiation
Riboflavin	Liver	–	Initiation
Minerals			
Calcium	Colon	–	Promotion?
Selenium	Breast, colon, liver	–	Initiation and/or promotion
Zinc	Esophagus	–	Initiation/progression
Miscellaneous Dietary Factors			
Alcohol	Liver, colon	+	Promotion
Methyl group deficiency	Liver	+	Promotion (initiation?)
Minor nonnutrient components of fruits and vegetables	Breast, stomach, colon	–	Initiation and/or promotion
Fiber	Colon	–	Promotion
Intestinal flora	Colon	±	Initiation/promotion?

Key: +, enhancement of carcinogenesis; –, inhibition of carcinogenesis.

when DMBA was given in multiple doses without TPA, retinoic acid failed to inhibit the development of papillomas. Several different retinoid analogs, administered in the diet after initiation with DMBA, acted to promote the development of papillomas (McCormick et al., 1987). Interestingly, mice on a severe vitamin A–deficient diet failed to develop visible tumors in the two-stage carcinogenesis protocol, but supplementation with retinoic acid after 12 weeks on the deficient diet resulted in the rapid development of papillomas by week 22 (DeLuca et al., 1989). Thus, the effects of retinoids on epidermal carcinogenesis in the mouse depend on the format of the carcinogenesis experiments and the structure of the retinoid employed. Furthermore, retinoids given orally inhibit the development of the stage of progression in multistage epidermal carcinogenesis in the mouse (DeLuca et al., 1994).

One of the most striking demonstrations of an effect of vitamin A on carcinogenesis in the rat is the inhibition of N-methyl-N-nitrosourea–induced bladder carcinogenesis by the synthetic retinoid 13-cis-retinoic acid (Sporn et al., 1977). In this case, administration of the retinoic acid derivative inhibited the incidence and extent of bladder cancer development even when its administration was initiated after cessation of carcinogen dosing. Administration of 13-cis-retinoate to animals given dimethylhydrazine inhibited the production of colonic neoplasms (Newberne and Suphakarn, 1977). Narisawa et al. (1996) have extended these investigations by

Table 8.9 Some Effects of Retinoids on Chemical Carcinogenesis

Site	Species	Agent	Retinoid	Effect	Reference(s)
Skin	Mice	DMBA	Vit. A analogs	↓	Bollag, 1971
	Mice	DMBA + TPA	Retinoic Ac	↑ or ↓	Hennings et al., 1982
	Mice	UV light	Retinoic Ac	↑	Forbes et al., 1979
Salivary glands	Hamsters	DMBA	Vit. A. def.	NE[a]	Chaudhny et al., 1961
		DMBA	13 cis ret. Ac	↓	Shklar et al., 1980
Mammary gland	Rats	DMBA	Ret. acetate	↓	Moon et al., 1976
	Rats	MNU	Ret. acetate + analogs	↓	Moon et al., 1977; Moon & McCormick, 1982
	Mice	DMBA	analogs	NE	Welsch et al., 1984
	Mice	None	Retinyl acetate	NE	Maiorana & Gullino, 1980
Forestomach	Hamsters	DMBA	Vit. A palmitate	↓	Chu & Malmgren, 1965
	Hamsters	BP	Vit. A palmitate	↓	Chu & Malmgren, 1965
Urinary bladder	Rats	BBN	Vit. A analogs	↓	Miyata et al., 1978; Sporn et al., 1977
	Mice	BBN	Vit. A + analogs	↓	Moon et al., 1982
	Rats	MNU	13 cis ret. Ac.	↓	Squire et al., 1977
	Rats	FANFT	Vit. A def.	↑	Cohen et al., 1976
	Rats	FANFT	Ret. palmitate	NE	Cohen et al., 1976
Lung	Rats	3MC	Vit. A def.	↑	Nettesheim et al., 1979
	Rats	3MC	Ret. acetate	NE	Nettesheim et al., 1979
	Hamsters	BP-FeO₃	Retinyl acetate	↑	Smith et al., 1975
Trachea	Hamsters	MNU	Vit. A analogs	↑	Stinson et al., 1981
Liver	Rats	AFB₁	Vit. A def.	↑	Newberne & Rogers, 1973
	Rats	DMAB	Ret. acid	↓	Dauod & Griffin, 1980
	Hamsters	BOP	Vit. A analogs	↑	Birt et al., 1983
Colon	Rats	AFB₁	Vit. A def.	↑ NE	Newberne & Suphakarn, 1977
	Rats	MNNG	Vit. A def.	↓	Narisawa et al., 1976
	Rats	DMH	13 cis ret. Ac	↓	Newberne & Suphakarn, 1977
	Rats	MNU	Vit. A analogs	NE	Silverman et al., 1981
Pancreas	Hamsters	BOP	Vit. A analogs	↑ NE	Birt et al., 1983
	Rats	Aza	Vit. A analogs	↓	Longnecker et al., 1982

Key: Def., deficiency; ret. Ac., retinoic acid; NE, negative; ↑, enhancement of carcinogenesis; ↓, inhibition of carcinogenesis.
Adapted from Birt, 1986, with permission of author and publisher.

demonstrating the inhibition of the development of preneoplastic aberrant crypt foci in the intestine of rats following MNU administration. Later studies by Mack et al. (1990) and Sarkar et al. (1995) have further substantiated the inhibition of 3′-methyl-4-dimethylaminoazobenzene–induced hepatic neoplasia in the rat. Furthermore, the feeding of β-carotene in a multistage model of hepatocarcinogenesis in the rat significantly inhibited the development of preneoplastic altered hepatic foci (Moreno et al., 1995). In addition to the inhibitory effects of retinoids on DMBA- and MNU-induced mammary neoplasia in the rat, dietary retinyl acetate inhibited the development of mammary neoplasms induced by estrogen in female rats (Holtzman, 1988). The

inhibition of MNU-induced mammary carcinogenesis by retinyl acetate may be due to prevention of the progression of very early neoplastic lesions (Thompson and Becci, 1979). Thus, one
may conclude that, in general, retinoids tend to inhibit carcinogenesis of a variety of tissues in
rats and mice but to a lesser extent in hamsters. Most inhibitory effects of retinoids occur during
the stage of promotion, in part by an inhibition of DNA synthesis induced by the promoting
agent (Paulsen, 1984; Gendimenico et al., 1989). However, Dogra et al. (1984) reported that the
extent of binding of benzo[a]pyrene to lung DNA in vivo was about 2.5-fold higher in vitamin
A-deficient rats than in those receiving a normal amount of vitamin A. Other mechanisms by
which retinoids exert their effects may be directed by an alteration of the expression of specific
genes important in the stage of promotion, such as ornithine decarboxylase (Chapter 7; Verma et
al., 1979). Retinoids are also involved in the induction of transglutaminase in the epidermis
(Yuspa, 1982). This enzyme has been implicated in the process of apoptosis in a number of cell
populations (Fesus et al., 1996). Since retinoids are known to exert their effect on gene expression via the retinoid receptors (Chapter 3), it is likely that many of the effects of retinoids may be
mediated through such a mechanism. Furthermore, there are specific antagonisms between retinoic acid receptors and other transcriptional activators such as c-*jun* and c-*fos* (Yang-Yen et al.,
1991). An enhancement of the immune system by retinoids may also serve as an indirect mechanism for the inhibition of the development of preneoplastic and neoplastic lesions (Watson and
Moriguchi, 1985; Malkovsky et al., 1983).

Vitamins C and E. Several vitamins and at least one mineral, selenium, play significant
roles in the regulation of the metabolism of active oxygen radicals and related molecules within
cells. Vitamins C (ascorbate) and E (α tocopherol) are two of these, while retinoids also exhibit
antioxidant effects both in vivo and in vitro (cf. Krinsky, 1993). The structures of these three
vitamins and their relatives may be noted in Figure 8.8. Vitamin C is water soluble, while caroti-
noids and vitamin E are predominantly lipid-soluble. The action of vitamin E as an antioxidant
can be seen in Figure 8.9. In this figure, the interaction between vitamin C (ascorbate) and the
reaction of tocopherols with lipid peroxyl radicals can be noted: the tocopheroxyl radical interrupts the radical chain reaction, thereby preventing the chain propagation of lipid peroxidation
(Sies et al., 1992). Vitamin C is water-soluble and can also react with glutathione to regenerate
the vitamin, while reduced glutathione is reformed by its reductase. In this way the antioxidant
system exerts its effect through these two vitamins in both an aqueous and a lipid (membrane)
environment (Meister, 1994). While vitamin C has been shown to inhibit the development of a
number of different histogenetic types of neoplasms—including those of the colon, lung, kidney,
and epidermis (Birt, 1986; Chen et al., 1988)—high levels of sodium ascorbate act to enhance
the development of colon and bladder neoplasms in rodents (cf. Block and Schwarz, 1994). This
latter effect is perhaps not surprising, since ascorbic acid has been known for almost two decades to induce mutations in several different life forms (cf. Shamberger, 1984). On the other
hand, such investigations have also demonstrated the antimutagenic effects of this vitamin (cf.
Shamberger, 1984). The exact mechanisms for these divergent effects of the same molecule are
not totally clear at the present time but are probably related to a combination of dose and its
effectiveness as both an antioxidant and oxidant.

While administration of vitamin E, either by diet or topically, inhibits the development of
skin, forestomach, colon, and mammary neoplasms in rodents (Birt, 1986), Some questions have
been raised and discrepancies noted as to the effectiveness of this vitamin. Ura et al. (1987) reported an inhibition of the "selective" action of 2-acetylaminofluorene on DEN induction of altered hepatic foci in rat liver by dietary vitamin E, but this regimen had no effect on later stages
of the process, including progression. In contrast, Lii et al. (1997) were unable to find any effect
of vitamin E on the development of preneoplastic hepatic foci resulting from neonatal initiation
by DEN with subsequent phenobarbital promotion. Furthermore, Kolaja and Klaunig (1997) re-

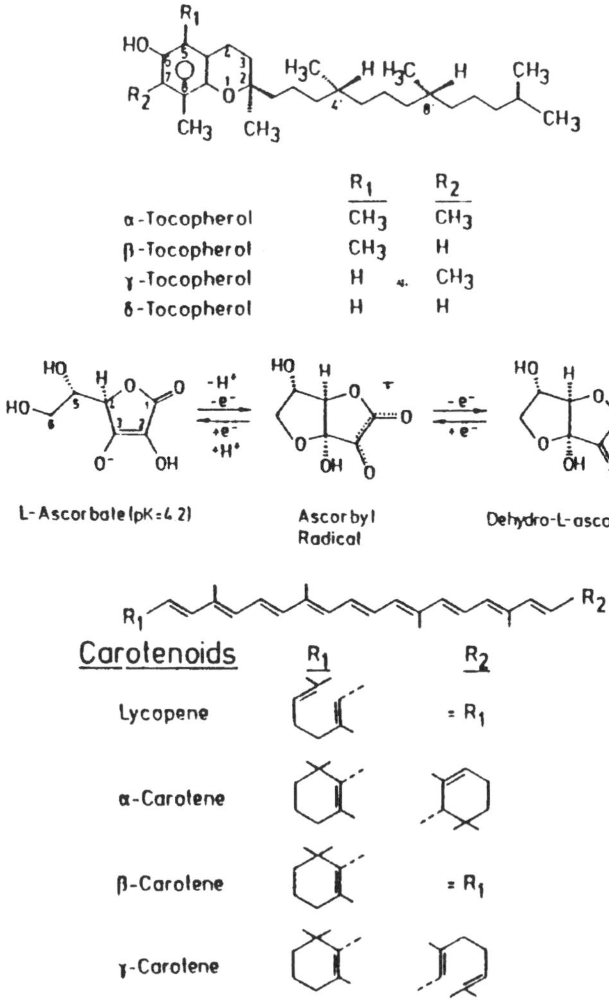

Figure 8.8 Structures of vitamins with antioxidant activity. The tocopherol series has the phytyl side chain (R_3). The radical function in the tocopheroxyl radical occurs at the hydroxyl of the chromane moiety. (Adapted from Sies and Stahl, 1995, with permission of authors and publisher.)

ported an enhancement of the growth of hepatic focal lesions in mice by both vitamin E supplementation and deficiency. In the azaserine induction of preneoplastic foci in rat pancreas, while the growth of acidophilic foci was inhibited in rats administered excess vitamins A and C, vitamin E exerted an inhibitory effect only on basophilic but not acidophilic foci (Woutersen and van Garderen-Hoetmer, 1988a). However, vitamin E as well as β-carotene inhibited the development of preneoplastic aberrant crypt foci in the colon of rats fed a high-fat, low-fiber diet (Shivapurkar et al., 1995). While the mechanisms of these discrepancies are not clear, both of these vitamins, C and E, may potentially inhibit "endogenous" carcinogenesis by inhibiting nitrosation of secondary amines ingested in the diet or produced in vivo (cf. Birt, 1986). In addition, both vitamins can inhibit mutagenesis, in vitro carcinogenesis, and the binding of active carcinogenic metabolites to cellular DNA as well as chromosomal breakage induced by chemical carcinogens (cf. Chen et al., 1988).

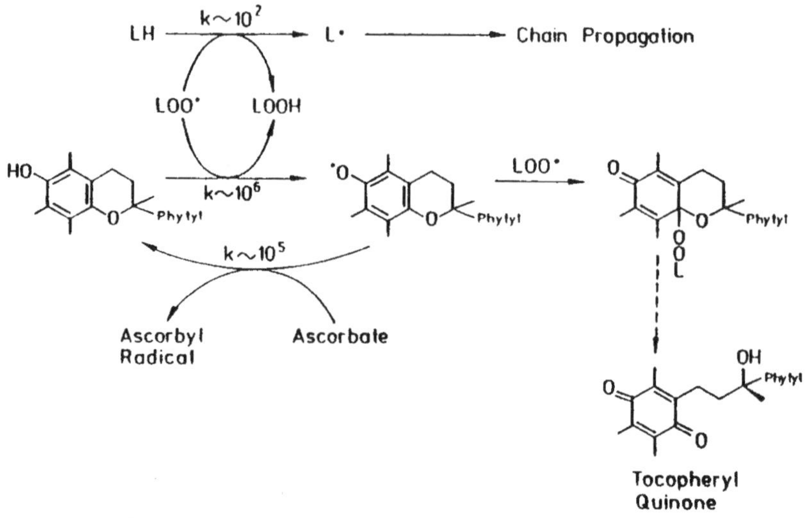

Figure 8.9   Action of vitamin E as an antioxidant in relation to lipid peroxides and subsequent oxidation by ascorbate. (Adapted from Sies et al., 1992, with permission of authors and publisher.)

Miscellaneous Vitamin Effects in Carcinogenesis.   One of the earliest effects of vitamins on carcinogenesis was reported by Morris and Robertson (1943), who observed that development of spontaneous mammary neoplasms was markedly depressed in C3H mice fed a riboflavin-deficient diet. This was in contrast to later studies demonstrating that riboflavin deficiency was accompanied by an increase in the effectiveness of carcinogenic azo dyes to induce hepatomas. This latter effect was probably due to the markedly diminished azo dye reductase activity seen in livers of riboflavin-deficient rats. Riboflavin is the cofactor of this enzyme, which metabolizes azo dyes to noncarcinogenic intermediates (cf. Miller and Miller, 1953). Similarly, folate deficiency, in both animal and human studies, has been associated with an increased risk for the development of neoplasms of the colon, cervix, lung, and brain (cf. Kim et al., 1997), but the role of folate in neoplastic development is not yet entirely clear (Glynn and Albanes, 1994). Cravo et al. (1992) reported the enhancement of the development of colonic neoplasia in rats treated with dimethylhydrazine that were folate deficient as compared with animals on control diets. Other studies have demonstrated that folate deficiency produces significant alterations in DNA and chromosome structure, including breakage, in both animals and humans in vivo (MacGregor et al., 1990; Blount et al., 1997). The active form of vitamin D, $1\alpha,25$-dihydroxyvitamin D_3, inhibits the proliferation of a variety of different neoplastic cells, both in vivo and in vitro (cf. Reichel et al., 1989). Administration of an analog of $1\alpha,25$-dihydroxyvitamin D_3 inhibited the development of colonic neoplasms induced by azoxymethane in rats when administered in the diet (Wali et al., 1995). The effects of this vitamin may be related to its regulation of the metabolism of calcium, whose effectiveness as an exogenous modifier is discussed below.

Minerals Effective as Exogenous Modifiers of Carcinogenesis.   Of the minerals known as exogenous modifiers of carcinogenesis, calcium is probably the most widespread in nature and exhibits the most varied functions in this category. The calcium ion is essential for cell replication and survival (Clapham, 1995). Within the cell, there are a large number of different calcium-binding proteins (Villereal and Palfrey, 1989) whose functions are modulated by calcium levels within the cell. These functions include muscle contraction, nerve transmission, membrane transport, signal transduction, and cell cycle progression (Clapham, 1995; Takuwa et al.,

1995). The reader is referred to the reviews cited for more details on the various functions of calcium and its binding proteins. Since regulation of the cell cycle is very important in carcinogenesis and neoplasia, it is not surprising to find that normal cells, and to a lesser extent neoplastic cells, exhibit varying degrees of inhibition of replication (Whitfield, 1992). Calcium added to the diet dramatically inhibited the development of neoplasms in rats administered 1,2-dimethylhydrazine in the presence or absence of vitamin E (McIntosh, 1992). In a separate study, Pence et al. (1995) demonstrated that calcium could effectively inhibit cholic acid promotion of azoxymethane-induced colon neoplasms. This finding is also reflected in the apparent inhibition of recurrences of adenomatous polyps in the human after polypectomy and after colorectal surgery for colorectal cancer (Duris et al., 1996). Thus, excess calcium may downregulate the stage of promotion in carcinogenesis of the colon and potentially other tissues through its regulatory effects on cell division and signal transduction.

Zinc is another mineral widespread in living systems and involved in numerous functions, including DNA replication, transcription, and a variety of peptidases and dehydrogenases (Wu and Wu, 1987; Coleman, 1992). In concert with these functions, especially those related to DNA synthesis and transcription, zinc deficiency inhibits the growth of a number of transplanted neoplasms in animals in vivo (cf. Walsh et al., 1994). In contrast, Fong et al. (1984) had previously reported that zinc deficiency enhanced the incidence of esophageal neoplasms induced by methylbenzylnitrosamine. This may be related to a direct effect of the deficiency in damaging the esophageal epithelium, with subsequent enhancement of replication of some epithelial cells. Very high levels of dietary zinc inhibited carcinogenesis by DMBA in hamsters and by azo dyes in livers of rats (cf. Walsh et al., 1994). Zinc deficiency induces thymic atrophy, which may be secondary to glucocorticoid-mediated apoptosis of thymocytes, thus potentially affecting the carcinogenic process indirectly (Fraker et al., 1995).

Another mineral micronutrient that has exhibited significant effects as an exogenous modifier of carcinogenesis is selenium. In living organisms, selenium is almost always associated with proteins which, in animal tissues, are almost exclusively in the form of selenocysteine (Burk and Hill, 1993). Selenocysteine has been termed the 21st amino acid in ribosome-mediated protein synthesis in both prokaryotes and eukaryotes. Selenocysteine is formed cotranslationally on a seryl tRNA with a UCA anticodon. The complementary mRNA codon is UGA. This codon is also a "stop" codon signifying the end of translation of an mRNA. It appears that the use of the selenocysteine tRNA in preference to the termination of translation depends on adjacent sequences within the mRNA (Stadtman, 1996; Böck et al., 1991). About a half dozen selenoproteins are known in mammals (Birk and Hill, 1993; Stadtman, 1996), but the protein that appears to be most significant in the function of selenium as an exogenous modifier of carcinogenesis is its presence in glutathione peroxidase. This enzyme participates in the elimination of potentially harmful active oxygen radicals and their products by mechanisms such as depicted in Figure 8.10.

The effects of selenium administration and selenium deficiency on carcinogenesis in several different types of tissues are seen in Table 8.10. Excess dietary inorganic selenium inhibits colon carcinogenesis induced in rats by bis(2-oxopropyl)nitrosamine (Birt et al., 1982), 1,2-dimethylhydrazine (Jacobs, 1983), and azoxymethane (Reddy et al., 1988). This inhibition can also occur with organic selenium compounds (Reddy et al., 1987), with the effects of this micronutrient occurring primarily during the stage of promotion (Reddy et al., 1988). In contrast, selenium deficiency either had no effect (Pence and Buddingh, 1985) or inhibited the incidence and development of colon tumors in rats after azoxymethane administration (Reddy and Tanaka, 1986).

In this last study, no interaction with vitamin E in the diet was seen. However, Woutersen and van Garderen-Hoetmer (1988b) demonstrated an inhibitory effect of dietary selenium on the

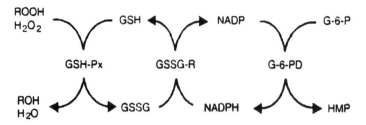

Figure 8.10 The glutathione redox cycle. ROOH/ROH: peroxy radical/alcohol. H$_2$O$_2$: hydrogen peroxide. GSH-Px: glutathione peroxidase. GSH/GSSG: reduced/oxidized glutathione. GSSG-R: glutathione reductase. NADPH/NADP: reduced/oxidized nicotinamide adenine dinucleotide phosphate. G-6-PD: glucose-6-phosphate dehydrogenase. G-6-P: glucose-6-phosphate. HMP: hexose monophosphate.

development of preneoplastic lesions in the pancreas of rats administered azaserine and in hamsters administered N-nitrosobis(2-oxopropyl)amine when animals were fed diets high in saturated fat. In rats initiated with aflatoxin B$_1$, those fed a diet deficient in selenium exhibited a significantly enhanced growth of preneoplastic foci in their livers as compared with livers of rats fed a normal amount of selenium. Rats fed a high-fat diet exhibited an inhibition of initiation by the administration of excess selenium (Baldwin and Parker, 1987). Excess organic and inorganic selenium also inhibited the development of preneoplastic foci in livers of animals administered either azoxymethane or aflatoxin B$_1$ respectively (Sugie et al., 1989; Milks et al., 1985), as well as a necrogenic dose of DEN followed by a partial hepatectomy (LeBoeuf et al., 1985). However, when initiation was carried out with a nonnecrogenic dose of DEN followed by promotion with phenobarbital, the addition of inorganic selenium to the diet actually enhanced the growth of preneoplastic lesions. In contrast, Dorado et al. (1985) were unable to demonstrate any effect of added dietary selenium in the format of the latter experiment. Reportedly, both inorganic and

Table 8.10 Effects of Selenium on Chemical Carcinogenesis

Site	Species	Agent	Effect	Reference(s)
Skin	Mice	uv light	↓	Overvad et al., 1985
	Mice	3MC	↓	Shamberger, 1970
	Mice	α-Pyrene	↓	Shamberger, 1970
Liver	Rat	DMAB	↓	Clayton & Baumann, 1949
	Rat	AAF	↓	Harr et al., 1972
	Rat	DEN	↓	LeBoeuf et al., 1985
Trachea	Hamster	MNU	NE[a]	Thompson & Becci, 1979
Lung	Rat	BOP	↓	Birt et al., 1982
Mammary gland	Mice	DMBA	↓	Medina & Shepherd, 1981
	Rat	DMBA	↓	Ip, 1981; Ip, 1983
	Rat	MNU	↓	Thompson & Becci, 1980
Colon	Rat	DMBA	↓	Jacobs et al., 1977
	Rat	BOP	↓	Birt et al., 1982
	Rat	AOM	↓	Soullier et al., 1981
Pancreas	Hamster	BOP	↓	Woutersen & van Garderen-
(high-fat diet)	Rat	Azaserine	↓	Hoetmer, 1988b

Key: NE, negative; ↓, inhibition of carcinogenesis.
Adapted from Birt, 1989, with permission of author and publisher.

organic forms of selenium administered in excess inhibited the development of mammary tumors in rats induced by either DMBA or MNU (Welsch et al., 1981; Ip and White, 1987), although a more recent study by Lane et al. (1990) did not find an inhibition by selenomethionine or selenocysteine. However, excess inorganic selenium did inhibit DMBA-induced mammary cancer development in mice. In the study by Ip and White (1987), vitamin E potentiated the effect of the inorganic but not the organic forms of selenium. In another study, Ip reported that administration of vitamin C in a similar experiment nullified the protective effect of inorganic selenite but had no effect on the inhibitory effect of selenomethionine on mammary carcinogenesis (Ip, 1986). Deficiencies of selenium together with a deficiency of vitamin E enhanced mammary carcinogenesis by MNU, but deficiencies of either single nutrient had no effect in altering the carcinogenic response (Thompson, 1991). In addition, Lijinsky et al. (1989) were unable to find an effect of dietary selenium on the induction of esophageal and bladder neoplasms in rats by two different nitrosamines.

The principal mechanism whereby selenium probably exerts its inhibitory effect on carcinogenesis is through its role as an essential component of the enzyme glutathione peroxidase, which is an essential part of the antioxidant defense system as described previously (Figures 8.8 and 8.9). The enzymatic activity of glutathione peroxidase is directly related to the concentration of selenium in blood (cf. Hocman, 1988a). Several of the studies noted above found an increased activity of glutathione peroxidase in several tissues in animals fed high levels of selenium in the diet (Birt et al., 1982; Reddy et al., 1987; Lane et al., 1990). In addition, feeding a combination of vitamin E and selenium to rats administered DMBA to induce mammary neoplasms inhibited lipid peroxidation occurring immediately after DMBA administration. This inhibition was directly correlated with an inhibition of mammary carcinogenesis (Takada et al., 1992). In addition to the effect of selenium on oxidant reactions, Medina and Morrison (1988) suggested several other possible mechanisms, including an alteration of carcinogen-DNA interactions, maintenance of intracellular glutathione levels, and effects on DNA and protein synthesis as well as gene expression. While a selenium-deficient diet reduced the level of cytochrome P450IA1, it did not affect its inducibility (Gairola and Chow, 1982). Conversely, administration of inorganic selenite to rats administered 1,2-dimethylhydrazine in vivo inhibited DNA alkylation significantly both in liver and in colon (Harbach and Swenberg, 1981). Dipple et al. (1986) found a similar inhibition of DMBA-deoxyadenosine adducts in fetal mouse cell cultures when administered 1 hour prior to but not 3 hours after the addition of the carcinogen. This study was somewhat at odds with an earlier investigation by Ip and Daniel (1985), who were unable to demonstrate any significant effect of DMBA-DNA binding in vivo in liver and mammary gland when excess inorganic selenite was administered. However, more recent investigations by Liu et al. (1991) showed a marked inhibition of total DMBA-DNA adducts after selenite supplementation of the diet for only 2 weeks. In addition, hepatic DNA of selenium-deficient rats exhibited a significant number of single-strand breaks shortly after injection of 2-acetylaminofluorene, but no effect of dietary selenium on DNA repair could be demonstrated (Wortzman et al., 1980). Thus, while most evidence argues that selenium exerts its inhibitory effect at the promotion stage of carcinogenesis, there is evidence that the initiation stage may also be affected by this mineral.

Other Minerals as Exogenous Modifiers of Carcinogenesis. Another relatively common mineral in living systems is iron and its salts. Feeding an excess level of iron in the diet resulted in increased mammary tumor incidence and lowered natural killer cell activity in rats (Spear and Sherman, 1992). Smith et al. (1993) also reported that injections of iron-dextran producing an iron overload caused a marked enhancement of the development of hepatic nodules in animals administered hexachlorobenzene, a hepatic carcinogen. Iron overload is known to induce tissue damage and increase the formation of reactive oxygen species (Okada, 1996). Iron deficiency enhanced lipid peroxidation in dimethylhydrazine-fed rats. This effect was also accompanied by an increase in liver glutathione peroxidase (Rao and Jagadeesan, 1996). Although these investigators did not carry the studies through to neoplasms, their findings, coupled with those cited above, argue that iron may serve as an exogenous modifier of carcinogenesis by altering lipid peroxidation and active oxygen formation. Deficiency of another mineral, copper, enhanced the formation of colonic neoplasms after dimethylhydrazine administration to rats (Greene et al., 1987; DiSilvestro et al., 1992). The mechanism for this effect is not clear at present.

Miscellaneous Dietary Factors in Carcinogenesis

Table 8.8 lists a number of miscellaneous dietary factors that act as exogenous modifiers of carcinogenesis. As noted, these are quite heterogeneous and some are as yet undefined, such as fiber, intestinal flora, and cruciferous vegetables. However, ethanol, and to a lesser extent diets deficient in methyl groups, are better defined in a chemical sense. In particular, ethanol as a dietary factor in carcinogenesis plays a very significant role not only in animals but also in humans (Chapter 11).

Ethanol. As further discussed in Chapter 11, the excessive intake of alcoholic beverages by humans has long been considered a significant risk factor for various types of cancer (Thomas, 1995; Longnecker and Enger, 1996), although a direct causal relationship has been questioned by some (cf. Rubin, 1996). Furthermore, epidemiological studies in the human have virtually all been carried out with dietary intake of ethanolic mixtures containing a variety of other substances, a number of which are known to be at least mutagenic if not carcinogenic (cf. Blot, 1992). In animal studies, however, it is possible to utilize the major organic constituent of alcoholic beverages, ethanol itself. Even in experimental studies, however, the demonstration of ethanol as an exogenous modifier of carcinogenesis has not been uniform (cf. Seitz and Simanowski, 1988; Garro and Lieber, 1990). Yet, there is sufficient evidence from a number of animal studies to indicate that, under some conditions, ethanol may act as an enhancer of experimental carcinogenesis by either a cocarcinogenic or promoting effect. Examples of such effects on carcinogenesis in several tissues of rats and mice may be seen in Table 8.11. In the rat, several different concentrations of ethanol in the drinking water enhance hepatocarcinogenesis induced by several different chemical agents. This fact—together with the effects noted in esophageal, gastric, and mammary carcinogenesis (Table 8.11)—tends to present experimental situations that may be analogous to the genesis of neoplasia in the same tissues in the human (Longnecker and Enger, 1996; Thomas, 1995). Singletary (1997) has reviewed the effect of ethanol in experimental mammary carcinogenesis and demonstrated that, in the mouse, spontaneous mammary carcinogenesis is little if at all affected by dietary ethanol. In the rat, however, most studies have indicated an enhancement of mammary carcinogenesis, with a few examples exhibiting no effect. Even the study noted in the table (Singletary et al., 1995) indicated that high concentrations of ethanol (30% of calories) exhibited no enhancing effect on mammary carcinogenesis induced by MNU, while ethanol intakes of 15% or 20% of calories exhibited a significant enhancement, primarily during the promotion stage. An interesting example of an exogenous modification of carcinogenesis by ethanol is that of the administration of DMN to C57BL mice, wherein the hepatocarcinogenic effect of the agent was essentially not altered by ethanol, but animals receiving the chemical carcinogen plus ethanol exhibited a dramatic incidence of olfactory neuroblastomas (Griciute et al., 1987).

In view of the widespread exposure to dietary ethanol, a variety of studies on the potential mechanisms of its toxicity have been carried out. A general survey of the genotoxicity of alcohol and its primary metabolite acetaldehyde (Bridges et al., 1987) concluded that ethanol is weakly mutagenic to bacteria and clastogenic to eukaryotic cells both in vivo and in vitro. The effect of

Table 8.11 Ethanol as an Exogenous Modifier of Experimental Carcinogenesis

Site	Species	Agent	Dose	Effect	Reference
Liver	Rat	Aflatoxin B$_1$	10% in H$_2$O	↑	Tanaka et al., 1989
	Rat	DEN	20% in H$_2$O	↑	Takada et al., 1986
	Rat	DEN	5% in H$_2$O	↑	Driver and McLean, 1986
	Rat	Ethynylestradiol norethindrone acetate	10% in H$_2$O	↑	Yamagiwa et al., 1991
Esophagus	Mouse	N-nitrosomethyl-benzylamine	30% in diet	↑	Eskelson et al., 1993
Mammary gland	Mouse	spontaneous	12% in H$_2$O	↓ latency	Schrauzer et al., 1979
	Rat	MNU	15 or 20% in diet	↑	Singletary et al., 1995
Olfactory organ	Mouse	OMN	80 mg twice weekly ig.	↑	Griciute et al., 1987
Lung	Mouse	DMN	1–10% in H$_2$O	↑	Anderson et al., 1992
Stomach	Rat	MNNG	0.5 mL IP every 2 days	↑	Iishi et al., 1989

Key: ↑, enhanced carcinogenesis; ↓ latency, decreased latency of appearance of neoplasms; ig.: intragastric

ethanol on germ cells was not clarified. However, ethanol with some degree of specificity induces cytochrome P450 2E1 in mammals (Tsutsumi et al., 1993). This cytochrome also activates several nitrosamines, including DMN and DEN, which may be important in its inhibitory and enhancing effects on carcinogenesis induced by these agents (Swann et al., 1984; Carlson, 1990). Further in line with this suggestion is the fact that lowering of the carboydrate intake, which would be expected to enhance xenobiotic metabolism in the liver (Hartshorn et al., 1979), together with ethanol ingestion enhanced the initiation of DEN hepatocarcinogenesis in rats (Yonekura et al., 1992). In addition to these factors, ethanol enhances lipid peroxidation and inhibits excisional DNA repair (cf. Garro and Lieber, 1990).

Dietary Deficiency of Methyl Groups and Carcinogenesis.   As discussed previously (Chapter 3), diets deficient in components involved in the utilization and production of methyl groups may, on prolonged administration, induce a development of liver neoplasms in rats (Mikol et al., 1983; Ghoshal and Farber, 1984; Nakae et al., 1992) as well as in mice (Yoshida et al., 1993). However, even prior to the demonstration of this direct dietary-deficient induction of neoplasia, the importance of methyl donors in the diet and the responses to chemical carcinogens was well known (cf. Rogers, 1995). Dietary methyl deficiency enhances the induction of hepatic neoplasia in rats by aflatoxin B$_1$, DEN, AAF, and several other chemicals. As noted above, folate deficiency can contribute substantially to the lack of normal methyl group metabolism (cf. Rogers, 1995).

The most obvious mechanism for the carcinogenic effect of methyl group deficiency is a lack of methylation of DNA or abnormalities in this process. This phenomenon has been shown in animals fed such methyl-deficient diets (Wainfan et al., 1989; Zapisek et al., 1992). These changes in nucleic acid methylation, which are accompanied by alterations in gene expression, are quite reversible on reintroduction of a normal diet (Christman et al., 1993). Correlations of alterations in the expression of specific proto-oncogenes have been noted in livers of rats fed a methyl-deficient diet (Dizik et al., 1991). In addition, methyl group–deficient diets induce alterations in nucleotide pools (James et al., 1992) and an increase in the level of uracil in hepatic DNA (Pogribny et al., 1997). An alternative or complementary mechanism of the effect of methyl-deficient diets is the enhanced lipid peroxidation (Yoshida et al., 1993) and deoxyguanosine hydroxylation of DNA occurring in hepatocytes of rats fed a methyl-deficient diet (Nakae et al., 1990). That such an oxidant effect of the diet is significant is also shown by the inhibitory effects of derivatives of vitamins C and E on the induction of preneoplastic lesions in livers of animals fed such diets (Mizumoto et al., 1994). Lombardi and associates (Lombardi and Smith, 1994) have studied the effect of choline deficiency and a more intense methyl-deficient diet on hepatocarcinogenesis, demonstrating a promoting action of such diets that may or may not be enhanced by phenobarbital (Shinozuka and Lombardi, 1980; Saito et al., 1990). Lombardi and associates have further argued that the promotion of endogenous initiated cells present within the livers of normal untreated rats can explain the promoting and carcinogenic effects of choline deficiency (Lombardi and Smith, 1994). Such a mechanism was also proposed by Sawada et al. (1990). Thus, while the mechanistic effects of methyl-deficient diets are quite varied, their effects on altering the stages of carcinogenesis appear to occur primarily at the stage of promotion through their enhancement of cell replication (Lombardi and Smith, 1994) and effects on DNA structure and gene expression. However, it is also reasonable to assume that the promutagenic and potentially clastogenic effects of the diets may enhance the transition from the stage of promotion to progression.

Minor Components of Fruits and Vegetables as External Modifiers of Carcinogenesis. That a high consumption of fruits and vegetables leads to a statistically significant protective effect on cancer incidence in a variety of sites in humans has been shown in a large number of studies (Block et al., 1992; Chapter 11). Wattenberg and associates (cf. Wattenberg and Loub, 1978) were among the first to investigate specific chemicals occurring within vegetables, notably cruciferous plants (cabbage, cauliflower, broccoli, etc.), that exerted a preventive effect on carcinogenesis. Since that time, with the advancement of knowledge in this area, Wattenberg (1985; 1992) has proposed a classification of minor nonnutrient inhibitors of carcinogenesis found in fruits and vegetables according to their action in relation to the carcinogenic process. The first category consists of compounds that prevent the formation of carcinogens from precursor substances either in vivo—e.g., ascorbate's prevention of the formation of nitroso compounds from the reactions of nitrites with appropriate amines—or prior to consumption of such compounds by the organism. Examples of the latter would be compounds preventing the formation of carcinogenic heterocyclic amines in meat products (Chapter 3) or those preventing the formation of urethane in alcoholic beverages and inhibiting the destruction of hydrazines in mushrooms (cf. Wattenberg, 1990). The second category of nonnutrient dietary inhibitors of carcinogenesis is that comprising so-called *blocking agents*. These agents inhibit metabolic activation of carcinogens and/or increase carcinogen detoxification by enhancing phase I and phase II pathways of xenobiotic metabolism (Chapter 3) in vivo. Those in the third category, *suppressing agents*, inhibit the development of the neoplastic process in cells previously exposed to carcinogenic agents. This category includes protease inhibitors (St. Clair et al., 1990; Hocman, 1992) and other dietary proteins (Papenburg et al., 1990; Messina et al., 1994), inhibitors of the arachidonic acid cascade (cf. Rao et al., 1993a), inositol hexaphosphate, and other chemicals (cf. Wattenberg, 1992). The structures of some of these blocking and suppressing agents are seen in Figure 8.11. Several of the phenolic chemicals seen in the figure act as blocking agents by enhancing the level of glutathione S-transferase activities. Benzyl isothiocyanate acts in a similar manner, while a large class of chemicals termed *glucosinolates*, occurring in cruciferous vegetables, induce these phase II activities and also act on phase I enzyme activities. The glucosinolates share a common basic molecular skeleton, containing a β-D-thioglucose grouping, a side chain, and a sulfonated oxime moiety. The various members of this group differ in the side chain

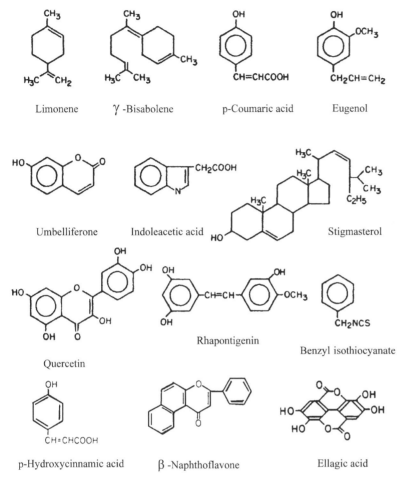

Figure 8.11   Chemical structures of some nonnutrient minor constituents of fruits and vegetables that can serve as exogenous modifiers of carcinogenesis. β-naphthoflavone is a synthetic congener, but the remaining structures are of naturally occurring substances.

(Verhoeven et al., 1997). Ellagic acid is, like several other chemicals noted in Figure 8.11, antimutagenic, occurring naturally in grapes, nuts, and strawberries (cf. Hayatsu et al., 1988). A number of other phenolic compounds found in tea and coffee also exert inhibitory effects on carcinogenesis (Dragsted et al., 1993). From this discussion, therefore, it becomes obvious that these nonnutrient minor constituents of fruits and vegetables use a number of different mechanisms for their inhibitory effects on carcinogenesis. However, these may be grouped primarily into effects on initiation (carcinogen activation) and the stage of promotion as emphasized by Wattenberg (1992).

Dietary Fiber as an Exogenous Modifier of Carcinogenesis.   Unlike most of the other exogenous modifiers considered in this chapter, studies on the effect of dietary fiber on carcinogenesis originated largely from human epidemiological investigations (cf. Howe et al., 1992). Since such investigations in the human did indicate a significant protective effect of dietary fiber from colon cancer, investigative studies to reproduce such effects in animals have been undertaken. Specific studies on the effect of various types of dietary fiber have indicated that poorly fermentable fibers such as wheat bran and cellulose are protective, while pectin and some other fermentable fiber supplements may have no effect or enhance chemically induced colon carcinogenesis in rodents (Jacobs, 1986; Bingham, 1990). In a recent study, Pierre et al. (1997) demonstrated that the administration of short-chain fructo-oligosaccharides to mice carrying the *min* mutation reduces the occurrence of colon tumors. Potential mechanisms for this inhibitory effect of fiber on colon carcinogenesis in animals (and by analogy in humans) include a reduction in fecal bile acid concentrations and an increase in the presence of short-chain fatty acids, particularly butyrate, as a result of fermentation of the fiber in the colon by bacteria (cf. Klurfeld, 1992). Cellulose fiber in particular has been demonstrated to prevent DNA damage by bile acids in an in vitro system (Cheah and Bernstein, 1990). As part of these mechanisms, it is now well known that changing the fiber content of the diet may also change the colonic microflora—e.g., germ-free rats exhibited a higher incidence of colon tumorigenesis than conventional rats when both were treated with azoxymethane by the intrarectal route (Reddy et al., 1975). In earlier studies, Popp and associates (Rickert et al., 1984) demonstrated that alteration in the fiber composition of the diet as well as in the microflora of the large intestine dramatically affected the carcinogenicity of 2,6-dinitrotoluene. In addition, lactic acid–fermenting bacteria, even when fed to animals, decreased the incidence of both preneoplastic and neoplastic lesions in mice administered dimethylhydrazine and other carcinogenic compounds (cf. Rafter, 1995).

EXOGENOUS MODIFIERS AND CANCER PREVENTION

Although the effective therapy of cancer is an ultimate goal of medical science, the prevention of cancer is, at our present state of knowledge, the most effective and, relatively, the most inexpensive mode of controlling this disease. The prevention of cancer has been discussed by a number of authors (Schottenfeld, 1981; Hirayama, 1992; Doll, 1996). Optimistically, our knowledge of the incidence of neoplasia in the human suggests that age-specific incidence rates might be reduced by as much as 80%, half of this reduction coming through the application of existing knowledge (Doll, 1996). In fact, such knowledge has already been applied to specific populations with significant results (Hirayama, 1992). As has been noted (Pitot, 1993), cancer prevention may occur passively or actively. Passive prevention of cancer involves a cessation or restriction of exposure to potentially carcinogenic influences, such as the cessation of smoking, dietary modification, and avoidance of excessive sunlight. Active cancer prevention involves a positive activity on the part of the individual by such things as vaccination against oncogenic viruses, dietary modification and supplements, or the administration of agents externally and/or internally that are known to prevent neoplastic development. This last subject is most pertinent to our discussion in this chapter.

Chemoprevention of Cancer by Exogenous Modifiers

Chemoprevention in relation to cancer is "the inhibition or reversal of carcinogenesis (before malignancy) by intervention with chemical agents" (Kelloff et al., 1996). From this definition it is obvious that the active prevention of neoplastic development by the administration of exogenous chemical modifiers of carcinogenesis is effective at the stages of initiation and/or promotion. However, because of the ubiquitous nature and occurrence of the stage of initiation in the mammalian population (Chapter 7), it may not be realistic at the present time to attempt to utilize chemicals to prevent the spontaneous initiation of cells. However, it is clear that a reduction in the number of initiated cells is feasible by a number of the agents noted earlier in this chapter. Thus, for chemoprevention to be effective in most cases, it must exert an effective inhibitory action on the stage of promotion. As developed earlier in this chapter, numerous examples of exogenous modifiers inhibiting the stage of promotion have been demonstrated. Furthermore, a combination of passive prevention formats such as those noted above, together with the administration of chemopreventive agents, may be the most effective approach to cancer prevention at this time.

In addition to the many naturally occurring exogenous modifiers that can serve as chemopreventive agents, a number of synthetic chemopreventive agents have now been developed from both human and animal studies. A number of these are listed in Table 8.12. Aspirin and other nonsteroidal anti-inflammatory drugs (NSAIDs), when administered for extended periods, have been shown to reduce the risk of colon cancer and polyps in humans (Giovannucci et al., 1995; Suh et al., 1993). As with dietary fiber (see above), the experiments in animals largely followed this observation in humans, and, as noted from the table, NSAIDs caused significant inhibition of both colon and bladder carcinogenesis as well as inhibition of the development of polyps in mice genetically prone to develop such lesions. Since NSAIDs appear to exert their effects by an

Table 8.12 Some Synthetic Chemopreventive Agents

Agent	Species	Site of neoplasm	Carcinogen	Effect	Reference
Aspirin and other NSAIDs	Rat	Colon	DMH	↓[a]	Davis and Patterson, 1994
	Mouse	Bladder	OH BBN	↓	Rao et al., 1996
	Mouse (min)	Intestine	Genetic mutation	↓	Jacoby et al., 1996
Diallylsulfide and organosulfur compounds	Rat	Colon	AOM	↓ (invasive cancers)	Reddy et al., 1993
	Rat	Forestomach	Anstolochic acid	↓	Hadjiolov et al., 1993
	Rat	Liver	DEN	↓ (pre-neoplastic foci)	Haber-Mignard et al., 1996
			Aflatoxin B_1	↓	
Difluoromethyl-ornithine	Rat	Bladder	BHBN	↓ (for 60 weeks)	Uchida et al., 1989
	Rat	Liver	DEN	↓	Kojima et al., 1993
	Mouse	Colon	DMH	↓	Tempero et al., 1989
Oltipraz	Rat	Liver	AFB_1	↓	Bolton et al., 1993
	Rat	Colon	AOM	↓	Rao et al., 1993b
Finasteride	Rat	Prostate	DMAB	↓	Tsukamoto et al., 1995
Tamoxifen	Hamster	Liver	Zeranol	↓	Coe et al., 1992
	Rat	Mammae	EMS	↓	Ueo et al., 1993
N-(4-Hydroxy-phenyl)retin-amide	Rat	Liver	DEN/AAF	↓	Mishkin et al., 1985
	Rat	Prostate	Spontaneous	↓	Pollard et al., 1991

[a]Inhibition of carcinogenesis.

inhibition of the prostaglandin pathway, their mechanisms may be similar to those noted in the different effects of ω3 and ω6 fatty acids (see above; Lands, 1992). The synthetic organosulfur compounds utilized in chemoprevention are analogous to those occurring naturally and presumably exert similar effects (cf. Wattenberg, 1992). Difluoromethylornithine (DFMO) is an effective inhibitor of the early steps in polyamine synthesis necessary for the stabilization and function of RNA and DNA (cf. Pegg, 1988). Thus, DFMO exerts its effects in the stages of initiation and promotion because of its inhibition of DNA synthesis and cell proliferation. When DFMO is given in the diet together with selenite, the inhibition of DMBA-induced mammary neoplasms in rats is inhibited to a much greater extent than if either chemopreventive agent is administered alone (Ip and Thompson, 1989). This and other studies thus suggest that chemoprevention may be more effective when more than one agent is administered, an effect analogous to the enhanced efficacy of combinations of chemotherapeutic drugs used in the treatment of cancer (Chapter 17). Oltipraz, which is actually an organosulfur compound, protects against chemically induced carcinogenesis in lung, trachea, forestomach, colon, breast, skin, liver, and urinary bladder in rodents (Kensler et al., 1992). Its effects also appear to involve both initiation and promotion. The synthetic steroid finasteride is known to inhibit the conversion of testosterone into dihydrotestosterone, and its administration significantly inhibits the chemical induction of prostatic carcinomas in rats induced by 3,2'-dimethyl-4-aminobiphenyl (DMAB). Tamoxifen alters the interaction of estrogen with its receptor and inhibits the development of neoplasia in tissues wherein estrogen plays a significant role in neoplastic development. Finally, as alluded to earlier in this chapter, a variety of synthetic retinoids have also been shown to be effective chemopreventive agents.

All of the synthetic exogenous modifiers noted in Table 8.12 exerted an inhibitory effect during the stage of promotion in chemical carcinogenesis. Several also alter the stage of initiation. This further reinforces the observation that the stages of neoplastic development most sensitive to prevention and modification of neoplastic development are initiation and promotion. Another critical target of such agents, whose importance becomes more evident in the next two chapters, is the transition of cells in the stage of promotion to the irreversible stage of progression.

REFERENCES

Agnew, L. R. C., and Gardner, W. U. The incidence of spontaneous hepatomas in C3H, C3H (low milk factor) and CBA mice and the effect of estrogen and androgen on the occurrence of these tumors in C3H mice. Cancer Res., *12*:757–761, 1952.

Akao, M., and Kuroda, K. Enhancing and inhibitory effects of some stilbene and steroid compounds on induction of hepatoma in rats fed 3'-methyl-4-(dimethylamino)azobenzene. Gann, *69*:375–382, 1978.

Albanes, D. Total calories, body weight, and tumor incidence in mice. Cancer Res., *47*:1987–1992, 1987.

Albert, R. E., Benjamin, S. A., and Shukla, R. Life span and cancer mortality in the Beagle dog and humans. Mech. Ageing Dev., *74*:149–159, 1994.

Anderson, L. M., Carter, J. P., Logsdon, D. L., Driver, C. L., and Kovatch, R. M. Characterization of ethanol's enhancement of tumorigenesis by *N*-nitrosodimethylamine in mice. Carcinogenesis, *13*:2107–2111, 1992.

Andervont, H. B. Studies on the occurrence of spontaneous hepatomas in mice of strains C3H and CBA. J. Natl. Cancer Inst., *11*:581–592, 1950.

Anisimov, V. N. Age-related mechanisms of susceptibility to carcinogenesis. Semin. Onc., *16*:10–19, 1989.

Appel, M. J., van Garderen-Hoetmer, A., and Woutersen, R. A. Effects of dietary linoleic acid on pancreatic carcinogenesis in rats and hamsters. Cancer Res., *54*:2113–2120, 1994.

Argus, M. F., Hoch-Ligeti, C., Arcos, J. C., and Conney, A. H. Differential effects of β-naphthoflavone and pregnenolone-16α-carbonitrile on dimethyl- nitrosamine-induced hepatocarcinogenesis. J. Natl. Cancer Inst., *61*:441–449, 1978.

Axelrad, A. Genetic resistance to Friend virus. Ann. N.Y. Acad. Sci., *567*:26–37, 1989.

Bal, D. G., and Foerster, S. B. Dietary strategies for cancer prevention. Cancer, *72*:1005–1010, 1993.

Baldwin, S., and Parker, R. S. Influence of dietary fat and selenium in initiation and promotion of aflatoxin B_1-induced preneoplastic foci in rat liver. Carcinogenesis, *8*:101–107, 1987.

Barrett, J. C., Annab, L. A., Alcorta, D., Preston, G., Vojta, P., and Yin, Y. Cellular senescence and cancer. Cold Spring Harbor Symp. Quant. Biol., *59*:411–418, 1994.

Beato, M. Transcriptional regulation of mouse mammary tumor virus by steroid hormones. Oncogenesis, *2*:195–210, 1991.

Bedigian, H. G., Copeland, N. G., Jenkins, N. A., Salvatore, K., and Rodick, S. *Emv-13* (*Akv-3*): a nonin-ducible endogenous ecotropic provirus of AKR/J mice. J. Virol., *46*:490–497, 1983.

Benson, D., Mitchell, N., and Dix, D. On the role of aging in carcinogenesis. Mutat. Res., *356*:209–216, 1996.

Berger, M. R. Synergism and antagonism between chemical carcinogens. *In*: J. C. Arcos, M. F. Argus, and Y.-t. Woo (Eds.), Chemical Induction of Cancer: Modulation and Combination Effects, pp. 23–49. Boston: Birkhäuser, 1995.

Berger, M. R., Schmähl, D., and Zerban, H. Combination experiments with very low doses of three genotoxic *N*-nitrosamines with similar organotropic carcinogenicity in rats. Carcinogenesis, *8*:1635–1643, 1987.

Best, S., Le Tissier, P., Towers, G., and Stoye, J. P. Positional cloning of the mouse retrovirus restriction gene *Fv1*. Nature, *382*:826–829, 1996.

Beth, M., Berger, M. R., Aksoy, M., and Schmähl, D. Comparison between the effects of dietary fat level and of calorie intake on methylnitrosourea-induced mammary carcinogenesis in female SD rats. Int. J. Cancer, *39*:737–744, 1987.

Bhatia, K. G., Cherney, B. W., Huppi, K., Magrath, I. T., Cossman, J., Sausville, E., Barriga, F., Johnson, B., Gause, B., Bonney, G., Neequayi, J., DeBernardi, M., and Smulson, M. A deletion linked to a poly(ADP-ribose) polymerase gene on chromosome 13q33-qter occurs frequently in the normal black population as well as in multiple tumor DNA. Cancer Res., *50*:5406–5413, 1990.

Bielschowsky, F. The role of hormonal factors in the development of tumours induced by 2-aminofluorene and related compounds. Acta Unio Int. Contra Cancrum, *17*:121–130, 1961.

Bingham, S. A. Mechanisms and experimental and epidemiological evidence relating dietary fibre (non-starch polysaccharides) and starch to protection against large bowel cancer. Proc. Nutr. Soc., *49*:153–171, 1990.

Bird, R. P., Yao, K., Lasko, C. M., and Good, C. K. Inability of low- or high-fat diet to modulate late stages of colon carcinogenesis in Sprague-Dawley rats. Cancer Res., *56*:2896–2899, 1996.

Birt, D. F. Update on the effects of vitamins A, C, and E and selenium on carcinogenesis. Proc. Soc. Exp. Biol. Med., *183*:311–320, 1986.

Birt, D. F. Fat and calorie effects on carcinogenesis at sites other than the mammary gland. Am. J. Clin. Nutr., *45*:203–209, 1987.

Birt, D. F. Effects of the intake of selected vitamins and minerals on cancer prevention. Magnesium, *8*:17–30, 1989.

Birt, D. F., Lawson, T. A., Julius, A. D., Runice, C. E., and Salmasi, S. Inhibition by dietary selenium of colon cancer induced in the rat by bis(2-oxopropyl)nitrosamine. Cancer Res., *42*:4455–4459, 1982.

Birt, D. F., Davies, M. H., Pour, P. M., and Salmasi, S. Lack of inhibition by retinoids of bis(2-oxopropyl)-nitrosamine-induced carcinogenesis in Syrian hamsters. Carcinogenesis, *4*:1215–1220, 1983.

Birt, D. F., Julius, A. D., White, L. T., and Pour, P. M. Enhancement of pancreatic carcinogenesis in ham-sters fed a high-fat diet *ad libitum* and at a controlled calorie intake. Cancer Res., *49*:5848–5851, 1989.

Birt, D. F., Kris, E. S., Choe, M., and Pelling, J. C. Dietary energy and fat effects on tumor promotion. Cancer Res., *52*:2035s–2039s, 1992.

Block, G., and Schwarz, R. Ascorbic acid and cancer: animal and cell culture data. *In*: Natural Antioxidants in Human Health and Disease, Chapter 2, pp. 129–155. New York: Academic Press, 1994.

Block, G., Patterson, B., and Subar, A. Fruit, vegetables, and cancer prevention: a review of the epidemiological evidence. Nutr. Cancer, *18*:1–29, 1992.

Blot, W. J. Alcohol and cancer. Cancer Res., *52*:2119s–2123s, 1992.

Blount, B. C., Mack, M. M., Wehr, C. M., MacGregor, J. T., Hiatt, R. A., Wang, G., Wickramasinghe, S. N., Everson, R. B., and Ames, B. N. Folate deficiency causes uracil misincorporation into human DNA and chromosome breakage: implications for cancer and neuronal damage. Proc. Natl. Acad. Sci. U.S.A., *94*:3290–3295, 1997.

Blunck, J. M., Lees, B. J., and Madsen, N. P. Prevention by chloramphenicol of suppressed hepatic azo reductase activity due to 3′-methyl-4-dimethylaminoazobenzene. Chem.-Biol. Interact., *4*:219–222, 1971/1972.

Böck, A., Forchhammer, K., Heider, J., Leinfelder, W., Sawers, G., Veprek, B., and Zinoni, F. Selenocysteine: the 21st amino acid. Mol. Microbiol., *5*:515–520, 1991.

Bollag, W. Therapy of chemically induced skin tumor of mice with vitamin A palmitate and vitamin A acid. Experientia, *27*:90–92, 1972.

Bollag, W. Prophylaxis of chemically induced benign and malignant epithelial tumors by vitamin A acid (retinoic acid). Eur. J. Cancer, *8*:689–693, 1972.

Bolton, M. G., Muñoz, A., Jacobson, L. P., Groopman, J. D., Maxuitenko, Y. Y., Roebuck, B. D., and Kensler, T. W. Transient intervention with olitpraz protects against aflatoxin-induced hepatic tumorigenesis. Cancer Res., *53*:3499–3504, 1993.

Boutwell, R. K. Caloric intake, dietary fat level, and experimental carcinogenesis. *In*: M. M. Jacobs (Ed.), Exercise, Calories, Fat, and Cancer, pp. 95–101. New York: Plenum Press, 1992.

Bridges, B. A. (Chairman), et al. (International Commission for Protection Against Environmental Mutagens and Carcinogens). Conclusions on the genotoxicity of alcohol and recommendations for further work. Mutat. Res., *186*:175–176, 1987.

Burk, R. F., and Hill, K. E. Regulation of selenoproteins. Annu. Rev. Nutr., *13*:65–81, 1993.

Burns, E. L., and Schenken, J. R. Spontaneous primary hepatomas in mice of strain C3H. II. The influence of breeding on their incidence. Cancer Res., *3*:691–692, 1943a.

Burns, E. L., and Schenken, J. R. Spontaneous primary hepatomas in mice of strain C3H. IV. A study of intracytoplasmic inclusion bodies and mitochondria. Cancer Res., *3*:697–701, 1943b.

Caderni, G., Luceri, C., Spagnesi, M. T., Giannini, A., Biggeri, A., and Dolara, P. Dietary carbohydrates modify azoxymethane-induced intestinal carcinogenesis in rats. J. Nutr., *124*:517–523, 1994.

Caderni, G., Lancioni, L., Luceri, C., Giannini, A., Lodovici, M., Biggeri, A., and Dolara, P. Dietary sucrose and starch affect dysplastic characteristics in carcinogen-induced aberrant crypt foci in rat colon. Cancer Lett., *114*:39–41, 1997.

Cameron, E., Bland, J., and Marcuson, R. Divergent effects of omega-6 and omega-3 fatty acids on mammary tumor development in C_3H/Heston mice treated with DMBA. Nutr. Res., *9*:383–393, 1989.

Cardeilhac, P. T., and Nair, K. P. C. Inhibition by castration of aflatoxin-induced hepatoma in carbon tetrachloride-treated rats. Toxicol. Appl. Pharmacol., *26*:393–397, 1973.

Carlson, G. P. Induction of *N*-nitrosodimethylamine metabolism in rat liver and lung by ethanol. Cancer Lett., *54*:153–156, 1990.

Carter, J. H., Carter, H. W., and Meade, J. Adrenal regulation of mammary tumorigenesis in female Sprague-Dawley rats: incidence, latency, and yield of mammary tumors. Cancer Res., *48*:3801–3807, 1988.

Chandra, M., and Frith, C. H. Spontaneous neoplasms in aged CD-1 mice. Toxicol. Lett., *61*:67–74, 1992a.

Chandra, M., and Frith, C. F. Spontaneous neoplasms in aged control Fischer 344 rats. Cancer Lett., *62*:49–56, 1992b.

Chang, T. K. H., and Bellward, G. D. Peripubertal androgen imprinting of rat hepatic cytochrome P450 2C11 and steroid 5α-reductase: pretranslational regulation and impact on microsomal drug activation. J. Pharmacol. Exp. Ther., *278*:1383–1391, 1996.

Chang, W.-C. L., Chapkin, R. S., and Lupton, J. R. Predictive value of proliferation, differentiation and apoptosis as intermediate markers for colon tumorigenesis. Carcinogenesis, *18*:721–730, 1997.

Chaudhny, A. P., Singer, L., Gorlin, R. S., and Vickers, R. A. Effects of vitamin A deficiency on experimental carcinogenesis in submandibular glands of hamsters. J. Dent. Res., 40:327–330, 1961.

Cheah, P. Y., and Bernstein, H. Colon cancer and dietary fiber: cellulose inhibits the DNA-damaging ability of bile acids. Nutr. Cancer, 13:51–57, 1990.

Chedid, A., Halfman, C. J ., and Greenberg, S. R. Hormonal influences on chemical carcinogenesis: studies with the aflatoxin B_1 hepatocarcinoma model in the rat. Dig. Dis. Sci., 25:869–874, 1980.

Chen, L. H., Boissonneault, G. A., and Glauert, H. P. Vitamin C, vitamin E and cancer. Anticancer Res., 8:739–748, 1988.

Chen, W., Zhou, Y., Nichols, J., Chung, K.-T., Hart, R. W., and Chou, M. W. Effect of dietary restriction on benzo[a]pyrene (BaP) metabolic activation and pulmonary BaP-DNA adduct formation in mouse. Drug Chem. Toxicol., 19:21–39, 1996.

Chou, M. W., and Chen, W. Food restriction reduces aflatoxin B_1 (AFB_1)-DNA adduct formation, AFB_1-glutathione conjugation, and DNA damage in AFB_1-treated male F344 rats and $B6C3F_1$ mice. J. Nutr., 127:210–217, 1997.

Christman, J. K., Sheikhnejad, G., Dizik, M., Abileah, S., and Wainfan, E. Reversibility of changes in nucleic acid methylation and gene expression induced in rat liver by severe dietary methyl deficiency. Carcinogenesis, 14:551–557, 1993.

Chu, E. W., and Malmgren, R. A. An inhibitory effect of vitamin A on the induction of tumors of forestomach and cervix in the Syrian hamster by carcinogenic polycyclic hydrocarbons. Cancer Res., 25:884–895, 1965.

Clapham, D. E. Calcium signaling. Cell, 80:259–268, 1995.

Clayton, C. C., and Baumann, C. A. Diet and azo dye tumors: effect of diet during a period when the dye is not fed. Cancer Res., 9:575–582, 1949.

Clinton, S. K., Truex, C. R., and Visek, W. J. Dietary protein, aryl hydrocarbon hydroxylase and chemical carcinogenesis in rats. J. Nutr., 109:55–62, 1979.

Clinton, S. K., Li, P. S., Mulloy, A. L., Imrey, P. B., Nandkumar, S., and Visek, W. J. The combined effects of dietary fat and estrogen on survival, 7,12-dimethylbenz(a)anthracene-induced breast cancer and prolactin metabolism in rats. J. Nutr., 125:1192–1204, 1995.

Coe, J. E., Ishak, K. G., Ward, J. M., and Ross, M. J. Tamoxifen prevents induction of hepatic neoplasia by zeranol, an estrogenic food contaminant. Proc. Natl. Acad. Sci. U.S.A., 89:1085–1089, 1992.

Cohen, L. A., Coi, K., Weisburger, J. H., and Rose, D. P. Effect of varying proportions of dietary fat on the development of N-nitrosomethylurea-induced rat mammary tumors. Anticancer Res., 6:215–218, 1986.

Cohen, S. M., Wittenberg, J. F., and Bryan, G. T. Effect of avitaminosis A and hypervitaminosis A on urinary bladder carcinogenicity of N-[4-(5-nitro-2-furyl)-2-thiazolyl] formamide. Cancer Res., 36:2334–2339, 1976.

Coleman, J. E. Zinc proteins: enzymes, storage proteins, transcription factors, and replication proteins. Annu. Rev. Biochem., 61:897–946, 1992.

Conybeare, G. Effect of quality and quantity of diet on survival and tumour incidence in outbred Swiss mice. Fd. Cosmet. Toxicol., 18:65–75, 1980.

Cravo, M. L., Mason, J. B., Dayal, Y., Hutchinson, M., Smith, D., Selhub, J., and Rosenberg, I. H. Folate deficiency enhances the development of colonic neoplasia in dimethylhydrazine-treated rats. Cancer Res., 52:5002–5006, 1992.

Daniel, F. B., DeAngelo, A. B., Stober, J. A., Pereira, M. A., and Olson, G. R. Chloroform inhibition of 1,2,-dimethylhydrazine-induced gastrointestinal tract tumors in the Fisher 344 rat. Fundam. Appl. Toxicol., 13:40–45, 1989.

Dauod, A. H., and Griffin, A. C. Effect of retinoic acid, butylated hydroxytoluene, selenium and sorbic acid on azo dye hepatocarcinogenesis. Cancer Lett., 9:299–304, 1980.

Davis, A. E., and Patterson, F. Aspirin reduces the incidence of colonic carcinoma in the dimethylhydrazine rat animal model. Aust. N.Z. J. Med., 24:301–303, 1994.

De Luca, L. M., Shores, R. L., Spangler, E. F., and Wenk, M. L. Inhibition of initiator-promoter–induced skin tumorigenesis in female SENCAR mice fed a vitamin A-deficient diet and reappearance of tumors in mice fed a diet adequate in retinoid or β-carotene. Cancer Res., 49:5400–5406, 1989.

De Luca, L. M., Darwiche, N., Celli, G., Kosa, K., Jones, C., Ross, S., and Chen, L.-C. Vitamin A in epithelial differentiation and skin carcinogenesis. Nutr. Rev., 52:S45–S52, 1994.

De Luca, L. M., Tarone, R., Huynh, M., Jones, C. S., and Chen, L.-C. Dietary retinoic acid inhibits mouse skin carcinogenesis irrespective of age at initiation. Nutr. Cancer, 25:249–257, 1996.

DeWille, J. W., Waddell, K., Steinmeyer, C., and Farmer, S. J. Dietary fat promotes mammary tumorigenesis in MMTV/v-Ha-ras transgenic mice. Cancer Lett., 69:59–66, 1993.

Dipple, A., Pigott, M. A., and Milner, J. A. Selenium modifies carcinogen metabolism by inhibiting enzyme induction. Biol. Trace Element Res., 10:153–156, 1986.

DiSilvestro, R. A., Greenson, J. K., and Liao, Z. Effects of low copper intake on dimethylhydrazine-induced colon cancer in rats. Proc. Soc. Exp. Biol. Med., 201:94–97, 1992.

Dizik, M., Christman, J. K., and Wainfan, E. Alterations in expression and methylation of specific genes in livers of rats fed a cancer promoting methyl-deficient diet. Carcinogenesis, 12:1307–1312, 1991.

Djuric, Z., Lu, M. H., Lewis, S. M., Luongo, D. A., Chen, X. W., Heilbrun, L. K., Reading, B. A., Duffy, P. H., and Hart, R. W. Oxidative DNA damage levels in rats fed low-fat, high-fat, or calorie-restricted diets. Toxicol. Appl. Pharmacol., 115:156–160, 1992.

Dogra, S. C., Khanduja, K. L., Gupta, M. P., and Sharma, R. R. Binding of benzo(a)pyrene to DNA in normal and vitamin A deficient rats. Indian J. Biochem. Biophys., 21:117–120, 1984.

Doll, R. Nature and nurture: possibilities for cancer control. Carcinogenesis, 17:177–184, 1996.

Dong, F., Brynes, R. K., Tidow, N., Welte, K., Löwenberg, B., and Touw, I. P. Mutations in the gene for the granulocyte colony-stimulating-factor receptor in patients with acute myeloid leukemia preceded by severe congenital neutropenia. N. Engl. J. Med., 333:487–493, 1995.

Dorado, R. D., Porta, E. A., and Aquino, T. M. Effects of dietary selenium on hepatic and renal tumorigenesis induced in rats by diethylnitrosamine. Hepatology, 5:1201–1208, 1985.

Dragsted, L. O., Strube, M., and Larsen, J. C. Cancer-protective factors in fruits and vegetables: biochemical and biological background. Pharmacol. Toxicol., 72:s116–s134, 1993.

Drinkwater, N. R. Effect of genetic susceptibility on tumor induction. In: J. C. Arcos, M. F. Argus, and Y.-t. Woo (Eds.), Chemical Induction of Cancer: Modulation and Combination Effects, pp. 451–472. Boston: Birkhäuser, 1995.

Driver, H. E., and McLean, A. E. M. Dose-response relationships for initiation of rat liver tumours by diethylnitrosamine and promotion by phenobarbitone or alcohol. Food Chem. Toxic., 24:241–245, 1986.

Dunning, W. F., Curtis, M. R., and Maun, M. E. The effect of added dietary tryptophan on the occurrence of 2-acetylaminofluorene-induced liver and bladder cancer in rats. Cancer Res., 10:454–459, 1950.

Duris, I., Hruby, D., Pekarkova, B., Huorka, M., Cernakova, E., Bezayova, T., and Ondrejka, P. Calcium chemoprevention in colorectal cancer. Hepatogastroenterology, 43:152–154, 1996.

Enzmann, H., Ohlhauser, D., Dettler, T., and Bannasch, P. Enhancement of hepatocarcinogenesis in rats by dietary fructose. Carcinogenesis, 10:1247–1252, 1989.

Eskelson, C. D., Odeleye, O. E., Watson, R. R., Earnest, D. L., and Mufti, S. I. Modulation of cancer growth by vitamin E and alcohol. Alcohol Alcohol, 28:117–125, 1993.

Etkind, P. R., Qiu, L., and Lumb, K. Dietary fat: gene expression and mammary tumorigenesis. Nutr. Cancer, 24:13–21, 1995.

Faris, R. A., and Campbell, T. C. Exposure of newborn rats to pharmacologically active compounds may permanently alter carcinogen metabolism. Science, 211:719–721, 1981.

Fernandes, G., Chandrasekar, B., Troyer, D. A., Venkatraman, J. T., and Good, R. A. Dietary lipids and calorie restriction affect mammary tumor incidence and gene expression in mouse mammary tumor virus/v-Ha-ras transgenic mice. Proc. Natl. Acad. Sci. U.S.A., 92:6494–6498, 1995.

Fernandes, G., Venkatraman, J. T., Turturro, A., Attwood, V. G., and Hart, R. W. Effect of food restriction on life span and immune functions in long-lived Fischer-344 × Brown Norway F_1 rats. J. Clin. Immunol., 17:85–95, 1997.

Fesus, L., Madi, A., Balajthy, Z., Nemes, Z., and Szondy, Z. Transglutaminase induction by various cell death and apoptosis pathways. Experientia, 52:942–948, 1996.

Feuers, R. J., Weindruch, R., and Hart, R. W. Caloric restriction, aging, and antioxidant enzymes. Mutat. Res., 295:191–200, 1993.

Fong, L. Y. Y., Lee, J. S. K., Chan, W. C., and Newberne, P. M. Zinc deficiency and the development of esophageal and forestomach tumors in Sprague-Dawley rats fed precursors of *N*-nitroso-*N*-benzyl-methylamine. J. Natl. Cancer Inst., *72*:419–425, 1984.

Forbes, P. D., Urbach, F., and Davies, R. E. Enhancement of experimental photocarcinogenesis by topical retinoic acid. Cancer Lett., *7*:85–90, 1979.

Fraker, P. J., Osati-Ashtiani, F., Wagner, M. A., and King, L. E. Possible roles for glucocorticoids and apoptosis in the suppression of lymphopoiesis during zinc deficiency: a review. J. Am. Coll. Nutr., *14*:11–17, 1995.

Freedman, L. S., Clifford, C., and Messina, M. Analysis of dietary fat, calories, body weight, and the development of mammary tumors in rats and mice: a review. Cancer Res., *50*:5710–5719, 1990.

Fukushima, S., Shibata, M.-A., Hirose, M., Kato, T., Tatematsu, M., and Ito, N. Organ-specific modification of tumor development by low-dose combinations of agents in a rat wide-spectrum carcinogenesis model. Jpn. J. Cancer Res., *82*:784–792, 1991.

Gairola, C., and Chow, C. K. Dietary selenium, hepatic arylhydrocarbon hydroxylase and mutagenic activation of benzo(a)pyrene, 2-aminoanthracene and 2-aminofluorene. Toxicol. Lett., *11*:281–287, 1982.

Gammal, E. B., Carroll, K. K., and Plunkett, E. R. Effects of dietary fat on mammary carcinogenesis by 7,12-dimethylbenz(*a*)anthracene in rats. Cancer Res., *27*:1737–1742, 1967.

Gao, P., and Chou, M. W. Effect of caloric restriction on hepatic nuclear DNA damage in male Fischer 344 rats treated with aflatoxin B$_1$. Toxicol. Lett., *61*:233–242, 1992.

Gardner, M. B., Rasheed, S., Pal, B. K., Estes, J. D., and O'Brien, S. J. *Akvr-1*, a dominant murine leukemia virus restriction gene, is polymorphic in leukemia-prone wild mice. Proc. Natl. Acad. Sci. U.S.A., *77*:531–535, 1980.

Garro, A. J., and Lieber, C. S. Alcohol and cancer. Annu. Rev. Pharmacol. Toxicol., *30*:219–249, 1990.

Gazdar, A. F., Oie, H., Lalley, P., Moss, W. W., Minna, J. D., and Francke, U. Identification of mouse chromosomes required for murine leukemia virus replication. Cell, *11*:949–956, 1977.

Gendimenico, G. J., Nair, X,. Bouquin, P. L., and Tramposch, K. M. Effects of retinoids on phorbol ester-stimulated epidermal DNA synthesis and hyperplasia in hairless mice. J. Invest. Dermatol., *93*:363–367, 1989.

Ghoshal, A. K., and Farber, E. The induction of liver cancer by dietary deficiency of choline and methionine without added carcinogens. Carcinogenesis, *5*:1367–1370, 1984.

Giovannucci, E., Egan, K. M., Hunter, D. J., Stampfer, M. J., Colditz, G. A., Willett, W. C., and Speizer, F. E. Aspirin and the risk of colorectal cancer in women. N. Engl. J. Med., *333*:609–614, 1995.

Globerson, A. T lymphocytes and aging. Int. Arch. Allergy Immunol., *107*:491–497, 1995.

Glynn, S. A., and Albanes, D. Folate and cancer: a review of the literature. Nutr. Cancer, *22*:101–119, 1994.

Goff, S. P. Operating under a gag order: a block against incoming virus by the *Fv1* gene. Cell, *86*:691–693, 1996.

Goodall, C. M., and Butler, W. H. Aflatoxin carcinogenesis: inhibition of liver cancer induction in hypophysectomized rats. Int. J. Cancer, *4*:422–429, 1969.

Grasl-Kraupp, B., Bursch, W., Ruttkay-Nedecky, B., Wagner, A., Lauer, B., and Schulte-Hermann, R. Food restriction eliminates preneoplastic cells through apoptosis and antagonizes carcinogenesis in rat liver. Proc. Natl. Acad. Sci. U.S.A., *91*:9995–9999, 1994.

Grasso, P., and Hardy, J. Strain difference in natural incidence and response to carcinogens. *In*: W. H. Butler and P. M. Newberne (Eds.), Mouse Hepatic Neoplasia, Chap. 6, pp. 111–132. Amsterdam: Elsevier, 1975.

Greene, F. L., Lamb, L. S., Barwick, M., and Pappas, N. J. Effect of dietary copper on colonic tumor production and aortic integrity in the rat. J. Surg. Res., *42*:503–512, 1987.

Griciute, L., Castegnaro, M., and Bereziat, J.-C. Influence of ethyl alcohol on carcinogenesis with *N*-nitrosodimethylamine. Cancer Lett., *13*:345–352, 1987.

Griffin, A. C., Rinfret, A. P., and Corsigilia, V. F. The inhibition of liver carcinogenesis with 3′-methyl-4-dimethylaminoazobenzene in hypophysectomized rats. Cancer Res., *13*:77–79, 1953.

Gross, L., and Dreyfuss, Y. Prevention of spontaneous and radiation-induced tumors in rats by reduction of food intake. Proc. Natl. Acad. Sci. U.S.A., *87*:6795–6797, 1990.

Gumprecht, L. A., Long, C. R., Soper, K. A., Smith, P. F., Haschek-Hock, W. M., and Keenan, K. P. The early effects of dietary restriction on the pathogenesis of chronic renal disease in Sprague-Dawley rats at 12 months. Toxicol. Pathol., *21*:528–537, 1993.

Günzburg, W. H., and Salmons, B. Factors controlling the expression of mouse mammary tumour virus. Biochem. J., *283*:625–632, 1992.

Haber-Mignard, D., Suschetet, M., Bergès, R., Astorg, P., and Siess, M.-H. Inhibition of aflatoxin B_1- and *N*-nitrosodiethylamine-induced liver preneoplastic foci in rats fed naturally occurring allyl sulfides. Nutr. Cancer, *25*:61–70, 1996.

Hadjiolov, D., Fernando, R. C., Schmeiser, H. H., Wießler, M., Hadjiolov, N., and Pirajnov, G. Effect of diallyl sulfide on aristolochic acid-induced forestomach carcinogenesis in rats. Carcinogenesis, *14*:407–410, 1993.

Harbach, P. R., and Swenberg, J. A. Effects of selenium on 1,2-dimethylhydrazine metabolism and DNA alkylation. Carcinogenesis, *2*:575–580, 1981.

Harley, J. W., Yetter, R. A., and Morse, H. C. III. A mouse gene on chromosome 5 that restricts infectivity of mink cell focus-forming recombinant murine leukemia viruses. J. Exp. Med., *158*:16–24, 1983.

Harr, J. R., Exon, J. H., Whanger, P. D., and Weswig, P. M. Effect of dietary selenium on *N*-fluorenyl-acetamide (FAA) induced cancer in vitamin E supplemented rats. Clin. Toxicol., *5*:187–194, 1972.

Hart, R. W., Chou, M. W., Feuers, R. J., Leakey, J. E. A., Duffy, P. H., Lyn-Cook, B., Turturro, A., and Allaben, W. T. Caloric restriction and chemical toxicity/carcinogenesis. Quality Assurance: Good Practice, Regulation, and Law, *1*:120–131, 1992.

Hartshorn, R. D., Demers, L. M., Sultatos, L. G., Vesell, E. S., Lang, C. M., and Hughes, H. C. Jr. Effects of chronic parenteral carbohydrate administration on hepatic drug metabolism in the rat. Pharmacology, *18*:103–111, 1979.

Hawrylewicz, E. J., Huang, H. H., Kissane, J. Q., and Drab, E. A. Enhancement of 7,12-dimethyl-benz(a)anthracene (DMBA) mammary tumorigenesis by high dietary protein in rats. Nutr. Rep. Int., *26*:793–806, 1982.

Hayatsu, H., Arimoto, S., and Negishi, T. Dietary inhibitors of mutagenesis and carcinogenesis. Mutat. Res., *202*:429–446, 1988.

Hei, T. K., and Sudilovsky, O. Effects of a high-sucrose diet on the development of enzyme-altered foci in chemical hepatocarcinogenesis in rats. Cancer Res., *45*:2700–2705, 1985.

Heller, T. D., Holt, P. R., and Richardson, A. Food restriction retards age-related histological changes in rat small intestine. Gastroenterology, *98*:387–391, 1990.

Hennings, H., Wenk, M. L., and Donahoe, R. Retinoic acid promotion of papilloma formation in mouse skin. Cancer Lett., *16*:1–5, 1982.

Herd, J. E., and Greene, F. E. Effects of perinatal exposure to benzo(a)pyrene on the aryl hydrocarbon hydroxylase system of adult rat liver. Biol. Neonate, *38*:291–299, 1980.

Hikita, H., Vaughan, J., and Pitot, H. C. The effect of two periods of short-term fasting during the promotion stage of hepatocarcinogenesis in rats: the role of apoptosis and cell proliferation. Carcinogenesis, *18*:159–166, 1997.

Hilkens, J., Colombatti, A., Strand, M., Nichols, E., Ruddle, F. H., and Hilgers, J. Identification of a mouse gene required for binding of Rauscher MuLV envelope gp70. Somat. Cell Genet., *5*:39–49, 1979.

Hiramatsu, Y., Takada, H., Yamamura, M., Hioki, K., Saito, K., and Yamamoto, M. Effect of dietary cholesterol on azoxymethane-induced colon carcinogenesis in rats. Carcinogenesis, *4*:553–558, 1983.

Hirayama, T. Life-style and cancer: from epidemiological evidence to public behavior change to mortality reduction of target cancers. J. Natl. Cancer Inst. Monogr., *12*:65–74, 1992.

Hoatlin, M. E., Kozak, S. L., Lilly, F., Chakraborti, A., Kozak, C. A., and Kabat, D. Activation of erythropoietin receptors by Friend viral gp55 and by erythropoietin and down-modulation by the murine *Fv-2^r* resistance gene. Proc. Natl. Acad. Sci. U.S.A., *87*:9985–9989, 1990.

Hocman, G. Chemoprevention of cancer: selenium. Int. J. Biochem., *20*:123–132, 1988a.

Hocman, G. Prevention of cancer: restriction of nutritional energy intake (joules). Comp. Biochem. Physiol., *91A*:209–220, 1988b.

Hocman, G. Chemoprevention of cancer: protease inhibitors. Int. J. Biochem., *24*:1365–1375, 1992.

Holtzman, S. Retinyl acetate inhibits estrogen-induced mammary carcinogenesis in female ACI rats. Carcinogenesis, *9*:305–307, 1988.

Howe, G. R., Benito, E., Castelleto, R., Cornée, J., Estève, J., Gallagher, R. P., Iscovich, J. M., Deng-ao, J., Kaaks, R., Kune, G. A., Kune, S., L'Abbé, K. A., Lee, H. P., Lee, M., Miller, A. B., Peters, R. K., Potter, J. D., Riboli, E., Slattery, M. L., Trichopoulos, D., Tuyns, A., Tzonou, A., Whittemore, A. S., Wu-Williams, A. H., and Shu, Z. Dietary intake of fiber and decreased risk of cancers of the colon and rectum: evidence from the combined analysis of 13 case-control studies. J. Natl. Cancer Inst., *84*:1887–1896, 1992.

Hunt, S. M., and Groff, J. L. Advanced Nutrition and Human Metabolism. St. Paul, MN: West, 1990.

Hunter, D. J., Spiegelman, D., Adami, H.-O., Beeson, L., van den Brandt, P. A., Folsom, A. R., Fraser, G. E., Goldbohm, A., Graham, S., Howe, G. R., Kushi, L. H., Marshall, J. R., McDermott, A., Miller, A. B., Speizer, F. E., Wolk, A., Yaun, S.-S., and Willett, W. Cohort studies of fat intake and the risk of breast cancer—a pooled analysis. N. Engl. J. Med., *334*:356–361, 1996.

Iishi, H., Tatsuta, M., Baba, M., and Taniguchi, H. Promotion by ethanol of gastric carcinogenesis induced by *N*-methyl-*N'*-nitro-*N*-nitrosoguanidine in Wistar rats. Br. J. Cancer, *59*:719–721, 1989.

Ingles, S. A., Ross, R. K., Yu, M. C., Irvine, R. A., La Pera, G., Haile, R. W., and Coetzee, G. A. Association of prostate cancer risk with genetic polymorphisms in vitamin D receptor and androgen receptor. J. Natl. Cancer Inst., *89*:166–170, 1997.

Ip, C. Prophylaxis of mammary neoplasia by selenium supplementation in the initiation and promotion phases of chemical carcinogenesis. Cancer Res., *41*:4386–4390, 1981.

Ip, C. Selenium mediated inhibition of mammary carcinogenesis. Biol. Trace Element Res., *5*:317–330, 1983.

Ip, C. Interaction of vitamin C and selenium supplementation in the modification of mammary carcinogenesis in rats. J. Natl. Cancer Inst., *77*:299–303, 1986.

Ip, C., and Daniel, F. B. Effects of selenium on 7,12-dimethylbenz(*a*)anthracene-induced mammary carcinogenesis and DNA adduct formation. Cancer Res., *45*:61–65, 1985.

Ip, C., and Thompson, H. J. New approaches to cancer chemoprevention with difluoromethylornithine and selenite. J. Natl. Cancer Inst., *81*:839–843, 1989.

Ip, C., and White, G. Mammary cancer chemoprevention by inorganic and organic selenium: single agent treatment or in combination with vitamin E and their effects on *in vitro* immune functions. Carcinogenesis, *8*:1763–1766, 1987.

Izbicki, J. R., Hamilton, S. R., Wambach, G., Harnisch, E., Wilker, D. K., Dornschneider, G., Eibl-Eibesfeldt, B,. and Schweiberer, L. Effects of androgen manipulations on chemically induced colonic tumours and on macroscopically normal colonic mucosa in male Sprague-Dawley rats. Br. J. Cancer, *61*:235–240, 1990.

Jacobs, L. R. Relationship between dietary fiber and cancer: metabolic, physiologic, and cellular mechanisms. Proc. Soc. Exp. Biol. Med., *183*:299–310, 1986.

Jacobs, M. M. Selenium inhibition of 1,2-dimethylhydrazine-induced colon carcinogenesis. Cancer Res., *43*:1646–1649, 1983.

Jacobs, M. M., Jansson, B., and Griffin, A. C. Inhibitory effects of selenium on 1,2-dimethylhydrazine and methylazoxymethanol acetate induction of colon tumors. Cancer Lett., *2*:133–138, 1977.

Jacoby, R. F., Marshall, D. J., Newton, M. A., Novakovic, K., Tutsch, K., Cole, C. E., Lubet, R. A., Kelloff, G. J., Verma, A., Moser, A. R., and Dove, W. F. Chemoprevention of spontaneous intestinal adenomas in the *Apc*[Min] mouse model by the nonsteroidal anti-inflammatory drug piroxicam. Cancer Res., *56*:710–714, 1996.

James, S. J., and Muskhelishvili, L. Rates of apoptosis and proliferation vary with caloric intake and may influence incidence of spontaneous hepatoma in C57BL/6 × C3H F_1 mice. Cancer Res., *54*:5508–5510, 1994.

James, S. J., Cross, D. R., and Miller, B. J. Alterations in nucleotide pools in rats fed diets deficient in choline, methionine and/or folic acid. Carcinogenesis, *13*:2471–2474, 1992.

Kamdem, L., Siest, G., and Magdalou, J. Differential toxicity of aflatoxin B_1 in male and female rats: relationship with hepatic drug-metabolizing enzymes. Biochem. Pharmacol., *31*:3057–3062, 1982.

Katayama, S., Ohmori, T., Maeura, Y., Croci, T., and Williams, G. M. Early stages of *N*-2-fluorenylaceta-mide-induced hepatocarcinogenesis in male and female rats and effect of gonadectomy on liver neoplastic conversion and neoplastic development. J. Natl. Cancer Inst., *73*:141–149, 1984.

Keenan, K. P., Smith, P. F., Hertzog, P., Soper, K., Ballam, G. C., and Clark, R. L. The effects of overfeeding and dietary restriction on Sprague-Dawley rat survival and early pathology biomarkers of aging. Toxicol. Pathol., *22*:300–315, 1994.

Keenan, K. P., Soper, K. A., Smith, P. F., Ballam, G. C., and Clark, R. L. Diet, overfeeding, and moderate dietary restriction in control Sprague-Dawley rats: I. Effects on spontaneous neoplasms. Toxicol. Pathol., *23*:269–286, 1995.

Keenan, K. P., Laroque, P., Soper, K. A., Morrissey, R. E., and Dixit, R. The effects of overfeeding and moderate dietary restriction on Sprague-Dawley rat survival, pathology, carcinogenicity, and the toxicity of pharmaceutical agents. Exp. Toxicol. Pathol., *48*:139–144, 1996.

Kelloff, G. J., Boone, C. W., Crowell, J. A., Nayfield, S. G., Hawk, E., Malone, W. F., Steele, V. E., Lubet, R. A., and Sigman, C. C. Risk biomarkers and current strategies for cancer chemoprevention. J. Cell. Biochem., *25S*:1–14, 1996.

Kendall, C. W., Janezic, S. A., Friday, D., and Rao, A. V. Dietary cholesterol enhances preneoplastic aberrant crypt formation and alters cell proliferation in the murine colon treated with azoxymethane. Nutr. Cancer, *17*:107–114, 1992.

Kensler, T., Styczynski, P., Groopman, J., Helzlsouer, K., Curphey, T., Maxuitenko, Y., and Roebuck, B. D. Mechanisms of chemoprotection by olitpraz. J. Cell. Biochem., *161*:167–172, 1992.

Kessler, L. G. The relationship between age and incidence of breast cancer. Cancer, *69*:1896–1903, 1992.

Kim, Y.-I., Pogribny, I. P., Basnakian, A. G., Miller, J. W., Selhub, J., James, S. J., and Mason, J. B. Folate deficiency in rats induces DNA strand breaks and hypomethylation within the p53 tumor suppressor gene. Am. J. Clin. Nutr., *65*:46–52, 1997.

Klurfeld, D. M. Dietary fiber-mediated mechanisms in carcinogenesis. Cancer Res., *52*:2055s–2059s, 1992.

Klurfeld, D. M., Aglow, E., Tepper, S. A., and Kritchevsky, D. Modification of dimethylhydrazine-induced carcinogenesis in rats by dietary cholesterol. Nutr. Cancer, *5*:16–23, 1983.

Klurfeld, D. M., Weber, M. M., and Kritchevsky, D. Inhibition of chemically induced mammary and colon tumor promotion by caloric restriction in rats fed increased dietary fat. Cancer Res., *47*:2759–2762, 1987.

Kodama, M., Kodama, T., and Kodama, M. The genesis of breast cancer is a two-step phenomenon. I. Differential effects of aging on the cancer incidence in the United Kingdom and Japan. Anticancer Res., *12*:145–152, 1992.

Kojima, T., Tanaka, T., Kawamori, T., Hara, A., and Mori, H. Chemopreventive effects of dietary D,L-α-difluoromethylornithine, an ornithine decarboxylase inhibitor, on initiation and postinitiation stages of diethylnitrosamine-induced rat hepatocarcinogenesis. Cancer Res., *53*:3903–3907, 1993.

Kolaja, K. L., and Klaunig, J. E. Vitamin E modulation of hepatic focal lesion growth in mice. Toxicol. Appl. Pharmacol., *143*:380–387, 1997.

Kolaja, K. L., Bunting, K. A., and Klaunig, J. E. Inhibition of tumor promotion and hepatocellular growth by dietary restriction in mice. Carcinogenesis, *17*:1657–1664, 1996.

Kozak, C. A., and Rowe, W. P. Genetic mapping of the ecotropic murine leukemia virus-inducing locus of BALB/c mouse to chromosome 5. Science, *204*:69–71, 1979.

Kozak, C. A., and Rowe, W. P. Genetic mapping of xenotropic murine leukemia virus-inducing loci in five mouse strains. J. Exp. Med., *152*:219–228, 1980.

Kozak, C. A., Villar, C. J., and Voytek, P. Genetic aspects of oncogenesis by murine leukemia viruses in wild mice. CRC Crit. Rev. Oncogenesis, *1*:127–144, 1989.

Krinsky, N. I. Actions of carotenoids in biological systems. Annu. Rev. Nutr., *13*:561–587, 1993.

Kristensen, V. N., Harada, N., Yoshimura, N., Haraldsen, E., Lonning, P. E., Erikstein, B., Karesen,

Kritchevsky, D. Dietary effects in experimental carcinogenesis: animal models. Comp. Anim. Nutr., *6*:174–185, 1988.

Kurachi, H., Okamoto, S., and Oka, T. Evidence for the involvement of the submandibular gland epidermal growth factor in mouse mammary tumorigenesis. Proc. Natl. Acad. Sci. U.S.A., *82*:5940–5943, 1985.

Laconi, E., Tessitore, L., Milia, G., Yusuf, A., Sarma, D. S. R., Todde, P., and Pani, P. The enhancing effect of fasting/refeeding on the growth of nodules selectable by the resistant hepatocyte model in rat liver. Carcinogenesis, *16*:1865–1869, 1995.

Lagopoulos, L., and Stalder, R. The influence of food intake on the development of diethylnitrosamine-induced liver tumours in mice. Carcinogenesis, *8*:33–37, 1987.

Lamartiniere, C. A. Neonatal diethylstilbestrol treatment alters aflatoxin B1-DNA adduct concentrations in adult rats. J. Biochem. Toxicol., *5*:41–46, 1990.

Lands, W. E. M. Biochemistry and physiology of n-3 fatty acids. FASEB J., *6*:2530–2536, 1992.

Lane, H. W., Teer, P., Dukes, J., Johnson, J., and White, M. T. The effect of four chemical forms of selenium on mammary tumor incidence in BALB/c female mice treated with 7-12-dimethylbenz[*a*]anthracene. Cancer Lett., *50*:39–44, 1990.

LeBoeuf, R. A., Laishes, B. A., and Hoekstra, W. G. Effects of dietary selenium concentration on the development of enzyme-altered liver foci and hepatocellular carcinoma induced by diethylnitrosamine or *N*-acetylaminofluorene in rats. Cancer Res., *45*:5489–5495, 1985.

Lee, K. T., and Goodall, C. M. Methylation of ribonucleic acid and deoxyribonucleic acid and tumour induction in livers of hypophysectomized rats treated with dimethylnitrosamine. Biochem. J., *106*:767–768, 1968.

Lemons, R. S., O'Brien, S. J., and Sherr, C. J. A new genetic locus, *Bevi*, on human chromosome 6 which controls the replication of baboon type C virus in human cells. Cell, *12*:251–262, 1977.

Leutzinger, Y., and Richie, J. P., Jr. The effect of animal age on tumor induction. *In*: J. C. Arcos, M. F. Argus, and Y.-t. Woo (Eds.), Chemical Induction of Cancer: Modulation and Combination Effects, pp. 373–395. Boston: Birkhäuser, 1995.

Lii, C.-K., Ko, J.-J., and Chen, H.-W. No inhibition of γ-glutamyl transpeptidase-positive foci by vitamin E with or without phenobarbital. Nutr. Cancer, *27*:200–205, 1997.

Lijinsky, W., Milner, J. A., Kovatch, R. M., and Thomas, B. J. Lack of effect of selenium on induction of tumors of esophagus and bladder in rats by two nitrosamines. Toxicol. Ind. Health, *5*:63–72, 1989.

Lijinsky, W., Riggs, C. W., and Walters, P. T. Lack of effect of carcinogen treatment on development of tumors arising spontaneously in Fischer 344 rats. J. Toxicol. Environ. Health, *39*:527–538, 1993.

Liu, J., Gilbert, K., Parker, H. M., Haschek, W. M., and Milner, J. A. Inhibition of 7,12-dimethylbenz(*a*)anthracene-induced mammary tumors and DNA adducts by dietary selenite. Cancer Res., *51*:4613–4617, 1991.

Loehrke, H., Schweizer, J., Dederer, E., Hesse, B., Rosenkranz, G., and Goerttler, K. On the persistence of tumor initiation in two-stage carcinogenesis on mouse skin. Carcinogenesis, *4*:771–775, 1983.

Lok, E., Scott, F. W., Mongeau, R., Nera, E. A., Malcolm, S., and Clayson, D. B. Calorie restriction and cellular proliferation in various tissues of the female Swiss Webster mouse. Cancer Lett., *51*:67–73, 1990.

Lombardi, B., and Smith, M. L. Tumorigenesis, protooncogene activation, and other gene abnormalities in methyl deficiency. J. Nutr. Biochem., *5*:2–9, 1994.

Longnecker, D. S., Curphey, T. J., Kuhlmann, E. T., and Roebuck, B. D. Inhibition of pancreatic carcinogenesis by retinoids in azaserine treated rats. Cancer Res., *42*:19–24, 1982.

Longnecker, M. P., and Enger, S. M. Epidemiologic data on alcoholic beverage consumption and risk of cancer. Clin. Chim. Acta, *246*:121–141, 1996.

Lotan, R. Effects of vitamin A and its analogs (retinoids) on normal and neoplastic cells. Biochim. Biophys. Acta, *605*:33–91, 1980.

Lotlikar, P. D. Effects of sex hormones on enzymic esterification of 2-(*N*-hydroxy-acetamido)fluorene by rat liver cytosol. Biochem. J., *120*:409–416, 1970.

Lotlikar, P. D., Enomoto, M., Miller, E. C., and Miller, J. A. The effects of adrenalectomy, hypophysectomy and castration on the urinary metabolites of 2-acetylaminofluorene in the rat. Cancer Res., *24*:1835–1844, 1964.

Lowenfels, A. B., Maisonneuve, P., DiMagno, E. P., Elitsur, Y., Gates, L. K., Jr., Perrault, J., Whitcomb, D. C., and the International Hereditary Pancreatitis Study Group. Hereditary pancreatitis and the risk of pancreatic cancer. J. Natl. Cancer Inst., *89*:442–446, 1997.

Lu, J., Jiang, C., Fontaine, S., and Thompson, H. J. *ras* may mediate mammary cancer promotion by high fat. Nutr. Cancer, *23*:283–290, 1995.

MacGregor, J. T., Schlegel, R., Wehr, C. M., Alperin, P., and Ames, B. N. Cytogenetic damage induced by folate deficiency in mice is enhanced by caffeine. Proc. Natl. Acad. Sci. U.S.A., *87*:9962–9965, 1990.

Mack, D. O., Reed, V. L., and Smith, L. D. Retinyl acetate inhibition of 3'-methyl-4-dimethyl-amino-azobenzene induced hepatic neoplasia. Int. J. Biochem., *22*:359–365, 1990.

Madhaven, T. V., and Gopalan, C. Effect of dietary protein on carcinogenesis of aflatoxin. Arch. Pathol., *85*:133–137, 1968.

Maiorana, A., and Gullino, P. M. Effect of retinyl acetate on the incidence of mammary carcinomas and hepatomas in mice. J. Natl. Cancer Inst., *64*:655–663, 1980.

Malkovsky, M., Dore, C., Hunt, R., Palmer, L., Chandler, P., and Medawar, P. B. Enhancement of specific antitumor immunity in mice fed a diet enriched in vitamin A acetate. Proc. Natl. Acad. Sci. U.S.A., *80*:6322–6326, 1983.

Masoro, E. J. Possible mechanisms underlying the antiaging actions of caloric restriction. Toxicol. Pathol., *24*:738–741, 1996.

Matsuura, B., Taniguchi, Y., and Ohta, Y. Effect of antiandrogen treatment on chemical hepatocarcinogenesis in rats. J. Hepatol., *21*:187–193, 1994.

McCormick, D. L., Bagg, B. J., and Hultin, T. A. Comparative activity of dietary or topical exposure to three retinoids in the promotion of skin tumor induction in mice. Cancer Res., *47*:5989–5993, 1987.

McIntosh, G. H. The influence of dietary vitamin E and calcium status on intestinal tumors in rats. Nutr. Cancer, *17*:47–55, 1992.

Medina, D., and Morrison, D. G. Current ideas on selenium as a chemopreventive agent. Pathol. Immunopathol. Res., *7*:187–199, 1988.

Medina, D., and Shepherd, F. Selenium-mediated inhibition of 7,12-dimethylbenz(a)anthracene-induced mouse mammary tumorigenesis. Carcinogenesis, *2*:451–455, 1981.

Meister, A. Glutathione-ascorbic acid antioxidant system in animals. J. Biol. Chem., *269*:9397–9400, 1994.

Melhem, M. F., Kunz, H. W., and Gill, T. J. III. Genetic control of susceptibility to diethylnitrosamine and dimethylbenzanthracene carcinogenesis in rats. Am. J. Pathol., *139*:45–51, 1991.

Merry, B. J., and Holehan, A. M. *In vivo* DNA synthesis in the dietary restricted long-lived rat. Exp. Gerontol., *20*:15–28, 1985.

Meruelo, D., and Bach, R. Genetics of resistance to virus-induced leukemias. Adv. Cancer Res., *40*:107–188, 1983.

Meruelo, D., and McDevitt, H. O. Recent studies on the role of the immune response in resistance to virus-induced leukemias and lymphomas. Semin. Hematol., *15*:399–419, 1978.

Messina, M. J., Persky, V., Setchell, K. D. R., and Barnes, S. Soy intake and cancer risk: a review of the *in vitro* and *in vivo* data. Nutr. Cancer, *21*:113–131, 1994.

Mikol, Y. B., Hoover, K. L., Creasia, D., and Poirier, L. A. Hepatocarcinogenesis in rats fed methyl-deficient, amino acid-defined diets. Carcinogenesis, *4*:1619–1629, 1983.

Milks, M. M., Wilt, S. R., Ali, I. I., and Couri, D. The effects of selenium on the emergence of aflatoxin B_1-induced enzyme-altered foci in rat liver. Fundam. Appl. Toxicol., *5*:320–326, 1985.

Miller, D. G. On the nature of susceptibility to cancer. The Presidential Address. Cancer, *46*:1307–1318, 1980.

Miller, J. A., and Miller, E. C. Carcinogenic azo dyes. Adv. Cancer Res., *1*:339, 1953.

Miller, J. A., Kline, B. E., Rusch, H. P., and Baumann, C. A. The carcinogenicity of *p*-dimethylaminoazobenzene in diets containing hydrogenated coconut oil. cancer Res., *4*:153–158, 1944.

Miller, R. A. The aging immune system: primer and prospectus. Science, *273*:70–74, 1996.

Minoura, T., Takata, T., Sakaguchi, M., Takada, H., Yamamura, M., Hioki, K., and Yamamoto, M. Effect of dietary eicosapentaenoic acid on azoxymethane-induced colon carcinogenesis in rats. Cancer Res., *48*:4790–4794, 1988.

Mishkin, S. Y., Farber, E., Ho, R., Mulay, S., and Mishkin, S. Tamoxifen alone or in combination with estradiol-17β inhibits the growth and malignant transformation of hepatic hyperplastic nodules. Eur. J. Cancer Clin. Oncol., *21*:333–341, 1985.

Miyata, Y., Tsuda, H., Matayoshi-Miyasato, K., Fukushima, S., Murasaki, G., Ogiso, T., and Ito, N. Effect of vitamin A acetate on urinary bladder carcinogenesis induced by N-butyl-n-(4-hydroxybutyl)nitrosamine in rats. Gann, 69:845–848, 1978.

Mizumoto, Y., Nakae, D., Yoshiji, H., Andoh, N., Horiguchi, K., Endoh, T., Kobayashi, E., Tsujiuchi, T., Shimoji, N., Denda, A., Tsujii, T., Nagao, M., Wakabayashi, K., and Konishi, Y. Inhibitory effects of 2-O-octadecylascorbic acid and other vitamin C and E derivatives on the induction of enzyme-altered putative preneoplastic lesions in the livers of rats fed a choline-deficient, L-amino acid-defined diet. Carcinogenesis, 15:241–246, 1994.

Mohr, U., and Lewkowski, J. P. The effect of diet on tumour development in animals. Exp. Pathol., 12:5–144, 1989.

Moon, R. C., and McCormick, D. L. Inhibition of chemical carcinogenesis by retinoids. J. Am. Acad. Dermatol., 6:809–814, 1982.

Moon, R. C., Grubbs, C. J., and Sporn, M. B. Inhibition of 7,12-dimethylbenz(a)anthracene–induced mammary carcinogenesis by retinyl acetate. Cancer Res., 36:2626–2630, 1976.

Moon, R. C., Grubbs, C. J., Sporn, M. B., and Goodman, D. G. Retinyl acetate inhibits mammary carcinogenesis induced by N-methyl-nitrosourea. Nature (London), 267:620–621, 1977.

Moon, R. C., McCormick, D. L., Becci, P. J., Shealy, Y. F., Frickel, F., Paust, J., and Sporn, M. B. Influence of 15 retinoic acid amides on urinary bladder carcinogenesis in the mouse. Carcinogenesis, 3:1469–1472, 1982.

Moreno, F. S., Wu, T.-S., Penteado, M. V. C., Rizzi, M. B. S. L., Jordão, A. A. Jr., Almeida-Muradian, L. B., and Dagli, M. L. Z. A comparison of β-carotene and vitamin A effects on a hepatocarcinogenesis model. Int. J. Vitam. Nutr. Res., 65:87–94, 1995.

Morris, H. P., and Robertson, W. V. B. Growth rate and number of spontaneous mammary carcinomas and riboflavin concentration of liver, muscle, and tumor of C3H mice as influenced by dietary riboflavin. J. Natl. Cancer Inst., 3:479, 1943.

Mulay, A. S., and O'Gara, R. W. Effect of hormonal status on incidence and morphology of hepatomas in rats fed N,N-dimethyl-p-(m-tolylazo)aniline. J. Natl. Cancer Inst., 29:567–581, 1962.

Muskhelishvili, L., Turturro, A., Hart, R. W., and James, S. J. π-Class glutathione-S-transferase–positive hepatocytes in aging B6C3F1 mice undergo apoptosis induced by dietary restriction. Am. J. Pathol., 149:1585–1591, 1996.

Nakae, D., Yoshiji, H., Maruyama, H., Kinugasa, T., Denda, A., and Konishi, Y. Production of both 8-hydroxydeoxyguanosine in liver DNA and γ-glutamyltransferase-positive hepatocellular lesions in rats given a choline-deficient, L-amino acid-defined diet. Jpn. J. Cancer Res., 81:1081–1084, 1990.

Nakae, D., Yoshiji, H., Mizumoto, Y., Horiguchi, K., Shiraiwa, K., Tamura, K., Denda, A., and Konishi, Y. High incidence of hepatocellular carcinomas induced by a choline deficient L-amino acid defined diet in rats. Cancer Res., 52:5042–5045, 1992.

Narisawa, T., Reddy, B. S., Wong, C.-Q., and Weisburger, J. H. Effect of vitamin A deficiency on rat colon carcinogenesis by N-methyl-N-nitro-N-nitrosoguanidine. Cancer Res., 36:1379–1383, 1976.

Narisawa, T., Fukaura, Y., Hasebe, M., Ito, M., Aizawa, R., Murakoshi, M., Uemura, S., Khachik, F., and Nishino, H. Inhibitor effects of natural carotenoids, α-carotene, β-carotene, lycopene and lutein, on colonic aberrant crypt foci formation in rats. Cancer Lett., 107:137–142, 1996.

Nettesheim, P., Snyder, C., and Kim, J. C. S. Vitamin A and the susceptibility of respiratory tract tissues to carcinogenic insult. Environ. Health Perspect., 29:89–93, 1979.

Newberne, P. M., and Connor, M. Effects of sequential exposure to aflatoxin B$_1$ and diethylnitrosamine on vascular and stomach tissue and additional target organs in rats. Cancer Res., 40:4037–4042, 1980.

Newberne, P. M., and Rogers, A. E. Rat colon carcinomas associated with aflatoxin and marginal vitamin A. J. Natl. Cancer Inst., 50:439–448, 1973.

Newberne, P. M., and Suphakarn, V. Preventive role of vitamin A in colon carcinogenesis in rats. Cancer, 40:2553–2556, 1977.

Newberne, P. M., Weigert, J., and Kula, N. Effects of dietary fat on hepatic mixed-function oxidases and hepatocellular carcinoma induced by aflatoxin B$_1$ in rats. Cancer Res., 39:3986–3991, 1979.

Nutter, R. L., Kettering, J. D., Aprecio, R. M., Weeks, D. A., and Gridley, D. S. Effects of dietary fat and protein on DMH-induced tumor development and immune responses. Nutr. Cancer, 13:141–152, 1990.

O'Brien, S. J. *Bvr-1*, a restriction locus of a type C RNA virus in the feline cellular genome: identification, location, and phenotypic characterization in cat X mouse somatic cell hybrids. Proc. Natl. Acad. Sci. U.S.A., *73*:4618–4622, 1976.

O'Connor, T. P., and Campbell, T. C. The contribution of animal experiments to knowledge of the relationship between diet and cancer risk in humans. Cancer Surv., *6*:573–583, 1987.

O'Connor, T. P., Roebuck, B. D., Peterson, F. J., Lokesh, B., Kinsella, J. E., and Campbell, T. C. Effect of dietary omega-3 and omega-6 fatty acids on development of azaserine-induced preneoplastic lesions in rat pancreas. J. Natl. Cancer Inst., *81*:858–863, 1989.

Odaka, T. Inheritance of susceptibility to Friend mouse leukemia virus. Separate genetic control of two viruses in Friend virus preparation. Int. J. Cancer, *11*:567–574, 1973.

Odaka, T., Ikeda, H., Yoshikura, H., Moriwaki, K., and Suzuki, S. *Fv-4*: gene controlling resistance to NB-tropic Friend murine leukemia virus. Distribution in wild mice, introduction into genetic background of BALB/c mice, and mapping of chromosomes. J. Natl. Cancer Inst., *67*:1123–1127, 1981.

Okada, S. Iron-induced tissue damage and cancer: the role of reactive oxygen species-free radicals. Pathol. Int., *46*:311–332, 1996.

Overvad, K., Thorling, E. B., Bjerring, P., and Ebbesen, P. Selenium inhibits UV light induced skin carcinogenesis in hairless mice. Cancer Lett, *27*:163–170, 1985.

Pahlavani, M. A., and Richardson, A. The effect of age on the expression of interleukin-2. Mech. Ageing Dev., *89*:125–154, 1996.

Papenburg, R., Bounous, G., Fleiszer, D., and Gold, P. Dietary milk proteins inhibit the development of dimethylhydrazine-induced malignancy. Tumor Biol., *11*:129–136, 1990.

Pariza, M. W., Hargraves, W. A., Benjamin, H., Christou, M., Jefcoate, C. R., Storkson, J., Albright, K., Kraus, D., Sharp, P., Boissonneault, G. A., and Elson, C. E. Modulation of carcinogenesis by dietary factors. Environ. Health Perspect., *67*:25–29, 1986.

Pashko, L. L., and Schwartz, A. G. Inhibition of 7,12-dimethylbenz[*a*]anthracene-induced lung tumorigenesis in A/J mice by food restriction is reversed by adrenalectomy. Carcinogenesis, *17*:209–212, 1996.

Paulini, K., Beneke, G., Körner, B., and Enders, R. The relationship between the latent period and animal age in the development of foreign body sarcomas. Beitr. Pathol. Bd., *154*:161–169, 1975.

Paulsen, J. E. Effects of exogenous putrescine on the retinoic acid-induced reduction of 12-O-tetradecanoyl-phorbol-13-acetate-stimulated putrescine accumulation and rate of DNA synthesis in the hairless mouse epidermis. Virchows Arch. B. Cell. Pathol., *46*:199–204, 1984.

Pegg, A. E. Polyamine metabolism and its importance in neoplastic growth and as a target for chemotherapy. Cancer Res., *48*:759–774, 1988.

Pence, B. C., and Buddingh, F. Effect of dietary selenium deficiency on incidence and size of 1,2-dimethylhydrazine-induced colon tumors in rats. J. Nutr., *115*:1196–1202, 1985.

Pence, B. C., Dunn, D. M., Zhao, C., Landers, M., and Wargovich, M. J. Chemopreventive effects of calcium but not aspirin supplementation in cholic acid-promoted colon carcinogenesis: correlation with intermediate endpoints. Carcinogenesis, *16*:757–765, 1995.

Peto, R., Roe, F. J. C., Lee, P. N., Levy, L., and Clack, J. Cancer and ageing in mice and men. Br. J. Cancer, *32*:411–426, 1975.

Phelouzat, M.-A., Arbogast, A., Laforge, T., Quadri, R. A., and Proust, J. J. Excessive apoptosis of mature T lymphocytes is a characteristic feature of human immune senescence. Mech. Ageing Dev., *88*:25–38, 1996.

Pierre, F., Perrin, P., Champ, M., Bornet, F., Meflah, K., and Menanteau, J. Short-chain fructo-oligosaccharides reduce the occurrence of colon tumors and develop gut-associated lymphoid tissue in *min* mice. Cancer Res., *57*:225–228, 1997.

Pitot, H. C. Multistage carcinogenesis—genetic and epigenetic mechanisms in relation to cancer prevention. Cancer Detect. Prev., *17*:567–573, 1993.

Pitot, H. C., Barsness, L., Goldsworthy, T., and Kitagawa, T. Biochemical characterization of stages of hepatocarcinogenesis after a single dose of diethylnitrosamine. Nature, *271*:456–458, 1978.

Pogribny, I. P., Muskhelishvili, L., Miller, B. J., and James, S. J. Presence and consequence of uracil in preneoplastic DNA from folate/methyl deficient rats. Carcinogenesis, in press.

Pollard, M., and Luckert, P. H. Tumorigenic effects of direct- and indirect-acting chemical carcinogens in rats on a restricted diet. J. Natl. Cancer Inst., 74:1347–1349, 1985.

Pollard, M., Luckert, P. H., and Sporn, M. B. Prevention of primary prostate cancer in Lobund-Wistar rats by N-(4-hydroxyphenyl)retinamide. Cancer Res., 51:3610–3611, 1991.

Poole, T. M., and Drinkwater, N. R. Two genes abrogate the inhibition of murine hepatocarcinogenesis by ovarian hormones. Proc. Natl. Acad. Sci. U.S.A., 93:5848–5853, 1996.

Prasanna, H. R., Hart, R. W., and Magee, P. N. Effect of food restriction on the metabolism of dimethyl-nitrosamine (NDMA) in rats. Anticancer Res., 9:93–96, 1989.

Prentice, R. L., Pepe, M., and Self, S. G. Dietary fat and breast cancer: a quantitative assessment of the epidemiological literature and a discussion of methodological issues. Cancer Res., 49:3147–3156, 1989.

Prutkin, L. Modification of the effect of vitamin A acid on the skin tumor keratoacanthoma by applications of actinomycin D. Cancer Res., 31:1080–1086, 1971.

Radomski, J. L., Radomski, T., and MacDonald, W. E. Cocarcinogenic interaction between DL-tryptophan and 4-aminobiphenyl or 2-naphthylamine in dogs. J. Natl. Cancer Inst., 58:1831–1834, 1977.

Rafter, J. J. The role of lactic acid bacteria in colon cancer prevention. Scand. J. Gastroenterol., 30:497–502, 1995.

Randerath, K., Hart, R. W., Zhou, G.-D., Reddy, R., Danna, T. F., and Randerath, E. Enhancement of age-related increases in DNA I-compound levels by calorie restriction: comparison of male B-N and F-344 rats. Mutat. Res., 295:31–46, 1993.

Rao, C. V., Desai, D., Simi, B., Kulkarni, N., Amin, S., and Reddy, B. S. Inhibitory effect of caffeic acid esters on azoxymethane-induced biochemical changes and aberrant crypt foci formation in rat colon. Cancer Res., 53:4182–4188, 1993a.

Rao, C. V., Rivenson, A., Katiwalla, M., Kelloff, G. J., and Reddy, B. S. Chemopreventive effect of olitpraz during different stages of experimental colon carcinogenesis induced by azoxymethane in male F344 rats. Cancer Res., 53:2502–2506, 1993b.

Rao, G., Xia, E., Nadakavukaren, M. J., and Richardson, A. Effect of dietary restriction on the age-dependent changes in the expression of antioxidant enzymes in rat liver. J. Nutr., 120:602–609, 1990.

Rao, J., and Jagadeesan, V. Lipid peroxidation and activities of antioxidant enzymes in iron deficiency and effect of carcinogen feeding. Free Radic. Biol. Med., 21:103–108, 1996.

Rao, K. V. N., Detrisac, C. J., Steele, V. E., Hawk, E. T., Kelloff, G. J., and McCormick, D. L. Differential activity of aspirin, ketoprofen and sulindac as cancer chemopreventive agents in the mouse urinary bladder. Carcinogenesis, 17:1435–1438, 1996.

Rao, M. S., Jago, M. V., and Reddy, J. K. Effect of calorie restriction on the fate of hyperplastic liver nodules induced by concurrent administration of lasiocarpine and thioacetamide. Human Toxicol., 2:15–26, 1983.

Reddy, B. S., Narisawa, T., Wright, P., Vukusich, D., Weisburger, J. H., and Wynder, E. L. Colon carcinogenesis with azoxymethane and dimethylhydrazine in germ-free rats. Cancer Res., 35:287–290, 1975.

Reddy, B. S., and Sugie, S. Effect of different levels of omega-3 and omega-6 fatty acids on azoxymethane-induced colon carcinogenesis in F344 rats. Cancer Res., 48:6642–6647, 1988.

Reddy, B. S., and Tanaka, T. Interactions of selenium deficiency, vitamin E, polyunsaturated fat, and saturated fat on azoxymethane-induced colon carcinogenesis in male F344 rats. J. Natl. Cancer Inst., 76:1157–1162, 1986.

Reddy, B. S., Sugie, S., Maruyama, H., El-Bayoumy, K., and Marra, P. Chemoprevention of colon carcinogenesis by dietary organoselenium, benzylselenocyanate, in F344 rats. Cancer Res., 47:5901–5904, 1987.

Reddy, B. S., Sugie, S., Maruyama, H., and Marra, P. Effect of dietary excess of inorganic selenium during initiation and postinitiation phases of colon carcinogenesis in F344 rats. Cancer Res., 48:1777–1780, 1988.

Reddy, B. S., Rao, C. V., Rivenson, A., and Kelloff, G. Chemoprevention of colon carcinogenesis by organosulfur compounds. Cancer Res., 53:3493–3498, 1993.

Reichel, H., Koeffler, H. P., and Norman, A. W. The role of the vitamin D endocrine system in health and disease. N. Engl. J. Med., *320*:980–991, 1989.

Reuber, M. D. Influence of hormones on *N*-2-fluorenyldiacetamide-induced hyperplastic hepatic nodules in rats. J. Natl. Cancer Inst., *43*:445–452, 1969.

Ricco, J.-B., Franco, D., Morin, J., Decloitre, F., and Bismuth, H. Modification of 3′-methyl-4-dimethyl-aminoazobenzene carcinogenesis of rat liver and carcinogen metabolism by portacaval anastomosis. Cancer Res., *37*:4500–4505, 1977.

Rickert, D. E., Butterworth, B. E., and Popp, J. A. Dinitrotoluene: acute toxicity, oncogenicity, genotoxicity, and metabolism. Crit. Rev. Toxicol., *13*:217–234, 1984.

Risser, R. Friend erythroleukemia antigen. A viral antigen specified by spleen focus-forming virus and differentiation antigen controlled by the *Fv-2* locus. J. Exp. Med., *149*:1152–1167, 1979.

Roebuck, B. D. Effects of high levels of dietary fats on the growth of azaserine-induced foci in the rat pancreas. Lipids, *21*:281–284, 1986.

Roebuck, B. D. Dietary fat and the development of pancreatic cancer. Lipids, *27*:804–806, 1992.

Roebuck, B. D., Baumgartner, K. J., and MacMillan, D. L. Caloric restriction and intervention in pancreatic carcinogenesis in the rat. Cancer Res., *53*:46–52, 1993.

Rogers, A. E. Methyl donors in the diet and responses to chemical carcinogens. Am. J. Clin. Nutr., *61*:659S–665S, 1995.

Rogers, A. E., Zeisel, S. H., and Groopman, J. Diet and carcinogenesis. Carcinogenesis, *14*:2205–2217, 1993.

Ronai, Z., Lau, Y., and Cohen, L. A. Dietary N-3 fatty acids do not affect induction of Ha-*ras* mutations in mammary glands of NMU-treated rats. Mol. Carcinog., *4*:120–128, 1991.

Ross, M. H., and Bras, G. Influence of protein under- and overnutrition on spontaneous tumor prevalence in the rat. J. Nutr., *103*:944–963, 1973.

Rubin, E. The questionable link between alcohol intake and cancer. Clin. Chim. Acta, *246*:143–148, 1996.

Ruggeri, B. A., Klurfeld, D. M., Kritchevsky, D., and Furlanetto, R. W. Caloric restriction and 7,12-dimethylbenz(*a*)anthracene-induced mammary tumor growth in rats: alterations in circulating insulin, insulin-like growth factors I and II, and epidermal growth factor. Cancer Res., *49*:4130–4134, 1989.

Russo, I. H., Koszalka, M., and Russo, J. Effect of human chorionic gonadotropin on mammary gland differentiation and carcinogenesis. Carcinogenesis, *11*:1849–1855, 1990.

Russo, I. H., and Russo, J. Mammary gland neoplasia in long-term rodent studies. Environ. Health Perspect., *104*:938–967, 1996.

Saito, R., Chandar, N., Janosky, J. E., and Lombardi, B. No enhancement by phenobarbital of the hepatocarcinogenicity of a choline-devoid diet in the rat. Res. Commun. Chem. Pathol. Pharmacol., *69*:197–207, 1990.

Sarkar, N. H., Fernandes, G., Telang, N. T., Kourides, I. A., and Good, R. A. Low-calorie diet prevents the development of mammary tumors in C3H mice and reduces circulating prolactin level, murine mammary tumor virus expression, and proliferation of mammary alveolar cells. Proc. Natl. Acad. Sci. U.S.A., *79*:7758–7762, 1982.

Sarkar, A., Mukherjee, B., and Chatterjee, M. Inhibition of 3′-methyl-4-dimethylaminoazobenzene-induced hepatocarcinogenesis in rat by dietary β-carotene: changes in hepatic anti-oxidant defense enzyme levels. Int. J. Cancer, *61*:799–805, 1995.

Sato, A., Nakajima, T., Koyama, Y., Shirai, T., and Ito, N. Dietary carbohydrate level as a modifying factor of 3′-methyl-4-dimethylaminoazobenzene liver carcinogenesis in rats. Gann, *75*:665–671, 1984.

Sawada, N., Poirier, L., Moran, S., Xu, Y.-H., and Pitot, H. C. The effect of choline and methionine deficiencies on the number and volume percentage of altered hepatic foci in the presence or absence of diethylnitrosamine initiation in rat liver. Carcinogenesis, *11*:273–281, 1990.

Schmitt, F. C. L., Estevao, D., Kobayasi, S., Curi, P., and de Camargo, J. L. V. Altered foci of hepatocytes in rats initiated with diethylnitrosamine after prolonged fasting. Food Chem. Toxicol., *31*:629–636, 1993.

Schottenfeld, D. The epidemiology of cancer: an overview. Cancer, *47*:1095–1108, 1981.

Schrauzer, G., McGinness, J., Ishmael, D., and Bell, L. Alcoholism and cancer. I. Effects of long-term exposure to alcohol on spontaneous mammary adenocarcinoma and prolactin levels in C3H/St mice. J. Stud. Alcohol, *40*:240–246, 1979.

Schulsinger, D. A., Root, M. M., and Campbell, T. C. Effect of dietary protein quality on development of aflatoxin B_1–induced hepatic preneoplastic lesions. J. Natl. Cancer Inst., *81*:1241–1245, 1989.

Schulte-Hermann, R., and Parzefall, W. Failure to discriminate initiation from promotion of liver tumors in a long-term study with the phenobarbital-type inducer α-hexachlorocyclohexane and the role of sustained stimulation of hepatic growth and monooxygenases. Cancer Res., *41*:4140–4146, 1981.

Schwartz, A. G., and Pashko, L. L. Food restriction inhibits [^{3}H] 7,12-dimethylbenz(a)anthracene binding to mouse skin DNA and tetradecanoylphorbol-13-acetate stimulation of epidermal [^{3}H] thymidine incorporation. Anticancer Res., *6*:1279–1282, 1986.

Schwartz, A. G., and Pashko, L. L. Role of adrenocortical steroids in mediating cancer-preventive and age-retarding effects of food restriction in laboratory rodents. J. Gerontol., *49*:B37–B41, 1994.

Seitz, H. K., and Simanowski, U. A. Alcohol and carcinogenesis. Ann. Rev. Nutr., *8*:99–119, 1988.

Shamberger, R. J. Relationship of selenium to cancer. I. Inhibitory effect of selenium on carcinogenesis. J. Natl. Cancer Inst., *44*:931–936, 1970.

Shamberger, R. J. Genetic toxicology of ascorbic acid. Mutat. Res., *133*:135–159, 1984.

Shibuya, T., Niho, Y., and Mak, T. W. Erythroleukemia induction by Friend leukemia virus. A host gene locus controlling early anemia or polycythemia and the rate of proliferation of late erythroid cells. J. Exp. Med., *156*:398–414, 1982.

Shimada, M., Murayama, N., Yamazoe, Y., Kamataki, T., and Kato, R. Further studies on the persistence of neonatal androgen imprinting on sex-specific cytochrome P-450, testosterone and drug oxidations. Jpn. J. Pharmacol., *45*:467–478, 1987.

Shinozuka, H., and Lombardi, B. Synergistic effect of a choline-devoid diet and phenobarbital in promoting the emergence of foci of γ-glutamyltranspeptidase-positive hepatocytes in the liver of carcinogen-treated rats. Cancer Res., *40*:3846–3849, 1980.

Shivapurkar, N., Tang, Z., Frost, A., and Alabaster, O. Inhibition of progression of aberrant crypt foci and colon tumor development by vitamin E and β-carotene in rats on a high-risk diet. Cancer Lett., *91*:125–132, 1995.

Shklar, G., Schwartz, J., Grau, D., Trickler, D. P., and Wallace, K. D. Inhibition of hamster buccal pouch carcinogenesis by 13 cts retinoic acid. Oral Surg. Oral Med. Oral Pathol., *50*:45–52, 1980.

Sidransky, H. Tryptophan and carcinogenesis: update on how tryptophan may act. Nutr. Cancer, *29*:181–194, 1997.

Sies, H., and Stahl, W. Vitamins E and C, β-carotene, and other carotenoids as antioxidants. Am. J. Clin. Nutr., *62*:1315S–1321S, 1995.

Sies, H., Stahl, W., and Sundquist, A. R. Antioxidant functions of vitamins. Vitamins E and C, beta-carotene, and other carotenoids. Ann. N.Y. Acad. Sci., *669*:7–20, 1992.

Silver, J. E., and Fredrickson, T. N. A new gene that controls the type of leukemia induced by Friend murine leukemia virus. J. Exp. Med., *158*:493–505, 1983.

Silverman, J., Katayama, S., Zelenakas, K., Lauber, J., Musser, T. K., Reddy, M., Levenstein, M. J., and Weisburger, J. H. Effect of retinoids on the induction of colon cancer in F344 rats by N-methyl-N-nitrosourea or by 1,2,-dimethylhydrazine. Carcinogenesis, *2*:1167–1172, 1981.

Singh, J., Hamid, R., and Reddy, B. S. Dietary fat and colon cancer: modulating effect of types and amount of dietary fat on *ras*-p21 function during promotion and progression stages of colon cancer. Cancer Res., *57*:253–258, 1997.

Singletary, K. Ethanol and experimental breast cancer: a review. Alcohol. Clin. Exp. Res., *21*:334–339, 1997.

Singletary, K., Nelshoppen, J., and Wallig, M. Enhancement by chronic ethanol intake of *N*-methyl-*N*-nitrosourea-induced rat mammary tumorigenesis. Carcinogenesis, *16*:959–964, 1995.

Skett, P., and Gustafsson, J.-Å. Imprinting of enzyme systems of xenobiotic and steroid metabolism. *In*: Hodgson, Bend, Philpot (Eds.), Reviews in Biochemical Toxicology, pp. 27–52. Amsterdam: Elsevier North Holland, 1979.

Smith, A. G., Carthew, P., Francis, J. E., Ricardo, J., Cabral, P., and Manson, M. M. Enhancement by iron of hepatic neoplasia in rats caused by hexachlorobenzene. Carcinogenesis, *14*:1381–1387, 1993.

Smith, D. M., Rogers, A. E., and Newberne, P. M. Vitamin A and benzo(a)pyrene carcinogenesis in the respiratory tract of hamsters fed a semisynthetic diet. Cancer Res., *35*:1485–1488, 1975.

Smith, G. S., and Walford, R. L. Influence of the H-2 and H-1 histocompatibility systems upon life span and spontaneous cancer incidences in congenic mice. Birth Defects: Original Article Series, *14*:281–312, 1978.

Solleveld, H. A., van Zwieten, M. J., Broerse, J. J., and Hollander, C. F. Effects of x-irradiation, ovariohysterectomy and estradiol-17β on incidence, benign/malignant ratio and multiplicity of rat mammary neoplasms—a preliminary report. Leuk. Res., *10*:755–763, 1986.

Soullier, B. K., Wilson, P. S., and Nigro, N. D. Effect of selenium on azoxymethane-induced intestinal cancer in rats fed high fat diet. Cancer Lett, *12*:343–348, 1981.

Soyka, L. F. Hepatic drug metabolizing enzyme activity and tumorigenesis in mice following perinatal exposure to benzo(a)pyrene. Pediatr. Pharmacol., *1*:85–96, 1980.

Spear, A. T., and Sherman, A. R. Iron deficiency alters DMBA-induced tumor burden and natural killer cell cytotoxicity in rats. J. Nutr., *122*:46–55, 1992.

Sporn, M. B., and Roberts, A. B. Role of retinoids in differentiation and carcinogenesis. Cancer Res., *43*:3034–3040, 1983.

Sporn, M. B., Squire, R. A., Brown, C. C., Smith, J. M., Wenk, M. L., and Springer, S. 13-Cis-retinoic acid: inhibition of bladder carcinogenesis in the rat. Science, *195*:487–489, 1977.

Squire, R. A., Sporn, M. B., Brown, C. C., Smith, J. M., Wenk, M. L., and Springer, S. Histopathological evaluation of the inhibition of rat bladder carcinogenesis by 13-cis retinoic acid. Cancer Res., *37*:2930–2936, 1977.

Stadtman, T. C. Selenocysteine. Annu. Rev. Biochem., *65*:83–100, 1996.

St. Clair, W. H., Billings, P. C., Carew, J. A., Keller-McGandy, C., Newberne, P., and Kennedy, A. R. Suppression of dimethylhydrazine-induced carcinogenesis in mice by dietary addition of the Bowman-Birk protease inhibitor. Cancer Res., *50*:580–586, 1990.

Steeves, R., and Lilly, F. Interactions between host and viral genomes in mouse leukemia. Ann. Rev. Genet., *11*:277–296, 1977.

Stenbäck, F., Peto, R., and Shubik, P. Initiation and promotion at different ages and doses in 2200 mice. II. Decrease in promotion by TPA with ageing. Br. J. Cancer, *44*:15–23, 1981.

Stinson, S. F., Reznik, G., and Donahoe, R. Effect of three retinoids on tracheal carcinogenesis with N-methyl-n-nitrosourea in hamsters. J. Natl. Cancer Inst., *66*:947–951, 1981.

Sugie, S., Reddy, B. S., El-Bayoumy, K., and Tanaka, T. Inhibition of dietary benzylselenocyanate of hepatocarcinogenesis induced by azoxymethane in Fischer 344 rats. Jpn. J. Cancer Res., *80*:952–957, 1989.

Suh, O., Mettlin, C., and Petrelli, N. J. Aspirin use, cancer, and polyps of the large bowel. Cancer, *72*:1171–1177, 1993.

Swann, P. F., Coe, A. M., and Mace, R. Ethanol and dimethylnitrosamine and diethylnitrosamine metabolism and disposition in the rat. Possible relevance to the influence of ethanol on human cancer incidence. Carcinogenesis, *5*:1337–1343, 1984.

Sylvester, P. W. Role of acute caloric-restriction in murine tumorigenesis. *In*: Dietary Fat and Cancer, pp. 517–528. New York: Alan R. Liss, 1986.

Takada, A., Nei, J., Takase, S., and Matsuda, Y. Effects of ethanol on experimental hepatocarcinogenesis. Hepatology, *6*:65–72, 1986.

Takada, H., Hirooka, T., Hatano, T., Hamada, Y., and Yamamoto, M. Inhibition of 7,12-dimethylbenz[*a*]anthracene-induced lipid peroxidation and mammary tumor development in rats by vitamin E in conjunction with selenium. Nutr. Cancer, *17*:115–122, 1992.

Takayama, S., Hasegawa, H., and Ohgaki, H. Combination effects of forty carcinogens administered at low doses to male rats. Jpn. J. Cancer Res., *80*:732–736, 1989.

Takizawa, S., and Hirose, F. Modification of renal tumorigenesis by gonadal ablation in rats treated with N-butylnitrosourea or dimethylnitrosamine. Hiroshima J. Med. Sci., *27*:247–252, 1978.

Takuwa, N., Zhou, W., and Takuwa, Y. Calcium, calmodulin and cell cycle progression. Cell. Signal., *7*:93–104, 1995.

Tamano, S., Hagiwara, A., Shibata, M.-A., Kurata, Y., Fukushima, S., and Ito, N. Spontaneous tumors in aging (C57BL/6N × C3H/HeN)F$_1$ (B6C3F$_1$) mice. Toxicol. Pathol., *16*:321–326, 1988.

Tanaka, T., Nishikawa, A., Iwata, H., Mori, Y., Hara, A., Hirono, I., and Mori, H. Enhancing effect of ethanol on aflatoxin B$_1$-induced hepatocarcinogenesis in male ACI/N rats. Jpn. J. Cancer Res., *80*:526–530, 1989.

Tannenbaum, A. Effects of varying caloric intake upon tumor incidence and tumor growth. Ann. N. Y. Acad. Sci., *49*:5–18, 1947.

Tannenbaum, A., and Silverstone, H. The genesis and growth of tumors. IV. Effects of varying the proportion of protein (casein) in the diet. Cancer Res., *9*:162–173, 1949.

Tatsuta, M., Iishi, H., Baba, M., and Nakaizumi, A. Inhibition by neurotensin of azaserine-induced carcinogenesis in rat pancreas. Int. J. Cancer, *47*:408–412, 1991.

Taylor, H. W., Lijinsky, W., Nettesheim, P., and Snyder, C. M. Alteration of tumor response in rat liver by carbon tetrachloride. Cancer Res., *34*:3391–3395, 1974.

Tempero, M. A., Nishioka, K., Knott, K., and Zetterman, R. K. Chemoprevention of mouse colon tumors with difluoromethylornithine during and after carcinogen treatment. Cancer Res., *49*:5793–5797, 1989.

Tessitore, L., Tomasi, C., Greco, M., Sesca, E., Laconi, E., Maccioni, O., Ramo, R., and Pani, P. A subnecrogenic dose of diethylnitrosamine is able to initiate hepatocarcinogenesis in the rat when coupled with fasting/refeeding. Carcinogenesis, *17*:289–292, 1996.

Thomas, D. B. Alcohol as a cause of cancer. Environ. Health Perspect., *103*:153–160, 1995.

Thompson, H. J. Effect of deficiencies of selenium and vitamin E alone or in combination on the induction of mammary carcinogenesis by 1-methyl-1-nitrosourea. Carcinogenesis, *12*:2175–2179, 1991.

Thompson, M. J., and Becci, P. J. Selenium inhibition of N-methyl-n-nitrosourea-induced mammary carcinogenesis in the rat. J. Natl. Cancer Inst., *65*:1299–1301, 1980.

Thompson, M. J., and Becci, P. J. Effect of graded dietary levels of selenium on tracheal carcinomas induced by 1-methyl-1-nitrosourea. Cancer Lett., *7*:215–219, 1979.

Tokumo, K., Umemura, T., Sirma, H., Gebhardt, R., Poirier, M. C., and Williams, G. M. Inhibition by gonadectomy of effects of 2-acetylaminofluorene in livers of male, but not female rats. Carcinogenesis, *14*:1747–1750, 1993.

Tsukamoto, S., Akaza, H., Imada, S., Koiso, K., Shirai, T., Ideyama, Y., and Kudo, M. Chemoprevention of rat prostate carcinogenesis by use of finasteride or casodex. J. Natl. Cancer Inst., *87*:842–843, 1995.

Tsutsumi, M., Matsuda, Y., and Takada, A. Role of ethanol-inducible cytochrome P-450 2E1 in the development of hepatocellular carcinoma by the chemical carcinogen, N-nitrosodimethylamine. Hepatology, *18*:1483–1489, 1993.

Tucker, M. J. The effect of long-term food restriction on tumours in rodents. Int. J. Cancer, *23*:803–815, 1979.

Uchida, K., Seidenfeld, J., Rademaker, A., and Oyasu, R. Inhibitory action of α-difluoromethylornithine on *N*-butyl-*N*-(4-hydroxybutyl)nitrosamine-induced rat urinary bladder carcinogenesis. Cancer Res., *49*:5249–5253, 1989.

Ueo, H., Matsuoka, H., Honda, M., Inoue, H., Takaki, R., and Akiyoshi, T. Chemopreventive effects of tamoxifen in ethyl methanesulphonate-induced rat mammary carcinogenesis. Cancer Lett., *71*:19–24, 1993.

Ura, H., Denda, A., Yokose, Y., Tsutsumi, M., and Konishi, Y. Effect of vitamin E on the induction and evolution of enzyme-altered foci in the liver of rats treated with diethylnitrosamine. Carcinogenesis, *8*:1595–1600, 1987.

Uwagawa, S., Tsuda, H., Inoue, T., Tagawa, Y., Aoki, T., Kagawa, M., Ogiso, T., and Ito, N. Enhancing potential of 6 different carcinogens on multi-organ tumorigenesis after initial treatment with N-methyl-N-nitrosourea in rats. Jpn. J. Cancer Res., *82*:1397–1405, 1991.

Van Duuren, B. L., Sivak, A., Katz, C., Seidman, I., and Melchionne, S. The effect of aging and interval between primary and secondary treatment in two-stage carcinogenesis on mouse skin. Cancer Res., *35*:502–505, 1975.

Venkatesan, N., Argus, M. F., and Arcos, J. C. Mechanism of 3-methylcholanthrene-induced inhibition of dimethylnitrosamine demethylase in rat liver. Cancer Res., *30*:2556–2562, 1970.

Verhoeven, D. T. H., Verhagen, H., Goldbohm, R. A., van den Brandt, P. A., and van Poppel, G. A review of mechanisms underlying anticarcinogenicity by brassica vegetables. Chem. Biol. Interact., *103*:79–129, 1997.

Verma, A. K., Shapas, B. G., Rice, H. M., and Boutwell, R. K. Correlation of the inhibition by retinoids of tumor promoter-induced mouse epidermal ornithine decarboxylase activity and of skin tumor promotion. Cancer Res., *39*:419–425, 1979.

Verma, A. K., Conrad, E. A., and Boutwell, R. K. Differential effects of retinoic acid and 7,8-benzoflavone on the induction of mouse skin tumors by the complete carcinogenesis process and by the initiation-promotion regimen. Cancer Res., *42*:3519–3525, 1982.

Vesselinovitch, S. D., and Mihailovich, N. The effect of gonadectomy on the development of hepatomas induced by urethan. Cancer Res., *27*:1788–1791, 1967.

Vesselinovitch, S. D., Itze, L., Mihailovich, N., Rao, K. V. N., and Manojlovski, B. Role of hormonal environment, partial hepatectomy, and dose of ethylnitrosourea in renal carcinogenesis. Cancer Res., *33*:339–341, 1973.

Villereal, M. L., and Palfrey, H. C. Intracellular calcium and cell function. Annu. Rev. Nutr., *9*:347–376, 1989.

Wachsman, J. T. The beneficial effects of dietary restriction: reduced oxidative damage and enhanced apoptosis. Mutat. Res., *350*:25–34, 1996.

Wade, A. E., Harley, W., and Bunce, O. R. The effects of dietary corn oil on the metabolism and mutagenic activation on *N*-nitrosodimethylamine (DMN) by hepatic microsomes from male and female rats. Mutat. Res., *102*:113–121, 1982.

Wainfan, E., Dizik, M., Stender, M., and Christman, J. K. Rapid appearance of hypomethylated DNA in livers of rats fed cancer-promoting, methyl-deficient diets. Cancer Res., *49*:4094–4097, 1989.

Wali, R. K., Bissonnette, M., Khare, S,. Hart, J., Sitrin, M. D., and Brasitus, T. A. 1α,25-Dihydroxy-16-ene-23-yne-26,27-hexafluorocholecalciferol, a noncalcemic analogue of 1α,25-dihydroxyvitamin D_3, inhibits azoxymethane-induced colonic tumorigenesis. Cancer Res., *55*:3050–3054, 1995.

Walsh, C. T., Sandstead, H. H., Prasad, A. S., Newberne, P. M., and Fraker, P. J. Zinc: health effects and research priorities for the 1990s. Environ. Health Perspect., *102*:5–46, 1994.

Ward, J. M. Increased susceptibility of livers of aged F344/NCr rats to the effects of phenobarbital on the incidence, morphology, and histochemistry of hepatocellular foci and neoplasms. J. Natl. Cancer Inst., *71*:815–823, 1983.

Warshawsky, D., Barkley, W., and Bingham, E. Factors affecting carcinogenic potential of mixtures. Fundam. Appl. Toxicol., *20*:376–382, 1993.

Wasan, H. S., Novelli, M., Bee, J., and Bodmer, W. F. Dietary fat influences on polyp phenotype in multiple intestinal neoplasia mice. Proc. Natl. Acad. Sci. U.S.A., *94*:3308–3313, 1997.

Watson, R. R., and Moriguchi, S. Cancer prevention by retinoids: role of immunological modification. Nutr. Res., *5*:663–675, 1985.

Wattenberg, L. W. Chemoprevention of cancer. Cancer Res., *45*:1–8, 1985.

Wattenberg, L. W. Inhibition of carcinogenesis by minor anutrient constituents of the diet. Proc. Nutr. Soc., *49*:173–183, 1990.

Wattenberg, L. W. Inhibition of carcinogenesis by minor dietary constituents. Cancer Res., *52*:2085s–2091s, 1992.

Wattenberg, L. W., and Loub, W. D. Inhibition of polycyclic aromatic hydrocarbon-induced neoplasia by naturally-occurring indoles. Cancer Res., *38*:1410–1413, 1978.

Weindruch, R. Effect of caloric restriction on age-associated cancers. Exp. Gerontol., *27*:575–581, 1992.

Weisburger, E. K., Grantham, P. H., and Weisburger, J. H. Differences in the metabolism of *N*-hydroxy-*N*-2-fluorenylacetamide in male and female rats. Biochemistry, *3*:808–811, 1964.

Wells, P., Aftergood, L., and Alfin-Slater, R. B. Effect of varying levels of dietary protein on tumor development and lipid metabolism in rats exposed to aflatoxin. J. Am. Chem. Soc., *53*:559–562, 1976.

Welsch, C. W. Relationship between dietary fat and experimental mammary tumorigenesis: a review and critique. Cancer Res., *52*:2040s–2048s, 1992.

Welsch, C. W., Goodrich-Smith, M., Brown, C. K., Greene, H. D., and Hamel, E. J. Selenium and the genesis of murine mammary tumors. Carcinogenesis, *2*:519–522, 1981.

Welsch, C. W., DeHoog, J. V., and Moon, R. C. Lack of an effect of dietary retinoids in chemical carcinogenesis of the mouse mammary gland: inverse relationship between mammary tumor cell anaplasia and retinoic efficacy. Carcinogenesis, *5*:1301–1304, 1984.

Welsch, C. W., House, J. L., Herr, B. L., Eliasberg, S. J., and Welsch, M. A. Enhancement of mammary carcinogenesis by high levels of dietary fat: a phenomenon dependent on ad libitum feeding. J. Natl. Cancer Inst., *82*:1615–1620, 1990.

Whitfield, J. F. Calcium signals and cancer. Crit. Rev. Oncogen., *3*:55–90, 1992.

Wortzman, M. S., Besbris, H. J., and Cohen, A. M. Effect of dietary selenium on the interaction between 2-acetylaminofluorene and rat liver DNA *in vivo*. Cancer Res., *40*:2670–2676, 1980.

Woutersen, R. A., and van Garderen-Hoetmer, A. Inhibition of dietary fat-promoted development of (pre)neoplastic lesions in exocrine pancreas of rats and hamsters by supplemental vitamins A, C and E. Cancer Lett., *41*:179–189, 1988a.

Woutersen, R. A., and van Garderen-Hoetmer, A. Inhibition of dietary fat promoted development of (pre)neoplastic lesions in exocrine pancreas of rats and hamsters by supplemental selenium and β-carotene. Cancer Lett., *42*:79–85, 1988b.

Wu, F. Y.-H., and Wu, C.-W. Zinc in DNA replication and transcription. Annu. Rev. Nutr., *7*:251–272, 1987.

Xia, E., Rao, G., van Remmen, H., Heydari, A. R., and Richardson, A. Activities of antioxidant enzymes in various tissues of male Fischer 344 rats are altered by food restriction. J. Nutr., *125*:195–201, 1995.

Yamagiwa, K., Higashi, S., and Mizumoto, R. Effect of alcohol ingestion on carcinogenesis by synthetic estrogen and progestin in the rat liver. Jpn. J. Cancer Res., *82*:771–778, 1991.

Yamamoto, R. S., and Weisburger, E. K. The role of hormones on digestive and urinary tract carcinogenesis. Recent Prog. Horm. Res., *33*:617–653, 1977.

Yamate, J., Tajima, M., Kudow, S., and Sannai, S. Background pathology in BDF_1 mice allowed to live out their life-span. Lab. Anim., *24*:332–340, 1990.

Yancik, R., and Ries, L. G. Cancer in the aged. An epidemiologic perspective on treatment issues. Cancer, *68*:2502–2510, 1991.

Yang-Yen, H.-F., Zhang, X.-k., Graupner, G., Tzukerman, M., Sakamoto, B., Karin, M., and Pfahl, M. Antagonism between retinoic acid receptors and AP-1: implications for tumor promotion and inflammation. New Biol., *3*:1206–1219, 1991.

Yonekura, I., Matsumoto, Y., Miura, K., and Sato, A. Ethanol ingestion combined with lowered carbohydrate intake enhances the initiation of diethylnitrosamine liver carcinogenesis in rats. Nutr. Cancer, *17*:171–178, 1992.

Yoshida, L. S., Miyazawa, T., Hatayama, I., Sato, K., Fujimoto, K., and Kaneda, T. Phosphatidylcholine peroxidation and liver cancer in mice fed a choline-deficient diet with ethionine. Free Radic. Biol. Med., *14*:191–199, 1993.

Yu, B. P. Aging and oxidative stress: modulation by dietary restriction. Free Radic. Biol. Med., *21*:651–668, 1996.

Yuspa, S. H., Ben, T., and Steinert, P. Retinoic acid induces transglutaminase activity but inhibits cornification of cultured epidermal cells. J. Biol. Chem., *257*:9906–9908, 1982.

Zapisek, W. F., Cronin, G. M., Lyn-Cook, B. D., and Poirier, L. A. The onset of oncogene hypomethylation in the livers of rats fed methyl-deficient, amino acid-defined diets. Carcinogenesis, *13*:1869–1872, 1992.

Zhao, L. P., Kushi, L. H., Klein, R. D., and Prentice, R. L. Quantitative review of studies of dietary fat and rat colon carcinoma. Nutr. Cancer, *15*:169–177, 1991.

Zuo, F., Kraus, R. J., Gulick, T., Moore, D. D., and Mertz, J. E. Direct modulation of simian virus 40 late gene expression by thyroid hormone and its receptor. J. Virol., *71*:427–436, 1997.

9
The Natural History of Neoplastic Development: Progression

The stages of *initiation* and *promotion* were discussed in Chapter 7 as the beginning processes leading to the ultimate development of cancer. However, it should be clear to the reader that many of the behavioristic characteristics of malignancy (Chapter 2) are not expressed in the stages of initiation and promotion. Thus, the cellular populations of these stages are rightfully said to represent *preneoplasia*. It is in the final stage of neoplastic development, the stage of *progression*, that neoplasia is expressed as a true clinical disease condition.

The transition from the early progeny of an initiated cell to the biologically malignant cell population is essential to the development of cancer in the host. In the human, the conversion of the reversible lesion of leukoplakia in the mouth to a frankly invasive malignant epidermoid carcinoma is an excellent example of such transition. A number of neoplasms may change from a low degree of malignancy to a rapidly growing, virulent, fatal neoplasm at some time in their development within the host. Collectively, these processes, especially the increasing growth rate, have been termed the *progression* of neoplasia.

Foulds (1954) was one of the first to recognize the importance of the development of neoplasia beyond the appearance of an initial gross tumor. He postulated that the early stages of initiation and promotion were really part of a larger and continuous process of progression. Later, Noble (1977) characterized progression as "the tendency for a cell to escape from its inherent limited capacity for proliferation."

Foulds (1964) suggested that tumor progression may be considered from at least two viewpoints. The first he termed the "independent progression of neoplasms," which meant that progression occurred independently in each of several different primary neoplasms in the same animal. The second component of progression he termed the "independent progression of characters," in which any one of a number of characteristics of a neoplasm changed (or progressed) independently of others. The "characters" referred to by Foulds included growth rate, invasiveness, metastatic frequency, hormonal responsiveness, and morphological characteristics. Many of the characteristics described by Foulds are a direct function of demonstrable changes in the genome of the cell or closely associated with them. Karyotypic alterations in neoplasms may be directly correlated with increased growth rate (Fisher et al., 1975; Wolman, 1983; van Echten et al., 1995), invasiveness (Bevacqua et al., 1988), metastatic potential and capability (Nicolson, 1987; Frost et al., 1987), hormone responsiveness (cf. Wolman, 1983), and morphological characteristics (Ritchie, 1970). Thus, the characters and their changes during progression as described by Foulds (1964) are a reflection of the genetic and karyotypic heterogeneity characteristically seen in the stage of progression both by karyotypic analyses and more detailed molecular studies (Heim, 1996; Sengstag, 1994). Concomitant with these changes, the karyotype of the cell population in the neoplasm changes as progression occurs. An example of such a change in karyotype may be seen in Figure 9.1, which depicts the normal karyotype of the rat at the top of the figure; the next three karyotypes are those of stem cell lines from early transplant generations 3 to 5 years later. At the bottom of the figure, the karyotype of the cell line 7 to 8 years after continued transplantation are seen. The increase in marker chromosomes (arrows) dramatically indicates the changing karyotypes, especially in the later transplant generations. In most instances, repeated transplantation results in more rapidly growing tumors with a higher degree of aneuploidy.

A similar karyotypic evolution has been described with successive passages of Chinese hamster cells explanted to cell culture as euploid cells, which progressed through various passages to a heteroploid tumorigenic cell line (Cram et al., 1983). Similarly, Kerler and Rabes (1996) have demonstrated the karyotypic evolution of a clonal rat liver cell line during the stage of progression in vivo as well as in vitro. In the human, a large number of examples of karyotypic evolution in vivo have been described (Jacoby et al., 1995; Atkin and Baker, 1969; Haapasalo et al., 1991; Norming et al., 1992; Sato et al., 1991; Hemmer and Schön, 1993; Morse et al., 1994). Nowell (1982, 1986) pointed out the importance of clonal evolution of cells exhibiting abnormal karyotypes both in relation to tumor cell heterogeneity and also to tumor progression, especially in various human leukemias such as chronic myelogenous leukemia. Yosida (1983) related invasiveness and metastatic capability of neoplastic cells—both characteristics of progression as noted by Foulds (see above) to the karyotypic evolution of neoplastic cells. Thus,

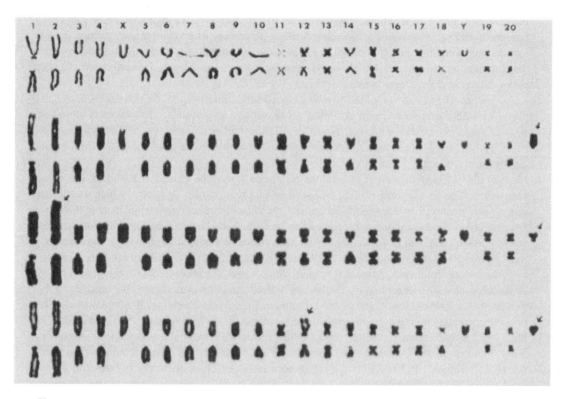

Figure 9.1 Karyotype of normal male rat (upper karyotype) with three karyotypes of serial transplantations from cell lines growing in 1961–62, 1965–67, and 1968–70. Arrows indicate the change in marker chromosomes in stem line cells of the neoplasms. (Adapted from Yosida, 1983, with permission of author and publishers.)

there is considerable evidence that progression is closely correlated with the appearance and subsequent evolution of karyotypic abnormalities in neoplastic cells, if not caused by them (cf. Nowell, 1990).

Kraemer and associates (1972) noted that, in a population of neoplastic cells exhibiting an extremely rapid growth rate and a high degree of aneuploidy, the DNA content of the average cell remained quite constant. Despite the constancy of the DNA content per cell, the population exhibited an extreme range of karyotype, extending at times from near diploid to hypotetraploidy. An example of this phenomenon, taken from the work of Kraemer and his associates (1972), is seen in Figure 9.2. In view of the myriad of karyotypes present in the population, they explained this phenomenon by postulating that the neoplastic cell had lost the ability to maintain a stable karyotype and that chromosomal components were interchanged with considerable frequency during successive cell cycles in this population. The changes seen do not reflect simply variation in numbers of chromosomes but also in their structure (Kraemer et al., 1974).

Although the exact mechanism of the phenomenon described by Kraemer and associates is not understood at the molecular level, the implications of such a phenomenon are clear. Some neoplastic cells in the stage of progression "shuffle" their chromosomes and components of their genome at some time during the cell cycle. It also appears from these studies (Kraemer et al., 1974) that cloning of a single cell from the HeLa heteroploid population results in a clone exhibiting the same DNA content as the original culture but also exhibiting a variety of karyotypes. If this conclusion is correct, then the heteroploid clone could only be accomplished by breakage and/or reconstitution of DNA strands during successive cell cycles, as well as aneuploidy, by mechanisms that are only incompletely understood at present (see below). More recently, Dues-

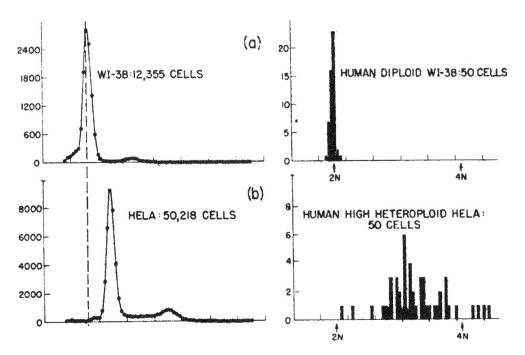

Figure 9.2 Auramine O-Feulgen-DNA distributions and chromosome number histograms of (a) normal human diploid WI-38 and (b) malignant HeLa cells in culture. The DNA content was determined by flow cytometry and the chromosome number by standard karyotyping. (Adapted from Kraemer et al., 1972, with permission of the authors and publisher.)

berg and associates (Duesberg et al., 1998; Rasnick and Duesberg, 1999) suggested a mechanism for the phenomenon described by Kraemer and reproduced in part by Duesberg. Their suggestion is that aneuploidy destabilizes the karyotype on the basis that it biases balance-sensitive mitosis proteins and organelles such as centrosomes, tubulin, etc. By their mechanism, aneuploidy tends to generate variations in chromosome number and evolution autocatalytically, resulting in karyotypic instability of neoplastic cells that is proportional to their degree of aneuploidy.

Although significant phenotypic heterogeneity has been described during the stage of promotion in hepatocarcinogenesis in the rat (Pitot et al., 1978; Peraino et al., 1984), significant biochemical homogeneity (Eriksson et al., 1983) and the lack of demonstrable genetic heterogeneity and instability characterize the stages of initiation and promotion (Chapter 7). Unlike the relatively limited phenotypic characteristics of cells in the stages of initiation and promotion, those in the stage of progression may undergo a continued evolution toward increased autonomy from host influences (Pitot, 1989). This process is accompanied by—or a reflection of—the continued evolution of karyotypic changes that accompanies the evolution of the stage of progression, as has been described in a variety of systems, both experimental (Aldaz et al., 1987; Sargent, 1996) and in the human (Nowell, 1986; Korabiowska et al., 1997).

THE BIOLOGY OF THE STAGE OF PROGRESSION

The growth of the progeny of initiated cells in the stage of promotion (preneoplastic cells) and their transition to the biologically malignant cell population constitute the major portion of the natural history of neoplastic development. We have already discussed the characteristics of the stages of initiation and promotion (Chapter 7). The transition of preneoplastic to neoplastic cells in the stage of progression may be considered the critical point in the development of neoplasia, although malignancy does not necessarily develop immediately after such transition. While the changes occurring during this transition may differ from tissue to tissue and proceed along a variety of pathways (see below), certain morphological and biological characteristics of the stage of progression can be delineated from studies of both experimental and human neoplasia. A listing of some of the major morphological and biological characteristics of the stage of progression may be seen in Table 9.1. Irreversibility of this stage is emphasized by the demonstrable alterations in the cellular genome—e.g., chromosomal translocations (Wolman, 1983), chromosomal deletions (Sato et al., 1991), gene amplification (Tlsty, 1996), and other structural DNA alterations (Malins et al., 1996) that are found within this stage. Such genomic changes clearly distinguish the stage of progression from the reversible preceding stage of promotion (Sargent et al., 1989; Aldaz et al., 1987; Balaban et al., 1986). Although the "reversibility" of the stage of

Table 9.1   Morphological and Biological Characteristics of the Stage of Progression During Carcinogenesis

---

Irreversible

Morphologically and molecularly discernible alterations in the cellular genome

Evolving karyotypic instability

Growth of cells in the stage of progression sensitive to environmental factors during early phase of this stage

Benign and malignant neoplasms observed in this stage

"Progressor" agents act to induce the transition of cells in the stage of promotion to that of progression

Spontaneous (fortuitous) induction of the stage of progression from the stage of promotion

---

promotion is accompanied by increased apoptotic rates (Chapter 7), the rate of apoptosis during the stage of progression varies dramatically with the histogenetic type of neoplasm (Staunton and Gaffney, 1995). Furthermore, as the stage of progression is extended into metastatic growth, cells may become increasingly resistant to apoptosis (Glinsky et al., 1997). As noted in Table 9.1, although cells in the stage of progression are not completely dependent for their existence on the continued presence of the promoting agent, promoting agents and other environmental factors may enhance the growth and genetic expression of cells in the stage of progression, especially early during the development of this stage. As growth of the neoplasm continues and karyotypic instability evolves, responses to environmental factors may be altered or lost (Noble, 1977; Welch and Tomasovic, 1985). Agents that act only to effect the transition of a cell from the stage of promotion to that of progression may properly be termed *progressor agents*. Some examples are seen in Table 9.2. Such agents would presumably have the characteristic of inducing chromosomal aberrations but may not necessarily be capable of initiation; in some cases, they may serve to enhance the clastogenesis associated with evolving karyotypic instability. Furthermore, the transition of the stage of progression from that of promotion frequently occurs as a spontaneous event even in studies involving chemical carcinogens that possess progressor agent activity (Luebeck and Moolgavkar, 1996; Cohen and Ellwein, 1990). In addition, there has been substantial evidence to demonstrate that the enhanced proliferation of cells in the stage of promotion does itself increase the likelihood of major genetic changes, resulting in demonstrable chromosomal alterations characteristic of the stage of progression (Ames and Gold, 1990b). Facilitation of the spontaneous transition from the stage of promotion to that of progression may occur, at least in part, through the mediation of active oxygen radicals, which occur commonly in the living cell (Chapter 3) and have been shown to be clastogenic in cells in vitro (Ochi and Kaneko, 1989; Emerit et al., 1991), as well as in the evolution of the stage of progression to the metastatic state in vivo (Malins et al., 1996).

The experimental demonstration of the stage of progression is somewhat more complex than that of initiation and promotion. In Figure 9.3 may be seen a general experimental format designed to demonstrate the effect of the administration of a progressor agent (lll) after a course of initiation and promotion with most of the appropriate controls. However, in this instance the end point that is quantitated is the number of neoplastic lesions (NL). In experimental systems, the most effective development of neoplasia involves the continued administration of the promoting agent even after application of the progressor agent has ceased. This might be expected, because cells early in the stage of progression respond to promoting agents, and this continuing proliferative response yields an increase in neoplastic lesions in the experimental system (Table 9.1). As noted, a lower yield of lesions, but usually still significantly different from the controls,

Table 9.2 Putative Progressor Agents in Carcinogenesis

Agent	Initiating Activity	Clastogenic Activity	Carcinogenic Activity
Arsenic salts	−	+	+
Asbestos fibers	?	+	+
Benzene	−	+	+
Benzoyl peroxide	−	+	±
Hydroxyurea	−	+	±
1,4-Bis[2-(3,5-dichloropyridyloxy)]-benzene	−	+	+
2,5,2′,5′-Tetrachlorobiphenyl	−	+	±

Modified from Pitot and Dragan, 1994.

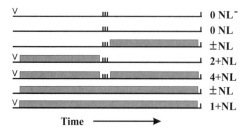

Figure 9.3 General experimental format for demonstration of the stage of progression and the effect of progressor agents in experimental systems. NL, neoplastic lesions; ±, occasional or infrequent; 1+, few; 2+, some; 4+, many; **III**, administration of progressor agent as single or several multiple doses; **V**, initiation; ■■■■■■, promoting agent dosing.

may be obtained without additional administration of the promoting agent. Because of the duration of the experiment, preneoplastic lesions occur to varying degrees in each of the experimental groups. The difficulty in such studies is the quantitation of the neoplastic lesions, which is usually carried out by determining the incidence and multiplicity of malignant tumors. However, premalignant lesions already in the stage of progression occur quite commonly (cf. Henson and Albores-Saavedra, 1986); thus the appropriate end point for the effect of progressor agents is the quantitation of such lesions. As yet, this has been extremely difficult to do, and thus quantitative analyses of the effects of progressor agents remain relatively crude.

CELL AND MOLECULAR MECHANISMS OF THE STAGE OF PROGRESSION

The stage of progression usually develops from cells in the stage of promotion but may develop directly from normal cells as a result of the administration of relatively high, cytotoxic doses of complete carcinogenic agents capable of inducing both initiation and progression. In addition, the incorporation into the genome of genetic information such as oncogenic viruses, the stable transfection of genetic material, or spontaneous chromosomal alterations may enhance the transition into the stage of progression. As previously noted in Table 9.1 and reemphasized in Table 9.3, the principal hallmark and characteristic of the stage of progression is that of evolving karyotypic instability. It is this molecular characteristic of cells in the stage of progression that potentially leads to multiple "stages" or changes in malignant cells that were first described by Foulds (1954) as "independent characteristics." As has been pointed out (cf. Harris, 1991), karyotypic changes are common if not ubiquitous in neoplastic cells in the stage of progression. A number of studies (Tlsty et al., 1993; Mäkelä and Alitalo, 1986; Sager et al., 1985) have emphasized the

Table 9.3 Some Cell and Molecular Mechanisms in the Stage of Progression

Genetic macrolesions (chromosomal translocations, deletions, gene amplification, recombination, gene conversion) resulting from evolving karyotypic instability

Irreversible changes in gene expression including fetal gene expression, altered MHC gene expression, and ectopic hormone production

Selection of neoplastic cells with genotypes/phenotypes for optimal growth in response to the cellular environment

Mutations in both alleles of one or more tumor suppressor genes

enhancement of gene amplification in neoplastic cells. Tlsty et al. (1989) demonstrated that the spontaneous rate of gene amplification in a number of neoplastic cell lines was almost 100 times the rate measured in nonneoplastic cells. In contrast, the frequencies of spontaneous point mutations have not generally been significantly different between normal and neoplastic cells (cf. Harris, 1991). Recently, however, with the demonstration that alterations in mismatch repair genes were responsible for increased incidences of several different types of neoplasms in affected individuals (Chapter 5), studies of micro- and minisatellite mutations have been undertaken in a variety of different neoplasms (Lothe, 1997; Speicher, 1995). This has led to the finding that, although 50% to 100% of neoplasms with mutations in mismatch repair genes exhibit mutations in micro- and minisatellites (Lothe, 1997), approximately 4% to 20% of spontaneous neoplasms of a variety of types exhibit similar "instability" (Speicher, 1995). The impact of this latter finding is softened by the demonstration that the frequency of microsatellite alterations in normal tissue is of the order of $1–5 \times 10^{-2}$, while that of the variation in minisatellite sequences may be as high as 10^{-1} in normal human tissues (Simpson, 1997). Of perhaps greater significance in the relationship of microsatellite mutations to the stage of progression is the proposal by Shibata et al. (1996) that the diversity of microsatellite mutations may be related to the number of replications and clonal expansions of the neoplasm during its development in the stage of progression.

Mutations in proto-oncogenes and tumor suppressor genes are relatively common in malignant neoplasms, both in the human (Yokota and Sugimura, 1993; Kiaris and Spandidos, 1995; Harris, 1996) and in the animal (Stowers et al., 1987; Jacks, 1996). In general, mutations can be identified in proto-oncogenes at early stages, including preneoplasia in the development of neoplastic disease (Burmer and Loeb, 1989; Ando et al., 1991; Ranaldi et al., 1995; Pellegata et al., 1994; Bauer-Hofmann et al., 1992). While many but not all proto-oncogene mutations can be seen in very early lesions, mutations in the p53 tumor suppressor gene in a variety of situations in both animals and the human are most readily identified during the stage of progression (Tamura et al., 1991; Navone et al., 1993; Tanaka et al., 1993; Donghi et al., 1993). In addition, abnormalities in the expression of the p16 tumor suppressor gene in melanomas are found frequently during the stage of progression but rarely in earlier stages (Reed et al., 1995). However, since karyotypic instability is unlikely to lead directly to point mutations in oncogenes and tumor suppressor genes, it is more likely that their appearance in malignant neoplasms reflects the selection of cells better suited to the growth environment of the neoplasm, such cells already having these mutations. Thus, the stage of progression is a function not only of evolving karyotypic instability but also of the selection of cells most suited for their aggressive replication and continued growth. Some cell and molecular mechanisms involved in the stage of progression are listed in Table 9.3. It should be noted that all of the characteristics in Table 9.3 can be directly associated with the evolving karyotypic instability, which may be considered the fundamental abnormality of this stage. Mechanisms associated with karyotypic instability are numerous and include disruption of the mitotic apparatus, alteration in telomere function (Ledbetter, 1992; Blackburn, 1994), inhibition of topoisomerase function (Cortés et al., 1993), DNA hypomethylation (Smith, 1998), DNA and genetic recombination (Chorazy, 1985; Murnane, 1990; Sengstag, 1994), gene amplification (Tlsty et al., 1993), gene conversion (Taghian and Nickoloff, 1997), and gene transposition (cf. Cheng and Loeb, 1993). As noted above, the relationship of alterations in mismatch repair with karyotypic instability is not entirely clear. Because of its unique role as "guardian of the genome," abnormalities in the p53 tumor suppressor gene may also contribute to evolving karyotypic instability (Sood et al., 1997). As Shackney and Shankey (1997) have pointed out, p53 abnormalities become appreciable in many developing neoplasms just prior to the transition from preinvasive to invasive malignancy. Thus, it appears that there are many pathways to the development of karyotypic instability in neoplastic cells in the stage of progression.

Mutational macrolesions (Table 7.6) resulting from chromosomal translocations, deletions, recombinations, and other karyotypic changes have been discussed in Chapter 6 in relation to the formation of fusion genes. Other examples of gene rearrangement occurring during the stage of progression may be seen in experimental and human myelomas, in which rearrangement of immunoglobulin genes mimics in part the normal rearrangement occurring in these genes during the maturation of antibody-producing plasma cells (Chapter 16). The small oncogenic DNA viruses whose genetic material is directly incorporated into that of the host cell may transform normal cells into neoplastic cells exhibiting the biological and molecular characteristics of progression (Rapp and Westmoreland, 1976). The T antigen, the product of the oncogene in such viruses, induces a large variety of chromosomal aberrations in transformed cells and may induce recombinational events in transformed and infected cells as well (cf. Fanning and Knippers, 1992). Some defective oncogenic RNA viruses lacking a specific transforming v-onc gene (Chapter 4) induce neoplasms in vivo only after a long latent period. Hayward et al. (1981) were among the first to demonstrate that—at least in specific cases—the delay is related to the requirement for the insertion of the DNA of the virus in an appropriate position in relation to the proto-oncogene, c-myc. Since that time, neoplasia resulting from retroviral integration into regions controlling the expression of specific cellular genes, termed *insertional mutagenesis*, has been described in a number of instances (Gray, 1991). Furthermore, Noori-Daloii et al. (1981) demonstrated the occurrence of gene amplification as well as structural alterations of the chromosomal region in which the insertion occurs. Other examples of such insertion occurring during the stage of progression have also been described (Breuer et al., 1989; Lazo and Tsichlis, 1988). Such findings further indicate that the stage of progression may occur very early in the natural history of many virus-induced neoplasms.

Gene amplification is another characteristic of the stage of tumor progression that may be directly related to karyotypic instability (Tlsty, 1996). With a number of drugs—including methotrexate (Sharma and Schimke, 1994), nitrogen mustards (Lewis et al., 1988), and etoposide (Campain et al., 1995)—amplification of the target gene(s) of the drug occurs, with resulting drug resistance due to the marked increase in the amount of gene product. As a result of this induced gene amplification, the neoplastic cell may become quite resistant to the effects of the drug (cf. Chapter 18). Gene amplification may also be induced by carcinogenic agents such as the tumor promoter tetradecanoyl phorbol acetate (Chapter 7), which is capable of stimulating amplifications of several genes in cultured cells, including folate reductase (Varshavsky, 1981), metallothionein I (Hayashi et al., 1983), and SV40 DNA in the host genome of transformed hamster embryo cells (Lavi, 1981).

The instability of the genome of the neoplastic cell in the stage of progression makes plausible an extension of the "promoter insertion theory" (Chapter 4) as a potential mechanism for many of the characteristics of progression, especially those related to growth and gene expression in this stage of development of neoplasms of viral, chemical, and physical origin. Furthermore, aneuploid cells, including those in the stage of progression, may be more likely to be able to incorporate exogenous DNA into their genome than are normal diploid cells (e.g., Coonrod et al., 1997). Numerous examples of "transfection" of genes into aneuploid cells with subsequent stable expression of genes in a small number of progeny have been described (cf. Graf, 1982). During the recent past, the transfection of genes isolated from neoplastic cells into appropriate recipient cells has been utilized as a method for identifying cellular oncogenes or transforming genes (cf. Cooper, 1982). Initially, studies by several laboratories identified a mutated Ha-*ras* proto-oncogene as the transforming gene occurring in both human and animal neoplasms (Chang et al., 1982; Parada et al., 1982). Later studies demonstrated that specific base changes in the normal Ha-*ras* proto-oncogene resulted in this transformation (Tabin et al., 1982). Since then a number of such transforming genes, not all of which are derivatives of proto-oncogenes, have been described (Table 9.4). Land et al. (1983) demonstrated that transfection of two different "transforming genes" into third-passage rat embryo fibroblasts resulted in the neoplastic transformation. Transfection of the genes separately failed to induce such transformation. The analogy between this phenomenon and that of the stages of promotion and progression in vivo is apparent. However, several studies have demonstrated that the transfection process itself can induce chromosome rearrangements and other types of mutations and epigenetic changes in recipient cells, leading to an induction of genomic instability in murine cells (Bardwell, 1989; Gilbert and Harris, 1988; Denko et al., 1994). Furthermore, transfection of a normal proto-oncogene into neoplastic cells in vitro enhanced karyotypic instability, so that the integration of the transfected gene occurred predominantly in aberrant chromosomes (de Vries et al., 1993). Thus, while the transfection of specific genes has many potential uses, the interpretation of the "transformation" of cells in culture and possibly also in vivo may be somewhat difficult in view of these latter experiments.

The continuing evolution of the stage of progression may also be related to irreversible changes in genetic expression. As noted above, alteration in methylation of the genome in neoplastic cells can occur as an early event in neoplastic development, possibly even preceding the stage of progression, and may continue during the stage of progression, resulting in altered gene expression (Smith, 1998; Makos et al., 1993). As noted in Table 9.3, such mechanisms, in addition to karyotypic instability, can lead to alterations in major groups of genes such as (1) those expressed during fetal life but not normally in the adult (Chapter 15), (2) repression and/or hyperexpression of genes involved in histocompatibility (Chapter 19), and (3) the ectopic production of hormones by neoplasms derived from cells that normally do not express such genes (Chapter 18). In addition, the expression of genes important in DNA synthesis, the cell cycle, and apoptosis may also be abnormal in neoplastic cells in the stage of progression, including cyclins (Imoto et al., 1997; Wani et al., 1997), telomerase (Shay and Wright, 1996), and the *bcl-2* gene (Chapter 6) (Bronner et al., 1995). Hyperexpression of the c-*myc* proto-oncogene reportedly is an example of the altered expression of a gene during the stage of progression, primarily as a result of the amplification of the proto-oncogene (Garte, 1993). Drug resistance in neoplasia

Table 9.4 Mutations in Genes Whose Transfection Leads to Cell Transformation

Gene	Mutation	Cell Type Transformed	Reference
neu (rat)	T → A (codon 664)	NIH3T3	Bargman et al., 1986
N-*ras* (mouse)	G → A (codon 12)	NIH3T3	cf. Guerrero and Pellicer, 1987
K-*ras* (mouse)	G → A (codon 2)	NIH3T3	cf. Guerrero and Pellicer, 1987
H-*ras* (mouse)	A → T (codon 61)	NIH3T3	Wiseman et al., 1986
trk 5 (human)	153 bp deletion	NIH3T3	Coulier et al., 1990
vav (mouse)	deletion of helix-loop-helix region	NIH3T3	Coppola et al., 1991
ect 2 (mouse)	truncation of 5′ 0.5 kb of cDNA	NIH3T3	Miki et al., 1993
fyn (human)	$try_{528} \to phe_{528}$	NIH3T3	Davidson et al., 1994
met (human)	$meth_{1268} \to threo_{1268}$	NIH3T3	Jeffers et al., 1997
kit (human)	T → A (codon 559)	B_2/F3	Hirota et al., 1998
rat (human)	$cys_{634} \to arg_{634}$	NIH3T3	Cote et al., 1995; Asai et al., 1995
fms (human)	$leu_{301} \to ser_{301}$	NIH3T3	Roussel et al., 1988

has also been directly associated with karyotypic instability, first by Terzi (1974) and more recently by Duesberg et al. (2001), who observed that a major mechanism of drug-resistant mutations in cell lines was characterized by and probably the result of karyotypic instability. More recently, Schnipper et al. (1989) noted that, in an artificial system dependent on drug resistance, the frequency of resistance increased with duration of exposure to the clastogenic large T antigen. Studies have also demonstrated that the expression of a gene can be affected by its location in the chromosome, as when a gene is moved close to a heterochromatic region. This is termed the *position effect* (cf. Pardue, 1991). Finally, in a recent study, Li et al. (1997), investigating a system of chemical transformation of Chinese hamster cells (Chapter 14) in culture, noted that aneuploidy correlated completely with the induction of cell transformation and presumed neoplasia in this system.

On the basis of our knowledge of tumor progression and its characteristics, one may thus propose the following definition of this stage in the development of neoplasia: *progression is that stage of neoplastic development characterized by the irreversible evolution of karyotypic instability, which results directly in mutational macrolesions, irreversible changes in gene expression, and the selection of neoplastic cells with genotypes/phenotypes optimal for growth in the immediate environment. These characteristics are further reflected by an increased growth rate, increased invasiveness, successful metastatic growth, and alterations in biochemical and morphological characteristics of the neoplasm.*

The latter part of the definition distinguishes the phase of progression from that of promotion, in which such major genetic changes have not been demonstrated. We have already noted (Chapter 6) gene rearrangements that occur during neoplastic development, many of these rearrangements being somewhat specific for individual types of neoplasms (Table 6.8). By the above definition, these neoplasms are thus in the stage of progression. Other examples of gene rearrangement occurring during the stage of progression are in experimental and human myelomas, in which rearrangement of immunoglobulin genes mimics in part the normal arrangement occurring in these genes during the maturation of antibody-producing plasma cells (Chapter 19).

The effect of the addition of exogenous genetic material, together with all of the apparatus needed for its expression, may be seen in virus-induced neoplasms, especially those resulting from RNA viruses. When the virus is nondefective, as with the Rous sarcoma virus, a stage of promotion cannot readily be discerned, since tumor production and growth are so rapid (Hanafusa, 1975). Similarly, many oncogenic DNA viruses, especially those whose genetic material is directly incorporated into that of the host cell, transform normal cells rapidly into neoplastic cells, which then exhibit many of the biological characteristics of progression (Rapp and Westmoreland, 1976). On the other hand, certain defective oncogenic RNA viruses, especially those lacking a transforming v-*onc* gene (Chapter 4), induce neoplasms only after a long latent period. In several instances, this delay is related to the requirement for the insertion of the DNA of the virus in an appropriate position in relation to proto-oncogenes (Chapter 4). Other DNA viruses that are clastogenic in human tissues include the hepatitis B virus (Simon et al., 1991), the human papillomavirus (Hashida and Yasumoto, 1991), the cytomegalovirus (Sakizli et al., 1981), and human polyomaviruses (Lazutka et al., 1996). Such oncogenic viruses that induce clastogenesis may be considered as progressor agents themselves.

CELLULAR REPLICATION, THE CELL CYCLE, AND THE STAGE OF PROGRESSION

We have already noted that the stages of initiation and promotion require cell replication for their expression. The stage of initiation requires "fixation" of the genetic changes in the initiated

cell by at least one round of cell replication (Chapter 7). The stage of tumor promotion is characterized by a selective promoter-induced replication of initiated cells into clonal colonies. In the
stage of progression, however, while cell replication is necessary for the ultimate growth of the
neoplasm, it is the aberrancies of the cell cycle that are inherent as the major characteristic of
this stage, karyotypic instability. The requirements for cell proliferation during the stages of carcinogenesis are summarized in Table 9.5.

The Cell Cycle

The events that occur during cellular division have for the past 125 years been a subject of fasci-
nation and intense study (Orlowski and Furlanetto, 1996; King et al., 1994). *Mitosis*, the process
of the division of the cytoplasm and the nucleus of a cell, and *meiosis*, the process of cellular
division leading to a 50% reduction in the number of chromosomes (Kleckner, 1996), have been
studied morphologically and biochemically in an attempt to dissect the functional components
leading up to and following this visible sign of cellular replication. From such investigations it
has become apparent that most dividing cells undergo a sequence of processes that have been
termed the *cell cycle* and that culminate in mitosis. As can be seen in Figure 9.4, the cell cycle is
divided into at least four separate components, with a fifth phase, G_0, consisting of cells that
appear to leave the normal cell cycle but can be induced to reenter the cycle by specific stimuli.
The tendency for liver cells to divide after partial hepatectomy may be an example of the stimulation of cells in G_0 to reenter the cycle. In addition, some cells, especially certain nerve cells of
the brain, may leave the cycle and never reenter it under any known circumstances. On the other
hand, neoplastic cells may undergo many normal cycles or alternatively leave the cell cycle and
enter G_0. This latter course may be due to major chromosomal abnormalities, with such affected
cells never reentering the cycle but rather ultimately dying. Other cells may remain in the G_0
state as dormant or latent neoplastic cells (Chapter 10).

Our understanding of the molecular mechanisms involved in the cell cycle and its regulation has become increasingly clear during the last decade. Figure 9.5 is a schematic of the cell
cycle, depicting the periods during which specific proteins and their complexes appear and disappear as well as external factors controlling the cell cycle at specific points. Key in driving and
regulating the cell cycle are the cyclins, of which at least eight have now been described (Noble
et al., 1997). The cyclins are bound to cyclin-dependent serine/threonine protein kinases designated CDKs and are essential for their activation. Association of the individual cyclins with specific CDKs as well as the regulation of CDKs by phosphorylation and/or inhibitor proteins timed
in their appearance at specific periods of the cell cycle results in regulated complexes that drive
the events of the cell cycle. While the concentration of cyclins varies during the cell cycle, as
noted in the figure, levels of the CDKs remain relatively constant. Cyclin levels increase in re-

Table 9.5 Cell Proliferation and Multistage Carcinogenesis

Stage	Cell Proliferation Requirements
Initiation	One to two cell cycles of target cell needed to "fix" the molecular initiation event
Promotion	Multiple cell cycles of initiated cell selectively induced by promoting agent(s)
Progression	Multiple cell cycles as a result of abnormalities in cell cycle components and/or effectors of the cycle

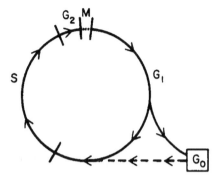

Figure 9.4 The cell cycle, indicating the periods of interphase (G_1), DNA synthesis (S), the period between the end of DNA synthesis and the beginning of mitosis (G_2), and the mitotic interval (M). The G_0 state is also depicted as a side extension of interphase, with the possibility that the G_0 cell may reenter the cycle (dashed line).

sponse to transcriptional activation and decrease following degradation through ubiquitination and proteosome function.

A number of factors external to the cycle itself and cyclin/CDK functions exist as regulators of the cell cycle through a variety of mechanisms. A major regulator of the cycle is the retinoblastoma tumor suppressor protein pRB (Chapter 5). This protein in its unphosphorylated state interacts with the E2F family of transcriptional factors (Chapter 7) to prevent transcription of critical components necessary for initiation of the cell cycle (Okayama et al., 1996). Cyclin D in association with one of its kinases (CDK4 or CDK6) as an active phosphorylation complex inactivates pRB by phosphorylation of the protein during G_1, such that at the restriction point (designated by the solid triangle in the G_1 phase of the cell cycle in Figure 9.5), the cell cycle is initiated and subsequent events are allowed to take place (Pardee, 1989). The cycle is controlled by other external proteins as well. The transcription of the inhibitor p16 is enhanced by growth factor inhibitors such as TGFβ as well as components of the E2F family. This latter mechanism acts as a negative feedback loop in regulating the cycle in normal cells. Members of the p16 family inhibit the action of the cyclin D/CDK4 or 6 complex by interfering with its formation, while p21, termed a "universal CDK inhibitor" (Sherr, 1994), and its family (p27, p57) inhibit CDK activity by forming a tertiary complex with the cyclin/CDK complex (Okayama et al., 1996). This latter family of inhibitors forms an inactive complex with the cyclin/CDK complex. The inhibitor p21 is directly regulated by the p53 tumor suppressor protein at the transcriptional level (Mowat, 1998), as noted in Figure 9.5.

With the exception of cyclin D in continuously cycling cells, the rapid disappearance of the cyclins during the cycle is the result of proteolysis mediated by the ubiquitin pathway, a process that has been well understood biochemically for several years (Ciechanover and Schwartz, 1998). Basically, the process involves the covalent attachment of several molecules of the small protein ubiquitin to a lysine on the substrate protein. This complex is directed to the proteosome, a complex proteolytic machine that degrades such polyubiquitinated protein into small peptides (Baumeister et al., 1998; Murray, 1995). Ubiquitination and proteolysis of the cyclins are enhanced by the presence of a specific sequence (the "destruction box") located near the N terminus of the protein, thus facilitating rapid destruction of the cyclin (cf. Klotzbücher et al., 1996). Concomitant with the destruction of cyclins, there is no further phosphorylation of pRB, which becomes dephosphorylated during the M phase as a result of the action of a protein phosphatase, with subsequent reactivation and sequestration of E2F (cf. Riley et al., 1994). Such a change in

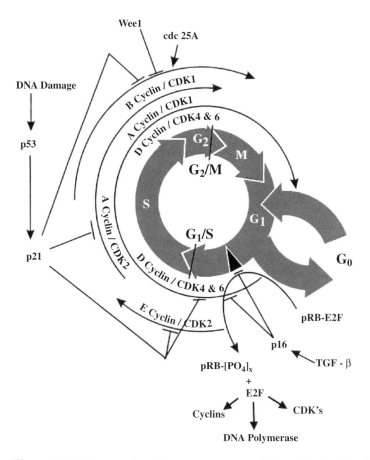

Figure 9.5 Diagram of regulatory components of the cell cycle. The "restriction point" or START (yeast) beyond which the cell is committed to complete the cycle is indicated by a dark triangle within the G_1 phase of the cycle. The G_1/S and G_2/M checkpoints are indicated by lines across the arrows at the end of G_1 and G_2 phases respectively. The single line arrows indicate the time during the cell cycle in which the cyclin/CDK complexes are individually active. The arrowheads indicate a positive effect of the molecular species indicated or of the cyclin/CDK complex. Short perpendicular lines at the end of specific signal lines indicate an inhibition of the underlined process. See text for description of individual molecular species.

the phosphorylation status also alters pRB interaction with a variety of other proteins involved in transcription, cell differentiation, and apoptosis (Herwig and Strauss, 1997; Whyte, 1995). Ubiquitination is also critical for the entrance into and cessation of mitosis. A specific protein complex termed the *anaphase promoting complex* has been described in eukaryotes from yeast to humans. Several of the proteins in this complex have been isolated and characterized. The function of the complex is to promote the transition from metaphase to anaphase by ubiquitinating mitotic cyclins and targeting them for destruction (Page and Hieter, 1997).

Regulation of the Cell Cycle—Checkpoints

In addition to the various components of the cell cycle and their regulation, the existence of surveillance systems that interrupt cell cycle progression when damage to the genome or spindle is detected or when cells have failed to complete an event has been described. These systems have been termed *checkpoints* (cf. Paulovich et al., 1997). The first checkpoint occurs in the region of the G_1/S boundary in the cell cycle, as noted in Figure 9.5. Functioning of this checkpoint is seen when DNA strand breaks induce G_1 arrest, thereby delaying the transition of cells from the G_1 phase to the S phase. Other types of DNA damage that may cause a G_1 arrest and function of the G_1/S checkpoint include mutations, DNA adducts, replicative gaps, etc. (Kaufmann and Paules, 1996). A major function of the G_1 arrest at this checkpoint is to allow DNA repair, primarily excisional repair, to function, thereby permitting the cell to continue through the cycle. One of the major mechanisms of the arrest is mediated by the p53 tumor suppressor gene that is activated by DNA damage. The enhanced expression of p53 allows for transactivation of other genes, paramount among which is the Waf1 or p21 gene, which we have noted as a general inhibitor of cyclin/CDK complexes. By this mechanism, the G_1 checkpoint can be activated and will continue to be activated until repair has occurred, p53 activation is eliminated, and p21 is destroyed by proteolysis, allowing the cycle to continue. However, if the damage is irreparable or too severe, p53 activation may enhance and initiate the process of apoptosis, thus eliminating a cell whose DNA alterations could not be repaired. The reader should also note that the alterations inducing the activation of the G_1 checkpoint are those we have already discussed as occurring during the process of initiation in carcinogenesis. Thus, if DNA repair is faulty or a cell carrying a mutation gets through the checkpoint, initiation is a potential result. Another potential checkpoint is that of S-phase replicon initiation (Kaufmann and Paules, 1996). Evidence for its existence comes from the fact that both chemical and physical damage to DNA that manages to escape the G_1/S checkpoint may lead to an inhibition of replicon initiation of DNA synthesis during the S period. It is not completely clear which genes are involved in this process, but it is likely that ε, one of the DNA polymerases, as well as the ataxia telangiectasia (AT) gene (Chapter 5), is active in this process. The other major checkpoint is that of the G_2/M boundary, which is activated by double-stranded DNA breaks and results in preventing the progression of the cycle through mitosis (Paulovich et al., 1997). This delay has been associated with an inhibition of the activity of CDK1, which is associated with cyclins A and B (cf. Kaufmann and Paules, 1996). Since repair of double-stranded DNA breaks is more complicated than that of simple excisional repair (Chapter 3), delay at the G_2/M checkpoint facilitates repair by increasing the time for repair to occur and by transcriptionally inducing gene expression concomitant with the inhibition of the activity of CDK1. An increase in the level of expression of cyclins A and B and of CDK1 occurs to compensate for the inhibition, possibly owing to phosphatase activity. However, if cells with unrepaired chromatin damage are driven into mitosis, the chance for major chromosomal abnormalities is great. Thus, failure of this checkpoint can lead to the induction of the stage of progression. A checkpoint at the spindle assembly has also been reported to occur in lower eukaryotes and quite probably occurs in mammals as well (Elledge, 1996).

THE CELL CYCLE IN NEOPLASIA

As yet, no irreversible abnormalities in the cell cycle have been demonstrated during the stage of promotion; however, the promoting agent phenobarbital does appear to affect one of the checkpoints in the cell cycle (Goldsworthy et al., 1999). During the stage of progression, both mutations in and altered regulation of cell cycle components have been described. A listing of genes, together with their abnormalities and the neoplasms in which such abnormalities are noted, is given in Table 9.6. Several of these genes, such as the retinoblastoma and p53 genes, have been discussed previously in relation to the genetic changes occurring in neoplasia (Chapters 5 and 6). From the table it can be noted, however, that several of the cyclins, most notably cyclin D_1, exhibit increased expression largely through the mechanism of amplification and translocation.

As noted from our previous discussion (Figure 9.5), one may readily understand that increased levels of these cyclins, especially when other factors regulating the cell cycle show abnormalities—e.g., p16, p53, and p21—can drive the enhanced replicative activity of neoplasms in the stage of progression. Most studies of p21 in human neoplasms have found few if any somatic mutations in this gene, although some polymorphisms in the gene have been described (cf. Gartel et al., 1996). The report by Jung et al. (1995) of an increased expression of p21 in a variety of cell lines from human gliomas suggests, just as with the increased transcription of cyclin A in leukemias (Paterlini et al., 1995), that amplification of the gene does occur in these neoplastic cells. The amplification of CDK4 noted in the number of gliomas and sarcomas (cf. Hall and Peters, 1996) would be expected to further the enhanced activity of the cycle by its association with cyclin D_1. The hBUB1 gene controls mitotic delay in response to spindle alterations. The protein product exhibits kinase activity and was found to be mutated in several colorectal cancer cell lines and associated with karyotypic instability (Cahill et al., 1998). Many of the alterations noted in the table are the result of processes probably occurring during the stage of progression concomitant with increased karyotypic instability. These include translocations, amplification, and deletions. Thus, a direct causative relation between the critical feature of the stage of progression, karyotypic instability, and deregulation of the cell cycle is readily understood from data such as those presented in Table 9.6.

Cell Proliferation and the Risk of Neoplastic Development

Although it has been long recognized that increased cell proliferation and neoplasia are related, it is only within the last decade that substantial emphasis has been placed on a potential role of cell proliferation itself in increasing the risk of neoplastic development (Croy, 1993). The present debate centers around whether cell proliferation itself is carcinogenic or whether it functions only as implied in our original definition of neoplasia (Chapter 2). Ames and colleagues (Ames and Gold, 1990a; Ames et al., 1993) have argued that mitogenesis is itself mutagenic and, in the presence of numerous real and potential opportunities for endogenous mutation, enhances the risk for mutation far more than seen in a quiescent cell. Furthermore, during cell

Table 9.6 Mutations and Altered Expression of Genes of the Cell Cycle in Neoplasia

Gene	Alteration	Neoplasm with Alteration	Reference
p53	Mutation	Lung, colon, liver, endometrium, etc.	Levine et al., 1991 Giaretti, 1997
RB	Mutation, deletion	Retinoblastoma, osteosarcoma	Schubert et al., 1994
Cyclin D_1	Translocation, amplification	Lymphomas, breast, esophagus, bladder	Hall and Peters, 1996
p16	Mutation, deletion	Melanoma, cholangioma, esophagus, gliomas	Hall and Peters, 1996
Cyclin E	Amplification, mutation	Stomach, breast	Akama et al., 1995 Keyomarsi et al., 1995
hBUB1	Mutation	Colorectal cancer lines	Cahill et al., 1998
Cyclin A	Increased transcription (amplification?)	Leukemias	Paterlini et al., 1995
p21	Increased expression	Gliomas	Jung et al., 1995
CDK4	Amplification	Gliomas and sarcomas	cf. Hall and Peters, 1996

Table 9.7 Enhancement of the Risk of Spontaneous Initiation and
Progression by Cell Proliferation

Increased risk of mutation during cell division
Enhanced chance for aneuploidy during mitosis
Enhancement of gene amplification at time of cell division (S phase)
Alteration of cytosine methylation during S phase

division, single-stranded DNA does not have the protection of base-pairing or histones and thus is more sensitive to damage than double-stranded DNA. Finally, these authors argue that cell division triggers mitotic recombination, gene conversion, and nondisjunction while allowing gene duplication and loss of 5-methylcytosine in DNA. A summary of these factors is seen in Table 9.7. All of these processes can be directly related to karyotypic abnormalities seen in the stage of progression. Similarly, cytotoxicity occurring at extremely high doses of agents being tested for carcinogenicity (Chapter 13) causes lysosomal breakdown, chromosome aberrations, and DNA double-strand breaks, all of which are again related to the characteristics of progressor agents (Bradley et al., 1987). Biological modeling of specific experimental systems has also led to the conclusion that rates of cell proliferation are integral if not the key factor in carcinogenesis of the rodent bladder induced by chemical carcinogens (Cohen and Ellwein, 1991a). Furthermore, a critical role for cell proliferation in carcinogenesis may be evidenced by the fact that a number of carcinogenic agents exhibit their carcinogenicity only when target cells are stimulated to divide and proliferate, usually as a result of toxicity induced by excessive doses of the test agent—e.g., exceeding the maximally tolerated dose (MTD) (Chapter 13). Furthermore, several studies (Table 9.8) have demonstrated a distinct correlation between the induction of cell proliferation as reflected in the labeling index (LI) and the development of neoplasia. Cunningham (1996) has similarly reported a positive association between increased cell proliferation and carcinogenesis.

On the other hand, several authors have argued that cell proliferation is not a major risk for neoplastic development (Weinstein, 1992; Farber, 1996; Melnick, 1992; Ward et al., 1993). In addition, arguments have been raised that chemical toxicity may not be a factor in the risk of

Table 9.8 Cell Proliferation Correlated with the Carcinogenic Effects of Chemicals

Chemical	Organ/Species	LI[a]		Tumors		Reference
		Low	High	Low Dose	High Dose	
Hexachlorobutadiene	Kidney/rat	?	+	?	+	Kociba et al., 1977; Stott et al., 1981
Chloroform	Liver/mouse (f)	–	+++	–	+++	Larson et al., 1994
Furan	Liver/mouse, rat	ND	+++	±	+++	Wilson et al., 1992
Methyl t-butyl ether	Kidney/rat (m)	+	+++	–	+++	Prescott-Matthews et al., 1997
FANFT (N-[4-(5-nitro-2-furyl)-2-thiazolyl]formamide	Bladder/rat (m)	–	+++	–	+++	Cohen and Ellwein, 1991b

[a]Labeling index

chemical carcinogenesis (Huff, 1993; Tennant et al., 1991; Hoel et al., 1988). Despite these reservations, however, it is difficult to argue that cell replication is not an inherent factor in carcinogenesis, although it is clear that a variety of other factors are also critical in the carcinogenic process. Furthermore, cell replication, as noted in the points made by Ames and colleagues (see above), enhances the risk of spontaneous initiation and progression as well as that induced by specific chemical, physical, or biological carcinogens. The enhanced cellular replication induced by promoting agents clearly suggests that a mutationally altered cell within an initiated clone has a greater risk of spontaneously entering the stage of progression than do normal cells derived from noninitiated cells. As seen above, cellular replication itself occurring during the stage of progression causes the continued evolution of karyotypic instability characteristic of and leading to greater degrees of malignancy.

CELLULAR REPLICATION RATES IN NEOPLASIA

In the natural history of neoplastic development, cellular replication plays a major role (Table 9.5), especially when the natural history of the replicating neoplastic cell population extends to its ultimate conclusion, the metastatic neoplastic cell. Certain populations of normal cells within the mammalian organism also undergo cellular replication, in some cases continuously, as in the bone marrow and intestinal epithelium, but in others more intermittently or only under specific circumstances, as in the liver following partial hepatectomy. In the epithelium of the bronchus, epidermis, and cervix, there is constant turnover and loss of cellular populations as the result of cell division from the basal or stem cells and subsequent migration and further cell replication (with final cell loss from the surface of the epithelium). It has been estimated that during the life span of an individual, the renewal of these epithelia represents between 10^{14} and 10^{16} cell divisions. Since the background mutation rate is 10^{-6} per gene per cell division, there is presumed to be some mechanism to eliminate or repair the numerous mutations that presumably occur in these cells during the lifetime of the individual. Theoretically, one or more such mutations might then lead to the conversion of a normal to an initiated cell. Subsequent mutation(s), spontaneous or induced, would transit the cell into the stage of progression.

Cairns (1975) has suggested that at least two mechanisms safeguard against such conversion. One mechanism involves the loss of cells that harbor such mutations through normal elimination such as desquamation or terminal differentiation. Second, it is theoretically possible that the daughter cell remaining in the stem cell population after division, the so-called immortal daughter cell, always receives the DNA molecules that represent the older of the two parental strands. In this way mutations occurring during replication would not collect in the stem cell population.

Although these ideas are unproven, they do have a counterpart in the development of cancer at several sites in the human. Oehlert (1973) and others have shown that the earliest changes seen in the development of neoplasia in the skin and bronchus are focal increased mitotic activity, loss of polarization, and breakdown of the structure of the epithelium. In the colon, where stem cells for the mucosal epithelium occur deep within the crypts, an increased rate of cell proliferation was noted in the deep region of the colonic crypts in aberrant crypts, putatively a preneoplastic lesion (Roncucci et al., 1993). However, earlier studies by Deschner (1982) suggested that an increased rate of DNA synthesis was seen in the upper (lumenal) region of crypts with colon cancer (isolated polyps) and familial polyposis. Since individual crypts were not examined, it is difficult to compare the two studies. In any event enhanced cell replication in certain regions of the crypt occurs very early during the development of these preneoplastic lesions in the genesis of colon cancer (Yamashita et al., 1994). In the case of carcinoma of the cervix, some early lesions, including carcinoma in situ and its precursors, have been shown to regress and disappear spontaneously, while others continue their development to carcinoma (Christopherson, 1977).

The growth characteristics of neoplasms in vivo have never been adequately investigated. Most scientists rely on a simple external measurement or on a determination from radiological studies to estimate the volume of a neoplasm (e.g., Greengard et al., 1985), considering such changes a function of time. Studies have also employed radioactive techniques either in vivo or in vitro, with labeled precursors of DNA, especially thymidine (for example, Newburger and Weinstein, 1980; Schiffer et al., 1979). On the basis of such investigations, the doubling time of the average human neoplasm, estimated as the time required to double the size of the tumor mass, has been reported to be between 50 and 60 days (Charbit et al., 1971). During the last decade, another method for determining cell proliferation in tissues, which has the advantage of not requiring prelabeling of the tissues with a precursor, is the immunohistochemical staining of a nuclear protein associated with cell proliferation, termed the *proliferating cell nuclear antigen* (PCNA). Analysis of PCNA expression in histological sections has been utilized for the estimation of growth fractions in neoplasms (Kamel et al., 1991; Gelb et al., 1992). PCNA functions as a processivity factor for DNA polymerase δ, the latter being the enzyme responsible for the replication of chromosomal DNA (Kelman, 1997). PCNA also interacts with cyclin D and p21 (Figure 9.5) and also appears to function in DNA repair (Kelman, 1997). More extensive measurements (Steel, 1977) have shown a variety of doubling times in a number of human tumors and their metastases. The values for such measurements for a number of histogenetic neoplasms of the human is seen in Table 9.9. From these data, adenocarcinomas of the colon appear to have the longest doubling times; metastatic lesions grow more rapidly. In most examples, human rectal cancer proliferates more slowly than normal rectal mucosa (Britton et al., 1975). In a more recent study of human tumor proliferation with bromodeoxyuridine administered in vivo to label DNA, Wilson (1991) found an enormous variation in the potential doubling time of several of the more common human carcinomas, ranging from a few days to more than 100 days in the case of lung cancers. An added complication is that apoptotic indices—the relative number of apoptotic bodies in a neoplasm—also vary in different neoplasms (Staunton and Gaffney, 1995). In general, apoptotic indices are greater than or similar to mitotic indices in neoplasms, but with exceptions such as melanoma and occasional metastatic lesions, where the rate of mitosis exceeds that of apoptosis. In malignant lymphomas, high apoptotic indices correlated significantly with overall lethality (Leoncini et al., 1993). However, most neoplasms are quite heterogeneous with respect to replicating cell populations (Nervi et al., 1982). As with normal tissues, it has been demonstrated that a small fraction of cells (the stem cells) are responsible for maintaining the integrity and continued survival of the neoplasm (cf. Trott, 1994; Chapter 14). By definition, a stem cell is capable of an indefinite number of divisions. For example, during the lifetime of a human being, a typical hematopoietic stem cell may divide some 2000 to 3000 times, with an exact stability of its genomic and functional integrity. It may be said that stem cells have a proliferative capacity that is equal or superior to that of virtually all neoplastic cells (Trott, 1994). As shown in Chapter 20, if any neoplastic stem cells survive therapy, a recurrence of growth of the neoplasm will occur. With a technique of quantitative transplantation, it has been demonstrated that the number of stem cells in the neoplasm varies from every cell being a potential stem cell to one stem cell per 10^5 to 10^6. Whereas stem cells of normal tissues (such as epithelia and bone marrow) exhibit restrained, orderly proliferation and differentiation, stem cells of neoplastic tissues exhibit a relative degree of autonomy, as exhibited in the entire neoplasm and in line with our original definition of neoplasia (Chapter 2).

Most experimental tumors in laboratory animals exhibit a growth pattern that is characterized by a declining rate of cell replication. Such growth has been regarded as an exponential

Table 9.9 Anatomic Site, Histological Type, and Volume Doubling Time of 780 Primary and Metastatic Human Tumors

Histological Type	Anatomic Site	No. of Tumors	Mean Volume Doubling Time (days)	95% Confidence Limits on Mean
Metastases observed in the lung				
Adenocarcinoma	Colon and rectum	56	94.86	84.1–107.1
	Breast	44	73.74	55.7–97.7
	Kidney	14	60.16	36.9–98.1
	Uterus	15	78.23	55.2–110.9
	Thyroid	16	67.22	43.9–102.9
	Ovary	4	33.30	
Squamous cell carcinoma	Head and neck	27	56.78	42.9–75.1
	Bladder	8	70.67	
	Lung	5	67.20	
Sarcoma	Fibrosarcoma	28	65.22	45.9–92.8
	Osteosarcoma	34	30.20	24.1–37.8
	Ewing sarcoma	9	17.55	
	Other sarcomata	30	42.91	31.8–58.0
Teratoma		80	30.25	25.2–36.4
Childhood tumors		4	19.71	
Melanoma		8	53.47	
Lymphoma		11	26.82	18.6–38.6
Metastases observed in lymph nodes				
	Carcinoma	9	41.63	
	Lymphosarcoma	5	19.80	
	Reticulum cell sarcoma	12	17.68	12.4–25.2
	Hodgkin disease	10	48.59	31.0–76.2
Primary bronchial neoplasms				
Carcinoma	Adenocarcinoma	64	148.30	121.0–181.0
	Squamous cell carcinoma	85	84.49	75.0–95.0
	Mixed	7	135.00	
	Undifferentiated	55	79.10	67.0–93.0
Primary adenocarcinoma of colon and rectum		19	632.00	426.0–938.0
Primary breast carcinoma		17	95.82	68.0–134
Primary bone sarcoma		6	68.50	
Lung metastases	All adenocarcinomata	159	77.8	69.3–87.3
	All squamous cell carcinoma	62	52.4	42.7–64.3
	All sarcomata	92	43.90	36.8–52.3
Lymph node metastases	All lymphomata	27	26.25	19.3–35.8
Primary lung carcinoma	All types	211	98.87	89.8–108.8

Modified from Steel, 1977.

growth function limited by an exponential retardation. As seen in Figure 9.6, the initial exponential growth of the neoplasm is characterized by successive mean generation times that increase according to an exponential equation, but growth is soon limited by an exponentially decreasing function. Laird (1965), in a comprehensive study of a large number of spontaneous, induced, and transplantable neoplasms in several species, showed that the number of cell doublings required for a neoplasm to grow unperturbed from a single cell to a predicted upper limit was essentially constant in the majority of systems studied in a specific species. In both animal and human, the smallest neoplasm likely to be detected by physical or radiological examination is about 1 g in weight, containing from 10^8 to 10^9 neoplastic cells. This lesion will be the result of about 30 doublings in cell number if it is clonally derived from a single neoplastic cell (Tannock, 1989). Another 10 doublings of the cells in the lesion will result in a potentially lethal tumor of approximately 1 kg. Therefore the period of neoplastic growth that is reasonably measurable represents only about one-quarter of the total development of the neoplasm itself. Obviously, this scenario

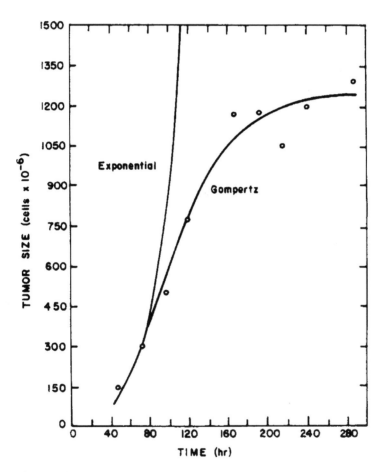

Figure 9.6   A plot of the growth of a murine neoplasm transplanted into a susceptible host. The theoretical Gompertz curve that best fits the data is shown, as is a single exponential curve, the latter constructed on the basis that the doubling time observed during the first interval measured remains constant throughout the growth of the tumor. (After Laird, 1965, with permission of the author and publisher.)

describes a neoplasm in the stage of progression, since, as we have already seen, cells in the stages of initiation and promotion represent different genetic populations incapable of the doubling pattern of the cell in the stage of progression.

The preceding description of tumor growth, however, does not take into account the potential for metastatic growth. Figure 9.7 shows a Gompertzian model of the growth of a mammary neoplasm in the human. The shaded region represents the variation in growth that could occur in the primary neoplasm (T) and in metastatic lesions (M). As discussed above, neoplastic lesions growing within the time frame and cell number are limited by the threshold of detection, and zero time would not be clinically or experimentally evident. Most important, one notes that at zero time, at which the neoplasm is first detected, one might predict that almost one-third of the metastatic lesions that will ultimately occur were initiated and present during the 12 months preceding the diagnosis (Tubiana, 1982).

This consideration of cell kinetics and cell proliferation in neoplasia has significant practical applications, as discussed later in the text (Chapter 20). In addition, from the model shown in Figure 9.7, it is obvious that a knowledge of the doubling times of neoplasms can also be related to the appropriate intervals between screening examinations that are necessary for the effective discovery of a neoplastic lesion before a cancer disseminates beyond the region of origin (Spratt, 1981).

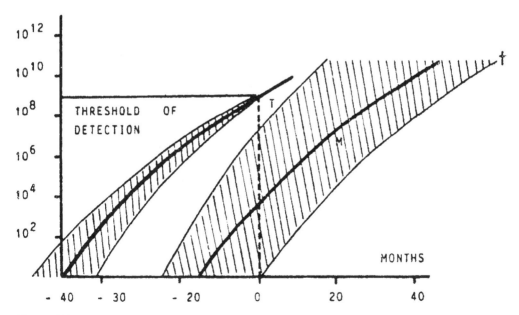

Figure 9.7 Gompertzian model of growth of human breast neoplasm. As predicted by the Gompertzian model, the doubling time of both the primary neoplasm (T) and the metastatic lesions (M) lengthens progressively with growth and time. The shaded areas represent the potential variation in the development of different lesions in different individuals, and the box labeled "threshold of detection" indicates the history of neoplastic growth prior to clinical or experimental detection. As noted, this model predicts that nearly one-third of the metastases eventually occurring were initiated during 12 months preceding the diagnosis. (Adapted from Tubiana, 1982, with permission of the author and publishers.)

CARCINOGEN CLASSIFICATION IN RELATION TO THE NATURAL HISTORY OF NEOPLASTIC DEVELOPMENT

With the division of the process of carcinogenesis into at least three distinct and sequential stages, it now becomes possible to place carcinogenic agents into various categories depending on their effecting one or more of the stages of initiation, promotion, and progression. Such a classification is given in Table 9.10. Agents that are capable of initiation and thus are true incomplete carcinogens are very rare if they exist at all. The "pure" initiating activity of certain chemicals in specific tissues has been reported (cf. DiGiovanni, 1992); but in most instances, at higher doses or in different tissues, such agents can be shown to be carcinogenic, usually acting as complete carcinogens. On the other hand, as we have seen from the experimental basis for a distinction between initiation and promotion, very low doses of complete carcinogens will act to initiate cells but cannot sustain the remainder of the carcinogenic process. This consideration is undoubtedly very important in carcinogenesis in the human, where most exposures to a carcinogenic agent are at extremely or relatively low levels. The list of promoting agents and putative promoting agents is, like complete carcinogens, growing steadily. Progressor agents in the strict sense of inducing the characteristics noted in Table 9.2 have been only tentatively identified (Table 9.2). Some agents, specifically initiating and progressor agents, possess as a primary aspect of their carcinogenic mechanism the ability to alter the structure of DNA and/or chromosomes. Such "genotoxic" effects of these agents have been linked directly to the induction of neoplasia. However, a number of chemicals when administered chronically to animals induce the development of neoplasia, but there is no evidence of their direct "genotoxic" action on target cells. Considering the effects of chemicals on the development of neoplasia via a multistage process, one may classify such agents as promoting agents acting to expand clones of spontaneously initiated cells. The consequent selective enhancement of cell replication in such initiated cell clones sets the stage for the spontaneous transition of an occasional cell into the stage of progression, as discussed above. However, this explanation of "nongenotoxic" carcinogenesis is likely to be oversimplified. Specifically, Tennant (1993) has demonstrated that, in a large series of whole-animal bioassays for carcinogenesis (Chapter 13), the frequencies of induced neoplasia by nonmutagenic carcinogens does not correlate well with the spontaneous rates of neoplastic development in a variety of tissues in control animals. A number of potentially indirect mechanisms for the action of nongenotoxic carcinogens—such as induction of oxidative stress, the permanent but nonmutagenic alteration of gene expression, or enhancement of intrachromosomal recombination (Schiestl, 1989)—may contribute to mechanisms involved in this process. Table

Table 9.10 Classification of Chemical Carcinogens in Relation to Their Action on One or More Stages of Carcinogenesis

Initiating agent (incomplete carcinogen)—a chemical capable only of initiating cells
Promoting agent—a chemical capable of causing the expansion of initiated cell clones
Progressor agent—a chemical capable of converting an initiated cell or a cell in the
    stage of promotion to a potentially malignant cell
Complete carcinogen—a chemical possessing the capability of inducing cancer from
    normal cells, usually possessing properties of initiating, promoting, and progressor
    agents

Table 9.11   Some Nonmutagenic Chemical Carcinogens

Compound	Species/Target Organ	Promoting Action
Benzene	Rat, mouse/zymbal gland	–
Butylated hydroxyanisole	Rat, hamster/forestomach	+
Chlorobenzilate	Rat/liver	+
Chloroform	Rat, mouse/liver	+
Clofibrate	Rat/liver	+
Dieldrin	Mouse/liver	+
Diethylhexyl phthalate	Rat/liver	±
p,p′-Dichlorodiphenyldichloroethylene	Rat/liver	+
1,4-Dioxane	Mouse, rat/liver, nasal turbinate	NT[a]
Furfural	Mouse/liver	+
Lindane	Mouse/liver	+
Methapyrilene	Rat/liver	+
Polychlorinated biphenyls	Rat, mouse/liver	+
Reserpine	Mouse/mammary tissue	NT
Saccharin	Rat/bladder	+
2,3,7,8-Tetrachlorodibenzo-p-dioxin	Rat/liver, lung	+
Trichloroethylene	Mouse/liver	+

[a]Not tested. +, effective; –, not effective; ±, weakly effective as a promoting agent.
Adapted from Pitot and Dragan, 1996, with permission of the publishers.

9.11 lists a representative sample of chemicals that are nonmutagenic as assessed by induction of mutations in bacteria or mammalian cells but which, on chronic administration, are carcinogenic in experimental systems. As indicated in the table, a number of these chemicals have been shown to be promoting agents, but some are not. Several of those that are not promoting agents may be classified as putative progressor agents, as evidenced by their effectiveness as clastogens in experimental systems (Table 9.2). A number of other chemicals (Tennant, 1993) have not been tested for their action at specific stages of carcinogenesis and thus cannot neatly be placed into the classification of Table 9.11.

Along with other mechanisms, agents that are not mutagenic or genotoxic may induce direct toxicity, with sustained tissue damage and subsequent cell proliferation. Both direct DNA damage and increased cell proliferation may lead to clastogenesis (Scott et al., 1991). The cell proliferation resulting from toxicity may selectively induce enhanced replication of an already damaged genome in the initiated cell population (Larson et al., 1994). Thus, while cell toxicity does not directly induce carcinogenesis, it is capable of indirectly enhancing the process (Bradley et al., 1987; Grasso et al., 1991). Since many agents that are tested at chronic doses induce at least a mild degree of toxicity, it has been argued that the format of the testing system leads to the induction of neoplasia. Thus, neoplastic development observed with the administration of test compounds may result from enhanced cell proliferation due to toxicity, associated with chronic high doses utilized, rather than from a direct carcinogenic effect of the agent (Ames and Gold, 1990b). However, several types of nonmutagenic chemical carcinogens have primarily a tumor-promoting type of effect, including agents that induce P450s, other mitogenic agents, and cytotoxic agents as well as many that act through receptor-mediated processes.

EVOLVING KARYOTYPIC INSTABILITY—BASIS FOR THE STAGE OF PROGRESSION

Just as the basis for the stage of *initiation* is *a simple mutation in one or more cellular genes controlling key regulatory pathways of the cell* and the basis for *promotion* is *the selective alteration of signal transduction pathways in the initiated cell*, the basis for the stage of *progression* is *evolving karyotypic instability*. In contrast to initiation and promotion, which do not exhibit any obvious patterns in their development, substantial evidence is now accumulating that the evolution of karyotypic changes, as the basis for the stage of progression, assumes certain patterns that appear to be tissue-specific.

Perhaps the first example of the tissue-specificity of karyotypic evolution in the stage of progression was exemplified by the Philadelphia chromosome, characteristically seen in more than 90% of cases of chronic myelogenous leukemia (Chapter 6). In the early development of this disease, essentially the only karyotypic abnormality seen in neoplastic cells is the 9:22 translocation, which constitutes the Philadelphia chromosome. However, as the disease evolves, numerous other karyotypic abnormalities become apparent, none of which are as common as the translocation resulting in the abnormal chromosome (Barton and Westbrook, 1994). Using this example in the human as a model, more recent investigations have not only demonstrated characteristic chromosomal abnormalities in tissue-specific neoplasms (Chapter 6, Table 6.8) but have also developed—from karyotypic studies in preneoplastic, neoplastic, and metastatic neoplasms—plausible schemes or patterns for the genetic and cytogenetic pathways of the stage of progression in specific tissues. Some examples of such patterns of karyotypic evolution are seen in Table 9.12. In several instances, the "early change" is assumed from the most consistent karyotypic findings in primary neoplasms and their benign counterparts. In the animal, it is possible to localize such changes to a much greater extent than in the human, as exemplified by karyotypic studies on the development of neoplasia in the mouse epidermis (Aldaz et al., 1989), hepatocyte in the rat (Sargent et al., 1997), and the plasmacytoma in the mouse (Ohno et al., 1979). It is of interest that two of these three examples are associated with a trisomic or duplicative change in specific chromosomes as the earliest alterations noted. Similar duplicative changes as early alterations can be noted in the genesis of several other animal and human neoplasms (Table 9.12). The "later changes" noted in the table are not meant to be inclusive, since—as these neoplasms develop further—subsequent chromosomal changes can be noted in many, but in others an apparently stable (Heim et al., 1988) and sometimes "normal" (Dutrillaux, 1995) karyotype may be maintained for the history of the neoplasm, especially in the human. In this latter instance, subtle alterations in other chromosomes likely exist, for in most instances, when such neoplasms are placed in cell culture, karyotypic evolution continues. The initial changes seen in the human in chronic myelogenous leukemia, Ewing sarcoma, and myxoid liposarcomas are translocations; while in the carcinomas indicated, the early lesions are more frequently represented by trisomic changes. For the process of colon carcinogenesis in the human, Fearon and Vogelstein have developed a genetic model that includes molecular changes during the early period of the stage of progression (adenomas and primary carcinomas), while changes in chromosomes 17 and 18 as well as other molecular changes occur late in the stage of progression, as noted in the table. A diagram of their model of colon carcinogenesis is shown in Figure 9.8. The terms in the boxes indicate the various morphological and biological characteristics of each succeeding step, with the indication of the stages of carcinogenesis in which each may be placed. Note that sequential karyotypic alterations in specific chromosomes are seen during the stage of progression (Fearon and Vogelstein, 1990). The loss of chromosome 22 in meningiomas is a frequent somatic mutation in this benign neoplasm (Chapter 6), but further development of

Table 9.12 Cell Type Patterns of Karyotypic Evolution in the Stage of Progression

Cell Type	Early Change	Later Change	Reference
Animal			
Epidermis (mouse)	+6, +7	+15, +6, –7	French et al., 1994
			Aldaz et al., 1989
Hepatocyte (rat)	+1q3.6-q4.2	–3q, –6p$_{ter}$	Sargent et al., 1997
Lymphoid (mouse)	+15	+17	Wiener et al., 1978
Mammary gland (rat)	+1q2.2-q4.3 or –1q2.1q3.1	–17, –18, –X, t (1′,2) (q2.2q2.2)	Aldaz et al., 1992
Plasmacytoma (mouse)	t (6;15) or t (12;15)	t (10–15)	Ohno et al., 1979
			cf. Miller and Miller, 1983
Human			
Chronic myelogenous leukemia	t (9;22) (q34;q11)	+8, +19 t(15:17)	Barton and Westbrook, 1994
Colon	+7	–1p, –18, –17	Bardi et al., 1995
			Bardi et al., 1993
			Herbergs et al., 1994
Ewing sarcoma	t (11;22) (q24;q12)	+8, t (1;16)	cf. Busam and Fletcher, 1997
Myxoid liposarcomas	t (12;16) (q13, p11)	+8, +1, –12	Turc-Carel et al., 1986
			Örndal et al., 1990
Lung carcinomas	–3p (14,2)-9p (LOH)	+7, –5q (13–21)	Whang-Peng et al., 1982
			Thiberville et al., 1995
			Miura et al., 1992
			Lee et al., 1987
Meningioma	–22	+1q, 20, –1p –18q, –9p (LOH)	Weber et al., 1997
Prostate carcinoma	+7q31, 5q	+1, +8, +12	Koivisto et al., 1996
			Jenkins et al., 1998
			Boland et al., 1995
Uterine cervix	+3q	?	Heselmeyer et al., 1996

the stage of progression results in a number of chromosomal and molecular alterations (Weber et al., 1997).

Thus, as emphasized in Chapter 6, the seemingly random karyotypic alterations occurring during the stage of progression are now more frequently being patterned as a sequence of changes that only become random during the established portion of the stage of progression. The apparent tissue specificity of many of the patterns of karyotypic evolution in the stage of progression seen in Table 9.12 is of great significance to our understanding of the development of this stage. However, the possible mechanisms for the evolution of karyotypic instability in neoplastic cells in relation to chromosomal alterations—coupled to the mutational events initiating carcinogenesis—remain as a primary dilemma in unraveling the mechanisms of carcinogenesis. The continued evolution and amplification of these genetic alterations are the result of the gradual alteration in mechanisms controlling the cell cycle. Unfortunately, our knowledge of these molecular mechanisms is still in its infancy, and it is unlikely that a rational, effective therapy for neoplasia in general will be found until we understand the molecular basis for karyotypic evolution in neoplasia. However, a number of other parallel processes and abnormalities result from evolving karyotypic instability. The next chapter focuses on several of the more important of these processes in the stage of progression.

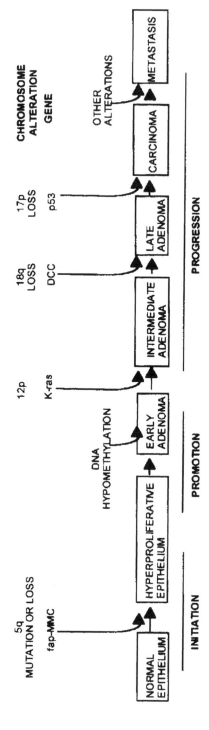

Figure 9.8 Multistep model of colon carcinogenesis in the human as proposed by Fearon and Vogelstein (1990). (Adapted with permission of the authors and publisher.)

REFERENCES

Akama, Y., Yasui, W., Yokozaki, H., Kuniyasu, H., Kitahara, K., Ishikawa, T., and Tahara, E. Frequent amplification of the cyclin E gene in human gastric carcinomas. Jpn. J. Cancer Res., 86:617–621, 1995.

Aldaz, C. M., Chen, A., Gollahon, L. S., Russo, J., and Zappler, K. Nonrandom abnormalities involving chromosome 1 and *Harvey-ras-1* alleles in rat mammary tumor progression. Cancer Res., 52:4791–4798, 1992.

Aldaz, C. M., Conti, C. J., Klein-Szanto, A. J. P., and Slaga, T. J. Progressive dysplasia and aneuploidy are hallmarks of mouse skin papillomas: relevance to malignancy. Proc. Natl. Acad. Sci. U.S.A., 84:2029–2032, 1987.

Aldaz, C. M., Trono, D., Larcher, F., Slaga, T. J., and Conti, C. J. Sequential trisomization of chromosomes 6 and 7 in mouse skin premalignant lesions. Mol. Carcinog., 2:22–26, 1989.

Ames, B. N., and Gold, L. S. Misconceptions on pollution and the causes of cancer. Angew. Chem. Int. Ed. Engl., 29:1197–1208, 1990a.

Ames, B. N., and Gold, L. S. Chemical carcinogenesis: too many rodent carcinogens. Proc. Natl. Acad. Sci. U.S.A., 87:7772–7776, 1990b.

Ames, B. N., Shigenaga, M. K., and Gold, L. S. DNA lesions, inducible DNA repair, and cell division: three key factors in mutagenesis and carcinogenesis. Environ. Health Perspect., 93:35–44, 1993.

Ando, M., Maruyama, M., Oto, M., Takemura, K., Endo, M., and Yuasa, Y. Higher frequency of point mutations in the c-K-*ras* 2 gene in human colorectal adenomas with severe atypia than in carcinomas. Jpn. J. Cancer Res., 82:245–249, 1991.

Asai, N., Iwashita, T., Matsuyama, M., and Takahashi, M. Mechanism of activation of the *ret* proto-oncogene by multiple endocrine neoplasia 2A mutations. Mol. Cell. Biol., 15:1613–1619, 1995.

Atkin, N. B., and Baker, M. C. Possible differences between the karyotypes of preinvasive lesions and malignant tumours. Br. J. Cancer, 23:329–336, 1969.

Balaban, G. B., Herlyn, M., Clark, W. H., Jr., and Nowell, P. C. Karyotypic evolution in human malignant melanoma. Cancer Genet. Cytogenet., 19:113–122, 1986.

Bardi, G., Johansson, B., Pandis, N., Bak-Jensen, E., Örndal, C., Heim, S., Mandahl, N., Andrén-Sandberg, Å., and Mitelman, F. Cytogenetic aberrations in colorectal adenocarcinomas and their correlation with clinicopathologic features. Cancer, 71:306–314, 1993.

Bardi, G., Pandis, N., Mitelman, F., and Heim, S. Karyotypic characteristics of colorectal tumors. *In*: S. R. Wolman and S. Sell (Eds.), Human Cytogenetic Cancer Markers, pp. 151–168. Totowa, NJ: Humana Press, 1995.

Bardwell, L. The mutagenic and carcinogenic effects of gene transfer. Mutagenesis, 4:245–253, 1989.

Bargmann, C. I., Hung, M.-C., and Weinberg, R. A. Multiple independent activations of the *neu* oncogene by a point mutation altering the transmembrane domain of p185. Cell, 45:649–657, 1986.

Barton, K., and Westbrook, C. A. Chronic myelogenous leukemia: a model for the genetic and biochemical basis of neoplasia. *In*: Biochemical and Molecular Aspects of Selected Cancers, pp. 1–17, Vol. 2. New York: Academic Press, 1994.

Bauer-Hofmann, R., Klimek, F., Buchmann, A., Müller, O., Bannasch, P., and Schwarz, M. Role of mutations at codon 61 of the c-Ha-*ras* gene during diethylnitrosamine-induced hepatocarcinogenesis in C3H/He mice. Mol. Carcinog., 6:60–67, 1992.

Baumeister, W., Walz, J., Zühl, F., and Seemüller, E. The proteasome: paradigm of a self-compartmentalizing protease. Cell, 92:367–380, 1998.

Bevacqua, S. J., Greeff, C. W., and Hendrix, M. J. C. Cytogenetic evidence of gene amplification as a mechanism for tumor cell invasion. Somat. Cell Mol. Genet., 14:83–91, 1988.

Blackburn, E. H. Telomeres: no end in sight. Cell, 77:621–623, 1994.

Boland, C. R., Sato, J., Appelman, H. D., Bresalier, R. S., and Feinberg, A. P. Microallelotyping defines the sequence and tempo of allelic losses at tumour suppressor gene loci during colorectal cancer progression. Nature Med., 1:902–909, 1995.

Bradley, M. O., Taylor, V. I., Armstrong, M. J., and Galloway, S. M. Relationships among cytotoxicity, lysosomal breakdown, chromosome aberrations, and DNA double-strand breaks. Mutat. Res., 189:69–79, 1987.

Breuer, M. L., Cuypers, H. T., and Berns, A. Evidence for the involvement of *pim*-2, a new common proviral insertion site, in progression of lymphomas. EMBO J., *8*:743–747, 1989.

Britton, D. C., Bone, G., Wright, N. A., and Camplejohn, R. S. Measurement of cell production rates in human gastro-intestinal cancer—a guide to treatment? Br. J. Surg., *62*:813–815, 1975.

Bronner, M. P., Culin, C., Reed, J. C., and Furth, E. E. The *bcl-2* proto-oncogene and the gastrointestinal epithelial tumor progression model. Am. J. Pathol., *146*:20–26, 1995.

Burmer, G. C., and Loeb, L. A. Mutations in the *KRAS2* oncogene during progressive stages of human colon carcinoma. Proc. Natl. Acad. Sci. U.S.A., *86*:2403–2407, 1989.

Busam, K. J., and Fletcher, C. D. M. The clinical role of molecular genetics in soft tissue tumor pathology. Cancer Metast. Rev., *16*:207–227, 1997.

Cahill, D. P., Lengauer, C., Yu, J., Riggins, G. J., Willson, J. K. V., Markowitz, S. D., Kinzler, K. W., and Vogelstein, B. Mutations of mitotic checkpoint genes in human cancers. Nature, *392*:300–303, 1998.

Cairns, J. Mutation selection and the natural history of cancer. Nature, *255*:197–200, 1975.

Campain, J. A., Slovak, M. L., Schoenlein, P. V., Popescu, N. C., Gottesman, M. M., and Pastan, I. Acquisition of multiple copies of a mutant topoisomerase IIα allele by chromosome 17 aneuploidy is associated with etoposide resistance in human melanoma cell lines. Somat. Cell Mol. Genet., *21*:451–471, 1995.

Chang, E. H., Furth, M. E., Scolnick, E. M., and Lowy, D. R. Tumorigenic transformation of mammalian cells induced by a normal human gene homologous to the oncogene of Harvey murine sarcoma virus. Nature, *297*: 479–483, 1982.

Cheng, K. C., and Loeb, L. A. Genomic instability and tumor progression: mechanistic considerations. Adv. Cancer Res., *60*:121–156, 1993.

Chorazy, M. Sequence rearrangements and genome instability. J. Cancer Res. Clin. Oncol., *109*:159–172, 1985.

Christopherson, W. M. Dysplasia, carcinoma in situ, and microinvasive carcinoma of the uterine cervix. Hum. Pathol., *8*:489–501, 1977.

Ciechanover, A., and Schwartz, A. L. The ubiquitin-proteasome pathway: the complexity and myriad functions of proteins death. Proc. Natl. Acad. Sci. U.S.A., *95*:2727–2730, 1998.

Cohen, S. M., and Ellwein, L. B. Proliferative and genotoxic cellular effects in 2-acetylaminofluorene bladder and liver carcinogenesis: biological modeling of the ED01 study. Toxicol. Appl. Pharmacol., *104*:79–93, 1990.

Cohen, S. M., and Ellwein, L. B. Genetic errors, cell proliferation, and carcinogenesis. Cancer Res., *51*:6493–6505, 1991a.

Cohen, S. M., and Ellwein, L. B. Cell proliferation and bladder tumor promotion. *In*: Chemically Induced Cell Proliferation: Implications for Risk Assessment, pp. 347–355. New York: Wiley-Liss, 1991b.

Coonrod, A., Li, F.-Q., and Horwitz, M. On the mechanism of DNA transfection: efficient gene transfer without viruses. Gene Ther., *4*:1313–1321, 1997.

Cooper, G. M. Cellular transforming genes. Science, *217*: 801–806, 1982.

Coppola, J., Bryant, S., Koda, T., Conway, D., and Barbacid, M. Mechanism of activation of the *vav* protooncogene. Cell Growth Diff., *2*:95–105, 1991.

Cortés, F., Piñero, J., and Ortiz, T. Importance of replication fork progression for the induction of chromosome damage and SCE by inhibitors of DNA topoisomerases. Mutat. Res., *303*:71–76, 1993.

Cote, G. J., Wohllk, N., Evans, D., Goepfert, H., and Gagel, R. F. RET proto-oncogene mutations in multiple endocrine neoplasia type 2 and medullary thyroid carcinoma. *In*: Baillière's Clinical Endocrinology and Metabolism, Vol. 9, No. 3, pp. 609–630. London: Baillière Tindall, 1995.

Coulier, F., Kumar, R., Ernst, M., Klein, R., Martin-Zanca, D., and Barbacid, M. Human *trk* oncogenes activated by point mutation, in-frame deletion, and duplication of the tyrosine kinase domain. Mol. Cell. Biol., *10*:4202–4210, 1990.

Cram, L. S., Bartholdi, M. F., Ray, F. A., Travis, G. L., and Kraemer, P. M. Spontaneous neoplastic evolution of Chinese hamster cells in culture: multistep progression of karyotype. Cancer Res,. *43*:4828–4837, 1983.

Croy, R. G. Role of chemically induced cell proliferation in carcinogenesis and its use in health risk assessment. Environ. Health Perspect., *101*:289–302, 1993.

Cunningham, M. L. Role of increased DNA replication in the carcinogenic risk of nonmutagenic chemical carcinogens. Mutat. Res., *365*:59–69, 1996.

Davidson, D., Fournel, M., and Veillette, A. Oncogenic activation of p59^{fyn} tyrosine protein kinase by mutation of its carboxy-terminal site of tyrosine phosphorylation, tyrosine 528. J. Biol. Chem., *269*:10956–10963, 1994.

Denko, N. C., Giaccia, A. J., Stringer, J. R., and Stambrook, P. J. The human Ha-*ras* oncogene induces genomic instability in murine fibroblasts within one cell cycle. Proc. Natl. Acad. Sci. U.S.A., *91*:5124–5128, 1994.

Deschner, E. E. Early proliferative changes in gastrointestinal neoplasia. Am. J. Gastroenterol., *77*:207–211, 1982.

de Vries, J. E., Kornips, F. H. A. C., Marx, P., Bosman, F. T., Geraedts, J. P. M., and ten Kate, J. Transfected *c-Ha-ras* oncogene enhances karyotypic instability and integrates predominantly in aberrant chromosomes. Cancer Genet. Cytogenet., *65*:35–43, 1993.

DiGiovanni, J. Multistage carcinogenesis in mouse skin. Pharmacol. Ther., *54*:63–128, 1992.

Donghi, R., Longoni, A., Pilotti, S., Michieli, P., Della Porta, G., and Pierotti, M. A. Gene p53 mutations are restricted to poorly differentiated and undifferentiated carcinomas of the thyroid gland. J. Clin. Invest., *91*:1753–1760, 1993.

Duesberg, P., Rausch, C., Rasnick, D., and Hehlmann, R. Genetic instability of cancer cells is proportional to their degree of aneuploidy. Proc. Natl. Acad. Sci. U.S.A., *95*:13692–13697, 1998.

Duesberg, P., Stindl, R., and Hehlmann, R. Origin of multidrug resistance in cells with and without multidrug resistance genes: chromosome reassortments catalyzed by aneuploidy. Proc. Natl. Acad. Sci. U.S.A., *98*:11283–11288, 2001.

Dutrillaux, B. Pathways of chromosome alteration in human epithelial cancers. Adv. Cancer Res., *67*:59–82, 1995.

Elledge, S. J. Cell cycle checkpoints: preventing an identity crisis. Science, *274*:1664–1672, 1996.

Emerit, I., Khan, S. H., and Esterbauer, H. Hydroxynonenal, a component of clastogenic factors? Free Radic. Biol. Med., *10*:371–377, 1991.

Eriksson, L., Ahluwalia, M., Spiewak, J., Lee, G., Sarma, D. S. R., Roomi, M. J., and Farber, E. Distinctive biochemical pattern associated with resistance of hepatocytes in hepatocyte nodules during liver carcinogenesis. Environ. Health Perspect., *49*:171–174, 1983.

Fanning, E., and Knippers, R. Structure and function of simian virus 40 large tumor antigen. Annu. Rev. Biochem., *61*:55–85, 1992.

Farber, E. Cell proliferation is not a major risk factor for cancer. Mod. Pathol., *9*:606, 1996.

Fearon, E. R., and Vogelstein, B. A genetic model for colorectal tumorigenesis. Cell, *61*:759–761, 1992.

Fearon, E. R., and Vogelstein, B. A genetic model for colorectal tumorigenesis. Cell, *61*:759–767, 1990.

Fisher, E. R., Shoemaker, R. H., and Sabnis, A. Relationship of hyperplasia to cancer in 3-methylcholanthrene-induced mammary tumorigenesis. Lab. Invest., *33*:33–42, 1975.

Foulds, L. The experimental study of tumor progression: a review. Cancer Res., *14*:327–339, 1954.

Foulds, L. Tumor progression and neoplastic development. *In*: O. Mühlbock and P. Emmelot (Eds.), Cellular Control Mechanisms and Cancer, pp. 242–255. Amsterdam: Elsevier, 1964.

French, J. E., Libbus, B. L., Hansen, L., Spalding, J., Tice, R. R., Mahler, J., and Tennant, R. W. Cytogenetic analysis of malignant skin tumors induced in chemically treated TG·AC transgenic mice. Mol. Carcinog., *11*:215–226, 1994.

Frost, P., Kerbel, R. S., Hunt, B., Man, S., and Pathak, S. Selection of metastatic variants with identifiable karyotypic changes from a nonmetastatic murine tumor after treatment with 2′-deoxy-5-azacytidine or hydroxyurea: implications for the mechanisms of tumor progression. Cancer Res., *47*:2690–2695, 1987.

Garte, S. J. The c-*myc* oncogene in tumor progression. Crit. Rev. Oncogen., *4*:435–449, 1993.

Gartel, A. L., Serfas, M. S., and Tyner, A. L. p21—negative regulator of the cell cycle. Proc. Soc. Exp. Biol. Med., *213*:138–149, 1996.

Gelb, A. B., Kamel, O. W., LeBrun, D. P., and Warnke, R. A. Estimation of tumor growth fractions in archival formalin-fixed, paraffin-embedded tissues using two anti-PCNA/cyclin monoclonal antibodies. Am. J. Pathol., *141*:1453–1458, 1992.

Giaretti, W. Aneuploidy mechanisms in human colorectal preneoplastic lesions and Barrett's esophagus. Is there a role for K-ras and p53 mutations? Anal. Cell. Pathol., *15*:99–117, 1997.

Gilbert, P. X., and Harris, H. The role of the *ras* oncogene in the formation of tumours. J. Cell Sci., *90*:433–446, 1988.

Glinsky, G. V., Glinsky, V. V., Ivanova, A. B., and Hueser, C. J. Apoptosis and metastasis: increased apoptosis resistance of metastatic cancer cells is associated with the profound deficiency of apoptosis execution mechanisms. Cancer Lett., *115*:185–193, 1997.

Graf, L. H. Jr. Gene transformation. Am. Sci., *70*:496–505, 1982.

Grasso, P., Sharratt, M., and Cohen, A. J. Role of persistent, non-genotoxic tissue damage in rodent cancer and relevance to humans. Annu. Rev. Pharmacol. Toxicol., *31*:253–287, 1991.

Gray, D. A. Insertional mutagenesis: neoplasia arising from retroviral integration. Cancer Invest., *9*:295–304, 1991.

Greengard, O., Head, J. F., Goldberg, S. L., and Kirschner, P. A. Biochemical measure of the volume doubling time of human pulmonary neoplasms. Cancer, *55*:1530–1535, 1985.

Guerrero, I., and Pellicer, A. Mutational activation of oncogenes in animal model systems of carcinogenesis. Mutat. Res., *185*:293–308, 1987.

Haapasalo, H., Atkin, N. B., Collan, Y., Pesonen, E., and Paljärvi, L. Tumour ploidy, morphometry, histological grading and clinical features in ovarian carcinoma: mutual relations. Anal. Cell. Pathol., *3*:261–271, 1991.

Hall, M., and Peters, G. Genetic alterations of cyclins, cyclin-dependent kinases, and Cdk inhibitors in human cancer. Adv. Cancer Res., *68*:67–108, 1996.

Hanafusa, H. Avian RNA tumor viruses. *In*: F. F. Becker (Ed.), Cancer—A Comprehensive Treatise, Vol. 2, Chap. 2, pp. 49–90. New York: Plenum Press, 1975.

Harris, C. C. Chemical and physical carcinogenesis: advances and perspectives for the 1990s. Cancer Res., *51*:5023s–5044s, 1991.

Harris, C. C. *p53* Tumor suppressor gene: from the basic research laboratory to the clinic—an abridged historical perspective. Carcinogenesis, *17*:1187–1198, 1996.

Hashida, T., and Yasumoto, S. Induction of chromosome abnormalities in mouse and human epidermal keratinocytes by the human papillomavirus type 16 E7 oncogene. J. Gen. Virol., *72*:1569–1577, 1991.

Hayashi, K., Fujiki, H., and Sugimura, T. Effects of tumor promoters on the frequency of metallothionein I gene amplification in cells exposed to cadmium. Cancer Res., *43*:5433–5436, 1983.

Hayward, W. S., Neel, B. G., and Astrin, S. M. Activation of a cellular *onc* gene by promoter insertion in ALV-induced lymphoid leukosis. Nature, *290*:475–480, 1981.

Heim, S. Clonal chromosome abnormalities in neoplastic cells: evidence of genetic instability? Cancer Surv., *28*:247–260, 1996.

Heim, S., Mandahl, N., and Mitelman, F. Genetic convergence and divergence in tumor progression. Cancer Res., *48*:5911–5916, 1988.

Hemmer, J., and Schön, E. Cytogenetic progression and prognosis in oral carcinoma: a DNA flow cytometric study on 317 cases. Int. J. Oncol., *3*:635–640, 1993.

Henson, D. E., and Albores-Saavedra, J. The Pathology of Incipient Neoplasia. Philadelphia: Saunders, 1986.

Herbergs, J., de Bruïne, A. P., Marx, P. T. J., Vallinga, M. I. J., Stockbrügger, R. W., Ramaekers, F. C. S., Arends, J. W., and Hopman, A. H. N. Chromosome aberrations in adenomas of the colon. Proof of trisomy 7 in tumor cells by combined interphase cytogenetics and immunocytochemistry. Int. J. Cancer, *57*:781–785, 1994.

Herwig, S., and Strauss, M. The retinoblastoma protein: a master regulator of cell cycle, differentiation and apoptosis. Eur. J. Biochem., *246*:581–601, 1997.

Heselmeyer, K., Schröck, E., du Manoir, S., Blegen, H., Shah, K., Steinbeck, R., Auer, G., and Ried, T. Gain of chromosome 3q defines the transition from severe dysplasia to invasive carcinoma of the uterine cervix. Proc. Natl. Acad. Sci. U.S.A., *93*:479–484, 1996.

Hirota, S., Isozaki, K., Moriyama, Y., Hashimoto, K., Nishida, T., Ishiguro, S., Kawano, K., Hanada, M., Kurata, A., Takeda, M., Tunio, G. M., Matsuzawa, Y., Kanakura, Y., Shinomura, Y., and Kitamura,

Y. Gain-of-function mutations of c-*kit* in human gastrointestinal stromal tumors. Science, *279*:577–580, 1998.

Hoel, D. G., Haseman, J. K., Hogan, M. D., Huff, J., and McConnell, E. E. The impact of toxicity on carcinogenicity studies: implications for risk assessment. Carcinogenesis, *9*:2045–2052, 1988.

Huff, J. Absence of morphologic correlation between chemical toxicity and chemical carcinogenesis. Environ. Health Perspect., *101*:45–54, 1993.

Imoto, M., Doki, Y., Jiang, W., Han, E. K.-H., and Weinstein, I. B. Effects of cyclin D1 overexpression on G1 progression-related events. Exp. Cell Res., *236*:173–180, 1997.

Jacks, T. Tumor suppressor gene mutations in mice. Annu. Rev. Genet., *30*:603–636, 1996.

Jacoby, R. F., Marshall, D. J., Kailas, S., Schlack, S., Harms, B., and Love, R. Genetic instability associated with adenoma to carcinoma progression in hereditary nonpolyposis colon cancer. Gastroenterology, *109*:73–82, 1995.

Jeffers, M., Schmidt, L., Nakaigawa, N., Webb, C. P., Weirich, G., Kishida, T., Zbar, B., and vande Woude, G. F. Activating mutations for the Met tyrosine kinase receptor in human cancer. Proc. Natl. Acad. Sci. U.S.A., *94*:11445–11450, 1997.

Jenkins, R. B., Qian, J., Lee, H. K., Huang, H., Hirasawa, K., Bostwick, D. G., Proffitt, J., Wilber, K., Lieber, M. M., Liu, W., and Smith, D. I. A molecular cytogenetic analysis of 7q31 in prostate cancer. Cancer Res., *58*:759–766, 1998.

Jung, J.-M., Bruner, J. M., Ruan, S., Langford, L. A., Kyritis, A. P., Kobayashi, T., Levin, V. A., and Zhang, W. Increased levels of p21[WAF1/Cip1] in human brain tumors. Oncogene, *11*:2021–2028, 1995.

Kamel, O. W., LeBrun, D. P., Davis, R. E., Berry, G. J., and Warnke, R. A. Growth fraction estimation of malignant lymphomas in formalin-fixed paraffin-embedded tissue using anti-PCNA/cyclin 19A2. Am. J. Pathol., *138*:1471–1477, 1991.

Kaufmann, W. K., and Paules, R. S. DNA damage and cell cycle checkpoints. FASEB J., *10*:238–247, 1996.

Kelman, Z. PCNA: structure, functions and interactions. Oncogene, *14*:629–640, 1997.

Kerler, R., and Rabes, H. M. Karyotype evolution of the clonal rat liver cell line CL 52 during progression in vitro and in vivo. Cancer Genet. Cytogenet., *87*:140–147, 1996.

Keyomarsi, K., Conte, D. Jr., Toyofuku, W., and Fox, M. P. Deregulation of cyclin E in breast cancer. Oncogene, *11*:941–950, 1995.

Kiaris, H., and Spandidos, D. A. Mutations of *ras* genes in human tumours. Int. J. Oncol., *7*:413–421, 1995.

King, R. W., Jackson, P. K., and Kirschner, M. W. Mitosis in transition. Cell, *79*:563–571, 1994.

Kleckner, N. Meiosis: how could it work? Proc. Natl. Acad. Sci. U.S.A., *93*:8167–8174, 1996.

Klotzbücher, A., Stewart, E., Harrison, D., and Hunt, T. The 'destruction box' of cyclin A allows B-type cyclins to be ubiquitinated, but not efficiently destroyed. EMBO J., *15*:3053–3064, 1996.

Kociba, R. J., Keyes, D. G., Jersey, G. C., Ballard, J. J., Dittenber, D. A., Quast, J. F., Wade, C. E., Humiston, C. G., and Schwetz, B. A. Results of a two year chronic toxicity study with hexachlorobutadiene in rats. Am. Ind. Hyg. Assoc. J., *38*:589–602, 1977.

Koivisto, P. A. Molecular cytogenetics of prostate cancer. Crit. Rev. Oncog., *7*:143–150, 1996.

Korabiowska, M., Brinckmann, U., Kellner, S., Brinck, U., Stachura, J., and Schauer, A. Differences of ploidy status in progression of head and neck melanomas. Int. J. Oncol., *10*:381–385, 1997.

Kraemer, P. M., Deaven, L. L., Crissman, H. A., and Van Dilla, M. A. DNA constancy despite variability in chromosome number. *In*: E. J. DuPraw (Ed.), Advances in Cell and Molecular Biology, pp. 47–108. New York: Academic Press, 1972.

Kraemer, P. M., Deaven, L. L., Crissman, H. A., Steinkamp, J. A., and Petersen, D. F. On the nature of heteroploidy. CSH Symp. Quant. Biol., *38*:133–144, 1974.

Laird, A. K. Dynamics of tumour growth: comparison of growth rates and extrapolation of growth curves to one cell. Br. J. Cancer, *19*:278–291, 1965.

Land, H., Parada, L. F., and Weinberg, R. A. Tumorigenic conversion of primary embryo fibroblasts requires at least two cooperating oncogenes. Nature, *304*:596–602, 1983.

Larson, J. L., Wolf, D. C., and Butterworth, B. E. Induced cytotoxicity and cell proliferation in the hepatocarcinogenicity of chloroform in female B6C3F$_1$ mice: comparison of administration by gavage in corn oil vs *ad libitum* in drinking water. Fundam. Appl. Toxicol., *22*:90–102, 1994.

Lavi, S. Carcinogen-mediated amplification of viral DNA sequences in simian virus 40-transformed Chinese hamster embryo cells. Proc. Natl. Acad. Sci. U.S.A., 78:6144–6148, 1981.

Lazo, P. A., and Tsichlis, P. N. Recombination between two integrated proviruses, one of which was inserted near c-*myc* in a retrovirus-induced rat thymoma: implications for tumor progression. J. Virol., 62:788–794, 1988.

Lazutka, J. R., Neel, J. V., Major, E. O., Dedonyte, V., Mierauskine, J., Slapsyte, G., and Kesminiene, A. High titers of antibodies to two human polyomaviruses, JCV and BKV, correlate with increased frequency of chromosome damage in human lymphocytes. Cancer Lett., 109:177–183, 1996.

Ledbetter, D. H. Minireview: Cryptic translocations and telomere integrity. Am. J. Hum. Genet., 51:451–456, 1992.

Lee, J. S., Pathak, S., Hopwood, V., Tomasovic, B., Mullins, T. D., Baker, F. L., Spitzer, G., and Neidhart, J. A. Involvement of chromosome 7 in primary lung tumor and nonmalignant normal lung tissue. Cancer Res., 47:6349–6352, 1987.

Leoncini, L., Del Vecchio, M. T., Megha, T., Barbini, P., Galieni, P., Pileri, S., Sabattini, E., Gherlinzoni, F., Tosi, P., Kraft, R., and Cottier, H. Correlations between apoptotic and proliferative indices in malignant non-Hodgkin's lymphomas. Am. J. Pathol., 142:755–763, 1993.

Levine, A. J., Momand, J., and Finlay, C. A. The p53 tumour suppressor gene. Nature, 351:453–455, 1991.

Lewis, A. D., Hickson, I. D., Robson, C. N., Harris, A. L., Hayes, J. D., Griffiths, S. A., Manson, M. M., Hall, A. E., Moss, J. E., and Wolf, C. R. Amplification and increased expression of alpha class glutathione *S*-transferase-encoding genes associated with resistance to nitrogen mustards. Proc. Natl. Acad. Sci. U.S.A., 85:8511–8515, 1988.

Li, R., Yerganian, G., Duesberg, P., Kraemer, A., Willer, A., Rausch, C., and Hehlmann, R. Aneuploidy correlated 100% with chemical transformation of Chinese hamster cells. Proc. Natl. Acad. Sci. U.S.A., 94:14506–14511, 1997.

Lothe, R. A. Microsatellite instability in human solid tumors. Mol. Med. Today, 3(2):61–68, February 1997.

Luebeck, E. G., and Moolgavkar, S. H. Biologically based cancer modeling. Drug Chem. Toxicol., 19:221–243, 1996.

Mäkelä, T. P., and Alitalo, K. Proto-oncogene amplification: role in tumour progression. Ann. Clin. Res., 18:290–296, 1986.

Makos, M., Nelkin, B. D., Reiter, R. E., Gnarra, J. R., Brooks, J., Isaacs, W., Linehan, M., and Baylin, S. B. Regional DNA hypermethylation at D17S5 precedes 17p structural changes in the progression of renal tumors. Cancer Res., 53:2719–2722, 1993.

Malins, D. C., Polissar, N. L., and Gunselman, S. J. Progression of human breast cancers to the metastatic state is linked to hydroxyl radical-induced DNA damage. Proc. Natl. Acad. Sci. U.S.A., 93:2557–2563, 1996.

Malins, D. C., Polissar, N. L., and Gunselman, S. J. Tumor progression to the metastatic state involves structural modifications in DNA markedly different from those associated with primary tumor formation. Proc. Natl. Acad. Sci. U.S.A., 93:14047–14052, 1996.

May, W. A., Gishizky, M. L., Lessnick, S. L., Lunsford, L. B., Lewis, B. C., Delattre, O., Zucman, J., Thomas, G., and Denny, C. T. Ewing sarcoma 11;22 translocation produces a chimeric transcription factor that requires the DNA-binding domain encoded by *FLI1* for transformation. Proc. Natl. Acad. Sci. U.S.A., 90:5752–5756, 1993.

Melnick, R. L. Does chemically induced hepatocyte proliferation predict liver carcinogenesis? FASEB J., 6:2698–2706, 1992.

Miki, T., Smith, C. L., Long, J. E., Eva, A., and Fleming, T. P. Oncogene *ect2* is related to regulators of small GTP-binding proteins. Nature, 362:462–465, 1993.

Miller, D. A., and Miller, O. J. Chromosomes and cancer in the mouse: studies in tumors, established cell lines, and cell hybrids. Adv. Cancer Res., 39:153–182, 1983.

Miura, I., Graziano, S. L., Cheng, J. Q., Doyle, A., and Testa, J. R. Chromosome alterations in human small cell lung cancer: frequent involvement of 5q. Cancer Res., 52:1322–1328, 1992.

Morse, H. G., Moore, G. E., Ortiz, L. M., Gonzalez, R., and Robinson, W. A. Malignant melanoma: from subcutaneous nodule to brain metastasis. Cancer Genet. Cytogenet., 72:16–23, 1994.

Mowat, M. R. A. p53 in tumor progression: life, death, and everything. Adv. Cancer Res., *74*:25–48, 1998.

Murnane, J. P. The role of recombinational hotspots in genome instability in mammalian cells. Bioessays, *12*:577–581, 1990.

Murray, A. Cyclin ubiquitination: the destructive end of mitosis. Cell, *81*:149–152, 1995.

Navone, N. M., Troncoso, P., Pisters, L. L., Goodrow, T. L., Palmer, J. L., Nichols, W. W., von Eschenbach, A. C., and Conti, C. J. p53 Protein accumulation and gene mutation in the progression of human prostate carcinoma. J. Natl. Cancer Inst., *85*:1657–1669, 1993.

Nervi, C., Badaracco, G., Maisto, A., Mauro, F., Tirindelli-Danesi, D., and Starace, G. Cytometric evidence of cytogenetic and proliferative heterogeneity of human solid tumors. Cytometry, *2*:303–308, 1982.

Newburger, A. E., and Weinstein, G. Cell proliferation patterns in human malignant melanoma in vivo. Cancer, *46*:308–313, 1980.

Nicolson, G. L. Tumor cell instability, diversification, and progression to the metastatic phenotype: from oncogene to oncofetal expression. Cancer Res., *47*:1473–1487, 1987.

Noble, M. E. M., Endicott, J. A., Brown, N. R., and Johnson, L. N. The cyclin box fold: protein recognition in cell-cycle and transcription control. Trends Biochem. Sci., *22*:482–487, 1997.

Noble, R. L. Hormonal control of growth and progression in tumors of Nb rats and a theory of action. Cancer Res., *37*:82–94, 1977.

Noori-Daloii, M. R., Swift, R. A., Kung, H.-J., Crittenden, L. B., and Witter, R. L. Specific integration of REV proviruses in avian bursal lymphomas. Nature, *294*:574–576, 1981.

Norming, U., Tribukait, B., Gustafson, H., Nyman, C. R., Wang, N., and Wijkström, H. Deoxyribonucleic acid profile and tumor progression in primary carcinoma in situ of the bladder: a study of 63 patients with grade 3 lesions. J. Urol., *147*:11–15, 1992.

Nowell, P. C. Genetic instability in cancer cells: relationship to tumor cell heterogeneity. *In*: A. H. Owens, D. S. Coffey, and S. B. Baylin (Eds.), Tumor Cell Heterogeneity, pp. 351–365. New York: Academic Press, 1982.

Nowell, P. C. Mechanisms of tumor progression. Cancer Res., *46*:2203–2207, 1986.

Nowell, P. C. Cytogenetics of tumor progression. Cancer, *65*:2172–2177, 1990.

Ochi, T., and Kaneko, M. Active oxygen contributes to the major part of chromosomal aberrations in V79 Chinese hamster cells exposed to N-hydroxy-2-naphthylamine. Free Radic. Res. Commun., *5*:351–358, 1989.

Oehlert, W. Cellular proliferation in carcinogenesis. Cell Tissue Kinet., *6*:325–335, 1973.

Ohno, S., Babonits, M., Wiener, F., Spira, J., Klein, G., and Potter, M. Nonrandom chromosome changes involving the Ig gene-carrying chromosomes 12 and 6 in pristane-induced mouse plasmacytomas. Cell, *18*:1001–1007, 1979.

Okayama, H., Nagata, A., Jinno, S., Murakami, H., Tanaka, K., and Nakashima, N. Cell cycle control in fission yeast and mammals: identification of new regulatory mechanisms. Adv. Cancer Res., *69*:17–62, 1996.

Orlowski, C. C., and Furlanetto, R. W. The mammalian cell cycle in normal and abnormal growth. Endocrinol. Metab. Clin. North Am., *25*:491–502, 1996.

Örndal, C., Mandahl, N., Rydholm, A., Nibert, M., Heim, S., Åkerman, M., and Mitelman, F. Chromosomal evolution and tumor progression in a myxoid liposarcoma. Acta Orthop. Scand., *61*:99–105, 1990.

Page, A. M., and Hieter, P. The anaphase promoting complex. Cancer Surv., *29*:133–150, 1997.

Parada, L. F., Tabin, C. J., Shih, C., and Weinberg, R. A. Human EJ bladder carcinoma oncogene is homologue of Harvey sarcoma virus *ras* gene. Nature, *297*:474–478, 1982.

Pardee, A. G1 events and regulation of cell proliferation. Science, *246*:603–608, 1989.

Pardue, M. L. Dynamic instability of chromosomes and genomes. Cell, *66*:427–431, 1991.

Paterlini, P., Suberville, A. M., Zindy, F., Melle, J., Sonnier, M., Marie, J. P., Dreyfus, F., and Bréchot, C. Cyclin A expression in human hematological malignancies: a new marker of cell proliferation. Cancer Res., *53*:235–238, 1993.

Paulovich, A. G., Toczyski, D. P., and Hartwell, L. H. When checkpoints fail. Cell, *88*:315–321, 1997.

Pellegata, N. S., Sessa, F., Renault, B., Bonato, M., Leone, B. E., Solcia, E., and Ranzani, G. N. K-*ras* and *p53* gene mutations in pancreatic cancer: ductal and nonductal tumor progress through different genetic lesions. Cancer Res., *54*:1556–1560, 1994.

Peraino, C., Staffeldt, E. F., Carnes, B. A., Ludeman, V. A., Blomquist, J. A., and Vesselinovitch, S. D. Characterization of histochemically detectable altered hepatocyte foci and their relationship to hepatic tumorigenesis in rats treated once with diethylnitrosamine or benzo[*a*]pyrene within one day after birth. Cancer Res., *44*:3340–3347, 1984.

Pitot, H. C. Progression: the terminal stage in carcinogenesis. Jpn. J. Cancer Res., *80*:599–607, 1989.

Pitot, H. C., and Dragan, Y. P. Chemical carcinogenesis. *In*: C. D. Klaassen (Ed.), Casarett and Doull's Toxicology—The Basic Science of Poisons, pp. 201–267. New York: McGraw-Hill, 1996.

Pitot, H. C., and Dragan, Y. P. Chemical induction of hepatic neoplasia. *In*: I. M. Arias, J. L. Boyer, N. Fausto, W. B. Jakoby, D. A. Schachter, and D. A. Shafritz (Eds.), The Liver: Biology and Pathobiology, 3rd ed., pp. 1467–1495. New York: Raven Press, 1994.

Pitot, H. C., Barsness, L., Goldsworthy, T., and Kitagawa, T. Biochemical characterization of stages of hepatocarcinogenesis after a single dose of diethylnitrosamine. Nature, *271*:456–458, 1978.

Prescott-Matthews, J. S., Wolf, D. C., Wong, B. A., and Borghoff, S. J. Methyl *tert*-butyl ether causes α2u-globulin nephropathy and enhanced renal cell proliferation in male Fischer-344 rats. Toxicol. Appl. Pharmacol., *143*:301–314, 1997.

Ranaldi, R., Gioacchini, A. M., Manzin, A., Clementi, M., Paolucci, S., and Bearzi, I. Adenoma-carcinoma sequence of colorectum. Prevalence of K-*ras* gene mutation in adenomas with increasing degree of dysplasia and aneuploidy. Diagn. Mol. Pathol., *4*:198–202, 1995.

Rapp, F., and Westmoreland, D. Cell transformation by DNA-containing viruses. Biochim. Biophys. Acta, *458*:167–211, 1976.

Rasnick, D., and Duesberg, P. H. How aneuploidy affects metabolic control and causes cancer. Biochem. J., *340*:621–630, 1999.

Reed, J. A., Loganzo, F. Jr., Shea, C. R., Walker, G. J., Flores, J. F., Glendening, J. M., Bogdany, J. K., Shiel, M. J., Haluska, F. G., Fountain, J. W., and Albino, A. P. Loss of expression of the *p16*/cyclin-dependent kinase inhibitor 2 tumor suppressor gene in melanocytic lesions correlates with invasive stage of tumor progression. Cancer Res., *55*:2713–2718, 1995.

Riley, D. J., Lee, E.Y.-H.P., and Lee, W.-H. The retinoblastoma protein: more than a tumor suppressor. Annu. Rev. Cell Biol., *10*:1–29, 1994.

Ritchie, A. C. The classification, morphology, and behaviour of tumours. *In*: H. W. Florey (Ed.), General Pathology, pp. 668–719. Philadelphia: Saunders, 1970.

Roncucci, L., Pedroni, M., Fante, R., Di Gregorio, C., and Ponz de Leon, M. Cell kinetic evaluation of human colonic aberrant crypts. Cancer Res., *53*:3726–3729, 1993.

Roussel, M. F., Downing, J. R., Rettenmier, C. W., and Sherr, C. J. A point mutation in the extracellular domain of the human CSF-1 receptor (c-*fms* proto-oncogene product) activates its transforming potential. Cell, *55*:979–988, 1988.

Sager, R., Gadi, I. K., Stephens, L., and Grabowy, C. T. Gene amplification: an example of accelerated evolution in tumorigenic cells. Proc. Natl. Acad. Sci. U.S.A., *82*:7015–7019, 1985.

Sakizli, M., Lüleci, G., and Günalp, A. Effect of cytomegalovirus on adult human chromosomes. Acta Virol., *25*:248–250, 1981.

Sargent, L. M., Dragan, Y. P., Sattler, G., Xu, Y.-H., Wiley, J., and Pitot, H. C. Specific chromosomal changes in albumin simian virus 40 T antigen transgenic rat liver neoplasms. Cancer Res., *57*:3451–3456, 1997.

Sargent, L., Dragan, Y., Xu, Y.-H., Sattler, G., Wiley, J., and Pitot, H. C. Karyotypic changes in a multistage model of chemical hepatocarcinogenesis in the rat. Cancer Res., *56*:2985–2991, 1996.

Sargent, L., Xu, Y.-h., Sattler, G. L., Meisner, L., and Pitot, H. C. Ploidy and karyotype of hepatocytes isolated from enzyme-altered foci in two different protocols of multistage hepatocarcinogenesis in the rat. Carcinogenesis, *10*:387–391, 1989.

Sato, T., Akiyama, F., Sakamoto, G., Kasumi, F., and Nakamura, Y. Accumulation of genetic alterations and progression of primary breast cancer. Cancer Res., *51*:5794–5799, 1991.

Schiestl, R. H. Nonmutagenic carcinogens induce intrachromosomal recombination in yeast. Nature, *337*:285–288, 1989.

Schiffer, L. M., Braunschweiger, P. G., Stragand, J. J., and Poulakos, L. The cell kinetics of human mammary cancers. Cancer, *43*:1707–1719, 1979.

Schnipper, L. E., Chan, V., Sedivy, J., Jat, P., and Sharp, P. A. Gene activation by induced DNA rearrangements. Cancer Res., *49*:6640–6644, 1989.

Schubert, E. L., Hansen, M. F., and Strong, L. C. The retinoblastoma gene and its significance. Ann. Med., *26*:177–184, 1994.

Scott, D., Galloway, S. M., Marshall, R. R., Ishidate, M. Jr., Brusick, D., Ashby, J., and Myhr, B. C. Genotoxicity under extreme culture conditions. Mutat. Res., *257*:147–204, 1991.

Sengstag, C. The role of mitotic recombination in carcinogenesis. Crit. Rev. Toxicol., *24*:323–353, 1994.

Shackney, S. E., and Shankey, T. V. Common patterns of genetic evolution in human solid tumors. Cytometry, *29*:1–27, 1997.

Sharma, R. C., and Schimke, R. T. The propensity for gene amplification: a comparison of protocols, cell lines, and selection agents. Mutat. Res., *304*:243–260, 1994.

Shay, J. W., and Wright, W. E. The reactivation of telomerase activity in cancer progression. Trends Genet., *12*:129–131, 1996.

Sherr, C. J. G1 phase progression: cycling on cue. Cell, *79*:551–555, 1994.

Shibata, D., Navidi, W., Salovaara, R., Li, Z.-H., and Aaltonen, L. A. Somatic microsatellite mutations as molecular tumor clocks. Nature Med., *2*:676–681, 1996.

Simon, D., London, T., Hann, H.-W. L., and Knowles, B. B. Chromosome abnormalities in peripheral blood cells of hepatitis B virus chronic carriers. Cancer Res., *51*:6176–6179, 1991.

Simpson, A. J. G. The natural somatic mutation frequency and human carcinogenesis. Adv. Cancer Res., *71*:209–240, 1997.

Smith, S. S. Stalling of DNA methyltransferase in chromosome stability and chromosome remodelling (review). Int. J. Mol. Med., *1*:147–156, 1998.

Sood, A. K., Skilling, J. S., and Buller, R. E. Ovarian cancer genomic instability correlates with p53 frameshift mutations. Cancer Res., *57*:1047–1049, 1997.

Speicher, M. R. Microsatellite instability in human cancer. Oncol. Res., *7*:267–275, 1995.

Spratt, J. S. The relationship between the rates of growth of cancers and the intervals between screening examinations necessary for effective discovery. Cancer Detect. Prev., *4*:301–305, 1981.

Staunton, M. J., and Gaffney, E. F. Tumor type is a determinant of susceptibility to apoptosis. Am. J. Clin. Pathol., *103*:300–307, 1995.

Steel, G. G. Cell population kinetics in relation to the growth and treatment of cancer. *In*: G. G. Steel (Ed.), Growth Kinetics of Tumours. New York: Oxford University Press, 1977.

Stott, W. T., Quast, J. F., and Watanabe, P. G. Differentiation of the mechanisms of oncogenicity of 1,4-dioxane and 1,3-hexachlorobutadiene in the rat. Toxicol. Appl. Pharmacol., *60*:287–300, 1981.

Stowers, S. J., Maronpot, R. R., Reynolds, S. H., and Anderson, M. W. The role of oncogenes in chemical carcinogenesis. Environ. Health Perspect., *75*:81–86, 1987.

Tabin, C. J., Bradley, S. M., Bargmann, C. I., Weinberg, R. A., Papageorge, A. G., Scolnick, E. M., Dhar, R., Lowy, D. R., and Chang, E. H. Mechanism of activation of a human oncogene. Nature, *300*:143–149, 1982.

Taghian, D. G., and Nickoloff, J. A. Chromosomal double-strand breaks induce gene conversion at high frequency in mammalian cells. Mol. Cell Biol., *17*:6386–6393, 1997.

Tamura, G., Kihana, T., Nomura, K., Terada, M., Sugimura, T., and Hirohashi, S. Detection of frequent *p53* gene mutations in primary gastric cancer by cell sorting and polymerase chain reaction single-strand conformation polymorphism analysis. Cancer Res., *51*:3056–3058, 1991.

Tanaka, S., Toh, Y., Adachi, E., Matsumata, T., Mori, R., and Sugimachi, K. Tumor progression in hepatocellular carcinoma may be mediated by *p53* mutation. Cancer Res., *53*:2884–2887, 1993.

Tannock, I. F. Principles of cell proliferation: cell kinetics. *In*: DeVita et al. (Eds.), Cancer—Principles and Practice of Oncology, Vol. 1, 3rd ed., pp. 3–13. Philadelphia: Lippincott, 1989.

Tennant, R. W. A perspective on nonmutagenic mechanisms in carcinogenesis. Environ. Health Perspect. Suppl., *101*:231–236, 1993.

Tennant, R. W., Elwell, M. R., Spalding, J. W., and Griesemer, R. A. Evidence that toxic injury is not always associated with induction of chemical carcinogenesis. Mol. Carcinogen., *4*:420–440, 1991.

Terzi, M. Chromosomal variation and the origin of drug-resistant mutants in mammalian cell lines. Proc. Natl. Acad. Sci. U.S.A., *71*:5027–5031, 1974.

Thiberville, L., Payne, P., Vielkinds, J., LeRiche, J., Horsman, D., Nouvet, G., Palcic, B., and Lam, S. Evidence of cumulative gene losses with progression of premalignant epithelial lesions to carcinoma of the bronchus. Cancer Res., *55*:5133–5139, 1995.

Tlsty, T. D. Gene amplification as marker for studying genomic instability. Methods Mol. Genet., *8*:388–401, 1996.

Tlsty, T. D., Margolin, B., and Lum, K. Differences in the rates of gene amplification in non-tumorigenic and tumorigenic cell lines as measured by Luria-Delbrück fluctuation analysis. Proc. Natl. Acad. Sci. U.S.A., *86*:9441, 1989.

Tlsty, T. D., Jonczyk, P., White, A., Sage, M., Hall, I., Schaefer, D., Briot, A., Livanos, E., Roelofs, H., Poulose, B., and Sanchez, J. Loss of chromosomal integrity in neoplasia. Cold Spring Harbor Symp. Quant. Biol., *58*:645–654, 1993.

Trott, K. R. Tumour stem cells: the biological concept and its application in cancer treatment. Radiother. Oncol., *30*:1–5, 1994.

Tubiana, M. L. H. Gray Medal Lecture: Cell kinetics and radiation oncology. Int. J. Radiat. Oncol., *8*:1471–1489, 1982.

Turc-Carel, C., Limon, J., Dal Cin, P., Rao, U., Karakousis, C., and Sandberg, A. A. Cytogenetic studies of adipose tissue tumors. II. Recurrent reciprocal translocation t(12; 16)(q13; p11) in myxoid liposarcomas. Cancer Genet. Cytogenet., *23*:291–299, 1986.

van Echten, J., van Gurp, R. J. H. L. M., Stoepker, M., Looijenga, L. H. J., de Jong, B., and Oosterhuis, J. W. Cytogenetic evidence that carcinoma in situ is the precursor lesion for invasive testicular germ cell tumors. Cancer Genet. Cytogenet., *85*:133–137, 1995.

Varshavsky, A. Phorbol ester dramatically increases incidence of methotrexate-resistant mouse cells: possible mechanisms and relevance to tumor promotion. Cell, *25*:561–572, 1981.

Wani, G., Noyes, I., Milo, G. E., and D'Ambrosio, S. M. Expression of molecular biomarkers in primary breast tumors implanted into a surrogate host: increased levels of cyclins correlate with tumor progression. Mol. Med., *3*:273–283, 1997.

Ward, J. M., Uno, H., Kurata, Y., Weghorst, C. M., and Jang, J.-J. Cell proliferation not associated with carcinogenesis in rodents and humans. Environ. Health Perspect., *101*:125–136, 1993.

Weber, R. G., Boström, J., Wolter, M., Baudis, M., Collins, V. P., Reifenberger, G., and Lichter, P. Analysis of genomic alterations in benign, atypical, and anaplastic meningiomas: toward a genetic model of meningioma progression. Proc. Natl. Acad. Sci. U.S.A., *94*:14719–14724, 1997.

Weinstein, I. B. Toxicity, cell proliferation, and carcinogenesis. Mol. Carcinogen., *5*:2–3, 1992.

Welch, D. R., and Tomasovic, S. P. Implications of tumor progression on clinical oncology. Clin. Exp. Metast., *3*:151–188, 1985.

Whang-Peng, J., Kao-Shan, C. S., and Lee, E. C. Specific chromosome defect associated with human small-cell lung cancer: deletion 3p(14-23). Science, *215*:181–182, 1982.

Whyte, P. The retinoblastoma protein and its relatives. Semin. Cancer Biol., *6*:83–90, 1995.

Wiener, F., Ohno, S., Spira, J., Haran-Ghera, N., and Klein, G. Chromosome changes (trisomies #15 and 17) associated with tumor progression in leukemias induced by radiation leukemia virus. J. Natl. Cancer Inst., *61*:227–232, 1978.

Wilson, D. M., Goldsworthy, T. L., Popp, J. A., and Butterworth, B. E. Evaluation of genotoxicity, pathological lesions, and cell proliferation in livers of rats and mice treated with furan. Environ. Mol. Mutagen., *19*:209–222, 1992.

Wilson, G. D. Assessment of human tumour proliferation using bromodeoxyuridine—current status. Acta Oncol., *30*:903–910, 1991.

Wiseman, R. W., Stowers, S. J., Miller, E. C., Anderson, M. W., and Miller, J. A. Activating mutations of the c-Ha-*ras* protooncogene in chemically induced hepatomas of the male B6C3 F_1 mouse. Proc. Natl. Acad. Sci. U.S.A., *83*:5825–5829, 1986.

Wolman, S. R. Karyotypic progression in human tumors. Cancer Metast. Rev., *2*:257–293, 1983.

Yamashita, N., Minamoto, T., Onda, M., and Esumi, H. Increased cell proliferation of azoxymethane-induced aberrant crypt foci of rat colon. Jpn. J. Cancer Res., *85*:692–698, 1994.

Yokota, J., and Sugimura, T. Multiple steps in carcinogenesis involving alterations of multiple tumor suppressor genes. FASEB J., *7*:920–925, 1993.

Yosida, T. H. Karyotype evolution and tumor development. Cancer Genet. Cytogenet., *8*:153–179, 1983.

10
Consequences of the Stage of Progression

In Chapter 9 were discussed the basic biological and molecular mechanisms of the stage of progression in the development of neoplasia. Unlike the stages of initiation and promotion, the stage of progression encompasses, for the most part, the clinical disease resulting from the presence and growth of neoplastic cells within the host. While the control or elimination of the stages of initiation and promotion are considered as methods of cancer prevention, the control of neoplastic disease during the stage of progression is almost entirely in the realm of therapy. Even early diagnosis of the disease in the stage of progression is not a form of prevention but rather a form of efficient therapy. The longer the stage of progression is allowed to develop, the less efficient become the therapeutic modalities used to treat this disease. It is the changes that occur during this stage of progression that dictate the way that neoplasia is diagnosed and treated.

Clonality of Neoplasms

Previous chapters discussed alterations in single cells (initiation) as well as in cellular populations (promotion), leading to the development of the stage of progression. Stem cells (Chapters 9 and 14), each of which may give rise to a clone of genetically identical cells, occur in both normal and neoplastic cellular growth. However, a question that has always intrigued investigators in the field of oncology is whether a neoplasm arises from a single cell or from multiple cells (a field) that have been transformed to neoplasia almost simultaneously, e.g., by viruses or germline genetic alterations. The answer to this question is by no means simple (Tanooka, 1988). In considering clonality, one must determine at what stage in the development of neoplasia the "founder" cell (not identical to a stem cell as defined in Chapter 14) occurs. Such a founder cell may be a normal cell that becomes initiated, and its progeny develop through the stage of promotion, with subsequent transition of a single cell in the clone to the stage of progression. Alternatively, the founder cell may be in the stage of promotion, which then gives rise to a clone in the stage of progression. Finally, since genetic abnormalities occur commonly during the stage of progression, subclones may appear, suggesting that the neoplasm is polyclonal in origin (Fey and Tobler, 1996; Woodruff, 1988). Usually the founder cells of neoplasms are those resulting from the transition of a cell in the stage of promotion to the stage of progression. However, preneoplastic lesions produced experimentally in the liver (Weinberg and Iannaccone, 1988) and the skin (Deamant and Iannaccone, 1987) are reportedly clonal.

Methods for Determining Clonality

The first indications that neoplasms were clonal came from cytogenetic and biochemical analyses. In chronic myelogenous leukemia, in which the leukemic cells all possess the Philadelphia chromosome, a monoclonal origin of the neoplasm would be expected. Myelomas and several types of lymphomas almost always produce only a single type of immunoglobulin. From our knowledge of immunobiology (Chapter 16), myelomas and lymphomas thus were felt to arise from a single cell or a very few cells. However, the most widely used method for the determination of a monoclonal or polyclonal origin of neoplasms depended on investigations of the isozymic forms of X-linked enzymes in cells.

In the normal mammalian female, early during embryonic development but after meiosis, one of the two X chromosomes in each cell is repressed (Figure 10.1). The mechanism of this repression is unknown, but it culminates, in the fully developed organism, in a mosaic cellular pattern consisting of a number of populations of cells expressing the genes on one X chromosome, while the remaining cellular populations of the organism express the genes on the other X chromosome. If an individual is heterozygous (different alleles or copies of the gene in each of the two chromosomes), then some cells will express one form of the gene and other cells the other form. In relation to the monoclonal derivation of neoplasms, some females are mosaic for two isozymic forms of the enzyme glucose-6-phosphate dehydrogenase, resulting from the repression of one or the other X chromosome in individual cells during early embryonic life, as stated by the Lyon hypothesis. Thus, if a neoplasm arising in such a mosaic individual contains only a single form of this enzyme, it is likely to have resulted from a single cell. On the other hand, it is difficult to rule out the possibility that the early neoplastic transformation occurred in many cells, but that then one or very few cells attained a growth advantage and overgrew the vast majority of the population. In studies with chimeric mice produced by the amalgamation of two

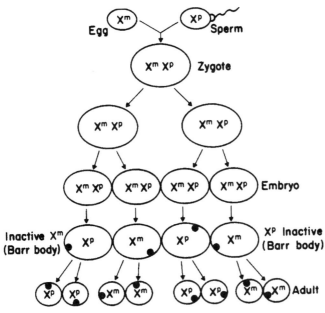

Figure 10.1 Diagrammatic representation of the Lyon hypothesis. The zygote (fertilized egg) is depicted as that of a female inheriting one X chromosome from the mother (X^m) and the other from the father (X^p). These chromosomes are passed to daughter cells, but at some early time in embryogenesis a difference occurs in the behavior of each of the two X chromosomes in each somatic cell, so that only one X chromosome remains active in each cell and its subsequent daughter cells. The other X chromosome is inactive and becomes the Barr body, as noted in the figure. Thus the adult female becomes a mosaic with a number of cells expressing the genes of X^p, while others express those of X^m. (After Fialkow, 1974, with permission of the author and publisher.)

embryos (allophenic mice), neoplasms of the skin induced in such animals exhibited an apparent clonal growth in that genetic markers characteristic of only one of the two parent embryos appeared in the neoplasms (Condamine et al., 1971). However, hepatomas produced in such animals were mosaic; that is, they possessed genetic characteristics of each of the parent embryos.

With the advent of newer methods of molecular biology, newer methods for the determination of clonality in cells have been developed. Table 10.1 lists more traditional methods, as described above, and a number that utilize techniques of molecular biology to analyze genetic alterations. The restriction fragment length polymorphism (RFLP) analyses have been discussed previously (Chapter 5). One may also combine the polymerase chain reaction with RFLP determination to increase the sensitivity of the analysis, such that the clonality of as few as 100 cells may be determined (Gilliland et al., 1991). While cells of a myeloma or lymphoma may be shown to be clonal by measuring the genetic structure of their immunoglobulin or T-cell receptor, owing to the production of only a single molecular species of these proteins by a lymphocyte, studies have demonstrated an apparent polyclonality of some lymphomas when the structure of the T-cell receptor gene is measured in these lesions (Ohno et al., 1997; Bignon et al., 1990). This phenomenon may be explained by arguing that the founder cell of each clone was produced during the stage of progression rather than in the transition from promotion to progression or earlier (Collins, 1997). DNA fingerprint analysis may also be somewhat variable, possibly owing to the appearance of subclones. Analysis of breakpoint cluster regions, as in the Philadelphia chromosome, is another method giving results similar to cytogenetic analysis but taking advantage of the unique, stable genetic alteration in the breakpoint region. Finally, the structures of the genomic termini of the Epstein-Barr virus (EBV) in episomes of infected cells may indicate whether the neoplasm arose from a very low multiplicity of infection (very few viral particles per target cell) or from a high multiplicity, with many cells being simultaneously infected and giving rise to a lymphoma (Chapter 12). Table 10.2 list data indicating the mono- or polyclonality of a variety of neoplasms of the human. As noted from the table, only two hereditary neoplasms, neurofibroma and trichoepithelioma, have been shown to be consistently polyclonal in origin, although recent studies have suggested polyclonality for several other neoplasms, both hereditary and spontaneous. These studies, which are now more than 20 years

Table 10.1 Methods of Clonality Determination

	Methods	
General Approach	Traditional	DNA
X-chromosome inactivation	G6PD isoenzymes Allophenic mice	X-linked RFLPs
Lymphocyte analysis	Immunoglobulin light chain analysis	Immunoglobulin and T-cell receptor gene analysis
Somatic mutation	Cytogenetic analysis	Detection of chromosome loss by RFLP analysis
		Detection of chromosome translocations by breakpoint cluster probes
		Detection of somatic mutations by DNA fingerprinting
		Detection of specific point mutations
Viral integration analysis		Analysis of genomic EBV termini

Adapted from Wainscoat and Fey, 1990, with permission of the authors and publisher.

Table 10.2 Single- or Multiple-Cell Origin of Tumors Determined with Immunoglobulin (Ig) and
Glucose-6-Phosphate Dehydrogenase (Glc-6-PD) Markers

	Marker	Single Cell (no. of specimens)	Multiple Cell (no. of specimens)
Myeloproliferative disorders			
Chronic myelocytic leukemia	Glc-6-PD	8	0
Polycythemia vera	Glc-6-PD	2	0
Lymphoproliferative disorders			
Acute "Burkitt-type"	Ig	6	0
leukemia	Ig	>150	Rare
"Hairy-cell" leukemia	Ig	2	0
Chronic lymphosarcoma leukemia	Ig	11	0
Reticulum cell sarcoma	Glc-6-PD	2	0
Burkitt lymphoma	Glc-6-PD	45	1
	Ig	92	1
Non-Hodgkin lymphoma	Glc-6-PD	4	0
	Ig	38	0
Chronic lymphocytic leukemia	Ig	K150	Rare
Multiple myeloma	Glc-6-PD	2	0
	Ig	Many	Rare
Carcinoma			
Nasopharynx (anaplastic)	Glc-6-PD	7	0
Cervix, preinvasive	Glc-6-PD	9	0
invasive	Glc-6-PD	30	0[c]
Ovary	Glc-6-PD	3	0
Palate	Glc-6-PD	4	0
Thyroid	Glc-6-PD	5	0
Melanoma	Glc-6-PD	2	0
Nephroblastoma	Glc-6-PD	2	0
Bronchioloalveolar lung carcinoma	X-linked RFLPs	0	3[e]
Papillary peritoneal carcinoma	p53	2	4[f]
Hereditary			
Neurofibroma	Glc-6-PD	0	14
Trichoepithelioma	Glc-6-PD	0	12(?)
Polyps in Gardner syndrome	Glc-6-PD	0	3[a]
Medullary thyroid carcinoma	Glc-6-PD	4	0[b]
Familial adenomatous polyposis adenomas	Y chromosome probes	4	13[d]
Endocrine			
Solitary thyroid adenoma	Glc-6-PD	22	0
Miscellaneous benign			
Leiomyoma of uterus	Glc-6-PD	184	0
Lipoma	Glc-6-PD	6	0
Salivary gland adenoma	Glc-6-PD	2	0
Ovarian teratoma	Glc-6-PD	39	0
Neurofibroma (sporadic)	Glc-6-PD	2	0

[a]Hsu et al., 1983
[b]Baylin et al., 1978
[c]Enomoto et al., 1997
[d]Novelli et al., 1996
[e]Barsky et al., 1994
[f]Muto et al., 1995
Modified from Fialkow, 1976.

old for the most part, were carried out on relatively large amounts of neoplastic tissue. More recent techniques have allowed the analysis of microdissected samples from morphologically distinct microscopic lesions. Such studies have in general confirmed the monoclonal origin of each distinctive lesion (Cheng et al., 1998).

Studies in experimental animals have indicated a clonal nature for some neoplasms (Collins and Fialkow, 1982); in other cases, however, chemicals have induced neoplasms of multicellular origin (Reddy and Fialkow, 1979). A follow-up analysis of the latter studies demonstrated that sarcomas induced by the subcutaneous injection of methylcholanthrene may develop as monoclonal or polyclonal neoplasms, depending on whether benzene or olive oil is the solvent vehicle in which the carcinogen is administered (Reddy and Fialkow, 1981). The same authors (Reddy and Fialkow, 1983) later showed that papillomas induced by a single painting of dimethylbenzanthracene, followed by promotion with TPA, are predominantly monoclonal in origin, whereas those neoplasms resulting from the repeated applications of the carcinogen itself exhibit a much higher incidence of polyclonal origins. A suggested explanation of these apparent discrepancies is that a relatively small dose of initiating agent may tend to induce more monoclonal neoplasms simply because fewer cells will be initiated, whereas relatively higher doses of an initiating agent will ultimately result in polyclonal neoplasms because of a greater chance of adjacent cells being initiated and developing together. However, Deamant and Iannaccone (1987) argued that the different observations of monoclonal or polyclonal neoplasms were the result of confounding by the presence of varying amounts of nonneoplastic dermal tissue. On the other hand, differences in growth rates and other factors such as nutrition (blood supply) and interaction among clones of neoplastic cells may result in the apparent monoclonality of a neoplasm even if the process of initiation was not clonal (cf. Woodruff, 1988; Chow and Rubin, 2000).

An alternative view of the clonality of neoplasms is that taken by Nowell (1976) and others on the clonal evolution of a neoplastic cell population, with neoplasms considered to evolve by the selection of one or more clones of cells during their natural developmental history. By this concept, the clonality of a neoplastic cell population in the stage of progression may simply be the result of the selective growth advantage of a clone of cells appearing during the natural history of development of the neoplasm, resulting in the overgrowth by this population. This has been recognized over the years by the demonstration of "stem" cell populations in neoplasms with a characteristic karyotype. Such clonal evolution can also account to a great degree for the progression of many neoplasms. It has also been suggested that diseases heretofore not classified as neoplastic in origin may exhibit clonal development of their basic pathological lesion and thus could possibly be related to the neoplastic transformation. This appears to be the case in atherosclerosis, as suggested by Benditt (1974), who demonstrated that the fibrous plaque seen in blood vessels in the early development of this disease is clonal, as shown by the use of X-linked markers.

Thus, the data (Table 10.2) in human neoplasia argue that most neoplasms are clonal in origin. However, this does not imply that their clonality arose at the stage of initiation but rather at the stage of progression. Preneoplastic lesions in the stage of promotion both in skin (Reddy and Fialkow, 1983) and in rat liver (Weinberg and Iannaccone, 1988) are clonal, presumably arising from single initiated cells. However, as discussed in Chapter 9, neoplastic lesions arise within preneoplastic lesions, presumably initiating a new clone, as evidenced both from different karyotypes and other markers of progression (Giaretti, 1997; Scherer et al., 1984). Apparently polyclonality may, in turn, result from high doses of the carcinogenic agent (Reddy and Fialkow, 1983), resulting in cells transiting into the stage of progression within a short time period. Therefore the clonal nature of both preneoplasia and neoplasia is an important aspect of our consideration of the natural history of neoplastic development.

THE ANATOMICAL EXTENSIONS OF NEOPLASIA

In Chapter 2 the distinctions between benign and malignant neoplasia were discussed, with the caveat that the distinction was largely artificial but convenient. In the context of the stages of neoplastic development, the imperfections of the behavioral classification of neoplasia become more apparent. While virtually all preneoplastic lesions may be considered as benign in the behavioristic classification, a significant number of benign lesions also occur during progression, such as adenomas of the thyroid, stomach, colon, ovary, and liver, as well as a few mesenchymal neoplasms (Henson and Albores-Saavedra, 1986). Still, the key distinction between benign and malignant neoplasms resides in their ability to extend beyond the primary growth by the process of invasion into adjacent tissues and to successfully metastasize, with resultant independent secondary growths. In recent years the characteristics and to some extent the mechanisms involved in the development of these anatomical extensions of neoplasia, invasion, and metastasis have been clarified.

Invasion

Initial considerations of the characteristics and mechanisms of invasive neoplastic growth argued that the increased mobility and rapidity of growth of the neoplastic cell, together with a capacity for proteolysis and a decrease in pH (possibly owing to the high glycolysis of the neoplasm; Chapter 15), were responsible for its ability to invade normal tissue (cf. Sylvén, 1968). Other mechanisms also were invoked to explain tumor cell invasion, including differences in intracellular osmotic pressure between normal and neoplastic cells, the degree of host reactions such as inflammation, the anatomical structure of the tissue being invaded, and the loss of "contact inhibition," a process whereby normal cells are inhibited in growth and motion by adjacent cells. All of these were thought to be factors in neoplastic cell invasion both in vivo and in vitro.

During the last decade, these descriptive characteristics and mechanisms of the process of neoplastic invasion of normal tissues have been greatly advanced by a better understanding of the molecular nature of cell-cell interaction in vivo as well as the interaction of cells with their immediate environment as defined by their surrounding extracellular matrix.

The Extracellular Matrix

In general terms, the extracellular matrix (ECM) consists of a mixture of macromolecules, ions, and substrates that are specific for any given tissue. The ECM thus provides a distinct environment for different cells of the organism (Scott-Burden, 1994). The ECM is largely made up of a complex blend of macromolecules, some of which, once formed, may exist for the life span of the organism (Hay, 1991). The macromolecules of the ECM largely but not entirely consist of fiber-forming elements (collagen and related molecules) and glycoprotein and proteoglycan "packing" components. A diagram of the ECM associated with vascular elements is given in Figure 10.2, in the upper part of which are depicted endothelial cells resting on a basement membrane. Basement membranes are heterogeneous, highly specialized, electron-dense structures constructed from components of a number of the extracellular matrix proteins. They vary from 20 to 200 nm in thickness and function to separate epithelia and endothelia from their underlying connective tissue. Basement membranes provide anchorage for adjacent cells as well as stimuli for cell differentiation, cell migration, and cell phenotype (Stanley et al., 1982; Weber, 1992).

Of the ECM molecules depicted in Figure 10.2, collagen is the predominant species, making up approximately one-third of the protein in the human body (cf. Scott-Burden, 1994). There are more than 14 different species of collagen molecules (van der Rest and Garrone, 1991), with

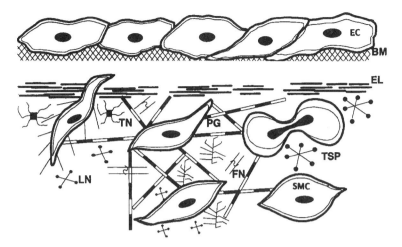

Figure 10.2 Diagrammatic representation of the ECM in association with vascular elements. Endothelial cells (EC) rest on a basement membrane (BM) of the internal vascular wall, whereas smooth muscle cells (SMC) are surrounded by molecules of the ECM. The internal elastic lamina (EL) acts as a fenestrated layer between the subendothelial intima and smooth muscle cells of the vascular medial layer. Molecules of the ECM shown schematically are tenascin (TN), proteoglycans (PG), laminin (LN), fibronectin (FN), thrombospondin (TSP), and collagen fibers which are depicted as large dashed lines. (Adapted from Scott-Burden, 1994, with permission of the author and publishers.)

type 1 collagen the predominant species in the ECM. The collagen structure is that of an extended triple helix bound together by numerous hydrogen bonds, some of which are dependent for their formation on posttranslational hydroxylation of proline and lysine catalyzed by a vitamin C (ascorbic acid)–dependent reaction. In addition, the collagen structure is further cemented by glycosylation of these and other hydroxyl groups, as well as oxidation of the ε-amino groups of lysine, some of which are oxidized by a copper-dependent lysyl oxidase and form covalent crosslinks with amino groups of adjacent collagen molecules, binding the multimolecular structure into strong, stress-resistant collagen fibers. Elastin—which is a key component of the ECM in pliable tissues such as vessels, alveolae of the lung, dermis, and intestine—has a structure somewhat similar to that of collagen, but with more hydrophobic domains that act as "coiled springs" and are related to the protein's elasticity.

A variety of glycoproteins and proteoglycans are associated with the ECM in normal tissues. The diagrammatic structures of several of these molecules are seen in Figure 10.3. The three glycoproteins shown—fibronectin, laminin, and SPARC—are generally representative of the glycoproteins existing in the ECM. All of the glycoproteins have various domains within the protein that interact selectively with cellular and matrix components, as indicated in the diagram. Fibronectin is composed of two nearly identical polypeptides linked by disulfide bridges and having a combined molecular weight near 450,000 (cf. Ruoslahti et al., 1982). The molecule is made up of a series of polypeptide repeats, as indicated in the figure (I, II, and III). Fibronectin monomers have varying numbers of these repeats, the number being dependent on differential splicing of fibronectin mRNA in various tissues. As a result, fibronectin monomers may exist in a wide diversity of molecular sizes. SPARC consists of a single polypeptide chain with four domains, as shown. In contrast, the laminin structure is more cruciform, consisting of three peptide chains linked together by disulfide bonding in the carboxyl half of the three peptides. Each of the three peptides is encoded by a different gene (cf. Scott-Burden, 1994), but no differential mRNA

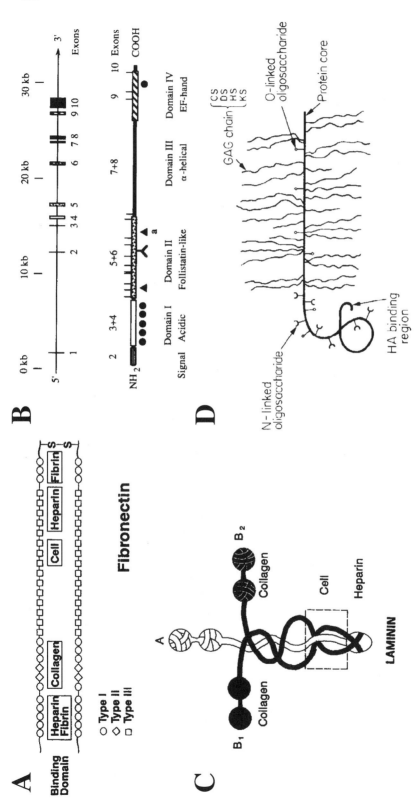

Figure 10.3 Diagrammatic structures of glycoproteins and proteoglycans of the extracellular matrix. The three different types of polypeptide repeats in fibronectin are noted as types I, II, and III in each of the two chains. (A) The domains are indicated in boxes. (B) The SPARC protein domains are indicated beneath the diagrammatic structure with an indication of the exons above the diagrammatic structure. (C) The association of the three peptide components of laminin are noted in addition to an indication of the regions binding collagen and the cell. (D) The generalized structure of this typical proteoglycan monomer shows the protein core and positions of the N-and O-linked oligosaccharides as well as the hyaluronic acid (HA) binding region. CS, chondroitin sulfate; DS, dermatan sulfate; HS, heparan sulfate; KS, keratan sulfate. Further details are given in the text. (Structures were adapted from the following: A, C: Scott-Burden, 1994; B: Lane and Sage, 1994; D: Wight, 1989 with permission of the authors and publishers.)

splicing has been reported, although at least seven different forms resulting from the association of different gene products have been reported (Timpl and Brown, 1994). Laminin and at least two other ECM glycoproteins, thrombospondin and tenascin, possess a large number of epidermal growth factor–like repeats in their structure. It has been theorized that cleavage of the molecule may produce active epidermal growth factor molecules affecting the growth of tissue (Chapter 14).

The proteoglycans consist of a protein backbone (core protein) that has many threonine and serine residues. To these hydroxyl groups are attached a series of long, linear carbohydrate chains termed *glycosaminoglycans*, which usually consist of a dimeric repeat structure of acid and amine structures of sugars (cf. Scott-Burden, 1994). Individual proteoglycans may bind to hyaluronic acid chains or in some cases may actually span membranes. A "link" protein may assist in this association, which leads to the formation of large aggregated molecules that largely fill the interstices of the ECM. It must be emphasized that the proteoglycans are an extremely diverse series of molecules, exhibiting the general structure shown in Figure 10.3 but having different oligosaccharides and core proteins, depending on the tissue and the species (Kjellén and Lindahl, 1991).

Cell Adhesion and Cell Behavior

While cells exist in the organism in various environments of extracellular matrix, both epithelial and mesenchymal cells interact directly with each other to form stable arrangements, as in epidermis and glandular and mucosal epithelium; they also undergo transient interactions involving lymphocytes in nodes and lymphoid organs, polymorphonuclear leukocytes, and macrophages. These cell-cell interactions form the basis for the architecture of tissues as well as their morphogenesis (Gumbiner, 1996). Both stable and transient cellular adhesions are the result of the interaction of ectoproteins of the plasma membrane interacting with each other on different or the same cell types as well as an interaction with the ECM. Diagrams of the structure of the four major molecular species of cell adhesion molecules are given in Figure 10.4. Each of these molecular species consists of a single transmembrane polypeptide with the exception of the integrins, which are heterodimers, an α and a β chain. The α subunit provides the molecular basis for ligand binding, while the β subunit is the major link to the cytoskeleton and signal transduction apparatus. At least 15 α subunits and 8 β subunits are known, giving rise to at least 19 different integrins (cf. Elangbam et al., 1997). Various members of the integrin family function in a variety of ways in different cell types, including embryogenesis, wound healing, and the immune response. These functions involve cell migration, cell-cell adhesion, and cell-ECM interaction, as well as signaling molecules, the latter primarily through the β integrins (LaFlamme and Aver, 1996). They are the most widely distributed adhesion molecules in mammalian organisms and possibly the most versatile (Faull, 1995). The extracellular heterodimeric portion of the molecule serves as a receptor for a variety of ligands, including collagen, laminin, fibronectin, fibrinogen, and several other cell adhesion proteins as well (Faull, 1995). The intracellular portion of these molecules, in turn, interacts with the cytoskeleton (Chapter 16) allowing for potential signal transduction mechanisms (see below).

The immunoglobulin family of molecules involved in cell adhesion are products of the immunoglobulin gene superfamily, which is discussed further in Chapter 17. Members of this family are linked to the plasma membrane as shown in Figure 10.4 and are involved in protein recognition, a process essential in the immune response (Chapter 19) as well as in cell adhesion. A short list of members of the immunoglobulin gene superfamily that are involved in cell adhesion is seen in Table 10.3. These adhesion molecules are expressed extensively on lymphocytes and other members of the immune system as well as in vascular endothelial cells and cells of the nervous system (Turner, 1992). One member of the family, NCAM, is a primary cell adhesion

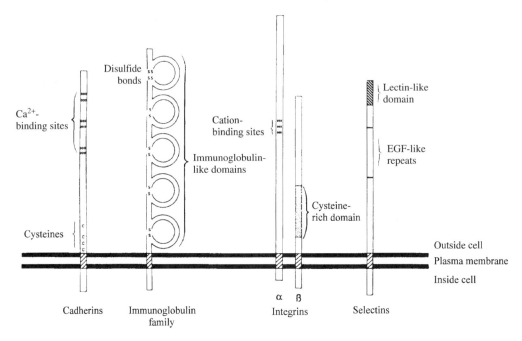

Figure 10.4 Diagrams of the molecular structure of families of cell adhesion molecules. See text for explanation. (Adapted from Garrod, 1993, with permission of the author and publisher.)

molecule that appears very early in development in all three germ layers and plays a very important role in the development of the central nervous system. Many other members of the family are involved in the relatively transient interaction of leukocytes, macrophages, and related cells in the vascular system during tissue injury, inflammation, and related processes. The selectins play a similar role in these processes in that they are expressed on the surface of endothelial cells, leukocytes, and platelets. These molecules influence the localization of circulating leukocytes on the endothelium at the site of inflammation. Members of this family are involved in a

Table 10.3 Adhesion Molecules of the Immunoglobulin Gene Superfamily

Immunoglobulin	Other Names	Ligand[a]
ICAM-1	CD54	$\alpha_L\beta_2$ (CD11a-CD18)
		$\alpha_M\beta_2$ (CD11b-CD18)
ICAM-2	CD102	$\alpha_L\beta_2$ (CD11a-CD18)
ICAM-3	CD50	$\alpha_L\beta_2$ (CD11a-CD18)
		$\alpha_M\beta_2$ (CD11b-CD18)
VCAM-1	CD106	$\alpha_4\beta_1$ (CD49d-CD29)
		$\alpha_4\beta_7$
PECAM-1	CD31	PECAM-1
MAdCAM-1		L-selectin, $\alpha_4\beta_7$

[a]The α and β ligands refer to various members of the integrin family. The term CD followed by a number indicates an immunologic classification to be discussed later (Chapter 17).

Adapted from Menger and Vollmar, 1996, with permission of the authors and publisher.

very early period of immune-inflammatory reactions as well as in the "homing" of lymphocytes to various places in the organism (Elangbam et al., 1997). The ligands for the selectins are carbohydrate moieties on protein molecules, such as mucins and sialated polysaccharide antigens on cell surfaces (Faull, 1995). A major contribution to cell-cell adhesion is made by calcium-dependent cadherins. These are simple transmembrane glycoproteins involved in establishing and maintaining intercellular connections through homophilic binding—i.e., a cadherin molecule on one cell binds to another cadherin molecule of the same type on an adjacent cell. The cytoplasmic domain of cadherins is linked to cellular components through catenins, proteins that are necessary for cadherin function (cf. Garrod, 1993). Three subclasses of cadherins have been recognized: epithelial (E)-cadherin or uvomorulin, placental (P)-cadherin, and neural (N)-cadherin (Elangbam et al., 1997). Cadherins function in cell-cell adhesion by clustering on the plasma membrane to form adhesion junctions. Interactions between cells involve the N-terminal cadherin repeat domain, potentially generating a "cadherin zipper," whose strength depends on the number of cadherin molecules involved in the adhesion junction (Klymkowsky and Parr, 1995). An excellent example of these adhesion junctions is seen in the skin, where a subgroup of cadherins termed the *desmosomal cadherins* localize to desmosomes in the skin and are linked to the keratin filament network, giving strength to the epidermal covering (Faull, 1995).

Several other adhesion molecules have been described, the most important of which is CD44, expressed on the surface of T lymphocytes (Chapter 19). This glycoprotein, which is a receptor for hyaluronic acid, regulates adhesion of these and other cells to endothelial cells and monocytes, a process that effects the recruitment of T lymphocytes to sites of inflammation (Elangbam et al., 1997). Since specific glycoproteins and mucins have now been shown to interact with individual selectins, one may also suggest that these proteins can act as adhesion molecules, at least with a transitory function (Menger and Vollmar, 1996).

Adhesion (Adherens) Junctions, Focal Adhesions, and Cell Signaling

As implied above, the structure of organisms and their tissues depends on the adhesion and interaction of cells to each other as well as of cells to basement membranes and the ECM. The cadherins are the major mediators of cell-cell adhesion, while the integrins mediate the attachment of cells to basement membranes and the ECM. Both the adherens junctions and the focal adhesions involve an intracellular interaction between the cytoplasmic portion of the adhesion molecule, cadherin or integrin, with cytoskeletal components (Chapter 16) and signal transduction pathways (Chapter 7). Figure 10.5 presents diagrammatic and hypothetical illustrations of an adherens junction and focal adhesions with their extracellular contacts and intracellular associations with protein species. The adherens junction diagrams the interaction or "zipper" intercellular contact zone between molecules of cadherens on one cell and those on another. Such interactions involve two dimers interacting in an antiparallel orientation through their adhesive binding surfaces, thus forming a continuous linear ribbon structure (Gumbiner, 1996; Aberle et al., 1996). These interactions also involve calcium-binding pockets that bridge and stabilize the successive structural repeats through coordination of acidic amino acid residues and align the domains into a rod shape (cf. Aberle et al., 1996). The cytoplasmic domains of the cadherins interact with catenins α and β and plakoglobin, which is closely related to β-catenin. These molecules, in turn, interact with the cytoskeleton, directly or indirectly—both microfilaments and intermediate filaments (Chapter 16). In addition, the catenins may complex with the product of the tumor suppressor gene, APC or adenomatous polyposis coli (Chapter 5; Polakis, 1997; Aberle et al., 1996). Certain functional ratios of cadherins, catenins, and the APC gene product seem to be necessary for the maintenance of a normal phenotype in epithelial cells (cf. Rosales et al., 1995). These complexes and/or another protein, p120[cas], are involved in protein phos-

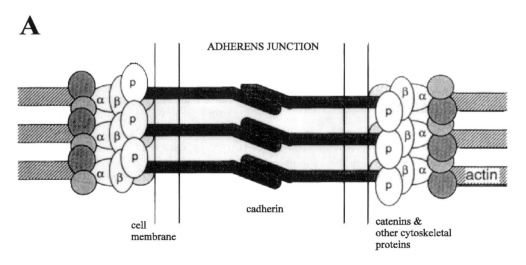

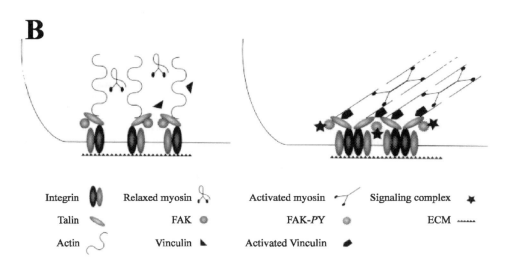

Figure 10.5 (A) A model illustration of the adherins junction showing the interaction of cadherins from two different cells. Each cadherin is associated through its intracellular component with the proteins α, α-catenin; β, β-catenin; p, plakoglobin (adapted from Takeichi et al., 1993, with permission of authors and publisher). (B) Focal adhesion assembly models showing on the left a quiescent cell adhering to the extra-cellular matrix (ECM). Interactions of integrins binding to the ECM in the extracellular component are noted. The integrins are linked to the cytoskeleton via proteins such as talin and others which are not shown. In the left portion of the figure integrins are shown under little tension with the myosin in a relaxed conformation. In the right-hand portion of the figure is seen myosin light chain phosphorylation stimulated in response to Rho (a member of the G protein family) activation. Myosin is shown as assembling into bipolar filaments generating tension on actin, resulting in clustering of the integrins bound to the ECM. This integrin clustering activates the focal adhesion kinase (FAK) leading to autophosphorylation (FAK-PY) and recruitment of other members of the signaling complex noted as a star. The model depicted is not meant to demonstrate all components of the assembly, but rather those of greater importance. (Adapted from Burridge et al., 1997, with permission of the authors and publisher.)

phorylation by cellular tyrosine kinases. Thus, catenin complexes appear to be involved in signal transduction pathways, but the exact mechanisms for this are not clear as yet. Takeichi et al. (1993) suggested that tyrosine phosphorylation of β-catenins may modulate their actions so as to loosen cell-cell contacts, causing a destabilization of the cadherin-cadherin interactions.

Focal adhesions (Figure 10.5) involve an interaction of cells with basement membranes and the ECM mediated by plasma membrane–spanning integrins. The cytoplasmic portion of the β integrin interacts with intracellular proteins such as talin and vinculin, as noted in the figure, which, in turn, associate with actin molecules of the microfilaments. In the figure, it is hypothesized that intracellular alterations leading to microfilament contraction cause a clustering of the integrin dimers, producing and strengthening focal adhesions and their interaction with the ECM and/or basement membranes (Figure 10.5). Also noted in the figure is the mediator of signal transduction, the focal adhesion kinase (FAK) (Burridge et al., 1997). This kinase interacts directly with the cytoplasmic tail of the β integrin subunit and also contains at least two SH2 binding domains (Chapter 7). It has been suggested (Clark and Brugge, 1995) that clustering of the integrins activates FAK, which in turn induces its autophosphorylation and subsequent binding to SH2 domains of signal transduction molecules such as Src and Grb2. A small GTP-binding protein, rho, appears to regulate the assembly of focal adhesions with actin fibers in response to growth factors (Ridley and Hall, 1992). This pathway may then continue the signal through ras to MAPK and the nucleus (Chapter 7). Thus, by alterations from the environment or from within the cell, adhesion molecules and the adhesive interaction of cells with each other and with the ECM and basement membranes can lead to dramatic alterations in gene expression within cells during normal development, hormonal alterations within the organism, or reaction to noxious external stimuli. Alterations in cell adhesion play a major role in the biological activity of neoplastic cells that invade and metastasize during the stage of progression.

Invasive Properties of Neoplastic Cells

Some pathologists have advanced the thesis, based primarily on studies of epithelial carcinoma in situ, that malignant neoplasia is characterized initially by invasion of neoplastic cells into and through the basement membrane (Figure 10.2). Despite reservations and exceptions to this observation, there is little question of the importance of the invasive properties of neoplastic cells in the stage of progression to the development of the disease. From knowledge of normal cell interactions with the extracellular matrix (ECM) and each other, as discussed above, similar interactions of neoplastic cells have been studied during the past two decades. Invasion deals predominantly with interactions of neoplastic cells with the ECM, while cell-cell interactions are somewhat more important in the mechanisms of metastases to be discussed later in this chapter; however, both interactions play roles in both invasion and metastases (Liotta, 1990).

Extracellular Matrix—Neoplastic Cell Interactions

A critical factor in the process of invasion is the interaction of neoplastic cells with the ECM. Thus, one would expect to see qualitative and quantitative alterations in the molecular species depicted in Figure 10.2. For carcinomas, interaction with the ECM and basement membranes involves primarily integrins and to a lesser extent selectins and immunoglobulin-like molecules. Integrin expression in normal epithelial cells is usually seen in a polarized pattern, while the integrin pattern in carcinomas is dispersed and discontinuous. Loss of expression or increased expression of some specific integrins may be seen in specific neoplastic cell types, leading to enhanced invasive and/or metastatic properties (Rosales et al., 1995). A loss or significant reduction in expression of the α5β1 integrin, which has a function as the "classical" fibronectin receptor, occurs in many transformed and neoplastic cells (cf. Juliano, 1993; Rosales et al., 1995). Fibronectin itself was first characterized as the large, external, transformation-sensitive (LETS) protein because it was lost from the surface of many transformed cells (Vaheri and Ruoslahti, 1975; Mautner and Hynes, 1977). The interaction of this integrin receptor with fibronectin involves recognition of a specific amino acid sequence, arginine-glycine-aspartate (RGD), that is also present in a number of other ECM proteins, including laminin, vitronectin, and collagen, type I (Yamada, 1991). Other recognition sequences are also present in several of these ECM proteins, allowing for the interaction with other integrins. Furthermore, the interaction of these ligands with specific integrins can be inhibited by specific synthetic peptides that contain these recognition sequences (Yamada, 1991; Stetler-Stevenson et al., 1993a). Overexpression of integrins such as $\alpha 5\beta 1$ leads to a reduction in malignant potential in animal systems as well as a reduction in cell proliferation (cf. Rosales et al., 1995; Varner and Cheresh, 1996). Interaction of integrins with their ligands may also alter apoptosis in either a positive or negative manner, depending on which integrin is involved (cf. Varner and Cheresh, 1996). These effects on cell proliferation and apoptosis are probably the result of the effect of integrin-ligand interaction, resulting in activation of the focal adhesion kinase and its substrates, as suggested in Figure 10.5 (cf. Rosales et al., 1995; Juliano, 1993). Rosales et al. (1995) have suggested that the loss of certain integrins from neoplastic cells, in particular $\alpha 1\beta 1$, may result in the elimination of a major "trigger" for apoptosis, the presence of unliganded integrin on cells that are not interacting with the ECM. Just as inhibition of apoptosis enhances tumor promotion, so this mechanism of the elimination of apoptosis of cells in the stage of progression would result in an enhancement of the development of this stage.

Protease Involvement in Invasion

While the interaction of neoplastic cells with the ECM via integrins is critical for the invasive properties of neoplastic cells, of equal importance is the ability of the neoplastic cell to destroy or alter physically the barriers posed to invasion by the ECM. Basement membranes are a critical component of these barriers, but they also include collagen and other components of the ECM. While noninvasive cells form focal adhesion contacts with the underlying ECM and tightly adhere via cell surface receptors, invasive cells produce membrane protrusions that actually invade the ECM (Monsky and Chen, 1993). But such physical invasion is not sufficient to allow a neoplastic cell to extend through a basement membrane or appreciably into the ECM. However, the invadopodia and membrane vesicles produced by the invading cell contain integral membrane proteases as well as receptors and activators for a variety of latent proteases. These include serine proteases, cathepsins, and a variety of matrix-metalloproteinases (MMPs). The principal serine protease involved in neoplastic invasion is the urokinase-type plasminogen activator (u-PA). This protease catalyzes the conversion of the inactive plasminogen to the active plasmin, a broad-spectrum protease that catalyzes the degradation of a variety of protein substrates. Plasminogen is found ubiquitously in the serum and interstitial fluids of mammals (Duffy, 1993; Mignatti and Rifkin, 1993). u-PA is synthesized as an inactive precursor peptide and secreted as such, as are all other proteases involved in the invasion of neoplastic cells with the exception of recently described membrane proteases. The precursor form of u-PA interacts with a membrane receptor on the surface of the cell that produced it or an adjacent cell and is then cleaved by either a membrane protease, a cathepsin, or by plasmin, the product of its catalytic function. In general, neoplasms produce higher levels of u-PA than corresponding normal cells, a fact that has been known for a number of decades (cf. Duffy, 1993). It is likely that the plasmin produced by the catalytic action of u-PA then functions in turn to activate (cleave the precursor form) other proteases involved in the process of invasion.

The largest group of proteases associated with the process of neoplastic invasion is the matrix metalloproteinase family. A recent listing of the members of this family and their domain structure is seen in Figure 10.6. Just as with u-PA, several of the MMPs are expressed at high levels in many neoplasms in vivo, giving further evidence of their importance in the process of invasion. However, regulation of the activity of such potent proteases is critical in order that the process be regulated in the whole organism. Thus, several tissue inhibitors of metalloproteinases (TIMP) have been described, and two members of this group, TIMP-1 and TIMP-2, are well characterized (Stetler-Stevenson et al., 1993b). Low levels of TIMP expression correlate with enhanced invasive and metastatic capabilities in neoplastic cells from both murine and human sources (cf. Stetler-Stevenson et al., 1996). Inhibitors of u-PA and cathepsins, which are known as serpins (serine proteinase inhibitors), have also been described (Pemberton, 1997) and perform a similar regulatory function with respect to the serine proteases involved in the invasive process. Evidence for a significant role of cathepsins, which include the lysosomal cysteine or aspartic proteinases classically described as functional at an acid pH optimum, in the invasive process is not so great as with u-PA and the MMPs. However, cathepsins have the capability of degrading many of the ECM proteins (Monsky and Chen, 1993) as well as activating u-PA and inactivating both the TIMPs and serpins. Because of their normal lysosomal compartmentation, it is likely that their effects in the invasive process occur secondarily as a result of apoptosis and necrosis of both normal and neoplastic cells.

Figure 10.7 is a diagram of the interactive functions of proteases and protease inhibitors in the ultimate modification of the extracellular matrix. The diagram indicates the changes in protease activation and inhibition as a cascade, analogous to the blood clotting protease cascade (Davie et al., 1991). By means of this cascade mechanism, a very tight control or regulation in ECM remodeling is maintained under normal conditions. However, alterations of protease and protease inhibitor concentrations by neoplastic cells can alter the cascade in favor of the invasive characteristic of the neoplastic cell.

Cadherins in the Invasive Process

While the process of invasion involved primarily direct interaction with the ECM through integrins and the simultaneous action of proteases, cell-cell adhesion must be altered to allow the invasive process to occur. Cadherins play a primary role in cell adhesion and thus will also play a role in invasion, especially in epithelial tissues, which normally exhibit considerable cell adhesion. In general, in malignant neoplasms, E-cadherin expression is reduced or abnormally localized (Mareel et al., 1994). The progression from benign to malignant neoplasia in mouse skin tumors induced by the two-stage protocol also exhibits a reduced expression of E-cadherin in the malignant but not the benign form (Ruggeri et al., 1992). A similar finding was reported by Perl et al. (1998) in transgenic pancreatic β-cell carcinogenesis. While Mareel et al. (1994) had suggested that mutations in cadherins had not been found in primary neoplasms, more recently Berx et al. (1996) have demonstrated a variety of different somatic mutations in the E-cadherin gene of infiltrating lobular breast carcinomas but not in breast cancers of other histopathological types. However, a variety of other potential mechanisms for decreased cadherin expression are known, including posttranslational modifications, alterations in catenins, and other interacting molecules as well as environmentally induced alterations in expression of the cadherin genes (Fish and Molitoris, 1994; Mareel et al., 1993). From these studies and a variety of others, both in vivo and in vitro, the cadherins have been labeled as *invasion/metastasis suppressor* molecules.

In addition to changes in cell-cell adhesion and interaction with the ECM, neoplastic cells must have the ability to locomote and migrate in order to express their invasive and metastatic properties. As indicated in Figure 10.5, changes at the focal adhesion through interaction of inte-

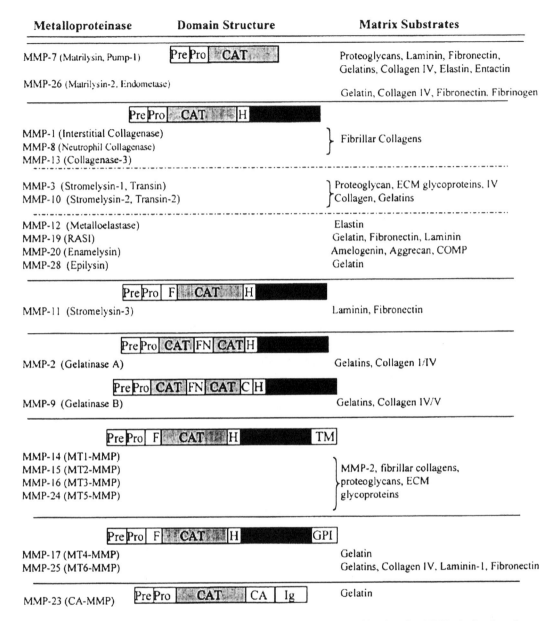

Metalloproteinase	Domain Structure	Matrix Substrates

MMP-7 (Matrilysin, Pump-1) — Proteoglycans, Laminin, Fibronectin, Gelatins, Collagen IV, Elastin, Entactin

MMP-26 (Matrilysin-2. Endometase) — Gelatin, Collagen IV, Fibronectin. Fibrinogen

MMP-1 (Interstitial Collagenase)
MMP-8 (Neutrophil Collagenase)
MMP-13 (Collagenase-3) — } Fibrillar Collagens

MMP-3 (Stromelysin-1, Transin)
MMP-10 (Stromelysin-2, Transin-2) — } Proteoglycan, ECM glycoproteins. IV Collagen, Gelatins

MMP-12 (Metalloelastase) — Elastin
MMP-19 (RASI) — Gelatin, Fibronectin, Laminin
MMP-20 (Enamelysin) — Amelogenin, Aggrecan, COMP
MMP-28 (Epilysin) — Gelatin

MMP-11 (Stromelysin-3) — Laminin, Fibronectin

MMP-2 (Gelatinase A) — Gelatins, Collagen I/IV

MMP-9 (Gelatinase B) — Gelatins, Collagen IV/V

MMP-14 (MT1-MMP)
MMP-15 (MT2-MMP)
MMP-16 (MT3-MMP)
MMP-24 (MT5-MMP) — } MMP-2, fibrillar collagens, proteoglycans, ECM glycoproteins

MMP-17 (MT4-MMP) — Gelatin
MMP-25 (MT6-MMP) — Gelatins, Collagen IV, Laminin-1, Fibronectin

MMP-23 (CA-MMP) — Gelatin

Figure 10.6 List and diagrams of the domain structure and classification for MMPs indicating the classes of this family based on the presence of similar domains. MT, membrane type; Pre, leader sequence; Pro, prodomain; CAT, catalytic domain; H, hinge domain; F, furin consensus site; FN, fibronectin-like domain; TM, transmembrane domain. (Adapted from Chambers and Matrisian, 1997, with permission of the authors and publisher.)

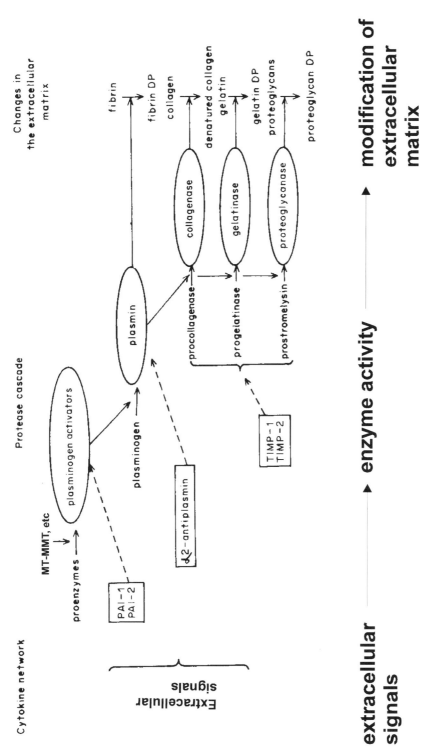

Figure 10.7 The protease cascade involved in extracellular matrix remodeling. The active proteases are noted in ellipses, while the protease inhibitors are indicated in rectangles. DP, degradation products; PAI, plasminogen activator inhibitor; TIMP, tissue-inhibitor of metalloproteinases. (Modified from Opedenakker and VanDamme, 1992, with permission of the authors and publisher.)

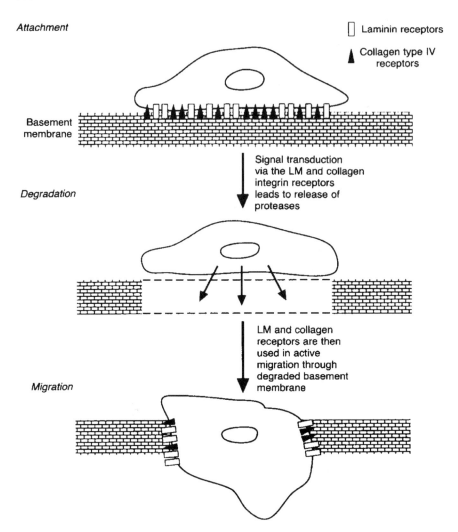

Figure 10.8 Schematic representation of the events involved in neoplastic cell invasion of basement membranes. LM, laminin. (Adapted from Dedhar, 1990, with permission of the author and publisher.)

grins with proteins and especially intracellular actin and myosin microfilaments can result in enhanced cell motility. Conversely, external factors may stimulate cellular motility through interaction with receptors and subsequent signal transduction pathways exerted through the focal adhesions. Among such external factors are the autocrine motility factor, a 55-kDa cytokine, which is produced by various neoplastic cells and in turn stimulates motility and organ-colonizing ability (Nabi et al., 1992). A number of other secreted cytokines that specifically induce cell motility, having molecular weights in the range of the autocrine motility factor and higher (up to 92 kDa), have also been described. One of these is the scatter factor/hepatocyte growth factor (SF/HGF). This growth factor interacts with the proto-oncogene c-*met*, which is its membrane receptor. SF/HGF may act as a mitogen or a motility factor (motogen) and also to induce or alter morphogenesis of both normal and neoplastic cells (cf. Ruiz and Gunthert, 1996). In both of these examples as well as others, alterations in cellular motility effected by these motogens are the result of signal transduction pathways that interact with intracellular molecules controlling motility by microfilaments via the focal adhesions as indicated above.

On the basis of the morphological characteristics of the process of invasion in vitro as well as our knowledge of the interaction of cells with the ECM, Liotta and his associates (Aznavoorian et al., 1993) proposed a model that was applicable both to neoplastic invasion as well as the initiation of successful metastatic growth. In Figure 10.8 may be seen a schematic representation of the events involved in the invasion of basement membranes by neoplastic cells; this representation may also be applied to invasion through endothelial basement membranes and even into the ECM itself. As noted, the step of attachment involves the interaction of integrins with the various components of the ECM in the basement membrane. The phase of degradation or local proteolysis involves the activation of u-PA and subsequently the MMPs. Finally, the process of migration through the altered ECM resulting from the first two steps completes the invasive process. The motility of the invading neoplastic cell is probably a function of signal transduction and the alteration of actin/myosin interactions (Figure 10.5) as well as the continued binding of integrin receptors with components of the ECM through focal adhesions and other surface structures interacting with specific components of the ECM. It is these components, which include the selectins, the cadherins, and members of the immunoglobulin superfamily on the surface of the cell, that play an even greater role in the successful development of metastatic lesions within the host, as described below.

METASTASIS AND METASTATIC GROWTH

Metastasis: Incidence and Mechanism

As noted earlier, a metastatic tumor is one that originates in and is physically separated from the primary neoplastic growth. The capacity of malignant tumors to metastasize is one of the major features of their lethality to the host.

Routes of Metastasis

Anatomically, a number of pathways for metastatic cells are possible. The most obvious is the blood circulation, in which neoplastic cells gain entrance to the vascular system by invasive and related processes and then are carried by the bloodstream to new sites, where they initiate growth. Usually this new growth begins in small capillaries, where neoplastic cells are caught and begin to invade through the capillary endothelium to initiate a new growth. It is obvious from a variety of studies that the number of cells that enter the bloodstream is far greater than the number that ever give rise to metastatic lesions. The phenomenon of "canceremia" or neoplastic cells in the blood has been studied in the past through the use of blood filtrates in which the number of neoplastic cells per milliliter of blood may be estimated. In advanced cases of neoplasia this number is quite high, whereas in early tumor growth there may be virtually no tumor cells within the blood vascular system. Recently, sensitive systems have been able to detect as few as one epithelial tumor cell per milliliter of whole blood (Denis et al., 1997; Komeda et al., 1995). In this study, the presence of neoplastic cells in the blood was generally correlated with the presence of metastatic lesions, but not entirely. With the polymerase chain reaction (PCR), patients exhibiting the presence of metastases showed a significantly higher level of the hepatocyte-specific alpha-fetoprotein mRNA in blood. Furthermore, from experimental studies, it would appear that only when a neoplasm reaches a certain critical size does it begin to shed cells into the bloodstream. Of the cells entering the bloodstream, considerably fewer than 0.01% ever give rise to any metastatic lesions (cf. Sellwood et al., 1969). Classical clinical observations have indicated that carcinomas metastasize more frequently via the lymphatic system, whereas sarcomas spread more commonly through the blood vascular system. However, the presence of numerous anastomoses between venous and lymphatic vessels tends to invalidate this concept (Fisher and Fisher, 1966).

Another common route of metastasis is the lymphatic system, in which the flow of neoplastic cells, although considerably slower than in the bloodstream, is probably of a similar magnitude. Some neoplasms may implant in other sites by mere physical movement from one site to another. This is commonly seen in certain ovarian or gastrointestinal neoplasms, with resultant implantation of neoplastic cells from one side of the peritoneal cavity to the other. A similar sort of implantation is probably the mechanism responsible for the appearance of accessory spleens or splenosis—i.e., intraabdominal splenic tissue separate from the spleen itself (Carr and Turk, 1992).

With the advent of numerous surgical techniques, a new pathway of metastasis has become apparent. If the surgeon is not careful, the operative knife may enter the neoplasm and become covered with living cells, which may be carried to and implanted at another site in the surgical field. This phenomenon has accounted for the reappearance of tumors in the operative site some months or years after the initial surgery. In addition, manipulation of the neoplasm during surgery may initiate both vascular and lymphatic metastatic lesions. However, now that these problems are apparent, most surgeons take extreme care to prevent the occurrence of such metastasis during curative resections by isolating the neoplastic lesion prior to extirpation and by thorough washing of the wound site.

In experimental oncology, the analog to surgical metastasis is the tumor transplant. Clearly, in the original behavioristic classification of neoplasms, the distinguishing feature of the metastatic capability of the malignant neoplasm is reflected in its transplantability. In some instances, however, it has been possible to transplant neoplasms that have not been shown to be behavioristically malignant in the original primary host. This further points out the artificiality of the behavioristic classification to the experimental oncologist.

Incidences and Sites of Metastases of Neoplasms

As stated previously, the number of metastatic cells that give rise to metastatic lesions is extremely small. Metastases usually appear in the adjacent lymph nodes or in the lung or liver, the site depending on where the tumor originates and its histogenetic origin. Certain neoplasms may have a predisposition, because of their anatomical location, to metastasize to certain organs. Cancer of the lung not uncommonly metastasizes to the brain, possibly because of neoplastic invasion into the pulmonary veins, from which metastatic cells may enter the carotid arteries and pass to the brain. Carcinoma of the breast regularly metastasizes to the adrenal glands, and carcinoma of the prostate frequently metastasizes to bones, particularly the vertebrae. Relatively few metastatic lesions occur in some organs—for example, the spleen and thymus. In the case of the thymus, this is probably because of its peculiar vascular system. Neoplastic cells may have difficulty in establishing metastatic lesions in the spleen because of its unique anatomical structure and its function in eliminating senescing or otherwise damaged cells (Bishop and Lansing, 1982). Figure 10.9 is a diagram of the organ distribution pattern of metastases from a variety of cancers.

Although the anatomical location of the organ in which metastases colonize can in many instances be explained by vascular connections of the primary tumor and adjacent lymphoid structures, in many circumstances the relative high incidence of metastasis of specific neoplasms to specific organs cannot be explained on this basis. Furthermore, it is possible, by using transplanted highly malignant murine neoplasms, to select variant metastatic cells that have a high predilection for growth in specific organs (Nicolson, 1978; Fidler et al., 1978). For example, clones of cells may be obtained from the parent neoplasm by repeated selection in vivo. These clones have a propensity for growth in the liver, the lung, or the brain. In recent years the mechanism for such organ selectivity has been studied rather intensively with respect to metastasis occurring through the vascular system. The critical tissue in organ-specific metastasis is the endothelium that lines the interior of blood/lymph vessels and the heart. The vascular endothelium provides a protective and antithrombogenic surface as well as acting as a vehicle for transport of various substances from or into the bloodstream. In this process the endothelium performs distinctive biological functions at different vascular sites and in individual organs (Fishman, 1982). Such functions appear to involve specific structural and chemical microdomains of the endothelial cell surface (cf. Pauli et al., 1990). Some of these domains may be expressed in an organotypic and vessel caliber–dependent fashion, whereas others are transient and regulated in a positive or negative manner depending on the functional needs of the tissue (cf. Pauli et al., 1990). The biochemical diversity of normal endothelial cells has been verified at the molecular level, demonstrating clear differences in carbohydrate and other moieties exposed on the surface of the cell. Included in these molecular arrays are the familiar cell adhesion molecules, integrins, cadherins, immunoglobulin superfamily members, selectins, and CD44. However, since the metastatic cell is floating freely within the bloodstream, lymph, or body cavities, the metastatic cell must find a suitable molecular interaction with an endothelial cell and subsequently utilize its invasive properties to extend through the vessel wall, through the basement membrane, and into the ECM in order to colonize the tissue. This process, which is quite analogous to that seen in Figure 10.8, is depicted in Figure 10.10, where the interaction is termed a "docking and locking" of the metastatic cell (Honn and Tang, 1992). Initial interaction of the neoplastic cell with the endothelium is likely to occur through members of the immunoglobulin superfamily, selectins and CD44, as well as interactions of these and other molecules with integrins. A variety of surface carbohydrate determinants on neoplastic cells as well as the endothelium appear to determine the initial aspects of successful metastasis (cf. Dennis and Laferte, 1987; Kannagi, 1997; McEver, 1997). The initial recognition or "docking" step depicted in Figure 10.10 occurs between the moving neoplastic cell and the underlying endothelial cell. This interaction is mediated by relatively weak and transient adhesive forces of carbohydrate-carbohydrate and/or carbohydrate-protein interactions involving primarily selectin recognition of carbohydrates and members of the immunoglobulin superfamily recognizing specific integrin receptors (Honn and Tang, 1992; Miyasaka, 1995). This process is very similar to "homing" of lymphocytes to specific areas of the organism (Roos, 1993). However, as with the altered genetic expression so characteristic of the stage of progression, neoplastic cells often employ ectopic expression of adhesion molecules to facilitate their interaction with endothelium and ultimately during the process of invasion (Tang and Honn, 1995). An excellent example of this is noted in the altered expression of CD44, the hyaluoranate receptor. This surface molecule contains 20 exons, and different tissues express different splice forms of the molecule. At least 20 different CD44 isoforms have been described based on alterations in the content of 10 variable exons occurring in the center of the molecule (Tuszynski et al., 1997). Malignant neoplasms express a wide variety of the splice variants, a number of which have been shown by transfection and other similar experiments to increase neoplastic cell growth and metastasis dramatically in vivo (Sleeman et al., 1995; Cooper and Dougherty, 1995).

In addition to the molecular species found in tissue-specific endothelial cells, certain tissues produce factors that stimulate the growth of metastatic neoplastic cells (cf. Nicolson, 1992). At times, neoplastic cells themselves may produce growth factors that can stimulate their own growth (autocrine growth). In other instances, experiments have demonstrated that both sponta-

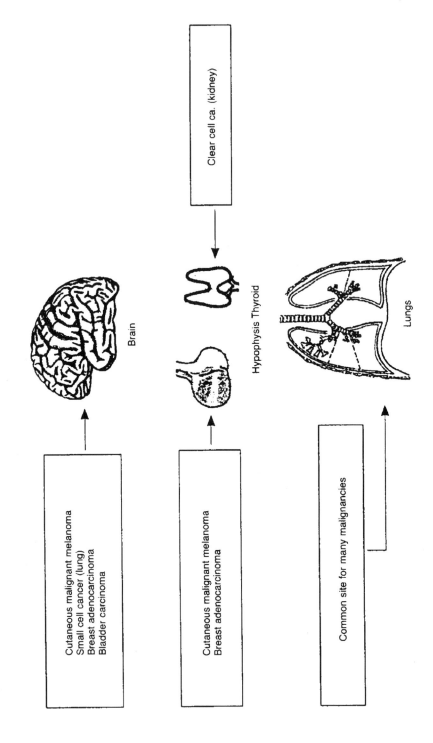

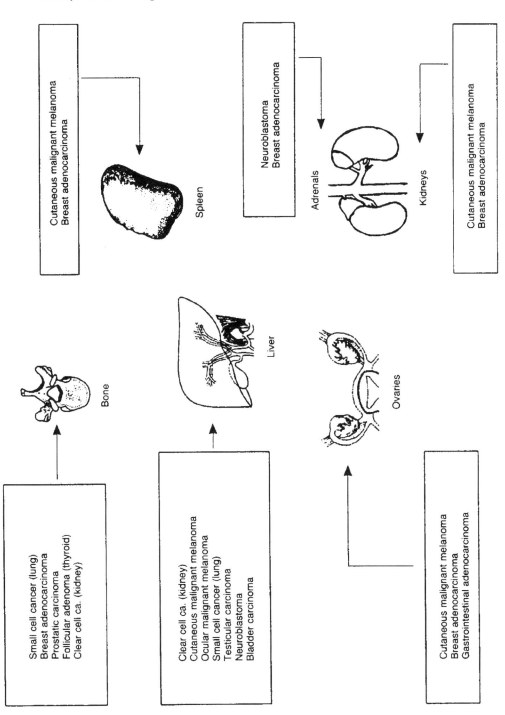

Figure 10.9 The distribution pattern of some neoplasms in relation to organ colonized. As noted in the text, direct vascular connections of the primary neoplasm with the target organ cannot fully explain the high incidence of metastasis in some organs. (Adapted from Rusciano and Burger, 1992, with permission of the authors and publisher.)

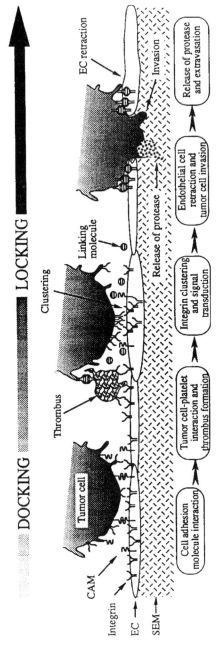

Figure 10.10 Artist's conception of the docking and locking hypothesis of initial metastatic colonization. In the "docking" phase, neoplastic cells within the vascular system interact initially with the surface of endothelial cells through carbohydrate-carbohydrate and/or carbohydrate-protein recognition interactions. Molecules involved at this stage are cell surface glycoproteins, selectins, or immunoglobulin cell adhesion molecules present on the neoplastic cells or the endothelial cell or both. Subsequently, platelet/coagulation interactions occur with the neoplastic cell leading to platelet aggregation, activation, and release reactions. At this time the neoplastic cell establishes stable bonds with the endothelial cell during the activation-dependent "locking" phase mediated largely by integrins and modulated by a host of mediators resulting from both activated platelets as well as the neoplastic cells. Thereafter, the metastatic cell induces retraction of the endothelial cell with subsequent release of proteases and extension into the extracellular matrix. EC, endothelial cell; CAM, cell adhesion molecules; SEM, subendothelial matrix. (Adapted from Honn and Tang, 1992, with permission of the authors and publisher.)

neous and transplanted metastatic neoplasms that are seen to metastasize frequently to specific tissues are also found to have their growth stimulated in vitro by extracts from those tissues to which they readily metastasize but not to other tissues (cf. Rusciano and Burger, 1992). An excellent example of tissue-specific growth enhancement of metastases is seen when prostatic adenocarcinoma metastasizes to the bone marrow, producing characteristic bone-forming (osteoblastic) lesions. The growth rate of these metastases is significantly more rapid than that of primary prostatic neoplasms. This effect appears to be due to the production in the bone marrow of a growth factor that is able to enhance specifically the growth of prostatic cancer cells (Chackal-Roy et al., 1989).

In most experimentally produced neoplasms, the animal is killed prior to the occurrence of metastatic lesions. Therefore it is not uncommon to find an animal harboring a histologically malignant neoplasm with no evidence of metastatic lesions. Were the animal to be allowed to die of the cancer, the incidence of metastatic lesions would be much higher in such experimental situations. Similarly, in the human, malignant neoplasms of the central nervous system rarely metastasize, since the lethal changes occurring in the confined space of the skull kill the host before the neoplasm has had an opportunity to express its metastatic capabilities (Alvord, 1976).

In the past it was felt that lymph nodes presented a barrier to the spread of metastatic cells (Cady, 1984). Several experimental findings have seriously questioned this concept and indicate that many neoplastic cells initially retained in lymph nodes maintain only a temporary residence there, and the nature of the neoplastic cells may be at least as great a determinant of their residence in lymph nodes as are the biological and mechanical properties of such structures (Fisher and Fisher, 1967; Kohno et al., 1979). Substantial evidence has accumulated that trauma may increase the number of metastatic cells (if such trauma is directed at the primary neoplasm) and may increase the chance of successful metastatic growth at a site distant from the primary neoplasm (Fisher et al., 1967).

The Pathogenesis of Metastasis

The overall pathogenesis of metastatic growth is a subject of concern to all individuals seeking a better understanding of the cause and control of cancer. It is usually the metastatic lesions of a primary neoplasm that are the direct or indirect cause of the demise of the patient with cancer. Since the first realization that metastatic neoplasia originated from a primary neoplasm (Chapter 1), the methods by which metastatic cells successfully colonize distant tissues have been investigated. Figure 10.11 is a diagram of the overall pathogenesis of metastatic lesions in a general sense.

Vascularization of a primary neoplasm involves an interesting interaction between neoplastic cells and the host, the latter supplying the vasculature—a topic discussed in Chapter 18. Invasion into the vascular system occurs by mechanisms that have already been discussed (Figure 10.8 and text). Neoplastic cells within the circulation interact with blood platelets, lymphocytes, and other circulating blood cells of the host. Fibrinogen and fibrin, its polymeric product, are likely to be related in a second, indirect manner to the formation of metastases (Malone et al., 1979). The interaction of neoplastic cells with platelets during and after their "docking" (Figure 10.10) is also a critical factor in the initial establishment of a metastatic clone. The "locking" or subsequent late phase of the process depicted in Figure 10.10 involves a firmer adhesion mediated by activation-dependent integrins and potential interaction with blood coagulation elements, especially blood platelets. Neoplastic cells in vitro exhibit the capability to cause platelet aggregation, which also involves surface carbohydrate-receptor interactions (Honn et al., 1992). The combination of platelet interaction with the neoplastic cell to form a minithrombus and the interaction of integrins with surface molecules on the endothelial cell stabilize the interaction of the neoplastic cell with the endothelial surface. Following this, there

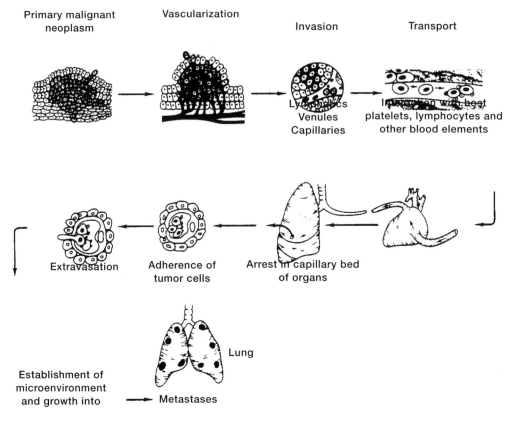

Figure 10.11   The pathogenesis of metastasis. Note that the extension from the primary neoplasm involves invasion into the vascular system and the subsequent development of metastases through the docking and locking mechanisms in Figure 10.10. (Adapted from Poste and Fidler, 1980, with permission of the authors and publishers.)

occurs both the release of proteases, as in the invasive process (Figure 10.8), as well as endothelial cell retraction to aid in the invasive process of the metastatic cell through the endothelial membrane. Furthermore, platelets release a variety of growth factors, including the platelet-derived growth factor (PDGF) and transforming growth factor-β (TGF-β) (Chapter 16), which can enhance growth of the metastatic clone. Subsequent to extravasation or invasion through the blood vessel wall, subsequent growth of the metastatic clone depends on a variety of complex interactions between the neoplastic cell population and that of the host. Paramount among these interactions is the development of blood vessels (angiogenesis) from normal host cells to supply the vasculature, oxygen, and nutrients to the developing neoplasm. This subject is considered more extensively as a complex host-tumor relationship in Chapter 18.

Genetic Mechanisms of Metastases

Virtually all successful metastatic lesions from primary neoplasms are aneuploid and in the stage of progression. It is, in fact, the karyotypic instability of neoplastic metastatic lesions that differentiate them from nonneoplastic metastatic cells. One must recall that certain normal tissues also have the capacity to metastasize. The placenta uniformly metastasizes during the last several months of pregnancy; in individuals who have died during this period, metastatic cells are found in the maternal pulmonary vasculature. Under normal circumstances, after parturition, metastatic placental cells die as a result of the alteration in the hormonal environment. Accessory spleens may be considered metastases from normal spleens. In certain cases of trauma, especially after fractures of bone, fat cells and other bone marrow elements may metastasize to other parts of the organism, sometimes with acute deleterious effects.

Just as karyotypic instability is probably the genetic basis for the altered phenotypes of neoplastic cells and affords them the advantage of invasion into adjacent tissues, metastatic cells that successfully invade and colonize secondary areas of the host do so because of their evolved genetic constitution. Karyotypic instability of neoplasms in the stage of progression results in a karyotypically heterogeneous neoplasm with cells of unequal metastatic potential (cf. Hart and Fidler, 1981). As already implied and seen in many of the examples used, genetic and epigenetic heterogeneity of neoplastic cells in the stage of progression can account for the complexity of many of the diverse properties of cancer (cf. Heppner and Miller, 1998). The incidence of spontaneous metastases in both primary and transplanted neoplasms is quite variable (Milas et al., 1983; Giavazzi et al., 1980). In the extreme, highly metastatic cells in experimental animals exhibit substantial increases in the rate of mutation (per cell generation) and may, even after cloning, generate metastatic variants at an apparent rate of about 10^{-5} per cell per generation (Cifone and Fidler, 1981; Harris et al., 1982). Neoplastic cells with fewer karyotypic and thus genetic changes have a lower incidence of successful metastatic growth, as evidenced by differences in gene amplification (Figure 10.12). In this figure, neoplasms exhibiting no metastasis show a lower degree of gene amplification than neoplasms exhibiting successful metastatic growth (Donovan-Peluso et al., 1991). It should also be noted that it is possible to select metastatic variants from neoplasms exhibiting little or no spontaneous metastatic activity in vivo (Frost et al., 1987). This finding has significant implications in the use of cytotoxic drugs capable of such metastatic selection in the therapy of neoplasia (Chapter 20).

Specific Genes Affecting Metastatic Potential

Although it is clear that genomic instability is the ultimate basis for the development of the stage of progression and its primary consequences, invasion and metastasis, one may ask whether specific genes and their products are involved in these last two processes. The critical nature of the expression of cell adhesion components, proteinases, and coagulation mechanisms of importance in invasion and metastasis has already been discussed. However, it is also apparent that specific genes and their products not directly involved in invasive and metastatic processes also influence, both directly and indirectly, these operations. Some of these genes are listed in Table 10.4, along with their functions and the correlation, either positive or negative, with metastatic potential. The Wnt-1 gene was found disrupted in several but not all primary mammary carcinomas in mice induced by the mouse mammary tumor virus through a mechanism of insertional mutagenesis (Chapters 4 and 8). However, no disruption or alteration of the gene was seen in any metastatic lesions, indicating that alteration of the gene either inhibited or was not relevant to the appearance of metastases (Sarkar, 1990). The mts-1 (p9Ka) gene, which codes for a calcium binding protein, is expressed at high levels in rat metastatic mammary tumor cell lines but not in benign neoplasms (cf. Ponta et al., 1994). In contrast, expression of the wild-type nm23 gene appears to inhibit the development of metastases, while mutation (Wang et al., 1993) or reduced levels of expression of the gene are related to an increased potential for metastases in most (Bevilacqua et al., 1989) but not all (Russell et al., 1997) carcinomas. In the case of the L-*myc* gene, a particular polymorphism was correlated with extensive metastases of lung cancer, especially

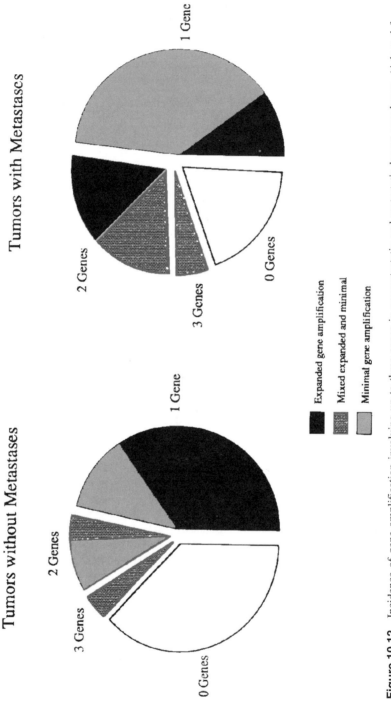

Figure 10.12 Incidence of gene amplification involving up to three genes in nonmetastatic and metastatic breast neoplasms. (Adapted from Donovan-Peluso et al., 1991, with permission of the authors and publisher.)

Table 10.4 Expressed Genes Correlated with Metastatic Potential

Gene	Function	Correlation	Reference
fucosyltransferase	Modification (fucosyla-tion) of surface proteins	–	Burger et al., 1982
int-1 (Wnt-1)	Glycoprotein (signaling, ECM)	+	Sarkar, 1990 Papkoff et al., 1987
L-myc	Transcription factor?	–	Kawashima et al., 1988 Ebralidze et al., 1989
mts-1 (p9Ka)	Ca^{2+}-binding protein	+	Dunnington et al., 1984
nm23	Nucleoside diphosphate kinase	–	Biggs et al., 1990 Bevilacqua et al., 1989
Vimentin/keratins	Intermediate filaments in cytoskeleton	+	Hendrix et al., 1992 Hendrix et al., 1996

Key: + indicates an enhanced expression of the gene, with an increase in metastases; – indicates that expression of the wild-type gene is seen in primary neoplasms that do not metastasize or metastasize infrequently.

adenocarcinomas in the human (Kawashima et al., 1988). Hendrix and associates (1992,1996) have also demonstrated a correlation of the expression of the intermediate filament proteins vimentin and keratins K8 and K18 (Chapter 16) with the metastatic potential of experimental melanoma cells. Higher levels of expression of these genes in transfected melanoma cells as well as other naïve neoplastic cells exhibited a higher degree of metastatic and invasive potential. Not listed in the table but of great significance is the suggestion by Glinsky et al. (1997) that metastatic cells exhibit a greater resistance to apoptosis than nonmetastatic neoplastic cells. Concomitant with this is a diminished level of nuclear calcium-dependent endonucleases and reduced activity of specific caspases.

Table 10.4 shows that most of the examples given are genes whose products function either in signal transduction pathways or as transcription factors, and all are associated with an interaction of the cell with its environment. Studies have also been undertaken wherein genes, especially those involved in signal transduction, are transfected into cells with a low metastatic potential to determine whether artificial disruption of signal transduction pathways would enhance metastatic growth. This was found to occur from studies by Liotta and colleagues (cf. Muschel and Liotta, 1988). Their investigations demonstrated that transfection of a mutant *ras* oncogene into mouse fibroblasts in culture resulted in increased expression of the transfected gene and enhanced expression of the endogenous *ras* gene. Both of these parameters correlated with a dramatic increase in metastatic growth of the transfected cells in vivo, usually in nude (immunocompromised, Chapter 19) mouse hosts. A striking example of this correlation is seen in Figure 10.13, where transfection of a mutant *ras* gene (EJ-ras) or wild-type *ras* (cHras) with the mutant v-*myc* oncogene into rat embryo fibroblasts showed a dramatic increase in lung metastases in nude mice and also a dramatic increase in the activity of collagenase. Transfection of the mutant EJ-*ras* gene, together with a viral oncogene E1A, resulted in no metastases or enhanced collagenase activity, although the resultant transfectants were tumorigenic in the immunocompromised host (Garbisa et al., 1987), suggesting that collagenase production was necessary for successful metastatic growth but not neoplasia. While these authors presented evidence that some of the transfectants exhibited little or no aneuploidy, other studies indicated that *ras* transfection of mouse cell lines resulted in enhanced aneuploidy of the metastatic cells (Ichikawa et al., 1990) and that *ras* transfection accelerates rather than initiates formation of

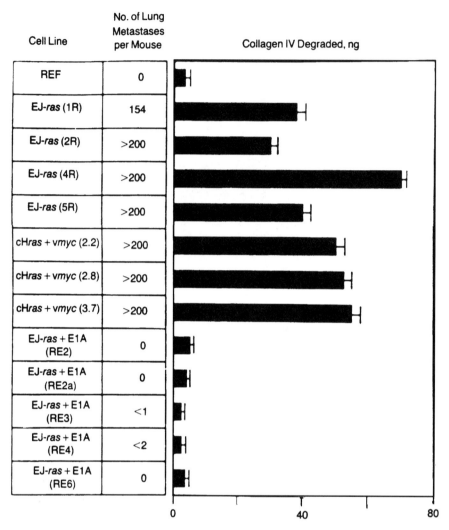

Figure 10.13 Transfection of the mutant oncogene EJ-*ras* or the wild-type proto-oncogene *cHras* with the viral oncogene v*myc* into diploid rat embryo fibroblasts (REFs) induces collagenase activity and metastasis formation. In contrast, transfection with mutant *ras* (EJ-*ras*) together with the adenovirus oncogene E1A eliminates the metastatic capability and increase in collagenase activity, but the cells remain fully neoplastic. The correlation between metastatic potential and expression of type IV collagenase is apparent. Numbers and letters in parentheses indicate the designation of the specific cell line under study. (Modified from Liotta and Kohn, 1990, with permission of the authors and publisher.)

metastases (Greig et al., 1985). Furthermore, in other rodent cells, transfection of the *ras* oncogene did not result in enhanced metastatic potential (Baisch et al., 1990; Tuck et al., 1990). As a further complication in the interpretation of such transfection experiments, Kerbel et al. (1987) reported that exposure of SP1, a nonmetastatic mouse mammary adenocarcinoma cell line, to calcium phosphate alone in the absence of DNA resulted in an increase in clones manifesting metastatic properties. Furthermore, transfection of DNA may induce chromosome rearrangements and other types of mutations as well as epigenetic changes in recipient cells (Bardwell, 1989).

That enhanced *ras* expression from either the endogenous gene or a transfected gene was not the only factor involved in enhanced metastatic capability of such cells was demonstrated by Ichikawa et al. (1992), who found that suppression of metastatic ability could occur by genetic means even in the presence of enhanced expression of the transfected *ras* oncogene. Furthermore, transfection of other oncogenes in NIH 3T3, the standard cell line utilized, also resulted in an enhanced potential for metastases (Egan et al., 1987; Greenberg et al., 1989). Transfection of p53 genomic clones into murine carcinoma cells exhibiting a low metastatic capacity led to an enhancement of the expression of the p53 protein together with increased metastatic potential of these cells (Pohl et al., 1988). In analogy to the original mutant *ras* oncogene studied by Liotta and colleagues, a single point mutation in the *met* proto-oncogene eliminated metastatic potential but not transformation to neoplasia of rat fibroblasts (Giordano et al., 1997). Although it is somewhat difficult to draw any general conclusions from these transfection experiments, it is clear that, under certain experimental circumstances, transfection of specific genes does enhance the metastatic potential of the cells being studied. In view of the functional characteristics of the small sample of endogenous genes that affect metastatic potential, as noted in Table 10.5, the types of genes used for the transfection experiments have functions overlapping with those indicated in the table, e.g., signal transduction. Thus, it is very likely not only that the metastatic phenotype is characterized by alterations in cell adhesion molecules and proteinases but also that alteration of signal transduction pathways plays a major role in the development of the successful metastatic phenotype.

Table 10.5 External Modulators of Metastatic Growth

Modulating Agent	Responsive System	Response	Reference
Angiostatin	Cell lines in mice	Inhibition	O'Reilly et al., 1994
Dietary components			
Linoleic acid (omega-6)	Primary murine mammary neoplasms	Enhancement	Erickson & Hubbard, 1990
Omega-3 fatty acids	Mammary cell lines in vivo	Inhibition	Rose et al., 1995
Retinoids	Murine melanoma B-16 in vivo	Inhibition	Edward and MacKie, 1989
Vitamin D$_3$	Lewis lung carcinoma in mice in vivo	Inhibition	Young et al., 1995
Hormones			
Melanocyte stimulating hormone	B-16 melanoma in vivo	Enhancement	Parker et al., 1991
Prostacyclins	Numerous systems	Inhibition	cf. Chen et al., 1992
Hypoxia	cell lines in mouse lung	Enhancement	Young et al., 1988
Ionizing radiation	Numerous systems	Enhancement	cf. von Essen, 1991
Peptides			
RGD congeners	B16 melanoma systems	Inhibition	Humphries et al., 1986 Saiki et al., 1989 Sheu et al., 1992
Laminin peptide	B16 melanoma lung colonization	Enhancement	Kanemoto et al., 1990

Modulation of Metastatic Growth

A number of factors, both internal and external, have been found to modify or alter metastatic growth. The genetic constitution of the metastatic cell may be considered among the internal factors altering metastatic potential with variable expression of genes, as indicated above. In addition to the genetic modulation of metastasis, there is also evidence that alteration in DNA methylation may affect the metastatic potential of neoplastic cells (Olsson and Forchhammer, 1984).

A number of external modulators of metastatic growth have been described. Representative examples of such modulators are given in Table 10.5. It should be noted from the table that the systems utilized to study the effects of such modulators on metastatic growth are somewhat artificial. In many instances the treatment occurs in vitro, with subsequent infusion of the cells into a suitable host animal. Angiostatin is a polypeptide fragment of plasminogen that bears some of the loop structures of the proprotease. This material blocks neovascularization of metastases in a model system. In analogy with tumor promotion (Chapter 8), omega-6 fatty acids enhance, while omega-3 fatty acids inhibit, metastatic growth of primary and transplanted neoplasms (Erickson and Hubbard, 1990; Rose et al., 1995). In similar artificial systems, both retinoids and vitamin D_3 inhibit the development of pulmonary metastases (Edward and MacKie, 1989; Young et al., 1995). The best example of hormonal effects on metastases is seen with the various prostacyclins, including prostaglandins (Chapter 8), in which, generally, inhibition of metastatic development in a variety of systems has been reported (cf. Chen et al., 1992). Cells subjected to hypoxia in vitro undergo anomalous DNA synthesis and karyotypic changes. Such cells, as expected, have a higher potential for metastatic growth (Young et al., 1988). In a similar vein, another potential progressor agent, ionizing radiation, enhances metastatic growth in a variety of different experimental systems, although the occurrence of such a phenomenon in the human has not been completely substantiated (cf. von Essen, 1991). As suggested from the earlier discussion of specific sequences in a variety of cell adhesion molecules and especially potential ligands for integrins and other cellular receptors, congeners of the tripeptide RGD generally inhibit the development of metastases in experimental systems. These effects presumably occur within the docking and locking pathway depicted in Figure 10.10. Interestingly, a synthetic peptide of 19 amino acids from the sequence of the A chain of laminin increases experimental metastasis in the murine melanoma system (Kanemoto et al., 1990). In an interesting report, Malins et al. (1996) presented data indicating that a greater than twofold increase in hydroxyl radical damage occurred in metastatic tumor DNA as compared with nonmetastatic tumor DNA.

From these few examples it is apparent that the development of metastases from a primary neoplasm is a very complex phenomenon both anatomically and at the cell and molecular levels. Although successful metastatic growth occurring clonally is a statistically uncommon phenomenon in an animal bearing a primary neoplasm, it actually takes only a single successful metastatic lesion to drastically worsen the prognosis of an individual with the disease. As discussed in Chapter 20, the primary difficulty in cancer therapy is the successful elimination of metastases, either by removal of the primary lesion before metastatic growth occurs or by some form of chemotherapy to curtail and ultimately eliminate the growth and spread of metastases.

The Dormancy of Neoplasia

Clinicians have known for some time that certain neoplasms may remain in the organism for many years without expressing their malignancy to any significant degree (cf. Berg et al., 1971).

An anatomical structure once known as the lateral aberrant thyroid has, in retrospect, been shown in many cases to be a very slowly growing metastatic carcinoma of the thyroid (Black, 1948). These tumors may remain in the host for decades, exhibiting little if any of their lethal potential (Seigal and Modan, 1981). Similar latent lesions of mammary glands may occur in association with carcinoma of the breast (Jensen et al., 1976). Such latent neoplastic cells are not to be confused with the recently termed "minimal residual disease," which occurs in both leukemias (Coustan-Smith et al., 1998) and carcinomas (Lindemann et al., 1992). Newer methods of molecular biology have allowed the detection of minimal residual disease at the cellular level by a variety of techniques involving the detection of specific nucleic acids and proteins (Hirsch-Ginsberg, 1998).

Fisher and Fisher (1959) demonstrated dormancy in tumor cells in an experiment in which more than 100 rats were inoculated with 50 cells of a highly malignant neoplasm. When the animals were left alone for 20 weeks, they did not show any clinical signs of the presence of malignant cells. However, when a surgical laparotomy was performed, this procedure alone was sufficient to stimulate malignant growth, with subsequent lethal consequences in all the operated animals, even when the inoculated cells had remained dormant in the animal for 3 months. The mechanism(s) for such an effect is still not clear, but recently Holmgren and associates (1995) demonstrated that when angiogenesis is inhibited (Chapter 18), lung micrometastases will remain dormant in mice until relief of the angiogenesis inhibition. In this case, neoplastic cells of the dormant micrometastases exhibited a greater than threefold higher incidence of apoptosis than those in metastases growing in animals not subjected to angiogenesis suppression. Another potential mechanism for this effect was suggested by Kodama and associates (1992), who found that experimental pulmonary metastases were facilitated in mice by hydrocortisone pretreatment, which they suggested as a substitute for the surgical stress that occurred in the Fisher and Fisher experiment. In any event, this experiment clearly demonstrates that neoplastic cells in the stage of progression, having already metastasized, may remain dormant in the host until some alteration within the internal environment of the host occurs, allowing such cells to continue their natural development in the stage of progression and leading ultimately to the destruction of the host. This critical interaction between the host and the neoplasm is discussed further in Chapters 17, 18, and 19.

THE REGRESSION OF NEOPLASIA

Experimental oncologists have known for years that some neoplasms may regress in vivo. This regression may be seen readily in tumors transplanted into new hosts. The host recognizes the tumor as foreign tissue and thus tends to reject it immunologically. In the human, examples of tumor regression are quite rare and many such examples may be explained on the basis of host immunity to the neoplasm, although in some instances such a mechanism may not explain the peculiar behavior of the neoplasm (O'Regan and Hirshberg, 1993). This is particularly true when certain types of neoplasms appear to differentiate into adult benign tissues after initially having demonstrated their malignant potential both morphologically and biologically (cf. Bolande, 1985). The mechanism for this phenomenon has not yet been explained, but it is unlikely that it is mutational. One of the earliest examples of a "controlled" reversion of differentiation of a neoplasm to normal tissue is seen in the plant. The crown gall tumors briefly discussed in Chapter 4 and several other plant neoplasms (including a teratoma) can, under controlled conditions, differentiate and produce a normal plant (Braun, 1972; Sacristán and Melchers, 1977). However, studies by Braun and Wood (1976) demonstrated that the differentiation of neoplastic plant cells to a normal phenotype may occur without the loss of the Ti-plasmid (Chapter 4), so that, under appropriate conditions such as those seen in cell culture, these cells will again express their neoplastic phenotype. Yang et al. (1980) have also shown that the generation of normal-appearing plants from a number of crown gall neoplasms is accompanied by the loss of Ti-plasmid sequences in the plant DNA; this indicates the necessity of the plasmid for the maintenance of the transformed state in vivo. Thus, the mechanism of the reversion of plant neoplasms to a normal phenotype may reflect changes in the genetic apparatus of the cell, including loss of oncogenic sequences (Yang et al., 1980) or changes in methylation of DNA, both mechanisms resulting in changes in the cellular production of auxins or plant hormones. Neoplastic plant cells are capable of producing their own supply of auxins, while nonneoplastic cells require exogenous sources of these regulatory substances (cf. Syôno and Fujita, 1994).

There have been a number of examples of regression resulting from differentiation of neoplastic cells of both benign and malignant neoplasms in experimental animals. Seilern-Aspang and Kratochwil (1962) demonstrated that carcinogen-induced epidermoid carcinoma in the newt in many instances will differentiate to normal-appearing cells, which ultimately disappear from the organism. Cooper and Pinkus (1977) have demonstrated that the intrauterine transplantation of basal cell carcinomas in the rat causes such cells to differentiate into keratinizing foci and cysts, with eventual complete loss of the malignant phenotype. Pierce (1974) was among the first to emphasize that both benign and malignant neoplasms commonly exhibited the capability for differentiation even to the point of terminal cell types incapable of further replication. As described in Chapter 5, Stewart and Mintz (1981), Papaioannou et al. (1975), Rossant and McBurney (1983), and others have demonstrated the differentiative capabilities of teratocarcinoma cells by their inoculation into developing blastocysts of genetically distinct animals, with subsequent development of chimeras composed of cells of both teratocarcinoma and host lineage, all of which exhibit a normal phenotype. Even in the adult, neoplastic cells may colonize their tissue of origin and differentiate morphologically into their normal adult counterpart, e.g., rat hepatocytes (Coleman et al., 1993). The induction of differentiation of neoplasms by chemicals is now a well-known phenomenon, usually occurring most readily in vitro (Freshney, 1985; Chapter 14). Such chemical induction of differentiation has been studied most extensively in hematopoietic and lymphoid tissues both in humans and experimental animals (Sachs, 1993). The potential for therapeutic intervention in neoplasia has even been realized in a few diseases, such as acute promyelocytic leukemia (Chapter 6; Breitman et al., 1994).

In the human, neuroblastoma of childhood, which in most cases is highly malignant and derived from neuroblasts of the adrenal medulla, may in a small percentage (about 7%) of all cases spontaneously regress either by differentiation to a benign ganglioneuroma or by disappearance of the neuroblastoma cell (Pahlman and Grotte, 1982). Evans (1982) has pointed out that it is mainly infants with an early stage of the disease who survive. In particular, almost 90% of patients exhibiting the clinical picture of a stage IV-S (De Bernardi et al., 1992) neuroblastoma survive free of their neoplasm with little or no therapeutic intervention. Spontaneous differentiation of neuroblastomas both in vivo and in vitro has been described both with and without treatment (Evans et al., 1976). A histologically related neoplasm, retinoblastoma, may also undergo spontaneous regression even in patients with the genotype for this disease (Gallie et al., 1982). Bolande (1985) has pointed out the potential significance of the regression, especially by the process of differentiation, of several types of malignant neoplasms in early life in the human, suggesting that specific repressive influences or factors of the internal environment may exert effects on neoplasms similar to those seen in the teratocarcinoma chimeras (see above).

A number of other rather common neoplasms in the adult human have been shown to regress spontaneously in rare instances (cf. Lewison, 1976). In the human, many primary lesions of malignant melanoma regress, reportedly as high as almost 60% (McGovern et al., 1983). However, the prognosis in patients with regressing primaries is usually less favorable than in those where no regression of the primary lesion is seen. Prehn (1996) has suggested that the reason for this is that the regression is the result of a relatively strong immune reaction, but that surviving neoplastic cells are more aggressive. However, Kelly et al. (1985) found no difference in prognosis between melanomas exhibiting regression and those that did not show such an effect. Interestingly, in miniature swine, regression of spontaneous melanoma occurs with nearly a 100% incidence (Oxenhandler et al., 1982). An interesting phenomenon has been described for renal cell carcinomas, in that removal of the primary tumor may lead to disappearance of pulmonary metastases (Markewitz et al., 1967; Fujita et al., 1988; Vogelzang et al., 1992). In addition, several isolated cases of spontaneous regression of hepatocellular carcinomas have been reported (cf. Kaczynski et al., 1998). In the special case of the chorionepithelioma, a malignant neoplasm of the placenta, spontaneous regression may be accounted for by host immunity, as the tumor tissue is actually foreign to the maternal immune system. In the male, a morphologically similar neoplasm that may arise from host tissues does not regress spontaneously.

The reader should keep in mind that spontaneous regressions of neoplasms in the human are exceedingly rare. However, the spontaneous regression of neoplasia in the human is now a well-documented albeit very sporadic phenomenon (Challis and Stam, 1990). A variety of theoretical mechanisms have been proposed to explain such occurrences (Stoll, 1992; Noda, 1993), including alterations in signal transduction, cell adhesion, and immunological, hormonal, and even "psychoneuroimmunological" mechanisms. With a few exceptions of demonstrable enhancement of immunological responses to specific neoplasms and the direct effect of chemicals on specific genes to induce differentiation, no satisfactory explanation has been forthcoming in cases where the diagnosis is clear. In the human, there have been at least two examples in which regression of neoplasms is a demonstrable component of their natural history. These include basal cell carcinoma (Curson and Weedon, 1979; Hunt et al., 1994) and intraepithelial neoplasia (carcinoma in situ) of the uterine cervix (Hanselaar et al., 1998). Differentiation of neoplastic cells, both in the human and in lower animals, has been described repeatedly, although in the vast majority of cases only a portion of the total neoplastic cell population differentiates to the terminal state. In some cases, differentiation, especially in lymphoid neoplasms, may result in a more malignant neoplasm (cf. Lynch, 1995). As discussed earlier (Chapter 7), preneoplastic lesions in the absence of promoting agents naturally regress, primarily through the mechanism of apoptosis. Regression of cells in the stage of progression, however, appears to use more varied mechanisms. The natural history of neoplastic development must take into account the potential for regression or differentiation of established neoplasms. Such considerations may alter our earlier considerations (Chapter 2) of the arbitrary nature of distinguishing benign from malignant neoplasms when viewed as dynamic processes traversing the stages of promotion and progression in neoplastic development. At least theoretically, some benign neoplasms may, in essence, be differentiated cell populations (such as the ganglioneuroma resulting from differentiation of the neuroblastoma) and thus will never develop beyond that stage. On the other hand, some lesions considered benign neoplasms may be cells in the stage of promotion, reflecting preneoplastic lesions (e.g., hepatic adenomas in patients receiving synthetic estrogens; Chapter 7). Unfortunately, it is not possible by means of histopathology to distinguish readily between benign neoplasms with the potential for progression to malignancy and those resulting from the differentiation of neoplastic cells. Further studies at the molecular level may allow a more definitive distinction.

Predicting the Stage of Progression—Prognosis

A patient always wants to know the outcome of his or her disease, whether treated or untreated. This desire is critical in patients suffering from cancer, both before and after treatment. Thus, a variety of biological, cellular, and molecular features of neoplastic development in the human have been studied, so that the patient may be informed of the most probable outcome of the disease with the greatest degree of accuracy. At the cellular level, malignant neoplasms in the human have been divided according to histological grade. The grade of a neoplasm is determined by its degree of anaplasia, both positional and cytological, although the latter characteristic usually predominates in the final determination of the grade of a malignant neoplasm. The grading of neoplasms by the pathologist can be done most easily with certain types of carcinomas, especially epidermoid carcinomas. A grade 1 carcinoma is a highly differentiated, slightly anaplastic carcinoma. At the other extreme, a grade 4 carcinoma is histologically very similar to a carcinosarcoma, a highly malignant, aneuploid, rapidly growing neoplasm. Grades 2 and 3 are intermediate stages, and their designation is obviously somewhat subjective. The histological grading of the tumor is always done by grading the most anaplastic histological areas of the neoplasm. In general, those neoplasms exhibiting lower grades offer the best prognosis, whereas high-grade malignancies offer a poorer prognosis.

In contrast to the histological grading of neoplasms by the pathologist, many histogenetic types of malignant neoplasms in the human have been subjected to the process of *staging* for the purposes of prognosis as well as therapy. The staging of neoplasms has been employed to characterize the lesion's invasive and extensive characteristics. For example, in the case of carcinoma of the cervix, a stage zero tumor would be a carcinoma in situ. Carcinoma in situ, of course, would not have invaded deeply into the cervix, although it might have invaded into the surrounding epithelium. Such intraepithelial invasion may also be seen in Paget disease of the nipple, which heralds a malignant neoplasm of the breast. One of the earlier examples of tumor staging was that of invasive cervical carcinoma. This scheme depended on whether the tumor was confined to the uterus (stage I), extended into neighboring regions such as the vagina and uterine ligaments (stage II), or showed distant metastases (stage III). The efficacy of therapy of a neoplasm will vary depending on the stage at which the neoplasm is first treated. However, in order to compare treatment regimens as to their effectiveness, it is important for the physician to make such comparisons at a specific stage.

The International Union Against Cancer in cooperation with the World Health Organization has recently devised a general method for the clinical staging or description of the extent of neoplastic disease in the human patient. This system has been termed the TNM system (Sobin et al., 1988). In general, it identifies the extent of disease by the use of three symbols:

T = extent of primary neoplasm
N = condition of regional lymph nodes
M = distant metastases

A typical example of such a classification is seen in Table 10.6. This system, unlike attempts to standardize the histological classification of neoplasms, has enjoyed general acceptance, with modifications necessitated by the histological type of neoplasm by most of the international medical community. It is already being used extensively for malignant neoplasms of the breast, oral cavity, urinary bladder, lung, and other organs. Besides the obvious significance of staging in relation to the medical prognosis of the disease itself, staging has found extensive usefulness in the therapy and management of various types of malignant neoplasms. One of the best examples of this is the complicated staging of Hodgkin disease, a specific type of malignant lymphoma seen in the human. The method of staging used for this disease is more complicated than

Table 10.6   TNM System of Clinical Staging of Neoplasia

Neoplasm	
T0	No evidence of primary tumor
TIS	Carcinoma in situ
T1, T2, T3, T4	Progressive increase in tumor size and involvement
TX	Tumor cannot be assessed
Nodes	
N0	Regional lymph nodes not demonstrably abnormal
N1, N2, N3, etc.	Increasing degrees of demonstrable abnormality of regional lymph nodes. (For many primary sites the subscript "a," e.g., $N1_a$, may be used to indicate that metastasis to the node is not suspected; and the subscript "b," e.g., $N1_b$, may be used to indicate that metastasis to the node is suspected or proved.)
NX	Regional lymph nodes cannot be assessed clinically
Metastasis	
M0	No evidence of distant metastasis
M1, M2, M3	Ascending degrees of distant metastasis, including metastasis to distant lymph nodes

the simple TNM system. Definitive therapy for each stage of the disease has now been designed and has resulted in cure rates for this neoplasm exceeding 90% (Moormeier et al., 1989).

With the refinement of cellular and molecular techniques, a variety of prognostic indicators have now been developed and are being employed more frequently, together with grading and staging, in the prognosis of neoplasia. Table 10.7 lists a variety of genetic alterations seen in neoplasms in relation to their predictive effectiveness in the prognosis of specific neoplasms. As noted in the table and as expected, both mutations and amplification or overexpression of proto-oncogenes and tumor suppressor genes result in a poorer prognosis. The fact that mutation in the p53 tumor suppressor gene in patients with colon carcinoma already exhibiting metastases indicates a more favorable response might suggest that such cells are more sensitive to some of the

Table 10.7   Molecular Indicators of Prognosis of Neoplasia

Neoplasm	Alteration	Prognostic Description	Reference
Breast	Mutant p53 expression	Poor	Allred et al., 1993
	c-*erb*B-2 amplification	Poor	Paterson et al., 1991
	int-2 amplification	Poor	Henry et al., 1993
Colon with metastases	Mutant p53 expression	Favorable	Belluco et al., 1996
Gastric	c-*erb*-2 overexpression	Poor	Yonemura et al., 1991
Liver	c-*myc* amplification	Poor	Abou-Elella et al., 1996
Lung	K-*ras* mutations	Poor	Mitsudomi et al., 1991
Non–small cell			Vega et al., 1996
Lymphoma			
B cell	p53 mutations	Poor	Ichikawa et al., 1997
Diffuse large cell	*bcl*-6 rearrangement	Favorable	Offit et al., 1994
Neuroblastoma	N-*myc* amplification	Poor	Bowman et al., 1997
	TRK overexpression	Favorable	Nakagawara et al., 1993

chemotherapeutic regimens utilized. The *bcl*-6 proto-oncogene is structurally related to a class of transcription factors involved in the regulation of cell proliferation, differentiation, and organ formation (cf. Offit et al., 1994). The TRK proto-oncogene is one component of the high-affinity nerve growth factor receptor in neuronal cells (cf. Nakagawara et al., 1993). However, it is difficult to explain the favorable prognostic features that result from rearrangement or overexpression of these two proto-oncogenes.

Not appreciated from the table is the growing evidence that multiple alterations in molecular species such as those depicted in Table 10.7 within the same cell almost always indicate a less favorable prognosis (Zheng et al., 1991; Henry et al., 1993). Again, this is to be expected, as karyotypic instability leads both to the selection of altered genotypes and the further amplification of a variety of proto-oncogenes. As yet, however, these molecular prognosticators (Table 10.7) are only a research tool. Not until many more analyses have been carried out on numerous patients with a variety of different neoplasms will it be possible to add molecular indicators of prognosis to the classical grading and staging methods that are in primary use today.

THE NATURAL HISTORY OF NEOPLASTIC DEVELOPMENT—A SUMMARY

Figure 10.14 presents a diagram of the natural history of neoplasia as the student may perceive it, beginning with the process of initiation, extending through the reversible promotion of the initiated cell to a visible tumor, followed by the natural progression of this tumor into a benign neoplasm and the ultimate expression of malignancy, that of distant metastases. At the bottom of the figure is the concomitant relationship of the cellular karyotype extending throughout this process. Exactly where in this scheme the progeny of initiated cells begin to exhibit the karyotypic abnormalities characteristic of the stage of progression will depend on the tissue of origin, the dose of the carcinogenic agent, and the rate of cell proliferation in the preneoplastic stages. Furthermore, it is important to remember that, although this diagram indicates the monoclonality of neoplasms, multiclonal neoplasms may well follow the same natural history, although in a somewhat more complicated manner, such as the coalescence of multiple clones during the stage of progression. The diagram does not show the potential for regression or dormancy during the stage of progression but rather represents the primary pathway of neoplastic development.

It should also be realized that not every neoplastic cell resulting from the transformation of a normal cell must follow this entire series of stages. Thus, complete carcinogens at very high doses may result in aneuploid neoplastic cellular populations on initial administration, such that the stages of initiation and promotion as defined in this text are bypassed. However, the development of the greater majority of human neoplasms is likely to progress through the natural history depicted in Figure 10.14.

An understanding of the natural history of neoplastic development is essential to our understanding of the mechanisms involved in the induction of neoplasia by chemical, physical, and biological agents as well as genetic factors. Table 9.10 gives a mechanistic classification of carcinogens as related to their specific actions during the individual stages of carcinogenesis. It is obvious from this classification that some chemicals may possess two of the classifications, such as promotion and progression or initiation and progression. It is, however, important to note that in this classification a complete carcinogen must have exhibited the capability of possessing initiating, promoting, and progressing capabilities by definition. The importance of this classification should be obvious to the student by now in that promoting agents given chronically over a long period of time, acting on spontaneously initiated cells, may mimic complete carcinogens and be classified as such in the absence of detailed mechanistic studies. On the other hand, progressor agents that truly do not have initiating capabilities would be dependent on their "com-

THE NATURAL HISTORY OF NEOPLASIA

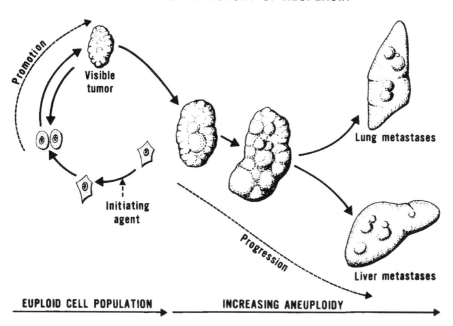

Figure 10.14   The natural history of neoplasia, beginning with the initiated cell after application of an initiating agent (carcinogen) followed by the potentially reversible stage of promotion to a visible tumor, with subsequent progression of this tumor to malignancy. The relation to karyotype is presented as a generalization on the lower arrows. The reader should again be cautioned that not all neoplastic cells undergo this entire natural history. It is theoretically possible, although this has not yet been definitively shown, that some neoplasms, such as those induced in animals by radiation or high doses of chemical carcinogens, may enter this sequence in the stage of progression, exhibiting aneuploidy, and thus bypass the early euploid cell stages.

plete carcinogenic" effects in the presence of promoted clones of cells. Since spontaneous promotion clearly occurs but takes considerable time in order to produce significant lesions, environmental progressor agents may be more carcinogenic in older individuals. Thus, an understanding of the mechanistic classification of carcinogens will lead not only to a better understanding of the mechanism of action of specific carcinogenic agents but also to an improvement in the modalities of both cancer prevention and cancer therapy.

REFERENCES

Aberle, H., Schwartz, H., and Kemler, R. Cadherin-catenin complex: protein interactions and their implications for cadherin function. J. Cell. Biochem., *61*:514–523, 1996.

Abou-Elella, A., Gramlich, T., Fritsch, C., and Gansler, T. c-*myc* amplification in hepatocellular carcinoma predicts unfavorable prognosis. Mod. Pathol., *9*:95–98, 1996.

Albores-Saavedra, H. The Pathology of Incipient Neoplasia. Philadelphia: Saunders, 1986.

Allred, D. G., Clark, G. M., Elledge, R., Fuqua, S. A. W., Brown, R. W., Chamness, G. C., Osborne, C. K., and McGuire, W. L. Association of p53 protein expression with tumor cell proliferation rate and clinical outcome in node-negative breast cancer. J. Natl. Cancer Inst., *85*:200–206, 1993.

Alvord, E. C., Jr. Why do gliomas not metastasize? Arch. Neurol., *33*:73, 1976.

Aznavoorian, S., Murphy, A. N., Stetler-Stevenson, W. G., and Liotta, L. A. Molecular aspects of tumor cell invasion and metastasis. Cancer, *71*:1368–1383, 1993.

Baisch, H., Collard, J., Zywietz, F., and Jung, H. No acquisition of metastatic capacity of R1H rhabdomyo-sarcoma upon transfection with c-Ha-*ras* oncogene. Invasion Metastasis, *10*:193–207, 1990.

Bardwell, L. The mutagenic and carcinogenic effects of gene transfer. Mutagenesis, *4*:245–253, 1989.

Barsky, S. H., Grossman, D. A., Ho, J., and Holmes, E. C. The multifocality of bronchioloalveolar lung carcinoma: evidence and implications of a multiclonal origin. Mod. Pathol., *7*:633–640, 1994.

Baylin, S. B., Hsu, S. H., Gann, D. S., Smallridge, R. C., and Wells, S. A., Jr. Inherited medullary thyroid carcinoma: a final monoclonal mutation in one of multiple clones of susceptible cells. Science, *199*:429–431, 1978.

Belluco, C., Guillem, J. G., Kemeny, N., Huang, Y., Klimstra, D., Berger, M. F., and Cohen, A. M. p53 Nuclear protein overexpression in colorectal cancer: a dominant predictor of survival in patients with advanced hepatic metastases. J. Clin. Oncol., *14*:2696–2701, 1996.

Benditt, E. P. Evidence for a monoclonal origin of human atherosclerotic plaques and some implications. Circulation, *50*:650–652, 1974.

Berg, J. W., Hajdu, S. I., and Foote, F. W. The prevalence of latent cancers in cancer patients. Arch. Pathol., *91*:183, 1971.

Berx, G., Cleton-Jansen, A.-M., Strumane, K., de Leeuw, W. J. F., Nollet, F., van Roy, F., and Cornelisse, C. E-cadherin is inactivated in a majority of invasive human lobular breast cancers by truncation mutations throughout its extracellular domain. Oncogene, *13*:1919–1925, 1996.

Bevilacqua, G., Sobel, M. E., Liotta, L. A., and Steeg, P. S. Association of low *nm23* RNA levels in human primary infiltrating ductal breast carcinomas with lymph node involvement and other histopatholog-ical indicators of high metastatic potential. Cancer Res., *49*:5185–5190, 1989.

Biggs, J., Hersperger, E., Steeg, P. S., Liotta, L. A., and Shearn, A. A *Drosophila* gene that is homologous to a mammalian gene associated with tumor metastasis codes for a nucleoside diphosphate kinase. Cell, *63*:933–940, 1990.

Bignon, Y.-J., Souteyrand, P., Roger, H., Fonck, Y., Bernard, D., Chassagne, J., Ramos, F., D'Incan, M., Chollet, P., Dastugue, B., and Plagne, R. Clonotypic heterogeneity in cutaneous T-cell lymphomas. Cancer Res., *50*:6620–6625, 1990.

Bishop, M. B., and Lansing, L. S. The spleen: a correlative overview of normal and pathologic anatomy. Hum. Pathol., *13*:334–342, 1982.

Black, B. M. Papillary adenocarcinoma of the thyroid gland, so-called lateral aberrant thyroid tumors. West. J. Surg., *56*:134–144, 1948.

Bolande, R. P. Spontaneous regression and cytodifferentiation of cancer in early life: the oncogenic grace period. Surv. Synth. Pathol. Res., *4*:296–311, 1985.

Bowman, L. C., Castleberry, R. P., Cantor, A., Joshi, V., Cohn, S. L., Smith, E. I., Yu, A., Brodeur, G. M., Hayes, F. A., and Look, A. T. Genetic staging of unresectable or metastatic neuroblastoma in infants: a pediatric oncology group study. J. Natl. Cancer Inst., *89*:373–380, 1997.

Braun, A. C. The relevance of plant tumor systems to an understanding of the basic cellular mechanisms underlying tumorigenesis. Prog. Exp. Tumor Res., *15*:165–187, 1972.

Braun, A. C., and Wood, H. N. Suppression of the neoplastic state with the acquisition of specialized func-tions in cells, tissues, and organs of crown gall teratomas of tobacco. Proc. Natl. Acad. Sci. U.S.A., *73*:496–500, 1976.

Breitman, T. R., Chen, Z.-X., and Takahashi, N. Potential applications of cytodifferentiation therapy in he-matologic malignancies. Semin. Hematol., *31*:18–25, 1994.

Burger, M. M., Tao, T. W., Finne, J., and Prieels, J.-P. The influence of membrane mutations on metastasis. Biosci. Rep., *2*:597–599, 1982.

Burridge, K., Chrzanowska-Wodnicka, M., and Zhong, C. Focal adhesion assembly. Trends Cell Biol., *7*:342–347, 1997.

Cady, B. Lymph node metastases. Arch. Surg., *119*:1067–1072, 1984.

Carr, N. J., and Turk, E. P. The histological features of splenosis. Histopathology, *21*:549–553, 1992.

Chackal-Roy, M., Niemeyer, C., Moore, M., and Zetter, B. R. Stimulation of human prostatic carcinoma cell growth by factors present in human bone marrow. J. Clin. Invest., *84*:43–50, 1989.

Challis, G. B., and Stam, H. J. The spontaneous regression of cancer. A review of cases from 1900 to 1987. Acta Oncol., *29*:545–550, 1990.

Chambers, A. F., and Matrisian, L. M. Changing views of the role of matrix metalloproteinases in metastasis. J. Natl. Cancer Inst., *89*:1260–1270, 1997.

Chen, Y. Q., Liu, B., Tang, D. G., and Honn, K. V. Fatty acid modulation of tumor cell-platelet-vessel wall interaction. Cancer Metastasis Rev., *11*:389–410, 1992.

Cheng, L., Song, S.-Y., Pretlow, T. G., Abdul-Karim, F. W., Kung, H.-J., Dawson, D. V., Park, W.-S., Moon, Y.-W., Tsai, M.-L., Linehan, W. M., Emmert-Buck, M. R., Liotta, L. A., and Zhuang, Z. Evidence of independent origin of multiple tumors from patients with prostate cancer. J. Natl. Cancer Inst., *90*:233–237, 1998.

Chow, M., and Rubin, H. Coculturing diverse clonal populations prevents the early-stage neoplastic progression that occurs in the separate clones. Proc. Natl. Acad. Sci. U.S.A., *97*:174–178, 2000.

Cifone, M. A., and Fidler, I. J. Increasing metastatic potential is associated with increasing genetic instability of clones isolated from murine neoplasms. Proc. Natl. Acad. Sci. U.S.A., *78*:6949–6952, 1981.

Clark, E. A., and Brugge, J. S. Integrins and signal transduction pathways: the road taken. Science, *268*:233–238, 1995.

Coleman, W. B., Wennerberg, A. E., Smith, G. J., and Grisham, J. W. Regulation of the differentiation of diploid and some aneuploid rat liver epithelial (stemlike) cells by the hepatic microenvironment. Am. J. Pathol., *142*:1373–1382, 1993.

Collins, R. D. Is clonality equivalent to malignancy: specifically, is immunoglobulin gene rearrangement diagnostic of malignant lymphoma? Hum. Pathol., *28*:757–759, 1997.

Collins, S. J., and Fialkow, P. J. Clonal nature of spontaneous AKR leukemia: studies utilizing the X-linked enzyme phosphoglycerate kinase. Int. J. Cancer, *29*:673–676, 1982.

Condamine, H., Custer, R. P., and Mintz, B. Pure-strain and genetically mosaic liver tumors histochemically identified with the β-glucuronidase marker in allophenic mice. Proc. Natl. Acad. Sci. U.S.A., *68*:2032–2036, 1971.

Cooper, D. L., and Dougherty, G. J. To metastasize or not? Selection of CD44 splice sites. Nature Med., *1*:635–637, 1995.

Cooper, M., and Pinkus, H. Intrauterine transplantation of rat basal cell carcinoma as a model for reconversion of malignant to benign growth. Cancer Res., *37*:2544–2552, 1977.

Coustan-Smith, E., Behm, F. G., Sanchez, J., Boyett, J. M., Hancock, M. L., Raimondi, S. C., Rubnitz, J. E., Rivera, G. K., Sandlund, J. T., Pui, C.-H., and Campana, D. Immunological detection of minimal residual disease in children with acute lymphoblastic leukaemia. Lancet, *351*:550–554, 1998.

Curson, C., and Weedon, D. Spontaneous regression in basal cell carcinomas. J. Cutan. Pathol., *6*:432–437, 1979.

Davie, E. W., Fujikawa, K., and Kisiel, W. The coagulation cascade: initiation, maintenance, and regulation. Biochemistry, *30*:10363–10370, 1991.

Deamant, F. D., and Iannaccone, P. M. Clonal origin of chemically induced papillomas: separate analysis of epidermal and dermal components. J. Cell Sci., *88*:305–312, 1987.

De Bernardi, B., Pianca, C., Boni, L., Brisigotti, M., Carli, M., Bagnulo, S., Corciulo, P., Mancini, A., De Laurentis, C., Di Tullio, M. T., Cordero di Montezemolo, L., Lanino, E., Clerico, A., Rogers, D. W., and Bruzzi, P. Disseminated neuroblastoma (stage IV and IV-S) in the first year of life. Cancer, *70*:1625–1633, 1992.

Dedhar, S. Integrins and tumor invasion. Bioessays, *12*:583–590, 1990.

Denis, M. G., Lipart, C., LeBorgne, J., LeHur, P.-A., Galmiche, J.-P., Denis, M., Ruud, E., Truchaud, A., and Lustenberger, P. Detection of disseminated tumor cells in peripheral blood of colorectal cancer patients. Int. J. Cancer, *74*:540–544, 1997.

Dennis, J. W., and Laferte, S. Tumor cell surface carbohydrate and the metastatic phenotype. Cancer Metastasis Rev., *5*:185–204, 1987.

Donovan-Peluso, M., Contento, A. M., Tobon, H., Ripepi, B., and Locker, J. Oncogene amplification in breast cancer. Am. J. Pathol., *138*:835–845, 1991.

Duffy, M. J. Urokinase-type plasminogen activator and malignancy. Fibrinolysis, *7*:295–302, 1993.

Dunnington, D. J., Kim, U., Hughes, C. M., Monaghan, P., and Rudland, P. S. Lack of production of myo-epithelial variants by cloned epithelial cell lines derived from the TMT-081 metastasizing rat mammary tumor. Cancer Res., *44*:5338–5346, 1984.

Ebralidze, A., Tulchinsky, E., Grigorian, M., Afanasyeva, A., Senin, V., Revazova, E., and Lukanidin, E. Isolation and characterization of a gene specifically expressed in different metastatic cells and whose deduced gene product has a high degree of homology to a Ca^{2+}-binding protein family. Genes Dev., *3*:1086–1093, 1989.

Edward, M., and MacKie, R. M. Retinoic acid-induced inhibition of lung colonization and changes in the synthesis and properties of glycosaminoglycans of metastatic B16 melanoma cells. J. Cell Sci., *94*:537–543, 1989.

Egan, S. E., Wright, J. A., Jarolim, L., Yanagihara, K., Bassin, R. H., and Greenberg, A. H. Transformation by oncogenes encoding protein kinases induces the metastatic phenotype. Science, *238*:202–204, 1987.

Elangbam, C. S., Qualls Jr., C. W., and Dahlgren, R. R. Cell adhesion molecules—update. Vet. Pathol., *34*:61–73, 1997.

Enomoto, T., Haba, T., Fujita, M., Hamada, T., Yoshino, K., Nakashima, R., Wada, H., Kurachi, H., Wakasa, K., Sakurai, M., Murata, Y., and Shroyer, K. R. Clonal analysis of high-grade squamous intra-epithelial lesions of the uterine cervix. Int. J. Cancer, *73*:339–344, 1997.

Erickson, K. L., and Hubbard, N. E. Dietary fat and tumor metastasis. Nutr. Rev., *48*:6–14, 1990.

Evans, A. E. Neuroblastoma: diagnosis and management. Curr. Concepts Oncol., *4*:10–20, 1982.

Evans, A. E., Gerson, J., and Schnaufer, L. Spontaneous regression of neuroblastoma. Natl. Cancer Inst. Monogr., *44*:49–54, 1976.

Faull, R. J. Adhesion molecules in health and disease. Aust. N.Z. J. Med., *25*:720–730, 1995.

Fey, M. F., and Tobler, A. Tumour heterogeneity and clonality—an old theme revisited. Ann. Oncol., *7*:121–128, 1996.

Fialkow, P. J. The origin and development of human tumors studied with cell markers. N. Engl. J. Med., *291*:26–35, 1974.

Fialkow, P. J. Clonal origin of human tumors. Biochim. Biophys. Acta, *458*:283–321, 1976.

Fidler, I. J., Gersten, D. M., and Hart, I. R. The biology of cancer invasion and metastasis. Adv. Cancer Res., *28*:149–250, 1978.

Fish, E. M., and Molitoris, B. A. Mechanisms of disease. N. Engl. J. Med., *330*:1580–1588, 1994.

Fisher, B., and Fisher, E. R. Experimental evidence in support of the dormant tumor cell. Science, *130*:918–919, 1959.

Fisher, B., and Fisher, E. R. The interrelationship of hematogenous and lymphatic tumor cell dissemination. Surg. Gynecol. Obstet., *122*:791–797, 1966.

Fisher, B., and Fisher, E. R. Barrier function of lymph node to tumor cells and erythrocytes. II. Effect of x-ray, inflammation, sensitization and tumor growth. Cancer, *20*:1914–1919, 1967.

Fisher, B., Fisher, E. R., and Feduska, N. Trauma and the localization of tumor cells. Cancer, *20*:23–30, 1967.

Fishman, A. P. Endothelium: a distributed organ of diverse capabilities. Ann. N.Y. Acad. Sci., *401*:1–8, 1982.

Freshney, R. I. Induction of differentiation in neoplastic cells. Anticancer Res., *5*:111–130, 1985.

Frost, P., Kerbel, R. S., Hunt, B., Man, S., and Pathak, S. Selection of metastatic variants with identifiable karyotypic changes from a nonmetastatic murine tumor after treatment with 2′-deoxy-5-azacytidine or hydroxyurea: implications for the mechanisms of tumor progression. Cancer Res., *47*:2690–2695, 1987.

Fujita, K., Kawamura, M., Murayama, T., and Narita, K. Complete remission of pulmonary metastases from renal cancer. Int. J. Immunother., *4*:57–61, 1988.

Gallie, B. L., Ellsworth, R. M., Abramson, D. H., and Phillips, R. A. Retinoma: spontaneous regression of retinoblastoma or benign manifestation of the mutation? Br. J. Cancer, *45*:513–521, 1982.

Garbisa, S., Pozzatti, R., Muschel, R. J., Saffiotti, U., Ballin, M., Goldfarb, R. H., Khoury, G., and Liotta, L. A. Secretion of type IV collagenolytic protease and metastatic phenotype: induction by transfection with c-Ha-*ras* but not c-Ha-*ras* plus Ad2-E1a. Cancer Res., *47*:1523–1528, 1987.

Garrod, D. R. Cell to cell and cell to matrix adhesion. Br. Med. J., *306*:703–705, 1993.

Giaretti, W. Aneuploidy mechanisms in human colorectal preneoplastic lesions and Barrett's esophagus. Is there a role for K-ras and p53 mutations? Anal. Cell. Pathol., *15*:99–117, 1997.

Giavazzi, R., Alessandri, G., Spreafico, F., Garattini, S., and Mantovani, A. Metastasizing capacity of tumour cells from spontaneous metastases of transplanted murine tumours. Br. J. Cancer, *42*:462–470, 1980.

Gilliland, D. G., Blanchard, K. L., Levy, J., Perrin, S., and Bunn, H. F. Clonality in myeloproliferative disorders: analysis by means of the polymerase chain reaction. Proc. Natl. Acad. Sci. U.S.A., *88*:6848–6852, 1991.

Giordano, S., Bardelli, A., Zhen, Z., Menard, S., Ponzetto, C., and Comoglio, P. M. A point mutation in the *MET* oncogene abrogates metastasis without affecting transformation. Proc. Natl. Acad. Sci. U.S.A., *94*:13868–13872, 1997.

Glinsky, G. V., Glinsky, V. V., Ivanova, A. B., and Hueser, C. J. Apoptosis and metastasis: increased apoptosis resistance of metastatic cancer cells is associated with the profound deficiency of apoptosis execution mechanisms. Cancer Lett., *115*:185–193, 1997.

Greenberg, A. H., Egan, S. E., and Wright, J. A. Oncogenes and metastatic progression. Invasion Metastasis, *9*:360–378, 1989.

Greig, R. G., Koestler, T. P., Trainer, D. L., Corwin, S. P., Miles, L., Kline, T., Sweet, R., Yokoyama, S., and Poste, G. Tumorigenic and metastatic properties of "normal" and *ras*-transfected NIH/3T3 cells. Proc. Natl. Acad. Sci. U.S.A., *82*:3698–3701, 1985.

Gumbiner, B. M. Cell adhesion: the molecular basis of tissue architecture and morphogenesis. Cell, *84*:345–357, 1996.

Hanselaar, A. G. J. M., Poulin, N., Pahlplatz, M. M. M., Garner, D., MacAulay, C., Matisic, J., LeRiche, J., and Palcic, B. DNA-cytometry of progressive and regressive cervical intraepithelial neoplasia. Anal. Cell. Pathol., *16*:11–27, 1998.

Harris, J. F., Chambers, A. F., Hill, R. P., and Ling, V. Metastatic variants are generated spontaneously at a high rate in mouse KHT tumor. Proc. Natl. Acad. Sci. U.S.A., *79*:5547–5551, 1982.

Hart, I. R., and Fidler, I. J. The implications of tumor heterogeneity for studies on the biology and therapy of cancer metastasis. Biochim. Biophys. Acta, *651*:37–50, 1981.

Hay, E. D. Extracellular Matrix. *In*: E. D. Hay (Ed.), Cell Biology of the Extracellular Matrix, pp. 1–4. New York: Plenum Press, 1991.

Hendrix, M. J. C., Seftor, E. A., Chu, Y.-W., Seftor, R. E. B., Nagle, R. B., McDaniel, K. M., Leong, S. P. L., Yohem, K. H., Leibovitz, A. M., Meyskens F. L. Jr., Conaway, D. H., Welch, D. R., Liotta, L. A., and Stetler-Stevenson, W. Coexpression of vimentin and keratins by human melanoma tumor cells: correlation with invasive and metastatic potential. J. Natl. Cancer Inst., *84*:165–174, 1992.

Hendrix, M. J. C., Seftor, E. A., Chu, Y.-W., Trevor, K. T., and Seftor, R. E. B. Role of intermediate filaments in migration, invasion and metastasis. Cancer Metastasis Rev., *15*:507–525, 1996.

Henry, J. A., Hennessy, C., Levett, D. L., Lennard, T. W. J., Westley, B. R., and May, F. E. B. *int*-2 Amplification in breast cancer: association with decreased survival and relationship to amplification of c-*erb*B-2 and c-*myc*. Int. J. Cancer, *53*:774–780, 1993.

Heppner, G. H., and Miller, F. R. The cellular basis of tumor progression. Int. Rev. Cytol., *177*:1–56, 1998.

Hirsch-Ginsberg, C. Detection of minimal residual disease: relevance for diagnosis and treatment of human malignancies. Annu. Rev. Med., *49*:111–122, 1998.

Holmgren, L., O'Reilly, M. S., and Folkman, J. Dormancy of micrometastases: balanced proliferation and apoptosis in the presence of angiogenesis suppression. Nature Med., *1*:149–153, 1995.

Honn, K. V., Tang, D. G., and Crissman, J. D. Platelets and cancer metastasis: a causal relationship? Cancer Metastasis Rev., *11*:325–351, 1992.

Honn, K. V., and Tang, D. G. Adhesion molecules and tumor cell interaction with endothelium and subendothelial matrix. Cancer Metastasis Rev., *11*:353–375, 1992.

Hsu, S. H., Luk, G. D., Krush, A. J., Hamilton, S. R., and Hoover, H. H., Jr. Multiclonal origin of polyps in Gardner syndrome. Science, *221*:951–953, 1983.

Humphries, M. J., Olden, K., and Yamada, K. M. A synthetic peptide from fibronectin inhibits experimental metastasis of murine melanoma cells. Science, *233*:467–470, 1986.

Hunt, M. J., Halliday, G. M., Weedon, D., Cooke, B. E., and Barnetson, R.StC. Regression in basal cell carcinoma: an immunohistochemical analysis. Br. J. Dermatol., *130*:1–8, 1994.

Ichikawa, T., Kyprianou, N., and Isaacs, J. T. Genetic instability and the acquisition of metastatic ability by rat mammary cancer cells following v-H-*ras* oncogene transfection. Cancer Res., *50*:6349–6357, 1990.

Ichikawa, T., Ichikawa, Y., and Isaacs, J. T. Genetic factors and suppression of metastatic ability of v-Ha-*ras*-transfected rat mammary cancer cells. Proc. Natl. Acad. Sci. U.S.A., *89*:1607–1610, 1992.

Ichikawa, A., Kinoshita, T., Watanabe, T., Kato, H., Nagai, H., Tsushita, K., Saito, H., and Hotta, T. Mutations of the p53 gene as a prognostic factor in aggressive B-cell lymphoma. N. Engl. J. Med., *337*:529–534, 1997.

Jensen, H. M., Rice, J. R., and Wellings, S. R. Preneoplastic lesions in the human breast. Science, *191*:295–297, 1976.

Juliano, R. L. The role of β_1 integrins in tumors. Cancer Biol., *4*:277–283, 1993.

Kaczynski, J., Hansson, G., Remotti, H., and Wallerstedt, S. Spontaneous regression of hepatocellular carcinoma. Histopathology, *32*:147–150, 1998.

Kanemoto, T., Reich, R., Royce, L., Greatorex, D., Adler, S. H., Shiraishi, N., Martin, G. R., Yamada, Y., and Kleinman, H. K. Identification of an amino acid sequence from the laminin A chain that stimulates metastasis and collagenase IV production. Proc. Natl. Acad. Sci. U.S.A., *87*:2279–2283, 1990.

Kannagi, R. Carbohydrate-mediated cell adhesion involved in hematogenous metastasis of cancer. Glycoconj. J., *14*:577–584, 1997.

Kawashima, K., Shikama, H., Imoto, K., Izawa, M., Naruke, T., Okabayashi, K., and Nishimura, S. Close correlation between restriction fragment length polymorphism of the L-*MYC* gene and metastasis of human lung cancer to the lymph nodes and other organs. Proc. Natl. Acad. Sci. U.S.A., *85*:2353–2356, 1988.

Kelly, J. W., Sagebiel, R. W., and Blois, M. S. Regression in malignant melanoma. A histologic feature without independent prognostic significance. Cancer, *56*:2287–2291, 1985.

Kerbel, R. S., Waghorne, C., Man, M. S., Elliott, B., and Breitman, M. L. Alteration of the tumorigenic and metastatic properties of neoplastic cells is associated with the process of calcium phosphate-mediated DNA transfection. Proc. Natl. Acad. Sci. U.S.A., *84*:1263–1267, 1987.

Kjellén, L., and Lindahl, U. Proteoglycans: structures and interactions. Annu. Rev. Biochem., *60*:443–475, 1991.

Klymkowsky, M. W., and Parr, B. The body language of cells: the intimate connection between cell adhesion and behavior. Cell, *83*:5–8, 1995.

Kodama, M., Kodama, T., Nishi, Y., and Totani, R. Does surgical stress cause tumor metastasis? Anticancer Res., *12*:1603–1616, 1992.

Kohno, K., Yamaguchi, T., and Takahashi, T. An experimental study of the spread of tumor cells through the lymph node. Tohoku J. Exp. Med., *127*:183–188, 1979.

Komeda, T., Fukuda, Y., Sando, T., Kita, R., Furukawa, M., Nishida, N., Amenomori, M., and Nakao, K. Sensitive detection of circulating hepatocellular carcinoma cells in peripheral venous blood. Cancer, *75*:2214–2219, 1995.

Kraemer, P. M., Deaven, L. L., Crissman, H. A., and Van Dilla, M. A. DNA constancy despite variability in chromosome number. *In*: E. J. DuPraw (Ed.), Advances in Cell and Molecular Biology, pp. 47–108. New York: Academic Press, 1972.

LaFlamme, S. E., and Auer, K. L. Integrin signaling. Semin. Cancer Biol., *7*:111–118, 1996.

Lane, T. F., and Sage, E. H. The biology of SPARC, a protein that modulates cell-matrix interactions. FASEB J., *8*:163–173, 1994.

Lewison, E. F. (Ed.) Conference on Spontaneous Regression of Cancer. J. Natl. Cancer Inst. Monograph 44. November 1976.

Lindemann, F., Schlimok, G., Dirschedl, P., Witte, J., and Riethmüller, G. Prognostic significance of micrometastatic tumour cells in bone marrow of colorectal cancer patients. Lancet, *340*:685–689, 1992.

Liotta, L. A. Cancer invasion and metastases. J.A.M.A., *263*:1123–1126, 1990.

Lynch, R. G. Differentiation and cancer: the conditional autonomy of phenotype. Proc. Natl. Acad. Sci. U.S.A., *92*:647–648, 1995.

Malins, D. C., Polissar, N. L., and Gunselman, S. J. Progression of human breast cancers to the metastatic state is linked to hydroxyl radical-induced DNA damage. Proc. Natl. Acad. Sci. U.S.A., *93*:2557–2563, 1996.

Malone, J. M., Wangensteen, S. L., Moore, W. S., and Keown, K. The fibrinolytic system. Ann. Surg., *190*:342–349, 1979.

Mareel, M., Bracke, M., Van Roy, F., and Vakaet, L. Expression of E-cadherin in embryogenetic ingression and cancer invasion. Int. J. Dev. Biol., *37*:227–235, 1993.

Mareel, M., Bracke, M., and Van Roy, F. Invasion promoter versus invasion suppressor molecules: the paradigm of E-cadherin. Mol. Biol. Rep., *19*:45–67, 1994.

Markewitz, M., Taylor, D. A., and Veenema, R. J. Spontaneous regression of pulmonary metastases following palliative nephrectomy. Cancer, *20*:1147–1154, 1967.

Mautner, V., and Hynes, R. O. Surface distribution of LETS protein in relation to the cytoskeleton of normal and transformed cells. J. Cell Biol., *75*:743–768, 1977.

McEver, R. P. Selectin-carbohydrate interactions during inflammation and metastasis. Glycoconj. J., *14*:585–591, 1997.

McGovern, V. J., Shaw, H. M., and Milton, G. W. Prognosis in patients with thin malignant melanoma: influence of regression. Histopathology, *7*:673–680, 1983.

Menger, M. D., and Vollmar, B. Adhesion molecules as determinants of disease: from molecular biology to surgical research. Br. J. Surg., *83*:588–601, 1996.

Mignatti, P., and Rifkin, D. B. Biology and biochemistry of proteinases in tumor invasion. Physiol. Rev., *73*:161–194, 1993.

Milas, L., Peters, L. J., and Ito, H. Spontaneous metastasis: random or selective? Clin. Exp. Metastasis, *1*:309–315, 1983.

Mitsudomi, T., Steinberg, S. M., Oie, H. K., Mulshine, J. L., Phelps, R., Viallet, J., Pass, H., Minna, J. D., and Gazdar, A. F. *ras* Gene mutations in non-small cell lung cancers are associated with shortened survival irrespective of treatment intent. Cancer Res., *51*:4999–5002, 1991.

Miyasaka, M. Cancer metastasis and adhesion molecules. Clin. Orthop., *312*:10–18, 1995.

Monsky, W. L., and Chen, W.-T. Proteases of cell adhesion proteins in cancer. Cancer Biol., *4*:251–258, 1993.

Moormeier, J. A., Williams. S. F., and Golomb, H. M. The staging of Hodgkin's disease. Hematol. Oncol. Clin. North Am., *3*:237–251, 1989.

Muschel, R., and Liotta, L. A. Role of oncogenes in metastases. Carcinogenesis, *9*:705–710, 1988.

Muto, M. G., Welch, W. R., Mok, S. C.-H., Bandera, C. A., Fishbaugh, P. M., Tsao, S.-W., Lau, C. C., Goodman, H. M., Knapp, R. C., and Berkowitz, R. S. Evidence for a multifocal origin of papillary serous carcinoma of the peritoneum. Cancer Res., *55*:490–492, 1995.

Nabi, I. R., Watanabe, H., and Raz, A. Autocrine motility factor and its receptor: role in cell locomotion and metastasis. Cancer Metastasis Rev., *11*:5–20, 1992.

Nakagawara, A., Arima-Nakagawara, M., Scavarda, N. J., Azar, C. G., Cantor, A. B., and Brodeur, G. M. Association between high levels of expression of the trk gene and favorable outcome in human neuroblastoma. N. Engl. J. Med., *328*:847–854, 1993.

Nicolson, G. L. Cell and tissue interactions leading to malignant tumor spread (metastasis). Am. Zool., *18*:71, 1978.

Nicolson, G. L. Paracrine/autocrine growth mechanisms in tumor metastasis. Oncol. Res., *4*:389–399, 1992.

Noda, M. Mechanisms of reversion. FASEB J., *7*:834–846, 1993.

Novelli, M. R., Williamson, J. A., Tomlinson, I. P. M., Elia, G., Hodgson, S. V., Talbot, I. C., Bodmer, W. F., and Wright, N. A. Polyclonal origin of colonic adenomas in an XO/XY patient with FAP. Science, *272*:1187–1190, 1996.

Nowell, P. C. The clonal evolution of tumor cell populations. Science, *194*:23–28, 1976.

Offit, K., Lo Coco, F., Louie, D. C., Parsa, N. Z., Leung, D., Portlock, C., Ye, B. H., Lista, F., Filippa, D. A., Rosenbaum, A., Ladanyi, M., Jhanwar, S., Dalla-Favera, R., and Chaganti, R. S. K. Rearrangement of the *bcl*-6 gene as a prognostic marker in diffuse large-cell lymphoma. N. Engl. J. Med., *331*:74–80, 1994.

Ohno, T., Stribley, J. A., Wu, G., Hinrichs, S. H., Weisenburger, D. D., and Chan, W. C. Clonality in nodular lymphocyte-predominant Hodgkin's disease. N. Engl. J. Med., *337*:459–465, 1997.

Olsson, L., and Forchhammer, J. Induction of the metastatic phenotype in a mouse tumor model by 5-azacytidine, and characterization of an antigen associated with metastatic activity. Proc. Natl. Acad. Sci. U.S.A., *81*:3389–3393, 1984.

Opdenakker, G., and Van Damme, J. Cytokines and proteases in invasive processes: molecular similarities between inflammation and cancer. Cytokine, *4*:251–258, 1992.

O'Regan, B., and Hirshberg, C. Spontaneous Remission: An Annotated Bibliography. Sausalito, CA: Institute of Noetic Science, 1993.

O'Reilly, M. S., Holmgren, L., Shing, Y., Chen, C., Rosenthal, R. A., Moses, M., Lane, W. S., Cao, Y., Sage, E. H., and Folkman, J. Angiostatin: a novel angiogenesis inhibitor that mediates the suppression of metastases by a Lewis lung carcinoma. Cell, *79*:315–328, 1994.

Oxenhandler, R. W., Berkelhammer, J., Smith, G. D., and Hook, R. R. Jr. Growth and regression of cutaneous melanomas in Sinclair miniature swine. Am. J. Pathol., *109*:259–269, 1982.

Pahlman, S., and Grotte, G. Are there two different forms of neuroblastoma? Z. Kinderchir., *35*:62–63, 1982.

Papaioannou, V. E., McBurney, M. W., Gardner, R. L., and Evans, M. J. Fate of teratocarcinoma cells injected into early mouse embryos. Nature, *258*:70–73, 1975.

Papkoff, J., Brown, A. M. C., and Varmus, H. E. The *int*-1 proto-oncogene products are glycoproteins that appear to enter the secretory pathway. Mol. Cell. Biol., *7*:3978–3984, 1987.

Parker, C., Whittaker, P. A., Weeks, R. J., Thody, A. J., and Sherbet, G. V. Modulators of metastatic behavior alter the expression of metastasis-associated genes MTS1 and NM23 in metastatic variants of the B16 murine melanoma. Clin. Biotechnol., *3*:217–222, 1991.

Paterson, M. C., Dietrich, K. D., Danyluk, J., Paterson, A. H. G., Lees, A. W., Jamil, N., Hanson, J., Jenkins, H., Krause, B. E., McBlain, W. A., Slamon, D. J., and Fourney, R. M. Correlation between c-*erb*B-2 amplification and risk of recurrent disease in node-negative breast cancer. Cancer Res., *51*:556–567, 1991.

Pauli, B. U., Augstin-Voss, H. G., El-Sabban, M. E., Johnson, R. C., and Hammer, D. A. Organ preference of metastasis. Cancer Metastasis Rev., *9*:175–189, 1990.

Pemberton, P. A. The role of serpin superfamily members in cancer. Cancer J., *10*:24–30, 1997.

Perl, A.-K., Wilgenbus, P., Dahl, U., Semb, H., and Christofori, G. A causal role for E-cadherin in the transition from adenoma to carcinoma. Nature, *392*:190–193, 1998.

Pierce, G. B. Neoplasms, differentiations and mutations. Am. J. Pathol., *77*:103–114, 1974.

Pitot, H. C. The Cell and Molecular Biology of Carcinogenesis: An Overview. *In*: Micotoxins, Cancer, and Health, G. A. Bray and D. H. Ryan (Eds.), pp. 103–125. Baton Rouge, LA: Louisiana State University Press, 1991.

Pohl, J., Goldfinger, N., Radler-Pohl, A., Rotter, V., and Schirrmacher, V. p53 increases experimental metastatic capacity of murine carcinoma cells. Mol. Cell. Biol., *8*:2078–2081, 1988.

Polakis, P. The adenomatous polyposis coli (APC) tumor suppressor. Biochim. Biophys. Acta, *1332*:F127–F147, 1997.

Ponta, H., Hofmann, M., and Herrlich, P. Recent advances in the genetics of metastasis. Eur. J. Cancer, *30A*:1995–2001, 1994.

Poste, G., and Fidler, I. J. The pathogenesis of cancer metastasis. Nature, *283*:139–146, 1980.

Prehn, R. T. The paradoxical association of regression with a poor prognosis in melanoma contrasted with a good prognosis in keratoacanthoma. Cancer Res., *56*:937–940, 1996.

Reddy, A. L., and Fialkow, P. J. Multicellular origin of fibrosarcomas in mice induced by the chemical carcinogen 3-methylcholanthrene. J. Exp. Med., *150*:878–887, 1979.

Reddy, A. L., and Fialkow, P. J. Effect of solvents on methylcholanthrene-induced carcinogenesis in mice. Int. J. Cancer, *27*:501–504, 1981.

Reddy, A. L., and Fialkow, P. J. Papillomas induced by initiation-promotion differ from those induced by carcinogen alone. Nature, *304*:69–71, 1983.

Ridley, A. J., and Hall, A. The small GTP-binding protein rho regulates the assembly of focal adhesions and actin stress fibers in response to growth factors. Cell, 70:389–399, 1992.

Roos, E. Adhesion molecules in lymphoma metastasis. Cancer Biol., 4:285–292, 1993.

Rosales, C., O'Brien, V., Kornberg, L., and Juliano, R. Signal transduction by cell adhesion receptors. Biochim. Biophys. Acta, 1242:77–98, 1995.

Rose, D. P., Connolly, J. M., Rayburn, J., and Coleman, M. Influence of diets containing eicosapentaenoic or docosahexaenoic acid on growth and metastasis of breast cancer cells in nude mice. J. Natl. Cancer Inst., 87:587–592, 1995.

Rossant, J., and McBurney, M. W. Diploid teratocarcinoma cell lines differ in their ability to differentiate normally after blastocyst injection. In: L. M. Silver, G. R. Martin, and S. Strickland (Eds.), Teratocarcinoma Stem Cells, pp. 625–633. Cold Spring Harbor, NY: Cold Spring Harbor Press, 1983.

Ruggeri, B., Caamano, J., Slaga, T. J., Conti, C. J., Nelson, W. J., and Klein-Szanto, A. J. P. Alterations in the expression of uvomorulin and Na$^+$, K$^+$-adenosine triphosphatase during mouse skin tumor progression. Am. J. Pathol., 140:1179–1185, 1992.

Ruiz, P., and Gunthert, U. The cellular basis of metastasis. World J. Urol., 14:141–150, 1996.

Ruoslahti, E., Pierschbacher, M., Hayman, E. G., and Engvall, E. Fibronectin: a molecule with remarkable structural and functional diversity. Trends Biochem. Sci., 7: 188–189, 1982.

Rusciano, D., and Burger, M. M. Why do cancer cells metastasize into particular organs? BioEssays, 14:185–194, 1992.

Russell, R. L., Geisinger, K. R., Mehta, R. R., White, W. L., Shelton, B., and Kute, T. E. nm23—Relationship to the metastatic potential of breast carcinoma cell lines, primary human xenografts, and lymph node negative breast carcinoma patients. Cancer, 79:1158–1165, 1997.

Sachs, L. Regulators of normal development and tumor suppression. Int. J. Dev. Biol., 37:51–59, 1993.

Sacristán, M. D., and Melchers, G. Regeneration of plants from "habituated" and "agrobacterium-transformed" single-cell clones of tobacco. Mol. Gen. Genet., 152:111–117, 1977.

Saiki, I., Iida, J., Murata, J., Ogawa, R., Nishi, N., Sugimura, K., Tokura, S., and Azuma, I. Inhibition of the metastasis of murine malignant melanoma by synthetic polymeric peptides containing core sequences of cell-adhesive molecules. Cancer Res., 49:3815–3822, 1989.

Sarkar, N. H. Genetic diversity of spontaneously developed primary and metastatic mammary tumor cells in mice. Cancer Commun., 2:379–386, 1990.

Scherer, E., Feringa, A. W., and Emmelot, P. Initiation-promotion-initiation. Induction of neoplastic foci within islands of precancerous liver cells in the rat. In: M. Börzsönyi, K. Lapis, N. E. Day, and H. Yamasaki (Eds.), Models, Mechanisms and Etiology of Tumour Promotion, pp. 57–66. Lyon: International Agency for Research on Cancer, 1984.

Scott-Burden, T. Extracellular matrix: the cellular environment. News Physiol. Sci., 9:110–115, 1994.

Seigal, A., and Modan, M. Latent carcinoma of thyroid in Israel: a study of 260 autopsies. Isr. J. Med. Sci., 17:249–253, 1981.

Seilern-Aspang, F., and Kratochwil, K. Induction and differentiation of an epithelial tumour in the newt (*Triturus cristatus*). J. Embryol. Exp. Morphol., 10:337–356, 1962.

Sellwood, R. A., Kuper, S. W. A., Payne, P. M., and Burn, J. I. Factors affecting the finding of cancer cells in the blood. Br. J. Surg., 56:649–652, 1969.

Sheu, J. R., Lin, C. H., Chung, J. L., Teng, C. M., and Huang, T. F. Triflavin, an Arg-Gly-Asp-containing antiplatelet peptide inhibits cell-substratum adhesion and melanoma cell-induced lung colonization. Jpn. J. Cancer Res., 83:885–893, 1992.

Sleeman, J., Moll, J., Sherman, L., Dall, P., Pals, S. T., Ponta, H., and Herrlich, P. The role of CD44 splice variants in human metastatic cancer. In: Cell Adhesion and Human Disease (Ciba Foundation Symposium 189), pp. 142–156. Chichester, UK: Wiley, 1995.

Sobin, L. H., Hermanek, P., and Hutter, R. V. P. TNM classification of malignant tumors. A comparison between the new (1987) and the old editions. Cancer, 61:2310–2314, 1988.

Stanley, J. R., Woodley, D. T., Katz, S. I., and Martin, G. R. Structure and function of basement membrane. J. Invest. Dermatol., 79:69s–72s, 1982.

Stetler-Stevenson, W. G., Aznavoorian, S., and Liotta, L. A. Tumor cell interactions with the extracellular matrix during invasion and metastasis. Annu. Rev. Cell Biol., 9:541–573, 1993a.

Stetler-Stevenson, W. G., Hewitt, R., and Corcoran, M. Matrix metalloproteinases and tumor invasion: from correlation and causality to the clinic. Cancer Biol., 7:147–154, 1996.

Stetler-Stevenson, W. G., Liotta, L. A., and Kleiner, Jr., D. E. Extracellular matrix 6: role of matrix metalloproteinases in tumor invasion and metastasis. FASEB J., 7:1434–1441, 1993b.

Stewart, T. A., and Mintz, B. Successive generations of mice produced from an established culture line of euploid teratocarcinoma cells. Proc. Natl. Acad. Sci. U.S.A., 78:6314–6318, 1981.

Stoll, B. A. Spontaneous regression of cancer: new insights. Biotherapy, 4:23–30, 1992.

Sylvén, B. Lysosomal enzyme activity in the interstitial fluid of solid mouse tumour transplants. Eur. J. Cancer, 4:463–474, 1968.

Syôno, K., and Fujita, T. Habituation as a tumorous state that is interchangeable with a normal state in plant cells. Int. Rev. Cytol., 152:265–299, 1994.

Takeichi, M., Watabe, M., Shibamoto, S., Ito, F., Oda, H., Uemura, T., and Shimamura, K. Dynamic control of cell-cell adhesion for multicellular organization. C.R. Acad. Sci. Paris, 316:818–821, 1993.

Tang, D. G., and Honn, K. V. Adhesion molecules and tumor metastasis: an update. Invasion Metastasis, 14:109–122, 1995.

Tanooka, H. Monoclonal growth of cancer cells: experimental evidence. Jpn. J. Cancer Res., 79:657–665, 1988.

Timpl, R., and Brown, J. C. The laminins. Matrix Biol., 14:275–281, 1994.

Tuck, A. B., Wilson, S. M., and Chambers, A. F. ras Transfection and expression does not induce progression from tumorigenicity to metastatic ability in mouse LTA cells. Clin. Exp. Metastasis, 8:417–431, 1990.

Turner, M. L. Cell adhesion molecules: a unifying approach to topographic biology. Biol. Rev., 67:359–377, 1992.

Tuszynski, G. P., Wang, T. N., and Berger, D. Adhesive proteins and the hematogenous spread of cancer. Acta Haematol., 97:29–39, 1997.

Vaheri, A., and Ruoslahti, E. Fibroblast surface antigen produced but not retained by virus-transformed human cells. J. Exp. Med., 142:530–535, 1975.

van der Rest, M., and Garrone, R. Collagen family of proteins. FASEB J., 5:2814–2823, 1991.

Varner, J. A., and Cheresh, D. A. Integrins and cancer. Curr. Opin. Cell Biol., 8:724–730, 1996.

Vega, F. J., Iniesta, P., Caldés, T., Sanchez, A., Lopez, J. A., de Juan, C., Diaz-Rubio, E., Torres, A., Balibrea, J. L., and Benito, M. Association of K-ras codon 12 transversions with short survival in non-small cell lung cancer. Int. J. Oncol., 9:1307–1311, 1996.

Vogelzang, N. J., Priest, E. R., and Borden, L. Spontaneous regression of histologically proved pulmonary metastases from renal cell carcinoma: a case with 5-year follow-up. J. Urol., 148:1247–1248, 1992.

von Essen, C. F. Radiation enhancement of metastasis: a review. Clin. Exp. Metastasis, 9:77–104, 1991.

Wainscoat, J. S., and Fey, M. F. Assessment of clonality in human tumors: a review. Cancer Res., 50:1355–1360, 1990.

Wang, L., Patel, U., Ghosh, L., Chen, H.-C., and Banerjee, S. Mutation in the nm23 gene is associated with metastasis in colorectal cancer. Cancer Res., 53:717–720, 1993.

Weber, M. Basement membrane proteins. Kidney Int., 41:620–628, 1992.

Weinberg, W. C., and Iannaccone, P. M. Clonality of preneoplastic liver lesions: histological analysis in chimeric rats. J. Cell Sci., 89:423–431, 1988.

Wight, T. N. Cell biology of arterial proteoglycans. Arteriosclerosis, 9:1–20, 1989.

Woodruff, M. F. A. Tumor clonality and its biological significance. Adv. Cancer Res., 50:197–229, 1988.

Yamada, K. M. Adhesive recognition sequences. J. Biol. Chem., 266:12809–12812, 1991.

Yang, F.-M., Montoya, A. L., Nester, E. W., and Gordon, M. P. Plant tumor reversal associated with the loss of foreign DNA. In Vitro, 16:87–92, 1980.

Yonemura, Y., Ninomiya, I., Yamaguchi, A., Fushida, S., Kimura, H., Ohoyama, S., Miyazaki, I., Endou, Y., Tanaka, M., and Sasaki, T. Evaluation of immunoreactivity for erbB-2 protein as a marker of poor short term prognosis in gastric cancer. Cancer Res., 51:1034–1038, 1991.

Yosida, T. H. Karyotype evolution and tumor development. Cancer Genet. Cytogenet., 8:153–179, 1983.

Young, M. R. I., Ihm, J., Lozano, Y., Wright, M. A., and Prechel, M. M. Treating tumor-bearing mice with vitamin D_3 diminishes tumor-induced myelopoiesis and associated immunosuppression, and reduces tumor metastasis and recurrence. Cancer Immunol. Immunother., *41*:37–45, 1995.

Young, S. D., Marshall, R. S., and Hill, R. P. Hypoxia induces DNA overreplication and enhances metastatic potential of murine tumor cells. Proc. Natl. Acad. Sci. U.S.A., *85*:9533–9537, 1988.

Zheng, J., Robinson, W. R., Ehlen, T., Yu, M. C., and Dubeau, L. Distinction of low grade from high grade human ovarian carcinomas on the basis of losses of heterozygosity on chromosomes 3, 6, and 11 and HER-2/*neu* gene amplification. Cancer Res., *51*:4045–4051, 1991.

11

Environmental Factors in the Etiology of Human Cancer—Chemical Agents and Processes

As noted in Chapter 1, the incidence of cancer at various tissue sites in humans varies greatly among countries and even within certain countries. Immigrants and especially their descendants tend to acquire the cancer incidences characteristic of their new habitats. The conclusion has been drawn that a high percentage, perhaps as much as 80%, of the more frequent and statistically important human neoplasms (of the bronchi, stomach, colon, breast, and others) have environmental factors, including lifestyle, as major components of their etiology. This has further led to a general agreement that at least 50% of all human cancers could be avoided if existing etiological knowledge were applied (cf. Tomatis et al., 1997). Differences in the exposure to carcinogenic radiations [other than solar ultraviolet (UV) light as the major cause of skin cancer], infectious disease, or hormonal factors do not appear sufficient to explain the geographical differences noted for most of the major cancers. Therefore a number of environmental chemicals, both synthetic and of natural occurrence, are under strong suspicion as carcinogens important in the etiology of much cancer in the human. Most notable among these are the chemicals in tobacco smoke. Asbestos and certain industrial chemicals have been implicated in some human cancers. However, contrary to some reports, present cancer incidence trends do not suggest a significantly rising age-adjusted incidence if lung cancer is factored out. Other than the continuing rise in bronchogenic carcinoma (resulting primarily from cigarette smoking) and the sharp decline in primary gastric carcinoma, little change has occurred in the incidences of major human neoplasms within the past 20 years. Suggestions that within the next decade as many as 25% of all cancers will result from occupational exposure to environmental agents have not been substantiated epidemiologically. These claims are based largely on a variety of theoretical projections. Although it is important to determine the most probable causes of cancer in humans with an aim of preventing this disease, it is very important to ensure that proposed preventive measures are based on scientific fact. *We must not let the fear of cancer infect our society with a cancer of fear.*

METHODS FOR THE DETERMINATION OF ETIOLOGICAL FACTORS IN HUMAN CANCER

"An ounce of prevention is worth a pound of cure." This well-known adage has become increasingly popular in relation to the prevention of cancer. Cairns (1975) has pointed out that more deaths from infectious disease have been prevented through measures such as vaccination, sani-

tary engineering, and widespread education and immunization of the population than by therapeutic measures, including the use of antibiotics. As our knowledge of the nature and causes of
cancer increases, many individuals have proposed that cancer prevention can become a reality
and be as effective as preventive programs against infectious diseases. One of the major bases
for this proposal is the estimation, originally suggested by Higginson, Doll, and others (cf. Higginson, 1979), that 80% to 90% of all human cancers are determined by environmental factors.
This estimate was derived by comparing the worldwide high and low cancer death rates for individual neoplasms (Table 1.1). The lowest cancer death rate was considered to be due to inherent
genetic and other "nonenvironmental factors," with the difference between the lowest and the
highest rates implicated as resulting from environmental agents. Even if the estimate were off by
100%, however, the environmentally induced cancers in the human would still be highly significant and, if prevented, could dramatically decrease the morbidity and mortality from cancer.

   One of the major known environmental causes of cancer in the human is smoking (Chapter 1). Unfortunately we have not taken sufficient advantage of this knowledge to decrease the
incidence of lung cancer, which is still increasing at a significant rate throughout the world. The
determination of the myriad of other environmental factors important in the causation of cancer
in the human is still a major problem. The most direct method for the determination of etiological factors in the causation of human cancer is the science of epidemiology. When epidemiological data are not available, scientists must rely on laboratory studies to aid in the determination
of such etiological factors.

Epidemiological Methodology

Epidemiology has been defined as the study of the distribution and determinants of health and
disease (Stewart and Sarfaty, 1978). Epidemiological methods seek to infer from observation
rather than experimentation. Epidemiological observations may take a number of forms (cf.
Rogan and Brown, 1979). Already in Chapter 1 one of the principal techniques of epidemiology
was discussed—that of surveys resulting in statistical findings of the incidence, morbidity, and
mortality of disease. In addition to such studies, the following are some of the general means of
obtaining epidemiological data:

   1. *Episodic observations.* The observation of isolated cases of cancer in relation to a spe-
      cific environmental factor has yielded clues in the past to cause-and-effect relation-
      ships. However, deductions must be carefully evaluated in properly designed studies.
   2. *Retrospective studies.* Investigations of the histories, habits, and other characteristics
      of groups of individuals who have developed a disease have been frequent sources of
      epidemiological data. This type of study is usually the first step in attempting to iden-
      tify causative factors. An important factor in such investigations is the use of case
      controls, and in many instances the suitable designation of such controls is the critical
      component in the study. Controls in case-control studies should be as similar as possi-
      ble in every way to the case population, differing only in the presence of the disease or
      condition in the cases. A study design of such a retrospective study is noted in Table
      11.1. In case-control studies, a number of patients with the disease under study
      (cases) are investigated in relation to another variable such as exposure to a chemical
      or dietary component. As noted in the table, one may readily determine the propor-
      tions of cases in controls that are exposed to the material. The calculation of the *odds
      ratio*, which is basically a cross-product ratio, may be related, sometimes very closely,
      to another parameter termed the *relative risk*, the risk in the exposed group/risk in the
      unexposed group (Rogan and Brown, 1979). An odds ratio that is close to one implies

Table 11.1 Retrospective Study Design[a]

	Selection	
	Cases (disease present)	Controls (disease absent)
Exposed	a	b
Not exposed	c	d
Totals	a + c	b + d
Proportions exposed	$\dfrac{a}{a+c}$	$\dfrac{b}{b+d}$
Odds ratio	$\dfrac{a \times d}{c \times b}$	

[a]Design of a retrospective (case-control) epidemiological study. The cases and controls, selected as shown, differ only in the presence or absence of the disease in question. This study attempts to relate exposure to a specific agent to the presence or absence of the disease. From these data as shown, one may calculate an odds ratio, which is important in determining both causation and risk.
Adapted from Goldberg, 1983, with permission of the author and publisher.

that there is no association between the chemical or component of interest and the disease being studied. An odds ratio less than one suggests a negative association between the two parameters, while an odds ratio greater than one implies a positive association. Increasing odds ratios connote an increase in exposure-related risk of having the disease (Goldberg, 1983). However, retrospective studies have a number of problems, such as the ability of the subject to recall previous environmental exposures, selection bias, and survivor bias (Lilienfeld, 1983).

3. *Prospective studies.* Prospective investigations involve analyses of the development of cancers in individuals with specific social habits, occupational exposures, etc. Such investigations require large populations, long follow-up periods (usually several years), and high follow-up rates for both controls and test groups. Many such investigations are presently under way in the United States and throughout the world.

Any one or all of these types of studies may be concerned with a single or with multiple factors involved in the causation of specific human cancers. Factors that lead to cancer or affect its development in humans are probably multifactorial in the vast majority of instances. Such factors include chemicals, radiations, genetic background, and biological agents and may be additive, synergistic, or antagonistic. Several agents may act at the same *stage* (that is, initiation or promotion) or at different stages.

Epidemiological studies can only identify factors that are different between two populations and that are sufficiently important in the etiology of the condition under study to play a determining role under the conditions of exposure. Furthermore, on the basis of epidemiological studies alone, it is usually very difficult to determine whether a specific chemical is or is not carcinogenic to the human. The reasons for this difficulty are the extended periods between first exposure and clinical occurrence of the neoplasm, the high background incidence for many cancers in the general population, the relatively imprecise knowledge of the nature of the exposure in most instances, exposures to multiple agents, and other confounding variables. Thus, many negative epidemiological studies must be considered as inconclusive for indicating the risk factor of relatively weak carcinogens or of low doses of carcinogens for inducing neoplastic disease in the human population.

In view of the fact that epidemiological studies in themselves are often insufficient to establish the carcinogenicity of an agent for humans, laboratory studies have been employed to complement or in some cases to supplant epidemiological observations where they exist. Many recent epidemiological investigations employ studies of biological markers such as DNA adducts, mutations in tumor suppressor genes and cellular oncogenes, genotypes for specific genes, and a variety of metabolites, proteins, and histopathological indications of preneoplasia as intermediate end points in a variety of studies (Perera, 1996). These and other methodologies are considered in Chapter 13, but at this point the discussion is restricted to a consideration of epidemiological data in determining the carcinogenicity of agents for humans. One of the pioneer agencies in the assessment of the carcinogenic risk of chemicals for humans has been the International Agency for Research on Cancer (IARC). In the recent preambles to monographs on the evaluation of carcinogenic risks to humans, IARC has defined the overall evaluation of the carcinogenicity to humans of an agent, mixture, or circumstance of exposure in the following manner (IARC Monographs, 1996):

Group 1—The agent (mixture) is carcinogenic to humans. The exposure circumstance entails exposures that are carcinogenic to humans.
This category is used when there is *sufficient evidence* of carcinogenicity in humans. Exceptionally, an agent (mixture) may be placed in this category when evidence in humans is less than sufficient but there is *sufficient evidence* of carcinogenicity in experimental animals and strong evidence in exposed humans that the agent (mixture) acts through a relevant mechanism of carcinogenicity.

Group 2
This category includes agents, mixtures, and exposure circumstances for which, at one extreme, the degree of evidence of carcinogenicity in humans is almost sufficient as well as those for which, at the other extreme, there are no human data but for which there is evidence of carcinogenicity in experimental animals. Agents, mixtures, and exposure circumstances are assigned to either group 2A (probably carcinogenic to humans) or group 2B (possibly carcinogenic to humans) on the basis of epidemiological and experimental evidence of carcinogenicity and other relevant data.

Group 2A—The agent (mixture) is probably carcinogenic to humans. The exposure circumstance entails exposures that are probably carcinogenic to humans.
This category is used when there is *limited evidence* of carcinogenicity in humans and sufficient evidence of carcinogenicity in experimental animals. In some cases, an agent (mixture) may be classified in this category when there is inadequate evidence of carcinogenicity in humans and *sufficient evidence* of carcinogenicity in experimental animals as well as strong evidence that the carcinogenesis is mediated by a mechanism that also operates in humans. Exceptionally, an agent, mixture, or exposure circumstance may be classified in this category solely on the basis of *limited evidence* of carcinogenicity in humans.

Group 2B—The agent (mixture) is possibly carcinogenic to humans. The exposure circumstance entails exposures that are possibly carcinogenic to humans.
This category is used for agents, mixtures, and exposure circumstances for which there is *limited evidence* of carcinogenicity in humans and less than *sufficient evidence* of carcinogenicity in experimental animals. It may also be used when there is *inadequate evidence* of carcinogenicity in humans but there is *sufficient evidence* of carcinogenicity in experimental animals. In some

instances, an agent, mixture, or exposure circumstance for which there is *inadequate evidence* of carcinogenicity in humans but *limited evidence* of carcinogenicity in experimental animals, together with supporting evidence from other relevant data, may be placed in this group.

Group 3—The agent (mixture or exposure circumstance) is not classifiable as to its carcinogenicity to humans.
This category is used most commonly for agents, mixtures, and exposure circumstances for which the evidence of carcinogenicity is inadequate in humans and inadequate or limited in experimental animals.

Exceptionally, agents (mixtures) for which the evidence of carcinogenicity is inadequate in humans but sufficient in experimental animals may be placed in this category when there is strong evidence that the mechanism of carcinogenicity in experimental animals does not operate in humans.

Agents, mixtures, and exposure circumstances that do not fall into any other group are also placed in this category.

Group 4—The agent (mixture) is probably not carcinogenic to humans.
This category is used for agents or mixtures for which there is *evidence suggesting lack of carcinogenicity* in humans and in experimental animals. In some instances, agents or mixtures for which there is *inadequate evidence* of carcinogenicity in humans but *evidence suggesting lack of carcinogenicity* in experimental animals, consistently and strongly supported by a broad range of other relevant data, may be classified in this group.

Despite the limitations of epidemiological studies in determining etiological factors for human cancer, under most circumstances an agent cannot be classified as carcinogenic for humans unless significant epidemiological evidence for its carcinogenic action in humans is available. From such evidence, a number of agents—chemical, physical, and biological—have been shown to be carcinogenic in humans. A recent detailed listing of such chemical carcinogens in the human has been presented by the National Toxicology Program of the U.S. government (Report on Carcinogens, 1998). The remainder of this chapter considers the majority of such agents classified as carcinogenic for the human at the present time.

CHEMICAL CARCINOGENESIS IN HUMANS

In Chapter 3 the experimental basis for the induction of cancer by chemicals of both exogenous and endogenous origin was considered. In a general sense, our knowledge of chemical carcinogenesis in the human can be traced to the observation by Ramazzini (cf. Wright, 1964) of the relatively high incidence of breast cancer in Catholic nuns (Chapter 1). Ramazzini proposed that breast cancer in this occupational group was the result of their lifestyle, and today there is good evidence to argue that endogenous hormonal interactions play a dominant role in the incidence of breast cancer, especially as related to the time of childbearing (Henderson et al., 1982). The first evidence for an exogenous chemical cause of cancer was described by Hill, who related the use of tobacco snuff to the occurrence of nasal polyps (Hill, 1761). Somewhat later, Pott demonstrated the causal relationship of soot to scrotal cancer in chimney sweeps (Chapter 3). Within the last century, a number of specific chemicals, industrial processes, and physiological conditions have been shown to be causally related to increased incidences of specific human cancers. This chapter focuses on the majority of such agents as listed by the IARC (Vainio et al., 1991) and reviewed by Doll and Peto (1981). For the sake of discussion we have divided these agents into those associated with lifestyle, with occupations, and with medical therapy and diagnosis.

Carcinogenic Chemical Agents and Related Factors Associated with Lifestyle

Table 11.2 is a listing, taken from the two references cited above, of those agents or conditions of lifestyle causally related to specific neoplasms in humans on the basis of epidemiological studies. The carcinogenicity of alcoholic beverages for human is related mostly to their action in association with another known carcinogenic agent. The combination of excessive alcohol ingestion and smoking markedly increases the risk of men and women for oral and laryngeal cancer compared with either of these two agents alone or in their absence (Herity et al., 1982; Day et al., 1993; Blot et al., 1994). The combination of ethanol ingestion in the form of alcoholic beverages and smoking also increased the risk of several cancers of the digestive tract, including the esophagus, rectum, and liver (Choi and Kahyo, 1991) in a cohort in Korea. Several studies have also implicated the combination in enhancing the development of premalignant lesions in the colon (Martiñez et al., 1995; Boutron et al., 1995) and in the esophagus (Castelletto et al., 1992). Cancer of the liver is associated with excessive alcohol consumption (Tuyns, 1979; Adami et al., 1992), and data reported by Ohnishi et al. (1982) suggest that habitual alcohol intake can promote the development of hepatocellular carcinoma in patients infected with the hepatitis B virus, a known oncogenic virus for the human liver (see below). Similarly, excessive intake of alcoholic beverages enhances the carcinogenic effect of the hepatitis C virus, an RNA virus oncogenic for human liver (Donato et al., 1997). While excessive ingestion of alcoholic beverages has also been associated with esophageal, rectal, and pancreatic cancer, a much more extensive series of investigations has been concerned with the potential relationship of alcoholic beverages and breast cancer. Although a causal relationship between alcohol ingestion and breast cancer has been disputed by some (Schatzkin and Longnecker, 1994), there is substantial epidemiological evidence from single and multiple studies for such an association (Smith-Warner et al., 1998). In Figure 11.1 may be seen a regression curve for the relationship between total alcohol intake per day and the risk of developing breast cancer. This study involved a pooled analysis of six prospective studies involv-

Table 11.2 Carcinogenic Factors Associated with Lifestyle

Chemical(s), Physiological Condition, or Process	Associated Neoplasm(s)	Evidence for Carcinogenicity[a]
Specific chemical agents		
Alcoholic beverages	Esophagus, liver, oropharynx, and larynx	Sufficient
Aflatoxins	Liver	Limited
Physiological conditions or processes		
Dietary intake (fat, protein, calories)	Breast, colon, endometrium, gallbladder	Sufficient
Salted fish (Chinese style)	Stomach	Sufficient
Reproductive history		
a. Late age at 1st pregnancy	Breast	Sufficient
b. Zero or low parity	Ovary	Sufficient
Sexual promiscuity	Cervix uteri	Sufficient
Tobacco smoking	Mouth, pharynx, larynx, lung, esophagus, bladder	Sufficient
Tobacco chewing (betel quid, etc.)	Mouth, pharynx	Sufficient

[a]This terminology refers to the IARC categorization and is based on the epidemiological findings in the IARC monographs and the review by Doll and Peto, 1981.

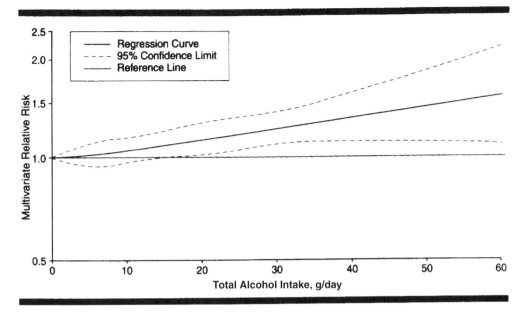

Figure 11.1   Nonparametric regression curve for the relationship between total alcohol intake and breast cancer. (From Smith-Warner et al., 1998, with permission of the authors and publisher.)

ing more than 300,000 women evaluated for up to 11 years. While there does appear to be some form of a threshold below 10 g/day, the relationship of significant risk to daily alcohol intake of 30 g or more appears very solid. Interestingly, consumption of alcoholic beverages reportedly is protective against the development of endometrial (Webster et al., 1989) and ovarian cancer (Gwinn et al., 1986). Although a variety of alcoholic beverages contain known chemical carcinogens, including nitrosamines (Tuyns and Griciute, 1980), and different forms of alcoholic beverages may have slightly different influences on the incidence of certain types of human cancer, most evidence suggests that the principal effect is due to the alcohol itself and is largely independent of the form in which it is drunk (Doll and Peto, 1981).

Aflatoxins and Other Dietary Contaminants

In 1960 more than 100,000 young turkeys died in England. Studies showed that the death of the birds was due to a contaminant present in the peanut meal, obtained from South Africa, in their diet. Comparable problems arose in eastern Africa at the same time. Careful chemical studies demonstrated that the offending agent belonged to a group of toxic metabolites termed the aflatoxins, which are produced by some strains of the ubiquitous mold *Aspergillus flavus*. Shortly thereafter, the carcinogenicity of purified aflatoxin B_1 was demonstrated in rodents, the most striking characteristic being its extremely high potency. Fifteen parts per billion of aflatoxin B_1 in the diet for approximately 1½ years produced hepatomas in all treated rats. In trout, one part or less per billion was effective as a carcinogen (Newberne and Butler, 1969).

Epidemiological studies have shown that the geographical regions in which there is extensive contamination of foodstuffs by aflatoxin are also the areas where the incidence of human liver cancer is relatively high. However, for the most part in these same areas, there is substantial prevalence of hepatitis B and/or C infections. Thus, at least one study has suggested that aflatoxin exposure in these areas has relatively little influence on the primarily virally induced hepatic neoplasms (Campbell et al., 1990). On the other hand, several studies have shown a direct association between the aflatoxin content of food and the frequency of hepatomas in the population. In parts of Africa and East Asia where aflatoxin is found in the diet, levels of 100 to 1000 parts per billion in individual foodstuffs are not unusual. Thus, unlike most other environmental carcinogenic agents for the human, the dose of aflatoxin to which the human is exposed greatly exceeds that known to produce cancer in experimental animals. As yet, however, because of the major role played by hepatitis B and C in the induction of human hepatic neoplasia (see below), the role of aflatoxin exposure in the causation of human hepatic neoplasia is somewhat uncertain.

Further evidence for the role of aflatoxin in inducing hepatic neoplasia comes from two sources. Several "markers" (Chapter 17) have now been developed and demonstrated to be directly related to aflatoxin exposure. In one study (Ross et al., 1992), a large number of Chinese patients were followed for several years. In those individuals exhibiting evidence both of hepatitis B virus infection and aflatoxin exposure as measured by a urinary marker, the aflatoxin-N^7-guanine adduct, a dramatic increase in the risk of developing liver cancer compared with the presence of either factor alone was noted. In addition, as we have noted in Chapter 6 (Figure 6.2), aflatoxin exposure has been related to a specific mutation at codon 249 in the p53 tumor suppressor gene (Hsu et al., 1991; Bressac et al., 1991). Further extension of these studies has demonstrated that patients from areas with high aflatoxin levels are more likely to exhibit the codon 249 mutation and other p53 mutations, especially transversion, than are patients from areas with low aflatoxin exposure (Lasky and Magder, 1997). However, other studies in nonhuman primates, as in the rat (Chapter 6), did not exhibit codon 249 mutations in p53 or, for the most part, in any other part of the gene investigated when animals were exposed to aflatoxin B_1 (Fujimoto et al., 1992). Furthermore, later investigations have suggested that many p53 gene mutations, which may be common in advanced hepatocellular carcinomas, occur as a late event during the stage of progression (Hsu et al., 1994). Thus, it appears that while some codon mutations in the p53 gene in hepatocytes may occur as an initiating event in hepatocellular carcinoma in the human, most mutations in this gene may be the result of selection during the stage of progression (Dragan and Pitot, 1994). The most likely scenario, however, is that high aflatoxin exposure to the human on a chronic basis may act as both an initiating and promoting stimulus which, in the presence of a viral infection involving clastogenic events (Hino et al., 1991), ultimately leads to the development of hepatocellular carcinoma. Although other mold toxins, such as sterigmatocystin (Gopalakrishnan et al., 1992), have been suggested as additional etiological factors in human liver cancer, their role in this disease has not been proven at the present time.

Other natural products—such as the pyrrolizidine alkaloids (McLean, 1970), which occur in extracts of various roots and leaves found in various parts of the world; cycasin, obtained from extracts of the cycad nut (Hoffmann and Morgan, 1984); and safrole (Borchert et al., 1973), a naturally occurring flavoring agent—have been shown to be carcinogenic for the liver in rodents. As yet there is no significant evidence that these materials cause hepatomas in humans, although the pyrrolizidine alkaloids have been implicated in the production of vascular disease of the liver in Jamaica and other West Indian countries (McLean, 1970). On the other hand, some natural products, as noted in Chapter 8 (Table 8.8), are inhibitory to the process of carcinogenesis, including even some naturally occurring mutagens (Stavric, 1984). A few edible plants have been found to contain or produce agents capable of inducing cancer in one or more species. Bracken fern is both a food delicacy and salad green in certain parts of the world. When fed to rats, this agent is a carcinogen for the bladder and intestine (Pamukcu et al., 1976). In areas of the world where cattle graze on bracken fern–containing pastures, these animals develop urinary bladder tumors.

An example of the induction of cancer in the human by naturally occurring dietary contaminants is described in several provinces of the People's Republic of China. In these locales, there is a positive correlation between the extremely high incidence of esophageal carcinoma and the consumption of pickled and otherwise moldy foodstuffs that contain carcinogenic nitrosamines (Singer et al., 1986; Li et al., 1986). Although the exact chemical structures of almost all of these dietary contaminants are unknown, at least one N-nitroso compound has been isolated from corn bread inoculated with fungi (Shixin et al., 1979) and from extracts of pickled vegetables. Moldy cornmeal fed to rats induces carcinoma and epithelial dysplasia of the forestomach. Since this latter structure is quite similar anatomically to the esophagus in the human, there is reason to argue for a causal relation of these contaminated foodstuffs to the high incidence of esophageal cancer in areas where such dietary contamination occurs.

Perhaps the most ubiquitous group of carcinogenic agents occurring "naturally" in the diet, primarily in cooked foods, are the heterocyclic amines, which have been described and studied by a number of investigators (cf. Sugimura et al., 1996). Figure 11.2, adapted from these authors (Sugimura et al., 1996), shows the structures of a number of mutagenic and carcinogenic heterocyclic amines that occur in heated foods. These substances apparently result from the pyrrolysis of amino acids and proteins. The chemistry of these reactions has been investigated and shown to occur in both crude and chemically characterized systems (Vuolo and Schuessler, 1985). The amount of these materials present in cooked food varies with the cooking method—i.e., broiling, frying, barbecuing, or microwaving—and the temperature of cooking above 150°C (Robbana-Barnat et al., 1996). Thus, one might expect that individuals consuming diets prepared in various ways will consume different levels of these carcinogenic amines; such a difference has been reported, for example, between Americans and Japanese (Nagao et al., 1996) as well as in specifically and carefully studied cohorts (Augustsson et al., 1997). Cancer potency estimates for the human have been placed as high as 1 in 10^3 or 10^4 for an average lifetime of cooked beef intake of approximately 0.5 lb/day (Bogen, 1994). On the other hand, Gold et al. (1994), in a very extensive study, have suggested that even the most potent of the heterocyclic amines offers a relatively low risk in the average American diet compared with other, less potent materials but which are consumed at much higher levels (e.g., ethyl alcohol). Epidemiological evidence suggests both a relationship between the methods of cooking meats and the daily consumption of meat in relation to the incidence of various cancers, especially colon cancer (cf. Felton et al., 1997).

A major area of concern in modern food technology is the addition of chemical agents to processed foods for flavor, coloring, and preservation. Also, additions to the human diet of potential carcinogens at low levels have been made inadvertently through the contamination of food sources by pesticides and industrial wastes. Examples of compounds that have been shown to be carcinogenic in experimental animals and that have entered the human diet are certain pesticides, DDT, and dieldrin as well as the industrial contaminant polychlorinated biphenyls. Specific additions to the human diet of agents that have been found to be carcinogenic at very high levels in experimental animals include the synthetic antioxidant butylated hydroxytoluene (BHT), the coloring agent red dye 2, and the artificial sweetener saccharin. Of these, saccharin created a national controversy in relation to the legal constraints of the Delaney amendment (Chapter 13) and the wishes of Congress and the public to keep this material on the market. Sodium nitrite has been used as a preservative in a wide variety of prepared meat products for many years. Although nitrites themselves are not carcinogenic, they have been shown in experimental animals to react with secondary amines both in the food and in the intestine to produce carcinogenic nitrosamines (Leaf et al., 1989). The demonstration of low levels of dimethylnitrosamine in fish meal treated with nitrite and the presence in flour of trace amounts of diethylnitrosamine, produced from drying the grain in a stream of exhaust gases containing oxides of nitrogen, are ample evidence that such compounds can be produced outside the living organism (cf. Gangolli et al., 1994). Furthermore, some experimental studies have demonstrated the production of a number of different malignancies of the gastrointestinal and respiratory tracts by the addition of nitrite and secondary or tertiary amines to the diet (Matsukura et al., 1977; Yoshida et al., 1993).

Studies have demonstrated that the major amount of nitrite in humans originates from endogenous sources, largely through the reduction of nitrates by oral bacteria ingested as components of vegetables and plant foodstuffs (Tannenbaum et al., 1978). The contribution of

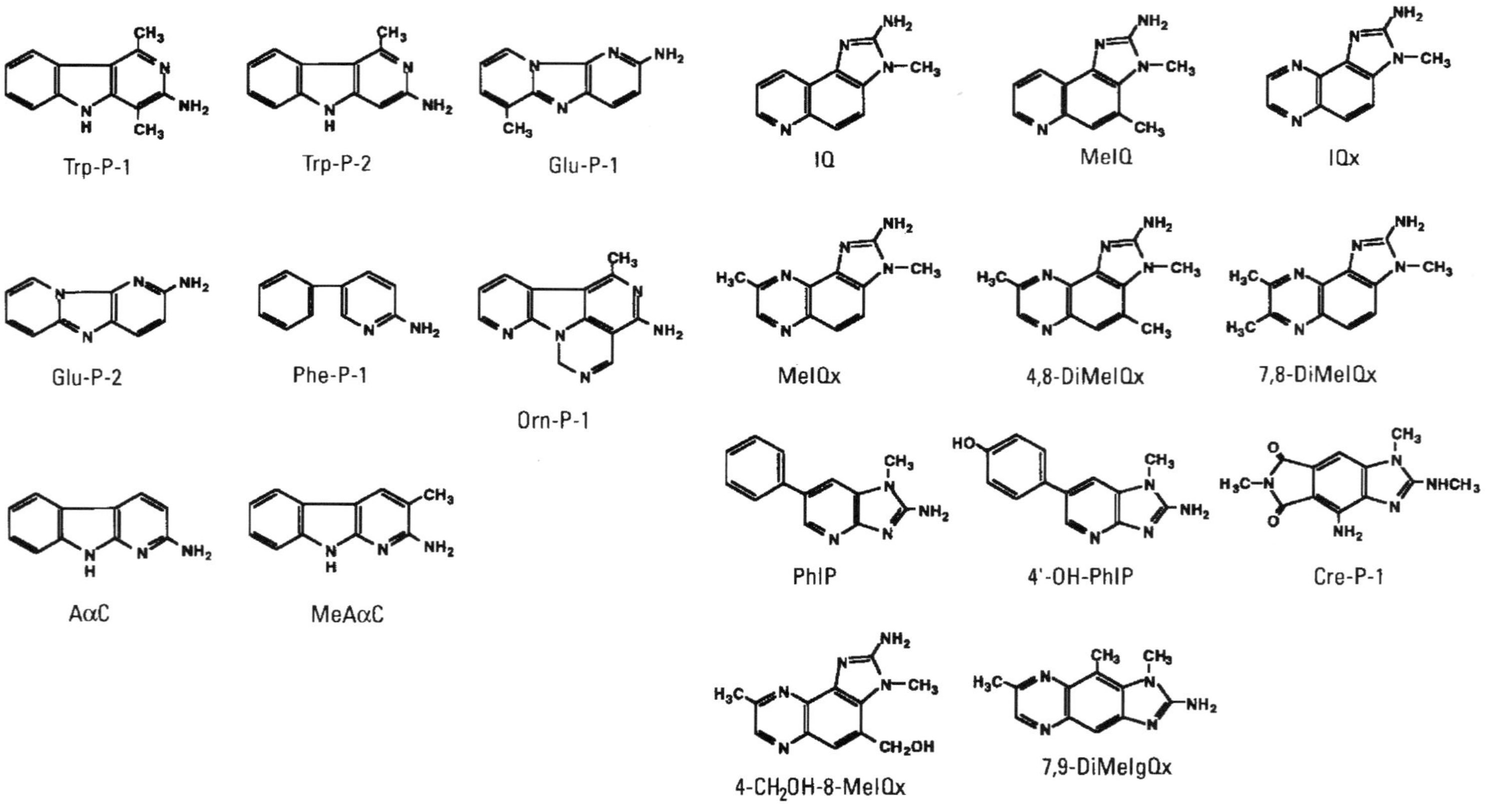

Figure 11.2 Structures of some mutagenic and carcinogenic heterocyclic amines. Abbreviations: Trp-P-1, 3-amino-1,4-dimethyl-5*H*-pyrido[4,3-*b*]indole; Trp-P-2, 3-amino-1-methyl-5*H*-pyrido[4,3-*b*]indole; Glu-P-1, 2-amino-6-methyldipyrido[1,2-*a*:3′,2′-*d*]imidazole; Glu-P-2, 2-aminodipyrido[1,2-*a*:3′,2′-*d*]imidazole; Phe-P-1, 2-amino-5-phenylpyridine; Orn-P-1, 4-amino-6-methyl-1*H*-2,5,10,10*b*-tetraazafluoranthene; A*α*C, 2-amino-9*H*-pyrido[2,3-*b*]indole; MeA*α*C, 2-amino-3-methyl-9*H*-pyrido[2,3-*b*]indole; IQ, 2-amino-3-methylimidazo[4,5-*f*]quinoline; MeIQ, 2-amino-3,4-dimethylimidazo[4,5-*f*]quinoline; IQx, 2-amino-3-methylimidazo[4,5-*f*]quinoxaline; MeIQx, 2-amino-3,8-dimethylimidazo[4,5-*f*]-quinoxaline; 4,8-DiMeIQx, 2-amino-3,4,8-trimethylimidazo[4,5-*f*]quinoxaline; 7,8-DiMeIQx, 2-amino-3,7,8-trimethylimidazo[4,5-*f*]quinoxaline; PhIP, 2-amino-1-methyl-6-phenylimidazo[4,5-*b*]pyridine; 4′-OH-PhIP, 2-amino-1-methyl-6-(4-hydroxyphenyl)imidazo[4,5-*b*]pyridine; Cre-P-1, 4-amino-1,6-dimethyl-2-methylamino-1*H*,6*H*-pyrrolo[3,4-*f*]benzimidazole-5,7-dione; 4-CH$_2$OH-8-MeIQx, 2-amino-4-hydroxymethyl-3,8-dimethylimidazo[4,5-*f*]quinoxaline; 7,9-DiMeIgQx, 2-amino-1,7,9-trimethylimidazo[4,5-*g*]quinoxaline. The following ten compounds have been proven to be carcinogenic: Trp-P-1, Trp-P-2, Glu-P-1, Glu-P-2, A*α*C, MeA*α*C, IQ, MeIQ, MeIQx, PhIP. (From Sugimura et al., 1996, with permission of the authors and publishers.)

exogenous nitrite to the total internal nitrite pool is only about 10%, thus raising significant questions as to what role if any nitrite preservatives and coloring agents have in the genesis of human cancer. Hartman has reported that the daily levels of nitrate ingestion in the 1970s showed a strong positive correlation with gastric cancer mortality in at least 12 countries (Hartman, 1983), and human exposure is still quite extensive (Bartsch et al., 1989). However, Pobel et al. (1995). in a case-controlled study in France, were unable to demonstrate any association between the intake of nitrate and nitrite and the increased risk of stomach cancer.

A few edible plants have been found to contain or produce agents capable of inducing cancer in one or more species. Bracken fern is both a food delicacy and salad green in certain parts of the world. When fed to rats, this agent is a carcinogen for the bladder and intestine (Pamukcu et al., 1976). In areas of the world where cattle graze on bracken fern–containing pastures, these animals develop urinary bladder tumors.

Nutritional Dietary Factors

Although dietary contaminants and alcohol in particular contribute significantly to the genesis of the cancer burden in the human population throughout the world, a factor that is probably more important in human carcinogenesis is the effect of dietary nutrients, both macro and micro. We have already noted in Chapter 8 that such dietary constituents demonstrably play major roles in both the spontaneous and induced development of neoplasia in lower animals. In one of the earlier, extensive studies of the effect of human diet on cancer development, Hoffman (1937) concluded that "overnutrition is common in the case of cancer patients to a remarkable and exceptional degree, and . . . overabundant food consumption unquestionably is the underlying cause of the root condition of cancer in modern life." Doll and Peto (1981) proposed that as many as one-third or more of human cancers were causatively associated with dietary nutrient factors. As seen from Table 11.2, the IARC has concluded—on the basis of epidemiological and experimental evidence—that dietary factors are a sufficient cause of human neoplasia, specifically those neoplasms listed in the table and potentially some more. There is ample experimental evidence to support this classification, as we saw from Chapter 8. While it is not possible in most instances to study the long-term incidence of cancer in individuals on balanced, restricted diets, inferences may be made from studies of relatively common human conditions such as obesity, weight gain, and body stature, where diet appears to play a significant role. In particular, obesity and a high body mass index (BMI), defined as the weight in kilograms of an individual divided by the square of his or her height in meters, are associated with increased mortality in men and women (Garfinkel, 1986; Manson et al., 1995). In middle-aged obese women who had never smoked, the relative risk of death from cancer and cardiovascular disease was 2.1 and 4.1 respectively (Manson et al., 1995). Similar trends had been seen earlier (Garfinkel, 1985). Obesity has been associated with increased risks of cancer of the breast, colon, endometrium, esophagus, liver, pancreas, and prostate (Osler, 1987; Ingram et al., 1989; Garfinkel, 1985; Møller et al., 1994b). Albanes et al. (1988) have also reported that short stature in both men and women is associated with a reduced risk of cancer, suggesting a role for nutrition early in life in human carcinogenesis. While these data on obesity and stature do not prove that dietary excesses and restriction are related respectively to increases and decreases in human cancer incidence, they are quite suggestive and clearly in line with data from experimental studies (Chapter 8).

Although it is difficult to study the overall effects of caloric restriction and excess on the incidence of human cancer, epidemiological and nutritional investigations directed toward specific nutrients, both macro and micro, have indicated a variety of associations, both positive and negative, with the development of specific human cancers. Table 11.3 gives a tabulation of many of the major nutritional dietary factors involved in site-specific human carcinogenesis. The incidence of bladder cancer is not affected by a variety of dietary factors, although Risch et al.

Table 11.3 Nutritional Dietary Factors in Human Carcinogenesis (Epidemiological Investigations)

Neoplasm	Causative	Preventive	References Human	References Animal
Bladder	Cholesterol (?)	Fruits/vegetables, Vit. C	Risch et al., 1988 La Vecchia et al., 1989 Nomura et al., 1991 Helzlsouer et al., 1989	Sporn et al., 1977 cf. Block, 1991
Breast	Red meat		Taniolo et al., 1994; Zheng et al., 1998	Hawrylewicz et al., 1982
	Dietary fat Dietary calories (energy)	Dietary fiber	Vatten et al., 1990 Howe et al., 1991 Rose, 1997 Wynder et al., 1997 Willett, 1997	Freedman et al., 1990
		Fruits/vegetables (fiber?)	Freudenheim et al., 1996 Rose, 1990	Zile et al., 1986 Rao et al., 1990 Cohen et al., 1996
Cervix		Antioxidant Micronutrients Fruit/vegetables	Herrero et al., 1991 Potischman, 1993 Brock et al., 1988 VanEenwyk et al., 1991	
Colon	Red meat Dietary fat		Potter & McMichael, 1986 Giovannucci et al., 1994 Willett et al., 1990 cf. Statland, 1992 Weinberg, 1994	Nutter et al., 1983 Zhao et al., 1991 Wasan et al., 1997
	Iron	Calcium Fiber	Newmark and Lipkin, 1992 Howe et al., 1992 Le Marchand et al., 1997	Pence et al., 1995 Jacobs, 1986
	Folate deficiency Bile acids	Fruits/vegetables	Matthew et al., 1997 Mason, 1994 cf. Cheah, 1990	Narisawa et al., 1996 Cravo et al., 1992 Weisburger et al., 1983 Rao et al., 1992

Site	Dietary factor	Protective factor	References
Endometrium	Meat	Fruit/vegetables	Zheng et al., 1995a; Levi et al., 1993; Sammon and Alderson, 1998
Esophagus	Corn (maize); Animal fat; Cholesterol	Vitamins A, C, E; Zn (?); Fruits and vegetables	van Rensburg, 1981; Launoy et al., 1998; Kaul et al., 1986; Zheng et al., 1995; Wahrendorf et al., 1988; Gao et al., 1994ab; Moerman et al., 1993; Zatonski et al., 1997; Odeleye et al., 1992; Fong et al., 1984
Gall bladder	High carbohydrate; High fat and oils (high energy)		Kato et al., 1989
Liver		Animal proteins; Fruits and vegetables; Dark green vegetables; Retinol (?)	Yu et al., 1995; He et al., 1997; Sarkar et al., 1995; Moreno et al., 1995
Lung	Cholesterol	Fruits and vegetables; Retinoids, Vit. E and C	Jain et al., 1990; Le Marchand et al., 1989; Yong et al., 1997; cf. Fontham, 1990; Menkes et al., 1986; Blot et al., 1994; Chiu et al., 1996; Kim et al., 1997; cf. Ong and Chytil, 1983; Gupta et al., 1990
Lymphoma/leukemia	Dietary fat; Animal protein)		Tallman et al., 1997
Ovary	Dietary meat; \Dietary β carotene	Retinoids	Mori and Miyake, 1988; Engle et al., 1991
Pancreas	Dietary calories (fat); Dietary meat		Silverman et al., 1998; Farrow and Davis, 1990; Ohba et al., 1996; cf. Roebuck, 1992

(table continues)

Table 11.3 (continued)

Neoplasm	Causative	Preventive	References	
			Human	Animal
Pancreas (continued)				
	Dietary cholesterol	Fruits and vegetables (vit. A, β carotene, se?)	Zatonski et al., 1991 Norell et al., 1986	Woutersen and van Garderen-Hoetmer, 1988 Roebuck et al., 1984
Prostate	Dietary fat (calories) (Dairy products)		cf. Giovannucci, 1998	cf. Wynder et al., 1994
	Dietary meat		Whittemore et al., 1995 Snowden et al., 1984 Talamini et al., 1992 Heshmat et al., 1985 Vlajinac et al., 1997	
		Vegetables (tomatoes) and fruit	Giovannucci et al., 1995	
			Ohno et al., 1988 Mills et al., 1989 Clinton et al., 1996	
		Carotenoids (lycopene)	Mettlin et al., 1989	Pollard et al., 1991 Slawin et al., 1993
Renal	Total energy intake		Mellemgaard et al., 1996 Wolk et al., 1996	
Stomach	Dietary salt		Nazario et al., 1993 Hirohata and Kono, 1997 You et al., 1988	Takahashi et al., 1994
	Dietary nitrate		Hartman, 1983	
		Dietary fruits and vegetables	Coggon et al., 1989 Graham et al., 1990	Maekawa et al., 1982
		(Vitamin C and β carotene)	Tuyns et al., 1992	Krinsky, 1994

(1988) reported that the daily intake of cholesterol was positively associated with a mild increase in risk of developing this neoplasm. On the other hand, consumption of green and yellow vegetables (G&YV) or increased vitamin C in women was associated with a significantly decreased risk of bladder cancer development (La Vecchia et al., 1989; Nomura et al., 1991). Although animal studies have not supported the cholesterol finding, investigations in animals have demonstrated effects of retinoids and vitamin C in preventing the development of experimental neoplasia (Sporn et al., 1977; cf. Block, 1991). Serum levels of selenium have also been shown to be inversely related to the incidence of bladder cancer in the human (Helzlsouer et al., 1989).

The evidence for diet as a major role in the incidence of gastrointestinal cancer in humans comes from studies of the lifestyle and dietary habits of particular societal groups. The Seventh Day Adventist population abstains from smoking and drinking, and about 50% of these individuals eat a largely vegetarian diet, avoiding the use of coffee, tea, hot condiments, and spices. General cancer mortality in this group is 30% to 50% lower than that in the general population for most cancer sites that are unrelated to smoking and drinking. In particular, cancers of the lower gastrointestinal tract are between 30% and 35% lower than in the controls. Another important source of evidence for the importance of diet in cancer incidence is the study of cancer incidence in migrants moving from one part of the world, where the incidence of a specific cancer is high or low, to another area, where the opposite is true. One of the most striking examples of this is seen in the dramatic decrease within only two generations in the incidence of stomach cancer in Japanese migrating to the United States, and the simultaneous marked increase in the incidence of colon cancer in this population on migration (cf. Liu et al., 1993). Willett (1990) has also presented evidence that human cancer risks are inversely correlated with the level of blood retinol and with the dietary content of β-carotene, both derivatives of vitamin A.

A number of studies both in animals (Hawrylewicz et al., 1982) and humans (Toniolo et al., 1994; Vatten et al., 1990) have indicated that diets high in protein or in "red meat" are associated with increased incidences of mammary neoplasia, but there has been considerable controversy on the role of dietary fat in enhancing mammary neoplasia, especially in humans. While a number of studies, including Howe et al. (1991) and Wynder et al. (1997), indicate a significant role for high fat diets in promoting the development of human breast cancer, a number of other investigations have not supported such a role. Rather, evidence suggests that the association is linked to total energy consumption rather than to levels of dietary fat per se (Willett, 1997). Figure 11.3 shows the now classic relationship between fat consumption and breast cancer deaths in a variety of countries (Carroll and Khor, 1975), on which are superimposed the more recent data of Willett et al. (1987). As can be noted, both fat consumption and calories from fat consumed are related directly to the death rate due to breast cancer.

Unfortunately, as pointed out by Schatzkin et al. (1989) and noted in the figure, the relative risk of breast cancer for women in the highest compared with the lowest fat-consuming groups would be only 1.5. Since animal studies support both viewpoints (Freedman et al., 1990; Rose, 1997), it is most likely that both the total energy content of the diet and dietary lipid itself play roles in the development of mammary cancer both in humans and in animals. In general, studies on the role of specific protective factors in mammary cancer development in humans have been conflicting. Freudenheim et al. (1996) described a study in humans that indicated that intake of fruits and vegetables decreased the risk of breast cancer development, and Rose (1990) reported that dietary fiber may have a protective effect because of its influence on estrogen metabolism and excretion or by other mechanisms. A protective effect of dietary fiber in N-methylnitrosourea–induced mammary cancer in rats has been published (Cohen et al., 1996), and several studies (Zile et al., 1986; Rao et al., 1990) have indicated an inhibitory effect of retinoids and antioxidant micronutrients in the development of experimental mammary neoplasia.

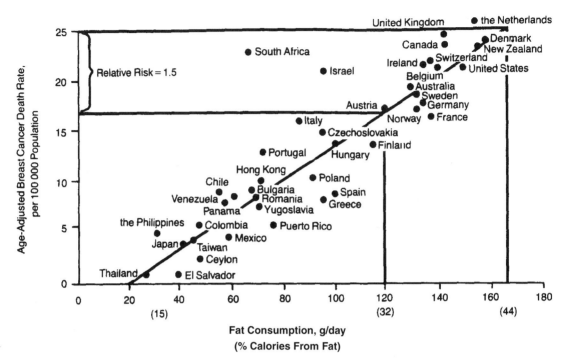

Figure 11.3 Relation between age-adjusted breast cancer mortality rates, per capita fat consumption, and percentage calories in the diet from fat (after Schatzkin et al., 1989, with permission of the authors).

In the case of colon carcinogenesis, the most convincing data in humans are the association of red meat in the diet with an increased risk of the development of colon cancer (Giovannucci and Goldin, 1997). As discussed earlier in this chapter and in the literature by Potter (1993) and others, this association may be directly related to the production of mutagens and heterocyclic amines (Figure 11.2) during the cooking process. A more controversial association is that of dietary fat with an increased incidence of colon cancer. One of the most detailed studies was that of Willett et al. (1990) among a large cohort of middle-aged and older women. This study demonstrated a positive association of the risk of colon cancer development with increased animal fat intake. Other studies (cf. Statland, 1992) have tended to confirm this finding, but another view is that neither case-control nor cohort studies have found that total fat composition of the diet increased the risk of colon cancer (Giovannucci and Goldin, 1997). Interestingly, at the experimental level, Nutter et al. (1983) reported that the feeding of beef protein to mice did not significantly affect the response of the intestines to 1,2-dimethylhydrazine–induced carcinogenesis. Unfortunately, the study did not indicate the actual treatment of the beef protein. On the other hand, dietary fat enhances experimental intestinal carcinogenesis, both chemically induced (Zhao et al., 1991) and genetically based (Wasan et al., 1997).

In four out of five prospective studies, an association has been noted between low serum cholesterol and an increased risk for colon cancer (cf. Burnstein, 1993). On the other hand, feeding of high-cholesterol diets to rodents during chemical induction of colon carcinogenesis significantly enhanced the number of colon neoplasms per animal (Hiramatsu et al., 1983; Makino et al., 1989). While the reasons for this association are not understood, it is likely that changes in bile acid metabolism may be the important factor. A number of epidemiological studies have revealed that fecal bile acid concentrations are elevated in populations having a high incidence of colon cancer, notably those consuming a high-fat, western-style diet (cf. Cheah, 1990). Bile acids have also been found to act as promoting agents in the experimental induction of colon carcinogenesis in animals (cf. Cheah, 1990). Recently, however, Narisawa et al. (1998) found that one bile acid, ursodeoxycholic acid, prevented N-methylnitrosourea–induced colon carcinogenesis in rats. Gupta and associates (1983) isolated from human feces and determined the structure of a number of hydrocarbon ethers, which they designated as fecapentaenes. These materials are evidently synthesized by bacteria within the colon and exhibit strong mutagenic activity (Kingston et al., 1990). However, their effectiveness as initiators or complete carcinogens in rats and mice has not been repeatedly verified in animals (Weisburger et al., 1990; Ward et al., 1988; Shamsuddin et al., 1991), and as yet the role of these unique mutagens in the induction of human colon cancer is not clear.

In a recent review, Weinberg (1994) reported that studies in animal models and relatively large groups of humans indicate a positive association of excessive iron with colorectal carcinogenesis. In contrast, administration of excessive calcium salts decreases the risk and development of colon cancer in both humans (Newmark and Lipkin, 1992) and animals (Pence et al., 1995). In the United Kingdom, a recent study indicated that patients selecting diets containing significantly less fruit and vegetables than were present in the diets of age-matched controls had an increased risk of developing colorectal cancer (Matthew et al., 1997). In experimental studies, Narisawa and associates (1996) had shown that a variety of natural carotenoids found in fruits and vegetables inhibited the development of preneoplastic aberrant crypt foci in the colons of rats receiving N-methylnitrosourea. There is now developing a substantial body of epidemiological data indicating a relationship between the status of the vitamin folic acid and the risk of developing colorectal neoplasia (Mason, 1994). These studies indicate that folate deficiency is related to an increased risk of colorectal neoplasia—a finding that is clearly supported by animal investigations (Mason, 1994; Cravo et al., 1992). Dietary fiber content has also been associated with a decreased risk of cancers of the colon and rectum in a number of epidemiological studies (Howe et al., 1992). This has been confirmed more recently (Le Marchand et al., 1997), where study of a cohort of a variety of ethnic groups indicated a strong, dose-dependent, inverse association in both sexes with fiber intake measured as crude fiber, dietary fiber, or nonstarch polysaccharides. Experimental evidence supports these findings (Jacobs, 1986), although experimental studies indicated that certain fibers were much more effective than others in such preventive effects. Matthew et al. (1997) reported that a group of patients at increased risk of colorectal cancer selected diets containing significantly less fruit and vegetables than those not at risk. This further supports the more general finding that diets high in fruits and vegetables tend to decrease the risk of a number of cancers (Hirayama, 1994).

Studies on the association of dietary factors with endometrial cancer, like cervical cancer, have not been extensive. In at least two studies (Zheng et al., 1995a; Levi et al., 1993), evidence was presented that consumption of various types of meats was associated with an increased risk of this disease. However, other investigations found either the reverse (Barbone et al., 1993) or no significant effect (Tzonou et al., 1996). The latter authors, studying a cohort in Greece, did present evidence that increased intake of monounsaturated fat, mostly olive oil, was somewhat protective. Few if any animal studies in this area have surfaced.

Carcinoma of the esophagus has long been known to be associated with smoking and alcohol abuse (Gao et al., 1994a; Launoy et al., 1997; Gammon et al., 1997). Dietary factors are also directly as well as indirectly related to the development of esophageal cancer in the human. At least two studies have demonstrated an increased risk of this lesion in populations consuming corn or maize as a predominant portion of their diet (Sammon and Alderson, 1998; van Rensburg, 1981). Sammon and Alderson (1998) have postulated that one possible mechanism concerns the presence of high concentrations of linoleic acid, a precursor of gastric prostaglandin synthesis, in maize. Together with other dietary abnormalities, this may lead to an increased concentration of prostaglandin E_2 in the gastric mucosa, with subsequent pyloric relaxation and related events leading to a greater reflux of gastric juices into the esophagus. It is this mechanism that is felt to be important in the development of a preneoplastic condition termed Barrett esophagus, the incidence of which has increased dramatically in North America and western Europe in recent years (Cameron, 1994). Approximately 10% of individuals with some degree of acid reflux in the esophagus suffer from this condition, the overall incidence of which may be in the neighborhood of 1 in 80 adults in the general population in these areas (cf. Cameron, 1994). Although esophageal cancer is a relatively uncommon cause of death in patients with Barrett esophagus (van der Burgh et al., 1996), patients with this condition have a 30- to 125-fold greater risk of developing esophageal cancer than the general population (cf. Cameron, 1994). Smoking and alcohol do not appear to be related to the predisposition of the changes seen in Barrett esophagus, but they are strongly associated with the development of adenocarcinoma in patients with established Barrett esophagus (Gray et al., 1993). Thus, diet, which in turn affects gastric acidity and reflux of gastric contents into the esophagus, may be related to an increased incidence of esophageal carcinoma. Increased intake of animal fat and cholesterol have also been related to an increased incidence of esophageal cancer (Launoy et al., 1998; Kaul et al., 1986). However, no significant associations were reported with total calories and esophageal cancer incidence (Brown et al., 1995), but salty and fried food intake was associated with increased risk (Gao et al., 1994b). The protective action of antioxidant vitamins such as A, C, and E, as well as fruits and vegetables, has been reported in several studies (Zheng et al., 1995b; Gao et al., 1994b; Brown et al., 1995; Launoy et al., 1998). At least one study in animals has shown a protective effect of vitamin E on nitrosamine-induced esophageal neoplasia in mice (Odeleye et al., 1992). Although one study involving dietary supplementation in a cohort in the People's Republic of China showed no specific effect of antioxidant vitamins and zinc on the prevalence of premalignant lesions of the esophagus, those individuals with large increases in these components in the blood were more likely to have a histologically normal esophagus at the end of the trial (Wahrendorf et al., 1988). In contrast, zinc deficiency in rats caused the development of a significantly higher incidence of esophageal and forestomach neoplasia in animals administered precursors of the carcinogen N-nitroso-N-benzylmethylamine (Fong et al., 1984). Thus, while diet may not directly be a major cause of esophageal cancer in the human, indirect effects leading to esophageal reflux and the significant potential for prevention indicate that diet plays an important role in the ultimate development of this disease in the human.

Cancer of the gallbladder is not uncommon in the human but is unusual in most animal species, even in experimental studies. In the human, studies have indicated that both a high-carbohydrate diet as well as one containing high levels of fats and oils and a high total energy intake are associated with an increased incidence of this disease (Moerman et al., 1993; Zatonski et al., 1997). These factors may also be related to the close association of biliary tract cancer and the presence of gallstones and obesity (cf. Tominaga and Kuroishi, 1994). In one Japanese study, intake of animal proteins and fats, as well as ingestion of fruits and vegetables, decreased the risk of gallbladder cancer (Kato et al., 1989). In contrast, our knowledge of dietary factors in the development of liver cancer, primarily hepatocellular carcinoma, comes from a knowledge of infectious agents. including the hepatitis B and C viruses (Chapter 12) and dietary contaminants such as aflatoxin (see above). Alcohol also plays a significant role in the development of cancer of this organ, but specific major dietary factors have not been studied extensively in the human. In one study (Yu et al., 1995), a low consumption of dark green vegetables was associated with an increased risk of hepatocellular carcinoma, as was a low serum retinol level. In animals a number of studies have shown the effects of specific dietary constituents on the development of liver neoplasia (Chapter 8). He et al. (1997) demonstrated that dietary extracts of carrots, tomatoes, and orange juice decreased the number of preneoplastic foci during initiation and also inhibited the growth of focal lesions during the stage of promotion. In general, administration of retinoids during hepatocarcinogenesis inhibits the process (Mack et al., 1990; Moreno et al., 1995; Gradelet et al., 1998). However, retinol itself reportedly enhanced carcinogenesis by 3′-methyl-4-dimethylaminoazobenzene (Ohkawa et al., 1991). Some studies actually indicated that β-carotene and related compounds were more effective than vitamin A and its derivatives in inhibiting the development of preneoplastic lesions in experimental hepatocarcinogenesis (Sarkar et al., 1995; Moreno et al., 1995). Similarly, vitamin E reportedly prevented the induction of preneoplastic enzyme-altered foci in rats (Ura et al., 1987), but it actually enhanced the growth of hepatic focal lesions in mice (Kolaja and Klaunig, 1997).

Dietary factors as causative of lung cancer have not been extensively investigated, since the primary cause of this disease is tobacco abuse. High dietary fat may increase the risk of lung cancer (Byers et al., 1987), and cholesterol intake was associated with significant increased risk in one investigation by Jain et al. (1990). Most studies of the relationship of dietary factors to lung cancer risk have been concerned with antioxidant vitamins and related dietary constituents both in the pure form and within fruits and vegetables. Le Marchand et al. (1989) demonstrated a strong inverse association between lung cancer risk and the intake of all vegetables, while another investigation (Yong et al., 1997) indicated a protective effect of both fruits and vegetables, especially those containing carotenoids. Ingestion of crude retinoids and carotenoids, especially β-carotene and vitamin E from fruits and vegetables as measured by serum levels of these components, indicated a protective action in decreasing the risk of lung cancer (Yong et al., 1997; Menkes et al., 1986; cf. Fontham, 1990). In contrast, two studies on vitamin E and β-carotene supplements to smokers demonstrated the absence of any preventive effect and found that β-carotene supplementation may slightly increase lung cancer incidence in cigarette smokers (Albanes et al., 1996; Omenn et al., 1996). An earlier study by Blot et al. (1994) in a different population suggested that supplementation with β-carotene, vitamin E, and selenium decreased the risk of lung cancer in smokers. In part, these discrepancies may be related to the fact that several reports indicate that vitamin E and carotenoids may exert their effects in patients who are relatively light smokers compared with those smoking heavily (Knekt, 1993; Yong et al., 1997). A preventive effect on the incidence of mesothelioma was also related to the intake of vegetables, especially cruciferous vegetables, whose consumption was inversely related to risk of this lesion in the lung induced by a different carcinogen—asbestos (Schiffman et al., 1988). Similarly, the prevalence of bronchial metaplasia, a preneoplastic condition, in asbestos-exposed workers was inversely related to the dietary intake of vitamin A (Mayne et al., 1998). Thus, similar dietary relationships have been noted for two entirely different histological types of neoplasms within the pulmonary cavity in the human. In nonsmokers, both men and women, dietary β-carotene, raw fruits and vegetables, and vitamin E supplements reduced the risk of lung cancer (Mayne et al., 1994).

While there are few if any data on the effect of diet on leukemias, myeloma, and sarcomas, at least one study (Chiu et al., 1996) did demonstrate that excessive dietary fat and animal protein increased the risk of non-Hodgkin lymphomas in older women. However, considerable data have accumulated, as noted earlier (Chapter 6), on the effect of retinoids, especially *trans*-retinoic acid (Tallman et al., 1997), in inhibiting the growth of acute promyelocytic leukemia. In this instance, administration of high levels of these retinoids induced differentiation with the potential for increased apoptosis of leukemic cells, the mechanism of which was discussed earlier (Figure 6.6). In a Japanese cohort, daily meat consumption was significantly associated with the occurrence of ovarian cancer (Mori and Miyake, 1988). The consumption of carrots and presumably β-carotene was found to be inversely associated with the risk of this neoplasm (Engle et al., 1991).

Several studies have indicated dietary factors as causative in the development of pancreatic cancer in the human. Increased intake of dietary meat as well as increased caloric intake reportedly enhance the risk of developing this lesion (Farrow and Davis, 1990; Ohba et al., 1996; Silverman et al., 1998). At least one study of a cohort from Poland indicated a strong positive association with the intake of cholesterol (Zatonski et al., 1991) as well as some positive association with dietary protein. However, Farrow and Davis (1990), studying a cohort in western Washington in the United States, did not find any effect of dietary cholesterol. In rodents, especially rats, dietary fat enhances or promotes the development of preneoplastic acinar lesions in the pancreas (cf. Roebuck, 1992). This is primarily true of dietary unsaturated fats of the omega-6 but not the omega-3 series (Chapter 8). Thus, promotion of these lesions by dietary fat appears only partly related to the high caloric content of the fat itself. Frequent consumption of fruits, vegetables (particularly carrots), and plant foods/protein lowered the risk of pancreatic cancer (Norell et al., 1986; Ohba et al., 1996). While no exactly comparable animal studies have been carried out, several investigations have demonstrated the inhibition of the development of preneoplastic foci in the pancreas of azaserine-treated rats by the administration of synthetic retinoids (Roebuck et al., 1984), β-carotene, and selenium (Woutersen and van Garderen-Hoetmer, 1988).

Just as with cancer of the breast, a major dietary factor in the development of prostatic carcinoma is dietary fat (Giovannucci, 1998; Whittemore et al., 1995), which finding is also reflected in the relationship of obesity to the risk of fatal prostate cancer (Snowdon et al., 1984). As in mammary cancer, there is also evidence that total energy intake is related to the development of preclinical prostate cancer (Meyer et al., 1997). However, not all investigations have supported these findings (e.g., Key et al., 1997). In a recent review, Giovannucci (1998) argued that the strongest correlation for a positive association of dietary factors with prostate cancer exists with dairy products, especially milk and high-fat milk. Just as in Figure 11.3, studies have demonstrated a quasilinear correlation between age-adjusted prostate cancer mortality and dietary animal fat (Rose et al., 1986). These workers have thus put the two relationships together and demonstrated an interesting quasilinear relationship between the age-adjusted mortality of prostate cancer and that of breast cancer in populations of a number of countries throughout the world (Figure 11.4). Dietary protein/meat intake has also been positively associated with an increased risk of prostate cancer in several studies (Heshmat et al., 1985; Talamini et al., 1992; Vlajinac et al., 1997). As with a large number of neoplastic cell types, fruits and vegetables and their constituents, especially carotenoids, have generally been found to play a protective role in the development of prostate cancer (Ohno et al., 1988; Mettlin et al., 1989; Mills et al., 1989). The single vegetable found most influential in several studies is the tomato, and within this vegetable the presence of the carotenoid lycopene appears to be a consistently effective inhibitor of the development of this lesion in humans (Giovannucci et al., 1995; Clinton et al., 1996). Although β-carotene and related carotenoids have been shown in some studies to be negatively associated with the risk of prostate cancer, other investigations have argued the opposite (Kolonel et al., 1988). Later investigations by this group in Hawaii (Le Marchand et al., 1991) have tempered their earlier findings, but several other studies have also shown a positive or no effect of vitamin A and related retinoids on the risk of prostate cancer (cf. Giovannucci, 1998). Interestingly, an inverse relationship between serum retinol and the risk of prostate cancer has been reported by at least two groups (Hsing et al., 1990; Hayes et al., 1988). In animal investigations, Wynder and associates (1994), in a review, have pointed out that the preponderance of studies on the effect of high fat intake in experimental prostate carcinogenesis have not reported any effect, although caloric restriction may cause a significant inhibition of tumor incidence. On

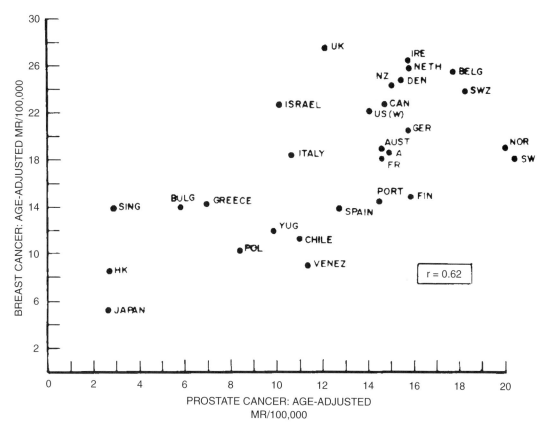

Figure 11.4 Relationship between breast and prostate cancer mortality rates for 30 countries for the years 1978–79. The axes indicate the age-adjusted mortality rate (MR) per 100,000 individuals. (Adapted from Rose et al., 1986, with permission of the authors and publishers.)

the other hand, synthetic retinoids fed in the diet can inhibit chemically (Pollard et al., 1991) and genetically induced prostate cancer in rodents (Slawin et al., 1993). In contrast to the extensive studies on the effect of diet on prostate cancer risk, relatively few investigations have been carried out on the effect of diet on the development of renal carcinoma. Two studies (Mellemgaard et al., 1996; Wolk et al., 1996) have indicated the importance of total dietary energy intake in the risk of renal cell carcinoma, but they found discrepant results on the protective effect of fruits and vegetables. These investigations included populations from Australia, Denmark, Sweden, and the United States.

Unlike many other neoplasms of the gastrointestinal tract and their related components, a major dietary factor associated with increased risk of gastric cancer is the high salt or sodium chloride content of ingested foods. This finding has been demonstrated in numerous investigations in the human, several of which are listed in the table and confirmed with experimental studies in rodents (Takahashi et al., 1994). In animals, the promoting or enhancing effect of sodium chloride on the development of gastric cancer can be related to a concentration-dependent tissue damage and subsequent cell proliferation in the stomach mucosa of the rodent (Charnley and Tannenbaum, 1985; Furihata et al., 1996). As a possible factor in these toxic effects of the salt, Takahashi et al. (1991) demonstrated that administration of sodium chloride is associated with enhanced lipid peroxidation in the gastric mucosa. In addition to gastric carcinogenesis, the development of nasopharyngeal carcinoma, while primarily related to infection with the Epstein-Barr virus (see below) has also been positively associated with a high-salt diet (Yu et al., 1986; Zou et al., 1994). The ingestion of sodium nitrate as a potential precursor of nitrite and subsequent nitrosation of secondary amines within the stomach (see above) have been argued to be potentially significant factors in the dietary causation of stomach cancer in the human (Hartman, 1983). However, other studies do not appear to bear this out (Pobel et al., 1995), and studies on the carcinogenicity of sodium nitrate in rats were negative (Maekawa et al., 1982). Pickled vegetables, which may also contain high levels of salt as well as possible carcinogenic nitrosamines (see above), have also been associated with an increased risk of gastric cancer (Ahn, 1997; Ramón et al., 1993). The relatively high incidence of gastric cancer in Iceland may be related to the high level of smoked fish consumed in that country. But as yet the dietary factors involved in the high morbidity and mortality rates of stomach cancer in Japan have not been clearly identified. The suggestion has been made that one reason for the decrease in gastric cancer seen in the United States over the past four decades is the addition of antioxidants to dairy products and other foods containing fat; however, this proposal has not been verified. As with other cancers of the gastrointestinal tract, consumption of fruits and vegetables is inversely associated with the incidence of stomach cancer in the human (Coggon et al., 1989; Graham et al., 1990; Tuyns et al., 1992). In mainland China, it appears that ingestion of Chinese cabbage, a staple food for lower income groups, may have an important role in reducing the risk of the development of stomach cancer (Hu et al., 1988). The components of fruits and vegetables that have been most closely associated with their preventive effect are ascorbic acid and β-carotene (Hansson et al., 1994; Kromhout and Bueno-de-Mesquita, 1997). The most important factor appears to be the concentration of vitamin C within the gastric juice rather than serum levels of ascorbate (Correa et al., 1998). In some animal studies (cf. Krinsky, 1994), administration of carotenoids may inhibit chemically induced development of gastric carcinoma.

General Considerations of Dietary Effects on Human Cancer Development

While the data in Table 11.3 are necessarily incomplete in their coverage of the literature, certain trends are clearly evident. Excess dietary meat—especially cooked meat, dietary fat, and excess dietary calories have been associated in a number of studies with an increased risk of a variety of human neoplasms. On the other hand, average increased intake of fruits and vegetables, as well as a number of the micronutrients found in these substances—e.g., vitamins A, C, E, and other carotenoids—are associated with a decreased risk of developing a variety of neoplasms in the human, especially when taken at somewhat increased levels compared with average consumption. Unique dietary factors include the possible effect of dietary cholesterol in increasing the risk of esophageal, lung, and pancreatic cancer and the effect of dietary salt on the development of stomach, nasopharyngeal, and esophageal cancer. Other dietary constituents that have been studied in relation to the risk of human cancer include milk and dairy products, studies that have been inconclusive for ovarian cancer risk (Mettlin and Piver, 1990; Cramer et al., 1989) but have suggested a relation to an increased risk of lymphoid neoplasia in at least one investigation (Ursin et al., 1990). More theoretical (Parodi, 1997) and experimental studies (Papenburg et al., 1990) have suggested that milk components may inhibit the development of neoplasia in humans and animals. Soy protein and its associated constituents, which make up major components of the human diet in certain parts of the world, especially southeast Asia, have been suggested as preventive for human cancer development (Persky and van Horn, 1995; Barnes, 1998), whereas animal studies, although predominantly supportive of these epidemiological indications, are by no means consistent (Messina et al., 1994; Sørensen et al., 1998). A more consistent inhibition of neoplasia in human and animals can be seen with the family of cruciferous vegetables. These include such common vegetables as horseradish, turnip, cabbage, brussels sprouts, cauliflower, broccoli, Chinese cabbage, radish, and mustard (cf. Verhagen et al., 1997). A number of epidemiological and animal studies have shown the effectiveness of cruciferous vegetables in inhibiting the development of a variety of human and animal neoplasms (cf. Nestle, 1997). The principal active ingredients in the inhibition of carcinogenesis are the glucosinolates and their hydrolysis products. These share a common basic skeleton containing a β-D-thioglucose grouping, a side chain, and a sulfonated oxime moiety but differ in their side chain. A general structure is as follows:

$$R - C \begin{array}{c} \diagup \; S - \beta - D \; glucose \\ \\ \diagdown \diagdown \; N - OSO_3^{\,-} \end{array}$$

These agents are active inducers of phase II xenobiotic metabolizing enzymes (Chapter 3). In addition, they are effective in preventing oxidative DNA damage both in humans (Verhagen et al., 1997) and in rodents (Deng et al., 1998). Another chemical commonly found in cruciferous vegetables, indole-3-carbinol, also inhibits experimental carcinogenesis, probably by a similar mechanism (Grubbs et al., 1995), but in some studies clear evidence for tumor-promoting activity of carcinogenesis by this compound has also been found (Dashwood, 1998). Thus, there is ample evidence to indicate the importance of a variety of dietary plants and their constituents in effectively inhibiting the development of neoplasia in mammalian organisms. It should be noted that such inhibition occurs predominantly at the stage of tumor promotion, as noted from the listing seen in Table 11.4. While the listing of types of neoplasia affected by these dietary factors is incomplete, as noted from Table 11.3, the neoplasms listed represent numerically the predominance of human neoplasia affected. Thus, as expected and readily noted from Table 11.3, preventing the dietary induction of human neoplasia by appropriate alternate dietary intake is not only feasible but, in most countries, readily or reasonably applicable. A number of studies have actually attempted to estimate the preventive potential of dietary alteration in the incidence of specific human neoplasms (cf. Miller et al., 1994). Table 11.5 summarizes a number of studies attempting to estimate potential preventive effects of dietary alterations on various neoplasms.

Thus, while one may be unwilling to accept the suggestion that 35% of human cancer is directly related to diet (Doll, 1992), there is increasing evidence that diet and related factors play

Table 11.4 Stages of Carcinogenesis at Which Dietary Factors Alter Cancer Incidence (Humans)

Dietary Component	Cancer Type	Change in Risk	Stage of Action
Calories	Breast, pancreas, prostate	+	Promotion
Protein	Colon, prostate	+	?
Fat	Breast, colon, prostate	+	Promotion
Vitamin A, β-carotene (retinoids)	Esophagus, lung, skin	–	Promotion
Cruciferous vegetables	Stomach, colon	–	Initiation, promotion
Alcoholic beverages	Rectum, breast, liver, larynx	+	Promotion

Key: +, increased risk; –, decreased risk.

Table 11.5 Estimates of Potential Effects of Dietary Change on the Incidence of Various Cancers

Site	Action	Potential Incidence Reduction PAR[a]	Potentially Preventable
Oropharynx, esophagus, and larynx	[Eliminate smoking and] reduce alcohol, increase fruit and vegetable consumption	[90%]	86%
Stomach	Reduce nitrite, cured meats and salt-preserved foods, increase fruit and vegetable consumption	68%	74%
Colon and rectum	Reduce fat and increase vegetables	50%	79%
Breast	Reduce fat and increase vegetables	27%	75%
	Reduce obesity (postmenopausal women)	12%	
Endometrium	Reduce obesity	30%	82%
Ovary	Reduce fat	?	66%
Prostate	Reduce fat	?	81%
Kidney	[Eliminate smoking], reduce fat	[30%]	98%
Lung	[Eliminate smoking], reduce fat and increase vegetables	[80%]	76%
Bladder	[Eliminate smoking], reduce dietary cholesterol	[60%]	73%
Pancreas	[Eliminate smoking], reduce calories and dietary cholesterol, increase vegetables	[50%]	70%
Liver	Reduce alcohol	30%	?

[a]PAR, population-attributable risk. Square brackets are used when some of the benefit derives from eliminating smoking. Estimates for males, except for breast, endometrium, and ovarian cancer. ? signifies that no estimate of effect is available.
Modified from Miller et al., 1994, with permission of authors and publisher.

a major role in the incidence of human cancer. However, this role is quite complex and in all likelihood does not result from the direct conversion of normal to neoplastic cells by dietary constituents but rather stems from an alteration in the development of cells within the organism that have the potential for neoplastic growth.

Reproductive and Sexual Behavior as Causative Factors in Human Cancer

That certain types of reproductive and sexual behavior alter the incidence of human cancer has been known since the time of Ramazzini (see above). Doll and Peto (1981) pointed out that pregnancy and childbirth seem to play a significant role in the prevention of cancers of the endometrium, ovary, and breast in that all of these conditions are less common in women who have borne children early than in those who have had no children. However, the risk factors for these various types of neoplasms do have some significant differences. These are noted in Table 11.6, where most of the risk factors are tabulated in relation to various physiological and pharmacological events.

As noted in the table, the two classic risk factors related to genital and mammary cancer in the female are alterations in the onset and cessation of menstruation—i.e., the time of menarche and of menopause. Menarche occurring at an early age (less than 13 years of age) is a significant

Table 11.6 Comparison of Hormonal Risk Factors for Cancers of the Endometrium, Ovary, Cervix, and Breast

	Endometrium	Ovary	Cervix	Breast
1. *Menstruation*				
Early age at menarche	+	0	0	+
Early age at natural or surgical menopause	–	–	0	–
Late age at natural menopause	+	?	0	+
Increasing years between menarche and menopause excluding pregnancies and duration of pregnancies and oral contraceptive use	+	?	?	+
2. *Pregnancy/intercourse*				
Married, never pregnant	+	+	–	+
Early age, first full-term pregnancy	0	0	0	–
Multiple full-term pregnancies	–	–	+	–
Age >35 1st full-term pregnancy	0	0	0	+
Age >35 last full-term pregnancy	–	0	+	?
Cumulative number of lactating months	0/+	0	?	–
Multiple sexual partners	?	?	+	?
3. *Obesity*				
Premenopausal women	+	?	?	–/+
Postmenopausal women	+	?	?	+
4. *Exogenous steroids*				
Estrogen/progestin oral contraceptives	–	–	+	+/?
Estrogen replacement without progestin	+	–/?	0	+
Estrogen replacement with progestin	+/–	–	0	+/?

Key: +, increased risk (> 1.0); –, decreased risk (< 1.0); 0, no risk relation established; ?, available data insufficient or equivocal.

risk factor for breast cancer development in later years (Titus-Ernstoff et al., 1998). While some earlier studies have suggested that early menarche may not be a risk factor, most indicate that such a circumstance does increase the risk of breast cancer as compared with menarche after age 15 (Adami et al., 1990). This increased risk is found only for cancer of the breast and endometrium and not for that of the ovary and cervix. Conversely, early age at menopause, whether natural or surgical, produces the opposite effect in both of these tissues as well as in the ovary, while late age at natural menopause exhibits an increased risk of endometrial and mammary cancer but not cervical neoplasia. As would be expected, increasing years between menarche and menopause also act to increase risk for both endometrial and breast cancer, but data are insufficient to determine the effects on ovarian and cervical cancer risk (Schottenfeld, 1995). Thus, menstrual parameters may affect the development of endometrial, ovarian, or breast cancer in various ways but do not seem to have a significant effect on cervical cancer risk. Although most cervical neoplasms are squamous cell carcinomas, a significant number of adenocarcinomas arising from the cervical canal of the uterus also occur. Interestingly, the risk factors for these lesions are more closely related to those for cancer of the cervix than to cancer of the endometrium (Kjaer and Brinton, 1993).

Perhaps more important than menstrual parameters in the risk of development of these hormonally influenced neoplasms are the effects of pregnancy and frequency of intercourse. As noted above, the nulliparity of Catholic nuns, which Ramazzini related to the high incidence of breast cancer in this population, affects not only this tissue but is also a risk factor for endometrial and ovarian cancer; however, nulliparity is significantly a negative or protective factor for cervical cancer risk. In contrast to the increased risk of mammary cancer in relation to an early menarchal age, the occurrence of the first full-term pregnancy at an early age (less than 20 years) confers a significant protection against the development of breast cancer but apparently has no relationship to risk of the other three neoplasms noted in Table 11.6. As also noted in the table, first full-term pregnancy occurring after age 35 results in a significantly increased risk of mammary neoplasia. In one analysis, this amounted to a 40% increase as compared with a first birth prior to age 20 years (Adami et al., 1990). However, Lambe et al. (1994) reported, in confirmation of other studies (Kvåle and Heuch, 1987; Kampert et al., 1988), that pregnancy transiently increases the risk of breast cancer but reduces the risk in later years. In women with two pregnancies, the short-term adverse effect of the second pregnancy is masked by the long-term protection imparted by the first pregnancy. Furthermore, women with many late pregnancies and those with a few widely spaced pregnancies exhibited a higher risk for the development of breast cancer than did nulliparous women in one study (Kvåle and Heuch, 1987). The observation of the protective effect of early pregnancy and the short-term increased risk followed by later protection may be related to mechanisms seen in rodents, such as those described by Russo and colleagues (cf. Russo et al., 1992), wherein pregnancy results in an alteration of the lobular structure of the breast, which in turn may modulate the susceptibility of the target cells for the initiation of mammary neoplasia (Russo and Russo, 1996). In contrast, these effects noted in the development of sporadic or nongenetically based breast cancer are not seen in a hereditary subset of breast cancers (Lynch et al., 1984), although a consistent increase in the risk of breast cancer was seen among women having a mother or sister with the disease that was exacerbated by first pregnancy (Colditz et al., 1996).

Multiple full-term pregnancies, except perhaps those occurring at a very late age, act as a protective sequence for endometrial, ovarian, and mammary cancer but not cervical cancer (Brinton et al., 1989). Lactation, especially for extensive periods, does act as a protective factor against the risk of breast cancer as reported in some but not all studies (cf. Adami et al., 1990; Newcomb et al., 1994; Enger et al., 1998). No definitive effect on the risk of endometrial, ovarian, or cervical cancer has been reported in relation to lactation, whether for long or short periods. In contrast, the incidence of cervical cancer, of both morphological types, is directly related to the number of sexual partners. This may be related to the risk seen with multiple full-term pregnancies, especially if they occurred with different sexual partners. The reason for this difference is most likely related to infections with the human papillomavirus (Chapter 12) (Schiffman and Brinton, 1995). This complicates our understanding of the role of other factors in this disease, including the age at first intercourse, smoking, and the use of oral contraceptives, as noted in the table (Harris et al., 1980).

DeWaard et al. (1964) were the first to describe the association between obesity and increased breast cancer risk. In women who are more than 50 lb overweight, the risk ratio is a factor of 10 to 1 (Rose, 1996). The risk of breast cancer resulting from a greater body mass is most significant in older women, while a reported decrease in relative risk of breast cancer occurs in younger women of large body size (Velentgas and Daling, 1994). The dramatic increase in risk of endometrial cancer as a result of increased body mass is probably related to the fact that the conversion of the precursor steroid androstenedione to estrone actually takes place in the stroma of fat cells. Thus, in obese women with more fat cells present, more estrone is produced, and one has a situation similar to the effect of unopposed estrogens administered exogenously and the high risk of endometrial cancer (Gambrell, 1994; see below). A similar effect has been postulated as the mechanism for the effect of a miscarriage or abortion late in reproductive life, followed by the lack of a subsequent full-term pregnancy. This effect may also result in the presence of "unopposed" estrogen leading to an increased risk of endometrial cancer (McPherson et al., 1996). The effect of abortion on breast cancer risk is equivocal (Adami et al., 1990), while such a procedure seems to be unrelated to ovarian cancer risk (cf. Daly, 1992).

Exogenous steroid hormones have been used specifically in medical practice for more than a half century. The initial use of the synthetic estrogen diethylstilbesterol to prevent early-term miscarriages resulted in a significant risk of vaginal and cervical cancer in offspring of women so treated (see below). With the advent of estrogens and progestins used in contraception, numerous studies were developed to study the effect of chronic administration of such agents on the development of neoplasms of the female reproductive tract and breast. As noted from Table 11.6, the modern oral contraceptive preparations combining estrogens and progestins serve to decrease the risk of endometrial and ovarian cancer (Rose, 1996; McGowan, 1989). In contrast, long-term users of oral contraceptives are at excess risk for the development of cervical cancer (Schiffman and Brinton, 1995). While the use of oral contraceptive preparations in younger women carries with it a significant increase in risk of breast cancer (Velentgas and Daling, 1994), the risk in older women is either nil (Velentgas and Daling, 1994) or equivocal (cf. Adami et al., 1990). However, several studies have indicated that postmenopausal estrogen replacement does significantly increase the risk of breast cancer in older women, especially when the treatment is continued for extended periods (Steinberg et al., 1991; Beral et al., 1997). A much more dramatic effect has been reported on the increased risk of endometrial cancer in women receiving unopposed estrogen therapy. The risk ratio for this effect ranges from six- to eightfold (Gordon et al., 1977; Antunes et al., 1979). Combining estrogen replacement therapy with progestins dramatically reduces the risk of endometrial cancer (Beresford et al., 1997), and the administration of progestins even years after unopposed estrogen tends to prevent the effect of the latter (Barrett-Connor, 1992). Exogenous steroids generally tend to decrease the risk of ovarian cancer—with one interesting exception, where replacement hormone use was associated with a threefold increased risk of a histological subset of ovarian neoplasms termed *endometrioid neoplasms* (Weiss et al., 1982; Daly, 1992). Estrogen replacement therapy does not affect cervical cancer risk (Persson, 1996). On the other hand, postmenopausal estrogen therapy plays a protective role in the development of colorectal cancer (Calle et al., 1995) and large colorectal adenomas (Grodstein et al., 1998). An interesting debate focuses on the effect of xenoestrogens—estrogenic chemicals occurring naturally in plants and animals—as well as side effects of pesticides and other chemicals on the risk of breast, testicular, and prostate cancers as well as other physiological processes (Crisp et al., 1998; Safe, 1998). As yet, however, this consideration has little or no epidemiological base but remains as a potential for future investigations.

Our knowledge of hormonal factors in the etiology of neoplasms of the male genital tract and male breast is far less advanced than that concerning the female. Table 11.7 shows some of the factors for which there is some evidence of a relationship with the development of these lesions. Our knowledge of prostate cancer, which is now the most common, potentially fatal neoplasm in the United States, is necessarily greater than that of testis or male breast. Furthermore, preneoplastic and premalignant lesions found in the prostate, benign prostatic hyperplasia, and occult prostatic carcinoma have been studied extensively in relation to their potential association with the development of prostate cancer. While benign prostatic hyperplasia is generally considered as having an etiology different from that of prostatic carcinoma (Griffiths et al., 1991), epidemiological studies have reported both an increased risk or no risk of invasive cancer in relation to the incidence of benign prostatic hyperplasia (Nomura and Kolonel, 1991). Occult prostatic cancer is extremely frequent throughout the world and increases in incidence with advancing age in the world male population. However, men in Japan and Taiwan have one of the lowest rates of clinically significant prostate cancer in the world; on the other hand, Japanese

Table 11.7 Hormonal Risk Factors for Cancers of the Prostate, Testes and Male Breast[a]

	Prostate	Testis	Male Breast
Endogenous hormones:			
Androgens	+		
Estrogens			+
Other hormones	+		
Specific drug therapy			+
Vasectomy	?	0	
Undescended testes	?	+	
Obesity	+		
Early puberty	–	+	
Sexual intercourse	+/–	0/+	– (?)
Related conditions			
Occult prostate cancer	+/0		
Benign prostatic hyperplasia	?		
Infections	+		+

[a]See key below Table 11.6 for definitions of symbols. Blanks indicate that no studies are available on that parameter for the neoplasm in question. See text for discussion and references.

men living in the continental United States exhibit an incidence of overt prostate cancer approaching that in Caucasian men in the United States. Similar associations are seen with black men in the United States compared with their counterparts in certain African nations (Wilding, 1995). The fact that prostate cancer patients become sexually active at an earlier age, have more sexual partners before marriage, have a higher fertility, and usually have a history of venereal disease compared with controls (Nomura and Kolonel, 1991; cf. Boyle and Zaridze, 1993) suggests an infectious agent involved in the causation of prostate cancer, in analogy to that seen in cervical cancer in the female (see above). Increased risk of prostate and testicular cancer has been seen in younger and older age groups respectively in at least two different studies (Mishina et al., 1985; Maden et al., 1993). Evidence of some of these parameters as associated with different risks for cancer of the male breast is less well known. However, endogenous hormones, especially androgens, appear to be associated with an increased risk for prostate cancer, while increases in circulating estrogens have been seen with male breast cancer (Calabresi et al., 1976). The best evidence for a role of endogenous androgens in the development of prostate cancer is seen in the fact that castration at an early age almost totally inhibits the development of prostate cancer as well as benign prostatic hyperplasia (cf. Nomura and Kolonel, 1991). High levels of circulating testosterone were also associated with an increased risk of prostate cancer in one study (Gann et al., 1996), but several other studies have been relatively inconsistent (Nomura and Kolonel, 1991; Wilding, 1995). In many men with occult prostate cancer, testosterone levels are low or normal despite a normal prostate-specific antigen (PSA) level (Morgentaler et al., 1996). This suggests that PSA levels, which are used extensively as biochemical markers in screening for the presence of prostate cancer (Chapter 17), may be altered by variations in serum androgen levels. During the last two decades, with the increasing popularity of vasectomy as a method for contraception, a number of studies have investigated the relation of this procedure to the risk of prostate and testicular cancer. While a very large study indicated that testicular cancer is not related to vasectomy (Møller et al., 1994a), studies on the relation of the operation to prostate cancer risk have demonstrated an increased risk (Zhu et al., 1996) or a possible protective effect (cf. Nomura and Kolonel, 1991). A major risk factor for testicular cancer, however, is the presence of an undescended testis, where the risk may be as high as eightfold or greater (Moss et al., 1986; Forman et al., 1994).

Both endogenous and exogenous hormones play significant roles in the incidence of human cancer, especially of the breast, prostate, endometrium, and ovary (Henderson et al., 1982; Key, 1995). Hormones are also likely to play some role in the development of other human cancers including those of the testis, thyroid, bone (Henderson et al., 1982), and of liver cell adenomas (Edmondson et al., 1976). It is also possible that endogenous hormones play a role in the development of other human neoplasms, but few or no definitive data are presently available. Furthermore, as can be seen from the relation of obesity to cancer incidence and endogenous hormone production, relations between dietary intake and endogenous hormonal levels may also effect an increased risk of various types of neoplasms. As yet, however, the complexity of these and other interactions in the genesis of human neoplasia has not been as well delineated as in animal studies. Still, it would be foolish to underestimate the importance of dietary and hormonal factors in the genesis of human neoplasia.

Tobacco Abuse as a Definitive Cause of Human Cancer

While diet and hormone alterations play major roles in the causation of human cancer, in most instances the exact mechanism resulting in such increased risk is not clear. In the abuse of tobacco and tobacco products through smoking, chewing, and related uses, a more definitive causative mechanism of human cancer has been clarified. Early observations in this century (cf. Hoffman, 1915) related cancer of the buccal cavity, and particularly of the lip, to smoking habits, especially with pipes. In this context, smoking was related to the use of the betel nut as a masticatory for chewing, a habit that has been known since the fourth century A.D. in different parts of the world (Sharan, 1996). Over time, the form of mastication of the betel nut has changed depending on the social circumstances. Thus, the betel nut may be used alone or as a quid along with a variety of ingredients including perfumes, stimulants, and different types of tobacco. Extracts of the quid have been shown to be carcinogenic in the mouse and other species (Bhide et al., 1979). Extracts of the nut itself contain alkaloids that have been shown to be mutagenic in bacteria (cf. Sharan, 1996). Recently, there has been a decline in betel quid chewing, especially in the young, and a concomitant decline in oral cancer (Reichart, 1995). Related uses of tobacco include its use as snuff and for chewing without the other additives of the betel quid. Chewing tobacco, a form of smokeless tobacco, while popular around 1900, decreased dramatically in use until about 25 years ago, at which time there was a marked increase in sales and production of smokeless tobacco, used both for chewing and for snuff dipping (holding cut tobacco between the cheek or lip and gingiva or beneath the tongue) (Connolly et al., 1986). This type of exposure to tobacco, as well as the betel quid, has been deemed as carcinogenic for humans by the IARC (IARC, 1985). While the IARC has deemed the evidence for human carcinogenicity of chewing tobacco as limited, alkaloids extracted from smokeless tobacco during its use give rise to potent carcinogenic N-nitrosamines such as NNK (Chapter 3) (Hoffmann and Hecht, 1988). Unfortunately, the use of smokeless tobacco today is most common in children and young adult males (Squier, 1988) as well as in young women who chronically dip snuff. In one study of this last population, the relative risk of oral and pharyngeal cancer approached 50-fold (Winn et al., 1981).

Tobacco smoking as a cause of lung and a variety of nonrespiratory cancers is largely a phenomenon of the twentieth century, especially the last two-thirds of the century. To a significant degree, this is probably the result of the ready availability and popularity of cigarettes. The mass production of cigarettes was made possible by the invention of the cigarette-rolling machine in the latter part of the nineteenth century, followed by the development of safety matches. The result of these inventions is seen by the fact that in 1880 smokers averaged 40 cigarettes per year, while in 1977 this average increased to 12,854 (Bartecchi et al., 1995). Concomitant with the increasing consumption of cigarettes was seen the increasing mortality from lung cancer (Figure 11.5). Tobacco abuse is the leading preventable cause of death in the United States, accounting for about 20% of total deaths (Bartecchi et al., 1994). This figure includes not only cancer but also respiratory and cardiovascular diseases caused by tobacco abuse. A further significant factor in the popularity and consumption of cigarettes is the extensive advertisement of their use. Cigarette marketing expenditures increased from $491 million in 1975 to $3274 million in 1988 (Bartecchi et al., 1995). An even more alarming statistic, estimated by Peto et al. (1996), is that some 3 million deaths a year are attributable to smoking now, and this figure will rise to 10 million per year in 30 to 40 years from now. This indicates that about 200 to 300 million of today's 3 billion adults can be expected eventually to die from tobacco abuse.

The results of tobacco abuse are not limited to its carcinogenic effects on the lung and upper respiratory tract. A significant proportion of a variety of other neoplasms can also be attributable to smoking in the United States (Figure 11.6). As with any chemical carcinogen, the risk of developing cancer of the lung and of the other organs noted in Figure 11.6 will vary with the number of cigarettes smoked per day. In a large study reviewing a number of reports, the relative risk of lung cancer versus the number of cigarettes smoked per day was essentially linear up to 40 cigarettes per day, which is as far as the study extended. However, the various reports differed in the relative risk seen from 10 to 40. Laryngeal cancer risk in a number of studies was even greater by far, but the spread was more extensive. For nonrespiratory cancers attributable to smoking, the relative risk was generally less than 10 for those who smoked 40 cigarettes per day (Dreyer et al., 1997). A more specific listing of the estimated cancer deaths caused by cigarette smoking in the United States in 1988 is seen in Table 11.8.

Not in the table, however, are at least two other types of neoplasms for which there is significant evidence of a causal relationship to tobacco abuse. One of these is hematopoietic cancer, including leukemias and to a lesser extent lymphomas. Since cigarette smoke contains benzene and is a source of ionizing radiation (polonium 210), both known causes of leukemia, it is quite possible that the two- to threefold excess of leukemias seen in smokers is related to their habit (cf. Newcomb and Carbone, 1992). A more alarming association is that described by Giovannucci and Martinez (1996) on the relation between smoking and cancers of the large bowel in U.S. men. In 1950, age-adjusted colorectal cancer incidence and mortality rates were similar in

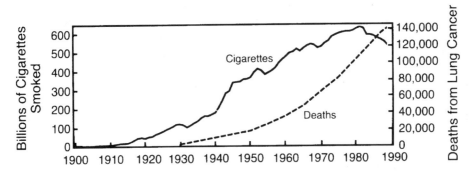

Figure 11.5 Relationship of cigarette consumption and total deaths from lung cancer in the United States 1900 to 1989. (Reprinted from an NIH publication entitled *Smoking, Tobacco and Cancer Program*, 1990.)

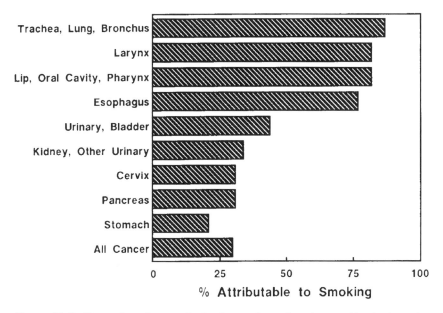

Figure 11.6 Proportion of cancer deaths that can be attributed to smoking in the United States in 1985. (Adapted from Newcomb and Carbone, 1992, with permission of the authors and publisher.)

U.S. men and women. By 1986, however, incidence rates were 34% higher and mortality rates 44% higher in men. These authors conclude that the increasing ratio of male to female mortality from colorectal cancer over the latter half of this century may have resulted from tobacco use by men earlier in the century. If this thesis is correct, as many as 20% of the large bowel cancers in men may be attributable to smoking during the last two decades. All of this information leads to the conclusion that tobacco abuse in general and cigarette smoking in particular are definable and thus preventable causes of approximately one-third of the cases of potentially fatal human cancer (Doll and Peto, 1981).

Table 11.8 Estimated Cancer Deaths Caused by Cigarette Smoking in the United States, 1998

Site	Males	Females	Total
Lung	83,321	50,987	134,308
Esophagus	6,970	2,002	8,972
Pancreas	3,626	4,619	8,245
Oral cavity	4,801	1,579	6,380
Bladder	3,679	1,402	5,081
Kidney	3,202	481	3,683
Larynx	2,706	769	3,475
Cervix		1,499	1,499
Total	108,305	63,338	171,643

From the National Cancer Institute, 1998.

Carcinogenic Agents Associated with Occupations

In 1713 Bernardino Ramazzini, of whom we have already spoken, published a text entitled *De Morbis Artificum*, or *Diseases of Workers*, which was translated in 1964 by Wright. It is in this text that Ramazzini describes the high incidence of mammary cancer in nuns, attributing it to their celibate life. However, the remainder of the book does not consider neoplastic disease to any extent in the more than 50 occupations described. Scrotal cancer in one-time chimney sweeps, described by Pott, was a later example of occupational cancer. During the nineteenth century, several reports of the association of specific cancers with mining, smelting, dyeing and lubrication processes and industries were reported. Unfortunately, in many instances, little was done for many years to protect the worker, a neglect of which we are still not entirely free today (Table 11.9).

The association of occupational exposure to asbestos and the subsequent development of bronchogenic carcinoma and mesothelioma have been well established (cf. Selikoff, 1978). However, in virtually all of the studies undertaken in this field, the highest incidence of bronchogenic carcinoma was found in those individuals exposed to asbestos who also had a history of cigarette smoking. In fact, risk ratios for the development of bronchogenic carcinoma of a

Table 11.9 Carcinogenic Risks Associated with Occupations

Chemical, process, or industry	Associated neoplasm(s)	Evidence for Carcinogenicity[a]
Acrylonitrile	Lung, colon, prostate	Limited
Arsenic	Lung	Sufficient
Asbestos	Lung, mesothelioma, gastrointestinal tract (?)	Sufficient
Manufacture of auramine	Bladder	Limited
Aromatic amines and nitroaromatics (aminobiphenyl, benzidine, 2-naphthylamine, 4-nitrobiphenyl)	Bladder	Sufficient
Benzene	Leukemia	Sufficient
Beryllium and its compounds	Lung	Limited
Bis(chloromethyl) ether	Lung	Sufficient
Boot and shoe manufacture and repair	Nasal carcinoma	Sufficient
Cadmium and its compounds	Lung, prostate (?)	Limited
Chromium and certain of its compounds	Lung, stomach, bone	Sufficient
Furniture manufacture (hardwood)	Nasal carcinoma	Sufficient
Hematite mining (underground)	Lung	Sufficient
Isopropyl alcohol manufacture	Cancer of paranasal sinuses	Sufficient
Nickel refining	Lung, nasal sinuses	Sufficient
Phenoxy herbicides, phenols, and polyhalogenated dioxins	Soft tissue sarcoma, lymphoma	Limited
Rubber industry (certain occupations)	Leukemia, bladder	Sufficient
Soot, tars, and oils	Skin, lung, bladder, gastrointestinal tract	Sufficient
Trichloroethylene	Liver and biliary tract	Limited
Vinyl chloride	Liver (angiosarcoma)	Sufficient

[a]See legend of Table 11.2.

large cohort of asbestos insulation workers in the United States and Canada as well as asbestos miners in Finland showed a dramatic increase in risk with smoking as compared with either smoking or asbestos exposure alone (Thiringer and Järvholm, 1980). This relationship can be seen in Table 11.10.

Hammond and Selikoff (1973) have suggested that this differential indicates the probable necessity for multiple environmental agents for the induction of bronchogenic carcinoma in the individuals exposed to asbestos. Carcinomas occurring in smokers exposed to asbestos exhibit a greater incidence of adenocarcinoma than those seen in smokers alone (Mollo et al., 1990; Johansson et al., 1992). In contrast, there appears to be little or no association between cigarette smoking and the occurrence of mesothelioma (Muscat and Wynder, 1991). Most pleural and peritoneal mesotheliomas in men can be attributed to exposure to asbestos, although such an association is less clear in women (Spirtas et al., 1994). The latency period from the first exposure to the diagnosis of mesothelioma may range from 20 to 45 years (Roggli, 1995; cf. Pisani et al., 1988). Asbestos fibers differ in structure. The predominant types are noted in Table 11.11, together with the evidence of their carcinogenicity in inducing mesotheliomas in the human (Pisani et al., 1988). Virtually all fiber types are carcinogenic (Huncharek, 1994) with the possible exception of anthophyllite (Meurman et al., 1974), as noted in the table. Further evidence in support of the direct carcinogenic effect of asbestos is the fact that mesotheliomas can be induced in rodents by appropriate exposure to this material (Wagner and Berry, 1969). Although other fibrous materials such as fiberglass have been shown to be carcinogenic in the rodent (Stanton et al., 1977), there is essentially no evidence to date that fiberglass causes human cancer.

The mechanism of asbestos carcinogenesis is unclear. However, asbestos fibers can cause cytogenetic effects in cell culture as well as "transformation" (Chapter 14) of Syrian hamster embryo cells in culture (Oshimura et al., 1984; Dopp et al., 1995). Hei et al. (1992) have also demonstrated that asbestos fibers may induce large deletions in hamster-derived cells in culture; this could be related to its clastogenic effects. In addition, asbestos fibers are able to generate reactive oxygen species in vitro, suggesting a molecular mechanism for the cytogenetic and transformation effects noted (Moyer et al., 1994). Although the mechanism of asbestos induction of cancer is as yet unknown, the demonstration that the type and size of fiber are important for the carcinogenicity of this material indicates that its carcinogenic action may be similar to that of "plastic film" carcinogenesis (Chapter 3). Several inorganic compounds and their primary elements have also been shown to be carcinogenic in the human (Table 11.9). There is only limited evidence that cadmium and its compounds are carcinogenic for the human, the best evidence being pulmonary carcinogenesis in epidemiological studies, where an actual dose-response relationship may exist (cf. Waalkes et al., 1992). The evidence is significantly less for a causative factor in human prostate cancer (Waalkes and Rehm, 1994). On the other hand, chromium compounds have been causally related to cancers of the respiratory system, especially the lung, as well as the stomach, bone, and the urogenital tract (cf. Cohen et al., 1993; Costa, 1997).

Table 11.10 Calculated Risk Ratios for Cancer of the Lung

Smoking	–	–	+	+	
Asbestos exposure	–	+	–	+	
Risk ratios:	1	4	11	91	(Selikoff et al., 1968)
	1.0	1.4	12	17	(Meurman et al., 1974)

Adapted from Thiringer and Järvholm, 1980, with permission of the authors and publisher.

Table 11.11   Types of Asbestos Fibers: Environmental Exposure
and Carcinogenicity

Type	Exposure	Mesothelioma Carcinogenicity
Crocidolite	Miners (South Africa)	High
	Factory workers	
Amosite	Miners	High
	Insulators	
	Factory workers	
Tremolite	Environmental (Greece)	High (?)
	As a contaminant in chrysotile	
Chrysotile	Miners (North America)	Low
	Insulators	
	Factory workers	
Anthophyllite	Miners (Finland)	None

As noted earlier (Chapter 3), there is substantial evidence for the interaction of chromium compounds with DNA, induction of protein-DNA crosslinks, and direct mutagenic effects on DNA
(cf. Cohen et al., 1993). Chromium compounds are clastogenic in humans and animals both in
vivo and in vitro (cf. Vainio and Sorsa, 1981). Exposure to nickel-containing dust in refineries
and other working environments is causally related to cancers of the respiratory tract, especially
the nose and lungs, after exposure periods extending from 5 to 25 years (cf. Magos, 1991). In
most instances such neoplastic development was associated with other evidence of toxicities,
such as chronic pulmonary irritation, rhinitis, and sinusitis.

A situation similar to the problem of asbestos exposure may be seen in underground hematite miners in several areas of Europe as well as in this country. Since iron oxide has not been
found to be carcinogenic in laboratory animals—although hematite dust enhances the carcinogenic activity of hydrocarbons in the lung—the exact agent or agents producing the increased
incidence of lung cancer in this occupational group have not yet been identified. Similarly,
workers in the furniture industry and related fields exposed to high levels of wood dust, especially from hardwood (Leclerc et al., 1994), are more prone to develop adenocarcinoma of the
nasal cavity and sinuses. A similar finding has been demonstrated for workers in the shoe industry in England; again, the offending agents are unknown. In previous years, during the manufac-
ture of isopropyl alcohol, oils were produced whose exact structure was not known but whose
presence was obviously related to the process. Workers in this industry had a significant increase
in cancer of the larynx and nasal cavity after chronic inhalation of these oils. Today the manufac-
turing process has been changed so that there is no risk to the worker.

One of the most interesting inorganic elements whose compounds have been shown to be
carcinogenic in the human is arsenic. As indicated in Chapter 3, the evidence for the carcinogenic effects of arsenic is far better in the human than in experimental animals. Only in the last
two decades has it been shown that arsenic compounds are carcinogenic in rodents, primarily if
not exclusively in the Syrian golden hamster, without the addition of other agents (Yamamoto et
al., 1987). More recently, a number of studies have demonstrated that organic arsenicals, especially methylated arsenicals, may act as promoting or progressor agents in several different experimental systems and species (Yamanaka et al., 1996; Hayashi et al., 1998; Yamamoto et al.,
1997; Germolec et al., 1997). Furthermore, in cells isolated from the Syrian hamster embryo and
explanted to tissue culture, arsenical compounds in the medium induced cell transformation

(Chapter 14) and cytogenetic effects (Lee et al., 1985). One of the earliest extensive reviews of arsenical cancer in the human was that of Neubauer (1947), in which he described clinical characteristics of cancer of the skin associated with ingestion of medicinals as well as occupational exposures. Since that time and especially during the last decade, there have been extensive epidemiological investigations on various exposures to arsenic compounds by a variety of environmental routes. A related environmental exposure to arsenic is in drinking water. One of the most extensively studied cohorts of individuals exposed to high levels of arsenic in drinking water was described in Taiwan (Chen et al., 1992). The concentration of arsenic in the well water was associated significantly with an increased risk for cancers of the liver, nasal cavity, lung, skin, bladder, and kidney in both males and females. While some have perhaps questioned the applicability of these findings to other situations, at least two other studies (Hopenhayn-Rich et al., 1996; Tsuda et al., 1995) have obtained similar evidence for the effect of arsenic in drinking water on the development of bladder and lung cancer. These findings have considerable practical importance in the United States, where a very large proportion of drinking water contains low levels of inorganic arsenic. However, a recent study by Buchet and Lison (1998) from Belgium has indicated that a low to moderate level of environmental exposure to inorganic arsenic (20 to 50 µg/L drinking water) does not seem to affect the causes of mortality in the exposed population. Generally, from these epidemiological studies, one may propose that inhaled arsenic induces primarily respiratory cancer, whereas ingested arsenic is associated with increased risk of cancer at multiple sites, including the skin and a variety of organs (Byrd et al., 1996). Furthermore, from the epidemiological investigations as well as experimental studies demonstrating the effective clastogenicity of arsenic and its compounds while producing an absence of point mutations (Stöhrer, 1991), as well as the effects on multistage carcinogenesis in animals, arsenicals may be more closely related to progressor agents (Chapter 9), exerting their effects at the late, progressor stage of the carcinogenic process (Brown and Chu, 1983).

The use of specific organic chemicals in industrial processes dates back to the middle of the last century; the carcinogenic effects of several of these chemicals have been completely or partially defined in the human species. The earliest of these were some aromatic amines used in the dye industry. In 1895, Rehn noted bladder neoplasms in three men working in a dye factory that used aniline as the basic ingredient for the preparation of fuchsin dyes (Rehn, 1895). Since that time, bladder neoplasms among aromatic amine workers have been referred to as "aniline tumors," although it is now known that the bladder carcinogen in Rehn's report was not aniline but 4-aminobiphenyl (Connolly and White, 1969). A related and also extensively produced chemical was β-naphthylamine, which was purified by distillation and sublimation in closed rooms during the last century. As noted in Figure 11.7, these distillation conditions resulted in the development of bladder cancer in virtually 100% of the individuals who worked in those rooms. While the danger to the human of the aromatic amines listed in Table 11.9 is now well known and considerable safety precautions are employed where such chemicals are used, there has still been some recent evidence that other aromatic amines, such as *o*-toluidine, may be a causal agents for bladder cancer in some industries (Ward et al., 1996).

A far more pervasive and common environmental chemical that has been designated as carcinogenic for the human is benzene. Although the clear carcinogenic effect of benzene in laboratory test animals has been demonstrated conclusively only within the last two decades, an association between exposure to benzene and leukemia has been known since before 1930 (Delore and Borgomano, 1928). In chronic bioassay studies, benzene induced neoplasms in a number of sites in both rats and mice (Huff et al., 1989). In the human, the toxicity for the hematopoietic system has been well documented, the most common effect being aplastic anemia (Smith, 1996). Although workers in the chemical and rubber industries may be exposed to greater concentrations of benzene for longer periods of time than the general population, expo-

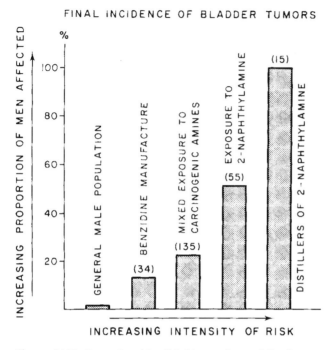

FINAL INCIDENCE OF BLADDER TUMORS

Figure 11.7   Increasing risk of bladder carcinoma following exposure to various aromatic amine carcinogens. Note the 100% incidence in those distilling 2-naphthylamine. (From Connolly and White, 1969, with permission of the authors and publisher.)

sure to benzene is pervasive (Figure 11.8). As noted in Figure 11.8, a typical smoker takes in roughly 2 mg of benzene per day, primarily from mainstream cigarette smoke. Nonsmokers inhale about one-tenth of this amount, predominantly from ambient air but also from automobile vapors (Wallace, 1996). Outdoor air contributes about 40% of the total benzene dose for nonsmokers, while the remainder involves primarily gasoline and automobile vapor emissions associated with automobile driving and maintenance as well as environmental tobacco smoke (ETS) exposures. As expected from its myelotoxicity, there is strong evidence that benzene induces leukemia, predominantly if not exclusively acute myelogenous leukemia, as noted from the combination of six studies reported by Lamm et al. (1989) (Figure 11.9). Although there is some suggestion that benzene may induce multiple myeloma (Goldstein, 1990), other studies have not borne out this suggestion (Wong, 1995).

Medinsky et al. (1994) have pointed out that acute myelogenous leukemia appears to involve repeated exposure to cytotoxic concentrations of benzene. Other studies (Wong, 1995; Schnatter et al., 1996) have demonstrated apparent thresholds of benzene exposure below which there is no evidence of neoplastic development. Smith (1996) has pointed out that benzene is not a "classic" chemical carcinogen in that it does not form a highly electrophilic metabolite on metabolism, and there is relatively little binding to DNA of radiolabeled benzene or its metabolites, although DNA adducts can be demonstrated by the ^{32}P-postlabeling technique (Bodell et al., 1996). However, both benzene and its metabolites induce chromosomal alterations in both humans and animals (cf. Snyder and Kalf, 1994). Chronic exposure to benzene induces breaks and translocations in specific chromosomes in vivo, which are significant at exposures of greater than 31 ppm (Figure 11.10) (Smith et al., 1998). Thus, while there has been much speculation as to the mechanism(s) of benzene carcinogenesis, it would appear that the known characteristics

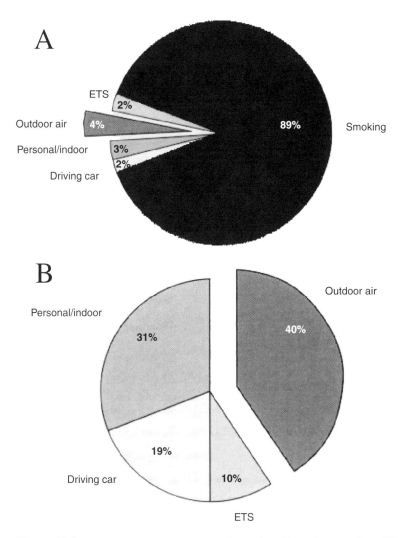

Figure 11.8 Sources of benzene exposure in smokers (A) and nonsmokers (B). A typical smoker takes in roughly 2 mg of benzene per day, while a nonsmoker typically inhales about 0.2 mg of benzene per day, assuming in the latter incidence an average exposure of 15 μg/m^3 and an alveolar respiration rate of 14 m^3/day. (Adapted from Wallace, 1996, with permission of the author and publisher.)

of this agent allow its classification as a progressor agent in human neoplastic development (Chapter 9).

Although the dioxins and polyhalogenated biphenyls induce neoplasms in experimental animals, it is important to note here the present controversy that suggests an effect of dioxins on the induction of soft tissue sarcomas. Hardell et al. (1995) have presented evidence that chronic exposure to phenoxy acids or chlorophenols is associated with significant increases in soft tissue sarcomas in Swedish workers, but others (cf. Bond and Rossbacher, 1993) were not able to confirm this in a similar study in Finland. Since these compounds are usually contaminated by dioxins and related toxic compounds, the argument has been made that such studies indicate the potential carcinogenicity of dioxins for humans. 2,3,7,8-Tetrachlorodibenzo-*p*-dioxin (TCDD)

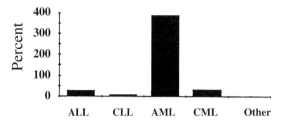

Figure 11.9 The percent observed/percent expected by type of leukemia for six studies as described by Lamm et al. (1989). ALL, acute lymphatic leukemia; CLL, chronic lymphatic leukemia; AML, acute myelogenous leukemia; CML, chronic myelogenous leukemia. (Reproduced with permission of the authors and publishers.)

and related halogenated compounds are pervasive environmental chemical contaminants which are of no practical or useful importance. TCDD and many of its congeners are minor by-products of a variety of synthetic processes utilized in the preparation of antiseptics and herbicides. They are also produced by incomplete combustion of a variety of halogen-containing organic chemicals and thus occur in stack exhausts and cigarette smoke. TCDD is extremely toxic to a variety of species (cf. Pohjanvirta and Tuomisto, 1994) and is carcinogenic on long-term exposure as well as being one of the most potent promoting agents known for experimental liver and skin cancer (Chapter 7; Lucier et al., 1993). In humans, the carcinogenic potential of TCDD has been confused by exposures that are almost always in association with multiple other chemicals and confounding effects such as smoking. However, the IARC has classified TCDD and phenoxy herbicides as carcinogenic to humans on the basis of limited evidence from epidemiological studies and sufficient evidence from animal studies (McGregor et al., 1998). An analysis of four Swedish studies was one of the bases for this decision, although other earlier investigations (Kang et al., 1987; Riihimäki et al., 1982) did not support such an association. Somewhat less clear is the association of non-Hodgkin lymphoma with herbicide and TCDD exposure, although the increasing incidence of this disease in a number of countries could be based, at least in part, on such chronic exposure (Zahm and Blair, 1992; Hardell et al., 1994). Still, because of the relative lack of genotoxic effects of TCDD in general and its extremely potent promoting action in experimental animals, its carcinogenic effects may be more closely related to this latter characteristic.

Unlike TCDD, the 2-carbon halogenated compounds trichloroethylene and vinyl chloride are produced and used extensively worldwide for a variety of occupational procedures. About a quarter of a million tons of trichloroethylene are produced in the world each year and used as a solvent in numerous industrial processes. The IARC (1995) has concluded that there is limited evidence in humans for the carcinogenicity of this compound, but a committee of the National Research Council in the United States (James et al., 1996) felt that the evidence both in humans and animals was less convincing, although they did choose to calculate a cancer risk based on estimates by the U.S. Environmental Protection Agency. A much less controversial subject is the association of malignant neoplasms of the liver with exposure to vinyl chloride, the monomer used in the production of a variety of plastics. A review by the IARC in 1975 reported on 43 cases of angiosarcoma found in 10 different countries throughout the world, all of the patients having a history of working with vinyl chloride. Hepatic angiosarcoma is an extremely rare neoplasm in humans, and thus the incidence seen in this group is far out of proportion to what might be expected in the general population. Cooper (1981) reviewed a population of 10,173 men whose jobs involved a probable exposure to vinyl chloride prior to January 1, 1973. In this

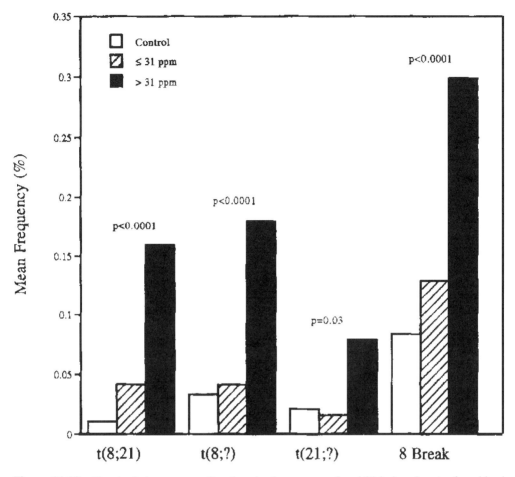

Figure 11.10 Structural chromosome alterations in chromosomes 8 and 21 in lymphocytes from blood of workers exposed to different levels of benzene in comparison with unexposed controls. The *p* values are significant for exposures at greater than 31 ppm. (Adapted from Smith et al., 1998, with permission of the authors and publishers.)

group, eight angiosarcomas were found, as well as a twofold increase in malignant neoplasms of the brain and other parts of the nervous system. Although the low incidence of these neoplasms in this large population suggests that vinyl chloride is a relatively weak carcinogen, the rarity of hepatic angiosarcoma in the general population strongly supports the causal relationship between the organic monomer and the induction of this mesenchymal neoplasm. In addition, vinyl chloride exposure induces other, somewhat uncommon pathologies in the liver, including extensive fibrosis, which may lead to portal hypertension (increased pressure within the portal venous system), splenomegaly, and hypertrophy and hyperplasia of both hepatocytes and hepatic and splenic mesenchymal cells (Thomas et al., 1975). Vinyl chloride is rapidly absorbed after respiratory exposure and is metabolized in the liver by the cytochrome P450 2E1 system to electrophilic metabolites, particularly chloroethyleneoxide and chloroacetaldehyde. These electrophiles react with DNA bases to form adducts, of which the etheno-base compounds (Figure 3.9) are highly persistent, with half-lives of more than 30 days (cf. Marion et al., 1996). Mutations in the *K-ras* and p53 genes occur in the livers of exposed individuals. The etheno adducts cause transition and transversion mutations in bacterial systems (Cheng et al., 1991; Marion et al., 1996).

The United States government has sponsored publications suggesting that occupational causes of neoplasia in humans may be responsible for as much as 20% of total cancer mortality, but Doll and Peto (1981) have presented compelling arguments that such is not the case. Their review of the presently available statistical and epidemiological evidence indicates that only about 4% of all cancer deaths in the United States can be attributed to occupational causes. Furthermore, the strict governmental regulation of actual and potential industrial health hazards promises to reduce this figure even further in the future (Chapter 13).

Carcinogenic Agents for the Human Associated with Medical Therapy and Diagnosis

In modern times the dictum of Hippocrates that a physician above all should do no harm to his or her patient has been modified to a consideration of the benefit to the patient in relation to the risk of the procedure or therapy involved. Many times the risk to the patient was unknown or unsuspected, and it was only at a later date that the risk factor became evident. Perhaps the best example of this was the administration of diethylstilbestrol to pregnant women in order to avert a threatened abortion. The benefit of such a procedure was obvious, but the risk did not become obvious until many years later, when a small percentage of the female offspring of mothers treated with this estrogenic analog during gestation developed vaginal carcinomas, usually shortly after puberty (Herbst, 1981) (Table 11.12). The incidence of clear cell adenocarcinoma

Table 11.12 Carcinogenic Risks of Chemical Agents Associated with Medical Therapy and Diagnosis

Chemical or Drug	Associated Neoplasms	Evidence for Carcinogenicity[a]
Alkylating agents (cyclophosphamide, melphalan)	Bladder, leukemia	Sufficient
Inorganic arsenicals	Skin, liver	Sufficient
Azathioprine (immunosuppressive drugs)	Lymphoma, reticulum cell sarcoma, skin, Kaposi sarcoma (?)	Sufficient
Chlornaphazine	Bladder	Sufficient
Chloramphenicol	Leukemia	Limited
Cyclosporine	Lymphoma, skin	Sufficient
Diethylstilbesterol	Vagina (clear cell carcinoma)	Sufficient
Estrogens:		
Premenopausal	Liver cell adenoma	Sufficient
Postmenopausal	Endometrium	Limited
Methoxypsoralen with ultraviolet light	Skin	Sufficient
Oxymetholone	Liver	Limited
Phenacetin	Renal pelvis (carcinoma)	Sufficient
Phenytoin (diphenylhydantoin)	Lymphoma, neuroblastoma	Limited
Radon	Lung	Sufficient
Tamoxifen	Endometrium	Sufficient
Thorotrast	Liver (angiosarcoma)	Sufficient

[a]See notes below Table 11.3.

of the vagina in women exposed to diethylstilbestrol in utero is about 1 per 1000 exposed mothers (Melnick et al., 1987). However, other abnormalities of the genital tract, especially a condition known as vaginal adenosis, occurred in about 70% of women exposed to diethylstilbestrol in utero (Johnson et al., 1979). While no carcinogenic effects were noted in male offspring exposed in utero, several anomalies of the genital tract have been described as well as possible modification of social behaviors in men exposed in utero (Mittendorf, 1995). Prenatal exposure of mice to diethylstilbestrol induces a variety of both neoplastic and developmental abnormalities in the genital tracts of both male and female offspring, some of which mimic those seen in the human (Newbold, 1995). Recently, there have been reports that women exposed to diethylstilbestrol in utero do have a moderately increased risk for developing breast cancer (Greenberg et al., 1984); this risk does not increase with time (Calle et al., 1996). Diethylstilbestrol may be metabolized to reactive forms, as shown by in vitro studies (Tsutsui et al., 1986; Gladek and Liehr, 1989). This alteration may lead to the formation of ^{32}P-postlabeled DNA adducts (Liehr et al., 1985), elevated 8-hydroxydeoxyguanosine levels in DNA in vivo (Roy et al., 1991), and DNA damage in germ cells in mice in vivo (Racine and Schmid, 1984). Diethylstilbestrol is clastogenic in a variety of systems (Birnboim, 1985), such as human leukocytes, and it induces aneuploidy in vivo and in vitro (Bishun et al., 1977). Interestingly, clear-cell adenocarcinomas of the vagina induced by diethylstilbesterol show no evidence for the induction of mutations in the K-*ras* or H-*ras* protooncogenes, the Wilms' tumor suppressor gene, the estrogen receptor gene, or the p53 tumor suppressor gene, but evidence of microsatellite instability was found in all of the neoplasms examined (Boyd et al., 1996). Thus, unlike natural estrogens, this synthetic estrogen may exert its effects by altering DNA and genomic structure during the stages of initiation and/or progression.

Other synthetic estrogens, primarily utilized as oral contraceptives, have been associated with the induction of liver cell adenomas when taken chronically by premenopausal women. The relation of risk of development of liver cell adenomas to the duration of the use of oral contraceptives is given in Table 11.13 (Edmondson et al., 1976). While some isolated cases have been reported as indicating an association between liver cell adenomas, dysplasia, and hepatocellular carcinoma (Tao, 1992), the epidemiological evidence to date is insufficient to conclude that there is a relation between carcinoma development and exposure to synthetic estrogens in oral contraceptives. Furthermore, studies have demonstrated that, upon withdrawal of the oral contraceptives, regression of adenomas and particularly a related lesion, focal nodular hyperplasia, occurs (Steinbrecher et al., 1981; Pain et al., 1991). Furthermore, the more recent preparations of oral contraceptives contain other steroids such as progestins, which seem to moderate the tendency for liver adenomas to develop. The potential relation between synthetic estrogens used in oral contraceptives and the development of breast cancer has been extensively investigated. In

Table 11.13 Duration of Use of Oral Contraceptives for 30 Case-Control Pairs

Duration (months)	Cases	Controls	Risk Ratio[a]
<12	6	15	1.0
13–36	4	8	1.3
37–60	7	7	2.5
61–84	4	2	5.0
85–108	3	1	7.5
>109	10	1	25.0

[a]Compared with use up to 1 year. Similar relative risks are obtained if a matched analysis is performed.

premenopausal women, there is some evidence for a slight increase in risk, again related to the length of use, as noted in Figure 11.11 (McGonigle and Huggins, 1991; Rookus and van Leeuwen, 1994). In postmenopausal women—in a study combining more than 50 epidemiological investigations—it was concluded that a small increase in the relative risk of breast cancer occurred within the first 10 years after cessation of the use of synthetic estrogens/progestins. Subsequently, the risk disappeared (Calle et al., 1996). A more striking phenomenon, however, is the relationship of unopposed (no progestins) estrogens and endometrial cancer in postmenopausal women. In this instance, the so-called hormonal replacement therapy was shown some years ago to be associated with a substantial (6- to 15-fold) risk for the development of endometrial carcinoma (Antunes et al., 1979). While the concomitant administration of progestin with the estrogen does not completely eliminate the risk (Beresford et al., 1997) of lingering effects of unopposed estrogen after administration has ceased, most carcinogenic effects of estrogens to the endometrium can be prevented by the addition of a progestin (Barrett-Connor, 1992).

More recently, on the basis of both clinical and experimental investigations, synthetic antiestrogens have come into play both for the therapy of breast cancer and for its prevention. At present the most commonly utilized antiestrogen is tamoxifen, which has a structure not unrelated to that of diethylstilbestrol (Chapter 3). This chemical has been shown to decrease the recurrence of breast cancer significantly after therapy. In addition, in a large clinical trial recently completed, tamoxifen decreased the risk of developing primary breast cancer in a high-risk population (Jordan, 1993; Fisher et al., 1998). Tamoxifen exhibits estrogen-antagonist activity in the breast and the hypothalamic-pituitary axis (Mandeville and Houde, 1994). However, in most other tissues, this chemical is a moderately active estrogen. Although in a large number of studies involving tamoxifen, in both therapeutic and preventive situations, little or no carcinogenic risk was demonstrated (Morgan, 1997), a significant number of investigations have indicated that tamoxifen therapy increases the risk of endometrial cancer sevenfold or more (Fisher et al., 1994; Morgan, 1997). Despite this finding, the benefit of using tamoxifen far exceeds this risk factor (Fisher et al., 1994; Assikis et al., 1996). Tamoxifen's carcinogenic action appears to be similar to that of diethylstilbestrol in that it and its congeners induce ^{32}P-postlabeled DNA adducts (Li et al., 1997). These antiestrogens are effective promoting agents in experimental systems (Dragan et al., 1995; Kim et al., 1996), and tamoxifen and its congenors induce aneuploidy in rodent tissues in vivo (Sargent et al., 1996). Thus, at least in some experimental systems, tamoxifen exhibits the characteristics of a complete carcinogen.

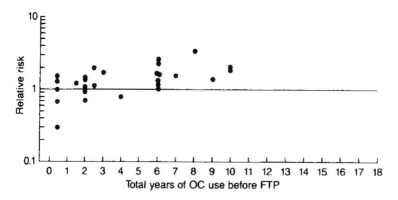

Figure 11.11   Breast cancer in women younger than 45 years of age: relative risk by total years of oral contraceptive use before first-term pregnancy in nine studies. OC, oral contraceptive; FTP, first-term pregnancy. (Adapted from Schlesselman, 1990, with permission of the author and publisher.)

Androgenic steroids in the form of synthetic congeners of testosterone, such as oxymetholone, have been used in the long-term therapy of aplastic anemia. A number of case reports of hepatocellular carcinomas have arisen in individuals treated for this and other conditions by this form of steroid (cf. Hoover and Fraumeni, 1981).

A number of agents known to damage DNA have been used in the therapy and diagnosis of various diseases, especially neoplasia. Alkylating agents are used primarily for the treatment of malignant neoplasms, and a number have been causally associated with the induction of a variety of leukemias and solid neoplasms, especially in children receiving intensive therapy for acute leukemia (Chapter 20). The induction of acute nonlymphocytic leukemia has been reported in adults receiving such chemotherapy, especially for Hodgkin disease (Swerdlow et al., 1992; Karp and Smith, 1997). Table 11.14 lists a number of chemotherapeutic agents used in the treatment of cancer that have been evaluated in the IARC monograph program. As noted from the table, almost all of these agents are alkylating agents, which are thus capable of reacting with DNA in their ultimate forms (Chapter 3).

The risk of development of a secondary leukemia does not increase linearly with time but rather exhibits a sharp peak or "critical window" of incidence, as noted in Figure 11.12. Al-

Table 11.14 Selected Chemotherapy Agents That Have Been Evaluated in the IARC Monographs Program

Agent	Mechanism of Action
Agents carcinogenic to humans (IARC group 1):	
N,N-Bis(2-chloroethyl)-2-naphthylamine (Chlornaphazine)	ALK
1,4-Butanediol dimethanesulfonate (Busulfan, Myleran)	ALK
Chlorambucil	ALK
(1-(2-)Chlorethyl)-3-(4-methylcyclohexyl)-1-nitrosourea (methyl-CCNU, semustine)	ALK
Cyclophosphamide	ALK
Melphalan	ALK
MOPP and other combined chemotherapy, including alkylating agents	ALK
Thio-TEPA [tris(1-aziridinyl)-phosphine]	ALK
Treosulphan	ALK
Agents probably carcinogenic to humans (IARC group 2A):	
Doxorubicin	INT, STR
Azacytidine	DNA MeI
Bischloroethyl nitrosourea (BCNU)	ALK
(1-(2-)Chloroethyl)-3-cyclohexyl-1-nitrosourea (CCNU)	ALK
Chlorozotocin	ALK
Cisplatin	ALK
Nitrogen mustard	ALK
Procarbazine hydrochloride	ALK
Agents possibly carcinogenic to humans (IARC group 2B):	
Bleomycin	STR
Darcarbazine	ALK
Mitomycin C	ALK
Uracil mustard	ALK

Key: ALK, DNA alkylation; INT, DNA intercalation; STR, DNA strand breakage; DNA MeI, DNA methylation inhibitor.
Modified from Boffetta and Kaldor, 1994, with permission of the authors and publisher.

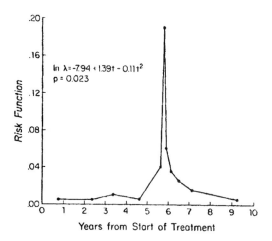

Figure 11.12 Risk function for the development of leukemia in patients with Hodgkin disease regardless of the type of treatment employed. The natural log transformation of the risk equation and the two-sided p value for the nonlinear term are noted in the figure. (Adapted from Blayney et al., 1987, with permission of the authors and publisher.)

though ionizing radiation is also utilized in the therapy of neoplasia, especially in association with chemotherapy at times, the carcinogenic effects of the chemotherapeutic agents can be distinguished from those of ionizing radiation (cf. Swerdlow et al., 1992; Reimer, 1982). More recently, newer therapeutic agents are being employed, and, although studies are yet incomplete, evidence strongly suggests that the effective platinum drugs as well as the topoisomerase inhibitors are carcinogenic (Greene, 1992; Karp and Smith, 1997). The topoisomerase inhibitors induce specific chromosomal abnormalities that are reflected in the ultimate neoplasms, usually leukemias, suggesting that such agents are primarily effecting the stage of progression.

There is no question of the association of lung cancer with chronic exposure to arsenic in industrial situations, but the exposure to arsenic compounds in the treatment of various diseases was widespread during the earlier parts of this century. Organic arsenicals were used to treat syphilis, and there is some evidence for an association with skin cancer in individuals receiving such treatment for prolonged periods. However, a much firmer association of skin as well as liver cancer with the chronic administration of Fowler's solution has now been well documented (Pershagen, 1981). This medicament, in the form of a solution of 1% potassium arsenite in aqueous alcohol, was used for the treatment of dermatitis, arthritis, and other conditions, including chronic leukemia. Since the material was often administered for years, some patients received many grams of arsenic during their period of treatment. An interesting study by Fierz (1966) reported a dose-response relationship between the development of skin cancer and the ingestion of Fowler's solution (Figure 11.13).

Chlornaphazine, which had been used to treat preleukemic conditions in humans, was shown to be carcinogenic for the bladder and today is no longer utilized in such therapy (IARC, 1982). Methoxypsoralen, which interacts with DNA, has been used in combination with ultraviolet light in the treatment of a skin condition known as psoriasis. Clear evidence of the induction of squamous cell carcinoma of the skin by this regimen has been reported (Stern and Laird, 1994). In addition, the administration of methotrexate, an analog of the vitamin folic acid, also increases the risk of skin cancer in patients with psoriasis treated by this antimetabolite. More recently, these same studies have indicated that the risk of malignant melanoma also increases in

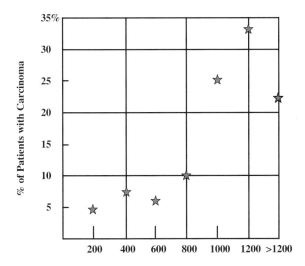

Figure 11.13   Percentage frequency of skin carcinoma as a function of the total dose of Fowler's solution. (After Fierz, 1966.)

patients who have been treated with ultraviolet light and methoxypsoralen for extended periods, usually involving more than 250 separate treatments (Stern et al., 1997). There has also been some epidemiological evidence that extensive exposure to fluorescent light may be a potential risk factor for melanoma (Walter et al., 1992), and there is an even greater risk from the use of sunlamps for tanning in a Swedish population, with a relative risk factor greater than 7 when such devices are used more than 10 times a year by young people (Westerdahl et al., 1994). These instances were in the absence of treatment with methoxypsoralen, indicating, as reiterated in the next chapter, the potential danger of ultraviolet and near-ultraviolet radiation in the development of skin cancer in the human.

A group of drugs has been utilized in the chemical immunosuppression of patients in preparation for transplantation of organs and tissues from one individual to another. The principal drug that has been associated with neoplasms in this group of patients is azathioprine. Although this drug and others used during clinical immunosuppression interact with DNA, it is not clear whether such compounds are actually carcinogenic in themselves or act by suppressing the natural resistance of the host to malignant cells already present. The predominant neoplasms appearing in such immunosuppressed patients are those derived from the skin and the immune system. In a study of more than 6000 individuals having had kidney transplant surgery in the United States, Hoover and Fraumeni (1973) reported dramatic increases in the risk for these two types of neoplasms; the most striking was reticulum cell sarcoma, the occurrence of which was 350 times greater than in the general population. A more recent series from England (London et al.,

1995) showed a somewhat different distribution of neoplasms in 70 of 918 renal transplant patients; 53% of these tumors were cutaneous in origin. The risk of developing these neoplasms of the skin, mostly squamous cell carcinomas, rose almost exponentially during a 20-year follow-up. It is reasonable to suggest that a major mechanism for the induction of neoplasia in immunosuppressed patients is the loss of host resistance to neoplastic cells that are already present but are normally prevented from expressing their neoplastic potential by immune mechanisms of the host. A marked increase in the incidence of Kaposi sarcoma has been seen in immunocompromised patients in this and other countries, especially male homosexuals with the acquired immunodeficiency syndrome (AIDS), a disease associated with marked immune dysfunction and loss of resistance to infectious agents (Kahn and Walker, 1998) (Chapter 12). These increases in neoplasms seen in immunosuppressed individuals may in part reflect the inability of the host to resist the development of neoplasia by immunological mechanisms, as discussed further in Chapter 19.

The association of leukemia with administration of the antibiotic chloramphenicol may be related to its depressive action on the bone marrow (IARC, 1982). Similarly, in 1987, the IARC classified the analgesic phenacetin as a cause of cancers of the renal pelvis, ureter, and bladder. Today this agent is not available as an over-the-counter analgesic in most western countries. There is little or no evidence that salicylates or acetaminophen exhibit any carcinogenic effects in the human. The association of lymphomas with the chronic administration of phenytoin for the control of epilepsy is very limited, with significant conflicting evidence (Olsen et al., 1989; Scoville and White, 1981). This drug induces lymphoid reactions that are at times difficult to distinguish from neoplasia, but there is limited evidence for its causal association with lymphoma, although the risk is probably much less than the benefit to the epileptic patient. An interesting but as yet unknown effect of administration of a known carcinogenic agent to humans for medicinal purposes was the use of ethylcarbamate (urethane) as a cosolvent in aqueous solutions of water-insoluble analgesics in Japan from 1950 through 1975 (Miller, 1991). No epidemiological follow-up was made of the use of some hundred million 2-mL ampules of 7% to 15% solutions of ethylcarbamate injected into patients between 1950 to 1975. Whether this and other medical treatments with potential carcinogens will alter cancer risk and incidence remains for future study.

Thus, it is clear that some forms of medical therapy and diagnosis are not without significant carcinogenic risk under certain circumstances. Chapter 13 presents a further discussion of the relation of benefit to risk in our society in the employment of known or suspected carcinogenic agents. In the final analysis, society and/or the individual must determine when one factor outweighs the other.

Multistage Chemical Carcinogenesis in the Human

The multistage nature of chemical carcinogenesis can be demonstrated in the human as it has been in the animal, although, for obvious reasons, not with the same degree of accuracy. Epidemiologists have utilized terms such as *late-stage carcinogens* to indicate agents such as asbestos and arsenic that exhibit effects after very long latent periods. The analogy of such terminology to progressor agents is obvious. It is also possible to classify, at least tentatively, chemical agents that have been shown to be carcinogenic in the human or have such a potential in relation to their action at one or more of the three stages of carcinogenesis. A number of agents considered in this chapter may be classified as effective promoting agents in the development of human neoplastic disease. Several other agents are potentially promoting agents in human carcinogenesis on the basis of experimental investigations. A compilation of the principal promoting agents for the human is given in Table 11.15 (Pitot, 1982). From this list and the information presented in

Table 11.15 Neoplasms Associated with Prolonged Contact with Promoting
Agents in the Environment

Agent	Resultant Neoplasm
Dietary fat	Mammary adenocarcinoma
High caloric intake	Increased cancer incidence in general
Cigarette smoke	Bronchogenic carcinoma (esophageal and bladder cancer)
Halogenated hydrocarbons (dioxin, PCBs)	Liver[a]
Phorbol esters	Esophageal cancer (?)
Saccharin	Bladder[a]
Phenobarbital	Liver[a]
Prolactin	Mammary adenocarcinoma[a]
Synthetic estrogens	Liver adenomas
Alcoholic beverages	Oral cancer
	Liver and esophageal cancer

[a]Promotion demonstrated in experimental animals, but not as yet in humans.
Adapted from Pitot, 1982, with permission of the publisher.

this chapter, it is apparent that the effects of chemicals in the environment on the incidence of human cancer are more likely to be related to the stages of tumor promotion and progression than to initiation.

Although not all such agents have been shown by epidemiological studies to be important factors in human cancer, a number clearly can be. We have already discussed some aspects of the importance of dietary caloric intake and dietary fat in the genesis of human cancer. In addition, experimental evidence has clearly indicated that dietary fat, especially unsaturated fatty acids, may act as a promoter in experimental mammary carcinogenesis and possibly in several other histogenetic types of neoplasms (cf. Carroll, 1980). Cigarette smoke is a complete carcinogen but contains many promoting agents, and epidemiological evidence argues that tumor promotion is a major factor in the development of pulmonary cancer in the human as a result of smoking (cf. Farber, 1981). Although there are numerous controversies over the relation of artificial sweeteners to human bladder cancer and of dioxins to human neoplasia, there is ample experimental evidence that both of these agents are promoters for bladder and liver cancer in experimental systems (cf. Pitot, 1982). As Berenblum (1978) has suggested, all endogenous hormones may be considered to be promoting agents, and the action of synthetic estrogens in inducing liver cell adenomas in the human, as well as in rodents argues for a promoting role of these compounds. Finally, epidemiological evidence that alcoholic beverages promote esophageal, gastric, and hepatic cancer in the human is substantial, although relatively little evidence has been uncovered to demonstrate their promoting action in animals (Lieber et al., 1979).

Several known chemicals shown to be carcinogenic to the human may be classified primarily as progressor agents. These include asbestos fibers, benzene, and arsenic on the basis of their clastogenic properties and relatively little evidence of their action as initiators. Unfortunately, it is difficult to prove the biological and molecular mechanisms involved in human carcinogenesis directly. However, animal studies have been utilized extensively in developing rationales for determining the carcinogenic risk of specific chemicals to humans. It is only logical that one should also consider the mechanisms similar to if not identical with those in several species including the human, and from this one can devise appropriate preventive and therapeutic measures for dealing with human chemical carcinogens.

REFERENCES

Adami, H.-O., Adams, G., Boyle, P., Ewertz, M., Lee, N. C., Lund, E., Miller, A. B., Olsson, H., Steel, M., Trichopoulos, D., and Tulinius, H. Chapter II. Breast Cancer Etiology. Report of a working party for the Nordic Cancer Union. Int. J. Cancer Suppl. 5:22–39, 1990.

Adami, H.-O., Hsing, A. W., McLaughlin, J. K., Trichopoulos, D., Hacker, D., Ekbom, A., and Persson, I. Alcoholism and liver cirrhosis in the etiology of primary liver cancer. Int. J. Cancer, 51:898–902, 1992.

Ahn, Y.-O. Diet and stomach cancer in Korea. Int. J. Cancer, 10:7–9, 1997.

Albanes, D., Heinonen, O. P., Taylor, P. R., Virtamo, J., Edwards, B. K., Rautalahti, M., Hartman, A. M., Palmgren, J., Freedman, L. S., Haapakoski, J., Barrett, M. J., Pietinen, P., Malila, N., Tala, E., Liippo, K., Salomaa, E.-R., Tangrea, J. A., Teppo, L., Askin, F. B., Taskinen, E., Erozan, Y., Greenwald, P., and Huttunen, J. K. α-Tocopherol and β-carotene supplements and lung cancer incidence in the alpha-tocopherol, beta-carotene cancer prevention study: effects of base-line characteristics and study compliance. J. Natl. Cancer Inst., 88:1560–1570, 1996.

Albanes, D., Jones, D. Y., Schatzkin, A., Micozzi, M. S., and Taylor, P. R. Adult stature and risk of cancer. Cancer Res., 48:1658–1662, 1988.

Antunes, C. M. F., Stolley, P. D., Rosenshein, N. B., Davies, J. L., Tonascia, J. A., Brown, C., Burnett, L., Rutledge, A., Pokempner, M., and Garcia, R. Endometrial cancer and estrogen use. Report of a large case-control study. N. Engl. J. Med., 300:9–13, 1979.

Assikis, V. J., Neven, P., Jordan, V. C., and Vergote, I. A realistic clinical perspective of tamoxifen and endometrial carcinogenesis. Eur. J. Cancer, 32A:1464–1476, 1996.

Augustsson, K., Skog, K., Jägerstad, M., and Steineck, G. Assessment of the human exposure to heterocyclic amines. Carcinogenesis, 18:1931–1935, 1997.

Barbone, F., Austin, H., and Partridge, E. E. Diet and endometrial cancer: a case-control study. Am. J. Epidemiol., 137:393–403, 1993.

Barnes, S. Evolution of the health benefits of soy isoflavones. Proc. Soc. Exp. Biol. Med., 217:386–392, 1998.

Barrett-Connor, E. Hormone replacement and cancer. Br. Med. Bull., 48:345–355, 1992.

Bartecchi, C. E., MacKenzie, T. D., and Schrier, R. W. The human costs of tobacco use. N. Engl. J. Med., 330:907–912, 1994.

Bartecchi, C. E., MacKenzie, T. D., and Schrier, R. W. The global tobacco epidemic. Sci. Am., 272:44–51, 1995.

Bartsch, H., Ohshima, H., Pignatelli, B., and Calmels, S. Human exposure to endogenous N-nitroso compounds: quantitative estimates in subjects at high risk for cancer of the oral cavity, oesophagus, stomach and urinary bladder. Cancer Surv., 8:335–362, 1989.

Beral, V., Bull, D., Doll, R., Key, T., Peto, R., and Reeves, G. Breast cancer and hormone replacement therapy: collaborative reanalysis of data from 51 epidemiological studies of 52,705 women with breast cancer and 108 411 women without breast cancer. Lancet, 350:1047–1059, 1997.

Berenblum, I. Guest editorial. Established principles and unresolved problems in carcinogenesis. J. Natl. Cancer Inst., 60:723–726, 1978.

Beresford, S. A. A., Weiss, N. S., Voigt, L. F., and McKnight, B. Risk of endometrial cancer in relation to use of oestrogen combined with cyclic progestagen therapy in postmenopausal women. Lancet, 349:458–461, 1997.

Bhide, S. V., Shivapurkar, N. M., Gothoskar, S. V., and Ranadive, K. J. Carcinogenicity of betel quid ingredients: feeding mice with aqueous extract and the polyphenol fraction of betel nut. Br. J. Cancer, 40:922–926, 1979.

Birnboim, H. C. DNA clastogenic activity of diethylstilbestrol. Biochem. Pharmacol., 34:3251–3257, 1985.

Bishun, N. P., Smith, N. S., Williams, D. C., and Raven, R. W. Carcinogenic and possible mutagenic effects of stilboestrol in offspring exposed in utero. J. Surg. Oncol., 9:293–300, 1977.

Blayney, D. W., Longo, D. L., Young, R. C., Greene, M. H., Hubbard, S. M., Postal, M. G., Duffey, P. L., and DeVita Jr., V. T. Decreasing risk of leukemia with prolonged follow-up after chemotherapy and radiotherapy for Hodgkin's disease. N. Engl. J. Med., *316*:710–714, 1987.

Block, G. Vitamin C and cancer prevention: the epidemiologic evidence. Am. J. Clin. Nutr., *53*:270S–282S, 1991.

Blot, W. J., Li, J.-Y., Taylor, P. R., and Li, B. Lung cancer and vitamin supplementation. N. Engl. J. Med., *331*:614, 1994.

Bodell, W. J., Pathak, D. N., Lévay, G., Ye, Q., and Pongracz, K. Investigation of the DNA adducts formed in B6C3F1 mice treated with benzene: implications for molecular dosimetry. Environ. Health Perspect., *104*:1189–1193, 1996.

Boffetta, P., and Kaldor, J. M. Secondary malignancies following cancer chemotherapy. Acta Oncol., *33*:591–598, 1994.

Bogen, K. T. Cancer potencies of heterocyclic amines found in cooked foods. Food Chem. Toxicol., *32*:505–515, 1994.

Bond, G. G., and Rossbacher, R. A review of potential human carcinogenicity of the chlorophenoxy herbicides MCPA, MCPP, and 2,4-DP. Br. J. Indust. Med., *50*:340–348, 1993.

Borchert, P., Miller, J. A., Miller, E. C., and Shires, T. K. 1′-Hydroxysafrole, a proximate carcinogenic metabolite of safrole in the rat and mouse. Cancer Res., *33*:590–600, 1973.

Boutron, M.-C., Faivre, J., Dop, M.-C., Quipourt, V., and Senesse, P. Tobacco, alcohol, and colorectal tumors: a multistep process. Am. J. Epidemiol., *141*:1038–1046, 1995.

Boyd, J., Takahashi, H., Waggoner, S. E., Jones, L. A., Hajek, R. A., Wharton, J. T., Liu, F.-s., Fujino, T., Barrett, J. C., and McLachlan, J. A. Molecular genetic analysis of clear cell adenocarcinomas of the vagina and cervix associated and unassociated with diethylstilbestrol exposure in utero. Cancer, *77*:507–513, 1996.

Boyle, P., and Zaridze, D. G. Risk factors for prostate and testicular cancer. Eur. J. Cancer, *29A*:1048–1055, 1993.

Bressac, B., Kew, M., Wands, J., and Ozturk, M. Selective G to T mutations of p53 gene in hepatocellular carcinoma from southern Africa. Nature, *350*:429–430, 1991.

Brinton, L. A., Reeves, W. C., Brenes, M. M., Herrero, R., de Britton, R. C., Gaitan, E., Tenorio, F., Garcia, M., and Rawls, W. E. Parity as a risk factor for cervical cancer. Am. J. Epidemiol., *130*:486–496, 1989.

Brock, K. E., Berry, G., Mock, P. A., MacLennan, R., Truswell, A. S., and Brinton, L. A. Nutrients in diet and plasma and risk of in situ cervical cancer. J. Natl. Cancer Inst., *80*:580–585, 1988.

Brown, C. C., and Chu, K. C. Implications of the multistage theory of carcinogenesis applied to occupational arsenic exposure. J. Natl. Cancer Inst., *70*:455–463, 1983.

Brown, L. M., Swanson, C. A., Gridley, G., Swanson, G. M., Schoenberg, J. B., Greenberg, R. S., Silverman, D. T., Pottern, L. M., Hayes, R. B., Schwartz, A. G., Liff, J. M., Fraumeni, J. F. Jr., and Hoover, R. N. Adenocarcinoma of the esophagus: role of obesity and diet. J. Natl. Cancer Inst., *87*:104–109, 1995.

Buchet, J. P., and Lison, D. Mortality by cancer in groups of the Belgian population with a moderately increased intake of arsenic. Int. Arch. Occup. Environ. Health, *71*:125–130, 1998.

Burnstein, M. J. Dietary factors related to colorectal neoplasms. Colorectal Cancer, *73*:13–28, 1993.

Byers, T. E., Graham, S., Haughey, B. P., Marshall, J. R., and Swanson, M. K. Diet and lung cancer risk: findings from the Western New York diet study. Am. J. Epidemiol., *125*:351–363, 1987.

Byrd, D. M., Roegner, M. L., Griffiths, J. C., Lamm, S. H., Grumski, K. S., Wilson, R., and Lai, S. Carcinogenic risks of inorganic arsenic in perspective. Int. Arch. Occup. Environ. Health, *68*:484–494, 1996.

Cairns, J. The cancer problem. Sci. Am., *233*:64–78, 1975.

Calabresi, E., De Giuli, G., Becciolini, A., Giannotti, P., Lombardi, G., and Serio, M. Plasma estrogens and androgens in male breast cancer. J. Steroid Biochem., *7*:605–609, 1976.

Calle, E. E., et al. (collaborative group on hormonal factors in breast cancer). Breast cancer and hormonal contraceptives: collaborative reanalysis of individual data on 53,297 women with breast cancer and

100,239 women without breast cancer from 54 epidemiological studies. Lancet, *347*:1713–1727, 1996a.

Calle, E. E., Mervis, C. A., Thun, M. J., Rodriguez, C., Wingo, P. A., and Heath, C. W. Jr. Diethylstilbestrol and risk of fatal breast cancer in a prospective cohort of US women. Am. J. Epidemiol., *144*:645–652, 1996b.

Calle, E. E., Miracle-McMahill, H. L., Thun, M. J., and Heath, C. W. Jr. Estrogen replacement therapy and risk of fatal colon cancer in a prospective cohort of postmenopausal women. J. Natl. Cancer Inst., *87*:517–523, 1995.

Cameron, A. J. Epidemiology of Barrett's esophagus. Gastroenterol. Clin. Biol., *18*:D3–D4, 1994.

Campbell, T. C., Chen, J., Liu, C., Li, J., and Parpia, B. Nonassociation of aflatoxin with primary liver cancer in a cross-sectional ecological survey in the People's Republic of China. Cancer Res., *50*:6882–6893, 1990.

Carroll, K. K. Lipids and carcinogenesis. J. Environ. Pathol. Toxicol., *3*:253–271, 1980.

Carroll, K. K., and Khor, K. T. Dietary fat in relation to tumorigenesis. Prog. Biochem. Pharmacol., *10*:308–353, 1975.

Castelletto, R., Muñoz, N., Landoni, N., Jmelnitzky, A., Crespi, M., Belloni, P., Chopita, N., and Teuchmann, S. Pre-cancerous lesions of the oesophagus in Argentina: prevalence and association with tobacco and alcohol. Int. J. Cancer, *51*:34–37, 1992.

Charnley, G., and Tannenbaum, S. R. Flow cytometric analysis of the effect of sodium chloride on gastric cancer risk in the rat. Cancer Res., *45*:5608–5616, 1985.

Cheah, P. Y. Hypotheses for the etiology of colorectal cancer—an overview. Nutr. Cancer, *14*:5–13, 1990.

Chen, C.-J., Chen, C. W., Wu, M.-M., and Kuo, T.-L. Cancer potential in liver, lung, bladder, and kidney due to ingested inorganic arsenic in drinking water. Br. J. Cancer, *66*:888–892, 1992.

Cheng, K. C., Preston, B. D., Cahill, D. S., Dosanjh, M. K., Singer, B., and Loeb, L. A. The vinyl chloride DNA derivative N^2,3-ethenoguanine produces G $\to$ A transitions in *Escherichia coli*. Proc. Natl. Acad. Sci. U.S.A., *88*:9974–9978, 1991.

Chiu, B. C.-H., Cerhan, J. R., Folsom, A. R., Sellers, T. A., Kushi, L. H., Wallace, R. B., Zheng, W., and Potter, J. D. Diet and risk of non-Hodgkin lymphoma in older women. J.A.M.A., *275*:1315–1321, 1996.

Choi, S. Y., and Kahyo, H. Effect of cigarette smoking and alcohol consumption in the etiology of cancers of the digestive tract. Int. J. Cancer, *49*:381–386, 1991.

Clinton, S. K., Emenhiser, C., Schwartz, S. J., Bostwick, D. G., Williams, A. W., Moore, B. J., and Erdman, J. W. Jr. *cis-trans* Lycopene isomers, carotenoids, and retinol in the human prostate. Cancer Epidemiol. Biomark. Prev., *5*:823–833, 1996.

Coggon, D., Barker, D. J. P., Cole, R. B., and Nelson, M. Stomach cancer and food storage. J. Natl. Cancer Inst., *81*:1178–1182, 1989.

Cohen, L. A., Zhao, Z., Zang, E. A., Wynn, T. T., Simi, B., and Rivenson, A. Wheat bran and psyllium diets: effects on *N*-methylnitrosourea–induced mammary tumorigenesis in F344 rats. J. Natl. Cancer Inst., *88*:899–907, 1996.

Cohen, M. D., Kargacin, B., Klein, C. B., and Costa, M. Mechanisms of chromium carcinogenicity and toxicity. Crit. Rev. Toxicol., *23*:255–281, 1993.

Colditz, G. A., Rosner, B. A., and Speizer, F. E. Risk factors for breast cancer according to family history of breast cancer. J. Natl. Cancer Inst., *88*:365–371, 1996.

Connolly, G. N., Winn, D. M., Hecht, S. S., Henningfield, J. E., Walker, B., Jr., and Hoffmann, D. The reemergence of smokeless tobacco. N. Engl. J. Med., *314*:1020–1027, 1986.

Connolly, J. G., and White, E. P. Malignant cells in the urine of men exposed to beta-naphthylamine. Can. Med. Assoc. J., *100*:879–882, 1969.

Cooper, W. C. Epidemiologic study of vinyl chloride workers: mortality through December 31, 1972. Environ. Health Perspect., *41*:101–106, 1981.

Correa, P., Malcom, G., Schmidt, B., Fontham, E., Ruiz, B., Bravo, J. C., Bravo, L. E., Zarama, G., and Realpe, J. L. Review article: antioxidant micronutrients and gastric cancer. Aliment Pharmacol. Ther., *12*:73–82, 1998.

Costa, M. Toxicity and carcinogenicity of Cr(VI) in animal models and humans. Crit. Rev. Toxicol., *27*:431–442, 1997.

Cramer, D. W., Willett, W. C., Bell, D. A., Ng, W. G., Harlow, B. L., Welch, W. R., Scully, R. E., and Knapp, R. C. Galactose consumption and metabolism in relation to the risk of ovarian cancer. Lancet, *2*:66–71, 1989.

Cravo, M. L., Mason, J. B., Dayal, Y., Hutchinson, M., Smith, D., Selhub, J., and Rosenberg, I. H. Folate deficiency enhances the development of colonic neoplasia in dimethylhydrazine-treated rats. Cancer Res., *52*:5002–5006, 1992.

Crisp, T. M., Clegg, E. D., Cooper, R. L., Wood, W. P., Anderson, D. G., Baetcke, K. P., Hoffmann, J. L., Morrow, M. S., Rodier, D. J., Schaeffer, J. E., Touart, L. W., Zeeman, M. G., and Patel, Y. M. Environmental endocrine disruption: an effects assessment and analysis. Environ. Health Perspect., *106*:11–56, 1998.

Daly, M. B. The epidemiology of ovarian cancer. Ovar. Cancer, *6*:729–738, 1992.

Dashwood, R. H. Indole-3-carbinol: anticarcinogen or tumor promoter in brassica vegetables? Chem. Biol. Interact., *110*:1–5, 1998.

Day, G. L., Blot, W. J., Austin, D. F., Bernstein, L., Greenberg, R. S., Preston-Martin, S., Schoenberg, J. B., Winn, D. M., McLaughlin, J. K., and Fraumeni, J. F. Jr., Racial differences in risk of oral and pharyngeal cancer: alcohol, tobacco, and other determinants. J. Natl. Cancer Inst., 85:465–473, 1993.

De Waard, F., Baanders-van Halewijn, E. A., and Huizinga, J. The bimodal age distribution of patients with mammary cancer. Cancer, *17*:141–151, 1964.

Delore, P., and Borgomano, C. Acute leukaemia following benzene poisoning. On the toxic origin of certain acute leukaemias and their relation to serious anaemias. J. Med. Lyon, *9*:227–233, 1928.

Deng, X.-S., Tuo, J., Poulsen, H. E., and Loft, S. Prevention of oxidative DNA damage in rats by Brussels sprouts. Free Radic. Res., *28*:323–333, 1998.

Doll, R. The lessons of life: keynote address to the nutrition and cancer conference. Cancer Res., *52*:2024s–2029s, 1992.

Doll, R., and Peto, R. The Causes of Cancer. Oxford, UK: Oxford University Press, 1981.

Donato, F., Tagger, A., Chiesa, R., Ribero, M. L., Tomasoni, V., Fasola, M., Gelatti, U., Portera, G., Boffetta, P., and Nardi, G. Hepatitis B and C virus infection, alcohol drinking, and hepatocellular carcinoma: a case-control study in Italy. Hepatology, *26*:579–584, 1997.

Dopp, E., Saedler, J., Stopper, H., Weiss, D. G., and Schiffmann, D. Mitotic disturbances and micronucleus induction in Syrian hamster embryo fibroblast cells caused by asbestos fibers. Environ. Health Perspect., *103*:268–271, 1995.

Dragan, Y. P., and Pitot, H. C. Aflatoxin carcinogenesis in the context of the multistage nature of cancer. *In*: The Toxicology of Aflatoxins: Human Health, Veterinary, and Agricultural Significance, pp. 179–206. New York: Academic Press, 1994.

Dragan, Y. P., Vaughan, J., Jordan, V. C., and Pitot, H. C. Comparison of the effects of tamoxifen and toremifene on liver and kidney tumor promotion in female rats. Carcinogenesis, *16*:2733–2741, 1995.

Dreyer, L., Winther, J. F., Pukkala, E., and Andersen, A. Tobacco smoking. APMIS (Acta Pathol Microbiol Immunol Scand) *105*(Suppl. 76):9–47, 1997.

Edmondson, H. A., Henderson, B., and Benton, B. Liver-cell adenomas associated with use of oral contraceptives. N. Engl. J. Med., *294*:470–472, 1976.

Enger, S. M., Ross, R. K., Paganini-Hill, A., and Bernstein, L. Breastfeeding experience and breast cancer risk among postmenopausal women. Cancer Epidemiol. Biomark. Prev., *7*:365–369, 1998.

Engle, A., Muscat, J. E., and Harris, R. E. Nutritional risk factors and ovarian cancer. Nutr. Cancer, *15*:239–247, 1991.

Farber, E. Chemical carcinogenesis and smoking. Can. J. Public Health, *72*:381–385, 1981.

Farrow, D. C., and Davis, S. Diet and the risk of pancreatic cancer in men. Am. J. Epidemiol., *132*:423–431, 1990.

Felton, J. S., Malfatti, M. A., Knize, M. G., Salmon, C. P., Hopmans, E. C., and Wu, R. W. Health risks of heterocyclic amines. Mutat. Res., *376*:37–41, 1997.

Fierz, U. Zürich: Katamnestische Untersuchungen über die Nebenwirkungen der Therapie von Haut-
    krankheiten mit anorganischem Arsen. Arch. Klin. Exp. Dermatol., *227*:286–290, 1966.

Fisher, B., Costantino, J. P., Redmond, C. K., Fisher, E. R., Wickerham, D. L., and Cronin, W. M. Endome-
    trial cancer in tamoxifen-treated breast cancer patients: findings from the National Surgical Adju-
    vant Breast and Bowel Project (NSABP) B-14. J. Natl. Cancer Inst., *86*:527–537, 1994.

Fisher, B., Costantino, J. P., Wickerham, D. L., Redmond, C. K., Kavanah, M., Cronin, W. M., Vogel, V.,
    Robidoux, A., Dimitrov, N., Atkins, J., Daly, M., Wieand, S., Tan-Chiu, E., Ford, L., Wolmark, N.,
    and other National Surgical Adjuvant Breast and Bowel Project Investigators. Tamoxifen for preven-
    tion of breast cancer: Report of the National Surgical Adjuvant Breast and Bowel Project P-1 Study.
    J. Natl. Cancer Inst., *90*:1371–1388, 1998.

Fong, L. Y. Y., Lee, J. S. K., Chan, W. C., and Newberne, P. M. Zinc deficiency and the development of
    esophageal and forestomach tumors in Sprague-Dawley rats fed precursors of *N*-nitroso-*N*-benzyl-
    methylamine. J. Natl. Cancer Inst., *72*:419–425, 1984.

Fontham, E. T. H. Protective dietary factors and lung cancer. Int. J. Epidemiol., *19*:S32–S42, 1990.

Forman, D., Pike, M. C., Davey, G., Dawson, S., Baker, K., Chilvers, C. E. D., Oliver, R. T. D., and Coup-
    land, C. A. C. Aetiology of testicular cancer: association with congenital abnormalities, age at pu-
    berty, infertility, and exercise. Br. Med. J., *308*:1393–1399, 1994.

Freedman, L. S., Clifford, C., and Messina, M. Analysis of dietary fat, calories, body weight, and the devel-
    opment of mammary tumors in rats and mice: a review. Cancer Res., *50*:5710–5719, 1990.

Freudenheim, J. L., Marshall, J. R., Vena, J. E., Laughlin, R., Brasure, J. R., Swanson, M. K., Nemoto, T.,
    and Graham, S. Premenopausal breast cancer risk and intake of vegetables, fruits, and related nutri-
    ents. J. Natl. Cancer Inst., *88*:340–348, 1996.

Fujimoto, Y., Hampton, L. L., Luo, L.-d., Wirth, P. J., and Thorgeirsson, S. S. Low frequency of *p53* gene
    mutation in tumors induced by aflatoxin B$_1$ in nonhuman primates. Cancer Res., *52*:1044–1046,
    1992.

Furihata, C., Ohta, H., and Katsuyama, T. Cause and effect between concentration-dependent tissue dam-
    age and temporary cell proliferation in rat stomach mucosa by NaCl, a stomach tumor promoter.
    Carcinogenesis, *17*:401–406, 1996.

Gambrell Jr., R. D. Pathophysiology and epidemiology of endometrial cancer. *In*: R. A. Lobo (Ed.), Treat-
    ment of the Postmenopausal Women: Basic and Clinical Aspects, pp. 355–362. New York: Raven
    Press, 1994.

Gammon, M. D., Schoenberg, J. B., Ahsan, H., Risch, H. A., Vaughan, T. L., Chow, W.-H., Rotterdam, H.,
    West, A. B., Dubrow, R., Stanford, J. L., Mayne, S. T., Farrow, D. C., Niwa, S., Blot, W. J., and
    Fraumeni, J. F. Jr. Tobacco, alcohol, and socioeconomic status and adenocarcinomas of the esopha-
    gus and gastric cardia. J. Natl. Cancer Inst., *89*:1277–1284, 1997.

Gangolli, S. D., van den Brandt, P. A., Feron, V. J., Janzowsky, C., Koeman, J. H., Speijers, G. J. A.,
    Spiegelhalder, B., Walker, R., and Wishnok, J. S. Nitrate, nitrite and *N*-nitroso compounds. Eur. J.
    Pharmacol., *292*:1–38, 1994.

Gann, P. H., Hennekens, C. H., Ma, J., Longcope, C., and Stampfer, M. J. Prospective study of sex hormone
    levels and risk of prostate cancer. J. Natl. Cancer Inst., *88*:1118–1126, 1996.

Gao, Y.-T., McLaughlin, J. K., Blot, W. J., Ji, B.-T., Benichou, J., Dai, Q., and Fraumeni, J. F. Jr. Risk
    factors for esophageal cancer in Shanghai, China. I. Role of cigarette smoking and alcohol drinking.
    Int. J. Cancer, *58*:192–196, 1994a.

Gao, Y.-T., McLaughlin, J. K., Gridley, G., Blot, W. J., Ji, B.-T., Dai, Q., and Fraumeni, J. F. Jr. Risk factors
    for esophageal cancer in Shanghai, China. II. Role of diet and nutrients. Int. J. Cancer, *58*:197–202,
    1994b.

Garfinkel, L. Overweight and cancer. Ann. Intern. Med., *103*:1034–1036, 1985.

Garfinkel, L. Overweight and mortality. Cancer, *58*:1826–1829, 1986.

Germolec, D. R., Spalding, J., Boorman, G. A., Wilmer, J. L., Yoshida, T., Simeonova, P. P., Bruccoleri, A.,
    Kayama, F., Gaido, K., Tennant, R., Burleson, F., Dong, W., Lang, R. W., and Luster, M. I. Arsenic
    can mediate skin neoplasia by chronic stimulation of keratinocyte-derived growth factors. Mutat.
    Res., *386*:209–218, 1997.

Giovannucci, E. Diet and other extrinsic factors influencing prostate cancer risk. *In*: J. G. Fortner and P. A. Sharp (Eds.), Accomplishments in Cancer Research, pp. 250–267. Philadelphia: Lippincott-Raven, 1998.

Giovannucci, E., and Goldin, B. The role of fat, fatty acids, and total energy intake in the etiology of human colon cancer. Am. J. Clin. Nutr., *66*:1564S–1571S, 1997.

Giovannucci, E., and Martínez, M. E. Tobacco, colorectal cancer, and adenomas: a review of the evidence. J. Natl. Cancer Inst., *88*:1717–1730, 1996.

Giovannucci, E., Ascherio, A., Rimm, E. B., Stampfer, M. J., Colditz, G. A., and Willett, W. C. Intake of carotenoids and retinol in relation to risk of prostate cancer. J. Natl. Cancer Inst., *87*:1767–1776, 1995.

Giovannucci, E., Rimm, E. B., Stampfer, M. J., Colditz, G. A., Ascherio, A., and Willett, W. C. Intake of fat, meat, and fiber in relation to risk of colon cancer in men. Cancer Res., *54*:2390–2397, 1994.

Gladek, A., and Liehr, J. G. Mechanisms of genotoxicity of diethylstilbestrol *in vivo*. J. Biol. Chem., *264*:16847–16852, 1989.

Gold, L. S., Slone, T. H., Manley, N. B., and Ames, B. N. Heterocyclic amines formed by cooking food: comparison of bioassay results with other chemicals in the Carcinogenic Potency Database. Cancer Lett., *83*:21–29, 1994.

Goldberg, R. J. Clinical uses of the epidemiologic approach. Hosp. Pract. Office edn. *18*(8):177–189, 1983.

Goldstein, B. D. Is exposure to benzene a cause of human multiple myeloma? Ann. N.Y. Acad. Sci., *609*:225–234, 1990.

Gopalakrishnan, S., Liu, X., and Patel, D. J. Solution structure of the covalent sterigmatocystin-DNA adduct. Biochemistry, *31*:10790–10801, 1992.

Gordon, J., Reagan, J. W., Finkle, W. D., and Ziel, H. K. Estrogen and endometrial carcinoma. An independent pathology review supporting original risk estimate. N. Engl. J. Med., *297*:570–571, 1977.

Gradelet, S., Le Bon, A.-M., Bergès, R., Suschetet, M., and Astorg, P. Dietary carotenoids inhibit aflatoxin B_1-induced liver preneoplastic foci and DNA damage in the rat: role of the modulation of aflatoxin B_1 metabolism. Carcinogenesis, *19*:403–411, 1998.

Graham, S., Haughey, B., Marshall, J., Brasure, J., Zielezny, M., Freudenheim, J.,West, D., Nolan, J., and Wilkinson, G. Diet in the epidemiology of gastric cancer. Nutr. Cancer, *13*:19–34, 1990.

Gray, M. R., Donnelly, R. J., and Kingsnorth, A. N. The role of smoking and alcohol in metaplasia and cancer risk in Barrett's columnar lined oesophagus. Gut, *34*:727–731, 1993.

Greenberg, E. R., Barnes, A. B., Resseguie, L., Barrett, J. A., Burnside, S., Lanza, L. L., Neff, R. K., Stevens, M., Young, R. H., and Colton, T. Breast cancer in mothers given diethylstilbestrol in pregnancy. N. Engl. J. Med., *311*:1393–1398, 1984.

Greene, M. H. Is cisplatin a human carcinogen? J. Natl. Cancer Inst., *84*:306–312, 1992.

Griffiths, K., Davies, P., Eaton, C. L., Harper, M. E., Turkes, A., and Peeling, W. B. Endocrine factors in the initiation, diagnosis, and treatment of prostatic cancer. *In*: K.-D. Voigt and C. Knabbe (Eds.), Endocrine Dependent Tumors, pp. 83–130. New York: Raven Press, 1991.

Grodstein, F., Martinez, E., Platz, E. A., Giovannucci, E., Colditz, G. A., Kautzky, M., Fuchs, C., and Stampfer, M. J. Postmenopausal hormone use and risk for colorectal cancer and adenoma. Ann. Intern. Med., *128*:705–712, 1998.

Grubbs, C. J., Steele, V. E., Casebolt, T., Juliana, M. M., Eto, I., Whitaker, L. M., Dragnev, K. H., Kelloff, G. J., and Lubet, R. L. Chemoprevention of chemically induced mammary carcinogenesis by indole-3-carbinol. Anticancer Res., *15*:709–716, 1995.

Gupta, I., Baptista, J., Bruce, W. R., Che, C. T., Furrer, R., Gingerich, J. S., Grey, A. A., Marai, L., Yates, P., and Krepinsky, J. J. Structures of fecapentaenes, the mutagens of bacterial origin isolated from human feces. Biochemistry, *22*:241–244, 1983.

Gupta, M. P., Khanduja, K. L., Koul, I. B., and Sharma, R. R. Effect of cigarette smoke inhalation on benzo[*a*]pyrene-induced lung carcinogenesis in vitamin A deficiency in the rat. Cancer Lett., *55*:83–88, 1990.

Gwinn, M. L., Webster, L. A., Lee, N. C., Layde, P. M., Rubin, G. L., and The Cancer and Steroid Hormone Study Group. Alcohol consumption and ovarian cancer risk. Am. J. Epidemiol., *123*:759–766, 1986.

Hammond, E. C., and Selikoff, J. J. Relation of cigarette smoking to risk of death of asbestos-associated disease among insulation workers in the United States. pp. 312–317. IARC Scientific Publications, No. 8. Lyon, France: IARC, 1973.

Hansson, L.-E., Nyrén, O., Bergström, R., Wolok, A., Lindgren, A., Baron, J., and Adami, H.-O. Nutrients and gastric cancer risk. A population-based case-control study in Sweden. Int. J. Cancer, 57:638–644, 1994.

Hardell, L., Eriksson, M., and Degerman, A. Exposure to phenoxyacetic acids, chlorophenols, or organic solvents in relation to histopathology, stage, and anatomical localization of non-Hodgkin's lymphoma. Cancer Res., 54:2386–2389, 1994.

Hardell, L., Eriksson, M., and Degerman, A. Meta-analysis of four Swedish case-control studies on exposure to pesticides as risk-factor for soft-tissue sarcoma including the relation to tumour localization and histopathological type. Int. J. Oncol., 6:847–851, 1995.

Harris, R. W. C., Brinton, L. A., Cowdell, R. H., Skegg, D. C. G., Smith, P. G., Vessey, M. P., and Doll, R. Characteristics of women with dysplasia or carcinoma in situ of the cervix uteri. Br. J. Cancer, 42:359–368, 1980.

Hartman, P. E. Review: putative mutagens and carcinogens in foods. I. Nitrate/nitrite ingestion and gastric cancer mortality. Environ. Mutagen, 5:111–121, 1983.

Hawrylewicz, E. J., Huang, H. H., Kissane, J. Q., and Drab, E. A. Enhancement of 7,12-dimethyl-benz(a)anthracene (DMBA) mammary tumorigenesis by high dietary protein in rats. Nutr. Rep. Int., 26:793–806, 1982.

Hayashi, H., Kanisawa, M., Yamanaka, K., Ito, T., Udaka, N., Ohji, H., Okudela, K., Okada, S., and Kitamura, H. Dimethylarsinic acid, a main metabolite of inorganic arsenics, has tumorigenicity and progression effects in the pulmonary tumors of A/J mice. Cancer Lett., 125:83–88, 1998.

Hayes, R. B., Bogdanovicz, J. F. A. T., Schroeder, F. H., de Bruijn, A., Raatgever, J. W., van der Maas, P. J., Oishi, K., and Yoshida, O. Serum retinol and prostate cancer. Cancer, 62:2021–2026, 1988.

He, Y., Root, M. M., Parker, R. S., and Campbell, T. C. Effects of carotenoid-rich food extracts on the development of preneoplastic lesions in rat liver and on in vivo and in vitro antioxidant status. Nutr. Cancer, 27:238–244, 1997.

Hei, T. K., Piao, C. Q., He, Z. Y., Vannais, D., and Waldren, C. A. Chrysotile fiber is a strong mutagenic in mammalian cells. Cancer Res., 52:6305–6309, 1992.

Helzlsouer, K. J., Comstock, G. W., and Morris, J. S. Selenium, lycopene, α-tocopherol, β-carotene, retinol, and subsequent bladder cancer. Cancer Res., 49:6144–6148, 1989.

Henderson, B. E., Ross, R. K., Pike, M. C., and Casagrande, J. T. Endogenous hormones as a major factor in human cancer. Cancer Res., 42:3232–3239, 1982.

Herbst, A. L. Clear cell adenocarcinoma and the current status of DES-exposed females. Cancer, 48:484–488, 1981.

Herity, B., Moriarty, M., Daly, L., Dunn, J., and Bourke, G. J. The role of tobacco and alcohol in the aetiology of lung and larynx cancer. Br. J. Cancer, 46:961–964, 1982.

Herrero, R., Potischman, N., Brinton, L. A., Reeves, W. C., Brenes, M. M., Tenorio, F., de Britton, R. C., and Gaitan, E. A case-control study of nutrient status and invasive cervical cancer. Am. J. Epidemiol., 134:1335–1346, 1991.

Heshmat, M. Y., Kaul, L., Kovi, J., Jackson, M. A., Jackson, A. G., Jones, G. W., Edson, M., Enterline, J. P., Worrell, R. G., and Perry, S. L. Nutrition and prostate cancer: a case-control study. Prostate, 6:7–17, 1985.

Higginson, J. Perspectives and future development in research on environmental carcinogenesis. In: A. C. Griffin and C. R. Shaw (Eds.), Carcinogens: Identification and Mechanisms, pp. 187–208. New York: Raven Press, 1979.

Hill, J. Cautions Against the Immoderate Use of Snuff, 2nd ed. London, 1761.

Hino, O., Tabata, S., and Hotta, Y. Evidence for increased in vitro recombination with insertion of human hepatitis B virus DNA. Proc. Natl. Acad. Sci. U.S.A., 88:9248–9252, 1991.

Hiramatsu, Y., Takada, H., Yamamura, M., Hioki, K., Saito, K., and Yamamoto, M. Effect of dietary cholesterol on azoxymethane-induced colon carcinogenesis in rats. Carcinogenesis, 4:553–558, 1983.

Hirayama, T. Lifestyle and mortality—the healthiest way to live. Homeostas. Health Dis., *35*:168–179, 1994.

Hirohata, T., and Kono, S. Diet/nutrition and stomach cancer in Japan. Int. J. Cancer, *10*:34–36, 1997.

Hoffman, F. L. The Mortality from Cancer Throughout the World. Newark, NJ: Prudential Press, 1915.

Hoffman, F. L. Cancer and Diet. Baltimore: Williams & Wilkins, 1937.

Hoffmann, D., and Hecht, S. S. Smokeless tobacco and cancer. ISI Atlas of Science. Pharmacology, *2*:46–50, 1988.

Hoffmann, G. R., and Morgan, R. W. Review: Putative mutagens and carcinogens in foods. V. Cycad azoxyglycosides. Environ. Mutagen., *6*:103–116, 1984.

Hoover, R., and Fraumeni, J. F. Jr. Risk of cancer in renal-transplant recipients. Lancet, *2*:55–57, 1973.

Hoover, R., and Fraumeni, J. F. Jr. Drug-induced cancer. Cancer, *47*:1071–1080, 1981.

Hopenhayn-Rich, C., Biggs, M. L., Fuchs, A., Bergoglio, R., Tello, E. E., Nicolli, H., and Smith, A. H. Bladder cancer mortality associated with arsenic in drinking water in Argentina. Epidemiology, *7*:117–124, 1996.

Howe, G. R., Benito, E., Castelleto, R., Cornée, J., Estève, J., Gallagher, R. P., Iscovich, J. M., Deng-ao, J., Kaaks, R., Kune, G. A., Kune, S., L'Abbé, K. A., Lee, H. P., Lee, M., Miller, A. B., Peters, R. K., Potter, J. D., Riboli, E., Slattery, M. L., Trichopoulos, D., Tuyns, A., Tzonou, A., Whittemore, A. S., Wu-Williams, A. H., and Shu, Z. Dietary intake of fiber and decreased risk of cancers of the colon and rectum: evidence from the combined analysis of 13 case-control studies. J. Natl. Cancer Inst., *84*:1887–1896, 1992.

Howe, G. R., Friedenreich, C. M., Jain, M., and Miller, A. B. A cohort study of fat intake and risk of breast cancer. J. Natl. Cancer Inst., *83*:336–340, 1991.

Hsing, A. W., Comstock, G. W., Abbey, H., and Polk, B. F. Serologic precursors of cancer. Retinol, carotenoids, and tocopherol and risk of prostate cancer. J. Natl. Cancer Inst., *82*:941–946, 1990.

Hsu, H.-C., Peng, S.-Y., Lai, P.-L., Chu, J.-S., and Lee, P.-H. Mutations of p53 gene in hepatocellular carcinoma (HCC) correlate with tumor progression and patient prognosis: a study of 138 patients with unifocal HCC. Int. J. Oncol., *4*:1341–1347, 1994.

Hsu, I. C., Metcalf, R. A., Sun, T., Welsh, J. A., Wang, N. J., and Harris, C. C. Mutational hotspot in the p53 gene in human hepatocellular carcinomas. Nature, *350*:427–428, 1991.

Hu, J., Zhang, S., Jia, E., Wang, Q., Liu, S., Lu, Y., Wu, Y., and Cheng, Y. Diet and cancer of the stomach: a case-control study in China. Int. J. Cancer, *41*:331–335, 1988.

Huff, J. E., Haseman, J. K., DeMarini, D. M., Eustis, S., Maronpot, R. R., Peters, A. C., Persing, R. L., Chrisp, C. E., and Jacobs, A. C. Multiple-site carcinogenicity of benzene in Fischer 344 rats and B6C3F$_1$ mice. Environ. Health Perspect., *82*:125–163, 1989.

Huncharek, M. Asbestos and cancer: epidemiological and public health controversies. Cancer Invest., *12*:214–222, 1994.

IARC Monographs. Evaluation of the carcinogenic risk of chemicals to humans. Supplement 4, Report of an ad hoc working group. Lyons, France: IARC, February 8–12, 1982.

IARC Monographs on the Evaluation of the Carcinogenic Risk of Chemicals to Humans: Tobacco Habits Other than Smoking; Betel-Quid and Areca-Nut Chewing; and Some Related Nitrosamines, Vol. 37. Lyon, France: IARC, 1985.

IARC Monographs on the Evaluation of Carcinogenic Risks to Humans: Analgesic Mixtures Containing Phenacetin. Updating of IARC Monographs Vols. 1 to 42, Suppl. 7, pp. 310–312. Lyon, France: IARC, 1987.

IARC Monographs on Trichloroethylene. 63: 75–158, 1995.

IARC Monographs on the Evaluation of Carcinogenic Risks to Humans: Some Pharmaceutical Drugs, Vol. 66. Lyon, France: IARC, 1996.

Ingram, D., Nottage, E., Ng, S., Sparrow, L., Roberts, A., and Willcox, D. Obesity and breast disease. The role of the female sex hormones. Cancer, *64*:1049–1053, 1989.

Jacobs, L. R. Relationship between dietary fiber and cancer: metabolic, physiologic, and cellular mechanisms. Proc. Soc. Exp. Biol. Med., *183*:299–310, 1986.

Jain, M., Burch, J. D., Howe, G. R., Risch, H. A., and Miller, A. B. Dietary factors and risk of lung cancer: results from a case-control study, Toronto, 1981–1985. Int. J. Cancer, *45*:287–293, 1990.

James, J. T., Kaplan, H. L., and Coleman, M. E. B11: Trichloroethylene. *In*: Spacecraft Maximum Allowable Concentrations for Selected Airborne Contaminants, Vol. 3, pp. 292–320. Washington, D.C.: National Academy Press, 1997.

Johansson, L., Albin, M., Jakobsson, K., and Mikoczy, Z. Histological type of lung carcinoma in asbestos cement workers and matched controls. Br. J. Ind. Med., *49*:626–630, 1992.

Johnson, L. D., Driscoll, S. G., Hertig, A. T., Cole, P. T., and Nickerson, R. J. Vaginal adenosis in stillborns and neonates exposed to diethylstilbestrol and steroidal estrogens and progestins. Obstet. Gynecol., *53*:671–679, 1979.

Jordan, V. C. A current view of tamoxifen for the treatment and prevention of breast cancer. Fourteenth Gaddum Memorial Lecture. University of Cambridge, January 1993. Br. J. Pharmacol., *110*:507–517, 1993.

Kahn, J. O., and Walker, B. D. Acute human immunodeficiency virus type 1 infection. N. Engl. J. Med., *339*:33–39, 1998.

Kampert, J. B., Whittemore, A. S., and Paffenbarger, R. S. Jr. Combined effect of childbearing, menstrual events, and body size on age-specific breast cancer risk. Am. J. Epidemiol., *128*:962–979, 1988.

Kang, H., Enziger, F., Breslin, P., Feil, M., Lee, Y., an Shepard, B. Soft tissue sarcoma and military service in Vietnam: a case-control study. J. Natl. Cancer Inst., *79*:693–699, 1987.

Karp, J. E., and Smith, M. A. The molecular pathogenesis of treatment-induced (secondary) leukemias: foundations for treatment and prevention. Semin. Oncol., *24*:103–113, 1997.

Kato, K., Akai, S., Tominaga, S., and Kato, I. A case-control study of biliary tract cancer in Niigata Prefecture, Japan. Jpn. J. Cancer Res., *80*:932–938, 1989.

Kaul, L., Nidiry, J. J., Charles-Marcel, Z., Enterline, J. P., and Brown, C. O. Diet and esophageal cancer: a case-control study. Nutr. Res., *6*:905–912, 1986.

Key, T. J. A. Hormones and cancer in humans. Mutat. Res., *333*:59–67, 1995.

Key, T. J. A., Silcocks, P. B., Davey, G. K., Appleby, P. N., and Bishop, D. T. A case-control study of diet and prostate cancer. Br. J. Cancer, *76*:678–687, 1997.

Kim, D. J., Han, B. S., Ahn, B., Lee, K. K., Kang, J. S., and Tsuda, H. Promotion potential of tamoxifen on hepatocarcinogenesis in female SD or F344 rats initiated with diethylnitrosamine. Cancer Lett., *104*:13–19, 1996.

Kim, D. J., Takasuka, N., Kim, J. M., Sekine, K., Ota, T., Asamoto, M., Murakoshi, M., Nishino, H., Nir, Z., and Tsuda, H. Chemoprevention by lycopene of mouse lung neoplasia after combined initiation treatment with DEN, MNU and DMH. Cancer Lett., *120*:15–22, 1997.

Kingston, D. G. I., Van Tassell, R. L., and Wilkins, T. D. The fecapentaenes, potent mutagens from human feces. Chem. Res. Toxicol., *3*:391–400, 1990.

Kjaer, S. K., and Brinton, L. A. Adenocarcinomas of the uterine cervix: the epidemiology of an increasing problem. Epidemiol. Rev., *15*:486–498, 1993.

Knekt, P. Vitamin E and smoking and the risk of lung cancer. Ann. N.Y. Acad. Sci., *686*:280–287, 1993.

Kolaja, K. L., and Klaunig, J. E. Vitamin E modulation of hepatic focal lesion growth in mice. Toxicol. Appl. Pharmacol., *143*:380–387, 1997.

Kolonel, L. N., Yoshizawa, C. N., and Hankin, J. H. Diet and prostatic cancer: a case-control study in Hawaii. Am. J. Epidemiol., *127*:999–1012, 1988.

Krinsky, N. I. Carotenoids and cancer: basic research studies. *In*: Natural Antioxidants in Human Health and Disease, pp. 239–261. New York: Academic Press, 1994.

Kromhout, D., and Bueno-de-Mesquita, H. B. Antioxidant vitamins and stomach cancer: the role of ecologic studies. Cancer Lett., *114*:333–334, 1997.

Kvåle, G., and Heuch, I. A prospective study of reproductive factors and breast cancer. II. Age at first and last birth. Am. J. Epidemiol., *126*:842–850, 1987.

La Vecchia, C., Negri, E., Decarli, A., D'Avanzo, B., Liberati, C., and Franceschi, S. Dietary factors in the risk of bladder cancer. Nutr. Cancer, *12*:93–101, 1989.

Lambe, M., Hsieh, C.-C., Trichopoulos, D., Ekbom, A., Pavia, M., and Adami, H.-O. Transient increase in the risk of breast cancer after giving birth. N. Engl. J. Med., *331*:5–9, 1994.

Lamm, S. H., Walters, A. S., Wilson, R., Byrd, D. M., and Grunwald, H. Consistencies and inconsistencies underlying the quantitative assessment of leukemia risk from benzene exposure. Environ. Health Perspect., *82*:289–297, 1989.

Lasky, T., and Magder, L. Hepatocellular carcinoma *p53* G>T transversions at codon 249: the fingerprint of aflatoxin exposure? Environ. Health Perspect., *105*:392–397, 1997.

Launoy, G., Milan, C. H., Faivre, J., Pienkowski, P., Milan, C. I., and Gignoux, M. Alcohol, tobacco and oesophageal cancer: effects of the duration of consumption, mean intake and current and former consumption. Br. J. Cancer, *75*:1389–1396, 1997.

Launoy, G., Milan, C., Day, N. E., Pienkowski, M. P., Gignoux, M., and Faivre, J. Diet and squamous-cell cancer of the oesophagus: a French multicentre case-control study. Int. J. Cancer, *76*:7–12, 1998.

Le Marchand, L., Hankin, J. H., Kolonel, L. N., and Wilkens, L. R. Vegetable and fruit consumption in relation to prostate cancer risk in Hawaii: a reevaluation of the effect of dietary beta-carotene. Am. J. Epidemiol., *133*:215–219, 1991.

Le Marchand, L., Hankin, J. H., Wilkens, L. R., Kolonel, L. N., Englyst, H. N., and Lyu, L.-C. Dietary fiber and colorectal cancer risk. Epidemiology, *8*:658–665, 1997.

Le Marchand, L., Yoshizawa, C. N., Kolonel, L. N., Hankin, J. H., and Goodman, M. T. Vegetable consumption and lung cancer risk: a population-based case-control study in Hawaii. J. Natl. Cancer Inst., *81*:1158–1164, 1989.

Leaf, C. D., Wishnok, J. S., and Tannenbaum, S. R. Mechanisms of endogenous nitrosation. Cancer Surv., *8*:323–334, 1989.

Leclerc, A., Martinez Cortes, M., Gérin, M., Luce, D., and Brugère, J. Sinonasal cancer and wood dust exposure: results from a case-control study. Am. J. Epidemiol., *140*:340–349, 1994.

Lee, T.-C., Oshimura, M., and Barrett, J. C. Comparison of arsenic-induced cell transformation, cytotoxicity, mutation and cytogenetic effects in Syrian hamster embryo cells in culture. Carcinogenesis, *6*:1421–1426, 1985.

Levi, F., Franceschi, S., Negri, E., and La Vecchia, C. Dietary factors and the risk of endometrial cancer. Cancer, *71*:3575–3581, 1993.

Li, D., Dragan, Y., Jordan, V. C., Wang, M., and Pitot, H. C. Effects of chronic administration of tamoxifen and toremifene on DNA adducts in rat liver, kidney, and uterus. Cancer Res., *57*:1438–1441, 1997.

Li, M.-H., Ji, C., and Cheng, S.-J. Occurrence of nitroso compounds in fungi-contaminated foods: a review. Nutr. Cancer, *8*:63–69, 1986.

Lieber, C. S., Seitz, H. K., Garro, A. J., and Worner, T. M. Alcohol-related diseases and carcinogenesis. Cancer Res., *39*:2863–2886, 1979.

Liehr, J. G., Randerath, K., and Randerath, E. Target organ-specific covalent DNA damage preceding diethylstilbestrol-induced carcinogenesis. Carcinogenesis, *6*:1067–1069, 1985.

Lilienfeld, A. M. Practical limitations of epidemiologic methods. Environ. Health Perspect., *52*:3–8, 1983.

Liu, M. C., Hai, A., and Huang, A. T. Cancer epidemiology in the Far East—contrast with the United States. Oncology, *7*:99–114, 1993.

London, N. J., Farmery, S. M., Will, E. J., Davison, A. M., and Lodge, J. P. A. Risk of neoplasia in renal transplant patients. Lancet, *346*:403–406, 1995.

Lucier, G., Clark, G., Hiermath, C., Tritscher, A., Sewall, C., and Huff, J. Carcinogenicity of TCDD in laboratory animals: implications for risk assessment. Toxicol. Ind. Health, *9*:631–668, 1993.

Lynch, H. T., Albano, W. A., Layton, M. A., Kimberling, W. J., and Lynch, J. F. Breast cancer, genetics, and age at first pregnancy. J. Med. Genet., *21*:96–98, 1984.

Mack, D. O., Reed, V. L., and Smith, L. D. Retinyl acetate inhibition of 3′-methyl-4-dimethyl-amino-azobenzene induced hepatic neoplasia. Int. J. Biochem., *22*:359–365, 1990.

Maden, C., Sherman, K. J., Beckmann, A. M., Hislop, T. G., Teh, C.-Z., Ashley, R. L., and Daling, J. R. History of circumcision, medical conditions, and sexual activity and risk of penile cancer. J. Natl. Cancer Inst., *85*:19–24, 1993.

Maekawa, A., Ogiu, T., Onodera, H., Furuta, K., Matsuoka, C., Ohno, Y., and Odashima, S. Carcinogenicity studies of sodium nitrite and sodium nitrate in F-344 rats. Food Chem. Toxicol., *20*:25–33, 1982.

Magos, L. Epidemiological and experimental aspects of metal carcinogenesis: physicochemical properties, kinetics, and the active species. Environ. Health Perspect., *95*:157–189, 1991.

Makino, M., Kaibara, N., and Koga, S. Enhanced induction by high-cholesterol diet of remnant gastric carcinogenesis by *N*-methyl-*N'*-nitro-*N*-nitrosoguanidine in rats. J. Natl. Cancer Inst., *81*:130–135, 1989.

Mandeville, R., and Houde, M. A critical review of the potential carcinogenicity of tamoxifen on steroid hormone-sensitive tissues. Cancer J., *7*:12–15, 1994.

Manson, J. E., Willett, W. C., Stampfer, M. J., Colditz, G. A., Hunter, D. J., Hankinson, S. E., Hennekens, C. H., and Speizer, F. E. Body weight and mortality among women. N. Engl. J. Med., *333*:677–685, 1995.

Marion, M.-J., De Vivo, I., Smith, S., Luo, J.-C., and Brandt-Rauf, P. W. The molecular epidemiology of occupational carcinogenesis in vinyl chloride exposed workers. Int. Arch. Occup. Environ. Health, *68*:394–398, 1996.

Martiñez, M. E., McPherson, R. S., Annegers, J. F., and Levin, B. Cigarette smoking and alcohol consumption as risk factors for colorectal adenomatous polyps. J. Natl. Cancer Inst., *87*:274–279, 1995.

Mason, J. B. Folate and colonic carcinogenesis: searching for a mechanistic understanding. J. Nutr. Biochem., *5*:170–175, 1994.

Matsukura, N., Kawachi, T., Sasajima, K., Sano, T., Sugimura, T., and Ito, N. Induction of liver tumors in rats by sodium nitrite and methylguanidine. Z. Krebsforsch., *90*:87–94, 1977.

Matthew, J. A., Fellows, I. W., Prior, A., Kennedy, H. J., Bobbin, R., and Johnson, I. T. Habitual intake of fruits and vegetables amongst patients at increased risk of colorectal neoplasia. Cancer Lett., *114*:255–258, 1997.

Mayne, S. T., Janerich, D. T., Greenwald, P., Chorost, S., Tucci, C., Zaman, M. B., Melamed, M. R., Kiely, M., and McKneally, M. F. Dietary beta carotene and lung cancer risk in U.S. nonsmokers. J. Natl. Cancer Inst., *86*:33–38, 1994.

Mayne, S. T., Redlich, C. A., and Cullen, M. R. Dietary vitamin A and prevalence of bronchial metaplasia in asbestos-exposed workers. Am. Soc. Clin. Nutr., *68*:630–635, 1998.

McGonigle, K. F., and Huggins, G. R. Oral contraceptives and breast disease. Fertil. Steril., *56*:799–819, 1991.

McGowan, L. Epidemiology of ovarian cancer. Oncology, *3*:51–62, 1989.

McGregor, D. B., Partensky, C., Wilbourn, J., and Rice, J. M. An IARC evaluation of polychlorinated dibenzo-*p*-dioxins and polychlorinated dibenzofurans as risk factors in human carcinogenesis. Environ. Health Perspect., *106*:755–760, 1998.

McLean, E. K. The toxic actions of pyrrolizidine (senecio) alkaloids. Pharmacol. Rev., *22*:429–476, 1970.

McPherson, C. P., Sellers, T. A., Potter, J. D., Bostick, R. M., and Folsom, A. R. Reproductive factors and risk of endometrial cancer. The Iowa Women's Health Study. Am. J. Epidemiol., *143*:1195–1202, 1996.

Medinsky, M. A., Schlosser, P. M., and Bond, J. A. Critical issues in benzene toxicity and metabolism: the effect of interactions with other organic chemicals on risk assessment. Environ. Health Perspect., *102*:119–124, 1994.

Mellemgaard, A., McLaughlin, J. K., Overvad, K., and Olsen, J. H. Dietary risk factors for renal cell carcinoma in Denmark. Eur. J. Cancer, *32A*:673–682, 1996.

Melnick, S., Cole, P., Anderson, D., and Herbst, A. Rates and risks of diethylstilbestrol-related clear-cell adenocarcinoma of the vagina and cervix. N. Engl. J. Med., *316*:514–516, 1987.

Menkes, M. S., Comstock, G. W., Vuilleumier, J. P., Helsing, K. J., Rider, A. A., and Brookmeyer, R. Serum beta-carotene, vitamins A and E, selenium, and the risk of lung cancer. N. Engl. J. Med., *315*:1250–1254, 1986.

Messina, M. J., Persky, V., Setchell, K. D. R., and Barnes, S. Soy intake and cancer risk: a review of the *in vitro* and *in vivo* data. Nutr. Cancer, *21*:113–131, 1994.

Mettlin, C. J., and Piver, M. S. A case-control study of milk-drinking and ovarian cancer risk. Am. J. Epidemiol., *132*:871–876, 1990.

Mettlin, C., Selenskas, S., Natarajan, N., and Huben, R. Beta-carotene and animal fats and their relationship to prostate cancer risk. Cancer, *64*:605–612, 1989.

Meurman, L. O., Kiviluoto, N., and Hakama, M. Mortality and morbidity among the working population of anthophyllite asbestos miners in Finland. Br. J. Ind. Med., *31*:105, 1974.

Meyer, F., Bairati, I., Fradet, Y., and Moore, L. Dietary energy and nutrients in relation to preclinical prostate cancer. Nutr. Cancer, *29*:120–126, 1997.

Miller, A. B., Berrino, F., Hill, M., Pietinen, P., Riboli, E., and Wahrendorf, J. Diet in the aetiology of cancer: a review. Eur. J. Cancer, *30A*:207–220, 1994.

Miller, J. A. The need for epidemiological studies of the medical exposures of Japanese patients to the carcinogen ethyl carbamate (urethane) from 1950 to 1975. Jpn. J. Cancer Res., *82*:1323–1324, 1991.

Mills, P. K., Beeson, W. L., Phillips, R. L., and Fraser, G. E. Cohort study of diet, lifestyle, and prostate cancer in Adventist men. Cancer, *64*:598–604, 1989.

Mishina, T., Watanabe, H., Araki, H ., and Nakao, M. Epidemiological study of prostatic cancer by matched-pair analysis. Prostate, *6*:423–436, 1985.

Mittendorf, R. Teratogen update: carcinogenesis and teratogenesis associated with exposure to diethylstilbestrol (DES) in utero. Teratology, *51*:435–445, 1995.

Moerman, C. J., Bueno de Mesquita, H. B., and Runia, S. Dietary sugar intake in the aetiology of biliary tract cancer. Int. J. Epidemiol., *22*:207–214, 1993.

Møller, H., Knudsen, L. B., and Lynge, E. Risk of testicular cancer after vasectomy: cohort study of over 73,000 men. Br. Med. J., *309*:295–299, 1994a.

Møller, H., Mellemgaard, A., Lindvig, K., and Olsen, J. H. Obesity and cancer risk: a Danish record-linkage study. Eur. J. Cancer, *30A*:344–350, 1994b.

Mollo, F., Piolatto, G., Bellis, D., Andrion, A., Delsedime, L., Bernardi, P., Pira, E., and Ardissone, F. Asbestos exposure and histologic cell types of lung cancer in surgical and autopsy series. Int. J. Cancer, *46*:576–580, 1990.

Moreno, F. S., Wu, T.-S., Penteado, M. V. C., Rizzi, M. B. S. L., Jordão, A. A., Jr., Almeida-Muradian, L. B., and Dagli, M. L. Z. A comparison of β-carotene and vitamin A effects on a hepatocarcinogenesis model. Int. J. Vit. Nutr. Res., *65*:87–94, 1995.

Morgan, R. W. Risk of endometrial cancer after tamoxifen treatment. Oncology, *11*:25–33, 1997.

Morgentaler, A., Bruning C. O. III, and DeWolf, W. C. Occult prostate cancer in men with low serum testosterone levels. J.A.M.A., *276*:1904–1906, 1996.

Mori, M., and Miyake, H. Dietary and other risk factors of ovarian cancer among elderly women. Jpn. J. Cancer Res., *79*:997–1004, 1988.

Moss, A. R., Osmond, D., Bacchetti, P., Torti, F. M., and Gurgin, V. Hormonal risk factors in testicular cancer. A case-control study. Am. J. Epidemiol., *124*:39–52, 1986.

Moyer, V. D., Cistulli, C. A., Vaslet, C. A., and Kane, A. B. Oxygen radicals and asbestos carcinogenesis. Environ. Health Perspect., *102*:131–136, 1994.

Muscat, J. E., and Wynder, E. L. Cigarette smoking, asbestos exposure, and malignant mesothelioma. Cancer Res., *51*:2263–2267, 1991.

Nagao, M., Wakabayashi, K., Ushijima, T., Toyota, M., Totsuka, Y., and Sugimura, T. Human exposure to carcinogenic heterocyclic amines and their mutational fingerprints in experimental animals. Environ. Health Perspect., *104*:497–501, 1996.

Narisawa, T., Fukaura, Y., Hasebe, M., Ito, M., Aizawa, R., Murakoshi, M., Uemura, S., Khachik, F., and Nishino, H. Inhibitory effects of natural carotenoids, α-carotene, β-carotene, lycopene and lutein, on colonic aberrant crypt foci formation in rats. Cancer Lett., *107*:137–142, 1996.

Narisawa, T., Fukaura, Y., Terada, K., and Sekiguchi, H. Prevention of N-methylnitrosourea–induced colon tumorigenesis by ursodeoxycholic acid in F344 rats. Jpn. J. Cancer Res., *89*:1009–1013, 1998.

National Cancer Institute. Tobacco Research Implementation Plan. Bethesda, MD: National Institutes of Health, 1998.

Nazario, C. M., Szklo, M., Diamond, E., Román-Franco, A., Climent, C., Suarez, E., and Conde, J. G. Salt and gastric cancer: a case-control study in Puerto Rico. Int. J. Epidemiol., *22*:790–797, 1993.

Nestle, M. Broccoli sprouts as inducers of carcinogen-detoxifying enzyme systems: clinical, dietary, and policy implications. Proc. Natl. Acad. Sci. U.S.A., *94*:11149–11151, 1997.

Neubauer, O. Arsenical cancer: a review. Br. J. Cancer, *1*:192–251, 1947

Newberne, P. M., and Butler, W. H. Acute and chronic effects of aflatoxin on the liver of domestic and laboratory animals: a review. Cancer Res., *29*:236–250, 1969.

Newbold, R. Cellular and molecular effects of developmental exposure to diethylstilbestrol: implications for other environmental estrogens. Environ. Health Perspect., *103*:83–87, 1995.

Newcomb, P. A., and Carbone, P. P. The health consequences of smoking. Cancer. Med. Clin. North Am., *76*:305–331, 1992.

Newcomb, P. A., Storer, B. E., Longnecker, M. P., Mittendorf, R., Greenberg, E. R., Clapp, R. W., Burke, K. P., Willett, W. C., and MacMahon, B. Lactation and a reduced risk of premenopausal breast cancer. N. Engl. J. Med., *330*:81–87, 1994.

Newmark, H. L., and Lipkin, M. Calcium, vitamin D, and colon cancer. Cancer Res., *52*:2067s–2070s, 1992.

Nomura, A. M. Y., and Kolonel, L. N. Prostate cancer: a current perspective. Am. J. Epidemiol., *13*:200–227, 1991.

Nomura, A. M. Y., Kolonel, L. N., Hankin, J. H., and Yoshizawa, C. N. Dietary factors in cancer of the lower urinary tract. Int. J. Cancer, *48*:199–205, 1991.

Norell, S. E., Ahlbom, A., Erwald, R., Jacobson, G., Lindberg-Navier, I., Olin, R., Törnberg, B., and Wiechel, K.-L. Diet and pancreatic cancer: a case-control study. Am. J. Epidemiol., *124*:894–902, 1986.

Nutter, R. L., Gridley, D. S., Kettering, J. D., Goude, A. G., and Slater, J. M. BALB/c mice fed milk or beef protein: differences in response to 1,2-dimethylhydrazine carcinogenesis. J. Natl. Cancer Inst., *71*:867–874, 1983.

Odeleye, O. E., Eskelson, C. D., Mufti, S. I., and Watson, R. R. Vitamin E protection against nitrosamine-induced esophageal tumor incidence in mice immunocompromised by retroviral infection. Carcinogenesis, *13*:1811–1816, 1992.

Ohba, S., Nishi, M., and Miyake, H. Eating habits and pancreas cancer. Int. J. Pancreatol., *20*:37–42, 1996.

Ohkawa, K., Abe, T., Hatano, T., Takizawa, N., Yamada, K., and Takada, K. The facilitated effect of retinol on rat hepatocarcinogenesis induced by 3′-methyl-4-dimethylaminoazobenzene. Carcinogenesis, *12*:2357–2360, 1991.

Ohnishi, K., Iida, S., Iwama, S., Goto, N., Nomura, F., Takashi, M., Mishima, A., Kono, K., Kimura, K., Musha, M., Kotota, K., and Okuda, K. The effect of chronic habitual alcohol intake on the development of liver cirrhosis and hepatocellular carcinoma: relation to hepatitis B surface antigen carriage. Cancer, *49*:672–677, 1982.

Ohno, Y., Yoshida, O., Oishi, K., Okada, K., Yamabe, H., and Schroeder, F. H. Dietary β-carotene and cancer of the prostate: a case-control study in Kyoto, Japan. Cancer Res., *48*:1331–1336, 1988.

Olsen, J. H., Boice Jr., J. D., Jensen, J. P. A., and Fraumeni, J. F. Jr. Cancer among epileptic patients exposed to anticonvulsant drugs. J. Natl. Cancer Inst., *81*:803–808, 1989.

Omenn, G. S., Goodman, G. E., Thornquist, M. D., Balmes, J., Cullen, M. R., Glass, A., Keogh, J. P., Meyskens, F. L., Jr., Valanis, B., Williams, J. H. Jr., Barnhart, S., Cherniack, M. G., Brodkin, C. A., and Hammar, S. Risk factors for lung cancer and for intervention effects in CARET, the beta-carotene and retinol efficacy trial. J. Natl. Cancer Inst., *88*:1550–1559, 1996.

Ong, D. E., and Chytil, F. Vitamin A and cancer. Vitam. Horm., *40*:105–144, 1983.

Oshimura, M., Hesterberg, T. W., Tsutsui, T., and Barrett, J. C. Correlation of asbestos-induced cytogenetic effects with cell transformation of Syrian hamster embryo cells in culture. Cancer Res., *44*:5017–5022, 1984.

Osler, M. Obesity and cancer. Danish Med. Bull., *34*:267–274, 1987.

Pain, J. A., Gimson, A. E. S., Williams, R., and Howard, E. R. Focal nodular hyperplasia of the liver: results of treatment and options in management. Gut, *32*:524–527, 1991.

Pamukcu, A. M., Ertürk, E., Yalciner, S., and Bryan, G. T. Histogenesis of urinary bladder cancer induced in rats by bracken fern. Invest. Urol., *14*:213–218, 1976.

Papenburg, R., Bounous, G., Fleiszer, D., and Gold, P. Dietary milk proteins inhibit the development of dimethylhydrazine-induced malignancy. Tumor Biol., *11*:129–136, 1990.

Parodi, P. W. Cows' milk fat components as potential anticarcinogenic agents. J. Nutr., *127*:1055–1060, 1997.

Pence, B. C., Dunn, D. M., Zhao, C., Landers, M., and Wargovich, M. J. Chemopreventive effects of calcium but not aspirin supplementation in cholic acid-promoted colon carcinogenesis: correlation with intermediate endpoints. Carcinogenesis, 16:757–765, 1995.

Perera, F. P. Molecular epidemiology: insights into cancer susceptibility, risk assessment, and prevention. J. Natl. Cancer Inst., 88:496–509, 1996.

Pershagen, G. The carcinogenicity of arsenic. Environ. Health Perspect., 40:93–100, 1981.

Persky, V., and van Horn, L. Epidemiology of soy and cancer: perspectives and directions. J. Nutr., 125:709S–712S, 1995.

Persson, I. Cancer risk in women receiving estrogen-progestin replacement therapy. Maturitas 23 (Suppl):S37–S45, 1996.

Peto, R., Lopez, A. D., Boreham, J., Thun, M., Heath, C. Jr., and Doll, R. Mortality from smoking worldwide. Br. Med. Bull., 52:12–21, 1996.

Pisani, R. J., Colby, T. V., and Williams, D. E. Malignant mesothelioma of the pleura. Mayo Clin. Proc., 63:1234–1244, 1988.

Pitot, H. C. The natural history of neoplastic development: the relation of experimental models to human cancer. Cancer, 49:1206–1211, 1982.

Pobel, D., Riboli, E., Cornée, J., Hémon, B., and Guyader, M. Nitrosamine, nitrate and nitrite in relation to gastric cancer: a case-control study in Marseille, France. Eur. J. Epidemiol., 11:67–73, 1995.

Pohjanvirta, R., and Tuomisto, J. Short-term toxicity of 2,3,7,8-tetrachlorodibenzo-p-dioxin in laboratory animals: effects, mechanisms, and animal models. Pharmacol. Rev., 46:483–549, 1994.

Pollard, M., Luckert, P. H., and Sporn, M. B. Prevention of primary prostate cancer in Lobund-Wistar rats by N-(4-Hydroxyphenyl)retinamide. Cancer Res., 51:3610–3611, 1991.

Potischman, N. Nutritional epidemiology of cervical neoplasia. J. Nutr., 123:424–429, 1993.

Potter, J. D. Colon cancer—do the nutritional epidemiology, the gut physiology and the molecular biology tell the same story? J. Nutr., 123:418–423, 1993.

Potter, J. D., and McMichael, A. J. Diet and cancer of the colon and rectum: a case-control study. J. Natl. Cancer Inst., 76:557–569, 1986.

Racine, R. R., and Schmid, B. P. DNA-damaging potential of diethylstilbestrol evaluated in the germ cell unscheduled DNA synthesis assay. Environ. Mutagen., 6:211–218, 1984.

Ramón, J. M., Serra, L., Cerdó, C., and Oromí, J. Dietary factors and gastric cancer risk. A case-control study in Spain. Cancer, 71:1731–1735, 1993.

Rao, A. R. N., Rao, A. R., Jannu, L. N., and Hussain, S. P. Chemoprevention of 7,12-dimethylbenz[a]anthracene-induced mammary carcinogenesis in rat by the combined actions of selenium, magnesium, ascorbic acid and retinyl acetate. Jpn. J. Cancer Res., 81:1239–1246, 1990.

Rao, A. V., Janezic, S. A., Friday, D., and Kendall, C. W. Dietary cholesterol enhances the induction and development of colonic preneoplastic lesions in C57BL/6J and BALB/cJ mice treated with azoxymethane. Cancer Lett., 63:249–257, 1992.

Rehn, L., Blasengeschwulste bei Fuchsin-Arbeitern. Arch. Klin. Chir., 50:600, 1895.

Reichart, P. A. Oral cancer and precancer related to betel and miang chewing in Thailand: a review. J. Oral Pathol. Med., 24:241–243, 1995.

Reimer, R. R. Risk of a second malignancy related to the use of cytotoxic chemotherapy. CA 32:286–292, 1982.

Riihimäki, V., Asp, S., and Hernberg, S. Mortality of 2,4-dichlorophenoxyacetic acid and 2,4,5-trichlorophenoxyacetic acid herbicide applicators in Finland. Scand. J. Work. Environ. Health, 8:37–42, 1982.

Risch, H. A., Burch, J. D., Miller, A. B., Hill, G. B., Steele, R., and Howe, G. R. Dietary factors and the incidence of cancer of the urinary bladder. Am. J. Epidemiol., 127:1179–1191, 1988.

Robbana-Barnat, S., Rabache, M., Rialland, E., and Fradin, J. Heterocyclic amines: occurrence and prevention in cooked food. Environ. Health Perspect., 104:280–288, 1996.

Roebuck, B. D. Dietary fat and the development of pancreatic cancer. Lipids, 27:804–806, 1992.

Roebuck, B. D., Baumgartner, K. J., Thron, C. D., and Longnecker, D. S. Inhibition by retinoids of the growth of azaserine-induced foci in the rat pancreas. J. Natl. Cancer Inst., 73:233–236, 1984.

Rogan, W. J., and Brown, S. M. Some fundamental aspects of epidemiology. A guide for laboratory scientists. Fed. Proc., *38*:1875–1879, 1979.

Roggli, V. L. Malignant mesothelioma and duration of asbestos exposure: correlation with tissue mineral fibre content. Ann. Occup. Hyg., *39*:363–374, 1995.

Rookus, M. A., van Leeuwen, F. E., for the Netherlands Oral Contraceptives and Breast Cancer Study Group. Oral contraceptives and risk of breast cancer in women aged 20–54 years. Lancet, *344*:844–851, 1994.

Rose, D. P. Dietary fiber and breast cancer. Nutr. Cancer, *13*:1–8, 1990.

Rose, D. P. Effects of dietary fatty acids on breast and prostate cancers: evidence from in vitro experiments and animal studies. Am. J. Clin. Nutr., *66*:1513S–1522S, 1997.

Rose, D. P., Boyar, A. P., and Wynder, E. L. International comparisons of mortality rates for cancer of the breast, ovary, prostate, and colon, and per capita food consumption. Cancer, *58*:2363–2371, 1986.

Rose, P. G. Endometrial carcinoma. N. Engl. J. Med., *335*:640–649, 1996.

Ross, R., Yuan, J.-M., Yu, M., Wogan, G. N., Qian, G.-S., Tu, J.-T., Groopman, J. D., Gao, Y.-T., and Henderson, B. E. Urinary aflatoxin biomarkers and risk of hepatocellular carcinoma. Lancet, *339*:943–946, 1992.

Roy, D., Floyd, R. A., and Liehr, J. G. Elevated 8-hydroxydeoxyguanosine levels in DNA of diethylstilbestrol-treated Syrian hamsters: covalent DNA damage by free radicals generated by redox cycling of diethylstilbesterol. Cancer Res., *51*:3882–3885, 1991.

Russo, J., and Russo, I. H. Experimentally induced mammary tumors in rats. Breast Cancer Res. Treat., *39*:7–20, 1996.

Russo, J., Rivera, R., and Russo, I. H. Influence of age and parity on the development of the human breast. Breast Cancer Res. Treat., *23*:211–218, 1992.

Safe, S. H. Interactions between hormones and chemicals in breast cancer. Annu. Rev. Pharmacol. Toxicol., *38*:121–158, 1998.

Sammon, A. M., and Alderson, D. Diet, reflux and the development of squamous cell carcinoma of the oesophagus in Africa. Br. J. Surg., *85*:891–896, 1998.

Sargent, L. M., Dragan, Y. P., Sattler, C., Bahnub, N., Sattler, G., Martin, P., Cisneros, A., Mann, J., Thorgeirsson, S., Jordan, V. C., and Pitot, H. C. Induction of hepatic aneuploidy *in vivo* by tamoxifen, toremifene and idoxifene in female Sprague-Dawley rats. Carcinogenesis, *17*:1051–1056, 1996.

Sarkar, A., Mukherjee, B., and Chatterjee, M. Inhibition of 3′-methyl-4-dimethylaminoazobenzene-induced hepatocarcinogenesis in rat by dietary β-carotene: changes in hepatic anti-oxidant defense enzyme levels. Int. J. Cancer, *61*:799–805, 1995.

Schatzkin, A., and Longnecker, M. P. Alcohol and breast cancer. Where are we now and where do we go from here? Cancer, *74*:1101–1110, 1994.

Schatzkin, A., Greenwald, P., Byar, D. P., and Clifford, C. K. The dietary fat-breast cancer hypothesis is alive. J.A.M.A., *261*:3284–3287, 1989.

Schiffman, M. H., and Brinton, L. A. The epidemiology of cervical carcinogenesis. Cancer, *76*:1888–1901, 1995.

Schiffman, M. H., Pickle, L. W., Fontham, E., Zahm, S. H., Falk, R., Mele, J., Correa, P., and Fraumeni, J. F. Jr. Case-control study of diet and mesothelioma in Louisiana. Cancer Res., *48*:2911–2915, 1988.

Schlesselman, J. J. Oral contraceptives and breast cancer. Am. J. Obstet. Gynecol., *163*:1379–1386, 1990.

Schnatter, A. R., Armstrong, T. W., Thompson, L. S., Nicolich, M. J., Katz, A. M., Huebner, W. W., and Pearlman, E. D. The relationship between low-level benzene exposure and leukemia in Canadian petroleum distribution workers. Environ. Health Perspect., *104*:1375–1379, 1996.

Schottenfeld, D. Epidemiology of endometrial neoplasia. J. Cell. Biochem., *23*:151–159, 1995.

Scoville, B., and White, B. G. Carcinogenicity of hydantoins: data, hypotheses, and public reviews. Psychopharmacol. Bull., *17*:195–197, 1981.

Selikoff, I. Asbestos and Disease. New York: Academic Press, 1978.

Selikoff, I., Hammond, C., and Churg, J. Asbestos exposure, smoking and neoplasia. J.A.M.A., *204*:104–110, 1968.

Shamsuddin, A. M., Ullah, A., Baten, A., and Hale, E. Stability of fecapentaene-12 and its carcinogenicity in F-344 rats. Carcinogenesis, *12*:601–607, 1991.

Sharan, R. N. Association of betel nut with carcinogenesis. Cancer J., *9*:13–19, 1996.

Shixin, L., Mingxin, L., Chuan, J., Mingyao, W., Yinglin, W., and Liang, H. A new N-nitroso compound, N-3-methylbutyl-N-1-methylacetonylnitrosamine, in corn-bread inoculated with fungi. Scientia Sinica, *22*:601, 1979.

Silverman, D. T., Swanson, C. A., Gridley, G., Wacholder, S., Greenberg, R. S., Brown, L. M., Hayes, R. B., Swanson, G. M., Schoenberg, J. B., Pottern, L. M., Schwartz, A. G., Fraumeni, J. F., Jr., and Hoover, R. N. Dietary and nutritional factors and pancreatic cancer: a case-control study based on direct interviews. J. Natl. Cancer Inst., *90*:1710–1719, 1998.

Singer, G. M., Chuan, J., Roman, J., Min-Hsin, L., and Lijinsky, W. Nitrosamines and nitrosamine precursors in foods from Linxian, China, a high incidence area for esophageal cancer. Carcinogenesis, *7*:733–736, 1986.

Slawin, K., Kadmon, D., Park, S. H., Scardino, P. T., Anzano, M., Sporn, M. B., and Thompson, T. C. Dietary fenretinide, a synthetic retinoid, decreases the tumor incidence and the tumor mass of *ras+myc*–induced carcinomas in the mouse prostate reconstitution model system. Cancer Res., *53*:4461–4465, 1993.

Smith, M. T. Overview of benzene-induced aplastic anaemia. Eur. J. Haematol., *57*:107–110, 1996.

Smith, M. T. The mechanism of benzene-induced leukemia: a hypothesis and speculations on the causes of leukemia. Environ. Health Perspect., *104*:1219–1225, 1996.

Smith, M. T., Zhang, L., Wang, Y., Hayes, R. B., Li, G., Wiemels, J., Dosemeci, M., Titenko-Holland, N., Xi, L., Kolachana, P., Yin, S., and Rothman, N. Increased translocations and aneusomy in chromosomes 8 and 21 among workers exposed to benzene. Cancer Res., *58*:2176–2181, 1998.

Smith-Warner, S. A., Spiegelman, D., Yaun, S.-S., van den Brandt, P. A., Folsom, A. R., Goldbohm, A., Graham, S., Holmberg,, L., Howe, G. R., Marshall, J. R., Miller, A. B., Potter, J. D., Speizer, F. E., Willett, W. C., Wolk, A., and Hunter, D. J. Alcohol and breast cancer in women. A pooled analysis of cohort studies. J.A.M.A., *279*:535–540, 1998.

Smoking, tobacco and cancer program: 1985–1989 status report. NIH publication no. 90-3107. Bethesda, MD: U.S. Department of Health and Human Services, 1990.

Snowden, D. A., Phillips, R. L., and Choi, W. Diet, obesity, and risk of fatal prostate cancer. Am. J. Epidemiol., *120*:244–250, 1984.

Snyder, R., and Kalf, G. F. A perspective on benzene leukemogenesis. Crit. Rev. Toxicol., *24*:177–209, 1994.

Sørensen, I. K., Kristiansen, E., Mortensen, A., Nicolaisen, G. M., Wijnands, J. A. H., van Kranen, H. J., and van Kreijl, C. F. The effect of soy isoflavones on the development of intestinal neoplasia in *Apc^{Min}* mouse. Cancer Lett., *130*:217–225, 1998.

Spirtas, R., Heineman, E. F., Bernstein, L., Beebe, G. W., Keehn, R. J., Stark, A., Harlow, B. L., and Benichou, J. Malignant mesothelioma: attributable risk of asbestos exposure. Occup. Environ. Med., *51*:804–811, 1994.

Sporn, M. B., Squire, R. A., Brown, C. C., Smith, J. M., Wenk, M. L., and Springer, S. 13-*cis*-retinoic acid: inhibition of bladder carcinogenesis in the rat. Science, *195*:487–489, 1977.

Squier, C. A. The nature of smokeless tobacco and patterns of use. CA, *38*:226–229, 1988.

Stanton, M. F., Layard, M., Tegeris, A., Miller, E., May, M., and Kent, E. Carcinogenicity of fibrous glass: pleural response in the rat in relation to fiber dimension. J. Natl. Cancer Inst., *58*:587–603, 1977.

Statland, B. E. Nutrition and cancer. Clin. Chem., *38*:1587–1594, 1992.

Stavric, B. Mutagenic flood flavonoids. Fed. Proc., *43*:2454–2458, 1984.

Steinberg, K. K., Thacker, S. B., Smith, S. J., Stroup, D. F., Zack, M. M., Flanders, W. D., and Berkelman, R. L. A meta-analysis of the effect of estrogen replacement therapy on the risk of breast cancer. J.A.M.A., *265*:1985–1990, 1991.

Steinbrecher, U. P., Lisbona, R., Huang, S. N., and Mishkin, S. Complete regression of hepatocellular adenoma after withdrawal of oral contraceptives. Dig. Dis. Sci., *26*:1045–1050, 1981.

Stern, R. S., and Laird, N. The carcinogenic risk of treatments for severe psoriasis. Cancer, *73*:2759–2764, 1994.

Stern, R. S., Nichols, K. T., and Väkevä, L. H. Malignant melanoma in patients treated for psoriasis with methoxsalen (psoralen) and ultraviolet A radiation (PUVA). N. Engl. J. Med., *336*:1041–1045, 1997.

Stewart, B. W., and Sarfaty, G. A. Environmental chemical carcinogenesis. Med. J. Aust., *1*:92–95, 1978.

Stöhrer, G. Arsenic: opportunity for risk assessment. Arch. Toxicol., *65*:525–531, 1991.

Sugimura, T., Nagao, M., and Wakabayashi, K. Carcinogenicity of food mutagens. Environ. Health Perspect., *104*:429–433, 1996.

Swerdlow, A. J., Douglas, A. J., Vaughan Hudson, G., Vaughan Hudson, B., Bennett, M. H., and MacLennan, K. A. Risk of second primary cancers after Hodgkin's disease by type of treatment: analysis of 2846 patients in the British National Lymphoma Investigation. Br. Med. J., *304*:1137–1143, 1992.

Takahashi, M., Hasegawa, T., Furukawa, F., Okamiya, H., Shinoda, K., Imaida, K., Toyoda, K., and Hayashi, Y. Enhanced lipid peroxidation in rat gastric mucosa caused by NaCl. Carcinogenesis, *12*:2201–2204, 1991.

Takahashi, M., Nishikawa, A., Furukawa, F., Enami, T., Hasegawa, T., and Hayashi, Y. Dose-dependent promoting effects of sodium chloride (NaCl) on rat glandular stomach carcinogenesis initiated with *N*-methyl-*N'*-nitro-*N*-nitrosoguanidine. Carcinogenesis, *15*:1429–1432, 1994.

Talamini, R., Franceschi, S., La Vecchia, C., Serraino, D., Barra, S., and Negri, E. Diet and prostatic cancer: a case-control study in northern Italy. Nutr. Cancer, *18*:277–286, 1992.

Tallman, M. S., Andersen, J. W., Schiffer, C. A., Appelbaum, F. R., Feusner, J. H., Ogden, A., Shepherd, L., Willman, C., Bloomfield, C. D., Rowe, J. M., and Wiernik, P. H. All-*trans*-retinoic acid in acute promyelocytic leukemia. N. Engl. J. Med., *337*:1021–1028, 1997.

Tannenbaum, S. R., Fett, D., Young, V. R., Land, P. D., and Bruce, W. R. Nitrite and nitrate are formed by endogenous synthesis in the human intestine. Science, *200*:1487–1489, 1978.

Tao, L.-C. Are oral contraceptive-associated liver cell adenomas premalignant? Acta Cytol., *36*:338–344, 1992.

Thiringer, G., and Järvholm, B. Smoking and lung cancer. Eur. J. Respir. Dis. Suppl. *107*, *61*:123–124, 1980.

Thomas, L. B., Popper, H., Berk, P. D., Selikoff, I., and Falk, H. Vinyl-chloride-induced liver disease. From idiopathic portal hypertension (Banti's syndrome) to angiosarcomas. N. Engl. J. Med., *292*:17–22, 1975.

Titus-Ernstoff, L., Longnecker, M. P., Newcomb, P. A., Dain, B., Greenberg, E. R., Mittendorf, R., Stampfer, M., and Willett, W. Menstrual factors in relation to breast cancer risk. Cancer Epidemiol. Biomark. Prev., *7*:783–789, 1998.

Tomatis, L., Huff, J., Hertz-Picciotto, I., Sandler, D. P., Bucher, J., Boffetta, P., Axelson, O., Blair, A., Taylor, J., Stayner, L., and Barrett, J. C. Avoided and avoidable risks of cancer. Carcinogenesis, *18*:97–105, 1997.

Tominaga, S., and Kuroishi, T. Biliary tract cancer. Cancer Surv., *19/20*:125–137, 1994.

Toniolo, P., Riboli, E., Shore, R. E., and Pasternack, B. S. Consumption of meat, animal products, protein, and fat and risk of breast cancer: a prospective cohort study in New York. Epidemiology, *5*:391–397, 1994.

Tsuda, T., Babazono, A., Yamamoto, E., Kurumatani, N., Mino, Y., Ogawa, T., Kishi, Y., and Aoyama, H. Ingested arsenic and internal cancer: a historical cohort study followed for 33 years. Am. J. Epidemiol., *141*:198–209, 1995.

Tsutsui, T., Suzuki, N., Maizumi, H., McLachlan, J. A., and Barrett, J. C. Alteration in diethylstilbestrol-induced mutagenicity and cell transformation by exogenous metabolic activation. Carcinogenesis, *7*:1415–1418, 1986.

Tuyns, A. J., and Griciute, L. L. Carcinogenic substances in alcoholic beverages. *In*: W. Davis, K. R. Harrap, and G. Stathopoulos (Eds.), Human Cancer: Its Characterization and Treatment, Advances in Tumour Prevention, Detection, and Characterization, Vol., 5 (International Congress Series, No. 484), pp. 130–136. Amsterdam: Excerpta Medica, 1980.

Tuyns, A. J., Kaaks, R., Haelterman, M., and Riboli, E. Diet and gastric cancer. A case-control study in Belgium. Int. J. Cancer, *51*:1–6, 1992.

Tuyns, A. J., Péquignot, G., and Abbatucci, J. S. Oesophageal cancer and alcohol consumption: importance of type of beverage. Int. J. Cancer, *23*:443–447, 1979.

Tzonou, A., Lipworth, L., Kalandidi, A., Trichopoulou, A., Gamatsi, I., Hsieh, C.-C., Notara, V., and Trichopoulos, D. Dietary factors and the risk of endometrial cancer: a case-control study in Greece. Br. J. Cancer, *73*:1284–1290, 1996.

Ura, H., Denda, A., Yokose, Y., Tsutsumi, M., and Konishi, Y. Effect of vitamin E on the induction and evolution of enzyme-altered foci in the liver of rats treated with diethylnitrosamine. Carcinogenesis, *8*:1595–1600, 1987.

Ursin, G., Bjelke, E., Heuch, I., and Vollset, S. E. Milk consumption and cancer incidence: a Norwegian prospective study. Br. J. Cancer, *61*:454–459, 1990.

Vainio, H., and Sorsa, M. Chromosome aberrations and their relevance to metal carcinogenesis. Environ. Health Perspect., *40*:173–180, 1981.

Vainio, H., Coleman, M., and Wilbourn, J. Carcinogenicity evaluations and ongoing studies: the IARC databases. Environ. Health Perspect., *96*:5–9, 1991.

van der Burgh, A., Dees, J., Hop, W. C. J., and van Blankenstein, M. Oesophageal cancer is an uncommon cause of death in patients with Barrett's oesophagus. Gut, *39*:5–8, 1996.

van Kaick, G., Lorenz, D., Muth, H., and Kaul, A. Malignancies in German thorotrast patients and estimated tissue dose. Health Physics, *35*:127–136, 1978.

van Rensburg, S. J. Epidemiologic and dietary evidence for a specific nutritional predisposition to esophageal cancer. J. Natl. Cancer Inst., *67*:243–251, 1981.

VanEenwyk, J., Davis, F. G., and Bowen, P. E. Dietary and serum carotenoids and cervical intraepithelial neoplasia. Int. J. Cancer, *48*:34–38, 1991.

Vatten, L. J., Solvoll, K., and Løken, E. B. Frequency of meat and fish intake and risk of breast cancer in a prospective study of 14,500 Norwegian women. Int. J. Cancer, *46*:12–15, 1990.

Velentgas, P., and Daling, J. R. Risk factors for breast cancer in younger women. Monogr. Natl. Cancer Inst., *16*:15–22, 1994.

Verhagen, H., de Vries, A., Nijhoff, W. A., Schouten, A., van Poppel, G., Peters, W. H. M., and van den Berg, H. Effect of Brussels sprouts on oxidative DNA-damage in man. Cancer Lett., *114*:127–130, 1997.

Vlajinac, H. D., Marinkoviæ, J. M., Iliæ, M. D., and Kocev, N. I. Diet and prostate cancer: a case-control study. Eur. J. Cancer, *33*:101–107, 1997.

Vuolo, L. L., and Schuessler, G. J. Review: putative mutagens and carcinogens in foods. VI. Protein pyrolysate products. Environ. Mutagen., *7*:577–598, 1985.

Waalkes, M. P., and Rehm, S. Cadmium and prostate cancer. J. Toxicol. Environ. Health, *43*:251–269, 1994.

Waalkes, M. P., Coogan, T. P., and Barter, R. A. Toxicological principles of metal carcinogenesis with special emphasis on cadmium. Crit. Rev. Toxicol., *22*:175–201, 1992.

Wagner, J. C., and Berry, G. Mesotheliomas in rats following inoculation with asbestos. Br. J. Cancer, *23*:567, 1969.

Wahrendorf, J., Muñoz, N., Jian-Bang, L., Thurnham, D. I., Crespi, M., and Bosch, F. X. Blood, retinol and zinc riboflavin status in relation to precancerous lesions of the esophagus: findings from a vitamin intervention trial in the People's Republic of China. Cancer Res., *48*:2280–2283, 1988.

Wallace, L. Environmental exposure to benzene: an update. Environ. Health Perspect., *104*:1129–1136, 1996.

Walter, S.D., Marrett, L. D., Shannon, H. S., From, L., and Hertzman, C. The association of cutaneous malignant melanoma and fluorescent light exposure. Am. J. Epidemiol., *135*:749–762, 1992.

Ward, E. M., Sabbioni, G., DeBord, D. G., Teass, A. W., Brown, K. K., Talaska, G. G., Roberts, D. R., Ruder, A. M., and Streicher, R. P. Monitoring of aromatic amine exposures in workers at a chemical plant with a known bladder cancer excess. J. Natl. Cancer Inst., *88*:1046–1052, 1996.

Ward, J. M., Anjo, T., Ohannesian, L., Keefer, L. K., Devor, D. E., Donovan, P. J., Smith, G. T., Henneman, J. R., Streeter, A. J., Konishi, N., Rehm, S., Reist, E. J., Bradford, W. W. III, and Rice, J. M. Inactivity of fecapentaene-12 as a rodent carcinogen or tumor initiator. Cancer Lett., *42*:49–59, 1988.

Wasan, H. S., Novelli, M., Bee, J., and Bodmer, W. F. Dietary fat influences on polyp phenotype in multiple intestinal neoplasia mice. Proc. Natl. Acad. Sci. U.S.A., *94*:3308–3313, 1997.

Webster, L. A., Weiss, N. S., and The Cancer and Steroid Hormone Study Group. Alcoholic beverage consumption and the risk of endometrial cancer. Int. J. Epidemiol., *18*:786–790, 1989.

Weinberg, E. D. Association of iron with colorectal cancer. Biometals, *7*:211–216, 1994.

Weisburger, J. H., Jones, R. C., Wang, C.-X., Backlund, J.-Y. C., Williams, G. M., Kingston, D. G. I., Van Tassell, R. L., Keyes, R. F., Wilkins, T. D., de Wit, P. P., van der Steeg, M., and van der Gen, A. Carcinogenicity tests of fecapentaene-12 in mice and rats. Cancer Lett., *49*:89–98, 1990.

Weisburger, J. H., Reddy, B. S., Barnes, W. S., and Wynder, E. L. Bile acids, but not neutral sterols, are tumor promoters in the colon in man and in rodents. Environ. Health Perspect., *50*:101–107, 1983.

Weiss, N., Lyon, J., Krishnamurthy, S., et al. Noncontraceptive estrogen use and the occurrence of ovarian cancer. J. Natl. Cancer Inst., *68*:95, 1982.

Westerdahl, J., Olsson, H., Måsbäck, A., Ingvar, C., Jonsson, N., Brandt, L., Jönsson, P.-E., and Möller, T. Use of sunbeds or sunlamps and malignant melanoma in southern Sweden. Am. J. Epidemiol., *140*:691–699, 1994.

Whittemore, A. S., Kolonel, L. N., Wu, A. H., John, E. M., Gallagher, R. P., Howe, G. R., Burch, J. D., Hankin, J., Dreon, D. M., West, D. W., Teh, C.-Z., and Paffenbarger, R. S. Jr. Prostate cancer in relation to diet, physical activity, and body size in blacks, whites, and Asians in the United States and Canada. J. Natl. Cancer Inst., *87*:652–661, 1995.

Wilding, G. Endocrine control of prostate cancer. Cancer Surv., *23*:43–62, 1995.

Willett, W. C. Nutritional Epidemiology. London: University Press, 1990.

Willett, W. C. Fat, energy and breast cancer. J. Nutr., *127*:921S–923S, 1997.

Willett, W. C., Stampfer, M. J., Colditz, G. A., Rosner, B. A., and Speizer, F. E. Relation of meat, fat, and fiber intake to the risk of colon cancer in a prospective study among women. N. Engl. J. Med., *323*:1664–1672, 1990.

Willett, W. C., Stampfer, M. J., Colditz, G. A., Rosner, B. A., Hennekens, C. H., and Speizer, F. E. Dietary fat and the risk of breast cancer. N. Engl. J. Med., *316*:22–28, 1987.

Winn, D. M., Blot, W. J., Shy, C. M., Pickle, L. W., Toledo, A., and Fraumeni, J. F. Jr. Snuff dipping and oral cancer among women in the southern United States. N. Engl. J. Med., *304*:745–749, 1981.

Wolk, A., Gridley, G., Niwa, S., Lindblad, P., McCredie, M., Mellemgaard, A., Mandel, J. S., Wahrendorf, J., McLaughlin, J. K., and Adami, H.-O. International renal cell cancer study. VII. Role of diet. Int. J. Cancer, *65*:67–73, 1996.

Wong, O. Risk of acute myeloid leukaemia and multiple myeloma in workers exposed to benzene. Occup. Environ. Med., *52*:380–384, 1995.

Woutersen, R. A., and van Garderen-Hoetmer, A. Inhibition of dietary fat promoted development of (pre)neoplastic lesions in exocrine pancreas of rats and hamsters by supplemental selenium and β-carotene. Cancer Lett., *42*:79–85, 1988.

Wright, W. C. Diseases of Workers. (Translation of De Morbis Artificum, 1713, by B. Ramazzini.) The History of Medicine Series. New York: New York Academy of Medicine, 1964.

Wynder, E. L., Cohen, L. A., Muscat, J. E., Winters, B., Dwyer, J. T., and Blackburn, G. Breast cancer: weighing the evidence for a promoting role of dietary fat. J. Natl. Cancer Inst., *89*:766–775, 1997.

Wynder, E. L., Rose, D. P., and Cohen, L. A. Nutrition and prostate cancer: a proposal for dietary intervention. Nutr. Cancer, *22*:1–10, 1994.

Yamamoto, A., Hisanaga, A., and Ishinishi, N. Tumorigenicity of inorganic arsenic compounds following intratracheal instillations to the lungs of hamsters. Int. J. Cancer, *40*:220–223, 1987.

Yamamoto, S., Wanibuchi, H., Hori, T.-a., Yano, Y., Matsui-Yuasa, I., Otani, S., Chen, H., Yoshida, K., Kuroda, K., Endo, G., and Fukushima, S. Possible carcinogenic potential of dimethylarsinic acid as assessed in rat in vivo models: a review. Mutat. Res., *386*:353–361, 1997.

Yamanaka, K., Ohtsubo, K., Hasegawa, A., Hayashi, H., Ohji, H., Kanisawa, M., and Okada, S. Exposure to dimethylarsinic acid, a main metabolite of inorganic arsenics, strongly promotes tumorigenesis initiated by 4-nitroquinoline 1-oxide in the lungs of mice. Carcinogenesis, *17*:767–770, 1996.

Yong, L.-C., Brown, C. C., Schatzkin, A., Dresser, C. M., Slesinski, M. J., Cox, C. S., and Taylor, P. R. Intake of vitamins E, C, and A and risk of lung cancer. Am. J. Epidemiol., *146*:231–243, 1997.

Yoshida, A., Harada, T., and Maita, K. Tumor induction by concurrent oral administration of ethylenethiourea and sodium nitrite in mice. Toxicol. Pathol., *21*:303–310, 1993.

You, W.-C., Blot, W. J., Chang, Y.-S., Ershow, A. G., Yang, Z.-T., An, Q., Henderson, B., Xu, G.-W., Fraumeni, J. F. Jr., and Wang, T.-G. Diet and high risk of stomach cancer in Shandong, China. Cancer Res., *48*:3518–3523, 1988.

Yu, M. C., Ho, J. H. C., Lai, S.-H., and Henderson, B. E. Cantonese-style salted fish as a cause of nasopharyngeal carcinoma: report of a case-control study in Hong Kong. Cancer Res., *46*:956–961, 1986.

Yu, M.-W., Hsieh, H.-H., Pan, W.-H., Yang, C.-S., and Chen, C.-J. Vegetable consumption, serum retinol level, and risk of hepatocellular carcinoma. Cancer Res., *55*:1301–1305, 1995.

Zahm, S. H., and Blair, A. Pesticides and non-Hodgkin's lymphoma. Cancer Res., *52*:5485s–5488s, 1992.

Zatonski, W. A., Lowenfels, A. B., Boyle, P., Maisonneuve, P., Bueno de Mesquita, H. B., Ghadirian, P., Jain, M., Przewozniak, K., Baghurst, P., Moerman, C. J., Simard, A., Howe, G. R., McMichael, A. J., Hsieh, C. C., and Walker, A. M. Epidemiologic aspects of gallbladder cancer: a case-control study of the SEARCH Program of the International Agency for Research on Cancer. J. Natl. Cancer Inst., *89*:1132–1138, 1997.

Zatonski, W., Przewozniak, K., Howe, G. R., Maisonneuve, P., Walker, A. M., and Boyle, P. Nutritional factors and pancreatic cancer: a case-control study from South-West Poland. Int. J. Cancer, *48*:390–394, 1991.

Zhao, L. P., Kushi, L. H ., Klein, R. D., and Prentice, R. L. Quantitative review of studies of dietary fat and rat colon carcinoma. Nutr. Cancer, *15*:169–177, 1991.

Zheng, W., Gustafson, D. R., Sinha, R., Cerhan, J. R., Moore, D., Hong, C.-P., Anderson, K. E., Kushi, L. H., Sellers, T. A., and Folsom, A. R. Well-done meat intake and the risk of breast cancer. J. Natl. Cancer Inst., *90*:1724–1729, 1998.

Zheng, W., Kushi, L. H., Potter, J. D., Sellers, T. A., Doyle, T. J., Bostick, R. M., and Folsom, A. R. Dietary intake of energy and animal foods and endometrial cancer incidence. The Iowa Women's Health Study. Am. J. Epidemiol., *142*:388–394, 1995a.

Zheng, W., Sellers, T. A., Doyle, T. J., Kushi, L. H., Potter, J. D., and Folsom, A. R. Retinol, antioxidant vitamins, and cancers of the upper digestive tract in a prospective cohort study of postmenopausal women. Am. J. Epidemiol., *142*:9565–960, 1995b.

Zhu, K., Stanford, J. L., Daling, J. R., McKnight, B., Stergachis, A., Brawer, M. K., and Weiss, N. S. Vasectomy and prostate cancer: a case-control study in a health maintenance organization. Am. J. Epidemiol., *144*:717–722, 1996.

Zile, M. H., Cullum, M. E., Roltsch, I. A., DeHoog, J. V., and Welsch, C. W. Effect of moderate vitamin A supplementation and lack of dietary vitamin A on the development of mammary tumors in female rats treated with low carcinogenic dose levels of 7,12-dimethylbenz(*a*)anthracene. Cancer Res., *46*:3495–3503, 1986.

Zou, X. N., Lu, S. H., and Liu, B. Volatile N-nitrosamines and their precursors in Chinese salted fish—a possible etological factor for NPC in China. Int. J. Cancer, *59*:155–158, 1994.

12

Environmental Factors in the Etiology of Human Cancer—Physical and Biological Agents

At our present state of knowledge, evidence argues that the majority of human neoplasms result from the chemical induction of neoplasia; however, it is clear that radiation, both ionizing and ultraviolet, as well as infectious agents also contribute as primary factors in the development of a significant proportion of human neoplasia. Just as with chemical carcinogenesis, in the human the basis of our knowledge of the physical and infectious causation of human cancer derives from both epidemiological and experimental findings. However, unlike many chemical carcinogens whose carcinogenic activity in the human is based either entirely on experimental findings [e.g., 2-acetylaminofluorene, dimethylnitrosamine, and ethyleneimine (Chapter 13)] or solely on epidemiological findings [e.g., organic arsenicals and ethanol (Chapter 11)], evidence for the ultraviolet and ionizing radiation–induced human neoplasia as well as a number of viruses as causative of human neoplasia is based solidly on both experimental and epidemiological evidence. This chapter looks at the epidemiological evidence of physical and infectious carcinogenesis in the human in the light of basic experimental findings, most of which have already been considered earlier in the text.

PHYSICAL CARCINOGENESIS IN HUMANS

It is likely that radiogenic neoplasms have occurred in humans sporadically since the dawn of civilization; but only in the 20th century, with the advent of our greater knowledge of the components of the electromagnetic spectrum and the existence of ionizing and ultraviolet radiation, have the cancer-inducing properties of these latter two agents been recognized. Although experiments in animals have shown us a great deal about the basic aspects of radiogenic neoplasia, epidemiological studies in humans have advanced our knowledge of radiogenic neoplasms to an almost equal or greater extent. The most unfortunate and at the same time the greatest single incidence of radiation-induced cancers in humans resulted from the atomic bomb explosions at Hiroshima and Nagasaki.

Ionizing Radiation Exposure

Today humans are exposed daily to both ionizing and ultraviolet radiation. Fortunately, when the sources of such radiation are recognized, exposure may often be voluntarily controlled to a much greater degree than was seen in the 1800s and early 1900s, during the days of Madame Curie,

Roentgen, radium dial painters, and the shoe-store x-ray machines. Figure 12.1 lists the common sources of exposure to ionizing radiation and the average dose per individual in millisieverts (Chapter 3) per year in this decade. As can be noted from the figure, natural sources of radiation, especially radon, a radioactive elemental gas that permeates the earth's surface, contribute to the majority of exposure of humans to ionizing radiation. Cosmic radiation is a much smaller but significant source, while medical irradiation, both therapeutic and diagnostic, is second only to radon in its contribution to this background radiation. Sources of medical therapeutic irradiation involve relatively high doses, but these are applied to only a small segment of the total population. On the other hand, diagnostic radiation is used quite extensively in all age groups in most western and many other countries but involves much lower doses of ionizing radiation. A much smaller source of ionizing radiation also applicable to specific portions of the population (much less than 1% of total human exposure) is that of occupational exposure from nuclear power plants. That 3% of total radiation exposures come from consumer products is somewhat misleading (Hoel, 1995). The main sources included in this category are building materials, water supplies, and agricultural products, which are not generally thought of as consumer products. Perhaps the best known consumer product involving radiation is cigarette smoke. Polonium 210, a radioactive element, is found in tobacco as a result of airborne radon decay deposited on the tobacco plants' leaves. However, the differences in estimates of radiation doses resulting from cigarette smoke are so disparate that the contribution of cigarette smoke to radiation carcinogenesis is quite uncertain (cf. Hoel, 1995).

Table 12.1 shows a ranking of those cancers associated with the carcinogenic effects of ionizing radiation (Boice et al., 1996). For those cancers most frequently associated with radiation, one may also find other factors involved, along with the overall risk, as noted in Table 12.2. While leukemia is frequently the earliest observed radiogenic cancer after exposure to ionizing radiation of the human, such neoplasms may be considered of relatively less importance, since the radiation effect dies out in a relatively short time. However, solid tumors induced by radiation develop much later, and the increased cancer risk evidently persists for most if not all of the lifetime of exposed individuals (Radford, 1983).

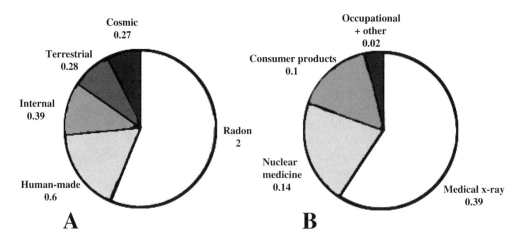

Figure 12.1 Average annual radiation exposure: A. effective total dose equivalent in millisieverts (mSr); B. breakout of human-made exposures in mSv. (Modified from Hoel, 1995, with permission of the author and publisher.)

Table 12.1   Risk Estimates of Various Human Cancers in Relation to Exposures to Ionizing Radiation

Type of Cancer	Range of Risk Estimates		Comment
	RR at 1 Gy	Excess Risk $\times 10^4$ PY-Gy	
Cancers Frequently Associated with Radiation, with Authoritative Risk Estimates			
Leukemia	1.3–6.2	0.5–2.9	Especially myeloid leukemia
Thyroid	1.6–31	3.0–13	Low mortality
Female breast	1.1–2.7	3.5–18	Little risk if exposed after 40 years of age
Cancers Occasionally Associated with Radiation, with Valid Risk Estimates			
Lung	1.0–1.6	0.0–1.7	Interaction with smoking uncertain
Stomach	1.0–1.7	0.0–4.7	Major A-bomb effect
Colon	1.0–1.9	0.0–3.0	Not seen after cervical cancer
Esophagus	1.3–1.6	0.3–0.5	
Bladder	1.1–2.3	0.1–1.0	Both low and high dose effect
Ovary	1.0–2.3	0.1–0.7	
Myeloma	1.0–3.3	0.0–0.3	Uncertainty which association causal
Cancers Rarely Associated with Radiation, with Uncertain Risk Estimates[a]			
Brain, meninges, and nervous system	1.0–5.9	0.0–1.1	Mainly after childhood exposures
Kidney	1.0–1.7	0.0–1.1	
Liver	1.0–1.5	0.0–1.6	Major Thorotrast effect (angiosarcoma and cholangiocarcinoma)
Salivary glands	1.1–1.7	0.1–0.2	Little evidence
Non-Hodgkin lymphoma	[b]	[b]	Little evidence, possible high dose effect
Skin	1.0–2.0	0.1–2.5	Effect may be limited to high doses (or ultraviolet necessary)
Rectum	1.0–1.2	0.0–0.1	Effect may be limited to high doses
Uterus	1.0–1.01	0.0–0.5	Effect may be limited to high doses
Bone	1.0–1.1	0.0–0.1	Effect may be limited to high doses (radium dial painters)
Connective tissues	[b]	[b]	Effect may be limited to high doses
Cancers Never or Sporadically Associated with Radiation, with No Risk Estimates[c]			
Chronic lymphocytic leukemia	[b]	[b]	Absent?
Pancreas	[b]	[b]	Little evidence
Hodgkin's disease	[b]	[b]	Little evidence
Prostate	[b]	[b]	Little evidence
Testis	[b]	[b]	Little evidence
Cervix	[b]	[b]	Little evidence
Certain childhood cancers[d]	[b]	[b]	Absent?
Supporting tissues of skeleton[e]	[b]	[b]	Little evidence

Note: Relative risks and rankings of cancers associated with exposure to ionizing radiation in relation to the strength of the associations found and the availability of reliable estimates of radiation risk per unit organ dose.
[a]Association is inconsistently found and/or available estimates of risk are highly uncertain.
[b]No reliable estimate available.
[c]Sites for which radiation-induced cancers have not been reported or confirmed.
[d]Retinoblastoma, Wilms' tumor, and other tumors of embryonic origin.
[e]Muscles, tendons, and synovial membranes of joints.
Adapted from Boice et al., 1996, with permission of the authors and publishers.

Table 12.2   Factors in Radiation Response in Three Radiogenic Cancers in the Human[a]

Factor	Leukemia	Thyroid	Lung
Age sensitivity	Fetus most sensitive	Peak at 4 years	?
Risk (no. cases/10^6/year/rad)	0.7–15	1–6	0.6–3
Average latent period (years)	7–13	10–15	15
Duration of excess risk[b] (years)	15	30	lifetime

[a]After Fry and Ainsworth, 1977.
[b]Data not precise.

Human Neoplasms Resulting from Exposure to Ionizing Radiation

Risk estimates for a variety of human cancers related to exposures to ionizing radiation are given in Table 12.1. Leading the list is leukemia, which has been the most frequent fatal cancer in a variety of situations. Perhaps most notable is the relatively high incidence of leukemia attributable to exposure to radiation from the atom bomb blasts of Hiroshima and Nagasaki (Shimizu et al., 1990). Leukemia was also a major result of x-ray treatment of ankylosing spondylitis in persons diagnosed between 1935 and 1957 in the United Kingdom (Weiss et al., 1995). Just as with the atom bomb survivors, the major risk of leukemia development occurred during the first 10 years following the first x-ray treatment, with risk decreasing rapidly to near zero thereafter. The incidence of chronic lymphocytic leukemia was not significantly affected by ionizing radiation, an effect also noted in the atomic bomb survivors (Ishimaru et al., 1979). Another dramatic relationship between therapeutic radiation and induction in human cancer is seen with external radiation of the head, neck, and upper thorax and the induction of benign and malignant neoplasms of the thyroid gland. As shown in Figure 12.2, an almost linear dose-response of ionizing radiation and the developing thyroid cancer is noted in individuals radiated prior to age 15, whereas older individuals do not exhibit a similar risk relationship (cf. Schneider and Ron, 1997). This finding emphasizes the sensitivity of young individuals, with relatively high rates of cell replication in a variety of tissues, during growing years. A similar relationship is also seen in the induction of female breast cancer by ionizing radiation, as noted from the fact that essentially all cases of breast cancer resulting from radiation after the atom bomb blasts occurred in premenopausal women under age 40 (Goodman et al., 1994). A similar effect was noted in patients receiving radiotherapy for breast cancer in relation to risk of developing cancer in the unaffected breast. The risk of cancer development in the second breast was significantly increased among women less than 45 years of age who underwent radiation therapy (Boice et al., 1992). Furthermore, children irradiated for various therapeutic reasons also exhibited an increased risk of breast cancer development (Modan et al., 1989; Hildreth et al., 1989). Another unfortunate example of radiation carcinogenesis in the human was that of workers who utilized pigments containing radium salts to paint the dials of watches and airplane instruments. Many of the people operating such industries and instructing the workers did not believe the radium-containing paint to be hazardous. Thus, many of these workers absorbed the radioactive ions by mouth from the practice of shaping a sharp point to the brush with their lips after dipping the brush in a solution of radium ions. Within 15 to 25 years after exposure, a significant number of these individuals developed osteogenic sarcomas from the deposition of the radioactive radium in their bones. In addition, a large number of carcinomas of the cranial sinuses also occurred (Rowland and Lucas, 1984). Many of the other radiogenic neoplasms listed in Table 12.1 as significantly associated with ionizing radiation exposure were identified in patients surviving the atom bomb blast. A

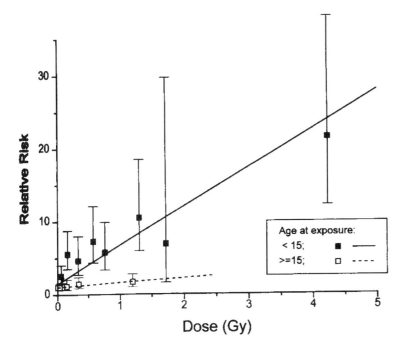

Figure 12.2 Dose-response curves for the development of thyroid cancer averaged from five cohort studies of childhood exposure (<15 years of age) and two studies of adult exposure (>15 years). (From Ron, 1996, with permission of the author and publisher.)

significant exception is the relatively rare phenomenon of postirradiation soft tissue sarcomas, which developed in a small percentage (less than 5%) of patients receiving relatively intensive doses of therapeutic radiation for a variety of reasons (Laskin et al., 1988; Brady et al., 1992; Bloechle et al., 1995). Osteogenic sarcomas and malignant fibrous histiocytomas predominate among these induced neoplasms, which usually have a very poor prognosis (Robinson et al., 1988).

Situational Exposures of Humans to Ionizing Radiation

As noted above, in a number of specific situations humans are exposed to excesses of ionizing radiation. The atom bomb blasts at Hiroshima and Nagasaki and medical therapy have accounted for a substantial part of such radiation.

Radon and Human Cancer

One of the more perplexing situations in which humans are exposed to low levels of ionizing radiation involves the ubiquitous element known as radon gas. The carcinogenic effects of this gas are most evident in underground miners, especially those in uranium mines, where substantial levels of radon gas occur. Figure 12.3 shows the relative risk of lung cancer for cohorts of miners for all exposures and for exposures restricted to under 600 WLM (working-level months). For all exposures, any deviation from linearity was not statistically significant (Lubin et al., 1995). The dashed line in the right-hand figure indicates a relative risk of 1.0. For residential radon exposure, living 30 years in a home with concentrations of radon gas at 1 and 4 pCi/L

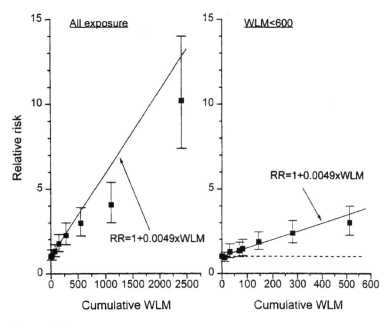

Figure 12.3 Relative risks (RR) of lung cancer for categories of working-level months (WLM) for all exposures to radon by underground miners and for exposures restricted to individuals of less than 600 WLM. For all exposures, deviation from linearity was not statistically significant. The dashed line indicates a relative risk of 1. For comparison, residential radon exposure, living 30 years in a home at 1 and 4 pCi/L is equivalent to about 6 and 24 WLM, respectively (from Lubin et al., 1995, with permission of the authors and publisher.)

is equivalent to about 6 and 24 WLM respectively. Thus, while the dose-response curve indicates that the very low levels of exposure over extended periods in homes carry a significant risk, it is almost impossible to determine unequivocally the actual carcinogenic risk of this environmental agent to the human at these extremely low doses. However, a study in Sweden (Pershagen et al., 1994) concluded that residential exposure to radon gas is an important cause of lung cancer in the general population, and a recent metanalysis of eight epidemiological studies on the long-term effects of exposure to indoor radon concentrations also concluded that this environmental agent was a factor in cancer induction in the human (Lubin and Boice, 1997). Furthermore, an earlier investigation (AMA, 1987) concluded that variations of radon levels in private dwellings in the United States are 100-fold or greater, with many homes exceeding the 4 pCi/L seen in the figure (AMA, 1987). Radon gas is clastogenic and mutagenic in experimental systems (Jostes, 1996). However, the total impact on the general population of exposure to this ubiquitous radioactive gas may never be completely known.

Occupational Exposures to Ionizing Radiation

Since medical therapy contributes significantly to the population burden of ionizing radiation (Figure 12.1), it is not surprising that workers who utilize sources of ionizing radiation, particularly radiologists, will show some excess risk for neoplasia. In fact, the first cancer that was attributed to the effects of ionizing radiation was on the hand of a radiologist, reported in 1902, and leukemia was first associated with chronic exposure to ionizing radiation by radiologists (cf. Boice et al., 1996). The incidence of leukemia in radiologists in the first half of this century was three to four times that in the general population, and skin cancer was also excessive in this group. However, since the middle of this century, such an association has dramatically decreased, in all likelihood because of the greater control and protection from sources of ionizing radiation used in medical practice. In part because of increased public concern, many studies have been carried out on workers at various nuclear installations and shipyards involved in the building of nuclear-powered vessels. In general, these studies have not indicated any significant risk of cancer in such installations in the United States (Boice et al., 1996). Even after accidental emissions, as at the Three Mile Island Nuclear Plant, subsequent follow-up has not indicated significant influence of this accident on cancer risk in the area (Hatch et al., 1990). However, in the accident occurring in the Chernobyl Nuclear Power Plant in the Soviet Union, excess cases of leukemias and thyroid cancers had already been diagnosed and verified by 1997 (Ivanov et al., 1997). Thus, an accident at a nuclear installation does carry a potential for significant risk of exposure and subsequent carcinogenesis. However, careful maintenance and protective and safety measures have essentially eliminated the environmental risk of ionizing radiation from these sources.

Medical Therapy and Diagnosis as Sources of Ionizing Radiation

The fact that therapeutic radiation poses a significant risk to the patient in most instances is recognized by all, but, as noted above, the benefit in most instances far outweighs the risk. Several examples of carcinogenesis resulting from therapeutic radiation have already been discussed. The association of subsequent cancers with treatment of cervical cancer, Hodgkin disease, and a number of childhood cancers has been described (cf. Boice, 1981), as well as the increased risk of cancer developing in the contralateral breast after radiation treatment for cancer in the affected breast (see above). In addition, a series of women who received radiation treatment for acute postpartum mastitis have also shown a significantly increased risk for developing breast cancer (Shore et al., 1986). In women who had received radiation therapy for breast cancer, there was an increased risk of lung cancer developing 10 years later even in nonsmokers, but a multiplicative effect was observed in smokers (Neugut et al., 1994).

Less apparent is the risk of cancer development from diagnostic radiation, in most instances for routine diagnoses. Diagnostic radiography was found to have only a small influence on the occurrence of leukemia and breast cancer in women so exposed (Evans et al., 1986) as well as in several studies investigating the radiation risk of mammography. Essentially no excess cancer risk was determined for this diagnostic procedure, especially in relation to the potential benefit obtained by mammographic screening (Feig, 1984). In addition to the relative safety of diagnostic x-rays, the use of radioactive iodine in determining abnormalities in the thyroid gland by techniques of nuclear medicine is not carcinogenic to the human, as evidenced in one large cohort subjected to these diagnostic procedures (Holm et al., 1988). On the other hand, Bross et al. (1979) argued that small subgroups in the general population are particularly sensitive to ionizing radiation, and this factor should be taken into account in determining safe exposures.

Furthermore, not all diagnostic radiation is free from risk. There is now substantial evidence that children irradiated in utero with ionizing radiation for diagnostic purposes have an excess risk of childhood cancer of about 40% (cf. Wakeford, 1995). Another series supporting this finding reported approximately a twofold increase in risk of childhood cancer after prenatal x-ray exposure (Harvey et al., 1985). The use of Thorotrast (Chapter 11) as an x-ray contrast medium for diagnosing the presence of lesions in the liver, kidney, and other solid organs has now clearly been associated with the development of angiosarcoma of the liver as well as leukemia from the alpha radiation given off by the decay of thorium (Andersson and Storm, 1992). There has also been a report that diagnostic radiation may increase the risk of salivary gland neoplasms (Preston-Martin et al., 1988). Still, despite these few examples of the sensitivity of the exposed individual (the fetus) and the chronic intense localized dose of radiation such as that from iodine 131, diagnostic radiation is a comparatively safe procedure in which the extensive benefits generally far outweigh the minimal risk.

Estimate of Risk of Human Cancer Due to Ionizing Radiation

While there is no question that substantial doses of radiation provide a considerable risk of carcinogenesis to the human being, estimating and predicting the risk of low doses of radiation is extremely difficult. It is made more difficult by the fact that there is no single unifying model that describes the dose-response effect when dealing with doses less than 100 rad. Moreover, because of the large number of subjects and the long time elapsing between irradiation and the appearance of cancer (for instance), studies on risk estimates are usually complicated by uncertainties about the size of the irradiation dose to affected individuals and the possible influence of factors other than radiation. For these reasons, estimates of risk are based on extrapolations from assumptions about dose-response relationships.

Some of the most extensive conclusions about the relative risk of ionizing radiation were developed from studies of survivors of the atomic bomb blasts at Hiroshima and Nagasaki. Figure 12.4 shows the relative risk for cancer at one grade of exposure for survivors from 1950 through 1985 (Shimizu et al., 1990). The overall incidence of cancer in Hiroshima and Nagasaki between 1958 and 1987 increased more than 40% in males and some 15% in females (Goodman et al., 1994). The rate of liver cancer has increased dramatically among males in these cohorts during the past 20 years, with a twofold increase in incidence in the past 10 years alone. How-

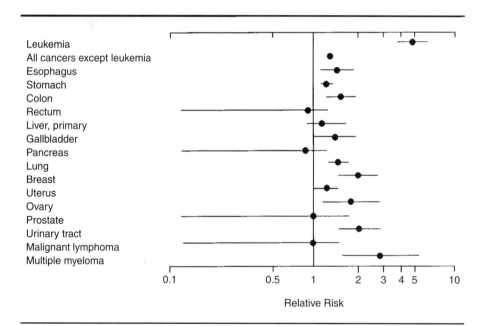

Figure 12.4 Relative risk for development of individual types of cancer at one Gy exposure with 90% confidence intervals for survivors of the atom bomb blasts at Hiroshima and Nagasaki from the years 1950 through 1985. (Adapted from Shimizu et al., 1990, with permission of the authors and publisher.)

ever, this finding undoubtedly involves a number of risk factors other than the radiation exposure. Interestingly, in children of atomic bomb survivors who were less than 20 years old between 1946 and 1982, the risk of cancer did not increase significantly as the parental gonadal dose increased (Yoshimoto, 1990).

The absolute risk from exposure to ionizing radiation for the development of neoplastic disease has always been considered as linear, with the absence of any threshold effect (Figure 12.3; Chapter 3). Recently, this concept was given substantial experimental reinforcement by the report by Hei et al. (1997) that the traversal through a cell by a single α particle has a low probability of being lethal to the cell, with over 80% survival following such an exposure, but the frequency of gene mutations is enhanced more than twofold over the background in these surviving cells. This clearly indicates that a single photon or particle can have mutational and potentially carcinogenic effects on a single cell (Hei et al., 1997). While it appears that almost all models of radiobiological cellular reactions conform approximately to a linear-quadratic dose-response relation at low, protracted doses (Sachs et al., 1997), an analysis of the dose-response curves for rates of several different types of cancer, especially leukemia, in survivors of the atom bomb blast indicated a U-shaped dose-response curve. Such a curve for leukemia deaths is seen in Figure 12.5 and follows the findings by Kondo (1990). While several reports have questioned these findings and conclusions (Little and Muirhead, 1997; Pierce and Vaeth, 1991), this hormesis (biphasic dose-response relationship) effect has been reported for some chemical carcinogens (Teeguarden et al., 1998; Parsons, 1994; Rossi, 1981). No obvious mechanism for such a "protective" effect of low doses of ionizing radiation is obvious; however, Makinodan and James (1990) have found that low doses of ionizing radiation potentiate responses in the immune system, which could in part explain this apparent protective effect of carcinogens.

The federal government and the National Academy of Sciences of the United States have been extremely concerned about the estimation of risks to ionizing radiation. Several reports of the National Research Council's Committee on the Biological Effects of Ionizing Radiations (BEIR) have been concerned with this subject in particular. The latest BEIR V report has validated previous estimates of radiation effects and risks with some claim that ionizing radiation is more hazardous than had been previously assumed. Despite the extensive efforts of many, the BEIR V report "illustrates that the data currently available about radiation effects are still too meager to define quantitative risk estimates at low exposures with absolute certainty" (Hendee, 1992).

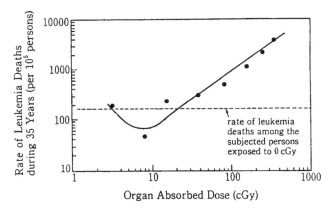

Figure 12.5   Dose-response relation of leukemia deaths among atom bomb survivors. (Adapted from Hattori, 1994, with permission of the author and publisher.)

Ultraviolet Radiation Exposure

Perhaps the greatest single risk of radiation exposure to the human being is not ionizing radiation, but rather exposure to ultraviolet light in sunlight. In the 1940s Rusch and his colleagues (Rusch et al., 1941) demonstrated the production of skin tumors in mice by ultraviolet radiation; the most carcinogenic wavelengths lay between 2900 and 3400 angstroms. As noted in Chapter 3, ultraviolet radiation spans the wavelengths of light between 2000 and 4000 angstroms. The span of the electromagnetic spectrum is generally divided into three regions: ultraviolet C (UVC) ranging from 2000 to 2900 angstroms (Å); ultraviolet B (UVB), ranging from 2900 to 3200 Å; and ultraviolet A (UVA), ranging from 3200 to 4000 Å (cf. Longstreth, 1988). UV radiation that reaches the earth's surface is almost entirely in the UVA and UVB region, since ozone in the stratosphere strongly absorbs UVC and to some extent UVB but not UVA. In experimental situations, neoplasms have been produced with a combination of UVA and UVB but not with UVA alone. These data have been interpreted to indicate that UVB is capable of initiation and possibly also tumor promotion, while UVA is essentially only a promoting agent (Elwood, 1984).

The most common neoplasms of the skin in the human are squamous cell carcinoma, basal cell carcinoma, and melanoma. Experimental induction of the former two lesions in the skin of rodents by UV radiation has been repeatedly demonstrated, but the induction of malignant melanoma in experimental animals by any means is a relatively unusual event. Similarly, as pointed out below, epidemiological evidence strongly indicates the carcinogenic effect of UV radiation in the induction of squamous and basal cell carcinomas of the skin; but the epidemiological evidence linking sunlight exposure to the development of malignant melanoma in the human is not quite so firm.

The Epidemiology of Ultraviolet-Induced Skin Cancer

According to Armstrong and Kricker (1996), at least six major lines of evidence support the proposition that sun exposure causes skin cancer (Table 12.3). Interestingly, the publication on sunlight and skin cancer of the International Agency for Research on Cancer (IARC) (1992) argues that the evidence was sufficient for both melanoma and nonmelanoma skin cancer (basal and squamous cell carcinomas of the skin), but was more substantial in support of a causative relationship between sun exposure and melanoma development. This is somewhat surprising in view of considerable literature, both before and after the IARC report, that does not indicate such a certain relationship between UV radiation and melanoma development (Urbach, 1997; Leffell and Brash, 1996; Elwood, 1996). In any event, there is no question that UV

Table 12.3 Categories of Epidemiological Evidence for the Causation of Skin Cancer by Sun Exposure

1. Skin cancers are more frequent in residents of areas of high ambient solar radiation.
2. Skin cancers are more frequent in sun-sensitive people.
3. Skin cancers occur mainly on sun-exposed areas of the body.
4. Skin cancers are more frequently seen in people having high sun exposure.
5. Skin cancers are more frequent in people with benign sun-related skin conditions.
6. Skin cancers are less likely to occur where the skin is protected against solar radiation by a variety of means.

Adapted from Armstrong and Kricker, 1996.

radiation in sunlight plays a major if not the predominant role in the development of skin cancer in the human.

Squamous and Basal Cell Skin Cancers

In conformance with the arguments expressed in Table 12.3, the incidence rates of squamous and basal cell carcinomas in whites increase significantly more dramatically than those of melanoma with increasing proximity to the equator and with increasing measured ambient UV radiation (cf. Armstrong and Kricker, 1996). Migrant studies, primarily from Australia, have demonstrated that the incidence and mortality rates of basal cell carcinoma and melanoma are higher in people born in countries with high ambient solar radiation than in migrants to these countries from areas with lower ambient solar radiation. The evidence for squamous cell carcinoma is similar but not so extensive. Furthermore, basal and squamous cell carcinomas are much more frequently found in areas of the body that are most frequently exposed to sun, mainly the head and neck, and to a lesser extent the shoulders and back (Armstrong and Kricker, 1996). Actual quantitation of exposure to sunlight is somewhat more difficult, but Kricker et al. (1995) have been able to develop a dose-response curve relating total sun exposure to the risk of development of basal cell carcinoma in an Australian cohort (Figure 12.6). When lifetime exposure is considered as in this figure, the quadratic model utilized showed an initial rise in the risk of basal cell cancer with increasing exposure of the site, with a peak at about 35,000 hours of exposure, followed by a fall. The interesting exception was the head and neck, while the trunk showed the greatest odds ratio of 2.4. The apparent inhibition of carcinogenesis by increasing sun exposure is suggestive of a hormetic effect (see above) perhaps different from that depicted in Figure 12.5. A benign lesion, which in some cases may be a precursor of squamous cell carcinoma, is the

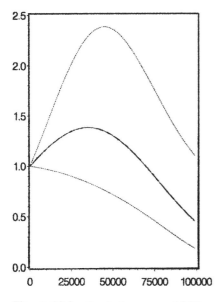

Figure 12.6 Quadratic curve and 95% confidence intervals for the continuous relationship between total hours of sun exposure and the development of basal cell carcinoma. In this model, the interaction between exposure and body site was not significant. Abscissa: total hours of sun exposure. Ordinate: odds ratio. (From Kricker et al., 1995, with permission of the authors and publisher.)

actinic or solar keratosis that also occurs predominantly if not almost exclusively on the head and neck, the back of the hands, and rarely the trunk.

Malignant Melanoma

Like the actinic keratosis mentioned above as a rare precursor lesion to squamous cell carcinoma, the pigmented nevus has been considered by some to be a benign form of melanoma or at least of collections of melanocytes. The incidence of both actinic keratoses and nevi is related to sun exposure, as demonstrated by the prevalence of nevi in young Australian children that is inversely proportional to the latitude of residence (Kelly et al., 1994) and by the fact that individuals with a history of severe sunburn in childhood have a significantly increased risk of nevus development (Dennis et al., 1996). In the United States, adults typically have fewer than 50 nevi, and the relative risk of melanoma increases by both nevus type and number (Tucker, 1998) (Table 12.4). As noted from the data presented in Table 12.4, the odds ratio for the development of melanoma is threefold in patients with more than 50 nevi. Dysplastic nevi have a much greater risk for melanoma development, as reflected in their distinctly abnormal morphology (Tucker, 1998). In addition to the number of nevi, sun exposure, and migrant history, genetic susceptibility (Chapter 5) and intermittent exposure to sunlight (Elwood, 1996) play significant roles in the development of malignant melanoma in the human. As indicated above, sun exposure during childhood increases the risk of melanoma development in the adult (Autier and Doré, 1998; Longstreth, 1988).

Table 12.4 Adjusted Estimated Relative Risks of Melanoma by Nevus Type and Number

No. of Nevi by Type	No. of Cases	No. of Controls	Adjusted[a] RR (95% CI)
Nevi >2 mm and <5 mm			
0–24	258	658	1.0
25–49	163	190	1.8 (1.3–2.5)
50–99	169	107	3.0 (2.1–4.4)
≥100	123	43	3.4 (2.0–5.7)
Nondysplastic nevi >5 mm			
0	239	507	1.0
1	135	224	0.9 (0.7–1.3)
2–4	188	195	1.3 (1.0–1.8)
5–9	86	51	1.7 (1.0–2.7)
≥10	65	21	2.3 (1.2–4.3)
Dysplastic nevi			
None	301	778	1.0
Indeterminate	72	127	1.0 (0.7–1.6)
1	64	50	2.3 (1.4–3.6)
2–4	121	33	7.3 (4.6–12)
5–9	45	15	4.9 (2.5–9.8)
≥10	55	6	12 (4.4–31)

Key: CI, confidence interval; RR, relative risk.
[a]Mutually adjusted and adjusted for age, gender, center, referral pattern, morphologic dysplastic nevi <5 mm, sunburns, freckles, solar damage, scars, nevus excisions, and family history of melanoma.
Adapted from Tucker (1998) with permission of author and publisher.

Somatic Mutations and Other Mechanisms Involved in the Ultraviolet Light Induction of Skin Cancer

As noted in Chapter 6, both chemical and physical carcinogens may initiate carcinogenesis by inducing somatic mutations in specific genes that are critical in the normal functioning of the cell. While such mutations have been described both in proto-oncogenes and tumor suppressor genes, it has been pointed out that proto-oncogenes require specific mutations for the "activation" of the protein (Chapter 6), but tumor suppressor genes may be inactivated by a considerably more extensive range of mutations. This latter effect leads to a greater propensity for mutations in tumor suppressor genes to retain the "signature" of the carcinogen involved. As noted in Chapter 3, UV light produces two relatively unique mutations in DNA, a pyrimidine-pyrimidine dimerization and a 6-4 linkage between two adjacent pyrimidines (Taylor, 1994). These changes lead to a $C \rightarrow T$ transition at dipyrimidine sites as well as tandem $CC \rightarrow TT$ mutations, which are highly characteristic of UVB and UVC radiation. Almost 90% of human squamous cell cancers exhibit such mutations in the p53 tumor suppressor gene (Leffell and Brash, 1996; Kraemer, 1997). Furthermore, actinic keratoses exhibit a similar high frequency of p53 mutations, which are the signature of UV exposure (cf. Kraemer, 1997). Jonason et al. (1996) found that normal-appearing skin in patients who did not have skin cancer contained clones of cells with characteristic UV-type p53 mutations. Such mutant cells usually occurred in clones of 60 to 3000 cells (Brash, 1997), quite reminiscent of the altered hepatic foci seen in rodent liver initiated with chemical carcinogens (Chapter 7). In older individuals, almost 1 epidermal cell in 20 on the face and hands exhibited a p53 UV-type mutation. Brash and colleagues have proposed that the relatively high incidence of such clones is due to the fact that normal squamous cells undergo apoptosis, especially in sunlight-damaged skin, whereas cells containing one allele of a mutated p53 tumor suppressor gene are more resistant to apoptosis. If the stem cell of such mutated clones is not eliminated by normal epidermal turnover, such mutated cells can remain in the epidermis for many years, with their progeny exhibiting the potential for developing into actinic keratoses, with 1 in 1000 of these lesions developing into squamous cell cancers (Figure 12.7; Kraemer, 1997; Brash, 1997).

In addition to somatic mutations in the p53 tumor suppressor gene, which appear to account for the majority of squamous cell cancers, about half of basal cell cancers but relatively few melanomas exhibit similar mutations. In these latter two instances, from our knowledge of the molecular genetics of hereditary syndromes involving abnormally high incidences of basal cell cancers (Gorlin syndrome) and malignant melanomas (familial melanoma syndrome) (Chapter 6; Brash, 1997), involvement of somatic mutations may be considerably more complex.

Immunological Factors in the Development of Skin Cancer in the Human

There has been some epidemiological evidence suggesting an association between the incidence of non-Hodgkin lymphoma and solar UV radiation in England and northern Europe (Bentham, 1996; Adami et al., 1995). While such an association has not been found in the United States (Hartge et al., 1996), alteration in the immune system by UV light, which is known to occur (Chapter 19), may possibly contribute to this increased incidence of this non-skin cancer. Furthermore, patients with immunological abnormalities do have a greater propensity for certain types of skin cancer, suggestive of a potential role for abnormalities in the skin immune system in development during both the promotion and progression stages of human skin cancer. This topic is discussed more extensively in Chapter 19.

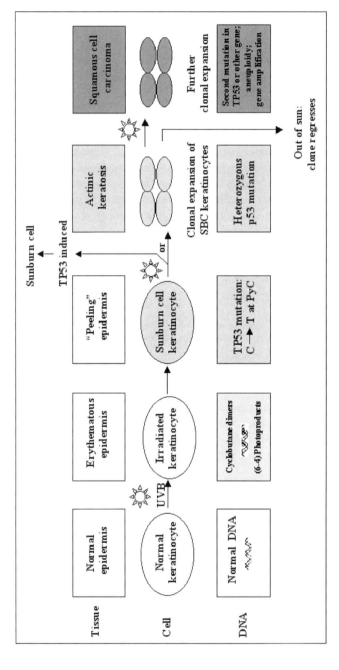

Figure 12.7 A model for genetic and cellular events leading to the development of squamous cell carcinoma of the skin in the human. Sunlight creates cyclobutane dimers and (6-4) photoproducts in DNA, some of which may cause mutations in the p53 tumor suppressor gene (TP53). One of the cellular phenotypes resulting from a TP53 mutation, resistance to sunlight-induced apoptosis, allows repeated sunlight exposure to select for TP53-mutated cells. An occasional one of these cells might incur the same mutagenic events resulting in mutation of the second TP53 allele thus totally altering the function of the gene product. (Adapted from Brash, 1997, with permission of author and publisher.)

Nonionizing, Nonultraviolet Radiation and Human Cancer

Unlike the solid scientific and epidemiological bases for the causal relationship between ionizing and UV radiation and the genesis of human cancer, the association of radio frequency, microwave, and visible radiation and magnetic fields with the causation of human cancer has been driven largely by legal, political, and social factors, with little or no scientific and epidemiological base. Perhaps the initial driving force attempting to relate exposure to such energy fields and long wavelengths was the mere fact that these represented some form of radiation, and some perhaps influential individuals made little or no distinction between such radiation and ionizing and UV radiation. As noted in Chapter 3, this is clearly not correct. Furthermore, Valberg et al. (1997) have argued with sound scientific basis that biological effects in humans from extremely low-frequency electromagnetic fields of the order of those found in residential environments are "implausible based on current understanding of physics and biology." There is little or no reproducible evidence that such radiation and magnetic fields induce any mutational damage to DNA in living cells in a direct manner, such as evident with exposure to ionizing and UV radiation. Furthermore, evidence of overall carcinogenic effects induced by radio frequency and/or microwave radiation and magnetic fields is predominantly negative and/or irreproducible (McCann et al., 1998; Kavet, 1996). A more reproducible effect of extremely low frequency (ELF) electromagnetic fields is on gene transcription in experimental studies, as listed in Table 12.5. Epidemiological investigations have in some areas been somewhat more reproducible, although in virtually all reported studies associations reported may well be due to factors and variables not controlled for or even considered in the investigation when one is looking for only a single association regardless of other factors (Lacy-Hulbert et al., 1998).

Many scientists in cancer research have viewed the publicity given to the potential of carcinogenesis by nonionizing, non-UV radiation and magnetic fields as excessive, misleading, and unscientific. However, the effects of electromagnetic fields on specific experimental systems of

Table 12.5   Effects of ELF Electromagnetic Fields on Gene Transcription in Vitro and in Vivo

System	Genes	Exposure/Time	Change	Reference
In Vitro				
Lymphoblastoid human cell line	c-*fos*, c-*jun*, c-*myc*, *PKC*	60 Hz/15 min 384 milligauss	Increase	Phillips et al., 1992
Hela S3 cells	c-*fos*	0.18–0.2 T/24 h	Increase	Hiraoka et al., 1992
HL-60 cell line (human leukemia)	c-*myc*, β-actin histone 2B	60 Hz/20 min 5.7 μT	Increase	Goodman et al., 1992
B-lineage lymphoid cells (human)	Lyn kinase	60 Hz/0–18 h	Increase	Uckun et al., 1995
Human lymphoma CEM cells	Ornithine decarboxylase	60 Hz/1 h	Increase	Byus et al., 1987
In Vivo				
Liver regeneration (rat)	Ornithine decarboxylase	50 Hz, 0.006 T 30 min/h–12 h	Increase	Ottani et al., 1984
Mammary tissue (rat)	Ornithine decarboxylase	50 Hz, 50 μT 6 weeks	Twofold increase	Mevissen et al., 1995
Mouse liver	Metallothionein	3–4.7T 6–48 h	Two- to threefold increase	Satoh et al., 1996

Adapted from Pitot, 1998, with permission of publisher. See Kaune (1993) for details on units of measurement.

the living cells or organism (Table 12.5) offer the potential that continued chronic exposure of humans and other mammals to such forms of energy may produce altered health effects, of which carcinogenesis is perhaps the least likely.

BIOLOGICAL CARCINOGENESIS IN THE HUMAN

As noted earlier, in Chapter 4, biological factors as causes of cancer in lower animals have been known since the beginning of the twentieth century and were suspected even earlier. However, it was not until the latter half of the twentieth century that infectious agents began to be significantly appreciated as causative factors in human cancer. Perhaps the scientific embarrassment engendered by the irreproducibility of Febiger's experiment (Chapter 4) led to an aversion of scientists to try and relate infectious agents to the development of the neoplastic process. This was true despite the suggestion from ancient times of an association between infection with species of platyhelminth worms, especially *Schistosoma haematobium*, and bladder cancer; this had been known or suspected for thousands of years beginning in ancient Egypt (cf. Elsebai, 1977; Hicks, 1983). That bacteria and viruses could cause human cancer was not substantially appreciated until the last four decades of the twentieth century.

Extracellular Parasites and Their Roles in the Causation of Human Cancer

The principal extracellular parasites causally associated with human cancer are species of worms, flukes, and bacteria. The specific species of each of these classes of organisms for which such an association has been determined by the IARC according to the criteria noted at the beginning of Chapter 11 are listed in Table 12.6. The IARC evaluation specifies whether there is sufficient evidence that the infection is carcinogenic or whether the evidence is limited, leading to possible or probable carcinogenesis.

In the class of helminths, *Schistosoma haematobium*, a parasitic worm that affects an estimated 200 million people in 74 countries, represents by far the greatest infestation potentially resulting in human cancer (IARC, 1994b). Eggs of the parasite, usually spread by human excre-

Table 12.6 Extracellular Parasites Causally Associated with Human Cancer

Species	Class	Regions of Infection	Associated Cancers	IARC Evaluation
Clonorchis sinensis	Helminth (fluke)	China, Vietnam	Hepatocellular carcinoma	Limited
Opisthorchis viverrini	Helminth (fluke)	Thailand, Eastern Europe, Russia	Hepatocellular carcinoma Cholangiocarcinoma	Sufficient
Schistosoma haematobium	Helminth (worm)	West and Central Africa, Egypt, Middle East	Bladder carcinoma	Sufficient
Schistosoma japonicum	Helminth (worm)	China, Indonesia	Liver, colorectal cancer	Limited
Helicobacter pylori	Bacteria	Worldwide	Gastric carcinoma Gastric lymphoma	Sufficient

Summarized from IARC Monograph 61, 1994.

ment, mature in an aqueous environment to a small multicellular larval form, which infects a specific species of snails. The larvae mature in the snail to a swimming form, termed cercariae, which then penetrate human skin, enter the vascular system, and metamorphose into young worms, which colonize in the host, especially in the bladder. The chronic infection may lead to bladder carcinoma by a mechanism that is not clear at present. However, studies by Rosin and Anwar (1992) demonstrated chromosomal changes in the urothelial cells of the bladder in patients with chronic infestations of *S. haematobium*. Since urine itself contains a number of growth factors, the combination of the promoting effect of such growth factors and the induced karyotypic abnormalities may lead to neoplasia. *Schistosoma japonicum* infestations have been associated with the development of liver and colorectal cancer, but the evidence for a direct causal association is relatively limited (IARC, 1994b).

Infestation of the human with liver flukes, another form of helminth, can also lead to the development of liver cancer. This is particularly true in the case of infections with *Opisthorchis viverrini*, which has an even more complicated life cycle, in which the development to the adult involves two intermediate hosts. In this instance the fluke infests the liver through the biliary system, in which the worms live and lay eggs that are excreted through the feces. As with schistosomes, there is no reproduction of the adult form within the human. Chronic infestation with this parasite can lead to the development of hepatocellular carcinoma and cholangiocarcinoma (IARC Monograph 61, 1994).

At present, the most widespread extracellular parasite causatively associated with the development of human cancer is the bacterium *Helicobacter pylori*. This species is one of a number of related bacterial species that infect a variety of different animal species. In 1984, Marshall and Warren (1984) identified the organism and called it *Campylobacter pylori* and associated its infection in the stomach with gastritis and peptic ulceration. Infection with the organism occurs worldwide and varies from 30% to 90% in patients over 55 years of age (IARC, 1994b). Chronic infection with the organism may induce chronic active inflammation of the gastric mucosa, which may ultimately lead to the loss of gastric glands and the establishment of atrophic gastritis with associated development of intestinal metaplasia and dysplasia (Kuipers, 1998). Other workers have shown that the bacterium is associated with early development of gastric cancer (Asaka et al., 1994; Endo et al., 1995), and Rugge and associates (1996) have suggested that chronic infection by *H. pylori* plays a role in the promotion of gastric carcinogenesis. In support of this last proposal is the finding by Peek et al. (1997) that infection by *H. pylori* increases gastric mucosal proliferation in relation to the severity of the gastritis induced. The increased proliferation was not accompanied by a parallel increase in apoptotic indices.

There is substantial evidence that lymphomas of the mucosa-associated lymphoid tissue (MALT) of the stomach are also causally related to infection with *H. pylori* (cf. Wotherspoon, 1998). The low-grade forms of these MALT lymphomas occur in association with infection with the bacterium and may completely disappear on successful eradication of the bacterial infection (cf. Wotherspoon, 1998). Furthermore, the early lesions of this disease appear to be monoclonal (Nakamura et al., 1998; Sorrentino et al., 1996). However, specific chromosomal alterations may occur in these lesions, suggesting a mechanism whereby some growths do not regress on eradication of the infection but continue as neoplasms (Banerjee et al., 1997).

Mechanisms of the effect of *H. pylori* on the gastric mucosa have been somewhat difficult to investigate because of the lack of experimental models. However, recently Honda et al. (1998) have demonstrated the development of *H. pylori*–induced gastric carcinoma in Mongolian gerbils. Establishment and maintenance of the infection in humans depends on the ability of the bacterium to attach to the gastric mucosa, which it does through a blood group antigen (protein) (Borén et al., 1993), and then to produce prodigious amounts of the enzyme urease, which catalyzes the formation of ammonia from urea, which is normally present at millimolar levels in body fluids. This expediency allows the organism to exist at a reasonable pH, since the ammonia neutralizes the gastric hydrochloric acid in the immediate area around the bacterium (Stark et al., 1995; Dunn et al., 1997). Ammonium ions and/or urease may also be toxic to adjacent gastric mucosal cells, as is a cytotoxin produced by the bacterium itself (Cover, 1996). In addition to these possible mechanisms, the bacterium does elicit an immune response by several mechanisms, including the release of the toxin mentioned above; the presence of the gene *cagA*, which is associated with virulence; the release of a lipopolysaccharide, albeit of relatively low immunogenic activity; and other factors that lead to a mucosal immune response that rarely may result in the elimination of the infection but much more commonly leads to a chronic, protracted gastritis with continued bacterial colonization (Dixon, 1994; Moran, 1996; Shimoyama and Crabtree, 1998). Host responses to such immunomodulatory factors include the development of mucosa-associated lymphoid follicles, whereas normal gastric mucosa exhibits no lymphoid accumulation (cf. Ferrero, 1997). In the final analysis, chronic infection with *H. pylori* may lead to chronic superficial gastritis, which then has a number of potential end points, as noted in Figure 12.8. Although, as pointed out in Chapter 3, chronic infections are relatively rare in our society today, chronic infections with *H. pylori* and parasitic helminths appear to be exceptions and may lead to neoplasia, just as was noted in chronic skin infections.

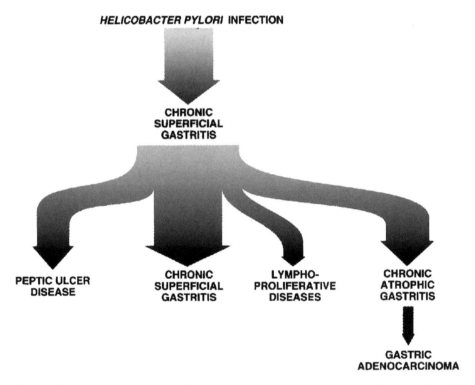

Figure 12.8 Infection with *Helicobacter pylori* progresses to chronic superficial gastritis within months in most infected individuals. Left untreated, this condition may persist for life in most people. A small number of individuals, however, may develop peptic ulcer disease, lymphoproliferative diseases including MALT lymphoma, or severe chronic atrophic gastritis, leading to adenocarcinoma of the stomach. (Adapted from Blaser, 1996, with permission of the author and publishers.)

Viruses as a Cause of Specific Human Cancers

Viruses were demonstrated to cause neoplasms in lower animals as early as 1909 (Ellermann and Bang, 1909). Several decades later, Gross reported the presence of a virus-like agent in mice capable of causing salivary gland carcinomas when inoculated into newborns (Gross, 1953). The association of viruses with human cancer was not seriously appreciated until a report by Epstein and associates (1964) described the presence of virus particles in lymphoblasts isolated from a lymphoma of the type originally reported by Dr. Dennis Burkitt (1958). Burkitt had observed that the lymphoma bearing his name occurred primarily in children in certain parts of Africa. Because of this, he proposed an infectious origin for the neoplasm (cf. Henle et al., 1979) based largely on this peculiar geographic distribution, which was similar to some other infectious diseases seen in Africa. Since the discovery of the Epstein-Barr virus (EBV) in 1964, there has been an almost exponential increase in the number of viruses shown to cause specific human cancers. Moreover, the number of people at risk from infections of such oncogenic viruses and subsequent risk of neoplasia is well into the millions throughout the world. Table 12.7 lists vi-

Table 12.7   Viruses and Human Cancer and Related Disease

	Human Cancer/Disease	IARC Classification
DNA Viruses		
Epstein-Barr virus (EBV)	Burkitt lymphoma	Sufficient
	Hodgkin disease	Sufficient
	Immunosuppression-related lymphoma	Sufficient
	Infectious mononucleosis	(C)
	Nasopharyngeal carcinoma	Sufficient
	Oral hairy leukoplakia	(C)
	Sinonasal T-cell lymphoma	Sufficient
Hepatitis viruses		
Hepatitis B	Hepatocellular carcinoma	Sufficient
Herpes simplex II virus	Carcinoma of cervix and vulva	(A)
Human papillomavirus	Warts	(C)
Types 16, 18	Carcinoma of anus, cervix, penis, oral cavity, esophagus, larynx, skin papillomas of esophagus, nasal cavity	Sufficient
Types 6, 11	Carcinoma of conjunctiva, eyelid, oral cavity, larynx, esophagus	Limited
Kaposi sarcoma herpes virus	Kaposi sarcoma and lymphoma of body cavities	Limited
Papovaviruses (JC, BK, SV40)	Progressive multifocal leukoencephalopathy (JC virus)	(C)
	Brain neoplasms and mesotheliomas (SV40)	(A) ?
RNA Viruses		
Hepatitis viruses		
Hepatitis C	Hepatocellular carcinoma	Sufficient
Human immunodeficiency virus (HIV)	AIDS	Sufficient
Human T-cell lymphotropic viruses (HTLV)	T-cell leukemia/lymphoma	Sufficient
	Tropical spastic paraparesis	(A)

Key: (C), causative; (A), associated; ?, questionable.
Table taken from data in IARC monographs (vol. 59, 1994; vol. 64, 1995; vol. 67, 1996; vol. 70, 1997) and references in text.

ruses known to be causative or at least associated with the development of a variety of human neoplasms as well as specific nonneoplastic diseases that may be indirectly associated with an increased development of neoplasia, such as the acquired immunodeficiency syndrome (AIDS). In the table, the IARC classification of carcinogenic risk is given where it has been published. Where the IARC has not made any definitive statements or the condition is not a neoplasm, the codes C for causative and A for associated are given. Each of these agents is considered briefly in the remainder of this chapter.

DNA Viruses and Human Cancer

Epstein-Barr Virus as a Cause of Human Disease

Worldwide infection with EBV is so widespread that by the third decade of life it is estimated that 80% to 100% of individuals have become carriers of the infection (IARC, 1997). In the United States, antibody to EBV occurs in about 10% of individuals in the neonatal period, rising to some 60% by 10 years of age (Evans and Niederman, 1989). In contrast, antibody to EBV is seen in nearly 90% to 100% of individuals less than 10 years of age in Africa as well as the East and West Indies. In parallel with these differences, the picture of EBV-induced disease differs significantly in the United States and these other regions of the world. Perhaps the most common disease induced by EBV in the United States is infectious mononucleosis, characterized by fever, sore throat, tonsillitis, lymphadenopathy, and splenomegaly. This self-limiting disease rarely has a protracted course, although some complications may occur (Sumaya, 1989; Okano and Gross, 1996). Primary EBV infection is usually asymptomatic, and infection occurs predominantly via salivary and urinary contact (cf. Gratama and Ernberg, 1995). Thus, in populations with high standards of hygiene, such as predominate in western cultures, primary EBV infections may not occur until late childhood or adolescence, at which time the potential for developing infectious mononucleosis appears to predominate in individuals with a relatively mature immune system. In contrast, in Third World countries, especially where classic Burkitt lymphoma predominates, extensive infections with the virus occur early in life, as noted by the antibody response, resulting in neoplastic development. This theory, while not yet proven, does take into account a number of the epidemiological and geographical characteristics of these diseases.

The clinical and histopathological characteristics of Burkitt lymphoma have allowed the distinction of at least two forms of the disease—that predominating in young children and affecting lymphoid tissue of the head and neck, with quite characteristic clinical features in association with the lymphadenopathy of the disease; and a second clinical form involving lymphoid structures in the abdominal cavity, seen in older children and adults (cf. Levin and Levine, 1998). In the first or "African" form of the disease, more than 95% of patients exhibit infection with the Epstein-Barr virus and infectious virus within the neoplasm. In the abdominal form, which is increasing in Africa along with socioeconomic improvements, only 10% to 30% of such neoplasms appear to be associated with the Epstein-Barr virus (IARC, 1997). There is also substantial evidence that malarial infestation, especially in the young, increases the risk of developing Burkitt lymphoma. The lymphoma is rare in regions in which malaria eradication campaigns have been successful. Another possible environmental factor in the pathogenesis of Burkitt lymphoma in Africa is the presence of and use of products from the plant *Euphorbia tirucalli* (IARC, 1997). The phorbol esters present in this plant have structures closely related to the phorbol esters used as tumor-promoting agents in experimental studies in mouse epidermal carcinogenesis (Chapter 7). Such agents can increase the ability of EBV to transform B lymphocytes and increase the likelihood of chromosomal alterations in such cells. The plant is endemic in areas of equatorial Africa where Burkitt lymphoma incidence is quite high.

EBV is also causally associated with the development of nasopharyngeal carcinoma, a disease with a remarkable racial and geographical distribution. In most parts of the world, the incidence is usually less than 1 per 100,000 persons per year (Parkin et al., 1997). However, in some provinces of mainland China, the rates may be as high as 25 to 40 per 100,000 person-years. The most common histological type of these neoplasms is undifferentiated carcinomas, with prominent lymphoid stroma accounting for up to 80% of the cases (Niedobitek et al., 1996). Squamous cell carcinomas with little or no lymphoid stroma make up the remaining percentage of these neoplasms. While the undifferentiated carcinomas with lymphoid stroma almost all exhibit detectable virus, a smaller percentage of the squamous cell carcinomas do so. Thus, even sporadic cases throughout the world of the undifferentiated carcinoma/lymphoid stroma type of nasopharyngeal carcinoma exhibit molecular evidence of EBV causation. To a greater extent than with Burkitt lymphoma, environmental factors appear to regulate the expression of the neoplastic state in that individuals living in endemic regions migrating to nonendemic regions exhibit a dramatic decrease in the incidence of nasopharyngeal carcinoma within the first generation (IARC, 1997). Several environmental factors, including the consumption of highly salted fish and other preserved foods, have been related to nasopharyngeal carcinoma incidence, specifically in the regions where this lesion is endemic. In addition, exposure to formaldehyde, tobacco smoke, alcohol, and various herbal preparations as well as host genetic factors have been implicated in this dramatic migratory effect on the incidence of nasopharyngeal carcinoma (Jeannel et al., 1999).

Hodgkin disease is a form of malignant lymphoma characterized by the presence of abnormal mononuclear cells and their multinucleated variants, termed Reed-Sternberg cells. In addition, the histological picture is quite heterogeneous and variable, with various classifications having been reported (Jackson and Parker, 1944; Lukes et al., 1966). The incidence of Hodgkin disease in western populations is largely bimodal with respect to age (Figure 12.9). Generally, few cases occur among children, but there is a rapid increase in incidence among teenagers, peaking at about age 25. The incidence then decreases to a plateau through middle age, after which rates increase with age to a second peak. In developing countries, Hodgkin disease in childhood is much more common, with the children at risk appearing to be of the lower social class. Epidemiological studies have suggested a role for the Epstein-Barr virus in the causation of Hodgkin disease, since infectious mononucleosis was found to be a significant risk factor for Hodgkin disease in the first 5 years after diagnosis of the former condition (cf. Levin and Levine, 1998). Furthermore, infectious mononucleosis usually occurs in young adulthood, in higher social classes with higher maternal education and lower housing density in childhood; in addition, smaller sibship size is another risk factor for young adulthood Hodgkin disease, all of these factors being indicative of a "late" exposure to an infectious agent (Mueller, 1996). Although a relationship between EBV and Hodgkin disease had been suspected for several decades, the breakthrough for such a causative association came from molecular epidemiology. Assays by a variety of techniques have demonstrated the EBV genome in neoplastic cells of about 30% to 50% of Hodgkin disease cases in western countries; but in South America and the Orient, this proportion may reach 60% to 100%. Thus, the infectious pattern for this disease is quite analogous to that for Burkitt lymphoma in the younger age groups, although the pathogenesis of the EBV induction of Hodgkin disease in older age groups is not clear.

Another relatively unusual neoplasm strongly associated with EBV infection is the sinonasal T-cell lymphoma, also known as lethal midline granuloma or reticulosis. EBV is present in most tumor cells of these neoplasms (IARC, 1997) but is found much less frequently in sinonasal B-cell lymphomas. This neoplasm indicates that EBV may colonize T cells as well as B cells, the latter characteristic of infectious mononucleosis and Burkitt lymphoma. Several other neoplasms have also been associated with EBV with molecular technologies, but for the most part at very low incidence. These include gastric adenocarcinoma and a variety of lymphoepithe-

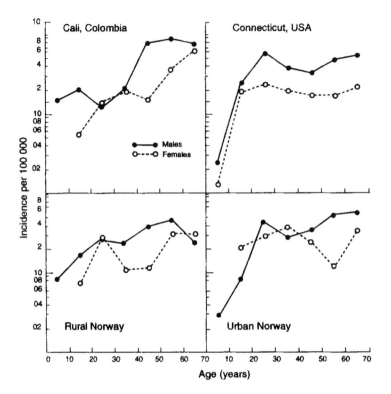

Figure 12.9 Age-specific incidence rates of Hodgkin disease per 100,000 population for each sex as noted in the areas listed in each of the four graphs. The inclusive years studied were as follows: Cali-Colombia, 1962–66; Connecticut, U.S.A., 1960–62; Rural Norway, 1964–66; Urban Norway, 1964–66. (Adapted from IARC, 1997, with permission of the authors and publisher.)

liomas seen in the human (Anagnostopoulos and Hummel, 1996). In addition, EBV may infect certain New World primates, particularly cotton-topped tamarins, with the resultant development of lymphomas (IARC, 1997).

Pathogenesis and Characteristics of EBV Infection in Humans

The Epstein-Barr virus is a member of the herpesvirus family and has also been designated as human herpesvirus 5 or HHV5. The DNA genome of the virus exists in the virion as a double-stranded linear molecule of 172 kb. Figure 12.10 gives an outline of the structure of the EBV genome in its latent or episomal form as it occurs in nonneoplastic lymphoblastoid cells found in all EBV-infected individuals and as it is also found within neoplastic cells of Burkitt lymphoma (Steven, 1997). Although a number of proteins are produced by the virus and more than 100 coded in the genome, within Burkitt lymphoma cells only the EBNA (EB virus nuclear antigen) 1 is expressed, while in nonneoplastic lymphoblastoid cells a variety of other proteins are expressed as well (cf. Steven, 1997). The proteins (9) expressed in the nonneoplastic, lymphoblastoid cells have a variety of functions involving cell signaling and evasion of the immune system.

The pathogenesis of EBV infection involves the specific molecular interaction between a major membrane antigen on the virus, gp350, and its specific binding to a receptor on the surface of B cells, CD21. CD21 is also a receptor for a component of the complement system involved in host immunity (Chapter 19). In cells not possessing this specific receptor but yet

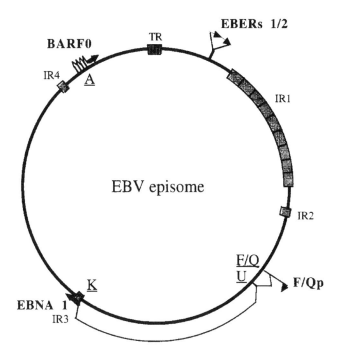

Figure 12.10 Structure of EBV DNA episome indicating patterns of gene transcription during latency in cells of Burkitt's lymphoma. The double-stranded, linear EBV genome within the virion is covalently closed within the episome by overlapping terminal repeat sequences (TR). The genome possesses four internal repeat regions (IR). In bold letters are shown the sites of transcription of genes expressed during the infection. EBV-encoded RNAs (EBERs) are noncoding transcripts which are abundantly expressed in all forms of viral latency. mRNAs are also expressed coding for a putative protein termed BARF0 and a promoter region termed F/Qp. EBNA 1 is the only protein actually shown to be expressed in Burkitt lymphoma cells. (From Steven, 1997; reproduced with permission of the author and publisher.)

capable of infection by EBV, it is thought that the virus is taken up by endocytosis or, in the case of epithelial cells, by interaction with antibodies and subsequently with specific receptors (Lin et al., 1997; Sixbey and Yao, 1992). A diagram of the initial pathogenesis of EBV infection is in Figure 12.11. Lymphoblastoid B cells that have been rendered "immortal" by infection with EBV continue to have a number of copies of the virus as episomes within their nuclei. These circles of episomal viral DNA are independent of the host genome but replicate appropriately during the cell cycle. Rarely, the EBV genome can also persist by integrating into chromosomal DNA (cf. IARC, 1997). Integration into host cell DNA is seen more commonly in cultured cell lines of lymphoid cells (Lawrence et al., 1988; Matsuo et al., 1984). The presence of the virus and its products drives the proliferation of these cells, but their number is controlled by the primary immune response of T cells (Chapter 19) in normal individuals. However, in carriers, a small number of lymphoblastoid EBV-infected B cells continue to survive and evade the immune system. In contrast, in primary infections where the proliferating B cells initially overcome the immune response, infectious mononucleosis may result, with the vast majority of cells in the blood being activated T cells programmed to eliminate EBV-infected cells. Sugden (1994) has reported that only one infectious particle of EBV is necessary for the infection of a single B cell to yield indefinitely proliferating, latently infected "immortalized" progeny. However, the mechanism of the transformation to neoplasia resulting in the various neoplasms noted in Table

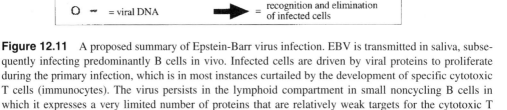

First infection
(eg. infectious mononucleosis)

Long-term infection
(eg. most healthy adults)

Figure 12.11 A proposed summary of Epstein-Barr virus infection. EBV is transmitted in saliva, subsequently infecting predominantly B cells in vivo. Infected cells are driven by viral proteins to proliferate during the primary infection, which is in most instances curtailed by the development of specific cytotoxic T cells (immunocytes). The virus persists in the lymphoid compartment in small noncycling B cells in which it expresses a very limited number of proteins that are relatively weak targets for the cytotoxic T cells. Infected B cells may also enter a productive cycle, leading to the release of infective virus in saliva. Both noncycling and proliferative cells are susceptible to the host immune surveillance. (From Steven, 1997, with permission of the author and publishers.)

12.7 is not absolutely clear. Whereas the number of viral episomes found in the lymphoblastoid B cells is relatively low (5 to 100 per cell) (Steven, 1997), in Burkitt lymphoma cells as well as in cells of nonneoplastic conditions such as oral "hairy" leukoplakia, 200 or more viral DNA molecules per cellular genome may be found in lymphoblastoid B cells (Greenspan et al., 1985).

The Immune System and the Development of EBV-Induced Neoplasms

The response to EBV infection by the development of neoplasms seen in young Africans and in people of several other underdeveloped countries—in contrast to the self-limiting infectious mononucleosis resulting from EBV infection in western countries having relatively high standards of hygiene—suggests that host immune functions may play a role in these differential responses to the same infectious agent. Support for such a thesis was forthcoming in the description by Purtilo and others of the very high incidence of lymphomas in patients with genetic immunodeficiencies, especially in a condition known as the X-linked lymphoproliferative syndrome (cf. Purtilo, 1981). In this condition, the development of infectious mononucleosis may lead to the further development of atypical lymphoproliferative disease and lymphomas; the latter condition occurs in up to 25% of affected individuals. Logically, one would also expect to find EBV-induced lymphomas in adults whose immune system has been significantly compromised. This is true in that organ-transplant recipients may develop EBV-induced lymphoproliferative disease, of which lymphomas are a significant portion (Lucas et al., 1997). Such EBV-induced diseases may occur in as many as 35% of transplant recipients, while in a series of pediatric liver transplants, the occurrence ranged from 9% to 14% (cf. Lucas et al., 1997; Renard et al., 1991; Malatack et al., 1991). Even in patients developing lymphomas without any clinical evidence of altered immune function, a significant number of EBV genomes may be found in the neoplastic cells (IARC, 1997; Aozasa et al., 1998). Another example of acquired immunodeficiency in the human is that of the disease AIDS. It has been reported that between 10% and 20% of individuals with AIDS will have B-cell lymphoma as either their initial or their subsequent AIDS-defining condition (Aboulafia, 1998). However, the presence of the Epstein-Barr virus within neoplastic cells of these lesions varies dramatically all the way to 100% in some series (IARC, 1997). The pathogenesis of non-Hodgkin lymphomas in AIDS patients appears to be similar to that of posttransplant lymphoproliferative disorders involving an initial EBV-driven proliferation of B cells, leading eventually to the outgrowth of fully malignant lymphomas (Gaidano and Dalla-Favera, 1995). It has also been suggested that a subtype of EBV, termed type 2, may be the predominant infectious agent in lymphomas arising in immunocompromised individuals (De Re et al., 1993). In any event, it is clear that the immune system plays a major role in the pathogenesis of EBV infection in the human, leading either to benign infections exhibiting little or no clinical abnormalities that make up the vast majority or to a variety of different neoplasms, predominantly those involving cells of the immune system. Strategies and attempts have also been developed to produce an effective vaccine against infection with the virus (Moss et al., 1996; Spring et al., 1996), but to date no general success has been achieved.

Hepatitis Viruses and Human Cancer—Hepatitis B

The first suggestion that the hepatitis B virus (HBV) might be related causally to genesis of human hepatocellular carcinoma (HCC) was made by Payet et al. (1956). Subsequently it was recognized that chronic viral hepatitis was a frequent sequela of HBV infection on the basis of the identification of viral surface antigens in patients with chronic viral hepatitis. Today it is estimated that there are nearly 300 million individuals chronically infected with HBV. A map indicating the areas where infection predominates is seen in Figure 12.12 (IARC, 1994a). Generally speaking, the highest incidence of HCC is also found in the areas exhibiting the highest incidence of chronic HBV hepatitis (Melnick, 1983). Furthermore, almost every patient with HCC in highly endemic areas (but not in the United States) exhibits serological and virological evidence of hepatitis B infection. Since it is not possible to eliminate chronic infection completely and the incubation period for the development of HBV-associated HCC may be as long as 30 years, the potential incidence of HCC as a result of this chronic infection is very high, approaching 40% in some areas (cf. Chisari and Ferrari, 1995). Today liver cancer ranks sixth of the most common, potentially fatal cancers in the world (Chapter 1). The reason for these distinctive differences in incidence of HBV infection and HCC is seen diagrammatically in Figure 12.13. In several Asian countries, notably Taiwan, hepatitis B is frequently passed from mother to infant, resulting in very early infections; almost all of these infants subsequently become

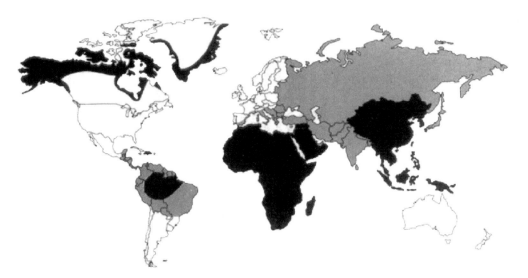

Figure 12.12 Geographical pattern of the prevalence of hepatitis B infection in the humans. Black: ≥8%, high; gray: 2% to 7.9%, intermediate; white: <2%, low. (From IARC Monograph 59, 1994, with permission of the publisher.)

chronic carriers. A similar phenomenon occurs in African countries, although the mode of initial transmission is not clear. In nonendemic countries, such as the United States and many European countries, the primary infection that occurs later in life seldom results in the chronic carrier state. HCC is a relatively unusual sequela of the carrier state in nonendemic areas; but in endemic areas such as Taiwan and parts of mainland China, the risk for developing HCC is 200-fold greater than in uninfected individuals (Buendia, 1992). This risk may be increased as much as eightfold if the infected individual is chronically exposed to aflatoxin B_1 as a contaminant in the diet (cf. Groopman et al., 1996). Vaccines against HBV are now readily available but somewhat expensive. Thus far, extensive vaccination programs have not been carried out in most countries with the exception of Taiwan, where there is evidence of the prevention of cancer by the vaccine when it is administered to children (cf. Wild and Hall, 1999).

Pathogenesis and Cell Biology of HBV Infection

HBV belongs to a group of hepatotropic DNA viruses known as the hepadnaviruses, which are found in a number of mammalian and avian species (Chapter 4). A diagram of the structure of the virus shows the major antigens (Ags) to which the host develops antibodies. The DNA genome is small, about 3200 bp, and occurs as a circular complete minus (–) strand with a complementary plus (+) strand that is incomplete (Chapter 4). As with other animal hepadnaviruses, the virion contains a DNA polymerase/reverse transcriptase that is utilized during its complex life cycle, as described in more detail in Chapter 4. Since the life cycle of the virus involves an RNA intermediate, as in retroviruses, one might expect to find integrated viral DNA in the host genome. This is true, although in many instances the integration of the viral genome into host cell DNA appears to involve rearrangement and recombination of the viral genome (Takada et al., 1990; Zhou et al., 1987). Other studies have indicated that incorporation of the viral genome into the host genome results in genetic instability of the host cell genome (Hino et al., 1991; Matsuzaki et al., 1997), indicating that virus infection in the hepatocyte may mimic the action of a progressor agent (Chapter 9). Although there is no known "oncogene" within the HBV

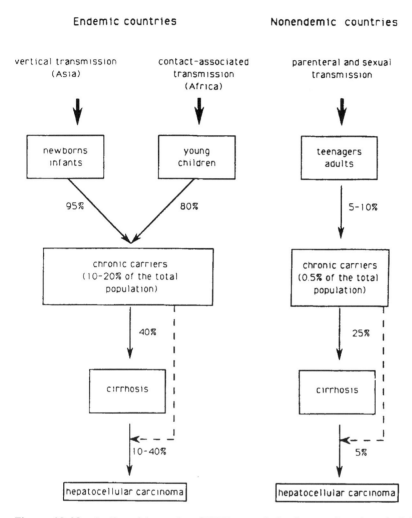

Endemic countries   Nonendemic countries

vertical transmission   contact-associated   parenteral and sexual
        (Asia)   transmission   transmission
                                  (Africa)

newborns   young   teenagers
infants   children   adults

95%   80%   5-10%

chronic carriers   chronic carriers
(10-20% of the total   (0.5% of the total
population)   population)

40%   25%

cirrhosis   cirrhosis

10-40%   5%

hepatocellular carcinoma   hepatocellular carcinoma

Figure 12.13 Outline of the modes of HBV transmission in countries where the infection is endemic as compared with where it is non-endemic. The rates of progression to chronicity and the HCC incidence in endemic and non-endemic regions are noted in the figure as % of the population affected. (Adapted from Buendia, 1992, with permission of the author and publisher.)

genome, an interesting gene termed the *X gene*, giving rise to a protein with a similar designation, occurs in all hepadnaviruses. Mutation of the X gene results in loss of viral replication in the animal host (cf. Yen, 1996). The X protein functions as a transcriptional transactivator for a number of cellular genes (cf. Koike and Takada, 1995) and may also be involved in the processes of cellular DNA repair (Feitelson and Duan, 1997; Prost et al., 1998) and signal transduction (Cong et al., 1997).

As noted above, chronic infection with HBV is a prolonged, lifelong process that may be dramatically modified by appropriate therapy (Hoofnagle and di Bisceglie, 1997; Terrault, 1996) but probably never completely cured. The natural history of HBV infection, leading ultimately to cirrhosis and/or hepatocellular carcinoma, is seen in Figure 12.15. Furthermore, it is quite likely that the immune response of the host to the chronic infection with HBV plays a major role

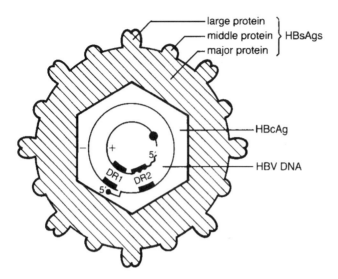

Figure 12.14   Diagrammatic structure of the hepatitis B virus. The envelope is noted as consisting of several proteins, which are the surface antigens to which antibodies are produced. The nucleocapsid core contains the partially double-stranded viral genome and the DNA polymerase/reverse transcriptase (large, filled circle). The boxes indicate the positions of direct repeats (DR1 and DR2). The core antigen protein (HbcAg) may also serve as an antigen for the host immune system. (Adapted from Blum et al., 1989, with permission of the authors and publisher.)

in the ultimate development of hepatocellular carcinoma. Transgenic mice that overproduce the hepatitis B virus large-envelope polypeptide and accumulate toxic quantities of hepatitis B surface antigen within the hepatocyte develop extensive, prolonged hepatocellular injury involving inflammation, regenerative hyperplasia, aneuploidy, and ultimately hepatocellular carcinoma (Chisari et al., 1989). This finding has implied that the immune response induced by HBV infection is perhaps equal to or more important in the development of hepatocellular carcinoma in the human than is the integration of the viral genome into the host DNA (Chisari and Ferrari, 1995). Thus, the immune response resulting in chronic viral hepatitis, cell proliferation, and apoptosis may be analogous to tumor promotion in rodent hepatocarcinogenesis (Chapter 7), and the progressor action of the virus transits such promoted cells into the stage of progression and malignant neoplasia in the human host.

Herpes Simplex Viruses and Human Cancer

In 1972 a report by Frenkel et al. (1972) demonstrated the presence of a portion of herpes simplex II viral DNA within a human cervical neoplasm. Since that time, a number of investigations have demonstrated the presence of fragments of the herpes simplex genome within human genital neoplasms (Macnab, 1987), but the significance of such findings in the genesis of human genital neoplasia is not clear, especially in view of the demonstrated importance of the human papilloma virus in the development of such neoplasms (see below). Transfection experiments both in vivo (Anthony et al., 1989) and in vitro (DiPaolo et al., 1990) have demonstrated the oncogenic potential of herpes simplex DNA in lower animals, but epidemiologic studies have not indicated that a direct causal association between herpes simplex virus infection and genital cancer occurs in the human (Melnick et al., 1976; Graham et al., 1982). Somewhat more recently, Di Luca et al. (1995) have proposed that herpes simplex virus may function as a "cooper-

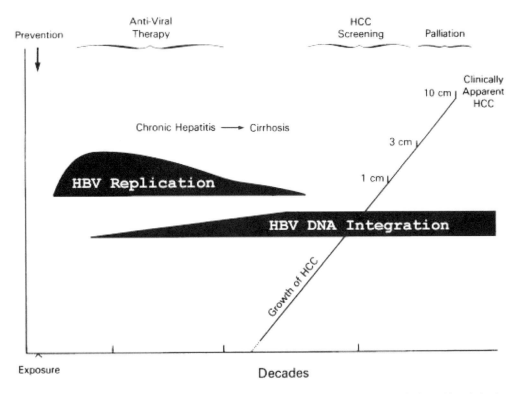

Figure 12.15 Diagram of the natural history of HBV infection leading to chronic hepatitis, cirrhosis, and hepatocellular carcinoma (HCC). Possible interventions are noted at the top of the figure. Note that while HBV replication occurs early in the disease, integration into DNA and the potential for genomic instability occur in parallel with the development of HCC. (Adapted from di Bisceglie et al., 1988, with permission of the authors and publisher.)

ating agent" in the development of human genital neoplasia. The virus might act as an initiator or a progressor or even to alter cellular and viral gene expression. As yet, however, these concepts are somewhat theoretical, and the actual role, if any, that herpes simplex virus infection may play in the development of human genital cancer is not clear.

Human Papillomaviruses and Human Cancer

As noted in Chapter 4, papillomaviruses infect a variety of vertebrate species including the human. More than 70 different strains of papillomavirus have been isolated from the human (IARC, 1995). Most of these viruses are associated with a number of human conditions, both benign and malignant. Table 12.8 lists some of the more common strains and their association with specific human diseases. As noted in the table, the most common strains causally associated with human cancer are types 16, 18, 31, and 45, while a number of other strains are associated with the development of benign lesions. The worldwide burden of human papillomavirus (HPV) infections is not known, but zur Hausen (1996) has pointed out that cervical cancer represents the second most frequent malignant neoplasm in women worldwide, corresponding to approximately 450,000 new cases per year or 5.8% of the global cancer incidence. If one accepts that more than 50% of anogenital cancers and 20% of oral, laryngeal, and nasal cancers contain

Table 12.8 Association of HPV Types with Various Clinical Lesions

Clinical lesion	HPV Types
Common warts (verruca vulgaris)	**2**, 4
Plantar warts	**1**
Flat warts	**3**, 10, 28, 41
Epidermodysplasia verruciformis	**5**, **8**, as well as 9, 12, 14, 15, 17, 19, 20–25, 36–38, 47, and 49
Butcher's warts	7
Condyloma acuminatum (genital warts)	**6**, **11**, 42, 43, 44
Laryngeal papillomatosis	**6**, **11**
LSIL or equivalent	Essentially all mucosotropic types (>24 types)
HSIL	Same as invasive cervical cancer
Invasive cervical cancers	**16**, **18**, **31**, 33, 35, 39, **45**, 51, 52, 56, 58, 59, 66, 67, and 68
Bowenoid high-grade dysplasia	Mainly 16
Invasive squamous cancer of other anogenital sites	Mainly 16

Key: LSIL, low grade squamous intraepithelial lesions; HSIL, high grade squamous intraepithelial lesions.
Boldface numbers indicate those types most commonly associated with the lesion.
Adapted from Stoler, 1996.

the high-risk HPV types, papillomavirus infections may be the cause of almost 10% of the worldwide cancer burden. The IARC (1995) has argued that more than 90% of all cervical cancers are caused by infection with various types of HPV. HPV infection is also quite common in immunocompromised patients such as those with AIDS or transplants. A high rate of association with HPV infections in the skin is seen in the rare, inherited disease known as epidermodysplasia verruciformis. Affected individuals are extremely sensitive to widespread HPV infection in the skin, leading initially to various types of skin warts and to the development of multiple cutaneous malignancies in about half of these infected patients (cf. Majewski and Jablonska, 1992). The genetic defects in the disease may involve two different genes, one of which is X-linked. The development of skin lesions also depends on cocarcinogenic effects of ultraviolet radiation and presumably some defect in the major histocompatibility complex and tumor necrosis factor locus and antigen presentation (Chapter 18). In homosexual men with AIDS, the relative risk of developing anorectal cancer associated with HPV may range up to 80% (IARC, 1995). Similarly, more than half in a series of renal transplant patients exhibiting nonmelanoma carcinomas of the skin had evidence of HPV infection in the neoplasms (Shamanin et al., 1996). As might be expected, human papillomaviruses are commonly found in normal skin of immunocompetent hosts (Astori et al., 1998).

By far the most common human neoplasm associated with HPV infection is carcinoma of the uterine cervix. The presence of HPV has been noted both in cervical dysplasia as well as in cervical intraepithelial neoplasia (CIN). Although HPV-associated cervical dysplasia and low-grade CIN may spontaneously regress (Kataja et al., 1989), persistent HPV infection is associated with persistent cervical dysplasia (Ho et al., 1995); in higher grades of CIN, the incidence of HPV infection increases (Bergeron et al., 1992). Other risk factors associated with cervical HPV infections include current smoking, warts in sexual partners, and increasing frequency of sexual intercourse per week, especially with different partners (Kataja et al., 1993; Tortolero-Luna, 1999).

Pathogenesis of HPV Infection

HPV is structurally very closely related to the lower animal papillomaviruses (Chapter 4). Unlike HCV (above), the viral genome is relatively stable, with only 1% of genomic variability originating over periods exceeding 10^5 years (cf. IARC, 1995). HPVs are highly specific for the human, but as yet it has not been possible to readily infect human cells in culture with HPV; consequently molecular investigations must be done with transfected cells or in artificial human transplants to athymic mice (Kreider et al., 1986). In preoplastic cervical dysplasia and many CINs, papillomaviruses occur in the circular episomal form; but in malignant neoplasms, integration of the viral genome into the host cell DNA is the rule. A diagram of the organization of the HPV genome and its pattern of integration is seen in Figure 12.16. In comparison with the genome of animal papillomaviruses (Chapter 4), the organization is quite similar, although the integration structure may vary in some neoplasms (Stoler, 1996). Of the genes noted in the figure, E5, E6, and E7 are associated with growth stimulation and the transformation process. L1 and L2 are capsid proteins, and the other E genes are concerned with viral replication and transcription (Chapter 4). Thus far, in vitro systems for infection of cells in culture and development of vaccines to HPV have not been developed. On the other hand, transgenic mice expressing one

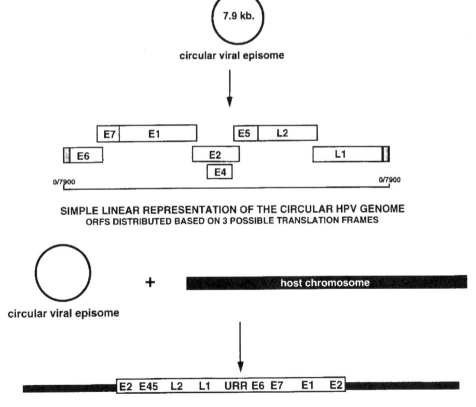

Figure 12.16 Organization of the HPV genome and pattern of its integration. In low-grade lesions the circular episomal form is dominant. In most neoplasms integration occurs randomly in the host genome, although the viral genome is usually disrupted in the E2 open reading frame, leading to loss of E2 protein transregulatory functions. (After Stoler, 1996, with permission of the author and publisher.)

or more of the critical genes have the potential to increase our knowledge of the pathogenesis and possible immunology of the virus infection (Griep and Lambert, 1994).

The natural history of the development of cervical cancer has been studied in several epidemiological investigations (cf. IARC, 1995; Melbye and Frisch, 1998). A peak incidence of HPV infection is observed among women aged 20 to 25 years, followed by another peak of high-grade cervical lesions 5 to 10 years later. The incidence of cancer of the cervix declines in women over 50 years of age, after which time increasing incidences of vulvar, penile, and anal cancer, many of which are associated with HPV infection, are seen (Figure 12.17). However, studies in both immunodeficient and immunocompetent women have indicated that HPV infection is followed by the development of dysplastic and intraepithelial neoplasia, the latter ultimately developing into invasive carcinoma. This model of HPV pathogenesis suggests that the virus may serve as a promoting agent during its episomal life, transforming into a progressor agent upon integration of the viral genome into the host cell genome (Kashyap and Das, 1998).

Human Herpesvirus 8 and Human Cancer

We have already seen the actual and potential role of herpesviruses in the causation of human cancer. EBV was among the first definitive human cancer-causing viruses, and the herpes simplex group has been suggested but not proven to have a role in the development of cervical cancer in the human. In 1994 Chang et al. demonstrated the presence of a human herpesvirus, now termed HHV-8 or Kaposi sarcoma–associated herpesvirus (KSHV), in all epidemiological forms of Kaposi sarcoma, an angiosarcoma found worldwide but most recently at an extremely high incidence in AIDS patients, which is 7000 times higher than in the non-AIDS population (Emmanoulides et al., 1996). HHV-8 genomes have also been consistently found in primary effusion lymphoma (PEL) and multicentric Castleman disease (MCD). Originally, PEL was confused with the form of Burkitt lymphoma seen in western nations, involving primarily

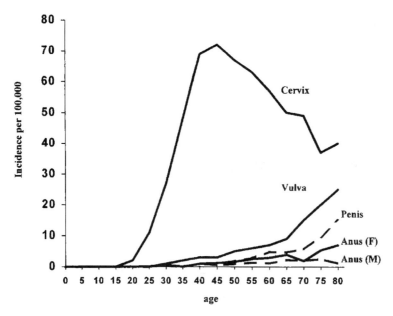

Figure 12.17   Age-specific incidence of cervical, vulvar, anal, and penile cancer in the Danish population. (After Melbye and Frisch, 1998, with permission of the authors and publisher.)

abdominal lymphoid structures. However, closer investigation revealed clear differences between the two and particularly in the viral genomes involved. The virus has also been found in several benign and malignant endothelial lesions in patients with Kaposi's sarcoma (Dictor et al., 1996). In addition, in other studies the presence of HHV-8 sequences was seen in premalignant Bowen disease (71.4%) and malignant squamous cell carcinoma (50%), as well as in 33.3% of actinic keratoses (Inagi et al., 1996). In addition, McDonagh et al. (1996) reported the presence of HHV-8 sequences in 29% of angiosarcomas in patients, most of whom were not immunocompromised. Transmission of HHV-8 in AIDS patients appears to be largely by sexual means. However, in Africa, both horizontal and vertical transmission of HHV-8 is quite common among young children (cf. Schulz, 1999). Although the presence of the virus in Kaposi sarcoma, PEL, and MCD argues very strongly that there is a causative association between infection and the neoplastic transformation, other data are also supportive of this argument. Flore et al. (1998) demonstrated the transformation of primary human endothelial cells by HHV-8 in vitro. In addition, the relationship of the presence of antibodies to HHV-8–associated latent nuclear antigens (see below) in relation to the development of Kaposi sarcoma strongly indicates a direct causative relationship (Figure 12.18).

HHV-8 Characterization and Pathogenesis of Virus Associated Human Neoplasms

The genome of HHV-8 consists of a 140.5-kb length of DNA unique coding region flanked by multiple G+C-rich 801-bp terminal repeat sequences (Russo et al., 1996). The genome contains a number of "pirated" genes that have very close cellular homologs in a manner analogous to that seen with retrovirally transduced oncogenes (Chapter 4). Table 12.9 lists several of these genes with their cellular homolog and possible function (Boshoff and Weiss, 1998). However, expression of the viral genome in Kaposi's sarcoma is quite limited (Zhong et al., 1996). One of the genes expressed is analogous to transforming proteins found in other herpesviruses and may be related to transformation by HHV-8 (Lee et al., 1998). Latently infected cells have multiple copies of circularized HHV-8 DNA maintained as episomes in a manner similar to that of EBV (cf. Ballestas et al., 1999). A latency-associated nuclear antigen appears to mediate the efficient

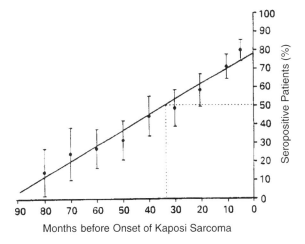

Figure 12.18 Estimated prevalence of serum antibodies against HHV-8–associated latent nuclear antigens in 40 patients with AIDS-associated Kaposi sarcoma in relation to the number of months prior to the diagnosis of the neoplasm. (After Gao et al., 1996, with permission of the authors and publisher.)

Table 12.9 Potential Functions of Pirated KSHV Genes

Viral Gene	Cellular Homolog	Possible Function
K1	—	Promote cellular growth
ORF 4	CD46	Complement regulation
K2	IL-6	Lymphocyte growth promotion
K4, K4.1 and K6	vMIP-I, -III	Paracrine growth and angiogenesis
ORF 16	Bcl-2	Prevents apoptosis
K9	IRF[a]	Promote growth, immunoregulatory
K12	—	? Transactivator
ORF 71	DED domain proteins	Prevent apoptosis
ORF 72	Cyclin D	Promote cellular growth
ORF 73 (LNA-1)	—	? Transactivator
ORF 74	IL-8 GPCR[b]	Promote cellular growth
K14	NCAM-like protein	Intercellular signaling

[a]Interferon regulatory family.
[b]G protein–coupled receptor homolog.
Adapted from Boshoff and Weiss, 1998, with permission of the authors and publisher.

persistence of extrachromosomal DNA of HHV-8 in the same way that the EBV nuclear antigen performs this function (Ballestas et al., 1999). As noted in Table 12.9, a number of the pirated genes code for proteins involved in cell growth and death. This may actually serve to modulate the growth of neoplastic, latently infected cells of Kaposi sarcoma and other HHV-8–induced neoplasms (Dittmer and Kedes, 1998). A model of the pathogenesis of Kaposi sarcoma is seen in Figure 12.19, indicating the production of various growth factors and related proteins in cells early during infection, with subsequent transformation to sarcoma cells and continued production of autocrine growth factor (Emmanoulides et al., 1996). HHV-8 may also induce lysis of infected cells with production of virus (Ensoli and Sirianni, 1998). This model of the pathogenesis of the development of Kaposi sarcoma after infection with HHV-8 is quite analogous to that for the development of Burkitt lymphoma after infection with EBV except for the fact that, based on present knowledge, it is unlikely that there is a high incidence of subclinical infections with HHV-8 in the general population throughout the world.

Papovaviruses in Relation to Human Disease

As noted in Table 12.7, herpes, hepatitis, and papilloma viruses constitute the major infectious causes of human neoplasms. However, the search for papovaviruses as etiological agents in human neoplasia was pursued intensively for several decades. The first indication for a role of papovaviruses in human disease was the observation by Zu Rhein and Chou (1965) of the presence of papovavirus-like particles in the nuclei of glial cells from patients with a rare demyelinating disease, progressive multifocal leukoencephalopathy (PML). Later studies by these workers and their colleagues (Padgett et al., 1971) allowed the cultivation of papovaviruses from the brain of a patient with PML. Subsequently, this virus has been termed the JC virus, and it is closely related to other papovaviruses such as the simian virus 40. The majority of patients with PML exhibit some impairment of the T-cell immune response (Chapter 18). As many as 4% of patients with AIDS will have PML, while up to 85% of all new cases of PML will have AIDS (cf. Tornatore et al., 1994). In PML, the JC virus infects oligodendrogliocytes, cells responsible for the myelination of nerve axons in the central nervous system. Destruction of these cells leads to

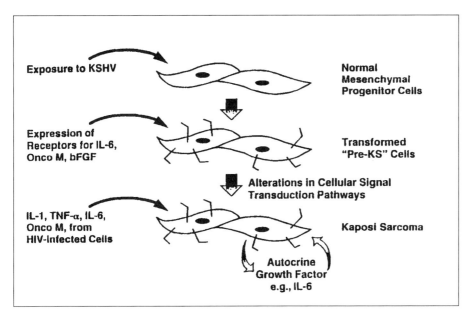

Figure 12.19 Model of the pathogenesis of Kaposi sarcoma. bFGF, basic fibroblast growth factor; IL, interleukin; KSHV, Kaposi sarcoma–associated herpesvirus; Onco M, oncostatin M; TNF-α, tumor necrosis factor-alpha. (From Emmanoulides et al., 1996, with permission of the authors and publisher.)

the loss of myelin in axons and disruption of normal function in the central nervous system (Aksamit, 1995).

The JC virus also induces a variety of neoplasms in rodents, especially hamsters, and can also infect a variety of cultured cells (Zu Rhein, 1987; cf. Major et al., 1992). In addition, brain tumors have been induced in monkeys inoculated with the JC virus (London et al., 1978). A closely related virus, the BK virus, is commonly present in normal individuals, but there is little or no evidence that the virus is involved in the causation of human disease (Wold et al., 1978). However, a recent study by Flægstad et al. (1999) detected BK virus DNA in all of a series of 18 human neuroblastomas.

In support of a potential role for papovaviruses in the causation of specific human neoplasms, some evidence has been reported for the presence of simian virus 40 DNA in several different types of human brain neoplasms (Krieg et al., 1981; Bergsagel et al., 1992; Martini et al., 1996) and in malignant mesotheliomas (Testa et al., 1998). At least one group (Bergsagel et al., 1992) has suggested that there may be a causal relationship between these viruses and the genesis of these brain tumors involving papovavirus genomes present in those human neoplasms. One possible source of infection is suggested to be through inadvertent inoculation of humans with the simian virus 40 that had contaminated vaccines against other viruses used between 1955 and 1963 (Carbone et al., 1997). However, Strickler et al. (1998) reported an extensive retrospective epidemiologic study that showed no association between exposure to simian virus 40-contaminated poliovirus vaccine and increased rates of brain neoplasms, sarcomas, or mesotheliomas.

Although the JC and BK virus, when infecting rodent cells, become incorporated into the DNA with subsequent transformation to the neoplastic state (cf. Major et al., 1992), JC virus in brains and kidneys of patients with PML is not integrated into the host cell genome (Grinnell et al., 1983). Thus, while there is no question that the JC virus causes PML, the relation, if any, of papovaviruses to the causation of human neoplasia remains an unanswered question with relatively little supporting data for such an association at the present time.

RNA Viruses and Human Cancer

Although the association of DNA viruses causally with human cancer has been known for more than four decades, it is only within the last 15 years or so that a causative association between specific RNA viruses and human neoplasia has been elucidated. The viruses involved are the hepatitis C virus and two retroviruses, human immunodeficiency virus and human T cell lymphotropic virus. Literally millions of humans are infected at the present time with these three different virus types, and the prospects for control and prevention are not bright at the present time.

Hepatitis Viruses and Human Cancer—Hepatitis C

While hepatitis B infection has been known or at least suspected as a cause of chronic viral hepatitis and HCC for nearly half a century, the nature of hepatitis C virus as a cause for the same two conditions has been reasonably understood only for the last decade. Prior to that time, patients with chronic viral hepatitis who did not exhibit evidence of hepatitis A or B infection were classified as infected with non-A, non-B (NANB) hepatitis virus (cf. Purcell, 1994). Cloning and sequencing of the hepatitis C virus genome, reported in 1989 (Choo et al., 1989), allowed for accelerated progress in our understanding of the nature of this virus and the pathogenesis of its effects in the human. The virus is quite infectious, with more than 50% of exposed individuals developing chronic infection. However, infection occurs almost entirely by the parenteral route with the most common mode of transmission involving transfusions and/or parenteral contact with blood products (Heintges and Wands, 1997). The proportions of the modes of viral infection are seen in Figure 12.20. Blood transfusion, illicit intravenous drug use, and similar high-risk behavior accounts for 90% of HCV infections. Prior to 1990, when blood testing for HCV

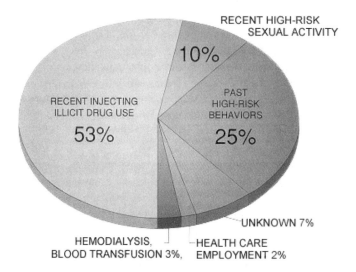

Figure 12.20 Risk factors associated with HCV infections in the human. (From Koff, 1998, with permission of the author and publisher.)

began nationally, the transmission from blood transfusions was probably proportionally much higher than seen in Figure 12.20 (Alter, 1997). Antibodies to viral proteins are indicative of viral infection. The prevalence of such antibodies in blood donors in the world is seen in Figure 12.21. Although very high levels of infection are noted in regions of Africa, the Ukraine, and Vietnam, other areas including western countries exhibit significant levels of infection in the general population. In Japan, where HCV infection in relation to HCC development has been investigated, the risk of HCC among HCV carriers was 30% for males between the ages of 45 and 64 years and 6% for females between the ages of 50 and 64 years (cf. Tanaka and Tsukuma, 1999). These studies indicate that HCV carriers have an extremely high probability of developing HCC, and their lifetime risk for this disease is comparable to or greater than the risk of HBV carriers. In addition to HCV infection as a cause of HCC, the virus has also been implicated in the pathogenesis of low-grade non-Hodgkin lymphomas, especially those producing extensive amounts of cryoglobulins, a specific form of immunoglobulin-like molecules (cf. Silvestri and Baccarani, 1997; Pozzato et al., 1996). HCV has been found in bone marrow and lymphoid cells of infected patients and may cause B-cell clonal expansion (Santini et al., 1998). Infections with both HBV and HCC have been found in patients with hepatocellular carcinoma, but usually representing a relatively small percentage of the total, 1.6% to 3% in two different series (Tanaka and Tsukuma, 1999; Hadziyannis et al., 1995).

Pathogenesis and Cell Biology of HCV Infection

Hepatitis C virus is a positive-strand RNA virus related to the flaviviruses on the basis of molecular and biophysical characteristics (cf. IARC, 1994). A diagrammatic characterization of the virion and its genome and genomic products is seen in Figure 12.22. After infection, the positive-strand RNA of the virus is translated by ribosomes producing the various proteins, including the RNA-dependent RNA polymerase necessary for the production of the minus strand and subsequent replication to produce the positive strand that interacts with the various structural proteins and is released from the cell by a budding mechanism (Koff, 1998). The core protein (p21,

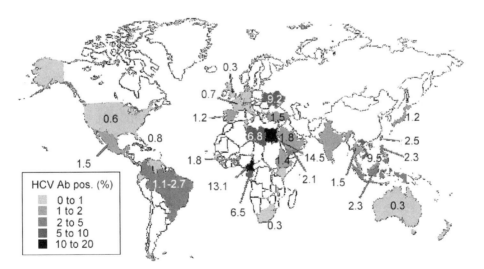

Figure 12.21 World map illustrating the prevalence of antibodies to hepatitis C virus (HCV) in blood donors measured by modern technologies. (From Heintges and Wands, 1997, with permission of the authors and publisher.)

Hepatitis C Virus

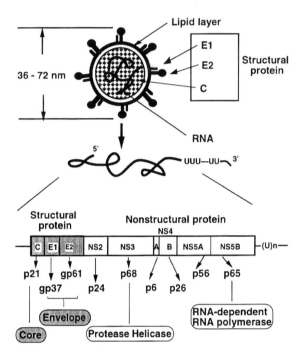

Figure 12.22 Schematic features of the HCV virion, its RNA, and functional products thereof. (After Esumi and Shikata, 1994; modified by authors with newer findings.

Figure 12.22) is the antigen inducing the predominant antigenic response in patients with hepatocellular carcinoma (Watanabe et al., 1991), and there is some evidence that this protein has the ability to transform rat fibroblasts in culture as well as to suppress apoptosis (cf. DiBisceglie, 1997). A number of different genotypes of the virus have been reported and are now classified into types I to VI with various subtypes (IARC, 1994). The host range or species specificity of HCV infection is limited to humans and chimpanzees. The nucleotide divergence of the various genotypes may be as high as 20%, and there is substantial evidence that the virus exhibits extreme genetic variability with an estimated rate of nucleotide change of 10^{-3} substitution/site year (cf. Bréchot, 1997). Such extreme genetic variability, which is comparable to that seen with the AIDS virus (see below), markedly reduces the effectiveness of the development of any vaccine for the virus infection. Still, the viral gene products are quite immunogenic and are associated with chronic infection of the target organ, the liver, ultimately leading to cirrhosis and HCC. Since the HCV genome does not integrate into the host cell genome but its gene products may serve to transactivate cellular genes (e.g., Ray et al., 1997), the virus serves the function of a complex promoting agent in inducing HCC.

Retroviruses and Human Cancer

Two retroviral types from each of two subfamilies, the lentiviruses and the oncoviruses, have been associated with human neoplasia. In the lentivirus subfamily of retroviruses (Chapter 4), human immunodeficiency virus types 1 and 2 (HIV-1; HIV-2) induce human diseases involving immunodeficiency and wasting syndromes. In the oncovirus subfamily, human T-cell lympho-tropic viruses (HTLV) types I and II have been associated causally or by association only, re-spectively (IARC, 1996), with human disease. In Figure 12.23 may be seen diagrammatic representations of the genomic structures of the HIV-1 virus and of HTLV-I. Because of exten-sive investigation, many of the functions of the various genes of HIV-1 are known, as evidenced from the figure. The *tax* and *rex* genes in HTLV-I may be considered as analogs of the *tat* and *rev* genes in HIV-1. Note that these viral genomes are significantly more complicated than those discussed in Chapter 4, involving a variety of oncogenes that had been transduced into a variety of retroviruses, both in the natural state and artificially. The analogous genes—such as *tat*, *rev*, *tax*, and *rex*—do not appear to have counterparts in the mammalian genome. Furthermore, HIV functions to kill specific cells of the immune system, causing a release of virus, while HTLV infection in cells stimulates cell growth while allowing the production of infectious virus.

HIV and Human Cancer

HIV is the cause of acquired immunodeficiency syndrome (AIDS), a slowly debilitating, almost always fatal, human disease. The disease has been recognized relatively recently as a specific entity, and in 1985 criteria for the diagnosis of AIDS were developed (cf. Purtilo et al., 1986). Since then, the disease has increased dramatically in numbers throughout the world. As of mid-1993, the estimated distribution of HIV infections in adults throughout the world is shown in Figure 12.24 (Merson, 1993). Although there is no definitive evidence that the HIV virus actu-ally transforms cells to neoplasia unaided by other viruses, the IARC has stated that infection with HIV-1 is carcinogenic to humans, while infection with HIV-2 is possibly carcinogenic to humans (IARC, 1996). We have already noted above the dramatic increase in Kaposi sarcoma seen in AIDS patients and resulting from infection and transformation of cells with HHV-8 (see above). A listing of neoplasms developing in AIDS patients at levels significantly higher than those of the average population is seen in Table 12.10. In general, "non-AIDS" cancers exhibit an increased risk of 1.9 in a large series of AIDS patients recently studied (Goedert et al., 1998). The vast majority of AIDS-related lymphomas are associated with EBV infections (Gaidano and Dalla-Favera, 1995). Increased incidences of many of the other neoplasms seen in the table may be related to infection with other potentially oncogenic herpesviruses or, more likely, with the dramatically compromised immune system, allowing the growth of neoplasms that otherwise might have been suppressed by a normal immune response (Chapter 18).

Characteristics and Pathogenesis of HIV and Its Infection

The genome of HIV as noted in Figure 12.23 has a number of genes and genetic elements that involve both viral replication and the virus's interaction with the infected cell. The predominant cell types infected by the virus through specific receptors are the "helper" (CD4) T cell (Chapter 18) and the macrophage (Greenberg, 1992). As a retrovirus, the DNA copy integrated into the cell genome may remain dormant in the cell for extended periods, but in most instances the in-fected cell produces an altered array of its normal products as a result of the infection as well as producing multiple new virions with the ultimate demise of the cell (Shearer, 1998). However, there is no firm evidence that HIV viruses actually transform cells that they infect, and thus the carcinogenic influence of the virus is indirect, compromising the immune system and allowing infection by a variety of other oncogenic viruses as well as the expression of neoplasms nor-mally suppressed by the host immune system (Chapter 18). Therapy of AIDS has been directed toward preventing viral replication by use of inhibitors of the reverse transcriptase and the pro-tease, both required for viral synthesis. While dramatic therapeutic effects have been obtained, the genetic variation of HIV ultimately results in the development of a resistant viral strain

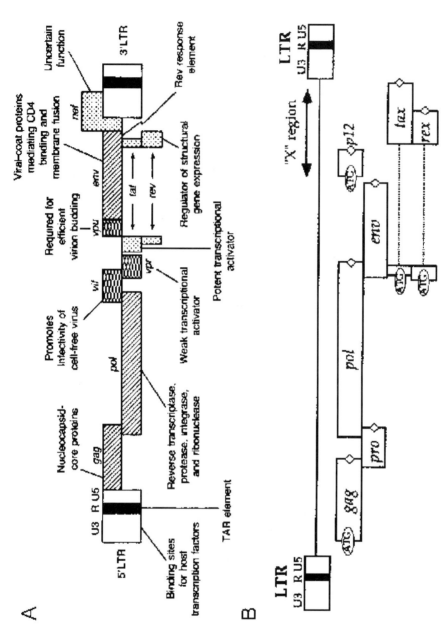

Figure 12.23 A. Genomic structure of HIV-1, indicating most of the known genes and their recognized primary functions. The 5' and 3' long terminal repeats (LTR) containing regulatory sequences recognized by various host transcription factors are also depicted. (Adapted from Greene, 1991, with permission of the author and publisher.) B. Genomic organization of HTLV-I. Long terminal repeats (LTR) and open reading frames are depicted with the translational start (ATG) and stop codons (diamonds) indicated. (X) denotes intragenic region containing multiple short open reading frames. (After Ferreira et al., 1997, with permission of the authors and publisher.)

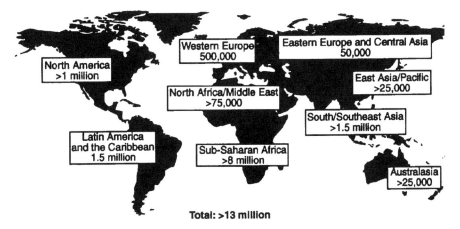

Figure 12.24 Estimated distribution of cumulative HIV infections in adults in various parts of the world as of mid-1993. (Adapted from Merson, 1993, with permission of the author and publisher.)

within the patient (Arts et al., 1998; Ridky and Leis, 1995). Since RNA viruses are deficient in specific proofreading mechanisms of the reverse transcriptase, replication errors that occur become immortalized, as can be seen in the genetic variation in viruses in patients in vivo (Hahn et al., 1986; Nowak et al., 1991). Mutation rates of the virus have been estimated at 3×10^{-4} to 3×10^{-5} per base per round of replication (Pezo and Wain-Hobson, 1997). Such rates of mutation are close to the maximum possible. Thus, it is not surprising that vaccines against the virus have been relatively unsuccessful in preventing infection in primates. These molecular facts bode ill for any lasting method of vaccination or therapeutic cure of the established disease, emphasizing the primary role of prevention in the control of AIDS in the world.

HTLV and Human Lymphomas

Like HIV infection, infection with HTLV is also worldwide, as noted in Figure 12.25. However, unlike HIV, sequence conservation is the rule in viral infections throughout the world, with the

Table 12.10 AIDS-Associated Malignant Neoplasms

	Relative Risk[a]
Kaposi sarcoma	310 (292–330)
Non-Hodgkin lymphoma	113 (104–123)
Angiosarcoma	37 (4–133)
Anal carcinoma	32 (12–69)
Leukemia	11 (3–28)
Hodgkin disease	7.6 (4–13)
Soft tissue sarcoma	7 (1.5–21)
Squamous cell carcinoma (unusual sites)	7 (1.4–20)
Multiple myeloma	4.5 (1–13)
Brain	3.5 (1.4–7)
Seminoma	3 (1.1–6)

[a]Average (range).
Adapted from Goedert et al., 1998.

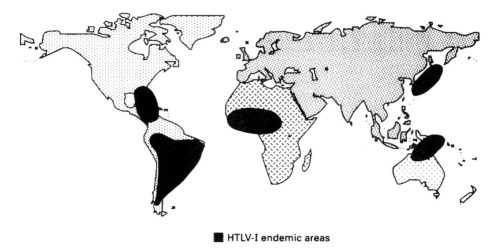

■ HTLV-I endemic areas

Figure 12.25 Worldwide distribution of HTLV-I. (Adapted from Wigdahl and Brady, 1996, with permission of the authors and publisher.)

overall nucleotide divergence of strains being only about 4%, depending on the region of the genome analyzed (cf. Ferreira et al., 1997). HTLV transmission occurs at birth due to infection in mothers or later in life through sexual contact, blood transfusion, and needle sharing, modes quite similar to the transmission of HIV infections. Like HIV, HTLV as a cause of human lymphomas was first reported less than two decades ago (Poiesz et al., 1980). While HIV has an incubation or latent period, usually of several years during which no clinical disease is evident, the incubation period for the development of adult T-cell leukemia/lymphoma after infection with HTLV is probably in the order of decades (Wiktor and Blattner, 1991). Generally, the clinical course of the disease is short, but several variants that induce a chronic disease picture have also been described (cf. Wiktor and Blattner, 1991).

HTLV-I–Associated Myelopathy/Tropical Spastic Paraparesis

In addition to the clear causal association of HTLV-I with adult T-cell leukemia/lymphoma in various parts of the world, in these same areas the virus has also been associated with a chronic progressive demyelinating disease that affects predominantly the spinal cord. This disease reportedly affects between 0.2% and 5% of HTLV-I infected individuals in endemic areas and is more frequent in women than in men (cf. Ferreira et al., 1997). The mechanism whereby some individuals develop tropical spastic paraparesis and not T-cell leukemia is not clear. However, there is some evidence suggestive of genetic factors that may be responsible for these differences (cf. Tajima and Takezaki, 1998). Typically, the onset of tropical spastic paraparesis is in the fourth decade of life, but transfusion of HTLV-I–infected blood may result in development of the condition within as little as 6 months (such a finding argues very strongly for a causative relationship between HTLV-I and tropical spastic paraparesis).

Pathogenesis of HTLV-Induced Lymphoma

HTLV-I efficiently transforms human primary lymphocytes of several varieties to neoplasia both in vivo and in vitro. However, leukemia develops in only a small portion of infected individuals after a long time. Thus, a variety of events in the infected host, including interaction with the immune system and genetic factors, probably play roles in the ultimate pathogenesis of the disease itself. Viral genes, particularly the *tax* gene, are capable of transactivating a variety of host cell genes, some of which are listed in Table 12.11. Notably, the genes transactivated include interleukin-2 (IL-2) and its receptors (IL-2Rα). This lymphokine (Chapter 18) working through its receptor is a critical growth factor for the lymphoid cells infected by the virus. Thus, the virus, in addition to transactivating many other genes, some of which are important in cell replication (PCNA, c-*fos*), places the cell in an autocrine mode of growth, i.e. producing both the growth factor IL-2 and its receptor within the same cell. In addition, Yoshida (1996) has presented evidence that the Tax protein is involved in binding to specific nuclear factors involved in cell cycle function. The virus integrates into the host genome randomly (Ohshima et al., 1998) and in so doing appears to induce substantial chromosomal abnormalities. However, because of the extended latent period of viral existence within the genomes of host cell lymphocytes and no obvious neoplastic expression, the viral infection may act initially as a promoting agent over an extended period, ultimately resulting in a transition to the stage of tumor progression and neoplasia. Preclinical studies in animal models involving lower primates and rabbits have suggested the feasibility of an HTLV-I vaccine, but as yet no human trials to test the efficacy of such vaccines have been undertaken (cf. IARC, 1996).

The Impact of Infectious Agents in the Causation of Human Cancer

Recently Parkin et al. (1999) made estimates of the global health burden of infection-associated cancers. Their conclusions were that approximately 15% of human neoplasms were caused by infectious agents worldwide as of 1990. This includes 10% of all lymphomas and leukemias, 70% of all liver cancers, 42% of gastric carcinomas, and 88% of carcinomas of the cervix and vulva worldwide. These authors estimated that 1.2 million cancer cases were attributable to infectious agents in the year 1990. Most of this burden was related to viral infections. Almost a third, 4.3% of the 14.8%, were related to infection with *Helicobacter* but only a small proportion to parasitic infections. Theoretically, with the development of appropriate vaccines and other therapeutic modalities, most such cancers could probably be prevented within the

Table 12.11 Cellular Genes Transactivated by HTLV-1 Tax

Cytokines	Receptors	Cell Cycle	Miscellaneous
IL-2	IL-2Rα	PCNA	Vimentin
IL-3		β-polymerase	c-*fos*
IL-1α		(repressive)	c-*sis*
GM-CSF			PTHrP
TGF-β1			Proenkephalin
NGF			β-globin
Act-2 cytokine			e-globin
TNF-α			egr-1 (Krox-24)
			egr-2 (Krox-20)
			Class I MHC
			Class II MHC
			IκB

Adapted from Wigdahl and Brady, 1996, with permission of the authors and publisher.

next decade, given the appropriate economic requirements. Just two decades ago, the percentage of cancers caused by infectious agents was considered to be less than 1%; but as our knowledge has increased, infectious agents clearly play a significant role in the worldwide burden of cancer.

The Causes of Human Cancer

As we have discussed in earlier chapters (Chapter 5 and 6), it is likely that less than 5% of human cancers are directly caused by genetic abnormalities. Genetic predisposition, on the other hand, plays a much greater role in the development of human cancer, but also requires environmental input. Thus, one may suggest that up to 90% of human cancer is caused by environmental factors. Figure 12.26 is a diagram of the various environmental causes of human cancer as originally proposed for the United States population by Doll and Peto (1981). Although this chart is more than two decades old, there is substantial evidence to support these proportional contributions. While the proportion of cancer due to infection is higher than depicted in the figure (see above), this change would not dramatically affect the overall distribution of causations. As we have noted in this and the previous chapter, environmental factors contributing to cancer causation are, at least theoretically if not practically, remediable. In fact, at least two-thirds of human cancer could be prevented by appropriate actions, individual and societal. Although cancer therapy, as we shall see later in the text, has made enormous strides during the last few decades, it is likely that our knowledge of the significant environmental factors in the causation of human cancer will lead to extensive programs of prevention in the near future.

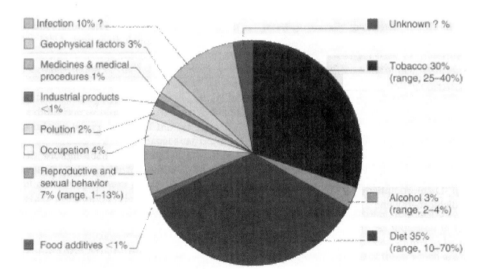

Figure 12.26 Proportions of cancer deaths attributed to various environmental factors. (After Doll and Peto, 1981.)

REFERENCES

Aboulafia, D. Epidemiology and pathogenesis of AIDS-related lymphomas. Oncology, *12*:1068–1078, 1998.

Adami, J., Frisch, M., Yuen, J., Glimelius, B., and Melbye, M. Evidence of an association between non-Hodgkin's lymphoma and skin cancer. Br. Med. J., *310*:1491–1495, 1995.

Aksamit, A. J. Jr. Progressive multifocal leukoencephalopathy: a review of the pathology and pathogenesis. Microsc. Res. Tech., *32*:302–311, 1995.

Alter, M. J. Epidemiology of hepatitis C. Hepatology, *26*:62S–65S, 1997.

AMA. Radon in homes. J.A.M.A., *258*:668–672, 1987.

Anagnostopoulos, I., and Hummel, M. Epstein-Barr virus in tumours. Histopathology, *29*:297–315, 1996.

Andersson, M., and Storm, H. H. Cancer incidence among Danish Thorotrast-exposed patients. J. Natl. Cancer Inst., *84*:1318–1325, 1992.

Anthony, D. D., Wentz, W. B., Reagan, J. W., and Heggie, A. D. Induction of cervical neoplasia in the mouse by herpes simplex virus type 2 DNA. Proc. Natl. Acad. Sci. U.S.A., *86*:4520–4524, 1989.

Aozasa, K., Ohsawa, M., Tomita, Y., and Kanno, H. Epstein-Barr virus and malignant lymphoma. Gann Monogr. Cancer Res., *45*:117–127, 1998.

Armstrong, B. K., and Kricker, A. Epidemiology of sun exposure and skin cancer. Cancer Surv., *26*:133–153, 1996.

Arts, E. J., Quiñones-Mateu, M. E., and Albright, J. L. Mechanisms of clinical resistance by HIV-I variants to zidovudine and the paradox of reverse transcriptase sensitivity. Drug Resist. Updates, *1*:21–28, 1998.

Asaka, M., Kimura, T., Kato, M., Kudo, M., Miki, K., Ogoshi, K., Kato, T., Tatsuta, M., and Graham, D. Y. Possible role of *Helicobacter pylori* infection in early gastric cancer development. Cancer, *73*:2691–2694, 1994.

Astori, G., Lavergne, D., Benton, C., Höckmayr, B., Egawa, K., Garbe, C., and de Villiers, E.-M. Human papillomaviruses are commonly found in normal skin of immunocompetent hosts. J. Invest. Dermatol., *110*:752–755, 1998.

Autier, P., and Doré, J.-F. Influence of sun exposures during childhood and during adulthood on melanoma risk. Int. J. Cancer, *77*:533–537, 1998.

Ballestas, M. E., Chatis, P. A., and Kaye, K. M. Efficient persistence of extrachromosomal KSHV DNA mediated by latency-associated nuclear antigen. Science, *284*:641–644, 1999.

Banerjee, S. K., Weston, A. P., Persons, D. L., and Campbell, D. R. Non-random loss of chromosome 3 during transition of *Helicobacter pylori*–associated gastric MALT to B-cell MALT lymphoma revealed by fluorescence in situ hybridization. Cancer Lett., *121*:83–90, 1997.

Bentham, G. Association between incidence of non-Hodgkin's lymphoma and solar ultraviolet radiation in England and Wales. Br. Med. J., *312*:1128–1131, 1996.

Bergeron, C., Barrasso, R., Beaudenon, S., Flamant, P., Croissant, O., and Orth, G. Human papillomaviruses associated with cervical intraepithelial neoplasia. Am. J. Surg. Pathol., *16*:641–649, 1992.

Bergsagel, D. J., Finegold, M. J., Butel, J. S., Kupsky, W. J., and Garcea, R. L. DNA sequences similar to those of simian virus 40 in ependymomas and choroid plexus tumors of childhood. N. Engl. J. Med., *326*:988–993, 1992.

Blaser, M. J. The bacteria behind ulcers. Sci. Am., *274*:104–107, 1996.

Bloechle, C., Peiper, M., Schwarz, R., Schroeder, S., and Zornig, C. Post-irradiation soft tissue sarcoma. Eur. J. Cancer, *31A*:31–34, 1995.

Blum, H. E., Gerok, W., and Vyas, G. N. The molecular biology of hepatitis B virus. Trends Genet., *5*:154–158, 1989.

Boice, J. D. Cancer following medical irradiation. Cancer, *47*:1081–1090, 1981.

Boice, J. D., Land, C. E., and Preston, D. L. Ionizing radiation. *In*: D. Schottenfeld and J. F. Fraumeni (eds.), Cancer Epidemiology and Prevention, 2nd ed., pp. 319–354. New York: Oxford University Press, 1996.

Boice Jr., J. D., Harvey, E. B., Blettner, M., Stovall, M., and Flannery, J. T. Cancer in the contralateral breast after radiotherapy for breast cancer. N. Engl. J. Med., *326*:781–785, 1992.

Borén, T., Falk, P., Roth, K. A., Larson, G., and Normark, S. Attachment of *Helicobacter pylori* to human gastric epithelium mediated by blood group antigens. Science, *262*:1892–1895, 1993.

Boshoff, C., and Weiss, R. A. Kaposi's sarcoma-associated herpesvirus. Adv. Cancer Res., *75*:57–86, 1998.

Brady, M. S., Gaynor, J. J., and Brennan, M. F. Radiation-associated sarcoma of bone and soft tissue. Arch. Surg., *127*:1379–1385, 1992.

Brash, D. E. Sunlight and the onset of skin cancer. Trends Genet., *13*:410–414, 1997.

Bréchot, C. Hepatitis C virus: molecular biology and genetic variability. *In*: Hepatitis C Virus: Genetic Heterogeneity and Viral Load, pp. 7–27. Paris: John Libbey Eurotext, 1997.

Bross, I. D. J., Ball, M., and Falen, S. A dosage response curve for the one rad range: adult risks from diagnostic radiation. Am. J. Public Health, *69*:130–136, 1979.

Buendia, M. A. Hepatitis B viruses and hepatocellular carcinoma. Adv. Cancer Res., *59*:167–226, 1992.

Burkitt, D. P. A sarcoma involving the jaws in African children. Br. J. Surg., *46*:218–223, 1958.

Byus, C. V., Pieper, S. E., and Adey, W. R. The effects of low-energy 60-Hz environmental electromagnetic fields upon the growth-related enzyme ornithine decarboxylase. Carcinogenesis, *8*:1385–1389, 1987.

Carbone, M., Rizzo, P., and Pass, H. I. Simian virus 40, poliovaccines and human tumors: a review of recent developments. Oncogene, *15*:1877–1888, 1997.

Chang, Y., Cesarman, E., Pessin, M. S., Lee, F., Culpepper, J., Knowles, D. M., and Moore, P. S. Identification of herpesvirus-like DNA sequences in AIDS-associated Kaposi's sarcoma. Science, *266*:1865–1869, 1994.

Chisari, F. V., and Ferrari, C. Hepatitis B virus immunopathogenesis. Annu. Rev. Immunol., *13*:29–60, 1995.

Chisari, F. V., Klopchin, K., Moriyama, T., Pasquinelli, C., Dunsford, H. A., Sell, S., Pinkert, C. A., Brinster, R. L., and Palmiter, R. D. Molecular pathogenesis of hepatocellular carcinoma in hepatitis B virus transgenic mice. Cell, *59*:1145–1156, 1989.

Choo, Q. L., Kuo, G., Weiner, A. J., Overby, L. R., Bradley, D. W., and Houghton, M. Isolation of a cDNA clone derived from a blood-borne non-A, non-B hepatitis genome. Science, *244*:359–362, 1989.

Cong, Y.-S., Yao, Y.-L., Yang, W.-M., Kuzhandaivelu, N., and Seto, E. The hepatitis B virus X-associated protein, XAP3, is a protein kinase C-binding protein. J. Biol. Chem., *272*:16482–16489, 1997.

Cover, T. L. The vacuolating cytotoxin of *Helicobacter pylori*. Mol. Microbiol., *20*:241–246, 1996.

Dennis, L. K., White, E., Lee, J. A. H., Kristal, A., McKnight, B., and Odland, P. Constitutional factors and sun exposure in relation to nevi: a population-based cross-sectional study. Am. J. Epidemiol., *143*:248–256, 1996.

De Re, V., Boiocchi, M., De Vita, S., Dolcetti, R., Gloghini, A., Uccini, S., Baroni, C., Scarpa, A., Cattoretti, G., and Carbone, A. Subtypes of Epstein-Barr virus in HIV-1–associated and HIV-1–unrelated Hodgkin's disease cases. Int. J. Cancer, *54*:895–898, 1993.

Di Bisceglie, A. M. Hepatitis C and hepatocellular carcinoma. Hepatology, *26*:34S–38S, 1997.

Di Bisceglie, A. M., Rustgi, V. K., Hoofnagle, J. H., Dusheiko, G. M., and Lotze, M. T. Hepatocellular carcinoma. Ann. Intern. Med., *108*:390–401, 1988.

Dictor, M., Rambech, E., Way, D., Witte, M., and Bendsöe, N. Human herpesvirus 8 (Kaposi's sarcoma-associated herpesvirus) DNA in Kaposi's sarcoma lesions, AIDS Kaposi's sarcoma cell lines, endothelial Kaposi's sarcoma simulators, and the skin of immunosuppressed patients. Am. J. Pathol., *148*:2009–2016, 1996.

Di Luca, D., Caselli, E., and Cassai, E. Herpes simplex virus as a cooperating agent in human genital carcinogenesis. *In*: G. Barbanti-Brodano et al. (Eds.), DNA Tumor Viruses: Oncogenic Mechanisms, pp. 281–293. New York: Plenum Press, 1995.

DiPaolo, J. A., Woodworth, C. D., Popescu, N. C., Koval, D. L., Lopez, J. V., and Doniger, J. HSV-2-Induced tumorigenicity in HPV16-immortalized human genital keratinocytes. Virology, *177*:777–779, 1990.

Dittmer, D., and Kedes, D. H. Do viral chemokines modulate Kaposi's sarcoma? Bioessays, *20*:367–370, 1998.

Dixon, M. F. Pathophysiology of *Helicobacter pylori* infection. Scand. J. Gastroenterol., *29* (Suppl 201):7–10, 1994.

Doll, R., and Peto, R. The causes of cancer—quantitative estimates of avoidable risks of cancer in the United States today. Oxford: Oxford, UK: University Press, 1981.

Dunn, B. E., Cohen, H., and Blaser, M. J. *Helicobacter pylori*. Clin. Microbiol. Rev., *10*:720–741, 1997.

Ellerman, V., and Bang, O. Experimentelle Leukamie bei Huhnern. Z. Hyg. Infekt., *62*:231–233, 1909.

Elsebai, I. Parasites in the etiology of cancer—bilharziasis and bladder cancer. CA, *27*:100–106, 1977.

Elwood, J. M. Initiation and promotion actions of ultraviolet radiation on malignant melanoma. *In*: M. Börzsönyi, K. Lapis, N. E. Day, and H. Yamasaki (Eds.), Models, Mechanisms and Etiology of Tumour Promotion, pp. 421–440. Lyon, France: International Agency for Research on Cancer, 1984.

Elwood, J. M. Melanoma and sun exposure. Semin. Oncol., *23*:650–666, 1996.

Emmanoulides, C., Miles, S. A., and Mitsuyasu, R. T. Pathogenesis of AIDS-related Kaposi's sarcoma. Oncology, *10*:335–341, 1996.

Endo, S., Ohkusa, T., Saito, Y., Fujiki, K., Okayasu, I., and Sato, C. Detection of *Helicobacter pylori* infection in earl stage gastric cancer. Cancer, *75*:2203–2208, 1995.

Ensoli, B., and Sirianni, M. C. Kaposi's sarcoma pathogenesis: a link between immunology and tumor biology. Crit. Rev. Oncog., *9*:107–124, 1998.

Epstein, M. A., Achong, B. G., and Barr, V. M. Virus particles in cultured lymphoblasts from Burkitt's lymphoma. Lancet *1*:702, 1964.

Esumi, M., and Shikata, T. Hepatitis C virus and liver diseases. Pathol. Int., *44*:85–95, 1994.

Evans, A. S., and Niederman, J. C. Epstein-Barr virus. *In*: A. S. Evans (Ed.), Viral Infections of Humans, 3rd ed., pp. 265–292. New York: Plenum Press, 1989.

Evans, J. S., Wennberg, J. E., and McNeil, B. J. The influence of diagnostic radiography on the incidence of breast cancer and leukemia. N. Engl. J. Med., *315*:810–815, 1986.

Feig, S. A. Radiation risk from mammography: is it clinically significant? Am. J. Roentgenol., *143*:469–475, 1984.

Feitelson, M. A., and Duan, L.-X. Hepatitis B virus x antigen in the pathogenesis of chronic infections and the development of hepatocellular carcinoma. Am. J. Pathol., *150*:1141–1157, 1997.

Ferreira Jr., O. C., Planelles, V., and Rosenblatt, J. D. Human T-cell leukemia viruses: epidemiology, biology, and pathogenesis. Blood Rev., *11*:91–104, 1997.

Ferrero, R. L. Immune responses to mucosal infection: the *Helicobacter pylori* paradigm. Res. Immunol., *148*:91–107, 1997.

Flægstad, T., Andresen, P. A., Johnsen, J. I., Asomani, S. K., Jørgensen, G.-E., Vignarajan, S., Kjuul, A., Kogner, P., and Traavik, T. A possible contributory role of BK virus infection in neuroblastoma development. Cancer Res., *59*:1160–1163, 1999.

Flore, O., Rafii, S., Ely, S., O'Leary, J. J., Hyjek, E. M., and Cesarman, E. Transformation of primary human endothelial cells by Kaposi's sarcoma-associated herpesvirus. Nature, *394*:588–592, 1998.

Frenkel, N., Roizman, B., Cassai, E., and Nahmias, A. A DNA fragment of herpes simplex 2 and its transcription in human cervical cancer tissue. Proc. Natl. Acad. Sci. U.S.A., *69*:3784–3789, 1972.

Fry, R. J. M., and Ainsworth, E. J. Radiation injury: some aspects of the oncogenic effects. Fed. Proc., *36*:1703–1707, 1977.

Gaidano, G., and Dalla-Favera, R. Molecular pathogenesis of AIDS-related lymphomas. Adv. Cancer Res., *67*:113–152, 1995.

Gao, S.-J., Kingsley, L., Hoover, D. R., Spira, T. J., Rinaldo, C. R., Saah, A., Phair, J., Detels, R., Parry, P., Chang, Y., and Moore, P. S. Seroconversion to antibodies against Kaposi's sarcoma-associated herpesvirus-related latent nuclear antigens before the development of Kaposi's sarcoma. N. Engl. J. Med., *335*:233–241, 1996.

Goedert, J. J., Coté, T. R., Virgo, P., Scoppa, S. M., Kingma, D. W., Gail, M. H., Jaffe, E. S., and Biggar, R. J. Spectrum of AIDS-associated malignant disorders. Lancet, *351*:1833–1839, 1998.

Goodman, M. T., Mabuchi, K., Morita, M., Soda, M., Ochikubo, S., Fukuhara, T., Ikeda, T., and Terasaki, M. Cancer incidence in Hiroshima and Nagasaki, Japan, 1958–1987. Eur. J. Cancer, *30A*:801–807, 1994.

Goodman, R., Bumann, J., Wei, L. X., and Shirley-Henderson, A. Exposure of human cells to electromagnetic fields: effect of time and field strength on transcript levels. Electromagnetobiology, *11*:19–28, 1992.

Graham, S., Rawls, W., Swanson, M., and McCurtis, J. Sex partners and herpes simplex virus type 2 in the epidemiology of cancer of the cervix. Am. J. Epidemiol., *115*:729–735, 1982.

Gratama, J. W., and Ernberg, I. Molecular epidemiology of Epstein-Barr virus infection. Adv. Cancer Res., *67*:197–255, 1995.

Greenberg, P. Immunopathogenesis of HIV infection. Hosp. Pract., ofc. edn. *27*(2):109–117, 121, 124, 1992.

Greene, W. C. The molecular biology of human immunodeficiency virus type 1 infection. N. Engl. J. Med., *324*:308–317, 1991.

Greenspan, J. S., Greenspan, D., Lennette, E. T., Abrams, D. I., Conant, M. A., Petersen, V., and Freese, U. K. Replication of Epstein-Barr virus within the epithelial cells of oral "hairy" leukoplakia, an AIDS-associated lesion. N. Engl. J. Med., *313*:1564–1571, 1985.

Griep, A. E., and Lambert, P. F. Role of papillomavirus oncogenes in human cervical cancer: transgenic animal studies. Proc. Soc. Exp. Biol. Med., *206*:24–34, 1994.

Grinnell, B. W., Padgett, B. L., and Walker, D. L. Distribution of nonintegrated DNA from JC papovavirus in organs of patients with progressive multifocal leukoencephalopathy. J. Infect. Dis., *147*:669–675, 1983.

Groopman, J. D., Scholl, P., and Wang, J.-S. Epidemiology of human aflatoxin exposures and their relationship to liver cancer. *In*: Genetics and Cancer Susceptibility: Implications for Risk Assessment, pp. 211–222. New York: Wiley-Liss, 1996.

Gross, L. Presence of leukemic agent in normal testes and ovaries of young mice of Ak line. Acta Haematol., *10*:18–26, 1953.

Hadziyannis, S., Tabor, E., Kaklamani, E., Tzonou, A., Stuver, S., Tassopoulos, N., Mueller, N., and Trichopoulos, D. A case-control study of hepatitis B and C virus infections in the etiology of hepatocellular carcinoma. Int. J. Cancer, *60*:627–631, 1995.

Hahn, B. H., Shaw, G. M., Taylor, M. E., Redfield, R. R., Markham, P. D., Salahuddin, S. Z., Wong-Staal, F., Gallo, R. C., Parks, E. S., and Parks, W. P. Genetic variation in HTLV-III/LAV over time in patients with AIDS or at risk for AIDS. Science, *232*:1548–1553, 1986.

Hartge, P., Devesa, S. S., Grauman, D., Fears, T. R., and Fraumeni, J. F. Jr. Non-Hodgkin's lymphoma and sunlight. J. Natl. Cancer Inst., *88*:298–300, 1996.

Harvey, E. B., Boice Jr., J. D., Honeyman, M., and Flannery, J. T. Prenatal x-ray exposure and childhood cancer in twins. N. Engl. J. Med., *312*:541–545, 1985.

Hatch, M. C., Beyea, J., Nieves, J. W., and Susser, M. Cancer near the Three Mile Island nuclear plant: radiation emissions. Am. J. Epidemiol., *132*:397–412, 1990.

Hattori, S. State of research and perspective on radiation hormesis in Japan. Belle Newslett., *3*:1–7, 1994.

Hei, T. K., Wu, L.-J., Liu, S.-X., Vannais, D., Waldren, C. A., and Randers-Pehrson, G. Mutagenic effects of a single and an exact number of alpha particles in mammalian cells. Proc. Natl. Acad. Sci. U.S.A., *94*:3765–3770, 1997.

Heintges, T., and Wands, J. R. Hepatitis C virus: epidemiology and transmission. Hepatology, *26*:521–526, 1997.

Hendee, W. R. Estimation of radiation risks. BEIR V and its significance for medicine. J.A.M.A., *268*:620–624, 1992.

Henle, W., Henle, G., and Lennette, E. T. The Epstein-Barr virus. Sci. Am., *241*:48–59, 1979.

Hicks, R. M. The canopic worm: role of bilharziasis in the aetiology of human bladder cancer. J. R. Soc. Med., *76*:16–22, 1983.

Hildreth, N. G., Shore, R. E., and Dvoretsky, P. M. The risk of breast cancer after irradiation of the thymus in infancy. N. Engl. J. Med., *321*:1281–1284, 1989.

Hino, O., Tabata, S., and Hotta, Y. Evidence for increased *in vitro* recombination with insertion of human hepatitis B virus DNA. Proc. Natl. Acad. Sci. U.S.A., *88*:9248–9252, 1991.

Hiraoka, M., Miyakoshi, J., Li, Y. P., Shung, B., Takebe, H., and Abe, M. Induction of c-*fos* gene expression by exposure to a static magnetic field in HeLaS3 cells. Cancer Res., *52*:6522–6524, 1992.

Ho, G. Y. F., Burk, R. D., Klein, S., Kadish, A. S., Chang, C. J., Palan, P., Basu, J., Tachezy, R., Lewis, R., and Romney, S. Persistent genital human papillomavirus infection as a risk factor for persistent cervical dysplasia. J. Natl. Cancer Inst., *87*:1365–1371, 1995.

Hoel, D. G. Ionizing radiation and cancer prevention. Environ. Health Perspect., *103*:241–243, 1995.

Holm, L.-E., Wiklund, K. E., Lundell, G. E., Bergman, N. Å., Bjelkengren, G., Cederquist, E. S., Ericsson, U.-B. C., Larsson, L.-G., Lidberg, M. E., Lindberg, R. S., Wicklund, H. V., and Boice, J. D. Jr. Thyroid cancer after diagnostic doses of iodine-131: a retrospective cohort study. J. Natl. Cancer Inst., *80*:1132–1138, 1988.

Honda, S., Fujioka, T., Tokieda, M., Satoh, R., Nishizono, A., and Nasu, M. Development of *Helicobacter pylori*–induced gastric carcinoma in Mongolian gerbils. Cancer Res., *58*:4255–4259, 1998.

Hoofnagle, J. H., and di Bisceglie, A. M. The treatment of chronic viral hepatitis. N. Engl. J. Med., *336*:347–356, 1997.

IARC. Monographs on the Evaluation of Carcinogenic Risks to Humans: Vol. 55, Solar and Ultraviolet Radiation. Lyon, France: IARC, 1992.

IARC. Monographs on the Evaluation of Carcinogenic Risks to Humans: Vol. 59, Hepatitis Viruses. Lyon, France: IARC, 1994a.

IARC. Monographs on the Evaluation of Carcinogenic Risks to Humans: Vol. 61, Schistosomes, Liver Flukes and *Helicobacter pylori*. Lyon, France: IARC, 1994b.

IARC. Monographs on the Evaluation of Carcinogenic Risks to Humans: Vol. 64, Human Papillomaviruses. Lyon, France: IARC, 1995.

IARC. Monographs on the Evaluation of Carcinogenic Risks to Humans: Vol. 67, Human Immunodeficiency Viruses and Human T-Cell Lymphotropic Viruses. Lyon, France: IARC, 1996.

IARC. Monographs on the Evaluation of Carcinogenic Risks to Humans: Vol. 70, Epstein-Barr Virus and Kaposi's Sarcoma Herpesvirus/Human Herpesvirus 8. Lyon, France: IARC, 1997.

Inagi, R., Kosuge, H., Nishimoto, S., Yoshikawa, K., and Yamanishi, K. Kaposi's sarcoma–associated herpesvirus (KSHV) sequences in premalignant and malignant skin tumors. Arch. Virol., *141*:2217–2223, 1996.

Ishimaru, T., Otake, M., and Ichimaru, M. Dose-response relationship of neutrons and gamma rays to leukemia incidence among atomic-bomb survivors in Hiroshima and Nagasaki by type of leukemia, 1950–1971. Radiat. Res., *77*:377–394, 1979.

Ivanov, V. K., Tsyb, A. F., Gorsky, A. I., Maksyutov, M. A., Rastopchin, E. M., Konogorov, A. P., Korelo, A. M., Biryukov, A. P., and Matyash, V. A. Leukaemia and thyroid cancer in emergency workers of the Chernobyl accident: estimation of radiation risks (1986–1995). Radiat. Environ. Biophys., *36*:9–16, 1997.

Jackson, H., and Parker, F. Hodgkin's disease. II. Pathology. N. Engl. J. Med., *231*:35–44, 1944.

Jeannel, D., Bouvier, G., and Hubert, A. Nasopharyngeal carcinoma: an epidemiological approach to carcinogenesis. Cancer Surv., *33*:125–155, 1999.

Jonason, A. S., Kunala, S., Price, G. J., Restifo, R. J., Spinelli, H. M., Persing, J. A., Leffell, D. J., Tarone, R. E., and Brash, D. E. Frequent clones of p53-mutated keratinocytes in normal human skin. Proc. Natl. Acad. Sci. U.S.A., *93*:14025–14029, 1996.

Jostes, R. F. Genetic, cytogenetic, and carcinogenic effects of radon: a review. Mutat. Res., *340*:125–139, 1996.

Kamihira, S., Nakasima, S., Oyakawa, Y., Moriuti, Y., Ichimaru, M., Okuda, H., Kanamura, M., and Oota, T. Transmission of human T-cell lymphotropic virus type I by blood transfusion before and after mass screening of sera from seropositive donors. Vox Sang, *52*:43–44, 1987.

Kashyap, V. ,and Das, B. C. DNA aneuploidy and infection of human papillomavirus type 16 in preneoplastic lesions of the uterine cervix: correlation with progression to malignancy. Cancer Lett., *123*:47–52, 1998.

Kataja, V., Syrjänen, K., Mäntyjärvi, R., Väyrynen, M., Syrjänen, S., Saarikoski, S., Parkkinen, S., Yliskoski, M., Salonen, J. T., and Castren, O. Prospective follow-up of cervical HPV infections: life table analysis of histopathological, cytological and colposcopic data. Eur. J. Epidemiol., *5*:1–7, 1989.

Kataja, V., Syrjänen, S., Yliskoski, M., Hippeläinen, M., Väyrynen, M., Saarikoski, S., Mäntyjärvi, R., Jokela, V., Salonen, J. T., and Syrjänen, K. Risk factors associated with cervical human papillomavirus infections: a case-control study. Am. J. Epidemiol., *138*:735–745, 1993.

Kaune, W. T. Introduction to power-frequency electric and magnetic fields. Environ. Health Perspect., *101*:73–81, 1993.

Kavet, R. EMF and current cancer concepts. Bioelectromagnetics, *17*:339–357, 1996.

Kelly, J. W., Rivers, J. K., MacLennan, R., Harrison, S., Lewis, A. E., and Tate, B. J. Sunlight: a major factor associated with the development of melanocytic nevi in Australian schoolchildren. J. Am. Acad. Dermatol., *30*:40–48, 1994.

Koff, R. S. Hepatitis C. Sci. Med., *5*:16–25, 1998.

Koike, K., and Takada, S. Biochemistry and functions of hepatitis B virus X protein. Intervirology, *38*:89–99, 1995.

Kondo, S. Rational risk estimation in relation to atomic bomb radiation. J. Radiat. Res., *31*:174–188, 1990.

Kraemer, K. H. Sunlight and skin cancer: another link revealed. Proc. Natl. Acad. Sci. U.S.A., *94*:11–14, 1997.

Kreider, J. W., Howett, M. K., Lill, N. L., Bartlett, G. L., Zaino, R. J., Sedlacek, T. V., and Mortel, R. In vivo transformation of human skin with human papillomavirus type 11 from condylomata acuminata. J. Virol., *59*:369–376, 1986.

Kricker, A., Armstrong, B. K., English, D. R., and Heenan, P. J. A dose-response curve for sun exposure and basal cell carcinoma. Int. J. Cancer, *60*:482–488, 1995.

Krieg, P., Amtmann, E., Jonas, D., Fischer, H., Zang, K., and Sauer, G. Episomal simian virus 40 genomes in human brain tumors. Proc. Natl. Acad. Sci. USA, *78*:6446–6450, 1981.

Kuipers, E. J. Review article: relationship between *Helicobacter pylori*, atrophic gastritis and gastric cancer. Aliment. Pharmacol. Ther., *12*:25–36, 1998.

Lacy-Hulbert, A., Metcalfe, J. C., and Hesketh, R. Biological responses to electromagnetic fields. FASEB J., *12*:395–420, 1998.

Laskin, W. B., Silverman, T. A., and Enzinger, F. M. Postradiation soft tissue sarcomas. Cancer, *62*:2330–2340, 1988.

Lawrence, J. B., Villnave, C. A., and Singer, R. H. Sensitive, high-resolution chromatin and chromosome mapping in situ: presence and orientation of two closely integrated copies of EBV in a lymphoma line. Cell, *52*:51–61, 1988.

Lee, H., Veazey, R., Williams, K., Li, M., Guo, J., Neipel, F., Fleckenstein, B., Lackner, A., Desrosiers, R. C., and Jung, J. U. Deregulation of cell growth by the K1 gene of Kaposi's sarcoma-associated herpesvirus. Nature Med., *4*:435–440, 1998.

Leffell, D. J., and Brash, D. E. Sunlight and skin cancer. Sci. Am., *275*:52–59, 1996.

Levin, L. I., and Levine, P. H. The epidemiology of Epstein-Barr virus-associated human cancers. Gann Monogr. Cancer Res., *45*:51–74, 1998.

Lin, C.-T., Lin, C.-R., Tan, G.-K., Chen, W., Dee, A. N., and Chan, W.-Y. The mechanism of Epstein-Barr virus infection in nasopharyngeal carcinoma cells. Am. J. Pathol., *150*:1745–1756, 1997.

Little, M. P., and Muirhead, C. R. Curvilinearity in the dose-response curve for cancer in Japanese atomic bomb survivors. Environ. Health Perspect., *105*:1505–1509, 1997.

London, W. T., Houff, S. A., Madden, D. L., Fuccillo, D. A., Gravell, M., Wallen, W. C., Palmer, A. E., Sever, J. L., Padgett, B. L., Walker, D. L., Zu Rhein, G. M., and Ohashi, T. Brain tumors in owl monkeys inoculated with a human polyomavirus (JC virus). Science, *201*:1246–1249, 1978.

Longstreth, J. Cutaneous malignant melanoma and ultraviolet radiation: a review. Cancer Metast. Rev., *7*:321–333, 1988.

Lubin, J. H., and Boice Jr., J. D. Lung cancer risk from residential radon: meta-analysis of eight epidemiologic studies. J. Natl. Cancer Inst., *89*:49–57, 1997.

Lubin, J. H., Boice Jr., J. D., Edling, C., Hornung, R. W., Howe, G. R., Kunz, E., Kusiak, R. A., Morrison, H. I., Radford, E. P., Samet, J. M., Tirmarche, M., Woodward, A., Yao, S. X., and Pierce, D. A. Lung cancer in radon-exposed miners and estimation of risk from indoor exposure. J. Natl. Cancer Inst., *87*:817–827, 1995.

Lucas, K. G., Pollok, K. E., and Emanuel, D. J. Post-transplant EBV induced lymphoproliferative disorders. Leuk. Lymph., *25*:1–8, 1997.

Lukes, R. J., Butler, J. J., and Hicks, E. B. Natural history of Hodgkin's disease as related to its pathologic picture. Cancer, *19*:317–344, 1966.

Macnab, J. C. M. Herpes simplex virus and human cytomegalovirus: their role in morphological transformation and genital cancers. J. Gen. Virol., *68*:2525–2550, 1987.

Majewski, S., and Jablonska, S. Epidermodysplasia verruciformis as a model of human papillomavirus-induced genetic cancers: the role of local immunosurveillance. Am. J. Med. Sci., *304*:174–179, 1992.

Major, E. O., Amemiya, K., Tornatore, C. S., Houff, S. A., and Berger, J. R. Pathogenesis and molecular biology of progressive multifocal leukoencephalopathy, the JC virus-induced demyelinating disease of the human brain. Clin. Microbiol. Rev., *5*:49–73, 1992.

Makinodan, T., and James, S. J. T cell potentiation by low dose ionizing radiation: possible mechanisms. Health Phys., *59*:29–34, 1990.

Malatack, J. J., Gartner, J. C., Urbach, A. H., and Zitelli, B. J. Orthotopic liver transplantation, Epstein-Barr virus, cyclosporine, and lymphoproliferative disease: a growing concern. J. Pediatr., *118*:667–675, 1991.

Marshall, B. J., and Warren, J. R. Unidentified curved bacilli in the stomach of patients with gastritis and peptic ulceration. Lancet, *1*:1311–1314, 1984.

Martini, F., Iaccheri, L., Lazzarin, L., Carinci, P., Corallini, A., Gerosa, M., Iuzzolino, P., Barbanti-Brodano, G., and Tognon, M. SV40 early region and large T antigen in human brain tumors, peripheral blood cells, and sperm fluids from healthy individuals. Cancer Res., *56*:4820–4825, 1996.

Matsuo, T., Heller, M., Petti, L., O'Shiro, E., and Kieff, E. Persistence of the entire Epstein-Barr virus genome integrated into human lymphocyte DNA. Science, *226*:1322–1325, 1984.

Matsuzaki, Y., Chiba, T., Hadama, T., Asaoka, H., Doy, M., Shoda, J., Tanaka, N., and Kinoshita, M. HBV genome integration and genetic instability in HBsAg-negative and anti-HCV–positive hepatocellular carcinoma in Japan. Cancer Lett., *119*:53–61, 1997.

McCann, J., Dietrich, F., and Rafferty, C. The genotoxic potential of electric and magnetic fields: an update. Mutat. Res., *411*:45–86, 1998.

McDonagh, D. P., Liu, J., Gaffey, M. J., Layfield, L. J., Azumi, N., and Traweek, S. T. Detection of Kaposi's sarcoma-associated herpesvirus-like DNA sequences in angiosarcoma. Am. J. Pathol., *149*:1363–1368, 1996.

Melbye, M., and Frisch, M. The role of human papillomaviruses in anogenital cancers. Cancer Biol., *8*:307–313, 1998.

Melnick, J. L. Hepatitis B virus and liver cancer. *In*: L. A. Phillips (Ed.), Viruses Associated with Human Cancer, pp. 337–366. New York: Marcel Dekker, 1983.

Melnick, J. L., Courtney, R. J., Powell, K. L., Schaffer, P. A., Benyesh-Melnick, M., Dreesman, G. R., Anzai, T., and Adam, E. Studies on herpes simplex virus and cancer. Cancer Res., *36*:845–856, 1976.

Merson, M. H. Slowing the spread of HIV: agenda for the 1990s. Science, *260*:1266–1268, 1993.

Mevissen, M., Kietzmann, M., and Löscher W. In vivo exposure of rats to a weak alternating magnetic field increases ornithine decarboxylase activity in the mammary gland by a similar extent as the carcinogen DMBA. Cancer Lett., *90*:207–214, 1995.

Modan, B., Alfandary, E., Chetrit, A., and Katz, L. Increased risk of breast cancer after low-dose irradiation. Lancet, *1*:629–631, 1989.

Moran, A. P. Pathogenic properties of *Helicobacter pylori*. Scand. J. Gastroenterol., *31* (Suppl 215) 22–31, 1996.

Moss, D. J., Schmidt, C., Elliott, S., Suhrbier, A., Burrows, S., and Khanna, R. Strategies involved in developing an effective vaccine for EBV-associated diseases. Adv. Cancer Res., *69*:213–245, 1996.

Mueller, N. Hodgkin's disease. *In*: D. Schottenfeld and J. F. Fraumeni, Jr. (Eds.), Cancer Epidemiology and Prevention, pp. 893–919. New York: Oxford University Press, 1996.

Nakamura, S., Aoyagi, K., Furuse, M., Suekane, H., Matsumoto, T., Yao, T., Sakai, Y., Fuchigami, T., Yamamoto, I., Tsuneyoshi, M., and Fujishima, M. B-cell monoclonality precedes the development of gastric MALT lymphoma in *Helicobacter pylori*–associated chronic gastritis. Am. J. Pathol., *152*:1271–1279, 1998.

Nazaroff, W. W., Feustel, H., Nero, A. V., Revzan, K. L., and Grimsrud, D. T. Radon transport into a detached one-story house with a basement. Atmos. Environ., *19*:31–46, 1985.

Nero, A. V., Schwehr, M. B., Nazaroff, W. W., and Revzan, K. L. Distribution of airborne radon-222 concentrations in U.S. homes. Science, *234*:992–997, 1986.

Neugut, A. I., Murray, T., Santos, J., Amols, H., Hayes, M. K., Flannery, J. T., and Robinson, E. Increased risk of lung cancer after breast cancer radiation therapy in cigarette smokers. Cancer, *73*:1615–1620, 1994.

Niedobitek, G., Agathanggelou, A., and Nicholls, J. M. Epstein-Barr virus infection and the pathogenesis of nasopharyngeal carcinoma: viral gene expression, tumour cell phenotype, and the role of the lymphoid stroma. Cancer Biol., *7*:165–174, 1996.

Nowak, M. A., Anderson, R. M., McLean, A. R., Wolfs, T. F. W., Goudsmit, J., and May, R. M. Antigenic diversity thresholds and the development of AIDS. Science, *254*:963–969, 1991.

Ohshima, K., Ohgami, A., Matsuoka, M., Etoh, K.-i., Utsunomiya, A., Makino, T., Ishiguro, M., Suzumiya, J., and Kikuchi, M. Random integration of HTLV-1 provirus; increasing chromosomal instability. Cancer Lett., *132*:203–212, 1998.

Okano, M., and Gross, T. G. Epstein-Barr virus-associated hemophagocytic syndrome and fatal infectious mononucleosis. Am. J. Hematol., *53*:111–115, 1996.

Ottani, V., Monti, M. G., Piccinini, G., Pernecco, L., Zaniol, P., Ruggeri, A., et al. Pulsed electromagnetic fields increase the rate of rat liver regeneration after partial hepatectomy. Proc. Soc. Exp. Biol. Med., *176*:371–377, 1984.

Padgett, B. L., Walker, D. L., Zu Rhein, G. M., Eckroade, R. J., and Dessel, B. H. Cultivation of papova-like virus from human brain with progressive multifocal leucoencephalopathy. Lancet, *1*:1257–1260, 1971.

Parkin, D. M., and Iscovich, J. Risk of cancer in migrants and their descendants in Israel: II. Carcinomas and germ-cell tumours. Int. J. Cancer, *70*:654–660, 1997.

Parkin, D. M., Pisani, P., Muñoz, N., and Ferlay, J. The global health burden of infection associated cancers. Cancer Surv., *33*:5–33, 1999.

Parsons, P. A. Radiation hormesis: an evolutionary expectation based upon exposure to background radiation. Belle Newsl., *3*:9–11, 1994.

Payet, M., Camain, R., and Pene, P. Primary liver cancer. Critical study of 240 cases. Rev. Int. Hepatol., *6*:1–20 (in French), 1956.

Peek Jr., R. M., Moss, S. F., Tham, K. T., Pérez-Pérez, G. I., Wang, S., Miller, G. G., Atherton, J. C., Holt, P. R., and Blaser, M. J. *Helicobacter pylori* cagA$^+$ strains and dissociation of gastric epithelial cell proliferation from apoptosis. J. Natl. Cancer Inst., *89*:863–868, 1997.

Pershagen, G., Åkerblom, G., Axelson, O., Clavensjö, B., Damber, L., Desai, G., Enflo, A., Lagarde, F., Mellander, H., Svartengren, M., and Swedjemark, G. A. Residential radon exposure and lung cancer in Sweden. N. Engl. J. Med., *330*:159–164, 1994.

Pezo, V., and Wain-Hobson, S. HIV genetic variation: life at the edge. J. Infect., *34*:201–203, 1997.

Phillips, J. L, Haggren, W., Thomas, W. J., Ishida-Jones, T., and Adey, W. R. Magnetic field-induced changes in specific gene transcription. Biochim. Biophys. Acta *1132*:140–144, 1992.

Pierce, D. A., and Vaeth, M. The shape of the cancer mortality dose-response curve for the A-bomb survivors. Radiat. Res., *126*:36–42, 1991.

Pitot, H. C. The progression of neoplasia, cell replication, and electromagnetic fields. Int. J. Toxicol., *17*:59–108, 1998.

Poiesz, B. J., Ruscetti, F. W., Gazdar, A. F., Bunn, P. A., Minna, J. D., and Gallo, R. C. Detection and isolation of type C retrovirus particles from fresh and cultured lymphocytes of a patient with cutaneous T-cell lymphoma. Proc. Natl. Acad. Sci. USA, *77*:7415–7419, 1980.

Pozzato, G., Mazzaro, C., Santini, G., and Burrone, O. Hepatitis C virus and non-Hodgkin's lymphomas. Leuk. Lymph., *22*:53–60, 1996.

Preston-Martin, S., Thomas, D. C., White, S. C., and Cohen, D. Prior exposure to medical and dental x-rays related to tumors of the parotid gland. J. Natl. Cancer Inst., *80*:943–949, 1988.

Prost, S., Ford, J. M., Taylor, C., Doig, J., and Harrison, D. J. Hepatitis B x protein inhibits p53-dependent DNA repair in primary mouse hepatocytes. J. Biol. Chem., *273*:33327–33332, 1998.

Purcell, R. H. Hepatitis C virus: historical perspective and current concepts. FEMS Microbiol. Rev., *14*:181–192, 1994.

Purtilo, D. T. Immune deficiency predisposing to Epstein-Barr virus-induced lymphoproliferative diseases: the X-linked lymphoproliferative syndrome as a model. Adv. Cancer Res., *34*:279–312, 1981.

Purtilo, D. T., Linder, J., and Volsky, D. J. Acquired immune deficiency syndrome (AIDS). Clin. Lab. Med., *6*:3–25, 1986.

Radford, E. P. Epidemiology of radiation-induced cancer. Environ. Health Perspect., *52*:45–50, 1983.

Ray, R. B., Steele, R., Meyer, K., and Ray, R. Transcriptional repression of p53 promoter by hepatitis C virus core protein. J. Biol. Chem., *272*:10983–10986, 1997.

Renard, T. H., Andrews, W. S., and Foster, M. E. Relationship between OKT3 administration, EBV seroconversion, and the lymphoproliferative syndrome in pediatric liver transplant patients. Transplant Proc., *23*:1473–1476, 1991.

Ridky, T., and Leis, J. Development of drug resistance to HIV-1 protease inhibitors. J. Biol. Chem., *270*:29621–29623, 1995.

Robinson, E., Neugut, A. I., and Wylie, P. Clinical aspects of postirradiation sarcomas. J. Natl. Cancer Inst., *80*:233–240, 1988.

Ron, E. Thyroid cancer. *In*: D. Schottenfeld and J. F. Fraumeni (eds.), Cancer Epidemiology and Prevention, 2nd ed, pp. 1000–1021. New York: Oxford University Press, 1996.

Rosin, M. P., and Anwar, W. Chromosomal damage in urothelial cells from Egyptians with chronic *Schistosoma haematobium* infections. Int. J. Cancer, *50*:539–543, 1992.

Rossi, H. H. The estimation of low-dose hazards by extrapolation from high doses. Yale J. Biol. Med., *54*:339–344, 1981.

Rowland, R. E., and Lucas Jr., H. F. Radium-dial workers. *In*: J. D. Boice, Jr. and J. F. Fraumeni, Jr. (Eds.), Radiation Carcinogenesis: Epidemiology and Biological Significance, pp. 231–240. New York: Raven Press, 1984.

Rugge, M., Cassaro, M., Leandro, G., Baffa, R., Avellini, C., Bufo, P., Stracca, V., Battaglia, G., Fabiano, A., Guerini, A., and di Mario, F. *Helicobacter pylori* in promotion of gastric carcinogenesis. Dig. Dis. Sci., *41*:950–955, 1996.

Rundo, J., and Toohey, R. E. Radon in homes and other technologically enhanced radioactivity. Proceedings of the Nineteenth Annual Meeting of the National Council on Radiation Protection and Measurements, pp. 16–26, April 6–7, 1983. Washington, D.C.: National Academy of Sciences, 1983.

Rusch, H. P., Kline, B. E., and Baumann, C. A. Carcinogenesis by ultraviolet rays with reference to wavelength and energy. Arch. Pathol., *31*:135–146, 1941.

Russo, J. J., Bohenzky, R. A., Chien, M.-C., Chen, J., Yan, M., Maddalena, D., Parry, J. P., Peruzzi, D., Edelman, I. S., Chang, Y., and Moore, P. S. Nucleotide sequence of the Kaposi sarcoma-associated herpesvirus (HHV8). Proc. Natl. Acad. Sci. U.S.A., *93*:14862–14867, 1996.

Sachs, R. K., Hahnfeld, P., and Brenner, D. J. The link between low-LET dose-response relations and the underlying kinetics of damage production/repair/misrepair. Int. J. Radiat. Biol., *72*:351–374, 1997.

Santini, G. F., Crovatto, M., Giannini, F., Bortolin, M. T., Mazzaro, C., and Invernizzi, F. Hepatitis C virus and immunoglobulin gene rearrangements: an early step in lymphomagenesis? Acta Haematol., *100*:117–122, 1998.

Satoh, M., Tsuji, Y., Watanabe, Y., Okonogi, H., Suzuki, Y., Nakagawa, M., and Shimizu, H. Metallothionein content increased in the liver of mice exposed to magnetic fields. Arch. Toxicol., *70*:315–318, 1996.

Schneider, A. B., and Ron, E. Radiation and thyroid cancer. Lessons from 46 years of study. *In*: L. E. Braverman (Ed.), Contemporary Endocrinology: Diseases of the Thyroid, pp. 265–286. Totowa, NJ: Humana Press, 1997.

Schulz, T. F. Epidemiology of Kaposi's sarcoma-associated herpesvirus/human herpesvirus 8. Adv. Cancer Res., *76*:121–160, 1999.

Shamanin, V., zur Hausen, H., Lavergne, D., Proby, C. M., Leigh, I. M., Neumann, C., Hamm, H., Goos, M., Haustein, U.-F., Jung, E. G., Plewig, G., Wolff, H., and de Villiers, E.-M. Human papillomavirus infections in nonmelanoma skin cancers from renal transplant recipients and nonimmunosuppressed patients. J. Natl. Cancer Inst., *88*:802–811, 1996.

Shearer, G. M. HIV-induced immunopathogenesis. Immunity, *9*:587–593, 1998.

Shimizu, Y., Schull, W. J., and Kato, H. Cancer risk among atomic bomb survivors. The RERF life span study. J.A.M.A., *264*:601–604, 1990.

Shimoyama, T., and Crabtree, J. E. Bacterial factors and immune pathogenesis in *Helicobacter pylori* infection. Gut, *43*:S2–S5, 1998.

Shore, R. E., Hildreth, N., Woodard, E., Dvoretsky, P., Hempelmann, L., and Pasternack, B. Breast cancer among women given x-ray therapy for acute postpartum mastitis. J. Natl. Cancer Inst., *77*:689–696, 1986.

Silvestri, F., and Baccarani, M. Hepatitis C virus-related lymphomas. Br. J. Haematol., *99*:475–480, 1997.

Sixbey, J. W., and Yao, Q.-Y. Immunoglobulin A-induced shift of Epstein-Barr virus tissue tropism. Science, *255*:1578–1580, 1992.

Sorrentino, D., Ferraccioli, G. F., DeVita, S., Avellini, C., Beltrami, C. A., Labombarda, A., Bernardis, V., De Biase, F., Trevisi, A., Pivetta, B., Boiocchi, M., and Bartoli, E. B-cell clonality and infection with *Helicobacter pylori*: implications for development of gastric lymphoma. Gut, *38*:837–840, 1996.

Spring, S. B., Hascall, G., and Gruber, J. Issues related to development of Epstein-Barr virus vaccines. J. Natl. Cancer Inst., *88*:1436–1441, 1996.

Stark, R. M., Greenman, J., and Millar, M. R. Physiology and biochemistry of *Helicobacter pylori*. Br. J. Biomed. Sci., *52*:282–290, 1995.

Steven, N. M. Epstein-Barr virus latent infection *in vivo*. Rev. Med. Virol., *7*:97–106, 1997.

Stoler, M. H. A brief synopsis of the role of human papillomaviruses in cervical carcinogenesis. Am. J. Obstet. Gynecol., *175*:1091–1098, 1996.

Strickler, H. D., Rosenberg, P. S., Devesa, S. S., Hertel, J., Fraumeni, J. F. Jr., and Goedert, J. J. Contamination of poliovirus vaccines with simian virus 40 (1955–1963) and subsequent cancer rates. J.A.M.A., *279*:292–295, 1998.

Sugden, B. Latent infection of B lymphocytes by Epstein-Barr virus. Virology, *5*:197–205, 1994.

Sumaya, C. V. Epstein-Barr virus and infectious mononucleosis: a review. J. Clin. Immunoassay, *12*:168–174, 1989.

Tajima, K., and Takezaki, T. Human T cell leukaemia virus type I. Cancer Surv., *33*:191–211, 1998.

Takada, S., Gotoh, Y., Hayashi, S., Yoshida, M., and Koike, K. Structural rearrangement of integrated hepatitis B virus DNA as well as cellular flanking DNA is present in chronically infected hepatic tissues. J. Virol., *64*:822–828, 1990.

Tanaka, H., and Tsukuma, H. Hepatitis C virus. Cancer Surveys, *33*:213–235, 1999.

Taylor, J.-S. Unraveling the molecular pathway from sunlight to skin cancer. Accounts Chem. Res., *27*:76–82, 1994.

Teeguarden, J. G., Dragan, Y. P., and Pitot, H. C. Implications of hormesis on the bioassay and hazard assessment of chemical carcinogens. Hum. Exp. Toxicol., *17*:254–258, 1998.

Terrault, N. A. Treatment of chronic hepatitis B and chronic hepatitis C. Rev. Med. Virol., *6*:215–228, 1996.

Testa, J. R., Carbone, M., Hirvonen, A., Khalili, K., Krynska, B., Linnainmaa, K., Pooley, F. D., Rizzo, P., Rusch, V., and Xiao, G.-H. A multi-institutional study confirms the presence and expression of simian virus 40 in human malignant mesotheliomas. Cancer Res., *58*:4505–4509, 1998.

Tornatore, C., Amemiya, K., Atwood, W., Conant, K., Major, E. O., and Berger, J. JC virus: current concepts and controversies in the molecular virology and pathogenesis of progressive multifocal leucoencephalopathy. Rev. Med. Virol., *4*:197–219, 1994.

Tortolero-Luna, G. Epidemiology of genital human papillomavirus. Hematol. Oncol. Clin. North Am., *13*:245–257, 1999.

Tucker, M. A. Nevi, sun exposure, and the risk of melanoma. *In*: S. A. Wells and P. A. Sharp (Eds.), Accomplishments in Cancer Research, pp. 162–168. New York: Lippincott, Williams & Wilkins, 1998.

Uckun, F. M., Kurosaki, T., Jin, J., Jun, X., Morgan, A., Takata, M., Bolen, J., and Luben, R. Exposure of B-lineage lymphoid cells to low energy electromagnetic fields stimulates Lyn kinase. J. Biol. Chem., *270*:27666–27670, 1995.

Urbach, F. Ultraviolet radiation and skin cancer of humans. J. Photochem. Photobiol. B, *40*:3–7, 1997.

Valberg, P. A., Kavet, R., and Rafferty, C. N. Can low-level 50/60 Hz electric and magnetic fields cause biological effects? Radiat. Res., *148*:2–21, 1997.

Wakeford, R. The risk of childhood cancer from intrauterine and preconceptional exposure to ionizing radiation. Environ. Health Perspect., *103*:1018–1025, 1995.

Watanabe, Y., Harada, S., Saito, I., and Miyamura, T. Prevalence of antibody against the core protein of hepatitis C virus in patients with hepatocellular carcinoma. Int. J. Cancer, *48*:340–343, 1991.

Weiss, H. A., Darby, S. C., Fearn, T., and Doll, R. Leukemia mortality after x-ray treatment for ankylosing spondylitis. Radiat. Res., *142*:1–11, 1995.

Wigdahl, B., and Brady, J. N. Molecular aspects of HTLV-I: relationship to neurological diseases. J. Neurovirol., 2:307–322, 1996.

Wiktor, S. Z., and Blattner, W. A. Epidemiology of human T-cell leukemia virus type I (HTLV-I). *In*: The Human Retroviruses, pp. 175–192. New York: Academic Press, 1991.

Wild, C. P., and Hall, A. J. Hepatitis B virus and liver cancer: unanswered questions. Cancer Surv., *33*:35–54, 1999.

Wold, W. S. M., Mackey, J. K., Brackmann, K. H., Takemori, N., Rigden, P., and Green, M. Analysis of human tumors and human malignant cell lines for BK virus-specific DNA sequences. Proc. Natl. Acad. Sci. U.S.A., *75*:454–458, 1978.

Wotherspoon, A. C. Gastric lymphoma of mucosa-associated lymphoid tissue and *Helicobacter pylori*. Annu. Rev. Med., *49*:289–299, 1998.

Yen, T. S. B. Hepadnaviral X protein: review of recent progress. J. Biomed. Sci., *3*:20–30, 1996.

Yoshida, M. Molecular biology of HTLV-I: recent progress. J. Acquir. Immune Defic. Syndr. Hum. Retrovirol., *13*:S63–S68, 1996.

Yoshimoto, Y. Cancer risk among children of atomic bomb survivors. J.A.M.A., *264*:596–600, 1990.

Zhong, W., Wang, H., Herndier, B., and Ganem, D. Restricted expression of Kaposi sarcoma–associated herpesvirus (human herpesvirus 8) genes in Kaposi sarcoma. Proc. Natl. Acad. Sci. U.S.A., *93*:6641–6646, 1996.

Zhou, Y.-z., Butel, J. S., Li, P.-j., Finegold, M. J., and Melnick, J. L. Integrated state of subgenomic fragments of hepatitis B virus DNA in hepatocellular carcinoma from mainland China. J. Natl. Cancer Inst., *79*:223–231, 1987.

zur Hausen, H. Papillomavirus infections—a major cause of human cancers. Biochim. Biophys. Acta, *1288*:F55–F78, 1996.

Zu Rhein, G. M. Human viruses in experimental neuro-oncogenesis. *In*: E. Grundmann (ed.), Cancer Campaign: Vol. 10, Experimental Neurooncology, Brain Tumor and Pain Therapy, pp. 19–46. Stuttgart, New York: Gustav Fischer, 1987.

Zu Rhein, G. M., and Chou, S. M. Particles resembling papova viruses in human cerebral demyelinating disease. Science, *148*:1477–1479, 1965.

13

Evaluation of Toxic and Carcinogenic Environmental Agents: Scientific and Societal Considerations and Their Role in Cancer Prevention

Definitive epidemiological observations and investigations are the surest way to relate a specific etiologic agent—chemical, physical, or biological—causally with human neoplasms, but epidemiological studies are still relatively insensitive for identifying causative factors in human cancer. Such studies can only identify factors that are different between two populations and that are sufficiently important to play a determining role under the conditions of exposure. Furthermore, on the basis of epidemiological studies, it is extremely difficult to determine whether a specific chemical is or is not carcinogenic to the human because of the extended lag period between exposure and clinical occurrence of a neoplasm, the high background incidence of many cancers in the general population, the relatively imprecise knowledge of the nature of the exposure in most instances, and a number of other confounding variables. Only under exceptional circumstances such as the induction of rare and infrequent neoplasms—e.g., vinyl chloride and angiosarcoma (Dannaher et al., 1981)—is it possible to identify an agent as carcinogenic solely by epidemiological studies when the incidence of cancer induced by that agent is less than 50% more than the occurrence of the resulting cancer in the general human population. Therefore, a "negative" result of an epidemiological investigation must be considered as inconclusive for determining whether or not a relatively weak carcinogenic agent has a role in the etiology of human neoplasia. How, then, is it possible to identify actual and potential carcinogenic agents in our environment by methods other than epidemiological studies? This question has been answered in part by relating the results of additional studies, usually carried out with experimental animals, to the problem of the etiology of human cancer and the risks of environmental agents to populations and/or specific individuals. It is from such studies that government agencies make decisions that ultimately regulate the production and use of—and accordingly the exposures of populations to—agents determined to be actually or potentially carcinogenic for the human.

The ultimate goal of such epidemiological and basic studies is the prevention of human cancer. As discussed in the last two chapters, there is today sufficient scientific knowledge to allow the prevention of more than 60% of human cancers. The failure to achieve such a goal is largely the result of personal and societal decisions well beyond the realm of science. However, since the prevention of disease is by far the most effective and inexpensive mode of health care, it is appropriate that there be a constant and sustained effort to utilize the ever-expanding knowledge of neoplasia to accomplish its control through cancer prevention.

PREVENTION OF HUMAN CANCER—ACTIVE AND PASSIVE

Cancer prevention in humans may in general be grouped into two approaches: active and passive. Table 13.1 supplies an outline of various methods of cancer prevention with an indication of the stage of carcinogenesis toward which the preventive measure is directed. The passive prevention of cancer involves the cessation of smoking, dietary restrictions, and modification of other personal habits such as those of a sexual nature. Active prevention of cancer development is usually accomplished by the administration of an agent to prevent infection by carcinogenic viruses and other organisms or by the intake of chemicals, nutrients, or other factors that may modify or prevent the action of carcinogenic agents. Theoretically, passive cancer prevention or the alteration of one's "carcinogenic" habits can be the most effective and unintrusive method of cancer prevention. However, for many individuals, passive prevention requires external persuasion, such as governmental regulation or peer pressure, to force an alteration of their habits. Obviously, in many instances such methods are doomed to failure. Active cancer prevention, which many consider a form of preventive "therapy," is likely to be the most effective method in this area.

Most of the examples noted in Table 13.1 have been discussed earlier in this text. Individuals with hereditary conditions involving alterations in specific oncogenes or tumor suppressor genes constitute a relatively small part of the population. However, genes that may modify the susceptibility of an individual to the development of certain types of neoplasms probably represent significant factors in the development of an important fraction of human cancers (Spitz and Bondy, 1993). In reviewing the table, one can see that most methods of cancer prevention are linked to action at the stage of promotion. Because this is the reversible stage of neoplastic development, such a finding is not surprising. However, since we still do not know all or even most of the causes of human cancer, the continued identification of agents, especially chemicals, that might induce human cancer is important. While the results of epidemiological studies, when exhibiting sufficient evidence for a causal relationship, may be considered the "gold standard," such detailed studies, even where feasible, for all the potentially carcinogenic agents existing and entering into our environment would be impossible. Therefore, during the last half century, as knowledge of the mechanisms of carcinogenesis increased, a significant effort backed by a

Table 13.1 Modes of the Prevention of Cancer

Mode	Stage
Passive	
Smoking cessation	Pr, Pg
Dietary restriction	Pr
Moderation of alcohol intake	Pr
Modification of sexual and reproductive habits	I, Pr
Avoidance of excessive ultraviolet exposure	I, Pr
Active	
Dietary modification and supplements	Pr
Vaccination against oncogenic viruses	I, Pr
Application of ultraviolet blocking agents in appropriate situations	I, Pr
Selective screening for certain preneoplastic lesions	I, Pr
Determination of genetic background in relation to neoplastic disease	I, Pr
Administration of antihormones	Pr

Key: I, initiation; Pr, promotion; Pg, progression.
After Pitot (1993).

number of governmental agencies throughout the world was directed toward the development of methods for the identification of potentially carcinogenic agents in the environment by a variety of different systems from bacteria to whole animals. This chapter deals with the identification, characterization, and ultimate estimation of human risk from chemical, biological, and physical agents.

IDENTIFICATION OF POTENTIAL CARCINOGENIC AGENTS

A major factor in determining the carcinogenic potential of an agent is its identification as being carcinogenic. While this statement appears obvious and even redundant, identification of a carcinogen is necessary but not sufficient for determining carcinogenic potential. Still, identification is the starting point and for this reason has received the most attention. Generally speaking, the various tests that have been applied to identifying agents with carcinogenic potential may be classified into several general areas. These are seen in Table 13.2. As noted in the table, the time involved in the assay has been arbitrarily separated into short, medium, and long. Short-term assays usually involve days to a few weeks for development of an end point; medium-term assays require weeks to some months but much less than a year. Long-term bioassays usually involve 1½ to 2 years of treatment of animals with a test agent. Each of these general categories consists of specific methods, and each is considered in somewhat greater detail below.

Short-Term Tests—Mutagenesis Assays

A variety of short-term tests, almost all of which are involved in direct or indirect assays of mutagenicity, both in vivo and in vitro, have now been developed and are used to aid in the identification of potential carcinogens. However, virtually all of these methods are of limited use in directly establishing the estimation of the risk that such chemicals pose for the human population. As seen in earlier chapters in this text (Chapters 5 and 6), a ubiquitous characteristic of neoplastic cells is the presence of a variety of different types of mutations. The fact that many but not all carcinogenic agents are mutagenic or may be metabolized to mutagenic forms further establishes the importance of mutations in the development of the neoplastic process. It is on this basis that short-term tests for mutagenicity were developed to identify potential carcinogenic agents on the basis of their capacity for inducing mutations in DNA in cells in vitro or in vivo.

Table 13.3 lists many of the more commonly used short-term tests for mutagenicity and thus carcinogenic potential. The most widely utilized of these mutagenicity assays was originally developed in *Salmonella typhimurium* by Bruce Ames and associates (Ames et al., 1975). In this assay, bacterial cells that are deficient in DNA repair and lack the ability to grow in the

Table 13.2 General Methods for Identification of Potential Carcinogens

Methods	Time Frame
Short term	
Mutagenesis assays	Several weeks
Transformation in cell culture	1–3 months
Medium term	
Qualitative and quantitative analysis of preneoplasia	2–8 months
Long term	
Chronic bioassay in animals	18–24 months

Table 13.3   Short-Term Tests for Mutagenicity

Test	End Point	Reference
Gene mutation assays in vitro		
Prokaryote mutagenesis in vitro (Ames test, etc.)	Back or forward mutations in specific bacterial strains	Maron & Ames, 1983
Mouse lymphoma thymidine kinase (TK)	Mutations in TK	Majeska & Matheson, 1990
Chinese hamster ovary (CHO) and V79 hypoxanthine guanine phosphoribosyl-transferase (HGPRT)	Mutations in HGPRT	Li et al., 1987
Gene mutation assays in vivo		
Dominant lethal assay	Death of fertilized egg in mammalian implanted species	Bateman, 1973 Lockhart et al., 1992
Sperm abnormality induction	Microscopically abnormal sperm	Wyrobek & Bruce, 1975
Mutation induction in transgenes in vivo		
LacZ$^-$ mouse	Mutations in LacZ$^-$ gene	Myhr, 1991
LacI mouse	Mutations in LacI gene	cf. Mirsalis et al., 1994
LacI rat	Mutations in LacI gene	de Boer et al., 1996
rpsL mouse	Mutations in rpsL gene	Gondo et al., 1996
Chromosomal alterations in vivo		
Heritable translocation test (mice)	Translocations induced in germ cells	Generoso et al., 1980
Rat bone marrow clastogenesis in vivo	Chromosomal aberrations in bone marrow cells in vivo	Ito et al., 1994
Micronucleus test	Appearance of micronuclei in bone marrow cells in vivo	Tinwell and Ashby, 1994 Heddle et al., 1983
Chromosomal alterations in vitro		
Mitotic recombination, mitotic crossing over, or mitotic gene conversion in yeast	Conversion of heterozygous alleles to homozygous state	Wintersberger & Klein, 1988
Induced chromosomal aberrations in cell lines	Visible alterations in karyotype	Galloway et al., 1985
Sister chromatid exchange	Visible exchange of differentially labeled sister chromatids	Latt, 1981 Murphy et al., 1992
Primary DNA damage		
DNA repair in vivo or in vitro	Unscheduled DNA synthesis and/or DNA strand breaks	Furihata & Matsushima, 1987
Rodent liver: unscheduled DNA synthesis induction	Unscheduled DNA synthesis in rodent liver cells in vivo and/or in vitro	Kennelly, 1995 Steinmetz et al., 1988

absence of histidine are treated with several dose levels of the test compound, after which reversion to the histidine-positive phenotype is ascertained. Because bacteria differ in their metabolic capabilities compared with mammals, a drug-metabolizing system is added to these assays. Specifically, the 9000 *g* supernatant (S9) that results from centrifuging a liver homogenate prepared from a rat treated with an inducer of multiple P-450s, such as Aroclor 1254, is used in combination with an NADPH regenerating system. The method for performing the *Salmonella* assay (the Ames assay) is described in Figure 13.1. Several different lines of *Salmonella* have been generated to permit the detection of point mutations (TA100, TA1535) and frameshift mutations (TA98, TA1537, TA1538), and the assay is continuously being refined. Typically, five dose levels of the test compound are used in addition to the solvent control. Activation-dependent and activation-independent positive control mutagenic substances are tested concurrently. Certain types of carcinogens are not detected by these bacterial mutagenicity assays, including hormonal carcinogens, metals, agents that have a multiple-target-organ mode of action, and agents with a nongenotoxic mode of action. This bacterial reverse mutation system, when performed in the presence of a mammalian S9 activation system, is, however, a very sensitive screen for the detection of many mutagenic agents.

In addition to the bacterial mutational assay, several in vitro mammalian cell mutation assays exist, including the mouse lymphoma L5178Y (MOLY) assay and the Chinese hamster ovary (CHO) assay. These mammalian mutagenicity assays use either the hypoxanthine-guanine phosphoribosyltransferase (HGPRT) or the thymidine kinase (TK) gene as the end point. The basis for these assays is seen in Figure 13.2. They are similar to the Ames assay in that the phenotypic expression of a mutation in a single-copy gene is compared in treated and untreated cells. These assays are frequently performed in the presence of an exogenous metabolizing source, such as an epithelial cell layer that has been irradiated. The mammalian mutation test systems are forward mutation assays in which the heterozygous state of a gene is used as a tool to detect genetic damage that might result in the loss of a phenotype, e.g., growth in the presence of a toxic compound. In CHO cells, the X-linked HPGRT locus is used as the target gene for analysis. This enzyme is important in purine salvage and allows the incorporation of toxic purine analogs such as 6-thioguanine and 8-azaguanine into DNA, resulting in inhibition of cell growth and/or cell death. Alternatively, a mutation in this gene that results in phenotype loss may permit colony formation in the presence of toxic analogs. Assays based on the forward mutation of TK are similar in that colony formation in the presence of a DNA-damaging agent is scored in the presence of a pyrimidine analog. Because these short-term tests are based on the premise that carcinogens damage DNA, their concordance with the chronic bioassay in vivo (see below) is only between 30% and 80%. In addition, the results of tests are coincident with each other and tend to detect the same types of carcinogens without providing the battery approach that has been suggested. Among the short-term mutagenicity tests that use mutation as the end point, the Ames assay has been the best studied and has been applied to the greatest number of compounds.

Gene Mutation Assays in Vivo

Until relatively recently, a measurement of mutational effects in vivo was rather difficult to perform. One of the more popular assays utilized in this area was the dominant lethal assay, in which male mice are exposed to a potential genotoxic stimulus and mated with untreated female mice; the percentage of pregnancies or number of implants is then determined (Lockhart et al., 1992). While the method is fairly easy to perform, relatively few carcinogenic agents have been studied by this method. Similarly, the production of sperm abnormalities in mice by the administration of chemical agents in vivo has not found general use as a short-term mutagenic assay (Wyrobek and Bruce, 1975).

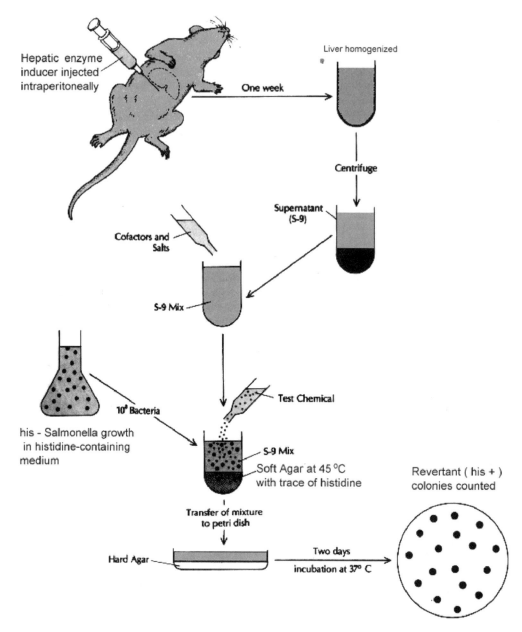

Figure 13.1 Scheme of the Ames test for mutagenesis of chemicals in *Salmonella* bacterial strains. The upper part of the figure outlines the preparation of the S-9 mixture of enzymes and particulates prepared from rodent liver taken from animals previously administered an agent to induce the concentration of such metabolizing enzymes. The *Salmonella*, which require histidine for their growth (his⁻), are grown in the presence of histidine, separated from the growth media, and added with the test chemical and S-9 mix as well as soft agar containing a trace of histidine, which allows the cells to undergo one or two divisions (required for mutation fixation). The S-9 and soft agar mix is transferred to a petri dish while still warm, incubated for several days, and the colonies that develop in the absence of histidine are counted. (Modified from McCann, 1983, with permission of the author and publisher.)

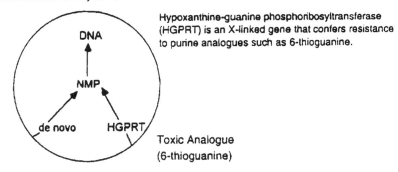

Mammalian Cell Lines Used for Gene Mutation Studies

Mouse lymphoma L5178Y	TK, HGPRT
CHO	HGPRT
V79 hamster cells	HGPRT

Selection of forward mutations by loss of HPGRT+ phenotype in V79 or chinese hamster ovary cells.

DNA

Hypoxanthine-guanine phosphoribosyltransferase (HGPRT) is an X-linked gene that confers resistance to purine analogues such as 6-thioguanine.

NMP

de novo   HGPRT

Toxic Analogue
(6-thioguanine)

Performed in the presence of an activation system or hepatic feeder layer

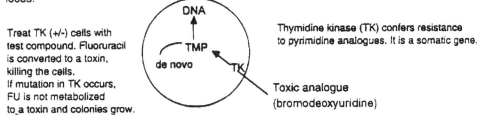

Selection of mutagen-induced TK -/- phenotype in TK+/- in mouse lymphoma assay (MOLY) in L5178Y cells. This assay detects forward mutations at the TK locus.

Treat TK (+/-) cells with test compound. Fluoruracil is converted to a toxin, killing the cells. If mutation in TK occurs, FU is not metabolized to a toxin and colonies grow.

DNA

TMP

de novo   TK

Thymidine kinase (TK) confers resistance to pyrimidine analogues. It is a somatic gene.

Toxic analogue
(bromodeoxyuridine)

Figure 13.2 Outline of chemically induced mutation in mouse cell lines with thymidine kinase (TK) or hypoxanthine-guanine phosphoribosyltransferase (HGPRT) as the target gene. (Reproduced from Pitot and Dragan, 1996, with permission of the authors and publisher.)

In recent years, with a variety of genetic tools available, genetically engineered cells and animals have been developed that have found use in short-term mutagenesis assays. The four examples given in Table 13.3 are those most commonly used for mutational analysis in vivo. The first three involve genetically engineered animals containing transgenes within which are components of the *lac* operon of *Escherichia coli*, a set of coordinately regulated genes involved in lactose metabolism. A schematic representation of the *lac* operon is seen in Figure 13.3. Some details of the function of the *lac* operon are given in the figure legend. Basically, the *lacI* and *lacZ* genes are the ones utilized in the mutational assays. As noted in the figure, mutations in the *lacI* gene will alter the regulation of expression of the *lacZ* gene, which codes for β-galactosidase activity. Thus, the transgene contains either one or the other of the operons. Mutations in the bacterial transgene are determined by the methods seen in Figure 13.4. In this technique,

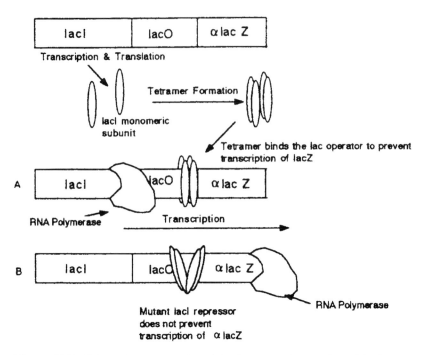

Figure 13.3 Schematic representation of the *lac* operon in *E. coli*. A. The *lacI* gene codes for protein that forms a homotetramer that binds to the *lacO* operator sequence. Binding of the repressor to *lacO* prevents transcription of *lacZ*. B. Transcription of *lacZ* occurs in the presence of the inducing agent, isopropyl-β-thiogalactoside (IPTG). Mutations of the *lacI* may result in partial or complete inactivation of the *lac* repressor, the *lacI* tetrameric protein. Furthermore, mutations in the *lacZ* gene may prevent interaction with the repressor or may be nonfunctional, resulting in no production of the structural gene, *lacZ*. (Reproduced from Provost et al., 1993, with permission of the authors and publisher.)

DNA is extracted from the tissue of interest, and because of the nature of the transgene, construct may be packaged into a bacterial virus, lambda, which then infects the bacteria, *E. coli,* on a lawn of bacterial growth on a dish as noted in the figure. By selecting appropriate bacterial strains and media, one can isolate mutant phage and analyze the sequence of the *lacI* or *lacZ* gene as appropriate. Thus, one may obtain both the number of mutations per unit DNA from the mouse or, more importantly, the actual sequence changes induced by the mutagenic action of the original agent. The *rpsL* transgene works by a similar mechanism but by a different metabolic pathway (Gondo et al., 1996).

Since several of the transgenic animals are commercially patented, this assay may entail some expense, but it is relatively versatile for an in vivo assay for mutagenic identification. However, its ability to detect nonmutagenic carcinogens is doubtful. Of interest is the fact that with at least one carcinogenic agent, ethylnitrosourea, the relative sensitivities of mutations induced in the *lacI* transgene and *hprt*, an endogenous gene, were essentially identical (Skopek et al., 1995). Species differences occur with different carcinogens in that, for example, aflatoxin B_1 treatment resulted in a much greater number of mutations in the *lacI* rat than in the *lacI* mouse (Dycaico et al., 1996). External ionizing radiation was not very mutagenic in the *lacZ* transgenic mouse (Takahashi et al., 1998), but of interest is the finding that the promoting agent phenobarbital enhanced mutation frequency in the livers of *lacZ* transgenic mice treated with diethylnitrosamine (Okada et al., 1997). While a significant number of spontaneous mutations occur in the

B6C3F₁ *lacI* Transgenic Mouse Mutagenicity Assay

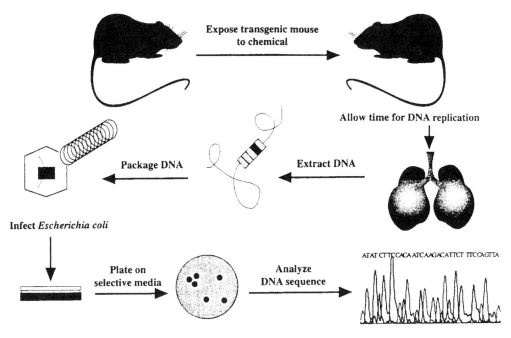

Figure 13.4 Sequence of steps utilized in the determination of the mutagenicity of chemicals in transgenic rodent mutagenicity assays in vivo. The details of the test are briefly discussed in the text or the reader may refer to the original article. (From Recio, 1995; reproduced with permission of the author and publisher.)

transgene, as yet this does not appear to be an insurmountable problem (de Boer et al., 1998). Thus, the potential for utilizing such transgenic models for the in vivo assay of mutagenesis is clearly bright. However, their effectiveness in identifying promoting and progressor agents has yet to be validated.

Chromosomal Alterations

As noted in Chapter 6, chromosomal alterations are extremely common if not ubiquitous in all malignant neoplasms, as was originally suggested by Boveri (1914). Therefore, the induction of chromosomal abnormalities by chemicals in relatively short-term in vivo and in vitro methodologies would logically be considered as an excellent test for carcinogenic potential. Although this has been true in general, the application of various tests for clastogenicity, aneuploidy, and chromatid alterations has not formed the basis for determining the potential carcinogenicity of chemicals. In part, the technology involved is more complicated and expensive than most of the gene mutation assays, and the molecular basis for at least one of the more common tests, that of sister chromatid exchange, is not fully understood. Theoretically, from considerations discussed in Chapter 9, short-term assays for the induction of clastogenicity and related abnormalities would allow the rapid identification of potential progressor agents.

Chromosomal alterations in vivo were studied in germ cells two decades ago by Generoso et al. (1980) in mice. As carried out by these workers, this procedure involves the administration of an agent to male mice shortly before breeding and subsequent examination of male offspring for sterility and/or chromosomal abnormalities in both germ and somatic cells. The test is somewhat complex, and thus far only a few very potent mutagenic agents have been found positive in it. A more commonly employed short-term test for clastogenesis is the micronucleus test, which measures induced clastogenesis in rodent bone marrow in vivo by morphological evaluation of micronuclei containing chromosome fragments in cell preparations from bone marrow (Heddle et al., 1983). However, this assay also has an occasional false positive, such as vitamin C (Tinwell and Ashby, 1994). With the LEC rat, which exhibits a defect in copper metabolism leading to hepatitis and hepatomas, an increased frequency of chromosome aberrations was seen in the bone marrow after administration of direct-acting alkylating agents that did not need metabolic activation (Ito et al., 1994). However, carcinogenic agents requiring metabolic activation, especially in the liver, induced fewer chromosomal abnormalities in the bone marrow of these rats than in normal rats.

Studies in vitro of chromosomal alterations have been carried out both in yeast and in cultured mammalian cells. In the former, various genetic end points are studied, the abnormalities seen being the result of chromosomal alterations (Wintersberger and Klein, 1988). In mammalian cell lines, most of the systems used the same lines as for the gene mutation assays, e.g., Galloway et al. (1985). Relatively few analyses of induced chromosomal alterations have been carried out in normal diploid cells in culture. This test is used much more extensively than most of the other short-term tests involving chromosomal alterations (cf. Ishidate et al., 1988). As might be expected, some discrepancies have arisen between the mutagenic and clastogenic effects of chemicals by these two different systems (cf. Ashby, 1988). Furthermore, chromosomal alterations in these cell lines are sensitive to oxidants (Gille et al., 1993; Shamberger et al., 1973; Kirkland et al., 1989), and preferential targets of chemicals in these aneuploid cell lines are chromosomes bearing amplified genes, already indicative of the karyotypic instability of the cell lines being used (Ottagio et al., 1993).

Another short-term test involving changes in chromosomal structure by mechanisms not entirely understood is the technique of "sister chromatid exchange" (SCE). During metaphase, sister chromatids, each of which is a complete copy of the chromosome, are bound together by mechanisms that involve specific proteins (Nasmyth, 1999). SCE reflects an interchange between DNA molecules within different chromatids at homologous loci within a replicating chromosome (Latt, 1981). The detection of SCEs requires methods of differentially labeling sister chromatids. The usual technique is to allow a cell to incorporate a label, usually a halogenated pyrimidine such as bromodeoxyuridine (BrdU), for one replication cycle and then letting it undergo a second replication cycle in which the presence of the labeled precursor is actually optional. Results of such a technique are seen in Figure 13.5. The degree of staining is noted by the shading of the boxes symbolizing the individual sister chromatids. The diagram in Figure 13.5 indicates the normal staining pattern that would be seen in the absence of SCE. In Figure 13.6 may be seen an example of cells in culture subjected to the technology seen in Figure 13.5, wherein several SCEs can readily be noted. Although the exact mechanism of this phenomenon is not understood, the frequency of induced SCEs has been related linearly to the induction of mutation in the same cell (Carrano and Thompson, 1982). On the other hand, clastogenic events do not parallel SCE formation (Galloway and Wolff, 1979). SCEs occur in normal individuals (Sinha et al., 1985), and the increased levels of SCEs induced in cultured cell lines many times disappear after a number of cell divisions in the absence of the inducing agent (Muscarella and Bloom, 1982). Increases in SCEs may also be induced in cell culture by altering amino acid levels (Zhang and Yang, 1992) and under conditions of nucleotide-pool imbalance (Kaufman, 1986). The procedure has been used in vivo as well as in vitro (DuFrain et al., 1984). In an extensive examination and comparison of the SCE method with cytogenetic changes, the two

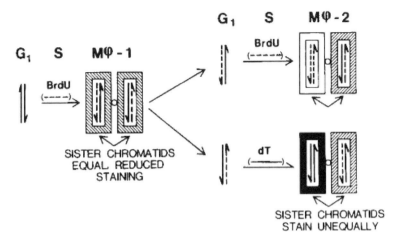

Figure 13.5 Sister chromatid differentiation by BrdU-dye techniques. Cells incorporate BrdU for one cycle shown on the left, followed by a second cycle of replication in which BrdU may be present or absent, the only difference being the intensity of labeling difference. Sister chromatids in metaphase chromosomes from such second-division cells will exhibit unequal staining intensity either by fluorescence or direct observation by visible light, depending on the stain utilized. Solid, hatched, and open areas around each rectangle symbolizing the sister chromatid represent intense, intermediate, and pale staining respectively. (Adapted from Latt, 1981 with permission of the author and publisher.)

methods were about 70% congruent, again indicating that clastogenesis and SCEs are not identical phenomena (Gebhart, 1981).

Primary DNA Damage

The measurement of DNA damage and repair induced by exogenous chemicals, both in vivo and in vitro, has been a relatively common technology used in short-term tests for potential carcinogenicity. The most generally utilized technology involves the analysis of nonreplicative DNA synthesis with appropriately labeled precursor nucleotides (cf. Harbach et al., 1991). More sophisticated techniques involve the measurement of DNA strand breakage by eluting DNA fragments from columns to which the DNA is bound with an alkaline solution (Sina et al., 1983; Miyamae et al., 1997). These techniques have been applied to a variety of tissues in cell culture, both primary and cell lines. Primary liver cell cultures have been among the most popular of the tissues utilized (Williams et al., 1989; Strom et al., 1981; Swierenga et al., 1991). While primary hepatocyte cultures have the advantage of an extensive endogenous metabolic apparatus, other workers have attempted to obviate the problem of metabolism of the agent to the active form by administration of the test chemical in vivo, with subsequent explantation of specific organ tissues to culture and measurement of unscheduled DNA synthesis in such cultures (cf. Furihata and Matsushima, 1987). Just as with all of the short-term tests indicated above, the use of DNA repair analysis has limitations, as evidenced by the fact that in an extensive investigation by Williams and associates (1989) of 167 chemicals testing negative, 44 were carcinogenic. This and the other points raised in this section demonstrate both the usefulness and limitations of short-term tests of mutagenicity and DNA damage for indicating potential carcinogenicity. Regulatory agencies have chosen to approach this problem by requiring a number of different tests to be performed during the study of a particular compound, and these data are taken into account with all of the other information, especially that developed by studies in vivo, as discussed below.

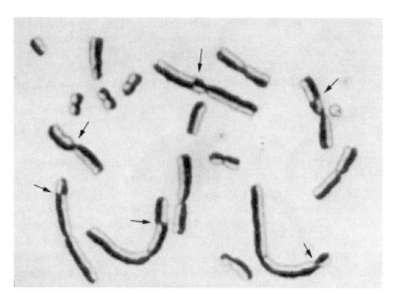

Figure 13.6 Example of Chinese hamster cells grown for two generations in BrdU and stained with Giemsa stain after appropriate treatments. The differential staining of the two sister chromatids can be readily noted, and the exchanges are indicated by arrows. (Adapted from Takayama and Sakanishi, 1977, with permission of the authors and publisher.)

Short-Term Tests—Transformation and Cell Culture

The phenomenon of carcinogenesis in cultured cells is discussed more extensively in Chapter 14. The terms *transformation* and *focus formation* in cultured cells, the basic end points of determining potential carcinogenicity by this technology, are defined in terms of their use and meaning in Chapter 14. As with other of the short-term tests listed in Table 13.3 and discussed above, determination of the "neoplastic" transformation in cultured cells has also taken the direction of the use of a primary (directly from the animal) culture system in which the cells are diploid and normal in all measurable respects. Another direction is the use of a number of cell lines exhibiting aneuploidy but having reasonably defined cultural characteristics. The techniques for the latter have been somewhat standardized (Dunkel et al., 1991), and an extensive degree of study has been carried out with primary Syrian hamster embryo (SHE) cells in primary culture for predicting the carcinogenic potential of a variety of chemicals (cf. Isfort et al., 1996; Barrett et al., 1984). While these techniques are relatively straightforward although somewhat more difficult to score in the SHE system, for the most part they suffer from the inability of the cells to metabolize test agents to their ultimate forms. In addition, given the expense required for the establishment and use of tissue culture methodology, this has been a less than popular short-term test for carcinogenic potential. On the other hand, perhaps more than most of the other short-term tests utilized, transformation to neoplasia in vitro in cell culture has found considerable usefulness in studying the basic cell and molecular aspects of the neoplastic transformation (Chapters 14 and 16).

Chronic Bioassays for Carcinogenicity—Medium- and Long-Term

The ability to induce neoplasia in lower animals has been the basis for our understanding of the pathogenesis of neoplasia. Early studies showing the induction of skin cancer in mice by coal tar derivatives and of liver cancer by organic dyes (Chapter 3) led to the establishment of model systems in these and other tissues, both for the investigation of cancer development and ultimately for testing of agents for their carcinogenic potential. The administration of chemicals in the diet for extended periods, pioneered in the 1930s by Yoshida and colleagues (Sasaki and Yoshida, 1935), formed the basis for the establishment of the chronic bioassay of carcinogenicity that is used today. This methodology was espoused by the National Cancer Institute some 30 years after Yoshida's findings (Hadidian et al., 1968), and almost 200 assays of chemicals for their carcinogenic potential by the prolonged feeding to animals was carried out over the next decade (Hottendorf and Pachter, 1985). Parallel to the use of this lifetime model of carcinogenesis in small rodents was the development of various organ-specific model systems, multistage models, and most recently the use of transgenic animals in carcinogen testing. A listing of these animal models is seen in Table 13.4.

Chronic 2-Year Bioassay

Today the gold standard for determining potential carcinogenic activity of a chemical is through the use of the chronic 2-year bioassay for carcinogenicity in rodents. This assay involves test groups of 50 rats and mice of both sexes and at two or three dose levels of the test agent. The

Table 13.4 Animal Models of Neoplastic Development

	End Point	References
Chronic 2-year bioassay	Tumors in all organs	Sontag, 1977
Tissue specific bioassays		
Liver, mouse	Hepatomas	Carmichael et al., 1997
Lung, mouse	Pulmonary adenomas	Shimkin and Stoner, 1975
Brain, rat	Gliomas	Kroh, 1995
Mammary gland, rat/mouse	Adenomas and carcinomas	Dunnick et al., 1995
Medium-term bioassays		
Ito model	Hepatic adenomas and carcinomas	Ito et al., 1989
Newborn mouse	Neoplasms in liver, lung, lymphoid organs	Fujii, 1991
Multistage models of neoplastic development		
Bladder, rat	Papillomas/carcinomas	Hicks, 1980
Colon, rat	Aberrant crypt polyp	Sutherland and Bird, 1994
Epidermis, mouse	Papillomas	DiGiovanni, 1992
Liver, rat	Altered hepatic foci	Pitot et al., 1996
Transgenic mice		
Knockout of p53 tumor suppressor gene ($p53^{\text{def}}$)	Tumors in heterozygous animals having normal phenotype	Donehower, 1996
v-Ha-*ras* with zetaglobin promoter; tandem insertion on chromosome 11 (TG.AC)	Induced transgene expression in skin leads to papilloma development	Spalding, 1993

animals should be susceptible but not hypersensitive to the tested effect. In general, two strains are typically used by regulatory agencies in the United States, the B6C3F1 mouse and the F344 rat. The format for the bioassay is seen in Figure 13.7. Quite simply, animals at about 8 weeks of age are placed on the test agent at the various doses for another 96 weeks of their lifespan. The test agent may be administered by dietary feeding, by gavage on a regular basis, or by inhalation in rather complex chambers. A variety of pretest analyses are carried out, such as those for acute toxicity, route of administration, and determination of the maximum tolerated dose (MTD). The use of the MTD has been challenged by many, arguing that the toxic effects of high doses of an agent can cause a replicative response in normal cells that could lead to an increase in neoplasia quite secondary to the effects of the agent itself (Cutler et al., 1997; Haseman and Lockhart, 1994). This is supported by the finding of a very high percentage, nearly half in some instances, of agents exhibiting no potential for mutagenicity but inducing neoplasia at the MTD (Gold et al., 1993). Furthermore, these two strains of rodents have a significant spontaneous tumor incidence, as can be noted in Table 13.5.

Because so many research dollars go into carcinogenicity testing and the data resulting from such studies are expected to be useful not only in hazard identification but also in risk estimation, an acceptable scientific protocol with quality assurance must be followed to produce scientifically and statistically valid data. A variety of factors relevant to the acceptable outcome of a carcinogenicity study are considered, including animal husbandry; the identity and purity of the test compound and identification of any contaminants; the homogeneity, stability, and physical properties of the test compound under various storage conditions; and the solubility, stability, and availability of the test compound in the solvent. In addition, the formulation should be either that which is to be administered to humans or that which permits bioavailability in the test organism. The environment of the rodent is also important, and care should be taken to control for sources of variability in the animals, their diet, and their housing. While the usual comparison in animal studies is the concurrent control, for a number of situations historical controls may be more appropriate (Haseman et al., 1997).

The underlying basis for risk extrapolation from animals to human is that the animal is a good model for human cancer development. In fact, 2-year bioassay models have been used to detect the compounds listed by the International Agency for Research on Cancer (IARC) (Vainio et al., 1991) as known human carcinogens. Also, most known human chemical carcinogens have a carcinogenic potential in animals that supports the results of epidemiological studies (Vainio et al., 1985). Exceptions include ethanol and arsenic. In addition, it has now become evident that some neoplastic responses to chemicals in animals are unique to the rodent and species as well as the sex involved. These include such responses as thyroid neoplasia (McClain, 1989), the induction of α_{2u}-globulin (Swenberg et al., 1985) resulting in renal neoplasms in male rats, and peroxisome proliferation (Ashby et al., 1994) associated with the induction of hepatic neoplasia in rats. In addition, a significant problem that has arisen in the continued use of the chronic bioassay is the requirement for ad libitum feeding. This results in animals, especially in rats, of extreme weight by the end of the 2 years; many will have died spontaneously prior to the end of

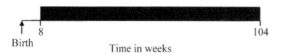

Figure 13.7 Diagram of format for chronic 2-year bioassay for carcinogenic potential.

Table 13.5 Spontaneous Tumor Incidence (Combined Benign and Malignant) in Selected Sites of the Two Species, B6C3F1 Mice and F344 Rats, Used in the NCI/NTP Bioassay

Site	B6C3F1 Mice		F344 Rats	
	Male	Female	Male	Female
Liver				
adenoma	10.3	4.0	3.4	3.0
carcinoma	21.3	4.1	0.8	0.2
Pituitary	0.7	8.3	24.7	47.5
Adrenal	3.8	1.0	19.4	8.0
Thyroid	1.3	2.1	10.7	9.3
Hematopoietic	12.7	27.2	30.1	18.9
Mammary gland	0	1.9	2.5	26.1
Lung	17.1	7.5	2.4	1.2

Adapted from Pitot and Dragan, 1996, with permission of publisher.

the test. Such complications are now being remedied by the use of dietary restriction in the chronic bioassay for the 2-year period. As shown in Chapter 8, this phenomenon reduces spontaneous cancer incidence and extends lifespan in rodents, and its usefulness in the refinement of the 2-year chronic bioassay is now becoming more appreciated (Keenan et al., 1996; Allaben et al., 1996).

The statistical analysis of results obtained in chronic bioassays has also been difficult when the analysis results in relatively few neoplasms in test animals. As can be seen from Table 13.6, a relatively high percentage of animals must bear tumors before a statistically significant result

Table 13.6 Percentage of Animals with Tumors (Rx) Administered a Test Agent Required to Obtain Statistical Significance When Compared with Control Animals with Tumors (Co)

Percent with Tumors in Control	Number of Animals		Percent with Tumors in Rx
	Control	+ Test Agent	
0	50	50	10
	100	50	6
	500	50	4
10	50	50	26
	100	50	22
	500	50	20
20	50	50	38
	100	50	34
	500	50	32
30	50	50	50
	100	50	46
	500	50	44

Adapted from Sontag, 1977.

can be obtained in the face of significant development of spontaneous lesions. Since the latter phenomenon is clearly a problem in these animals (Table 13.5), borderline results become a very difficult problem for regulatory agencies in determining whether or not a compound actually is carcinogenic in the assay or not. An exception to this is when a very unusual histogenetic type of neoplasm not seen spontaneously is found in the test animals at a significant, even very low level (Chu et al., 1981; Basu et al., 1996). The enumeration of all neoplasms versus those in specific tissues also can raise difficulties in interpretation of the bioassay. Despite these criticisms and problems, the chronic 2-year bioassay continues to be the major basis for regulatory action in this country and in many countries throughout the world.

Tissue-Specific Bioassays

During the performance of long-term bioassays, it became obvious that certain tissues in specific species exhibited neoplasms more frequently than others when a test agent was administered. From these observations, several tissue-specific bioassays were developed with the objective of a reasonably sensitive assay carried out in a shorter time than the usual chronic 2-year bioassay. The best-known tissue-specific assay is that utilizing the mouse liver. In a recent analysis of chronic bioassays carried out by the National Toxicology Program, Crump et al. reported that 108 of 390 studies indicated a positive carcinogenic response to the test chemical. In 81 of these studies, female mice exhibited significant increases in the incidence of hepatic neoplasms. As noted in Table 13.5, there is a high incidence of spontaneous hepatoma development in mice, more so in the male (Chapter 8). This has led to controversy in the interpretation of the significance of the development of mouse hepatomas, especially if they are the only statistically significant increased neoplastic response in the test animals. As a result of this controversy, the interpretation of the significance of the induction of mouse hepatic lesions has been called into question (cf. Dragan et al., 1998; Moch et al., 1996). A further complication of this assay is the fact that in at least one study, the majority of the chemicals testing positive exhibited no evidence of an ability to induce DNA damage or mutation (Carmichael et al., 1997).

Another tissue-specific bioassay that was developed by Shimkin and associates more than two decades ago (Shimkin and Stoner, 1975) is the development of pulmonary adenomas and carcinomas, primarily in strain A mice. The assay was shown to effectively identify a number of relatively potent carcinogenic agents, including a few inorganic carcinogens (Stoner et al., 1976). However, although the assay has not been generally accepted as a major component for the determination of carcinogenicity of chemicals, it has found usefulness in the determination of the molecular mechanisms of pulmonary carcinogenesis in this strain of animals (You et al., 1989; Nuzum et al., 1990). In addition, as noted from Table 13.4, induction of gliomas in the rat brain and of mammary neoplasms in both the rat and the mouse may exhibit potential for tissue-specific bioassays. There have also been attempts to utilize lower vertebrates in the development of tissue-specific bioassays, such as the rainbow trout embryo (Hendricks et al., 1980).

Medium-Term Bioassays

While tissue-specific bioassays were directed in part at decreasing the time required for the analysis of carcinogenic potential in vivo, at least two assays have been specifically designated as having reduced the time for the development of an end point. The one most intensively used today, primarily in Japan, is the model developed by Dr. Nobuyuki Ito and colleagues (Ogiso et al., 1990; Shirai, 1997). A diagram of the format for this assay is seen in Figure 13.8. The entire assay takes only 8 weeks, and the end point is nodules and focal lesions in the liver of rats that stain for glutathione S-transferase pi (GST-P). The initial "programming" of the liver by

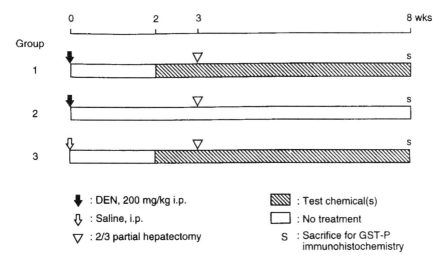

Figure 13.8 The medium-term liver bioassay protocol for identification of potentially carcinogenic agents. DEN, diethylnitrosamine; GST-P, glutathione S-transferase pi. (Reproduced from Shirai, 1997, with permission of the author and publisher.)

administration of a necrogenic dose of diethylnitrosamine poses some problems in that this dose by itself is carcinogenic, but only after a year or more. Furthermore, this high dose is also clastogenic to rat hepatocytes in vivo (Sargent et al., 1989). However, these authors and their colleagues have demonstrated a significant degree of correlation between long- and medium-term results, indicating the usefulness of this assay as a potential surrogate for the chronic bioassay (Ogiso et al., 1990). More recently these authors have used a slightly modified protocol in which five potent carcinogenic agents are administered for a 4-week period, followed by administration of the test chemical for a subsequent 24- to 32-week period (Ito et al., 1996). Unlike the assay depicted in Figure 13.7, this more complicated procedure may allow the detection of promoting and progressor agents as well as complete carcinogens in a variety of different tissues. However, outside of Japan these assay procedures have not been generally utilized.

The newborn mouse model of chemical carcinogenesis was initially described by Shubik and colleagues (Pietra et al., 1959) and later used extensively in studies of mouse hepatocarcinogenesis by Vesselinovitch and colleagues (1978). More recently, Fujii (1991) has utilized this procedure in the determination of the carcinogenic potential of 45 different chemicals with quite reasonable results. The end point of neoplasms in a variety of different tissues, including lung, liver, lymphoid and hematopoietic tissues, is determined within a 1-year period. The assay is relatively inexpensive, utilizing small amounts of the test materials. As yet, however, this assay has not found general usefulness in the determination of carcinogenic potential by regulatory agencies.

Multistage Models of Neoplastic Development

As previously noted, the original studies on multistage models of carcinogenesis were developed with the epidermis of the mouse (Chapter 7). It was not until some 40 years after those initial experiments that there was some attempt at standardization of the multistage model of carcinogenesis in mouse skin for the analysis of the carcinogenic potential of specific chemicals (Pereira, 1982). The format for such assays was essentially that described in Chapter 7 (Figure

7.1). Few refinements in the procedure were added with the exception of the use of a genetically susceptible strain of mice, the SENCAR strain, which is now utilized in such tests (Slaga, 1986). This system may also be extended to the potential analysis of progressor agents (Hennings et al., 1993; Warren et al., 1993).

Considerably later than the initial reports of the mouse skin system, Hicks et al. (1975) demonstrated the cocarcinogenic or promoting action of several agents in the development of bladder cancer in the rat. Subsequently, other promoting agents have been demonstrated with this or a related assay, some of which appear to be relatively unique to this tissue for both anatomical and chemical reasons (Cohen and Lawson, 1995; Ito and Fukushima, 1989). At about the same time as the initial report of the multistage bladder model of carcinogenesis, Peraino and associates (1977) reported a multistage model of carcinogenesis in the rat liver. This finding has led to the development of a number of models of multistage carcinogenesis in the rat liver. Solt and Farber (1976) reported a model somewhat analogous to that of Ito and colleagues, but with an aim directed primarily at studying mechanisms of hepatocarcinogenesis rather than utilizing it as an assay system for potential carcinogens. Shortly thereafter, Pitot et al. (1978) developed a model wherein initiation was performed with a nonnecrogenic dose of the initiating agent, subsequently followed by chronic administration of a promoting agent. The format of these two assay systems are noted in Figure 13.9. The end point of these systems is the quantitative analysis of altered hepatic foci measured by one of several enzymatic markers, the most sensitive being the expression of GST-P (Hendrich et al., 1987). Several studies have investigated the potential for such analyses in the detection of chemical carcinogens (Pereira and Stoner, 1985; Williams, 1989; Oesterle and Deml, 1990). A similar format has been used to study the preneoplastic aberrant crypt foci in the colon of animals administered potential carcinogens (Ghia et al., 1996). However, as yet all such assays utilizing preneoplastic end points have not found general usefulness in the identification of potential carcinogenic agents. It is possible that in the future such assays may be useful in distinguishing between agents exerting their carcinogenic effect primarily at one or another of the stages of carcinogenesis.

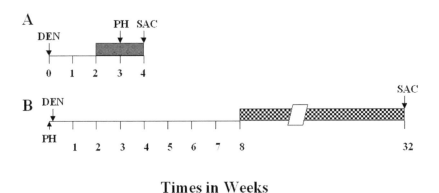

Times in Weeks

Figure 13.9 Formats of short-term models of multistage hepatocarcinogenesis in the rat. A. The Solt-Farber model, in which animals are administered a necrogenic dose of diethylnitrosamine followed 2 weeks later by the administration of 0.02% acetylaminofluorene (shaded bar) with a 70% partial hepatectomy performed after 1 week of AAF feeding and sacrifice 1 week following the surgery. B. The Pitot et al. (1978) model, in which a non-necrogenic dose (10 mg/kg) of DEN is administered 24 hours after a partial hepatectomy (PH), and animals are fed a normal diet for 8 weeks, at which time they are placed on a diet containing 0.05% phenobarbital for a subsequent 24 weeks and then sacrificed. The end point of both models is the quantitation of altered hepatic foci.

Transgenic and Knockout Mice as Models of Carcinogenesis

With the advent of the development of transgenic animals as well as gene targeting in mice (Chapter 5), recent efforts have been directed toward the development of animal models with specific genetic alterations that make them more susceptible to carcinogenesis by external agents. As noted from Table 13.4, the most popular of these are mice exhibiting one defective allele of the *p53* tumor suppressor gene and a transgenic mouse line (TG·AC) carrying a v-Ha-*ras* oncogene fused to a zeta globin promoter. A high frequency of a variety of spontaneous neoplasms develop in *p53*-deficient mice. The incidence of such tumors is noted in Figure 13.10. In general, all of the homozygous *p53*-defective mice develop neoplasms by 10 months of age, while the heterozygous mice have a 50% incidence by 18 months, with over 90% incidence by 2 years of age (Donehower, 1996). However, the heterozygous animals did not show an accelerated carcinogenesis of the liver, even when hepatocarcinogens were administered (Dass et al., 1999). In addition to this model system, which mimics the Li-Fraumeni syndrome in humans (Chapter 5), a large number of other gene-targeted mutations have been developed in mice but have not yet been utilized as model systems for identifying potential carcinogenic agents (Rosenberg, 1997).

The TG·AC transgenic mouse is one of a large number of potential transgenic mice and rats that might be considered for the study of the development of neoplasia in response to test agents. However, in most cases the expression of the transgene is targeted to a specific tissue, and thus one deals with a tissue-specific development of neoplasia (cf. Goldsworthy et al., 1994). The TG·AC transgenic mouse is very effective in the identification of potential promoting agents for the skin. Administration of the well-known skin-promoting agent, TPA (Chapter 7), could induce the development of papillomas after only three to ten applications (Spalding et al., 1993). These investigators also studied several other potential promoting and progressor agents,

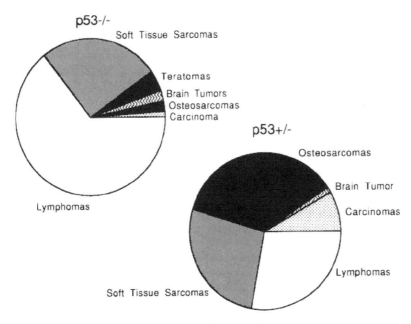

Figure 13.10 Tumor incidence of *p53*[−/−] and *p53*[+/−] mice. The relative frequency of each of the types of neoplasms is indicated by the proportionate size of the pie slice. (From Donehower, 1996, with permission of the author and publisher.)

all of which exhibited a short latency period and high incidence of papilloma induction. Thus, it is apparent that each of these genetic models of carcinogenesis has a role to play in the identification of potential carcinogenic agents. It will require considerable effort to validate each of the models with respect to tissue-specific carcinogenesis by complete carcinogens or by promoting and/or progressor agents (cf. Tennant, 1998).

EVALUATION OF CARCINOGENIC POTENTIAL

The multiple in vivo and in vitro tests described thus far in this chapter present the experimentalist or the regulator with an extensive amount of data from which to draw conclusions about the carcinogenic potential of the test agent. In addition, epidemiological studies (Chapters 11 and 12) provide perhaps the most definitive means of estimating the carcinogenic potential to humans from exposure to a specific agent. While such studies, if definitively positive, are the best evidence for the carcinogenic potential of an agent to the human, the evidence is usually obtained after an exposure has occurred in a population. In general, epidemiological studies can detect differences between populations only when there is approximately a twofold increase above the background incidence of neoplasia in the control population. Since many more agents than those classified as group 1 by IARC exhibit carcinogenic potential, the in vitro and in vivo tests described earlier have been used as surrogates in attempting to determine carcinogenic potential and risk to the human population. The results of such tests clearly offer qualitative information regarding the identification of agents exhibiting some potential hazard with respect to one or more aspects of the process of carcinogenesis as we know it today. Major difficulties remain in attempting to extrapolate in a scientific and meaningful way information obtained from in vitro and in vivo tests to an estimation of the potential risk of such agents to the human population as inducers of disease, especially neoplasia. As might be expected, a number of problems are involved in the scientific and practical application of information developed from short- and long-term tests to the estimation of human risk.

The Problem of Extrapolation

Since bacterial mutagenicity (Figure 13.1) is the most widely and extensively utilized test for estimating the qualitative carcinogenic potential of an agent, a number of investigations have been directed toward determining the relationship of bacterial mutagenesis and carcinogenesis of the same chemical, usually in rodents. An early graphical relationship of such a series of tests is seen in Figure 13.11. Obviously, considerably more efforts have been carried out since the publication of this in 1976 (Sugimura et al., 1976). However, the figure does place in rather definitive terms compounds that exhibit either carcinogenic and/or mutagenic activities. The indicated description of complete carcinogen, promoting agent, initiating agent, etc., is an exercise allowing the further classification of such agents in multistage carcinogenesis. In a far more extensive study, Tennant et al. (1987) related the results of bacterial mutagenicity to carcinogenic potential as determined in the chronic 2-year bioassay and found that the short-term assay detected only about half of the carcinogens as mutagens. These studies and a slightly later one by Ashby (1989) pointed again to the importance of using more than a single short-term assay in attempting to relate DNA structural alterations to potential carcinogenicity. Although the prediction of carcinogenic potential by the bacterial mutagenicity tests together with other short-term tests is in the neighborhood of 60% to 70%, it is somewhat surprising that interspecies extrapolation of carcinogenesis in rats and mice is not much greater than this. In an analysis by Gold et al. (1989), chronic bioassays for carcinogenic potential in either mice or rats were only about

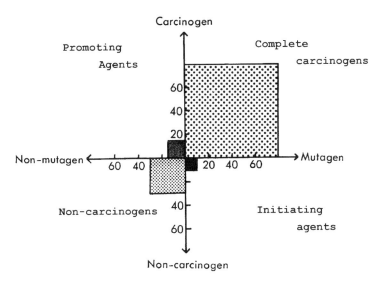

Figure 13.11 Graphical representation of mutagens and nonmutagens in relation to their known carcinogenic potential in animal tests. The labeling of the quadrants using the classification of Table 9.10 is a further potential extrapolation of these data. (After Sugimura et al., 1976, with permission of the authors and publisher.)

70% to 75% predictive of carcinogenicity in the other species. In a more recent study (Fung et al., 1993) of 379 chemicals tested by the National Cancer Institute/National Toxicology Program for carcinogenic potential, only slightly more than 50% of the chemicals tested exhibited carcinogenicity in at least one organ of one sex of one species. Less than half of these exhibited carcinogenic potential in both species tested, a situation most likely to be indicative of a carcinogenic hazard to humans.

Structure-Activity Relationships of Chemicals to Risk and Extrapolation

Although the Pullman's (Chapter 3) were among the first to attempt a structure-activity relationship of carcinogenic chemicals in relating this to predicting carcinogenicity in animals and potentially humans, this approach has been expanded during the last several decades. This is largely the result of various methodologies for the analysis of chemical structures and the extensive capability of data handling by computers and more modern technologies. Figure 13.11 depicts a summarized diagram of many of the "reactive forms" of chemical carcinogens. However, there are numerous other subtleties in structure that may be related to some carcinogenic potential. While it is beyond the scope of this text to consider this subject in detail, the student may be interested in reading several reviews of the subject using different approaches, such as those of Klopman and Rosenkranz, 1994; Enslein et al., 1994; and Zhang et al., 1996. Attempts have been made to predict carcinogenicity of nongenotoxic chemicals by structure-activity relationships (Lee et al., 1995) and distinguishing between genotoxic and nongenotoxic chemicals by similar methods (Cunningham et al., 1998). An extensive review of the implications of structure-activity relationships for cross species extrapolation in DNA damage and repair as related to mutagenesis and carcinogenesis has also been published (Vogel et al., 1996). In ideal circumstances, prediction of the carcinogenic action of a chemical by its structure is very much to be desired. In the final analysis, the prediction of the carcinogenic effect of specific structures in the human would be most useful, but as yet the biological effects of carcinogenic chemicals in the human are so diverse that no such ideal for extrapolation has been found.

Several other issues are also relevant to cross-species extrapolation, including differences in metabolism of chemical agents between the species. While metabolic schemes are qualitatively similar across species, significant quantitative differences, especially in metabolic rate, partly owing to elimination kinetics, are the rule. Exposure estimation is frequently based on the daily dose administered or on plasma concentration used as a surrogate for concentrations in the tissue. Using plasma concentrations for extrapolation across species assumes that each species responds in the same manner to any given dose of an agent. In the final analysis, it may be that the best basis for cross-species comparison is serum concentration expressed as milligrams per kilogram body weight, since this better predicts tissue concentration-response effects after chronic administration (Allen et al., 1988; Monro, 1992). Thus, it is clear that the problem of extrapolation of both short- and long-term tests to carcinogenic potential in the human is much less than perfect, suggesting an important need for reevaluation and reinterpretation of the tests currently in use. Needless to say, a program to develop better extrapolative end points should be a major priority.

The Dose-Response Problem

Another important component in the analysis of assays for carcinogenic potential, both in vivo and in vitro, is that of the dose-response to a particular test agent. Just as with radiation carcinogenesis (Chapter 3), the effectiveness of the induction of neoplasia by an agent is dependent on the dose of that agent administered to the test animal. The dose-response curves for the stage of initiation in rodent liver neoplasia were already noted in Chapter 7, as well as the dose-response of promoting agents in the mouse epidermal model of multistage carcinogenesis. The differences in the shapes of these two curves were discussed in that chapter and are considered again below.

Other factors may also influence a dose-response curve, such as the toxicity of the agent, the bioavailability of the agent, and the metabolic or pharmacokinetic characteristics of the agent within the living organism. A classic dose-response of a complete carcinogen and some of its ramifications are seen in Figure 13.12 (Druckrey et al., 1963). In this figure, curve 1 shows the relationship between the daily dose administered and the median total dose of animals developing carcinoma. Thus, the left ordinate indicates the sum of all doses administered up to a 50% tumor incidence, therefore relating the total dose to the tumor incidence. In this way the straight-line relationship, if extrapolated, would proceed through the origin. Curve 2 relates the daily dose of carcinogen to the median induction time of the appearance of the first neoplasm. While extrapolation of curve 1 through the origin indicates that there is no dose at which some incidence of neoplasms is not apparent, it should be noted that if the daily dose is less than 0.1 mg/kg, no experimental data points are available. Furthermore, extrapolation of curve 2 to this low-dose region indicates that at doses lower than 0.1 mg/kg, the rats used in this experiment and whose lifetime is approximately 1000 days will not live sufficiently long for carcinomas to appear. In the assay depicted in Figure 13.12, the animals were administered a carcinogenic agent at a constant rate in the diet. Littlefield and Gaylor (1985) noted that with another complete carcinogen, 2-acetylaminofluorene, both the dose rate and the total dose administered are important in the final analysis. These workers demonstrated that when the total doses of this test agent were similar, the higher dose rates with shorter time periods induced a higher prevalence of neoplasms.

The use of the maximal tolerated dose (MTD) has been criticized because of the toxicity it induces, paralleled by an increase in cell proliferation in a number of susceptible organs (Ames

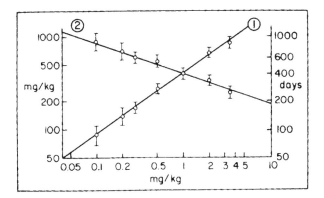

Figure 13.12   Dose-response relation seen in the chronic feeding of 4-dimethylaminostilbene to rats. 1. Relation between the daily dose and the median total dose for animals that developed carcinoma. 2. Relation between daily dose and median induction time. The abscissa shows the daily dose; the ordinate on the left is the total dose administered, and on the right is the time from the beginning of the experiment. All scales are logarithmic. (Modified from Druckrey et al., 1963.)

and Gold, 1990). At the other end of the dose-response curve, the problem of the presence or absence of a threshold (no-effect level) of a carcinogenic agent is still hotly debated. It has already been noted that, on theoretical grounds, agents capable of damaging DNA might not be expected to exhibit a threshold, whereas those exerting their effects through complicated receptor-mediated pathways, as with promoting agents, would be expected to exhibit a threshold of their effects (Aldridge, 1986). In addition, as briefly pointed out in the previous chapter (Chapter 12, Figure 12.5), carcinogenic agents, whether DNA-damaging or not, may exhibit a lower than control effect at very low doses (Kitchin et al., 1994; Teeguarden et al., 1998). Despite these observations, as well as the data depicted in Figure 13.12 and our knowledge of the mechanism of action of promoting agents, regulatory agencies have in general not seen fit to alter the philosophy that carcinogenic agents do not have threshold dose levels. As outlined below, this philosophy has permeated much of the regulatory action taken to date with respect to agents shown to be carcinogenic in any form of life.

In most epidemiological studies it has not been possible to determine the doses of the agents to which humans have been exposed, and only occasional, rather crude retrospective dose-response curves are available. However, a summary was made by the Meselson Committee (1975) of dose levels of several known human carcinogens that appear to be carcinogenic for certain human populations. These estimated levels were compared with levels of these agents known to produce neoplasms in animals (Table 13.7). They show that the cumulative doses required per unit of body weight for tumor induction in the human and in experimental animals are of the same order of magnitude for four of the six agents. However, a more detailed comparison would require a correction for the short observation time in many of the studies on humans (as in the case of diethylstilbestrol and vinyl chloride), since many cancers in humans do not appear for 20 to 30 years after exposure. In addition, both vinyl chloride and diethylstilbestrol cause a very rare neoplasm in humans that is not usually seen in experimental animals. Thus, the effective doses of several agents known to be carcinogenic for humans and rodents are not markedly dissimilar in the two species. If this conclusion can be extended to other chemical carcinogens in the human environment, then both the qualitative and quantitative extrapolations of such findings in the animal to the human situation have some degree of validity.

Table 13.7 Approximate Total Doses for Tumor Induction in Humans and Experimental Animals

Agent	Human		Animal	
	Dose and Organ	Incidence (%)	Dose, Species, and Organ	Incidence[a] (%)
Benzidine	50–200 mg/kg[b] (bladder)[c]	22–50	10,000 mg/kg[b] (mouse liver)[c]	67
			50–100 mg/kg (rat mammary gland)	50–80 (2)[a]
Chlornaphazine	2000 mg/kg (bladder)	16.0	75–4800 mg/kg (mouse lung)	40–100 (38)
Diethylstilbestrol	0.5–300 mg/kg (vaginal and cervical adenocarcinoma)	0.2	2–13 mg/kg (male mouse mammary gland)	4–27
			400 mg/kg (newborn female mouse cervix and vagina)	33
Aflatoxin B_1	0.1 mg/kg (liver)	0.5	1.25–6.0 mg/kg (mouse liver)	23–100 (3)
			0.3–1.5 mg/kg (rat liver)	19–100
Vinyl chloride	70,000 mg/kg (liver)	0.2	30,000 mg/kg (mouse lung and mammary gland)	25, lung 13, mammary
			40,000 mg/kg (rat kidney and liver)	9, kidney 6, liver
Cigarette smoke	From 1000 cigarettes/kg (lung)	2.5	From 400 cigarettes per kilogram (mouse lung)	4.9 (1.3)
			From 6000 cigarettes per kilogram (hamster larynx)	6

[a]Tumor incidence in control groups of animals, given in parentheses. When not designated, control incidence was 0 or not stated.
[b]The average dose of the group(s).
[c]The organ affected and species (for the animals) are noted in parentheses.
Meselson Committee, 1975.

The Problem of the Potency of Carcinogenic Agents

It should be apparent by now that not all carcinogenic agents are equally effective in inducing neoplasia, i.e., they exhibit differing carcinogenic potencies. The potency of an agent to induce neoplasia has been simply defined as the slope of the dose-response curve for induction of neoplasms (Choy, 1996). However, such a definition has generally not been the basis for estimates of carcinogenic potency based on data from chronic bioassays with continuous administration of the agent. In Table 13.8 may be seen a listing of some methods for the measurement of the potency of carcinogens, beginning with the early study by Iball (1939) resulting in the Iball Index, which was used for a number of years thereafter. The relationship of Meselson and Russell (1977) may also be derived from the results of bacterial mutagenesis assays. The potency relationship developed by Crouch and Wilson (1979) is dependent on a linear, no-threshold extrapolation of the animal bioassay result, giving the slope as β in the equation seen in the table (Barr, 1985). The TD_{50} has been extensively used, and values were recently compiled by Gold and Zeiger (1997) for a large number of chemicals. The range of carcinogenic potencies developed from such a relationship may be seen in Figure 13.13. Tennant and his associates (1997) have modified the TD_{50} potency relationship, using a different fraction of animals that develop neoplasms. The T_{25} is defined by these workers as the chronic dose rate in mg/kg of body weight per day that will give 25% of the animals neoplasms at a specific tissue site, after correction for spontaneous incidence, within the standard lifetime of the test species. As expected, since the relationship is basically the same as that noted in Table 13.8 except for only half the percentage, the T_{25} values are usually roughly one-half those of the TD_{50} values. Pepelko (1991) has pointed out one of the difficulties of these absolute potency measurements in that differences in solubility, bioavailability, and some other pharmacokinetic parameters do cause considerable variability in some of the potency values reported.

While the four relationships noted in the table under "absolute" do analyze carcinogenic potency of a chemical from the data on the bioassay of that chemical alone, Glass and associates (1991) proposed a relative potency relationship that has some degree of flexibility and may have some application in risk assessment different from the absolute analyses. Pitot et al. attempted to determine indices relating the stages of initiation and promotion to the potency of the agents inducing such stages. In the case of the initiation index, which is relatively straightforward, the values obtained are absolute. In the case of the promoting index, the value is always given in relation to the nontreated control, which does develop focal lesions from endogenous promotion of spontaneously initiated hepatocytes (Chapter 7). These measures of initiating and promoting potencies have been applied only to multistage hepatocarcinogenesis in the rat. But it is quite feasible to extend such analyses to multistage carcinogenesis in a number of other solid organs where the immediate results of initiation can be quantitated and the relative growth of lesions from the initiated cell population can be determined with some degree of accuracy (Pitot et al., 1987).

Carcinogenic Potencies Across Species

Although the parameter of carcinogenic potency is not of major concern to regulatory agencies, there have been a number of attempts at relating this parameter to carcinogenesis in the human. In 1989 Crump attempted to relate the potency of carcinogens in mice and humans, using a potency calculation somewhat similar to the T_{25} (Dybing et al., 1997), but did not find a great deal of concordance. Their results are seen in Figure 13.14, with the key for the chemical symbols in the figure legend. These authors suggest several reasons for lack of concordance, a major one being that confirmed human carcinogens have not been adequately studied in many animal models. However, they concluded, on the basis of the data seen in Figure 13.14, that animal and

Table 13.8 Some Methods for the Measurement of the Potency of Carcinogens

Relationship	Description	Reference
Absolute		
Carcinogenic (Iball) index = $\dfrac{\text{\% of tumors (animals with)}}{\text{average latent period in days}}$	The percentage number of tumor-bearing animals was calculated from the total number of animals used in the particular assay or from the total number of animals surviving at the time the first tumor became manifest (Hueper, 1963).	Iball, 1939
$K = \dfrac{\ln 2}{D_{1/2}}$	$D_{1/2}$ is the total animal dose which gives a 50% incidence of cancer after a 2-year exposure. K is defined as potency.	Meselson and Russell, 1977
$R = -\ln (1-p) = \alpha + \beta d$	R = potency where p is the probability of developing cancer at dose d, and α and β are derived constants.	Crouch and Wilson, 1979
$TD_{50} = \log(2)/b$	The TD_{50} (carcinogenic potency) of a chemical is defined as the dose rate (mg/kg body weight/day, b) which, if administered chronically for a standard period, would halve the probability of an animal remaining without any neoplasia (Bernstein, 1985).	Peto et al., 1984
Relative		
Relative potency = $\dfrac{\text{dose of a reference compound needed to produce a specific effect in a particular bioassay (reference dose)}}{\text{dose of a test compound needed to produce the same magnitude of the same effect in the same bioassay (test dose)}}$	The relative potency of a given agent is defined as the ratio of the dose of that chemical required to induce carcinogenesis in a particular bioassay, relative to the dose of another (reference) agent required to produce the same outcome in the same type of bioassay.	Glass et al., 1991
Multistage		
Initiation index = #AHF/liver/mmole/kg body weight	Index based on administration of a single dose of initiating agent in mmole/kg body weight.	Pitot et al., 1987
Promotion index = $V_f/V_c \times \text{mmol}^{-1} \times \text{weeks}^{-1}$	V_f is the total volume fraction (%) occupied by AHF in the livers of rats treated with the test agent, and V_c is the total volume of AHF in control animals, which have only been initiated. The dose rate of administration of the promoting agent is expressed as millimoles/week.	Pitot et al., 1987

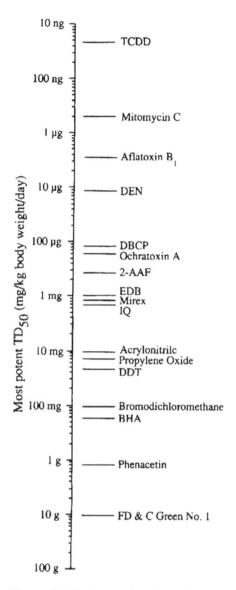

Figure 13.13   Range of carcinogenic potency as determined by the TD_{50} potency relationship of Peto et al. (1984). (Adapted from Gold et al., 1998, with permission of the authors and publisher.)

human potencies as measured by them were strongly correlated. Somewhat earlier than the data presented in Figure 13.14 was the study of Gold et al. (1987), who applied the TD_{50} potency index from animal studies to a number of chemicals having chronic occupational exposure for U.S. workers. They proposed the use of the TD_{50} to develop an index termed the permitted exposure/rodent potency (PERP), which does not estimate absolute risks directly, but rather is indicative of relative hazards for the substances to exposed workers. In a more recent study, Dedrick and Morrison (1992) related the carcinogenicity of several alkylating agents in causing leukemia in patients treated for cancer compared with the potency of these agents to induce neoplasms in

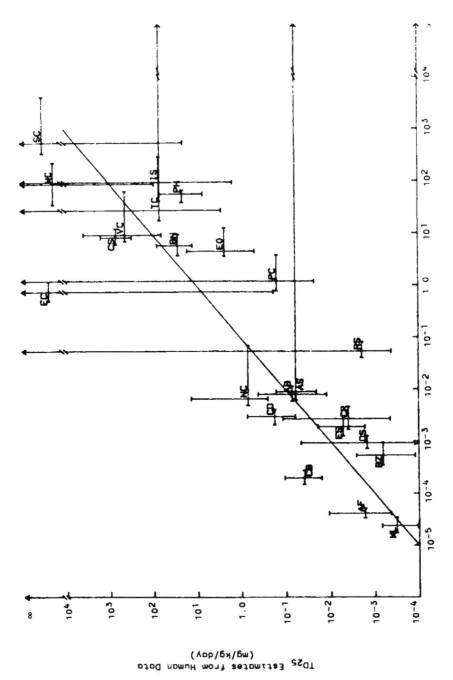

Figure 13.14 Human TD_{25} estimates versus animal TD_{25} estimates obtained from a log-log plot with data from any experiment, regardless of route of exposure. The best estimate of the animal TD_{25} is plotted for each chemical, with the vertical lines extending from that point representing the upper and lower bounds for the human TD_{25} and the horizontal lines representing the corresponding bounds for the animal TD_{25}. The chemicals that were studied are listed as follows, with the abbreviations seen in the figure:

Abbreviation	Chemical	Abbreviation	Chemical	Abbreviation	Chemical
AF	Aflatoxin	CS	Cigarette smoke	NC	Nickel
AS	Arsenic	DS	Diethylstilbestrol	PC	PCBs
AB	Asbestos	EC	Epichlorohydrin	H	Phenacetin
BN	Benzene	ES	Estrogens	RS	Reserpine
BZ	Benzidine	EO	Ethylene oxide	SC	Saccharin
CD	Cadmium	IS	Isoniazid	TC	Trichloroethylene
CB	Chlorambucil	ML	Melphalan	VC	Vinyl chloride
CR	Chromium	MC	Methylene chloride		

(Adapted from Crump, 1989, with permission of author and publisher.)

rats and mice. In general, a good correlation among species was observed when the carcinogenic potency was based on the total lifetime exposure.

RELATION (EXTRAPOLATION) OF BIOASSAY DATA TO HUMAN RISK

Campbell (1980) suggested the thesis that the risk (R) of some agent or event can be estimated as a function of the product of the probability (P) of the event and the severity of the harmfulness of the event or agent (H):

$$R = P \times H$$

From the simplest viewpoint, the risk-taker may accept harm of greater severity (high value of H) only if the probability of occurrence (P) is very low. Conversely, events that are only modestly harmful (low value of H) may be acceptable at higher levels of frequency or probability. From this argument, safety may be taken as a measure of acceptability of some degree of risk.

Table 13.9, taken from the work of Oser (1978) and Upton (1980), lists the risk of death classified in relation to specific activities. From this table, all of the activities listed exhibit some degree of risk or probability (P) of death or harm (H). The important point to note is that the probability of risk per million persons per year ranges from 0.1 for lightning striking to 20,000 in the case of motorcycling. A careful person presumably compares the risks of any event to his or her health with the benefits that will potentially accrue before making a decision. Relatively few people may actually do this, and even when they do, precisely what index is chosen as the indicator of relative safety is a function of the value judgment of each individual.

As to the risk of cancer, the harm (H) is considered by most lay persons to be extremely great. In view of this concern by the public, the U.S. government through its regulatory agencies, such as the Environmental Protection Agency (EPA), the Food and Drug Administration (FDA), and others, has assumed a major role in practical considerations of human risk from environmental agents. Two theorems are the basis for the estimations of human risk from carcinogenic agents in the environment.

1. A threshold (no-effect) level for a carcinogenic agent cannot be determined with any degree of accuracy.
2. All carcinogenic agents produce their effects in an irreversible manner, so that the actions of small amounts of carcinogenic agents in our environment are additive— producing a "carcinogenic burden" for the average individual during his or her lifetime.

These bases may be considered as default assumptions that are utilized if there is not sufficient evidence to alter these assumptions. Recent guidelines by the EPA have indicated that at least one regulatory agency is beginning to consider and even include in their final disposition of the regulation of a chemical data that may alter these default assumptions (Page et al., 1997). Since the presence of thresholds of promoting agents as well as their reversibility has already been noted (Chapter 7), such data may become useful in consideration of regulation of chemicals in the future. However, the gold standard chronic 2-year bioassay that is utilized as the mainstay in regulation of both industrial and pharmaceutical chemicals does not distinguish between initiating, promoting, and progressor agents; it will require substantial additional studies to give cause to alter the default assumptions. As noted above, scientific risk estimation should be carried out with the full knowledge of the action of the carcinogenic agent as a complete carcinogen, or as having a major action at one or more of the stages of carcinogenesis.

Table 13.9 Risk of Death, by Type of Activity

Activity	Risk of Death per Million Persons per Year
Travel	
Motorcycling	20,000
Pedestrian	40
Automobile	20–30
Airplane	9
Sports	
Car racing	1,200
Rock climbing	1,000
Canoeing	400
Skiing	170
Power boating	30
Swimming (recreational)	19–30
Bicycling	10
Eating and drinking	
Alcohol—one bottle of wine/day	75
Alcohol—one bottle of beer/day	20
Low-level radiation	
Coal mining (black lung disease, 1969)	8,000
Nuclear plant worker (0.8 rem/year, average) (radiation-induced cancer)	80
Airline pilot (0.3 rem/year, average) (radiation-induced cancer)	30
Grand Central Station (40 hours/week, 0.12 rem/year)	12
Jet air travel, general population (0.47 mrem/year) (radiation-induced cancer)	0.047
Miscellaneous	
Smoking 20 cigarettes/day	2,000–5,000
Pregnancy	230
Abortion after 14 weeks	70
Contraceptive pills	20
Home accidents	12
Vaccination against smallpox	3
Earthquakes (California)	1.7
Hurricanes	0.4
Lightning	0.1

After Oser, 1978, and Upton, 1980.

The extrapolation of bioassay data to human risk estimation is one of the most difficult problems that has faced society and will face us for years to come as numerous new chemicals enter the environment. In attempting to predict the behavior of a chemical in the human from data obtained from bioassays, a number of factors should be considered in extrapolation of bioassay data to human risk (Kraybill, 1978). These include:

- Reproducibility of experimental data
- Tumor incidence in experimental animals on a dose-dependent basis
- Relative approximation of experimental dose to that of human exposure
- Acceptable design and statistical evaluation of bioassay

- Consensus on interpretation of histopathological changes
- Availability of biochemical, metabolic, and pharmacokinetic data to be considered in final decision making

Not included in these factors proposed more than two decades ago is a knowledge of the action of the agent as an initiating, promoting, or progressor agent. Unfortunately, not all of these factors are taken into account when regulatory decisions are made at the governmental level concerning specific compounds in our environment. Newer requirements for more extensive studies of compounds that would satisfy these factors are a goal to be achieved but as yet not attained.

Another consideration in determination of human risk is whether or not the estimation is qualitative or quantitative. Qualitative risk estimation is much easier to develop based on qualitative analyses of the variety of bioassay procedures utilized. As noted in Chapter 11, the IARC as well as regulatory agencies throughout the world take very seriously the qualitative finding of induction of neoplasia in one or two species of animals as a qualitative indication of risk of carcinogenicity to the human. However, quantitative risk analysis is much more difficult. In fact, a number of epidemiologists have refused to make such quantitative relationships on the basis of animal data and would only use data in the human to carry out such estimates. Still, as we have seen from the utilization of various "safe" doses of carcinogenic agents and a variety of other factors, quantitative risk assessment has been and is being applied to human risk situations of specific chemicals and mixtures. Paramount in such considerations are the use of mathematical models in which, making a variety of assumptions, one may develop quantitative risk estimates for the human. Some of these models are considered below.

STATISTICAL ESTIMATES OF HUMAN RISK FROM BIOASSAY DATA BY USING MATHEMATICAL MODELS

The statistical analyses of whole-animal bioassay data have employed over the years a number of mathematical models in an attempt to relate experimental data to the human situation, especially for the purposes of quantitating human risk insofar as is possible. As Gaylor and Shapiro (1979) have pointed out, "There is no choice but to extrapolate." This means, in essence, that because of the insensitivity of epidemiologic studies and the number and quantity of actual and potential carcinogens in our environment, one must make every attempt possible to relate data from bioassay studies to the human condition, especially the potential risk to the public. Most of these mathematical models have as a basic tenet the assumption that carcinogenic agents lack a threshold, act irreversibly, and have effects that are additive. Equations for some of the more commonly used models are given in Table 13.10. None of these models can prove or disprove the existence of a threshold of response, and none can be completely verified on the basis of biological argument; however, the models have been useful in data evaluation and are presently being used by some federal agencies in extrapolating experimental data to the human risk situation. One of the most commonly used techniques is the log-probit model. In the earlier use of this model, the procedure was to regard every agent as carcinogenic. On this assumption, one must determine some "safe" dosage level at which the risk calculated would not exceed some very small level such as 1 in 100,000,000 or 10^{-8}.

The linear multistage model, first proposed by Armitage and Doll (1954), incorporates the idea of multiple steps into a statistical approach for risk analysis. This multistage model (Figure 13.15) incorporates one aspect of the pathogenesis of neoplastic development, that of multiple stages, but cell cycle-dependent processes, the dynamics of cell kinetics, birth rate, and death

Table 13.10 Mathematical Models Used in the Extrapolation of the
Risk of Carcinogenic Agents to the Human

	Equation for the Probability (P) of Tumor Induction at Dose d
One-hit (linear) model	$P(d) = 1 - e^{(-\lambda d)}$
Multihit (k-hit) model	$P(d) = 1 - \sum_{i=0}^{k-1} (\lambda d)^i e^{-\lambda d}/i!$
Multistage model	$P(d) = 1 - \exp[-(\alpha_1 + \beta_1 d) \ldots (\lambda_k + \beta_k d)]$
Extreme-value model	$P(d) = 1 - \exp[-\exp(\alpha + \beta \log d)]$
Log-probit model	$P(d) = \Phi[\alpha + \beta \log_{10}(d)]$

rate are not considered. Furthermore, the transition from one stage to the next is considered irreversible. Despite these deficiencies, the linearized multistage model is one of the most commonly utilized models at the present time. At a low dose, the multistage model is used to fit the observed tumor incidence data to a polynomial of the dose as noted in Table 13.10. The linear multistage model is not appropriate for estimating low-dose carcinogenic potency for many chemicals. In most cases, the dose response of high doses of testing differs substantially from the considerably lower doses for exposure. Pharmacokinetic and pharmacodynamic models provide information that can help bridge the gap between the high dose and low dose scenarios (Anderson, 1989). A second problem is associated with extrapolation of lifetime exposure of animals to the MTD of a compound to the less than lifetime exposure common for humans. This problem has been addressed by the EPA through the use of the Weibull model (Hanes and Wedel, 1985), which assumes that risk is greater when encountered at a younger age, and, once exposure occurs, risk continues to accrue despite the cessation of exposure. However, observations in humans and experimental animals have demonstrated that in many cases risk decreases after exposure ceases, as would be true if the agent were a promoting agent.

More recently, biomathematical modeling of cancer risk assessment has been used in an attempt to relate such models more closely to the biological characteristics of the pathogenesis of neoplasia. The best known of these biologically based models is that described originally by Moolgavkar, Venzon, and Knudson, termed the MVK model (Moolgavkar, 1986). This model, which is depicted in Figure 13.15, reproduces quite well the multistage characteristics of neoplastic development with μ_1, the rate at which normal cells are converted to "intermediate" cells (initiated cells), and μ_2, the rate at which intermediate cells are converted to neoplastic (N) cells. These rates model the rates of initiation and progression in multistage carcinogenesis, while the stage of promotion represents the expansion of the intermediate cell population, which is a function of α_2, the rate of division of "intermediate cells," and β_2, the rate of differentiation and/or death of intermediate cells. Other factors in the model that are also true in biology are the rate of replication and cell death of normal or stem cells. While this model originally was developed to explain certain epidemiological characteristics of breast cancer incidence and mortality in humans (Moolgavkar, 1986), it has found potential application in a variety of multistage models including that of rat liver (Luebeck et al., 1991). Application of the model to risk assessment problems has not found wide use, but this may change in the next few years (Anderson et al., 1992). In addition, integration of biological data, including pharmacokinetic and pharmacodynamic parameters, should aid in the development of a more biologically based risk assessment model.

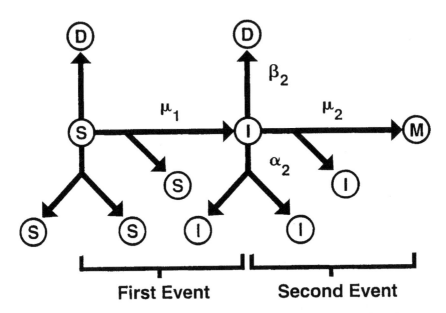

Figure 13.15 The Armitage and Doll (upper) and MKV (lower) models of multistage carcinogenesis. In the former, the number of stages is unspecified (T_k), and the transition between them is irreversible. In the MKV model, the fates of stem cells (S) and intermediate (I) cells are death (D) or proliferation. Rarely, I cells undergo μ_2 to malignancy (M). The rates of replication (α_2) and apoptosis (β_2) for I cells are indicated, and similar rates for S cells are implied. μ_1 and μ_2 are the rates of the first genetic event (initiation) and the second genetic event (progression). (Adapted from Pitot and Dragan, 1996, with permission of the authors and publishers.)

REGULATION OF CARCINOGENIC RISK AT THE FEDERAL LEVEL

At least four federal agencies have as their primary responsibility the regulation of risk. These agencies include the Consumer Product Safety Commission (CPSC), the EPA, the U.S. Food and Drug Administration (FDA), and the Occupational Safety and Health Administration (OSHA). At least two types of regulations affect risk analysis; these include regulations similar to the Clean Water Act, which imposes technology-based standards that are dictated by the best available technology, and the Clean Air Act, which imposes health- or risk-based standards to protect human health by providing an ample margin of safety. A number of laws have been passed that control exposure to carcinogens in food, drugs, and the environment (Table 13.11). Perhaps the most controversial is the Food, Drug, and Cosmetic Act of 1938, including the 1958 amendment known as the Delaney Amendment. The Delaney Amendment was passed to curtail any possible use of additives in food and drugs that had been demonstrated to induce cancer in humans or animals. This law ignores the presence of endogenous or endogenously produced compounds that have carcinogenic action. For example, nitrites are effective bactericidal agents when used at low levels as food additives, but nitrites are produced extensively in vivo during normal metabolism of nitrogenous compounds, especially when nitrates are present in the diet (Rogers, 1982). High doses of nitrites given with secondary amines result in the formation of nitrosamines, which are carcinogenic in rodents (Rogers, 1982). Thus, a number of difficulties are encountered when food and additives are regulated with strict adherence to the Delaney Amendment.

Besides science, a major driving force in legislative actions concerning the regulation of carcinogenic or potentially carcinogenic chemicals in the environment is the benefit obtained from such regulation. The saccharin-cyclamate debates were an interesting example of this (Kraybill, 1976). Saccharin is carcinogenic at a very high dose in rat uroepithelium (Anderson et al., 1988). After considerable debate, the U.S. Congress passed a law permitting the use of this "carcinogenic" compound as an artificial sweetener because of its low cost and benefit to a variety of individuals, especially diabetics. Recently, the courts rejected the use of two food colorings in drugs and cosmetics on the basis of an interpretation of the Delaney Amendment as prohibitive of the use of additives even when only minimal risk can be demonstrated. The EPA faces a difficult situation in the regulation of pesticides when it attempts to balance the requirement of the Federal Insecticide, Fungicide, and Rodenticide Act (FIFRA), which requires a balance of risk and benefit in the application of pesticides to raw agricultural products, and the zero tolerance for carcinogens in processed foodstuffs mandated by the Delaney Amendment. OSHA is responsible for regulating workers' exposure to potential toxins, including carcinogens. The statutes require that feasibility be considered in concert with lack of effect on workers' health. In

Table 13.11 Selected Federal Laws for Regulation of Toxic and Carcinogenic Agents

Name of Act and Year Passed and Amended	Area of Concern
Food Drug and Cosmetic Act (FDC): 1906, 1938, amended 1958 (Delaney), 1960, 1962, 1968, 1976, 1980, 1984, 1986, 1987, 1990, 1992	Food, drugs, cosmetics, food additives, color additives, new drugs, animal feed additives, medical devices.
Federal Insecticide, Fungicide, and Rodenticide Act (FIFRA): 1948, amended 1972, 1975, 1976	Pesticides
Clean Air Act: 1970, amended 1974, 1977, 1978, 1980, 1981, 1982, 1983, 1990	Air pollutants
Clean Water Act: 1972, amended 1977–1983, 1987, 1988, 1990, 1992; originally the Federal Water Control Act	Water pollutants
Occupational Safety and Health Act (OSHA): 1970, amended 1974, 1978, 1979, 1982, 1990, 1992	Workplace exposure to toxicants
Toxic Substances Control Act (TOSCA): 1976, amended 1981, 1983, 1984, 1986, 1988, 1990, 1992	Hazardous chemicals not covered elsewhere, including pre-market review

Adapted from Office of Science and Technology Policy, 1986.

the case of *Industrial Union Department v American Petroleum Institute*, the Supreme Court found that the allowable levels of a compound (i.e., benzene) could be established only if a significant risk from exposure could be demonstrated and that this risk could be lessened by a change in practice. In the final analysis, a significant proportion of risk to the average citizen is based on the perception of risk.

International Aspects of Environmental Regulation

Other countries have both preceded and followed legal actions in the United States in regulating noxious and carcinogenic agents that can and do occur in the human environment. The United Kingdom passed a Clean Air Act some three decades ago, well before such legislation appeared in the United States (cf. Hall, 1976). This same nation passed legislation regulating pollution in natural waters within the country at about the same time as similar legislation was enacted in the United States. The European Common Market has also advanced several programs in the area of environmental pollution, especially as related to air and water environments. More generally, they have established an environmental program that concerns itself with the impact of factors involving alterations in the environment, waste disposal, and educational programs (cf. Johnson, 1976). Other countries throughout the world have recognized the importance of controlling potentially damaging agents and have acted accordingly.

RISK-BENEFIT CONSIDERATIONS IN THE REGULATION OF ACTUAL AND POTENTIAL CARCINOGENIC ENVIRONMENTAL HAZARDS

We have briefly reviewed the methods for determining the actual and potential carcinogenic agents in our environment, methods for the estimation of risk to the human population of such agents, and the governmental approach to the regulation of such agents in our environment. An equally important consideration includes somewhat undefined concepts such as benefit-risk analysis, cost-effectiveness, and risk-cost analysis in the regulation of hazardous agents in our environment. These concepts are concerned with such traditional regulatory terms as "safe," "lowest feasible," and "best practicable technology."

Some of the regulatory legislation leaves no latitude for considerations of benefit versus risk. This is the case with the Delaney Amendment, a simplistic legal statement that can create major problems when the regulatory agencies are faced with obeying the law. Problems also arose with respect to nitrite, since the benefits of removing nitrites as preservatives in packaged meats were balanced against the risk of bacterial contamination, especially by *Clostridium botulinum*, in nonpreserved packaged products. Federal regulatory agencies decided that these data were insufficient to ban nitrites under the Delaney clause, and thus nitrite continues to be widely used as a preservative, although at lower levels.

Attempts have been made to quantitate and characterize risks versus benefits. One way is to consider risks to the environment and to health as opposed to risks to society and to general aspects of health. It is evident that reduction in risk from direct exposure to an environmental factor will, at some level of additional cost of control, create new risks to society in terms of increased costs of products, availability of services, personal freedoms, employment, and so on. This relation is shown in Figure 13.16. In controlling risks to the environment and to health, there is a point beyond which the benefits to society and the individual begin to decrease because of the cost, both financial and otherwise, incurred in reducing risk toward actual zero. As implied previously, there are very rare instances in which actual zero risk is obtained in any cir-

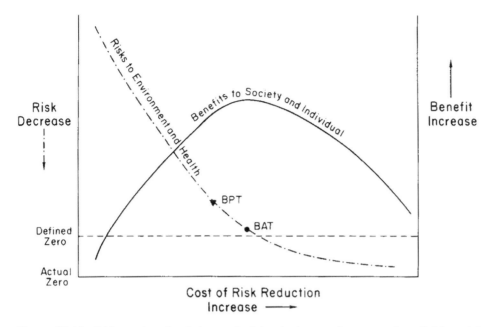

Figure 13.16 Risk-cost-benefit relation emphasizing the impact of cost control on all risks and demonstrating the loss of benefit beyond a certain cost of risk reduction. BPT, best practicable technology; BAT, best available technology. (Modified from Blair and Hoerger, 1979.)

cumstance. The points for best practicable technology (BPT) and for best available technology (BAT) are seen on the risk curve. Clearly BPT in risk reduction is less costly than BAT.

More extensive risk-benefit analyses have been published, such as those of Moll and Tihansky (1977), in which dollar values have been estimated for each life that could potentially be saved by eliminating a specific agent from the environment. They also point out that the risks of specific agents in industrial situations may be far greater than those to society as a whole. An example is asbestos, which, though clearly hazardous to some industrial workers, causes little or no hazard at the levels of exposure of the population in general. In this respect, Samuels (1979) has pointed to the potential fallacy in many benefit-risk determinations unless one takes into consideration the concept of *necessary risk*, especially as related to occupational and industrial hazards. This concept stresses the importance of making every effort to eliminate hazardous agents in our environment that are important to society by replacing them with equally useful but less hazardous or nonhazardous components. If this cannot be done and a necessary risk is present, this consideration must be balanced against the benefits.

REFERENCES

Aldridge, W. N. The biological basis and measurement of thresholds. Annu. Rev. Pharmacol. Toxicol., 26:39–58, 1986.

Allaben, W. T., Turturro, A., Leakey, J. E. A., Seng, J. E., and Hart, R. W. FDA points-to-consider documents: the need for dietary control for the reduction of experimental variability within animal assays and the use of dietary restriction to achieve dietary control. Toxicol. Pathol., 24:776–781, 1996.

Allen, B., Crump, K., and Shipp, A. Correlation between carcinogenic potency of chemicals in animals and humans. Risk Anal., 8:531–561, 1988.

Ames, B. N., and Gold, L. S. Chemical carcinogenesis: too many rodent carcinogens. Proc. Natl. Acad. Sci. U.S.A., 87:7772–7776, 1990.

Ames, B. N., McCann, J., and Yamasaki, E. Methods for detecting carcinogens and mutagens with the Salmonella/mammalian-microsome mutagenicity test. Mutat. Res., 31:347–364, 1975.

Anderson, M. E. Tissue dosimetry, physiologically based pharmacokinetic modeling, and cancer risk assessment. Cell Biol. Toxicol., 5:405–415, 1989.

Anderson, M. E., Krishnan, K., Conolly, R. B., and McClellan, R. O. Mechanistic toxicology research and biologically-based modeling: partners for improving quantitative risk assessments. Chem. Indust. Inst. Toxicol., 12:1–7, 1992.

Anderson, R., Lefever, F., and Mauer, J. Comparison of the responses of male rats to dietary sodium saccharin exposure initiated during nursing with responses to exposure initiated to weaning. Food Chem. Toxicol., 26:899–907, 1988.

Armitage, P., and Doll, R. The age distribution of cancer and a multi-stage theory of carcinogenesis. Br. J. Cancer, 8:1–12, 1954.

Ashby, J. An opinion on the significance of the 19 non-clastogenic gene-mutagens reported by Tennant et al. (1987). Mutagenesis, 3:463–465, 1988.

Ashby, J. Origins of current uncertainties in carcinogen/mutagen screening. Environ. Mol. Mutagen., 16:51–59, 1989.

Ashby, J., Brady, A., Elcombe, C. R., Elliott, B. M., Ishmael, J., Odum, J., Tugwood, J. D., Kettle, S., and Purchase, I. F. H. Mechanistically-based human hazard assessment of peroxisome proliferator-induced hepatocarcinogenesis. Hum. Exp. Toxicol., 13:S1–S117, 1994.

Barr, J. T. The calculation and use of carcinogenic potency: a review. Regul. Toxicol. Pharmacol., 5:432–459, 1985.

Barrett, J. C., Hesterberg, T. W., and Thomassen, D. G. Use of cell transformation systems for carcinogenicity testing and mechanistic studies of carcinogenesis. Pharmacol. Rev., 36:53S–70S, 1984.

Basu, A. P., Gaylor, D. W., and Chen, J. J. Estimating the probability of occurrence of tumor for a rare cancer with zero occurrence in a sample. Regul. Toxicol. Pharmacol., 23:139–144, 1996.

Bateman, A. J. The dominant lethal assay in the mouse. Agents Actions, 3(2):73–76, 1973.

Blair, E. H., and Hoerger, F. D. Risk/benefit analysis as viewed by the chemical industry. Ann. N.Y. Acad. Sci., 329:253–262, 1979.

Boveri, T. Zur Frage der Entstehung Maligner Tumoren. Jena: Gustav Fischer, 1914.

Campbell, T. C. Chemical carcinogens and human risk assessment. Fed. Proc., 39:2467–2484, 1980.

Carmichael, N. G., Enzmann, H., Pate, I., and Waechter, F. The significance of mouse liver tumor formation for carcinogenic risk assessment: results and conclusions from a survey of ten years of testing by the agrochemical industry. Environ. Health Perspect., 105:1196–1203, 1997.

Carrano, A. V., and Thompson, L. H. Sister chromatid exchange and gene mutation. Cytogenet. Cell Genet., 33:57–61, 1982.

Choy, W. N. Principles of genetic toxicology. In: A. M. Fan and L. W. Chang (Eds.), Toxicology and Risk Assessment. Principles, Methods, and Applications, pp. 25–36. New York: Marcel Dekker, 1996.

Chu, K. C., Cueto, C., Jr., and Ward, J. M. Factors in the evaluation of 200 National Cancer Institute carcinogen bioassays. J. Toxicol. Environ. Health, 8:251–280, 1981.

Cohen, S. M., and Lawson, T. A. Rodent bladder tumors do not always predict for humans. Cancer Lett., 93:9–16, 1995.

Crouch, E., and Wilson, R. Interspecies comparison of carcinogenic potency. J. Toxicol. Environ. Health, 5:1095–1112, 1979.

Crump, K. Correlation of carcinogenicity potency in animals and humans. Cell Biol. Toxicol., 5:393–403, 1989.

Cunningham, A. R., Rosenkranz, H. S., Zhang, Y. P., and Klopman, G. Identification of "genotoxic" and "non-genotoxic" alerts for cancer in mice: the carcinogenic potency database. Mutat. Res., 398:1–17, 1998.

Cutler, N. R., Sramek, J. J., Greenblatt, D. J., Chaikin, P., Ford, N., Lesko, L. J., Davis, B., and Williams, R. L. Defining the maximum tolerated dose: investigator, academic, industry and regulatory perspectives. J. Clin. Pharmacol., *37*:767–783, 1997.

Dannaher, C. L., Tamburro, C. H., and Yam, L. T. Occupational carcinogenesis: the Louisville experience with vinyl chloride-associated hepatic angiosarcoma. Am. J. Med., *70*:279–287, 1981.

Dass, S. B., Bucci, T. J., Heflich, R. H., and Casciano, D. A. Evaluation of the transgenic *p53*$^{+/-}$ mouse for detecting genotoxic liver carcinogens in a short-term bioassay. Cancer Lett., *143*:81–85, 1999.

de Boer, J. G., Erfle, H., Holcroft, J., Walsh, D., Dycaico, M., Provost, S., Short, J., and Glickman, B. W. Spontaneous mutants recovered from liver and germ cell tissue of low copy number *lacI* transgenic rats. Mutat. Res., *352*:73–78, 1996.

de Boer, J. G., Provost, S., Gorelick, N., Tindall, K., and Glickman, B. W. Spontaneous mutation in *lacI* transgenic mice: a comparison of tissues. Mutagenesis, *13*:109–114, 1998.

Dedrick, R. L., and Morrison, P. F. Carcinogenic potency of alkylating agents in rodents and humans. Cancer Res., *52*:2464–2467, 1992.

DiGiovanni, J. Multistage carcinogenesis in mouse skin. Pharmacol. Ther., *54*:63–128, 1992.

Donehower, L. A. The p53-deficient mouse: a model for basic and applied cancer studies. Semin. Cancer Biol., *7*:269–278, 1996.

Dragan, Y., Klaunig, J., Maronpot, R., and Goldsworthy, T. Mechanisms of susceptibility to mouse liver carcinogenesis. Toxicol. Sci., *41*:3–7, 1998.

Druckrey, H., Schmähl, D., and Dischler, W. Dosis-Wirkungs-Beziehungen bei der Krebserzeugung durch 4-Dimethylamino-stilben bei Ratten. Z. Krebsforsch., *65*:272–288, 1963.

DuFrain, R. J., McFee, A. F., Linkous, S., Jennings, C. J., and Lowe, K. W. In vivo SCE analysis using bromodeoxyuridine, iododeoxyuridine, and chlorodeoxyuridine. Mutat. Res., *139*:57–60, 1984.

Dunkel, V. C., Rogers, C., Swierenga, S. H. H., Brillinger, R. L., Gilman, J. P. W., and Nestmann, E. R. Recommended protocols based on a survey of current practice in genotoxicity testing laboratories: III. Cell transformation in C3H/10T1/2 mouse embryo cell, BALB/c 3T3 mouse fibroblast and Syrian hamster embryo cell cultures. Mutat. Res., *246*:285–300, 1991.

Dunnick, J. K., Elwell, M. R., Huff, J., and Barrett, J. C. Chemically induced mammary gland cancer in the National Toxicology Program's carcinogenesis bioassay. Carcinogenesis, *16*:173–179, 1995.

Dybing, E., Sanner, T., Roelfzema, H., Kroese, D., and Tennant, R. W. T25: a simplified carcinogenic potency index: description of the system and study of correlations between carcinogenic potency and species/site specificity and mutagenicity. Pharmacol. Toxicol., *80*:272–279, 1997.

Dycaico, M. J., Stuart, G. R., Tobal, G. M., de Boer, J. G., Glickman, B. W., and Provost, G. S. Species-specific differences in hepatic mutant frequency and mutational spectrum among lambda/*lacI* transgenic rats and mice following exposure to aflatoxin B$_1$. Carcinogenesis, *17*:2347–2356, 1996.

Enslein, K., Gombar, V. K., and Blake, B. W. Use of SAR in computer-assisted prediction of carcinogenicity and mutagenicity of chemicals by the *TOPKAT* program. Mutat. Res., *305*:47–61, 1994.

Fujii, K. Evaluation of the newborn mouse model for chemical tumorigenesis. Carcinogenesis, *12*:1409–1415, 1991.

Fung, V. A., Huff, J., Weisburger, E. K., and Hoel, D. G. Predictive strategies for selecting 379 NCI/NTP chemicals evaluated for carcinogenic potential: scientific and public health impact. Fund. Appl. Toxicol., *20*:413–436, 1993.

Furihata, C., and Matsushima, T. Use of in vivo/in vitro unscheduled DNA synthesis for identification of organ-specific carcinogens. CRC Crit. Rev. Toxicol., *17*:245–277, 1987.

Galloway, S. M., and Wolff, S. The relation between chemically induced sister-chromatid exchanges and chromatid breakage. Mutat. Res., *61*:297–307, 1979.

Galloway, S. M., Bloom, A. D., Resnick, M., Margolin, B. H., Nakamura, F., Archer, P., and Zeiger, E. Development of a standard protocol for in vitro cytogenesis testing with Chinese hamster ovary cells: comparison of results for 22 compounds in two laboratories. Environ. Mutagen., *7*:1–51, 1985.

Gaylor, D. W., and Shapiro, R. E. Extrapolation and risk estimation for carcinogenesis. Adv. Med. Toxicol., *1*:65–87, 1979.

Gebhart, E. Sister chromatid exchange (SCE) and structural chromosome aberration in mutagenicity testing. Hum. Genet., *58*:235–254, 1981.

Generoso, W. M., Bishop, J. B., Gosslee, D. G., Newell, G. W., Sheu, C.-J., and von Halle, E. Heritable translocation test in mice. Mutat. Res., *76*:191–215, 1980.

Ghia, M., Mattioli, F., and Mereto, E. A possible medium-term assay for detecting the effects of liver and colon carcinogens in rats. Cancer Lett., *105*:71–75, 1996.

Gille, J. J. P., van Berkel, C. G. M., and Joenje, H. Mechanism of hyperoxia-induced chromosomal break-age in Chinese hamster cells. Environ. Mol. Mutagen., *22*:264–270, 1993.

Glass, L. R., Easterly, C. E., Jones, T. D., and Walsh, P. J. Ranking of carcinogenic potency using a relative potency approach. Arch. Environ. Contam. Toxicol., *21*:169–176, 1991.

Gold, L. S., and Zeiger, E. (Eds.). Handbook of Carcinogenic Potency and Genotoxicity Databases. Boca Raton, FL: CRC Press, 1997.

Gold, L. S., Backman, G. M., Hooper, N. K., and Peto, R. Ranking the potential carcinogenic hazards to workers from exposures to chemicals that are tumorigenic in rodents. Environ. Health Perspect., *76*:211–219, 1987.

Gold, L. S., Bernstein, L., Magaw, R., and Slone, T. H. Interspecies extrapolation in carcinogenesis: predic-tion between rats and mice. Environ. Health Perspect., *81*:211–219, 1989.

Gold, L. S., Manley, N. B., Slone, T. H., Garfinkel, G. B., Rohrbach, L., and Ames, B. N. The fifth plot of the carcinogenic potency database: results of animal bioassays published in the general literature through 1988 and by the National Toxicology Program through 1989. Environ. Health Perspect., *100*:65–135, 1993.

Gold, L. S., Slone, T. H., and Ames, B. N. What do animal cancer tests tell us about human cancer risk?: Overview of analyses of the carcinogenic potency database. Drug Metab. Rev., *30*:359–404, 1998.

Goldsworthy, T. L., Recio, L., Brown, K., Donehower, L. A., Mirsalis, J. C., Tennant, R. W., and Purchase, I. F. H. Transgenic animals in toxicology. Fund. Appl. Toxicol., *22*:8–19, 1994.

Gondo, Y., Shioyama, Y., Nakao, K., and Katsuki, M. A novel positive detection system of in vivo muta-tions in *rpsL (strA)* transgenic mice. Mutat. Res., *360*:1–14, 1996.

Hadidian, Z., Fredrickson, T. N., Weisburger, E. K., Weisburger, J. H., Glass, R. M., and Mantel, N. Tests for chemical carcinogens. Report on the activity of derivatives of aromatic amines, nitrosamines, quinolines, nitroalkanes, amides, epoxides, aziridines, and purine antimetabolites. J. Natl. Cancer. Inst., *41*:985–1036, 1968.

Hall, T. W. Environmental regulation: an international view. I. Britain. Chem. Soc. Rev., *5*:431–440, 1976.

Hanes, B., and Wedel, T. A selected review of risk models: one hit, multihit, multistage, probit, Weibull, and pharmacokinetic. J. Am. Coll. Toxicol., *4*:271–278, 1985.

Harbach, P. R., Rostami, H. J., Aaron, C. S., Wiser, S. K., and Grzegorczyk, C. R. Evaluation of four meth-ods for scoring cytoplasmic grains in the in vitro unscheduled DNA synthesis (UDS) assay. Mutat. Res., *252*:139–148, 1991.

Haseman, J. K., and Lockhart, A. The relationship between use of the maximum tolerated dose and study sensitivity for detecting rodent carcinogenicity. Fund. Appl. Toxicol., *22*:382–391, 1994.

Haseman, J. K., Boorman, G. A., and Huff, J. Value of historical control data and other issues related to the evaluation of long-term rodent carcinogenicity studies. Toxicol. Pathol., *25*:524–527, 1997.

Heddle, J. A., Hite, M., Kirkhart, B., Mavournin, K., MacGregor, J. T., Newell, G. W., and Salamone, M. F. The induction of micronuclei as a measure of genotoxicity. A report of the U.S. Environmental Pro-tection Agency Gene-Tox Program. Mutat. Res., *123*:61–118, 1983.

Hendrich, S., Campbell, H. A., and Pitot, H. C. Quantitative stereological evaluation of four histochemical markers of altered foci in multistage hepatocarcinogenesis in the rat. Carcinogenesis, *8*:1245–1250, 1987.

Hendricks, J. D., Wales, J. H., Sinnhuber, R. O., Nixon, J. E., Loveland, P. M., and Scanlan, R. A. Rainbow trout (*Salmo gairdneri*) embryos: a sensitive animal model for experimental carcinogenesis. Fed. Proc., *39*:3222–3229, 1980.

Hennings, H., Glick, A. B., Greenhalgh, D. A., Morgan, D. L., Strickland, J. E., Tennenbaum, T., and Yuspa, S. H. Critical aspects of initiation, promotion, and progression in multistage epidermal car-cinogenesis. Proc. Soc. Exp. Biol. Med., *202*:1–18, 1993.

Hicks, R. M. Multistage carcinogenesis in the urinary bladder. Br. Med. Bull., *36*:39–46, 1980.

Hicks, R. M., Wakefield, J. St. J., and Chowaniec, J. Evaluation of a new model to detect bladder carcinogens or co-carcinogens; results obtained with saccharin, cyclamate and cyclophosphamide. Chem.-Biol. Interact., *11*:225–233, 1975.

Hottendorf, G. H., and Pachter, I. J. Review and evaluation of the NCI/NTP carcinogenesis bioassays. Toxicol. Pathol., *13*:141–146, 1985.

Iball, J. The relative potency of carcinogenic compounds. Am. J. Cancer, *35*:188–190, 1939.

Isfort, R. J., Kerckaert, G. A., and LeBoeuf, R. A. Comparison of the standard and reduced pH Syrian Hamster Embryo (SHE) cell in vitro transformation assays in predicting the carcinogenic potential of chemicals. Mutat. Res., *356*:11–63, 1996.

Ishidate Jr., M., Harnois, M. C., and Sofuni, T. A comparative analysis of data on the clastogenicity of 951 chemical substances tested in mammalian cell cultures. Mutat. Res., *195*:151–213, 1988.

Ito, N., and Fukushima, S. Promotion of urinary bladder carcinogenesis in experimental animals. Exp. Pathol., *36*:1–15, 1989.

Ito, N., Imaida, K., Hasegawa, R., and Tsuda, H. Rapid bioassay methods for carcinogens and modifiers of hepatocarcinogenesis. CRC Crit. Rev. Toxicol., *19*:385–415, 1989.

Ito, N., Hasegawa, R., Imaida, K., Hirose, M., and Shirai, T. Medium-term liver and multi-organ carcinogenesis bioassays for carcinogens and chemopreventive agents. Exp. Toxicol. Pathol., *48*:113–119, 1996.

Ito, Y., Fujie, K., Matsuda, S., Takahashi, R., and Maeda, S. Long-Evans A and C rat strains susceptible to clastogenic effects of chemicals in the bone marrow cells. Jpn. J. Cancer Res., *85*:26–31, 1994.

Johnson, S. P. Environmental regulation: an international view. II. European economic community. Chem. Soc. Rev., *5*:441–451, 1976.

Kaufman, E. R. Induction of sister-chromatid exchanges by the replication of 5-bromouracil-substituted DNA under conditions of nucleotide-pool imbalance. Mutat. Res., *163*:41–50, 1986.

Keenan, K. P., Laroque, P., Ballam, G. C., Soper, K. A., Dixit, R., Mattson, B. A., Adams, S. P., and Coleman, J. B. The effects of diet, *ad libitum* overfeeding, and moderate dietary restriction on the rodent bioassay: the uncontrolled variable in safety assessment. Toxicol. Pathol., *24*:757–768, 1996.

Kennelly, J. C. Design and interpretation of rat liver UDS assays. Mutagenesis, *10*:215–221, 1995.

Kirkland, D. J., Marshall, R. R., McEnaney, S., Bidgood, J., Rutter, A., and Mullineux, S. Aroclor-1254-induced rat-liver S9 causes chromosomal aberrations in CHO cells but not human lymphocytes: a role of active oxygen? Mutat. Res., *214*:115–122, 1989.

Kitchin, K. T., Brown, J. L., and Setzer, R. W. Dose-response relationship in multistage carcinogenesis: promoters. Environ. Health Perspect. Suppl., *1*:255–264, 1994.

Klopman, G., and Rosenkranz, H. S. Approaches to SAR in carcinogenesis and mutagenesis. Prediction of carcinogenicity/mutagenicity using MULTI-CASE. Mutat. Res., *305*:33–46, 1994.

Kraybill, H. Food chemicals and food additives. *In*: P. Newberne (Ed.), Trace Substances and Health, A Handbook, Part I, pp. 245–318. New York: Marcel Dekker, 1976.

Kraybill, H. F. Proper perspectives in extrapolation of experimental carcinogenesis data to humans. Food Technol., *32*:62–64, August, 1978.

Kroh, H. Chemical neuroncogenesis of the central nervous system. J. Neuropathol. Exp. Neurol., *54*:(Suppl.) 48S–49S, 1995.

Latt, S. A. Sister chromatid exchange formation. Annu. Rev. Genet., *15*:11–55, 1981.

Lee, Y., Buchanan, B. G., Mattison, D. M., Klopman, G., and Rosenkranz, H. S. Learning rules to predict rodent carcinogenicity of non-genotoxic chemicals. Mutat. Res., *328*:127–149, 1995.

Li, A. P., Carver, J. H., Choy, W. N., Hsie, A. W., Gupta, R. S., Loveday, K. S., O'Neill, J. P., Riddle, J. C., Stankowski, L. F. Jr., and Yang, L. L. A guide for the performance of the Chinese hamster ovary cell/hypoxanthine guanine phosphoribosyl transferase gene mutation assay. Mutat. Res., *189*:135–141, 1987.

Littlefield, N. A., and Gaylor, D. W. Influence of total dose and dose rate in carcinogenicity studies. J. Toxicol. Environ. Health, *15*:545–560, 1985.

Lockhart, A.-M. C., Piegorsch, W. W., and Bishop, J. B. Assessing overdispersion and dose-response in the male dominant lethal assay. Mutat. Res., *272*:35–58, 1992.

Luebeck, E., Moolgavkar, S., Buchman, A., and Schwarz, M. Effects of polychlorinated biphenyls in rat liver: quantitative analysis of enzyme-altered foci. Toxicol. Appl. Pharmacol., *111*:469–484, 1991.

Majeska, J. B. and Matheson, D. W. Development of an optimal S9 activation mixture for the L5178 TK± mouse lymphoma mutation assay. Environ. Mol. Mutagen., *16*:311–319, 1990.

Maron, D. M., and Ames, B. N. Revised methods for the Salmonella mutagenicity test. Mutat. Res., *113*:173–215, 1983.

McCann, J. In vitro testing for cancer-causing chemicals. Hosp. Pract., ofc. edn. *18*(9):73–85, 1983.

McClain, R. M. The significance of hepatic microsomal enzyme induction and altered thyroid function in rats: implications for thyroid gland neoplasia. Toxicol. Pathol., *17*:294–306, 1989.

Meselson, M., Chairman. Pest control: an assessment of present and alternative technologies. Volume 1, Contemporary Pest Control Practices and Prospects: The Report of the Executive Committee. Washington, D.C.: National Academy of Sciences, 1975.

Meselson, M., and Russell, K. Carcinogenic and mutagenic potency. *In*: H. H. Hiatt, J. D. Watson, and J. A. Weinstein (Eds.), Origins of Human Cancer. Cold Spring Harbor, NY: Cold Spring Harbor Laboratory, 1977.

Mirsalis, J. C., Monforte, J. A., and Winegar, R. A. Transgenic animal models for measuring mutations *in vivo*. Crit. Rev. Toxicol., *24*:255–280, 1994.

Miyamae, Y., Iwasaki, K., Kinae, N., Tsuda, S., Murakami, M., Tanaka, M., and Sasaki, Y. F. Detection of DNA lesions induced by chemical mutagens using the single-cell gel electrophoresis (Comet) assay. 2. Relationship between DNA migration and alkaline condition. Mutat. Res., *393*:107–113, 1997.

Moch, R. W., Dua, P. N., and Hines, F. A. Problems in consideration of rodent hepatocarcinogenesis for regulatory purposes. Toxicol. Pathol., *24*:138–146, 1996.

Moll, K. D., and Tihansky, D. P. Risk-benefit analysis for industrial and social needs. Am. Ind. Hyg. Assoc. J., *38*:153–161, 1977.

Monro, A. What is an appropriate measure of exposure when testing drugs for carcinogenicity in rodents? Toxicol. Appl. Pharmacol., *112*:171–181, 1992.

Moolgavkar, S. H. Carcinogenesis modeling: from molecular biology to epidemiology. Annu. Rev. Public Health, *7*:151–169, 1986.

Murphy, S. A., Tice, R. R., Smith, M. G., and Margolin, B. H. Contributions to the design and statistical analysis of in vivo SCE experiments. Mutat. Res., *271*:39–48, 1992.

Muscarella, D. E., and Bloom, S. E. The longevity of chemically induced sister chromatid exchanges in Chinese hamster ovary cells. Environ. Mutagen., *4*:647–655, 1982.

Myhr, B. C. Validation studies with MutaMouse: a transgenic mouse model for detecting mutations in vivo. Environ. Mol. Mutagen., *18*:308–315, 1991.

Nasmyth, K. Separating sister chromatids. Trends Biochem. Sci., *24*:98–104, 1999.

Nuzum, E. O., Malkinson, A. M., and Beer, D. G. Specific Ki-*ras* codon 61 mutations may determine the development of urethan-induced mouse lung adenomas or adenocarcinomas. Mol. Carcinog., *3*:287–295, 1990.

Oesterle, D., and Deml, E. Detection of chemical carcinogens by means of the "rat liver foci bioassay." Exp. Pathol., *39*:197–206, 1990.

Office of Science and Technology Policy: Chemical carcinogens: a review of the science and its associated principles. U.S. Interagency Staff Group on Carcinogens. Environ. Health Perspect., *67*:201–282, 1986.

Ogiso, T., Tatematsu, M., Tamano, S., Hasegawa, R., and Ito, N. Correlation between medium-term liver bioassay system data and results of long-term testing in rats. Carcinogenesis, *11*:561–566, 1990.

Okada, N., Honda, A., Kawabata, M., and Yajima, N. Sodium phenobarbital-enhanced mutation frequency in the liver DNA of *lacZ* transgenic mice treated with diethylnitrosamine. Mutagenesis, *12*:179–184, 1997.

Oser, B. L. Benefit/risk: Whose? What? How much? Food Technol., *32*:55–58, August, 1978.

Ottagio, L., Bonatti, S., Cavalieri, Z., and Abbondandolo, A. Chromosomes bearing amplified genes are a preferential target of chemicals inducing chromosome breakage and aneuploidy. Mutat. Res., *301*:149–155, 1993.

Page, N. P., Singh, D. V., Farland, W., Goodman, J. I., Conolly, R. B., Andersen, M. E., Clewell, H. J., Frederick, C. B., Yamasaki, H., and Lucier, G. Implementation of EPA revised cancer assessment guidelines: incorporation of mechanistic and pharmacokinetic data. Fundam. Appl. Toxicol., *37*:16–36, 1997.

Pepelko, W. E. Effect of exposure route on potency of carcinogens. Reg. Toxicol. Pharmacol., *13*:3–17, 1991.

Peraino, C., Fry, R. J. M., and Staffeldt, E. Effects of varying the onset and duration of exposure to phenobarbital on its enhancement of 2-acetylaminofluorene-induced hepatic tumorigenesis. Cancer Res., *37*:3623–3627, 1977.

Pereira, M. A. Mouse skin bioassay for chemical carcinogens. J. Am. Coll. Toxicol., *1*:47–74, 1982.

Pereira, M. A., and Stoner, G. D. Comparison of rat liver foci assay and strain A mouse lung tumor assay to detect carcinogens: a review. Fundam. Appl. Toxicol., *5*:688–699, 1985.

Peto, R., Pike, M. C., Bernstein, L., Gold, L. S., and Ames, B. N. The TD_{50}: a proposed general convention for the numerical description of the carcinogenic potency of chemicals in chronic-exposure animal experiments. Environ. Health Perspect., *58*:1–8, 1984.

Pietra, G., Spencer, K., and Shubik, P. Response of newly born mice to a chemical carcinogen. Nature, *183*:1689, 1959.

Pitot, H. C. Multistage carcinogenesis—genetic and epigenetic mechanisms in relation to cancer prevention. Cancer Detect. Prev., *17*:567–573, 1993.

Pitot, H. C., and Dragan, Y. P. Chemical carcinogenesis. *In*: C. D. Klaasen (Ed.), Casarett and Doull's Toxicology—The Basic Science of Poisons, pp. 201–267. New York: McGraw-Hill, 1996.

Pitot, H. C., Barsness, L., Goldsworthy, T., and Kitagawa, T. Biochemical characterization of stages of hepatocarcinogenesis after a single dose of diethylnitrosamine. Nature, 271:456–458, 1978.

Pitot, H. C., Goldsworthy, T. L., Moran, S., Kennan, W., Glauert, H. P., Maronpot, R. R., and Campbell, H. A. A method to quantitate the relative initiating and promoting potencies of hepatocarcinogenic agents in their dose-response relationships to altered hepatic foci. Carcinogenesis, 8:1491–1499, 1987.

Pitot, H. C., Dragan, Y. P., Teeguarden, J., Hsia, S., and Campbell, H. Quantitation of multistage carcinogenesis in rat liver. Toxicol. Pathol., *24*:119–128, 1996.

Provost, G. S., Kretz, P. L., Hamner, R. T., Matthews, C. D., Rogers, B. J., Lundberg, K. S., Dycaico, M. J., and Short, J. M. Transgenic systems for in vivo mutation analysis. Mutat. Res., *288*:133–149, 1993.

Recio, L. Transgenic animal models and their application in mechanistically based toxicology research. Chem. Ind. Inst. Toxicol., *15*:1–7, 1995.

Rogers, A. Nitrosamines. *In*: P. Newberne (Ed.), Trace Substances and Health: A Handbook, Part 2, pp. 47–80. New York: Marcel Dekker, 1982.

Rosenberg, M. P. Gene knockout and transgenic technologies in risk assessment: the next generation. Mol. Carcinog., 20:262–274, 1997.

Samuels, S. W. The fallacies of risk/benefit analysis. Ann. N.Y. Acad. Sci., *329*:267–273, 1979.

Sargent, L., Xu, Y.-H., Sattler, G. L., Meisner, L., and Pitot, H. C. Ploidy and karyotype of hepatocytes isolated from enzyme-altered foci in two different protocols of multistage hepatocarcinogenesis in the rat. Carcinogenesis, *10*:387–391, 1989.

Sasaki, T., and Yoshida, T. Experimentelle Erzeuqung des Lebercarcinoms durch Fütterung mit o-Amidoazotoluol. Virchow's Arch. Abt. A Pathol. Anat., *295*:175–200, 1935.

Shamberger, R. J., Baughman, F. F., Kalchert, S. L., Willis, C. E., and Hoffman, G. C. Carcinogen-induced chromosome breakage decreased by antioxidants. Proc. Natl. Acad. Sci. U.S.A., *70*:1461–1463, 1973.

Shimkin, M. B., and Stoner, G. D. Lung tumors in mice: application to carcinogenesis bioassay. Adv. Cancer Res., *21*:1–58, 1975.

Shirai, T. A medium-term rat liver bioassay as a rapid *in vivo* test for carcinogenic potential: a historical review of model development and summary of results from 291 tests. Toxicol. Pathol., *25*:453–460, 1997.

Sina, J. F., Bean, C. L., Dysart, G. R., Taylor, V. I., and Bradley, M. O. Evaluation of the alkaline elution/rat hepatocyte assay as a predictor of carcinogenic/mutagenic potential. Mutat. Res., *113*:357–391, 1983.

Sinha, A. K., Linscombe, V. A., Gollapudi, B. B., Jersey, G. C., and Park, C. N. Analysis of sister chromatid exchanges in lymphocytes cultured from 71 healthy men. Cell Biol. Toxicol., *1*:333–342, 1985.

Skopek, T. R., Kort, K. L., and Marino, D. R. Relative sensitivity of the endogenous *hprt* gene and *lacI* transgene in ENU-treated Big Blue™ B6C3F1 mice. Environ. Mol. Mutagen., *26*:9–15, 1995.

Slaga, T. J. SENCAR mouse skin tumorigenesis model versus other strains and stocks of mice. Environ. Health Perspect., *68*:27–32, 1986.

Solt, D., and Farber, E. New principle for the analysis of chemical carcinogenesis. Nature, *263*:702–703, 1976.

Sontag, J. M. Aspects in carcinogen bioassay. *In*: H. Hiatt, J. Watson, and J. Winsten (Eds.), Origins of Human Cancer, pp. 1327–1338. Cold Spring Harbor, NY: Cold Spring Harbor Laboratory, 1977.

Spalding, J. W., Momma, J., Elwell, M. R., and Tennant, R. W. Chemically induced skin carcinogenesis in a transgenic mouse line (TG·AC) carrying a v-Ha-ras gene. Carcinogenesis, *14*:1335–1341, 1993.

Spitz, M. R., and Bondy, M. L. Genetic susceptibility to cancer. Cancer, *72*:991–995, 1993.

Steinmetz, K. L., Green, C. E., Bakke, J. P., Spak, D. K., and Mirsalis, J. C. Induction of unscheduled DNA synthesis in primary cultures of rat, mouse, hamster, monkey, and human hepatocytes. Mutat. Res., *206*:91–102, 1988.

Stoner, G. D., Shimkin, M. B., Troxell, M. C., Thompson, T. L., and Terry, L. S. Test for carcinogenicity of metallic compounds by the pulmonary tumor response in strain A mice. Cancer Res., *36*:1744–1747, 1976.

Strom, S., Kligerman, A. D., and Michalopoulos, G. Comparisons of the effects of chemical carcinogens in mixed cultures of rat hepatocytes and human fibroblasts. Carcinogenesis, *2*:709–715, 1981.

Sugimura, T., Sato, S., Nagao, M., Yahagi, T., Matsushima, T., Seino, Y., Takeuchi, M., and Kawachi, T. Overlapping of carcinogens and mutagens. *In*: P. N. Magee et al. (Eds.), Fundamentals in Cancer Prevention, pp. 191–215. Baltimore: University Park Press, 1976.

Sutherland, L. A. M., and Bird, R. P. The effect of chenodeoxycholic acid on the development of aberrant crypt foci in the rat colon. Cancer Lett., *76*:101–107, 1994.

Swenberg, J. A., Richardson, F. C., Boucheron, J. A., and Dyroff, M. C. Relationships between DNA adduct formation and carcinogenesis. Environ. Health Perspect., *62*:177–183, 1985.

Swierenga, S. H. H., Bradlaw, J. A., Brillinger, R. L., Gilman, J. P. W., Nestmann, E. R., and San, R. C. Recommended protocols based on a survey of current practice in genotoxicity testing laboratories: I. Unscheduled DNA synthesis assay in rat hepatocyte cultures. Mutat. Res., *246*:235–253, 1991.

Takahashi, S., Kubota, Y., and Sato, H. Mutant frequencies in *lacZ* transgenic mice following the internal irradiation from ^{89}Sr or the external γ-ray irradiation. J. Radiat. Res., *39*:53–60, 1998.

Takayama, S., and Sakanishi, S. Differential Giemsa staining of sister chromatids after extraction with acids. Chromosoma (Berl.), *64*:109–115, 1977.

Teeguarden, J. G., Dragan, Y. P., and Pitot, H. C. Implications of hormesis on the bioassay and hazard assessment of chemical carcinogens. Hum. Exp. Toxicol., *17*:254–258, 1998.

Tennant, R. W. Evaluation and validation issues in the development of transgenic mouse carcinogenicity bioassays. Environ. Health Perspect., *106*:473–476, 1998.

Tennant, R. W., Spalding, J. W., Stasiewicz, S., Caspary, W. D., Mason, J. M., and Resnick, M. A. Comparative evaluation of genetic toxicity patterns of carcinogens and noncarcinogens: strategies for predictive use of short-term assays. Environ. Health Perspect., *75*:87–95, 1987.

Tinwell, H., and Ashby, J. Comparative activity of human carcinogens and NTP rodent carcinogens in the mouse bone marrow micronucleus assay: an integrative approach to genetic toxicity data assessment. Environ. Health Perspect., *102*:758–762, 1994.

Upton, A. C. Radiation injury: past, present and future. *In*: R. B. Hill and J. A. Terzian (Eds.), Topics in Environmental Pathology: Elements of a Curriculum for Students of Medicine. Bethesda, MD: Assoc. Univ. Res. Education Path., 1980.

Vainio, H., Hemminki, K., and Wilbourn, J. Data on the carcinogenicity of chemicals in the IARC Monographs programme. Carcinogenesis, *6*:1653–1665, 1985.

Vainio, H., Coleman, M., and Wilbourn, J. Carcinogenicity evaluations and ongoing studies: the IARC databases. Environ. Health Perspect., *96*:5–9, 1991.

Vesselinovitch, S. D., Mihailovich, N., and Rao, K. V. N. Morphology and metastatic nature of induced hepatic nodular lesions in C57BL × C3H F_1 mice. Cancer Res., *38*:2003–2010, 1978.

Vogel, E. W., Nivard, M. J. M., Ballering, L. A. B., Bartsch, H., Barbin, A., Nair, J., Comendador, M. A., Sierra, L. M., Aguirrezabalaga, I., Tosal, L., Ehrenberg, L., Fuchs, R. P. P., Janel-Bintz, R., Maenhaut-Michel, G., Montesano, R., Hall, J., Kang, H., Miele, M., Thomale, J., Bender, K., Engelbergs, J., and Rajewsky, M. F. DNA damage and repair in mutagenesis and carcinogenesis: implications for structure-activity relationships for cross-species extrapolation. Mutat. Res., *113*:177–218, 1996.

Warren, B. S., Naylor, M. F., Winberg, L. D., Yoshimi, N., Volpe, J. P. G., Gimenez-Conti, I., and Slaga, T. J. Induction and inhibition of tumor progression. Proc. Soc. Exp. Biol. Med., *202*:9–15, 1993.

Williams, G. M. The significance of chemically-induced hepatocellular altered foci in rat liver and application to carcinogen detection. Toxicol. Pathol., *17*:663–674, 1989.

Williams, G. M., Mori, H., and McQueen, C. A. Structure-activity relationships in the rat hepatocyte DNA-repair test for 300 chemicals. Mutat. Res., *221*:263–286, 1989.

Wintersberger, U., and Klein, F. Yeast-mating-type switching: a model system for the study of genome rearrangements induced by carcinogens. Ann. N.Y. Acad. Sci., *534*:513–520, 1988.

Wyrobek, A. J., and Bruce, W. R. Chemical induction of sperm abnormalities in mice. Proc. Natl. Acad. Sci. U.S.A., *72*:4425–4429, 1975.

You, M., Candrian, U., Maronpot, R. R., Stoner, G. D., and Anderson, M. W. Activation of the Ki-*ras* protooncogene in spontaneously occurring and chemically induced lung tumors of the strain A mouse. Proc. Natl. Acad. Sci. U.S.A., *86*:3070–3074, 1989.

Zhang, Y. P., Sussman, N., Macina, O. T., Rosenkranz, H. S., and Klopman, G. Prediction of the carcinogenicity of a second group of organic chemicals undergoing carcinogenicity testing. Environ. Health Perspect., *104*:1045–1050, 1996.

Zhang, Z., and Yang, J. Effects of amino acids on sister-chromatid exchanges. Mutat. Res., *280*:279–283, 1992.

14

The Natural History of the Development of Neoplasia in Cultured Cells and Tissues

Although the explantation of cells from a multicellular organism into an extraorganismal environment, that is, tissue culture, had been known since the beginning of this century, it was not until the early 1940s that Earle and associates (cf. Earle and Nettleship, 1943) attempted to induce the neoplastic transformation in cultured mammalian cells. These now classic experiments, which were carried out by the addition of polycyclic hydrocarbons to cultures of mouse fibroblasts, were monitored by the inoculation of treated and untreated cell cultures into host animals. Unfortunately the results of these experiments were ambiguous, since neoplasms arose in the test animals whether treated or control cultured cells were inoculated. As a result, the question of the feasibility of carcinogenesis in vitro lay dormant for almost two decades. However, the cells from these experiments have been maintained, even up to the present day, as the L cell line (cf. Jackson, 1991).

TECHNIQUES OF TISSUE CULTURE

It is not the objective of this text to present an extensive discussion of the methodology of cell and organ culture. The interested student is referred to the bibliographic references (e.g., Nardone, 1987; Celis and Celis, 1994). However, it is important to understand the difference between organ culture and cell culture. In the former, fragments of organs or even whole organs are removed from the organism, and their viability and organization are maintained in an artificial environment. While larger samples of tissue usually did not survive more than a few days, organ culture of fragments of colon (Shamsuddin et al., 1978), mouse mammary glands (Iyer and Banerjee, 1981), and embryonic rat pancreas (Parsa and Marsh, 1976) could be maintained for some period of time in culture. During this time the microscopic anatomy of the tissue was retained, remaining essentially identical with that seen in the organ in vivo.

On the other hand, cell culture involves the isolation and/or dispersion of cells from organs and tissues, with their subsequent cultivation as cellular populations with little regard to their original morphology and functionality. Such cell cultures may be cloned, that is, single cells are isolated and allowed to proliferate to a visible colony. Quantitative measurements and genetic studies may be performed relatively easily with cell cultures provided that the cells either are available in significant quantity or replicate quite readily in the culture environment. The term *primary culture* indicates those cells obtained directly from the animal and cultured in the specific system under study. The terms *secondary* and *transfer cultures* refer to the subsequent cultivation of cells, with the inoculum taken from cells already in culture. In Figure 14.1, a cutaway

A. Organ Culture

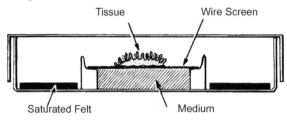

B. Cell Culture

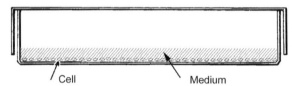

Figure 14.1   Diagram of tissue culture as organ culture (A) and cell culture (B). In the organ culture system shown, a fragment of whole tissue rests on a wire screen through which the medium permeates. For cell culture, suspensions of cells are plated on the surfaces of petri dishes, allowed to attach, and then covered with appropriate media. (The example in A is taken from Trier, 1976, with permission of the author and publisher.)

diagram of an organ and a cell culture in a petri dish may be noted. The major distinction is the special structure required to maintain the tissue in its organoid form while assuring access of sufficient nutrients from the medium for maintenance of viability. Cell cultures, on the other hand, usually consist of a monolayer of cells or small cell colonies, at most only a few cells in thickness, lying entirely within the environment of the liquid medium. A variety of other configurations for organ cultures have also been described (cf. Anderson and Jenkinson, 1998; Minuth et al., 1996). Cell cultures may also be maintained as suspensions of cells (e.g., Himmelfarb et al., 1969) or as multicellular spheroids (e.g., Korff and Augustin, 1998).

In general, cells within organ cultures maintain most of the genetic and functional capabilities of comparable cells in vivo. In cell culture, however, especially of tissues from certain types of animals such as rodents, the natural history of cells transferred and cultivated for long periods is that of karyotypic and biochemical changes, usually in the direction of increased aneuploidy and decreased biochemical differentiation. Certain terminologies have been developed for certain types of cell cultures and their progeny (Schaeffer, 1990). A *cell line* arises from a primary culture at the time of the first successful secondary or subculture. The cell line cultures thus should consist of lineages of cells originally present in the primary culture. Cell lines are termed *finite* or *continuous* if the history and potential of the line is known. If this is not known, then the term *line* will suffice. A *cell strain* may be derived either from a primary culture or from a cell line by the selection or cloning of cells having specific properties or markers. Thus, descriptions of cell strains should also include any specific features of the strain. As with cell lines, the terms *finite* or *continuous* are used as prefixes if the history and potential of the culture is known; otherwise, the term *strain* by itself is sufficient. Obviously, cell lines and strains may be derived from organ cultures as well. Cells from strains or lines may be frozen at liquid air temperatures and maintained in this state for years with relatively efficient recovery of viability on thawing. A few primary cell cultures have also been successfully maintained in this way, but organ cultures do not readily survive such treatment.

The media in which organ and cell cultures are maintained or stimulated to grow have been quite complex, consisting of numerous nutrients of known composition as well as, in most instances, numerous materials of unknown chemical composition such as serum, partial protein hydrolysates, and tissue extracts. During the last several decades, a number of chemically defined media have been developed for use with primary cultures as well as for the growth and maintenance of cell lines and cell strains. While the vast majority of these media are effective for cells that are derived from neoplasms or have a significant number of characteristics of neoplasia, several such media have been utilized for normal cell lines. These include human diploid fibroblasts (Bettger et al., 1981), human epidermal keratinocytes (Tsao et al., 1982), and human lymphocytes (Shive and Matthews, 1988). A number of other cell lines may also be maintained in defined media (Taub, 1990). The defined media may contain a number of proteins, growth factors, and other nutrients that presumably occur at some level in the serum, plasmid, or other organismal fluid that is used in nondefined culture media (Barnes, 1987; Bjare, 1992).

In addition to the composition of the medium, which is critical for cell growth and maintenance, the matrix on which the cells are cultured has become of increasing significance during the last two decades. Prior to this time most cultures with the exception of organ cultures were maintained on glass or plastic as the substratum. In 1975, Michalopoulos and Pitot described the primary culture of parenchymal hepatic cells from rats on collagen membranes. This technology allowed considerably longer maintenance times as well as enhanced biochemical and morphological differentiation of these cells in primary culture. During the next decade or more, similar or related technologies were developed to culture a variety of mesenchymal (cf. Kleinman et al., 1981) and differentiated epithelial tissues (e.g., Montesano et al., 1983; Yang et al., 1979; Yang et al., 1982; Chambard et al., 1981). Reid and associates (Rojkind et al., 1980) demonstrated the importance of the presence of extracellular matrix molecules (Chapter 10) in maintaining epithelial cells in a morphologically and biochemically differentiated state for extended periods of weeks or months (cf. Reid and Jefferson, 1984). A combination of extracellular components and collagen gels could effect the same result (Lin et al., 1997). Other variations in substratum for epithelial cell culture included the "sandwich" technique, with the matrix present on both sides of the epithelial sheet (Kern et al., 1997; Beken et al., 1997), and cocultivation of hepatocytes with littoral cells from the same organ (Namieno et al., 1996; Guguen-Guillouzo et al., 1983). A number of other very sophisticated technologies have been utilized for the culture of a variety of different cell types, both in microscopic and very large instruments, the latter allowing for the culture of large numbers of cells useful as molecular biological reagents and/or the production of specific protein products.

Differentiation in Cell Culture—Stem Cells

Although organ cultures maintain a relatively highly differentiated state of the cells for limited periods of time, until recently most cell lines, even after explantation in vitro for a few weeks, lost many differentiated characteristics that the tissue may have had in the whole animal. While there are exceptions to this statement, such as keratinocyte cultures (cf. Linge, 1996) and the growth of cells on specific substrata or "scaffolds" (Freed and Vunjak-Novakovic, 1998), the majority of cell lines and strains maintained in culture show relatively few differentiated characteristics, morphologically or molecularly. This problem has now been surmounted by the demonstration of the differentiation of cultures of embryonic stem cells (ES cells; Chapter 5) into a variety of different tissue types in vitro and in vivo (O'Shea, 1999). Stem cells may be defined as cells exhibiting extensive self-renewal properties extending throughout the life of the organism while at the same time retaining the ability to generate differentiated progeny (cf. Hollands, 1997; Morrison et al., 1997). It has now become apparent, within the last decade, that such ES cells exhibit the potential to differentiate along different tissue lines as a result of the presence of a variety of different factors, usually polypeptides, that regulate differentiation into various lineages (cf. Pedersen, 1999). Thus, with appropriate manipulation it is possible to generate cells of the hematopoietic (Dieterlen-Lièvre, 1997), immune (Chen and Mok, 1995), and neural (Brüstle et al., 1999) systems. Stem cells of the epidermis and gastrointestinal tract derived from adult tissues have also been isolated (Jones, 1997). A diagram of the procedure used for generating stem cells from the early embryo with their potential for transplantation in vivo is seen in Figure 14.2. While in the past it has been possible to maintain certain differentiated characteristics by careful control of a variety of culture conditions (Wolffe and Tata, 1984; Watt, 1991), the ability to characterize, isolate, and culture both ES cells and stem cells from adult tissues from which differentiated tissues arise offers great potential not only for a study of the mechanisms of differentiation but also for the practical application of organ transplantation and replacement (Pedersen, 1999; Thomson et al., 1998).

CARCINOGENESIS IN ORGAN CULTURES

Attempts at the induction of neoplasia in organ cultures were made in a reasonably systematic way by Heidelberger (1973) after the earlier studies of Lasnitzki (1963). Heidelberger attempted to induce carcinomas in organ culture of rat prostate by the addition of carcinogenic polycyclic hydrocarbons to the cultures. Although significant morphological changes occurred, including squamous metaplasia and cytological anaplasia, no neoplasms were produced when the cultures exhibiting such changes were inoculated into suitable mouse hosts. Later studies by Lasnitzki (1976) in this system demonstrated that retinoids added to the cultures could reverse the morphological effects produced by 10 days of incubation with a polycyclic hydrocarbon.

As an extension of these investigations, several investigators have developed an in vitro–in vivo format for carcinogenesis in organ cultures. Basically, the cultures are exposed to carcinogen for a specific time and then directly reimplanted into syngeneic hosts in order to study the development of neoplasia in vivo in the inoculated host. One example of such a system is the use of mouse mammary epithelial cells exposed to carcinogens and then implanted into the mammary fat pads. In such a system, morphological neoplasms of the mammary gland developed (Iyer and Banerjee, 1981; Rivera et al., 1981). In earlier studies, Laws and Flaks (1966) produced a similar effect by treating embryonic mouse lung tissue in organ culture with methylcholanthrene for 8 days and subsequent implantation into the flank of syngeneic mice. In more than half of the tissues implanted in vivo, pulmonary adenomas and related lesions developed from the implanted tissue. A difficulty of these experiments was the question of whether or not the original carcinogen had been completely removed from the cultures prior to their inoculation into suitable hosts. Obviously, if this removal had not occurred, one would be dealing merely with carcinogenesis in vivo.

IN VIVO–IN VITRO CARCINOGENESIS

With the refinement of tissue culture methodology, it is now possible to place cells from a variety of different tissues into culture. With such techniques, several systems have been devised in which the stage of initiation has been induced in vivo in appropriate animals, with the stages of promotion and progression allowed to continue primarily in vitro. Laerum and Rajewsky (1975)

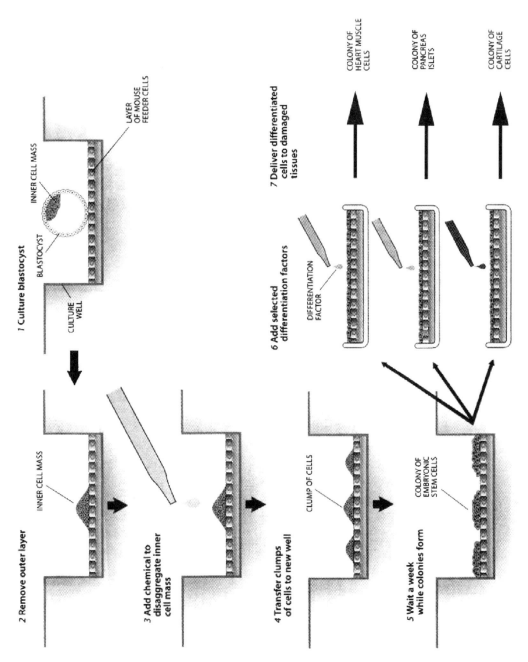

Figure 14.2   General procedure for isolation, growth, and differentiation of embryonic stem cells and their potential use in replacement strategies of missing or damaged cells of the organism. (Adapted from Pedersen, 1999, with permission of the author and publisher.)

described the transplacental initiation of fetal brain with ethylnitrosourea, with the subsequent culture of cells of the central nervous system begun several days after initiation. This led to a characteristic series of phenotypic alterations in the cultured cells, climaxed after some months by the demonstration of their neoplastic potential on inoculation into appropriate hosts, with the production of neoplasms. Figure 14.3 is a diagrammatic representation of the in vivo–in vitro system involving the initiation of cells in the fetal central nervous system by ethylnitrosourea given to the pregnant dam, the carcinogen reaching its target by the transplacental route. This is followed by cell culture of fetal brain tissue. The subsequent phenotypic stages of changes in

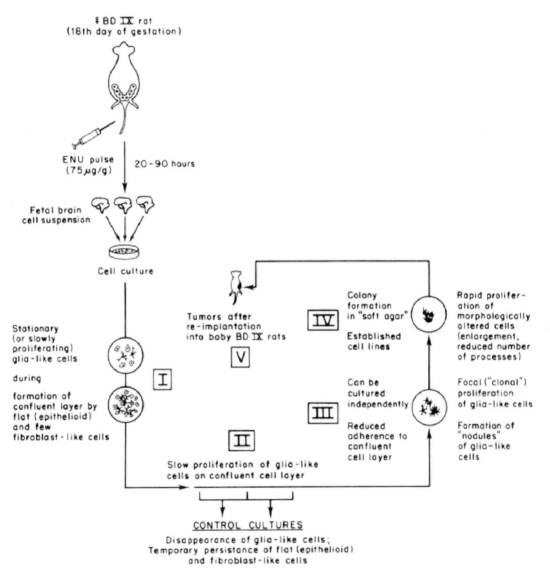

Figure 14.3 Diagrammatic representation of the in vivo–in vitro system for "pulse" carcinogenesis by ethylnitrosourea (ENU) in fetal brain cells. (After Laerum and Rajewsky, 1975, with permission of the authors and publisher.)

cells from animals treated with ethylnitrosourea in utero are also represented, along with the demonstration that neoplasms occurred after reimplantation of cells maintained in culture for 6 to 7 months. Control cultures do not exhibit the phenotypic changes seen in the figure and essentially cease growing after a week or so in culture (Laerum and Rajewsky, 1975). Chronic treatment of the cultures of fetal rat brain cells exposed to ethylnitrosourea in utero resulted in a dramatic acceleration of the morphological changes seen later in control cultures (Kokunai et al., 1986). Similar morphological findings were reported with rat kidney cells isolated from animals within 24 hours after a single carcinogenic dose of dimethylnitrosamine (Hard et al., 1977). In this instance, however, while phenotypic changes occurred in culture, no demonstration of neoplasms resulting from the inoculation of such altered cells into suitable hosts was reported. In contrast, x-irradiation of pregnant Syrian hamsters with the subsequent culture of cells from the irradiated embryos resulted in cell lines that gave rise to neoplasms when inoculated into appropriate Syrian hamster hosts (Borek et al., 1977).

Nettesheim and his colleagues (1981) developed an excellent system for following the morphological and biological changes during neoplastic development in rodent respiratory tract epithelium. In this system, initiation and early stages of promotion are induced in segments of trachea implanted subcutaneously in vivo. Subsequent isolation of epithelial cells from the trachea and culture of such cells show morphological alterations as well as the induction of neoplasms when these cells are inoculated into appropriate hosts. Although these systems have not been used widely by other investigators, they represent a potentially powerful tool with which to dissect both the early and late changes occurring during carcinogenesis in vivo and in vitro.

NEOPLASTIC "TRANSFORMATION" IN CELL CULTURE

It was almost 20 years after the pioneering studies of Earle and associates that Berwald and Sachs (1963) demonstrated the "transformation" of hamster embryo cells growing in cell cultures. These investigators utilized cells dissociated from hamster embryos by proteolytic digestion and dispersion of the cells, essentially as single cells. These cells were plated directly onto feeder layers of cells (normal cells having had their growth arrested by radiation or chemical means) in appropriate containers, usually petri dishes, at relatively low density (number of cells per plate) and were allowed to attach and grow. After seeding, appropriate carcinogenic agents were administered either in the medium or as ionizing radiation. The cultures were allowed to grow for 8 to 10 days, and the resultant colonies were fixed and stained. A diagram of the procedure is shown in Figure 14.4. Transformed cell colonies were identified by specific morphological characteristics distinguishing transformed from control or solvent-treated cells. The morphological characteristics demonstrated were those of small fusiform cells that grew in an irregular, random criss-cross pattern and did not appear to exhibit contact inhibition of movement or growth, as was found in untreated control cells in culture (Figure 14.5). The lack of "spontaneous" transformation in Syrian hamster embryo (SHE) cells as compared with the relative frequency of spontaneous transformation in mouse (Sanford et al., 1970) and rat cells in culture (Morel-Chany et al., 1985) was apparently critical to the success of this system. On the other hand, human fibroblastic cells rarely exhibited the morphologic transformation characteristics seen in Figure 14.4 (Hayflick, 1977). The mechanism of such spontaneous morphological transformation is not clear, although Rubin and associates (Rubin et al., 1990; Ellison and Rubin, 1992) have proposed several mechanisms based on studies of aneuploid cell lines. "Transformation" of such cell lines is discussed later in this chapter. That "morphological transformation" itself may not be a reflection of neoplastic transformation was seen by the studies of Evans et al. (1972), demonstrating that sera from different species and even different sexes

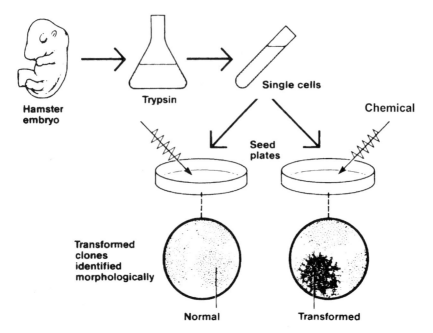

Figure 14.4 Protocol for the assay of morphological transformation of hamster embryo cells by chemicals or radiation. Midterm hamster embryos were removed from pregnant uteri, minced, enzymatically dissociated, and seeded as single cells on feeder layers (normal cells having had their growth arrested by radiation or chemical means). The newly seeded cells are treated with either radiation or chemicals, and the resultant colonies developing from the hamster embryo cells (normal and transformed) are scored after 8 to 10 days of incubation. (Adapted from Hall and Hei, 1986, with permission of the authors and publisher.)

within the same species resulted in different rates and yields of morphological transformation in culture as well as neoplastic development on inoculation of 10^6 or more cells into an appropriate mouse host.

Some of the characteristics of the experiments by Berwald and Sachs were quite interesting, especially the fact that the incidence of transformation was extremely high, exceeding 80% in some experiments. This argued rather strongly that the mechanism of the transformation by chemicals was not a simple mutation, because of the high incidence of conversion. These authors also demonstrated the transformation in vitro of hamster embryo cells (Borek and Sachs, 1968) and of human cells (Borek, 1980) by x-irradiation and by infection with oncogenic papovaviruses (cf. Sachs, 1974).

Studies by Huberman et al. (1976) indicated that cell transformation in culture is due to a mutagenic event in view of the constant ratio of transformation to mutation to ouabain resistance induced by carcinogenic hydrocarbons in vitro. While these studies did indicate an approximate 20-fold greater rate of transformation than of mutation, studies by Barrett and Ts'o (1978) indicated that morphological transformation in primary SHE cell cultures occurred with a frequency from 20 to 500 times higher than mutation at two different loci. This finding strongly suggests that the two processes are not identical. A review by Parodi and Brambilla (1977) of much of the literature on the relation between mutation and transformation in cell culture concluded that there was "an absolute difference between structural mutations and transformation." Furthermore, Elmore et al. (1983) demonstrated that increased mutation rates were not a necessary factor in carcinogen-induced transformation of human fibroblasts. Similarly, Kaden et al. (1989)

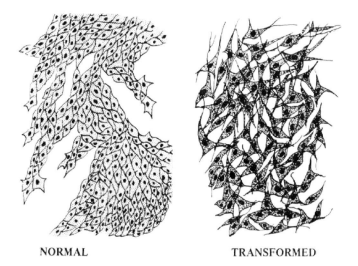

NORMAL   TRANSFORMED

Figure 14.5 An artist's conception of the microscopic appearance of normal and transformed cells in culture. The single-cell layer of spindle cells is characteristic of normal cells, which ultimately exhibit contact inhibition of replication, whereas transformed cells exhibit cytologic anaplasia and "piling up" of one cell on another, with lack of contact inhibition of replication.

found no simple correlation between spontaneous mutation rate and the malignant phenotype in Chinese hamster embryo fibroblast lines. The same conclusion had been drawn for the chemical and radiation induction of transformation in the mouse C3H/10T1/2 fibroblast cell line (Landolph and Heidelberger, 1979; Chan and Little, 1982). However, the fact that some structural alteration in DNA is associated with the neoplastic transformation in vitro was evidenced by the finding of Barrett et al. (1978) that ultraviolet irradiation of cells that had incorporated the base analog bromodeoxyuridine into their DNA were transformed. Neither of these two perturbations alone induced this transformation. Since it is well known that bromodeoxyuridine incorporation into mammalian cell DNA induces mutations by itself and that mutagenesis is markedly enhanced by the ultraviolet irradiation of such treated cells, these authors concluded that transformation resulted, at least in part, from the ultraviolet-induced structural alteration in DNA containing bromodeoxyuridine. Double-stranded DNA breaks induced by electroporated restriction enzymes induced morphological transformation in a mouse cell line, C3H10T1/2 (Borek et al., 1991). Transformation of SHE cells is also accompanied in many instances by the induction of aneuploidy. This is especially notable with both the synthetic estrogen diethylstilbestrol (Tsutsui et al., 1983) and asbestos fibers (Oshimura et al., 1984; Dopp et al., 1995). The normal estrogen, 17β-estradiol, was also effective in inducing both cell transformation and numerical chromosome changes in SHE cells (Tsutsui et al., 1987). However, male sex hormones, both synthetic and natural, exhibited only a very weak transforming effect on SHE cells (Lasne et al., 1990). While diethylstilbestrol may induce mutations at some but not all loci studied, no DNA adducts occurred in SHE cells at concentrations up to 10 µg/mL (Hayashi et al., 1996). Changes in the ^{32}P-postlabeling pattern of DNA adducts did occur in SHE cells in the presence of estradiol and some of its metabolites (Hayashi et al., 1996). Thus, while there is evidence that DNA damage can be correlated with morphological transformation, the quantitative relationships between mutation and transformation are not identical.

Studies by Heidelberger (1973) with the prostate system confirmed and extended these investigations. In Heidelberger's studies, the organ cultures treated with hydrocarbons were dispersed into cell suspensions and transformed cell lines were produced. DiPaolo et al. (1971a) confirmed the findings of Berwald and Sachs and demonstrated that, by inhibiting the cellular toxicity of carcinogenic hydrocarbons in hamster embryo cell cultures with various noncarcinogenic chemicals, one may dissociate the transforming property from the toxic metabolic property of carcinogenic hydrocarbons (DiPaolo et al., 1971b). The cytotoxicity of carcinogenic polycyclic hydrocarbons for cell cultures appears to depend on the presence and inducibility of the microsomal aryl hydroxylase complex, the regulation of which is mediated through the product of the *Ah* locus (Chapter 7). Utilizing human mammary epithelial cells, Stampfer et al. (1981) demonstrated that inhibition of growth of such cells was 50 to 100 times more sensitive to the presence of benzo[*a*]pyrene than were cultured fibroblasts. Nebert and associates (cf. Benedict et al., 1972) have shown that the metabolism of the hydrocarbon is necessary for cytotoxicity in that the inhibitors of hydrocarbon metabolism also inhibit the toxicity. Furthermore, Peterson and associates (1979) have demonstrated that the mutagenic lesion(s) produced by carcinogenic agents in cell culture is not associated with the cytotoxicity of the agent. On the other hand, Poiley et al. (1980) demonstrated that in a large number of normal hamster embryo cell preparations, those cells that were consistently more easily transformed by polycyclic hydrocarbons had consistently higher levels of aryl hydrocarbon hydroxylase and that the enzyme could be induced to a higher level by treatment with appropriate agents.

In addition to the systems mentioned above, which are concerned primarily with mesenchymal cell transformation, a number of differentiated epithelial cell types derived either from endoderm or ectoderm (Chapter 2) have been reported. These include cells derived from rat liver (e.g., Borenfreund et al., 1975; Montesano et al., 1980; Williams et al., 1973), mouse mammary epithelial cells (Miyamoto et al., 1988), rat tracheal epithelial cells (Thomassen et al., 1983), rat bladder (Hashimoto and Kitagawa, 1974), rabbit bladder (Summerhayes et al., 1981), and epidermal keratinocytes (Slaga et al., 1978; Yuspa et al., 1983b; Fusenig and Boukamp, 1998). In primary cultures of hepatocytes, the usual chemical hepatocarcinogens may not be effective for their conversion to proximate and ultimate forms because of the loss of phase I activity (Guillouzo, 1986). On the other hand, polycyclic hydrocarbons and alkylating agents as well as aflatoxin (Schaeffer and Heintz, 1978) and ethionine (Brown et al., 1983) did reportedly induce "transformation" of rat liver epithelial cells in culture. Perhaps the best-characterized of the epithelial transformations in vitro is that of keratinocytes, both rodent and human. Fusenig and Boukamp (1998), on the basis of studies of a spontaneously immortalized cell line obtained from normal human keratinocytes maintained in culture for an extended period, have proposed a multistage model for the development of normal keratinocytes into malignant neoplastic cells because of changes seen both in vivo and in vitro (Figure 14.6). Such a series of alterations are analogous to those seen in the stage of progression in both human and rodent neoplastic development (Table 9.12, Figure 9.8). In this model, however, the conversion of the immortal cell (HaCaT) occurring spontaneously in normal keratinocyte cultures to a "benign cell" requires transfection with the H-*ras* cellular oncogene. A major finding allowing for such experiments was the demonstration that high levels of calcium ions induced terminal differentiation of mouse epidermal keratinocytes, but continued maintenance may occur at decreased calcium concentrations. Treatment with several different types of chemical carcinogens induced the formation of cells that were resistant to the high calcium-induced differentiation of the keratinocytes (Kilkenny et al., 1985).

In general, transformation of mouse keratinocytes by a variety of chemical agents may be readily accomplished, but the transformation of human cells (either mesenchymal or epithelial) to cells capable of neoplastic growth in immunosuppressed animal hosts has met with much less success (McCormick and Maher, 1988; Kuroki and Huh, 1993; Holliday, 1996). Previous results demonstrating the growth of human cells in soft agar (anchorage independence; see below) may

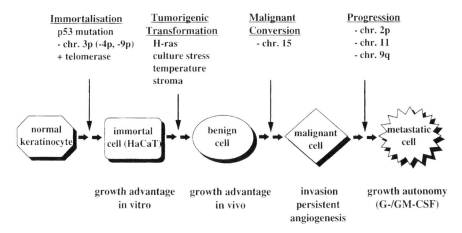

Figure 14.6 Schematic for "stages" of the transformation of normal human keratinocytes to metastatic cells in vivo. The conversion of the immortal cell to the benign cell requires transfection of the H-*ras* cellular oncogene as well as several other cultural characteristics noted in the figure. The steps thereafter can be demonstrated in vivo as well as in a special model in vitro system of these authors. (Adapted from Fusenig and Boukamp, 1998, with permission of the authors and publisher.)

not be a good method to characterize chemically induced transformation of human cells in vitro (Peehl and Stanbridge, 1981). On the other hand, several investigators (Milo et al., 1996; Gruenert et al., 1995; Stampfer and Bartley, 1985) have reported transformation and the formation of immortalized cell lines from both mesenchymal and epithelial human cells. Grafström (1990) reviewed such studies in human epithelial tissues in vitro. The mechanism for this peculiar "resistance" of human cells to transformation in vitro, despite the ability of such cells to metabolize polycyclic hydrocarbons and even form DNA adducts with their ultimate forms, is still not completely understood.

CRITERIA FOR NEOPLASTIC TRANSFORMATION IN VITRO

One of the critical points in the study of transformation in vitro is that it is obviously impossible to utilize the usual in vivo criteria of carcinogenesis to identify neoplastic cells. The morphologic changes seen initially by Berwald and Sachs (1963) were claimed to be the result of oncogenesis; however, such claims could be substantiated only if the cells could grow as neoplasms in a suitable host. Thus, there has been much discussion of the criteria for the neoplastic transformation in vitro. No universal criteria have been generally accepted, although many scientists in the field may have agreed on a number of characteristics (Katsuta and Takaoka, 1973). The more important of these criteria are listed in Table 14.1.

Few if any neoplastic cell populations in vitro exhibit all of the criteria indicated in Table 14.1. Furthermore, after initiation in vitro, transformed cells may acquire one or more of the characteristics shown as a function of time in culture after initiation. Barrett and Ts'o (1978) demonstrated in hamster embryo fibroblasts that the temporal acquisition during transformation in vitro of many of the characteristics listed in Table 14.1 was not simultaneous. Rather, morphological transformation (criterion 4) and the production of plasminogen activator (Chapter 16) occurred soon after the treatment with the carcinogen, whereas the growth of transformed cells in soft agar (criterion 3) usually occurred more than 30 population doublings after exposure to

Table 14.1   Criteria for Neoplastic Transformation in Vitro

Mesenchymal Cells	Epithelial Cells
1. Production of biologically malignant neoplasms in vivo by inoculation of 10^6 or fewer cells into syngeneic or immunodeficient hosts, in the absence of neoplasms produced by inoculation of comparable numbers of cells not treated with the "transforming" agent. Some "transformed" cell lines do not conform to this criterion, and some embryonic cells injected into immunosuppressed or syngeneic hosts will grow to the size of a gross tumor. The time of growth of transformed cells to detectable size in the syngeneic host may vary tremendously.	1. Same criteria as for mesenchymal cells.
2. "Immortality" of transformed cells in culture. This is characteristic of many biologically neoplastic cells, although in some instances those having immortality in vitro do not give rise to tumors in vivo.	2. Same criteria as for mesenchymal cells.
3. Growth of transformed cells in soft agar. With the exception of some mouse cell strains, e.g., Heidelberger's strain C3H/10T1/2 and transformed mouse prostate cells, transformed cells exhibiting this characteristic also produce neoplasms on inoculation into a suitable host. On the other hand, a number of biologically neoplastic tissues grown in vivo will not grow in soft agar in culture.	3. Many but not all epithelial cells transformed in vitro exhibit the capacity to grow in soft agar.
4. Colonies of transformed cells exhibit morphologic and growth characteristics in culture different from those of normal cells grown in culture. Nontransformed cells grow in an "ordered" way, whereas transformed cells tend to "pile up," with criss-cross patterns and a higher degree of pleomorphism. However, this criterion relates only to fibroblastic cells grown in culture. So few epithelial cells have been transformed in culture that morphological criteria of transformation for epithelial cells have not been determined accurately.	4. Often epithelial cells transformed in vitro do not exhibit morphological differences that are dramatically different from normal, but in many instances a greater degree of pleomorphism is seen in transformed epithelial cells compared with their nontransformed counterparts.

5. Loss of "contact inhibition" of cell replication under specific conditions of media and plating and increase in saturation density by transformed cells. A significant number of nontransformed cells in culture demonstrate no contact inhibition.

6. Reduced requirement for serum and growth factors compared with untransformed cells. This characteristic is less pronounced in transformed human cells since normal human cells can grow in lower serum levels.

7. Transformed cells in many, but not all, instances may be agglutinated by plant lectins. Not all agglutinated cells, however, demonstrate biological neoplasia in vivo.

8. Cells transformed by chemicals or viruses in culture exhibit antigenic alterations. "Spontaneous transformants" show no antigenic alterations.

9. Transformed cells may show karyotypic changes. However, cell lines that produce no tumors in vivo may be quite aneuploid, as are many "revertants" in culture.

10. Transformed cells usually have a greater efficiency of cloning than nontransformed cells.

11. Transformed cells usually exhibit a loss of bordered cytoplasmic actin and myosin, as exhibited by a loss of parallel arrays of microfilaments.

5. This characteristic is inconsistently seen in transformed epithelial cells, depending on the cell line and the tissue of origin; in some cell lines the piling up of cells occurs, whereas in others the monolayer growth pattern is maintained.

6. Decreased requirement compared with normal epithelial cells in liver; has not been sufficiently studied in a variety of systems.

7. Same criteria as for mesenchymal cells.

8. Many, but not all, epithelial cells transformed in vitro exhibit alterations in their antigenicity.

9. Same criteria as for mesenchymal cells.

10. Transformed epithelial cells usually have a much greater capability of growth in vitro from single or a few cells.

11. Most epithelial cells transformed in vitro exhibit alterations in their cytoskeletal structure, but this finding is inconsistent and not characteristic of all epithelial cells transformed in vitro.

These characteristics were obtained in a slightly modified form from reports by Fusenig et al., 1982; Borek, 1979; and Pitot, 1974.

the carcinogen. In a sense, this indicates that an analogy can be drawn between the progression of carcinogenesis in vivo and the full expression of cell transformation in vitro (Table 14.2).

Most investigators in oncology would probably agree that the criterion in Table 14.1 that is paramount for proving that a cell has been transformed to the neoplastic state in vitro is the formation of a neoplasm in vivo on inoculation of the putative transformed cultured cells (criterion 1). Other than this criterion, the characteristic most frequently correlated with the neoplastic potential of cells in vivo that had been transformed in vitro is their ability to grow in soft agar (Freedman and Shin, 1974; Weinstein et al., 1976) or exhibit "anchorage independence." As noted above, a major exception to this are human cells that may be "transformed" to anchorage independence but yet do not exhibit neoplastic potential in vivo (Peehl and Stanbridge, 1981). Furthermore, Kaplan and Ozanne (1983) argued that anchorage-independent growth is a function of the total concentration of growth factors in the medium to which these cells can respond. Thus, this criterion becomes a function of both the concentration of growth factors in the medium and the presence of their receptors on the surface of the cell, transformed or nontransformed.

Immortalization of cells in culture, i.e. the ability to continue replication beyond a finite number of doublings, a characteristic of normal cells (Hayflick, 1997), is seen with many, but not all, cells transformed in vivo or in vitro. The finite life span of most normal cells in vitro may be in some ways analogous to aging and the finite life span in vivo (Macieira-Coelho, 1993; Smith and Pereira-Smith, 1996). The process of immortalization in vitro probably involves specific genetic alterations linked to chromosomal changes, although "epigenetic" mechanism(s) cannot be ruled out in some instances (Trott et al., 1995).

Several workers have shown that "normal" cells or those transformed in vitro but exhibiting only a few of the criteria (Table 14.1) may grow as neoplasms in vivo when inoculated together with supporting structures—for example, glass beads (Boone, 1975), plastic plates (Sanford et al., 1980), or gelatin sponge (Okada et al., 1992). Barrett (1980) found that primary cultures of hamster embryo cells may be transformed to a stage in which neoplasms are produced in vivo only when the cultured cells are inoculated with polymer supports (Table 14.2). Several model cell lines that are aneuploid but commonly used in transformation studies in vitro, for instance C3H/10T1/2 and 3T3 mouse lines, exhibit such behavior (Boone and Jacobs, 1976); this indicates that all or some of these cell lines are beyond the stage of initiation. Furthermore, such cell lines may be transformed by alterations in the density of the cell culture (Haber and Thilly, 1978; Rubin et al., 1995), alkalinity of the medium (Oberleithner et al., 1991), polyamines (Tabib and Bachrach, 1998), anoxia (Anderson et al., 1989) and glass fibers (Whong et al., 1999), conditions that are unlikely to or have not induced transformation in primary cultures. On the basis of such findings, studies of the neoplastic transformation in vitro should be

Table 14.2 Characteristics of Stages in Syrian Hamster Embryo (SHE) Cell Transformation to Neoplasia

Normal SHE (GSHE)[a]	Immortalization (FOL[+])	"Tumorigenic" (ST[−])
Diploid	Aneuploid	Aneuploid
Low fibrinolytic activity	Enhanced fibrinolytic activity	Enhanced fibrinolytic activity
Anchorage dependent	Anchorage dependent	Anchorage independent
Nontumorigenic in suspension	Nontumorigenic in suspension	Tumorigenic in suspension
Nontumorigenic when attached to plastic substrate	Tumorigenic when attached to plastic substrate	Tumorigenic when attached to plastic substrate

[a]( ) = designations by Barrett (1980). Reproduced with permission of author and publisher.

carried out with cells of known genotype and phenotype, ideally shortly after primary explanta-tion and while still euploid.

It is clear that the ultimate standard of the neoplastic transformation is still the establish-ment of malignant neoplasms in vivo, but all of the characteristics listed above (Table 14.1) ap-ply to transformed cells in vitro, and, taken together, they strongly support the identification of a clone of cells transformed in vitro as biologically neoplastic. Still, with the possible exception of neoplasms induced on inoculation in vivo, no single criterion can mark a cell transformed in culture as biologically neoplastic.

CELL TRANSFORMATION AND THE NATURAL HISTORY OF NEOPLASTIC DEVELOPMENT IN VITRO

The definition of neoplasia noted in Chapter 2 was developed from observations of neoplastic disease in vivo. The criteria of transformation in cell culture listed in Table 14.1 did not define neoplastic disease in vitro but rather described a number of its characteristics. While neoplasia in vivo and cell transformation in vitro exhibit many apparent dissimilarities, considerable effort has been expended in trying to identify analogies in the natural history of the development of the neoplastic process in vivo and in vitro. We have already noted the changes spontaneously occur-ring in SHE cells transformed with chemical carcinogens or ionizing radiation (Table 14.2). However, a number of studies have been directed toward more controlled investigations of po-tential "stages" occurring during the development of cell transformation in vitro.

Initiation (Fixation)

As discussed earlier (Chapter 7), there is substantial evidence that the stage of initiation requires that division of the cell susceptible to the carcinogenic agent occur while the carcinogenic agent is present. This phenomenon was perhaps even more definitively demonstrated in cell culture with chemical carcinogenesis of SHE cells (Berwald and Sachs, 1963). These authors demon-strated that, unless the carcinogen remained in the culture medium for a period at least equiva-lent to that of a single cell cycle of the cells being treated, no transformation would occur. This finding led to the demonstration in cell culture that at least one round of cell division was neces-sary for the neoplastic transformation to be "fixed" (cf. Kakunaga, 1975). A similar phenome-non held true for both DNA tumor virus- and x-irradiation–induced transformation in cell culture, although the latter effect appeared to require two cell generations (Borek and Sachs, 1968). Sachs (1974) had suggested that possibly two cell divisions are required to fix transfor-mation by chemicals in cell culture as well. In the C3H/10T1/2 cell line, "transformation" is most efficient when the carcinogen is applied just prior to the onset of DNA synthesis in cultures synchronized for this parameter (Jones et al., 1977; Grisham et al., 1980).

In several instances, transformation induced by known carcinogens (such as polycyclic hydrocarbons) indicated that this process in vitro follows the kinetics of a single-hit phenome-non, exhibiting no threshold (cf. DiPaolo et al., 1971a), that is, lacking a "no-effect" level of the carcinogenic agent (Chapter 13). However, in the C3H10T1/2 cell line, the frequency of initia-tion or formation of foci by chemical carcinogens was found to decrease with increasing cell density of the culture (Huband et al., 1985). Furthermore, polycyclic hydrocarbons (such as benzo[a]pyrene) are themselves capable of inducing quiescent, confluent cultures of hamster embryo cells to enter DNA synthesis, after which cell transformation becomes apparent (Mironescu and Love, 1974).

Promotion

The first relatively clear demonstration of distinct stages in the transformation of cells in culture was the report by Mondal and Heidelberger (1976) of cells of the C3H/10T1/2 mouse line that were initiated with ultraviolet radiation and promoted with TPA (Table 14.3). Later studies by Sanchez et al. (1986), using N-methyl-N′-nitro-N-nitrosoguanidine (MNNG) as an initiating agent for the C3H10T1/2 cell line followed by promotion with TPA, induced numerous foci of morphologically transformed cells. Removal of TPA from the medium of such dishes containing foci resulted in regression of up to 84% of the foci and loss of morphological transformation. Stages in the induction of transformation in this cell line by chemicals (Lillehaug and Djurhuus, 1982) and ionizing radiation (Han and Elkind, 1982) have also been reported (Table 14.4). In addition, apparent steps in the transformation of other cell lines have also been identified (Thomassen and DeMars, 1982; Table 14.4). The JB6 mouse epidermal cell line (Colburn et al., 1982) has been used to identify genes potentially involved in the stage of tumor promotion in vitro as well as more broadly (Lerman et al., 1987). Transformed foci may be induced in this cell line by several different promoting agents.

In primary cultures, the natural history of neoplastic development has been best defined in the hamster embryo cell transformation system (Barrett and Ts'o, 1978). After initiation by either chemicals (Poiley et al., 1979) or radiation (DiPaolo et al., 1981), a clear promoting effect by TPA could be demonstrated in hamster embryo cells. Poiley et al. (1979) demonstrated that TPA could act as either an inhibitor or a promoting agent, depending on the length of time between initiation and the first addition of the promoting agent. Furthermore, Rivedal and Sanner (1982) demonstrated that reversal of the timing of the initiation and promotion stages resulted in no significant enhancement of transformation frequency in this system. Using this same system, Rivedal and Sanner (1981) demonstrated that several metal salts—including nickel sulfate, cadmium acetate, and potassium chromate—could act to promote the transformation of hamster

Table 14.3 Transformation of C3H/10T1/2 Cells by Ultraviolet Light and Tetradecanoylphorbol Acetate (TPA)[a]

Treatment Schedule	Plating Efficiency %	No. of Dishes with Foci/Total No. of Dishes	% Dishes with Foci	Transformation Frequency[b]
0.5% Acetone	19	0/23	0	0
TPA (0.1 μg mL^{-1})	20	0/12	0	0
Ultraviolet, 10 erg mm^{-2}	19	0/12	0	0
Ultraviolet, 10 erg mm^{-2} + TPA				
48 h[c]	19	3/12	25	0.08
72 h	19	5/12	42	0.18
Ultraviolet, 25 erg mm^{-2}	17	0/16	0	0
Ultraviolet, 25 erg mm^{-2} – TPA				
48 h	18	10/12	83	0.83
72 h	18	11/12	92	0.69

[a]The concentration of TPA used was 0.1 μg mL^{-1}.
[b]Percentage of transformed foci per surviving cell plated.
[c]Time after irradiation when TPA was added. Altered colonies or foci were enumerated 8–10 days after ultraviolet irradiation.
Adapted from Mondal and Heidelberger, 1976.

Table 14.4 Promotion of Cell Transformation in Vitro

	Initiating Agent	Promoting Agent	Reference
Primary Cells			
SHE	Methylcholanthrene	TPA	Poiley et al., 1979
	X-irradiation	TPA	DiPaolo et al., 1981
	—	Mezerein	Tu et al., 1992
	—	Estrogen	Hayashi et al., 1996
	Benzo[a]pyrene	Ni^{2+}, Cd^{2+}, and chromate salts	Rivedal and Sanner, 1981
	Benzo[a]pyrene	NaF	Jones et al., 1988
	Benzo[a]pyrene	pH 6.7	Kerckaert et al., 1996
Rat tracheal epithelium	N-methyl-N′-nitro-N-nitrosoguanidine (MNNG)	TPA	Steele et al., 1984
Mouse mammary organ culture	7,12-dimethyl-benz[a]anthracene	TPA	Mehta and Moon, 1986
Cell Lines			
C3H/10T1/2 mouse cells	MNNG	TPA	Boreiko et al., 1986
	MNNG	Mezerein	
	MNNG	TCDD	Abernethy et al., 1985
	Methylcholanthrene	Tri-n-butyltin	Parfett and Pilon, 1993
Mouse BALB/c-3T3	MNNG	TPA	Tsuchiya and Umeda, 1997
	Methylcholanthrene	Transforming growth factor β	Hamel et al., 1988
	Methylcholanthrene	1α, 25-Dihydroxy-vitamin D$_3$	Sasaki et al., 1986
	Methylcholanthrene	Tumor necrosis factor α	Komori et al., 1993
Mouse JB6 epi-dermal cell line	—	TPA	Colburn et al., 1982
		Mezerein	
		Epidermal growth factor	
WB-344 rat liver epithelial cell line	—	Transforming growth factor β	Zhang et al., 1994
Ei5 rat liver epithe-lial cell line	—	Transforming growth factor α	Tsao and Zhang, 1992

embryo cells initiated by benzo[a]pyrene. That spontaneously initiated cells may occur in these cultures was reported by Nakano and Ts'o (1981), who found subpopulations of cells lacking contact inhibition of cell division and anchorage dependence for growth in cell cultures established from hamster embryos. Sodium fluoride acts as a promoter in this system but was also shown to induce transformation in SHE cells in the absence of other initiating agents (Tsutsui et al., 1984). Two other promoting agents, mezerein (Tu et al., 1992) and diethylstil-bestrol (Hayashi et al., 1996), can induce transformation in cultured SHE cells as well. As pointed out by Boyd and Barrett (1990), these agents induce DNA damage, principally clastogenic effects suggesting that SHE cells are either quite sensitive to progressor agents or do in fact have a significant population of spontaneously initiated cells. In fact, Ueo et al. (1990) found that early-passage, normal diploid SHE cells contained a transient subpopulation of cells lacking density-dependent inhibition of cell division and presumably capable of forming morphologically transformed colonies. The interesting effect of lowered pH as a promoting agent in this system described by LeBoeuf and colleagues (cf. Kerckaert et al., 1996) may be explained by a concomitant increase in cell division caused by such lowered pH. Interestingly, the non–phorbol ester tumor promoter, okadaic acid, does not promote morphological transformation in SHE cells, although it is quite effective in mouse epidermis in vivo (Rivedal et al., 1990). In addition to the other examples of initiation/promotion systems in primary cultures, stages in the neoplastic development of other cell types in primary culture have been reported for the mouse submandibular gland epithelium (Wigley, 1983), rat embryo cells (Chouroulinkov and Lasne, 1978), and mouse epidermal cells (Yuspa et al., 1981). When hepatocytes were initiated in vivo and continued on several carcinogens for 6 to 12 weeks, TPA did not stimulate DNA synthesis or promote growth of primary cultures obtained from such livers (Kayano et al., 1982). In contrast, studies by Kaufmann et al. (1988) demonstrated that phenobarbital induced a proliferation of foci in primary cell culture from animals treated with methyl(acetoxymethyl)nitrosamine and then explanted to primary culture. These authors suggested that the proliferation of putatively initiated hepatocytes required the presence of the promoting agent as shown in vivo from other studies (Chapter 7). Kopelovich (1981) has shown that fibroblasts cultured from individuals genetically predisposed to colorectal cancer are less sensitive to the toxic effects of the promoting agent TPA, and Friedman et al. (1984) demonstrated that in cultures of colonic epithelial cells, TPA stimulated DNA synthesis in cells derived from patients with familial polyposis but not in control individuals. Later studies (Antecol, 1988) did not appear to substantiate these findings.

From all of these studies it becomes apparent that transformation of cells in culture may exhibit identifiable stages of initiation and promotion, with a number of the characteristics seen in these stages in vivo (cf. Boyd and Barrett, 1990). Some of the differences in vivo versus in vitro may be related either to the genetic constitution of the cells under study, e.g., cell lines, or the heterogeneity of the primary cultures utilized, e.g., SHE cells. In either event, the similarities are much greater than the differences, arguing that studies of the multistage nature of neoplastic development as seen in cell culture may have significant application to an understanding of mechanisms occurring both in vivo and in vitro in these individual stages. Because of the ability to control the cellular environment in vitro, cell culture may offer significant advantages as long as the investigator maintains a close association of findings in vitro with those in vivo.

Actions of Promoting Agents in Vitro

The number of multistage models of carcinogenesis in vitro has increased significantly over the past decade or more, and studies on the effects of promoting agents in a variety of cell systems have been quite extensive. Most of these studies have been directed toward the effects of TPA on cultured cells, both normal and neoplastic. A number of these effects of phorbol esters on cells in culture are listed in Table 14.5. Some of the effects of promoting agents, not necessarily phorbol esters, have been discussed in previous chapters. As noted from the table, TPA has a variety of effects in a variety of cell systems. The list of effects of TPA in a variety of cell cultures that are noted in Table 14.5 is by no means exhaustive. Some of the changes, such as induction of ornithine decarboxylase and enhanced cell division, can also be demonstrated in vivo during the stage of promotion, but TPA inhibited DNA synthesis and induction of ornithine decarboxylase in primary cultures of human epidermal cells (Chida and Kuroki, 1984). The effects on gene

Table 14.5 Effects of Phorbol Diester Tumor Promoters on Cells in Culture

Effects	Response	Cell Type	Reference
Biochemical			
Uptake of small molecules			
Sugars	Increased	Chick embryo fibroblasts—primary	Yamanishi et al., 1983
Choline	Increased	C3H10T1/2 cell line	Lijian et al., 1988
DNA strand breaks, chromosomal damage	Increased		Birnboim, 1982
Prostaglandin synthesis	Increased	Rat liver (C-9) cell line	Levine, 1988
Gene amplification	Increased	Mouse 3T6 mouse line	Barsoum and Varshavsky, 1983
Histone phosphorylation	Increased	BALB/C mouse spleno-cytes—primary	Patskan and Baxter, 1985
Lipid reorganization of plasma membrane	Increased	MDCK canine kidney cell line	Packard et al., 1984
Reorganization of actin filaments	Increased	FL human amnion cell line	Sastrodihardjo et al., 1987
DNA synthesis	Increased	3T3 mouse cell line	Dicker and Rozengurt, 1980
DNA synthesis	Decreased/ increased	Human skin fibroblasts—primary	Kopelovich and Chou, 1984; Oesch et al., 1988
Gap junctional intercellular communication	Inhibited	Several cell types	cf. Yamasaki and Fitzgerald, 1988
Signal transduction	Altered	Rat hepatoma cell line	O'Brien et al., 1991
		DDT$_1$MF-2 smooth muscle cell line	Leeb-Lundberg et al., 1985
		Rat hepatocytes—primary	González-Espinosa and García-Sáinz, 1995
			Caro et al., 1992
Gene expression			
Enzyme induction			
Ornithine decarboxylase	Increased	H35 rat hepatoma cell line	Goodman et al., 1988
		Rat hepatocytes—primary	Warholm, 1992
Transglutaminase	Increased	Mouse epidermal cells—primary	Yuspa et al., 1983a
Protein tyrosine phosphatase	Increased	NIH 3T3 mouse cells	Elson and Leder, 1995
Purine nucleoside phosphorylase	Increased	Human thymocytes—primary	Martinez-Valdez and Cohen, 1988
Cytochrome P4501	Increased	H35 hepatoma cell lines	Roesch and Wiebel, 1990
c-*fos* and c-*myc* proto-oncogenes	Increased	HU 1752 human urothelial cell line	Skouv et al., 1987
Biological			
Cellular morphology	Altered	Many different cell types	cf. Diamond et al., 1978
Cell division	Increased	Many cell types	cf. Diamond et al., 1978
DNA synthesis in low calcium Ca^{2+} medium	Increased	Mouse keratinocytes—primary	Yuspa et al., 1983b

(table continues)

Table 14.5   (continued)

Effects	Response	Cell Type	Reference
Biological (continued)			
Expression of mutations	Increased	V79-H3 Chinese hamster cell line	Tsuda, 1981
Terminal differentiation	Inhibited or stimulated	Erythroleukemia cell lines	Fibach et al., 1979; Loten and Sachs, 1979
		Myeloid leukemia—primary	
Herpesvirus, retrovirus, and EB virus synthesis	Increased	Several cell types	cf. Diamond et al., 1978
Malignant transformation by chemicals, radiation, or oncogenic viruses	Increased	Variety of cell types	cf. Diamond et al., 1978

expression as indicated by enzyme induction in the table are quite extensive and appear to be mediated through a specific consensus sequence in DNA, TGAC(G)TCA. This same sequence is involved in the AP-1 transcription activator complex involving the transcription factors, *jun* and *fos*, both of which are proto-oncogenes (cf. Szabo et al., 1991). Changes in cell morphology resulting from alterations in intracellular cytoskeletal elements such as actin (Rifkin et al., 1979) are reversible on removal of the promoting agent from the culture. A further discussion of alterations in cytoskeletal elements in cultured cells is presented in Chapter 16. However, it is important to point out that the vast majority of the effects of TPA noted in Table 14.5 are completely reversible on removal of the agent from the medium.

In addition to TPA, the effects of phenobarbital, a commonly used promoting agent in multistage hepatocarcinogenesis (Chapter 7), have also been studied with respect to its effects in cultured cells, predominantly in hepatocytes (Table 14.6). In general, in adult hepatocytes in culture, phenobarbital may transiently stimulate DNA synthesis under certain conditions (Yusof and Edwards, 1990); but on continued cultivation in the presence of this agent, DNA synthesis is usually inhibited (Manjeshwar et al., 1992; Miyazaki et al., 1998). In neonatal hepatocytes, on the other hand, an increase in cell growth was reported (Armato et al., 1985). A striking effect of phenobarbital on rat hepatocytes is its inhibition of the proliferative effects of a variety of growth factors (Meyer et al., 1989; Tsai et al., 1991). The increases noted in the smooth endoplasmic reticulum and cytochrome P450 2B1/2 reflect effects that are noted in livers of animals treated with phenobarbital in vivo.

The effects of a number of other promoting agents effective in multistage epidermal carcinogenesis in the mouse and hepatocarcinogenesis in the rat have also been studied, but the description of such effects is beyond the scope of this text. The examples given in Tables 14.5 and 14.6 are of two of the more commonly studied promoting agents in these systems. Their effects are manifold, a number of which can also be noted in vivo. However, the use of cell culture affords a much more controlled environment in which to study the direct effects of these tumor promoting agents on specific cell types.

TPA Alteration of Cell Differentiation

One of the more interesting effects of the phorbol diesters is their ability to modulate differentiation. TPA inhibits the induced differentiated expression of erythroid functions in murine erythroleukemia cells (Fibach et al., 1979); it also inhibits morphological differentiation in cultured

Table 14.6 Effects of Phenobarbital on Cells in Culture

Effects	Response	Cell Type	Reference
Biochemical			
Growth factor responses	Decrease	Rat hepatocytes—primary	Meyer et al., 1989 Tsai et al., 1991
Reorganization of cytoskeletal components	Increase	Rat liver epithelial cell lines	Decloitre et al., 1990
Gap junctional intercellular communication	Decrease	Mouse hepatocytes—primary	Ruch and Klaunig, 1988
Smooth endoplasmic reticulum proliferation	Increase	Neonatal rat hepatocytes—primary	Guillouzo et al., 1978
Gene expression			
Enzyme induction			
Glutathione S-transferase	Increase	Rat hepatocytes—primary	Vandenberghe et al., 1991
Cytochrome P450-2B1/2	Increase	Rat hepatocytes—primary	Sidhu and Omiecinski, 1998
Biological			
Cell growth and division	Decrease	Rat hepatocytes—primary	Miyazaki et al., 1998
	Increase	Neonatal rat hepatocytes—primary	Armato et al., 1985
Survival	Increase	Rat hepatocytes—primary	Miyazaki et al., 1990

mouse neuroblastoma cells (Ishii et al., 1978), but it induces normal differentiation in mouse and human myeloid leukemia cells (Lotem and Sachs, 1979). Although TPA inhibited granulocytic colony growth in cultures of human hematopoietic cells in vitro (Aye and Dunne, 1983), administration of TPA to patients with lowered blood counts resulting from cancer chemotherapy caused an increase in the peripheral white blood counts (Han et al., 1998). Terminal differentiation may also be induced acutely by administration of TPA to normal primary epithelial cells (Willey et al., 1984). Phorbol esters are also capable of activating or inducing the production and synthesis of several types of oncogenic viruses including EBV (Lin et al., 1983), mouse mammary tumor virus (Arya, 1980), and type C retroviruses (Hellman and Hellman, 1981).

TPA and Promoting Agent Effects on Gap Junctional Intercellular Communication (GJIC)

Cells, both in vivo and in vitro, communicate with each other or allow the direct transport of small molecules from one cell to another through the mediation of structures known as gap junctions. These structures, depicted in Figure 14.7, consist of hexameric channel structures known as connexons. Each protein subunit of the connexon is termed a *connexin*. Connexons from adjacent cells directly interact to produce a channel or pore between two cells as noted in the figure. Generally, the connexins in any connexon are identical or homotypic. In general, in vivo homotypic connexons are the rule, and interactions between cells to produce gap junctions result in the structure shown in Figure 14.7C, which involves interactions between homotypic or identical connexins. However, heterotypic interactions both within connexons and in gap junctions have also been described (Bruzzone et al., 1996). The pore or channel produced on opening of the gap junction as noted in Figure 14.7B allows the passage of molecules up to approximately 1000 Da in molecular mass (Kumar and Gilula, 1996). Thus, signaling molecules such as cyclic AMP,

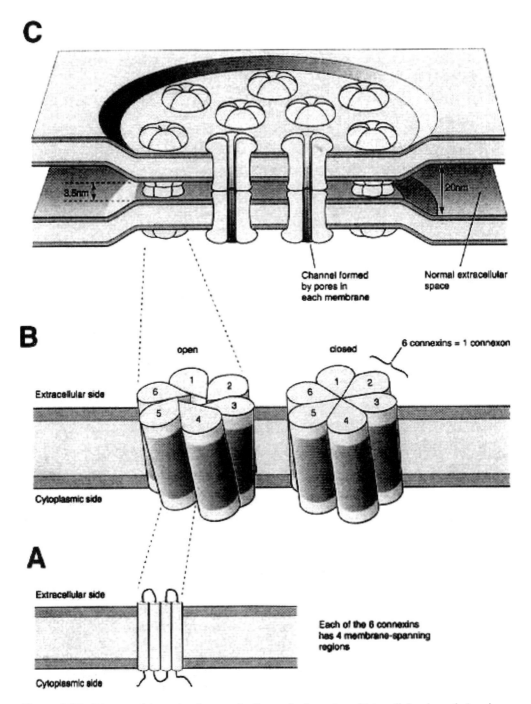

Figure 14.7   Diagram of the molecular steps leading to the formation of intercellular channels (gap junctions). A. Connexins are seen to oligomerize in a hexameric structure. B. The connexon is transported and inserted into the plasma membrane. C. Connexons from adjacent cells interact to form complete intercellular channels clustered in specialized membrane regions, the gap junctions. (From Bruzzone et al., 1996, with permission of the authors and publisher.)

many drugs, ions, and nutrients may pass through the channel occurring in the gap junction (Figure 14.7). The connexins themselves are members of a large multigene family occurring differentially in tissues (Table 14.7).

Studies on the inhibitory effects of promoting agents on GJIC in vitro were first reported almost simultaneously by two different laboratories (Murray and Fitzgerald, 1979; Yotti et al., 1979) and later by Trosko and others (Trosko et al., 1980). Since that time, considerable work has extended these earlier investigations with a variety of cultured cells, both primary and cell lines, and numerous different promoting agents whose effectiveness in the second stage of carcinogenesis has been demonstrated in vivo (cf. Yamasaki and Fitzgerald, 1988; Yamasaki et al., 1999). Transformed foci of mouse cells exhibit GJIC between transformed cells but do not appear to communicate through GJIC with surrounding nontransformed cells (cf. Yamasaki et al., 1999). In general, transformed cells in culture appear to have a decreased GJIC as compared to their normal counterparts (cf. Yamasaki, 1990). However, other examples have been reported of neoplastic cells in culture exhibiting increased GJIC correlated with their increased growth rate (Asamoto et al., 1994). In Table 14.8 is seen a listing (not exhaustive) of a number of examples of promoting agents whose effectiveness has been established in vivo, and their effects on GJIC in cultured cells, both primary and cell lines.

As noted in the table, not all promoting agents inhibit GJIC. The concentrations utilized in culture may not reflect those seen in vivo, and in some instances there is evidence that the effects in vitro may not be replicated in vivo (Kam and Pitts, 1988) but in other instances such replication has been demonstrated (Tateno et al., 1994). Notably trichloroethylene inhibits GJIC in mouse hepatocytes but not in rat hepatocytes in primary cultures (Table 14.8). Similar effects were known with the promoting agent saccharin, which was found to inhibit GJIC in the V-79 Chinese hamster cell line (Trosko et al., 1980) but not in human fibroblasts (Mosser and Bols, 1983). Furthermore, it appears that the conditions of the culture may alter the effectiveness of the agent to affect GJIC (Miller et al., 1987). Although TCDD does inhibit GJIC in primary rat hepatocyte cultures, it had no effect in the V-79 Chinese hamster cell line (Lincoln et al., 1987).

Table 14.7 Connexin Multigene Family

Greek Letter Nomenclature	Molecular Mass Nomenclature	Predicted Molecular Mass (kDa)	Examples of Organs with Expression
α1	Cx43	43.0	Heart
α2	Cx38	37.8	Embryo
α3	Cx46	46.0	Lens
α4	Cx37	37.6	Lung
α5	Cx40	40.4	Lung
α6	Cx45	45.7	Heart
α7	Cx33	32.9	Testis
α8	Cx50	49.6	Lens
β1	Cx32	32.0	Liver
β2	Cx26	26.5	Liver
β3	Cx31	31.0	Skin
β4	Cx31.1	31.1	Skin
β5	Cx30.3	30.3	Skin

Adapted from Kumar and Gilula, 1996, with permission of authors and publisher. The protein size in general is deduced from that predicted from the connexin cDNA.

Table 14.8   Effects of Promoting Agents on Gap Junctional Intercellular Communication (GJIC) in Cell Culture

Agent	Cell type	Effect	Effective concentration/time	Method[b]	Reference
Amobarbital (liver)[a]	Rat hepatocytes—primary	Inhibition	0.25 mM/14 days	Microinjection dye coupling	Ren and Ruch, 1996
Cholic acid (colon)	V-79 Chinese hamster cell line	None	50–200 γ/mL/7 days	Metabolic cooperation	Noda et al., 1981
Chlorobenzilate (liver)	V-79 Chinese hamster cell line	Inhibition	10–25 μM/3 days	Metabolic cooperation	Flodström et al., 1990
DDT (1,1-Bis[4-chlorophenyl]-2,2,2-trichloroethane) (liver)	Mouse hepatocytes—primary	Inhibition	0.1–10 γ/mL/8 h	Metabolic cooperation	Ruch and Klaunig, 1986
Diethylstilbestrol (liver)	V-79 Chinese hamster cell line	None	0/081–0.1 γ/mL/8 days	Metabolic cooperation	Barrett et al., 1983
Epidermal growth factor (liver)	T51B rat liver epithelial cell line	Inhibition	25 ng/mL/1 h	Microinjection dye coupling	Lau et al., 1992
α-Linolenate (mammary gland)	WB-F344 rat liver epithelial cell line	Inhibition	50 μM/2 days	Photobleaching	Hasler et al., 1991
Litocholic acid (colon)	V-79 Chinese hamster cell line	Inhibition	5–20 γ/mL/7 days	Metabolic cooperation	Noda et al., 1981
Okadaic acid (epidermis)	BALB/c 3T3 mouse cell line	None	1–10 γ/mL/12 days	Microinjection dye coupling	Katoh et al., 1990
Phenobarbital (liver)	Mouse hepatocytes—primary	Inhibition	500 γ/mL/4 h	Microinjection dye coupling	Ruch and Klaunig, 1988

Polybrominated biphenyl (liver)	V-79 Chinese hamster cell lines	Inhibition	5–10 γ/mL/2 days	Metabolic cooperation	Trosko et al., 1981
TCDD (2,3,7,8-tetra-chlorodibenzo-p-dioxin) (liver)	Rat hepatocytes—primary	Inhibition	10^{-8}–10^{-14}M/2 days	Microinjection dye coupling	Baker et al., 1995
TPA (epidermis)	BALBc/3T3 mouse cell line	Inhibition	1–10 ng/mL/4 h	Microinjection dye coupling	Yamasaki et al., 1985
Trichloroethylene (liver)	Mouse hepatocytes—primary	Inhibition	10^{-4}–10^{-5}M/3 h	Microinjection dye coupling	Klaunig et al., 1989
Trichloroethylene (liver)	Rat hepatocytes—primary	None	10^{-4}–10^{-5}M/3 h	Microinjection dye coupling	Klaunig et al., 1989

[a]Tissues in parentheses denote those in which the agent is effective as a promoter of carcinogenesis in vivo.

[b]The three principal methods indicated in this column are standard in most laboratories. The reader is referred to the individual reference for the specific method involved. In brief, the microinjection involves injection of a single cell with a fluorescent dye, then determining its migration to adjacent cells with a fluorescence microscope. Metabolic cooperation involves either prelabeling a cell population with a radioactive precursor, mixing it with an unlabeled population, and determining transference to the unlabeled cell population or, alternatively, in cells exhibiting mutations, making them resistant to base analogs. Inhibition of metabolic cooperation is measured as the increased recovery in cocultures of resistant and sensitive cells in a medium containing the analog. Photobleaching involves microinjection dye coupling with a very sophisticated instrument, as noted in the reference.

As noted in the table, the time during which the culture is exposed to the agent varies extensively from 1 hour to 2 weeks. This has suggested several different mechanisms, some of which must act relatively rapidly while others may exert their effects over more extended periods, raising the possibility of alterations in gene expression. As noted in Table 14.5, acidic pH could act as a promoting agent in the SHE cell transformation system. Ruch et al. (1990) demonstrated that acidic pH actually inhibited GJIC in these cells, thus possibly relating the two effects. Other studies have implicated phosphorylation of the connexins and their assembly as alterations being affected by promoting agents in cultured cells (Asamoto et al., 1991; Matesic et al., 1994). An effect both on connexin phosphorylation and alteration in connexin expression by TPA in mouse primary keratinocytes has also been noted (Brissette et al., 1991). Epidermal growth factor effects may involve the signal transduction pathway of this ligand with its receptor activating intracellular protein kinases (Kanemitsu and Lau, 1993). TPA downregulates E-cadherin in mouse keratinocytes (Jansen et al., 1996).

Some have argued that the inhibition of GJIC by promoting agents in vitro is a ubiquitous characteristic of promoting agents. However, even the incomplete listing of Table 14.8 indicates that a significant number of exceptions to this putative generalization occur. Still, the importance of GJIC in intercellular associations, the reversibility of the effects of promoting agents on connexin expression, e.g., Neveu et al. (1990), and the large number of examples where such an inhibition does occur (Table 14.8) argue that while modulation of GJIC by promoting agents may not be ubiquitous to all, it probably plays a very significant role in the development and maintenance of this stage in many instances.

Modulation of the Neoplastic Transformation in Vitro

Several studies (Grisham et al., 1980; Jones et al., 1976; McCormick and Bertram, 1982) have shown that the initiation of the neoplastic transformation in vitro is likely to be most effective at or near the interface of the G_1 and S phases of the cell cycle. As with the natural history of neoplastic development in vivo (Chapter 8), the stages of initiation and promotion may be modulated during carcinogenesis in vitro. As noted in Table 14.9, a variety of materials are effective in inhibiting transformation itself as well as altering the stages of initiation and promotion where such stages can be effectively identified. In primary cultures, most investigations have been carried out on the SHE cell system. Agents such as butylated hydroxytoluene and other antioxidants as well as cortisone act in a manner similar to that seen in vivo (Chapter 8). In contrast, fatty acids such as stearic acid and its derivatives, which have been found to enhance the stage of promotion in vivo, inhibit transformation of these cells in vitro (Embleton and Noy, 1991). Selenite ions added to mouse mammary gland organ culture were found to have opposite effects depending on their concentration in the culture (Chatterjee and Banerjee, 1982).

By use of cell lines, particularly the C3H10T1/2, a variety of inhibitors of transformation have been identified. A very interesting effect is the inhibition of transformation by various protease inhibitors (Kennedy, 1985) that also alter the effectiveness of modulators of protein kinase C during the transformation process (Umans and Kennedy, 1992). As noted in the table, several other agents such as ascorbate, aspirin, and β-carotene, which do inhibit development of the stage of promotion in vivo (Chapter 8), are also effective in this cell line in inhibiting morphological transformation. Unlike the effects in SHE cells, cortisone did not alter transformation induced by ionizing radiation in C3H10T1/2 cells (Kennedy and Weichselbaum, 1981). Arrest of proliferation of this cell line in isoleucine-free medium with subsequent replacement of this amino acid and exposure to MNNG causes an enhancement of transformation, probably by effecting a more efficient rate of initiation because of increased cell cycling on release of the nutritional block (Grisham et al., 1979). Borek et al. (1983) noted the dependence of transformation

Table 14.9 Modulation of Cell Transformation in Culture

Cell type	Transforming Agent	Modulating Agent	Effect	Stage	Reference
Primary cultures					
Syrian hamster embryo cells	Benzo[a]pyrene	Butylated hydroxytoluene	Inhibition	Initiation	Potenberg et al., 1986
			Enhancement	Promotion	
	Benzo[a]pyrene + TPA	Caffeine	Inhibition	Transformation	Rivedal and Sanner, 1985
	Benzo[a]pyrene	Ca^{2+} at 0.01 mM	Inhibition	Transformation	Evans and Boynton, 1982
	Benzo[a]pyrene + TPA	Cortisone	Inhibition	Initiation	Greiner and Evans, 1982
			Inhibition	Promotion	Rivedal., 1982
	3-Methylcholanthrene + TPA	Derivatives of stearic acid	Inhibition	Transformation	Embleton and Noy, 1991
Mouse mammary gland organ culture	7,12-Dimethylbenz[a]-anthracene	SeO_3^-	Enhancement $[10^{-8} - 10^{-2} \text{ M}]$	Transformation	Chatterjee and Banerjee, 1982
			Inhibition $[10^{-6} - 10^{-5} \text{ M}]$	Transformation	
Cell lines					
C3H10T1/2	Ionizing radiation	Antipain (protease inhibitors)	Inhibition	Transformation	Kennedy, 1985
	3-Methylcholanthrene	Ascorbate	Inhibition	Transformation	Benedict et al., 1980
	Ionizing radiation	Aspirin	Inhibition	Transformation	Radner and Kennedy, 1990
	3-Methylcholanthrene	β-carotene	Inhibition	Transformation	Pung et al., 1988
	Ionizing radiation	Cortisone	Enhancement	Transformation	Kennedy and Weichselbaum, 1981
	N-methyl-N′-nitro-N-nitrosoguanidine (MNNG)	Isoleucine-free medium	Enhancement	Transformation (initiation)	Grisham et al., 1979
	Ionizing radiation	Polyprenoic acid	Inhibition	Transformation	Borek et al., 1986
	Benzo[a]pyrene	Triiodothyronine	Enhancement	Transformation	Borek et al., 1983
	3-Methylcholanthrene	Triphenylmethane	Inhibition	Transformation	Cooney et al., 1992
3T3 cell line	—	Mg^{2+} deprivation	Inhibition	Transformation	Rubin et al., 1981
	3-Methylcholanthrene + TPA	3-nitro-2,4,6-trihydroxy-benzamide	Inhibition	Promotion	Semba et al., 1993

of C3H10T1/2 cells on the presence of triiodothyronine (T3). Complete removal of this hormone from the medium resulted in virtually complete loss of transformation effectiveness by ionizing radiation and chemical carcinogens. Addition of T3 back to the cultures restored transformation effectiveness.

Thus, while there are clear similarities between the modulation of transformation and the stages of initiation and promotion in vitro and in vivo, there are also significant differences. Until clearer definitions of the stages of initiation and promotion in vitro are obtained and the relationship of morphological transformation to the neoplastic transformation is understood, it will be difficult to rectify these differences between the in vivo and in vitro systems.

Progression

Since the principal characteristic of the stage of progression in morphological terms is the appearance of benign and malignant neoplasms, an analogous stage in cell culture would require some evidence that such cells are truly neoplastic. Thus, to be in the stage of progression cells in the process of cell transformation in vitro would have as an absolute characteristic the formation of neoplasms in vivo.

However, as noted in Chapter 9, the principal cellular and molecular characteristic of the stage of progression is that of evolving karyotypic instability and accompanying aneuploidy. Thus, one may reasonably argue that cells in culture undergoing transformation and exhibiting karyotypic instability are in the stage of progression. At our present state of knowledge this is probably an oversimplification. There are a number of aneuploid cell lines with relatively stable karyotypes that do not appear to develop into neoplasms when inoculated into an appropriate host. This also is not a true test unless one always reinoculates the transformed culture presumed to be in the stage of progression into the host from which it arose. Since this is not always possible, the lack of response or takes on reinoculation of "transformed" cells in vivo may be the result of immune responses in the host, the lack of appropriate circumstances in the host to allow growth of the inoculated cells, or the production by the cultured cells of a product detrimental to the host or to which the host responds excessively. The immunobiology of the host–tumor relationship is discussed later in the text (Chapter 19); there are very few neoplastic cell populations producing materials toxic to the species from which they arose. On the other hand, it has been pointed out earlier that the use of a variety of supports such as sponges, plastic films, etc., does allow the growth of cells in vivo as neoplastic cells when otherwise they would not grow (Boone et al., 1979; Sanford et al., 1980).

In parallel with the evolution of the stage of progression in vivo, one would expect to find some degree of karyotypic evolution in cell transformation as well. Table 14.10 gives a collection of several studies indicating that, both in chemically induced and spontaneous transformation, a time-dependent pattern of karyotypic changes evolves in the cells. Thus, one could argue by analogy that such cells are in the stage of progression, exhibiting its primary characteristic, karyotypic instability. Further evidence for this characteristic of the stage of progression in cell transformation in culture can be seen from the studies by Tlsty and her associates (1989) demonstrating that the rate of spontaneous gene amplification in transformed cells is significantly higher than that seen in nontransformed cells. Even in cell lines, it is possible to demonstrate an evolution of genomic instability when one compares nontransformed 3T3 mouse cells to those transformed by chemicals, radiation, or spontaneously (Honma et al., 1994). Mamaeva (1998) has emphasized the significance of karyotypic evolution in cells in culture, arguing that there are certain generalities that one may apply to the karyotypes of transformed and permanent cell lines. These include the nonrandom character of numerical and structural chromosome changes in cell lines of different histogenesis, the loss of one of the sex chromosomes during prolonged

Table 14.10   Patterns of Karyotypic Evolution in Cell Transformation in Vitro

Cell Type	Carcinogen	Early Change	Other Changes	References
Chinese hamster embryo cell line	Spontaneous	$3q^+$	6^-, 10^+	Shimizu et al., 1995
Rat tracheal epithelial cells (from primary)	MNNG	4^+, 7^+, 11^+	3^-	Endo et al., 1990
SHE cells, primary	$NaHSO_3$	13^-	$5q^-$	Popescu and DiPaolo, 1988
	Diethylstilbestrol	11^+	19^+	Ozawa et al., 1989
Salivary gland epithelial cell lines	Spontaneous	2^-, 12^-	9^-, 13^+	Cowell and Wigley, 1982
WCHE/5 Chinese hamster cell line	Spontaneous	?	5^+	Cram et al., 1983

cultivation, a similarity of the total chromosome material in all cells of the line despite their karyotypic heterogeneity, and retention of, as a minimum, disomy in all autosomes in most cell lines. Several of these characteristics echo the earlier findings of Kraemer et al. (1972) in comparing karyotypes of an established neoplastic cell line with those of normal cells (Chapter 9).

It is also possible to identify "progressor" agents in cell transformation. Hojo et al. have reported that cyclosporine induces many of the characteristics of the stage of tumor progression in a nontransformed cell line (Hojo et al., 1999). The SV40 T antigen of itself is capable of driving karyotypic instability, which precedes neoplastic transformation in human diploid fibroblasts (Ray et al., 1990). Furthermore, Li et al. (1997) demonstrated that transformation of primary cultures of Chinese hamster embryo cells by chemicals or spontaneous transformation resulted in essentially 100% of transformed cells exhibiting aneuploidy. These authors have argued that in this transformation process aneuploidy is the cause rather than a consequence of the transformation event itself. Thus, it would appear that, while the initial transformation event as originally described by Berwald and Sachs (1965) and further delineated by Barrett and his colleagues may not involve in all instances karyotypic alterations, events following transformation almost always lead to a stage in in vitro carcinogenesis that is completely analogous to the stage of progression in vivo. The alternative is the reversion of the transformed cell to a normal phenotype or its loss by apoptosis, which is considered below.

Loss or Modification of Malignant Potential as an Alternative Stage in the Natural History of Neoplastic Transformation in Vitro

An interesting finding resulting from studies of the neoplastic transformation in vitro is the phenomenon of the reversion from the transformed to the normal state after the initial exposure of cells to a carcinogenic agent. Rabinowitz and Sachs (1970) found that the incidence of the reversion from the morphologically transformed state to that of a morphologically normal cellular appearance and life span in chemical or radiation transformation was exceedingly high, usually in the range of 81% to 93%, although such reversion occurred in only 5% of polyoma-transformed SHE cells. Many of these reversion variants reacquire characteristics of normal cells, such as a limited life span in vitro (Rabinowitz and Sachs, 1970). Such a high rate of reversion did not support the concept that the transformation process was the result of a single gene mutation, but it did not rule out the role of chromosomal changes in the genesis of cell transformation in culture. Such revertants occur even in virus-transformed cells, and the reverted cells still possess viral information within their DNA. Sachs and associates (Hitotsumachi et al., 1972) demonstrated that most if not all reverted cells exhibit significant karyotypic abnormalities, usually characterized by some degree of polyploidy. They proposed a model that implies that the balance of gene dosage for the expression and suppression of the neoplastic transformation is critical in the formation of revertants. These concepts may be considered a forerunner of our knowledge of tumor suppressor genes, and later studies by Koi and Barrett (1986) supported this concept in suggesting that loss of tumor-suppressive function was then involved in the development of the stage of progression in SHE cell transformation. In addition, a number of instances of "transient" reversion of the transformed phenotype have been seen with the application of a variety of agents to specific cell culture systems. Examples of this include cycloheximide in human cell transformation (Cho and Rhim, 1979), chemically defined media in C3H/10T1/2 cells (Tomei and Bertram, 1978), interferon treatment of C3H10T1/2 cells (Brouty-Boyé and Gresser, 1981), and variation in cell density of different cell lines (Brouty-Boyé et al., 1980; Bempong and Myers, 1985). Reversion of the transformed phenotype in transformed NIH3T3 cell line was accomplished by the tumor-promoting agent okadaic acid (Sakai et al., 1989). Within 1 week of removal of the okadaic acid, the morphology of the cells reverted to the malignant phenotype. Suggesting that signal transduction is involved in some of these transient alterations, several reports have demonstrated the morphological reversion of transformed cells in vitro by the addition of cyclic AMP or its congenors (Johnson et al., 1971; Krystosek and Puck, 1990).

In addition to the "spontaneous" or transient reversion of cells transformed in culture, induction of such reversions or, in most cases, terminal differentiation has been described for a number of neoplasms cultured in vitro. Table 14.11 lists several such examples, together with the various chemicals and culture conditions inducing such reversion or terminal differentiation. We have already noted the effect of TPA in inducing and inhibiting differentiation of various cells in culture. The examples given in Table 14.11 extend this to other agents, several of which are not promoting agents, demonstrating a greater variety of chemicals inducing this effect in cell culture.

Even more extensively studied examples of the induction of terminal differentiation in neoplastic cells in culture are those of various leukemic cells, both primary and cell lines obtained from both human and animal sources. In Table 14.12 may be seen the rather extensive list of chemical agents capable of inducing differentiation in a human myeloid cell line (HL-60) and in the Friend erythroleukemia cell line from the mouse. The HL-60 cell line has been studied in

Table 14.11 Induced Differentiation in Cultured Neoplastic Cells

Cell Type	Agent	Reference
Breast cancer cell line, human	TPA, mycophenolic acid	Bacus et al., 1990
Choriocarcinoma cell line, human	Methotrexate	Friedman and Skehan, 1979
Colon carcinoma, human	N,N-dimethylformamide	Dexter et al., 1979
	Hexamethylene bisacetamide	Schroy et al., 1989
Hodgkin cell line, human	Extracellular matrix	Hsu et al., 1987
Melanoma cell lines, mouse	3-Acetamidobenzamide	Durkacz et al., 1992
human	Mycophenolic acid	Kiguchi et al., 1990
Osteosarcoma cell line, human	1,25-Dihydroxyvitamin D_3	Bonewald et al., 1992
Rhabdomyosarcoma, rat cell line	Retinoic acid, dimethylformamide	Gerharz et al., 1989
Small cell lung cancer cell lines, human	Retinoic acid	Doyle et al., 1989

Table 14.12 Induction of Differentiation in Cultured Leukemia Cell Lines

Cultured Neoplastic Cell Line	Inducers	Terminally Differentiated Cell Type
Myeloid leukemia (human)	Arginase hexamethylene bisacetamide, dimethylsulfoxide, genistein, hypoxanthine, actinomycin D,L-ethionine, tunicamycin, alkyl lysophospholipids, 1α,25-dihydroxy vitamin B_3, tetradecanoylphorbol acetate, retinoic acid, methotrexate, topoisomerase inhibitors, N-acetylspermidine, 4-hydroxynonenal	Macrophage or granulocyte
Friend erythroleukemia (mouse)	Dimethylsulfoxide, butyrate, 5-azacytidine, 6-thioguanine, hypoxanthine actinomycin D, hexamethylene bisacetamide, pyridine N-oxide, dimethylformamide, bromodeoxyuridine, high-K^+ medium, puromycin aminonucleoside, N-methyl-nicotinamide, L-histindinol	Orthochromatic normoblast

many laboratories (cf. Hozumi, 1983; Collins, 1987), while the Friend erythroleukemia cell line from the mouse has also been extensively investigated (cf. Rifkind et al., 1978). The HL-60 cell line has the interesting variation that cells may differentiate either to macrophages or granulocytes, some agents inducing transformation of the former (e.g., TPA), others the latter or both. HL-60 cells induced to differentiate to granulocytes apparently died subsequently via apoptosis (Martin et al., 1990).

It is significant that a number of chemotherapeutic drugs are among those inducing differentiation of leukemic and other neoplastic cell types. These include topoisomerase inhibitors (Nakaya et al., 1991), actinomycin D, methotrexate, and several base analogs. The potential importance of such findings with respect to the chemotherapy of cancer are discussed in Chapter 20.

Mechanistic Studies of Induced Differentiation

Since the changes that accompany induced differentiation of neoplastic cells are quite extensive (Olsson et al., 1996), a number of findings have suggested a variety of potential mechanisms involved in the induction of differentiation of cells in culture. Alterations in DNA methylation have been found during the induced differentiation of Friend erythroleukemia cells (Vizirianakis and Tsiftsoglou, 1996). Interestingly, the DNA methylation inhibitor, 5-azacytidine, is not a very effective inducer of differentiation of the Friend erythroleukemia system (Christman, 1984). Other studies using these cell lines suggest that alterations in membrane structure (Lyman et al., 1976), protein kinase C activation (Aihara et al., 1991), and alterations in the expression of a cyclic AMP–dependent protein kinase (Tortora et al., 1991) are indicative of significant effects in alterations of signal transduction pathways as components of the induced differentiation process. A role for heat-shock proteins and their interaction with the signal transduction pathway as components of the differentiation program has been suggested (Whitesell et al., 1994). Sachs (1993) and his associates have studied the effects of growth factors and cytokines that are normally involved in the regulation of erythroid and granulocyte maturation. These workers have suggested that reversion and induction of differentiation may occur in appropriate cell types even in the presence of significant genetic abnormalities such as chromosomal alterations. That active oxygen radicals may be involved in this process as well is suggested by the report by Barrera et al. (1991) of the induction of differentiation of HL-60 cells by 4-hydroxynonenal, a major product of lipid peroxidation. Although all of these various items of information do not make a clear picture as yet, the establishment of the phenomenon of the induction of differentiation of neoplastic cells in vitro and the several model systems in which mechanisms of this effect can be studied have opened the way to the potential use of such technologies in the therapy of human neoplasia (Chapter 20).

GENETIC STUDIES OF THE NEOPLASTIC TRANSFORMATION IN VITRO

Because one of the principal mechanisms involved in the neoplastic transformation is presumed to be that of specific structural alterations in the cellular genome, cell culture potentially offers a system in which to study directly genetic alterations causally related to or associated with the neoplastic transformation. Just as studies on the genetics of cell transformation by oncogenic viruses allowed the demonstration of temperature-sensitive mutants (Chapter 4), it has also been possible to isolate such mutants in cells transformable in culture. However, the examples of such identification have thus far been in cell lines, and it is somewhat difficult to equate such findings with those involving specific mutations in viral *onc* genes. Both in a line of epithelial cells derived from rat liver (Yamaguchi and Weinstein, 1975) and in the C3H/10T1/2 cell line (Boreiko and Heidelberger, 1980), mutants have been isolated that behave like transformed cells at temperatures of 33° to 36°C, whereas at 40°C such alterations are lost. Colburn and associates (Lerman et al., 1986) have identified genes, termed pro 1 and pro 2, that specify the sensitivity to the induction of transformation by TPA in a mouse epidermal cell line called JB6. Homologs of these genes have also been identified in human neoplasia, but only the pro 1 homolog was able to confer sensitivity to TPA-induced transformation and transfected into JB6 cells. Related studies by Bouck and diMayorca (1982) with a mouse cell line have suggested that transformation by a papovavirus is expressed as a dominant trait, whereas transformation by chemicals is indicative of a recessive trait. Other studies have partially characterized or postulated genes associated with neoplastic transformation in vitro in a human squamous cell carcinoma cell line (Li et al., 1995) and SHE cell transformation respectively (Preston et al., 1994). Of recent interest is the report by Hahn et al. (1999) of the induced transformation of normal human epithelial and fibroblast cells in primary culture by the transfection with retroviral vectors of three different genes, telomerase (Chapter 15), the SV40 large T antigen, and an oncogenic allele of the H-*ras* proto-oncogene. These authors suggested that the ectopic expression of these three genes resulted in the direct conversion of normal to neoplastic cells in vitro. These latter studies are some of the few that have been carried out on the genetics of the neoplastic transformation in primary cell cultures.

Somatic Cell Hybridization as a Tool to Study Mechanisms of the Neoplastic Transformation in Vitro

With the discovery of the phenomenon of somatic cell hybridization or cell fusion, the potential for genetic studies on somatic cells, especially neoplastic cells, was realized, at least theoretically. In this process (shown diagrammatically in Figure 14.8), two cells from the same or different species are fused, usually in the presence of inactivated Sendai virus, certain lipids, polyethylene glycol, or electrofusion (Široký and Cervenka, 1990) , resulting in the formation of a single cell with two nuclei. This is termed a *heterokaryon* when cells of two different types or

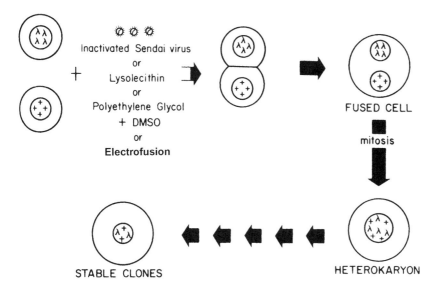

Figure 14.8 Outline of the fusion of somatic cells in the laboratory. The chromosomes of each of the two cells arising from two different species are denoted by + and λ. After fusion of the cells and subsequent mitosis, the heterokaryon is seen to contain the chromosomes of both cells, but subsequent replication results in stable clones with a reduced number of chromosomes.

species are fused. If cells of the same type are fused, the product is termed a *homokaryon*. The binucleate hetero- or homokaryon contains all of the genetic apparatus from each of the two original cells. After DNA synthesis, mitosis occurs with a mixing of the chromosomes from each of the two nuclei and subsequent formation of a single nucleus containing most or all of the chromosomes from the two donor cells. As the hetero- or homokaryon continues to undergo successive cell divisions, generally chromosomes of one or the other of the donor cell nuclei are lost until a relatively stable karyotype is obtained, usually consisting of virtually all of the chromosomes of one donor cell and one or only a few chromosomes from the other. By suitable chromosome identification one can determine the origin of each of the chromosomes of the heterokaryon.

Ephrussi (1965) and Harris (1972) and their associates were among the first to utilize this technique in an attempt to determine whether or not the inheritance of the malignant state in such heterokaryons acted as a dominant or recessive trait. In some of their studies on the fusion between malignant and nonmalignant cells, malignancy behaved like a recessive character, although fusion of a variety of malignant cells failed to demonstrate any complementation of the supposed genetic trait, since all such resulting heterokaryons were malignant (Wiener et al., 1974). When fusion of normal cells with virally transformed cells occurred, the resulting heterokaryon was neoplastic if it possessed integrated viral information within its genome (Croce et al., 1975). While a number of other studies demonstrated that hybrids produced within the same or different species sometimes were neoplastic, the careful studies of Stanbridge and associates reproduced the earlier investigations of Ephrussi and Harris studying the fusion of normal and neoplastic cells of the same or different tissues (cf. Stanbridge, 1984). The suppression of tumorigenicity occurred even in hybrids in which the neoplastic cell possessed activated oncogenes (Geiser et al., 1986). In some instances, the suppression of malignancy in the hybrid involves the production of gene products involved in terminal differentiation (Harris and Bramwell, 1987). In an extension of these investigations, Howell and Sager (1978), using techniques of mass fusion of whole cells with enucleated cytoplasm to form "cybrids," have shown that the suppression of tumor-forming ability may be cytoplasmically transmitted in specific cybrids. This finding was further supported by the studies of Israel and Schaeffer (1988), using normal and transformed cells derived from an original single clone.

Harris and his associates (Jonasson et al., 1977) also showed that if a normal–malignant hybrid lost many of its chromosomes, the neoplastic state would reappear; this indicates that the normal cells may contain specific suppressors of malignancy. Sachs and associates (Hitotsuma-chi et al., 1972) have suggested similar mechanisms, even relating the suppressor function to specific chromosomes within hamster cells (see above). More recently Sasabe and Inana (1991) have demonstrated that the suppression of malignancy in hybrids between a retinoblastoma cell line and a "nontransformed" NIH 3T3 resulted in cells of a nontransformed phenotype. These authors suggested that the normal retinoblastoma gene from the nontransformed cells was responsible for this change.

In general, these findings using homo- and heterokaryons of normal and neoplastic cells are compatible with the presence of tumor suppressor genes in situations where the transformed or malignant phenotype is suppressed in the heterokaryon. On the other hand, cell fusion of normal and neoplastic cells has found an interesting application in the production of monoclonal (uniquely specific) antibodies directed toward specific antigens (see Chapter 19). This technique, pioneered by Kohler and Milstein (1976), involves the fusion of normal antibody-producing cells obtained from the spleen or lymph nodes of animals immunized against certain antigens with malignant myeloma cells (cf. Westerwoudt, 1985). Specific clones of cells resulting from the fusion can be isolated and their antibody production determined. After cloning and isolation, the resulting homokaryon (termed a *hybridoma*) can be grown in appropriate animals or in cell culture for the production of specific monoclonal antibodies. This technique, a by-product of attempts to determine whether neoplasia is a dominant or recessive trait by the method of cell fusion, has revolutionized our ability to produce large amounts of monospecific antibodies for research and clinical use.

CELL CULTURE AS A TOOL IN OUR UNDERSTANDING OF CARCINOGENESIS AND CANCER

The transformation of cells in culture to the neoplastic state, both spontaneously and induced by chemical, physical, and biological agents, exhibits many similarities to carcinogenesis in vivo. In this chapter an effort has been made to emphasize the more important examples of close analogies between the carcinogenic process in vitro and in vivo. It is through a more careful study of the mechanisms of such analogies that a better understanding of the process of carcinogenesis may be forthcoming. On the other hand, an understanding of the mechanisms of the differences between the carcinogenic process in vivo and that in vitro may be equally rewarding.

REFERENCES

Abernathy, D. J., Greenlee, W. F., Huband, J. C., and Boreiko, C. J. 2,3,7,8-Tetrachlorodibenzo-*p*-dioxin (TCDD) promotes the transformation of C3H/10T1/2 cells. Carcinogenesis, *6*:651–653, 1985.

Aihara, H., Asaoka, Y., Yoshida, K., and Nishizuka, Y. Sustained activation of protein kinase C is essential to HL-60 cell differentiation to macrophage. Proc. Natl. Acad. Sci. U.S.A., *88*:11062–11066, 1991.

Anderson, G., and Jenkinson, E. J. Use of explant technology in the study of *in vitro* immune responses. J. Immunol. Methods, *216*:155–163, 1998.

Anderson, G. R., Stoler, D. L., and Scarcello, L. A. Normal fibroblasts responding to anoxia exhibit features of the malignant phenotype. J. Biol. Chem., *264*:14885–14892, 1989.

Antecol, M. H. Oncogenic potential in fibroblasts from individuals genetically predisposed to cancer. Mutat. Res., *199*:293–311, 1988.

Armato, U., Andreis, P. G., and Romano, F. The stimulation by the tumour promoters 12-O-tetradecanoylphorbol-13-acetate and phenobarbital of the growth of primary neonatal rat hepatocytes. Carcinogenesis, 6:811–821, 1985.

Asamoto, M., Oyamada, M., El Aoumari, A., Gros, D., and Yamasaki, H. Molecular mechanisms of TPA-mediated inhibition of gap-junctional intercellular communication: evidence for action on the assembly or function but not the expression of connexin 43 in rat liver epithelial cells. Mol. Carcinog., 4:322–327, 1991.

Asamoto, M., Takahashi, S., Imaida, K., Shirai, T., and Fukushima, S. Increased gap junctional intercellular communication capacity and connexin 43 and 26 expression in rat bladder carcinogenesis. Carcinogenesis, *15*:2163–2166, 1994.

Aye, M. T., and Dunne, J. V. Opposing effects of 12-O-tetradecanoylphorbol 13-acetate on human myeloid and lymphoid cell proliferation. J. Cell. Physiol., *114*:209–214, 1983.

Bacus, S. S., Kiguchi, K., Chin, D., King, C. R., and Huberman, E. Differentiation of cultured human breast cancer cells (AU-565 and MCF-7) associated with loss of cell surface *HER-2/neu* antigen. Mol. Carcinog., *3*:350–362, 1990.

Baker, T. K., Kwiatkowski, A. P., Madhukar, B. V., and Klaunig, J. E. Inhibition of gap junctional intercellular communication by 2,3,7,8-tetrachlorodibenzo-*p*-dioxin (TCDD) in rat hepatocytes. Carcinogenesis, *16*:2321–2326, 1995.

Barnes, D. Serum-free animal cell culture. Biotechniques, *5*:534–540, 1987.

Barrera, G., di Mauro, C., Muraca, R., Ferrero, D., Cavalli, G., Fazio, V. M., Paradisi, L., and Dianzani, M. U. Induction of differentiation in human HL-60 cells by 4-hydroxynonenal, a product of lipid peroxidation. Exp. Cell Res., *197*:148–152, 1991.

Barrett, J. C. A preneoplastic stage in the spontaneous neoplastic transformation of Syrian hamster embryo cells in culture. Cancer Res., *40*:91–94, 1980.

Barrett, J. C., and Ts'o, P. O. P. Relationship between somatic mutation and neoplastic transformation. Proc. Natl. Acad. Sci. U.S.A., *75*:3297–3301, 1978.

Barrett, J. C., McLachlan, J. A., and Elmore, E. Inability of diethylstilbestrol to induce 6-thioguanine-resistant mutants and to inhibit metabolic cooperation of V79 Chinese hamster cells. Mutat. Res., *107*:427–432, 1983.

Barsoum, J., and Varshavsky, A. Mitogenic hormones and tumor promoters greatly increase the incidence of colony-forming cells bearing amplified dihydrofolate reductase genes. Proc. Natl. Acad. Sci. U.S.A., *80*:5330–5334, 1983.

Beken, S., Tytgat, T., Pahernik, S., Koebe, H.-G., Vercruysse, A., and Rogiers, V. Cell morphology, albumin secretion and glutathione *S*-transferase expression in collagen gel sandwich and immobilization cultures of rat hepatocytes. Toxicol. in Vitro, *11*:409–416, 1997.

Bempong, M. A., and Myers, J. A. Phenotypic reversion of cultured mouse adenocarcinoma cells: mediation by cell density and chemical exposure. J. Am. Coll. Toxicol., *4*:79–90, 1985.

Benedict, W. F., Gielen, J. E., and Nebert, D. W. Polycyclic hydrocarbon-produced toxicity, transformation, and chromosomal aberrations as a function of aryl hydrocarbon hydroxylase activity in cell cultures. Int. J. Cancer, 9:435–451, 1972.

Benedict, W. F., Wheatley, W. L., and Jones, P. A. Inhibition of chemically induced morphological transformation and reversion of the transformed phenotype by ascorbic acid in C3H/10T½ cells. Cancer Res., *40*:2796–2801, 1980.

Berwald, Y., and Sachs, L. *In vitro* transformation of normal cells to tumor cells by carcinogenic hydrocarbons. J. Natl. Cancer Inst., *35*:641–661, 1963.

Bettger, W. J., Boyce, S. T., Walthall, B. J., and Ham, R. G. Rapid clonal growth and serial passage of human diploid fibroblasts in a lipid-enriched synthetic medium supplemented with epidermal growth factor, insulin, and dexamethasone. Proc. Natl. Acad. Sci. U.S.A., 78:5588–5592, 1981.

Birnboim, H. C. DNA strand breakage in human leukocytes exposed to a tumor promoter, phorbol myristate acetate. Science, 215:1247–1249, 1982.

Bjare, U. Serum-free cell culture. Pharmacol. Ther., 53:355–374, 1992.

Bonewald, L. F., Kester, M. B., Schwartz, Z., Swain, L. D., Khare, A., Johnson, T. L., Leach, R. J., and Boyan, B. D. Effects of combining transforming growth factor β and 1,25-dihydroxyvitamin D_3 on differentiation of a human osteosarcoma (MG-63). J. Biol. Chem., 267:8943–8949, 1992.

Boone, C. W. Malignant hemangioendotheliomas produced by subcutaneous inoculation of Balb/3T3 cells attached to glass beads. Science, 188:68–70, 1975.

Boone, C. W., and Jacobs, J. B. Sarcomas routinely produced from putatively nontumorigenic Balb/3T3 and C3H/10T1/2 cells by subcutaneous inoculation attached to plastic platelets. J. Supramol. Struct., 5:131–137, 1976.

Boone, C. W., Vembu, D., White, B. J., Takeichi, N., and Paranjpe, M. Karyotypic, antigen, and kidney-invasive properties of cell lines from fibrosarcomas arising in C3H/10T½ cells implanted subcutaneously attached to plastic plates. Cancer Res., 39:2172–2178, 1979.

Boreiko, C., and Heidelberger, C. Isolation of mutants temperature-sensitive for expression of the transformed state from chemically transformed C3H/10T1/2 cells. Carcinogenesis, 1:1059–1073, 1980.

Boreiko, C. J., Abernethy, D. J., Sanchez, J. H., and Dorman, B. H. Effect of mouse skin tumor promoters upon [^{3}H]uridine exchange and focus formation in cultures of C3H/10T1/2 mouse fibroblasts. Carcinogenesis, 7:1095–1099, 1986.

Borek, C. Malignant transformation in vitro: criteria, biological markers, and application in environmental screening of carcinogens. Radiat. Res., 79:209–232, 1979.

Borek, C. X-ray-induced in vitro neoplastic transformation of human diploid cells. Nature, 283:776–778, 1980.

Borek, C., and Sachs, L. The number of cell generations required to fix the transformed state in x-ray–induced transformation. Proc. Natl. Acad. Sci. U.S.A., 59:83–85, 1968.

Borek, C., Pain, C., and Mason, H. Neoplastic transformation of hamster embryo cells irradiated in utero and assayed in vitro. Nature, 266:452–454, 1977.

Borek, C., Guernsey, D. L., Ong, A., and Edelman, I. S. Critical role played by thyroid hormone in induction of neoplastic transformation by chemical carcinogens in tissue culture. Proc. Natl. Acad. Sci. U.S.A., 80:5749–5752, 1983.

Borek, C., Ong, A., and Muto, Y. Inhibition of radiogenic and chemically induced transformation in C3H10T-1/2 cells by a polyprenoic acid (E-5166). Jpn. J. Cancer Res., 77:5–8, 1986.

Borek, C., Ong, A., Morgan, W. F., and Cleaver, J. E. Morphological transformation of 10T1/2 mouse embryo cells can be initiated by DNA double-strand breaks alone. Mol. Carcinog., 4:243–247, 1991.

Borenfreund, E., Higgins, P. J., Steinglass, M., and Bendich, A. Properties and malignant transformation of established rat liver parenchymal cells in culture. J. Natl. Cancer Inst., 55:375–384, 1975.

Bouck, N., and diMayorca, G. Chemical carcinogens transform BHK cells by inducing a recessive mutation. Mol. Cell. Biol., 2:97–105, 1982.

Boyd, J. A., and Barrett, J. C. Genetic and cellular basis of multistep carcinogenesis. Pharmacol. Ther., 46:469–486, 1990.

Brissette, J. L., Kumar, N. M., Gilula, N. B., and Dotto, G. P. The tumor promoter 12-O-tetradecanoylphorbol-13-acetate and the ras oncogene modulate expression and phosphorylation of gap junction proteins. Mol. Cell. Biol., 11:5364–5371, 1991.

Brouty-Boyé, D., and Gresser, I. Reversibility of the transformed and neoplastic phenotype. I. Progressive reversion of the phenotype of x-ray-transformed C3H/10T1/2 cells under prolonged treatment with interferon. Int. J. Cancer, 28:165–173, 1981.

Brouty-Boyé, D., Tucker, R. W., and Folkman, J. Transformed and neoplastic phenotype: reversibility during culture by cell density and cell shape. Int. J. Cancer, 26:501–507, 1980.

Brown, J. D., Wilson, M. J., and Poirier, L. A. Neoplastic conversion of rat liver epithelial cells in culture by ethionine and S-adenosylethionine. Carcinogenesis, 4:173–177, 1983.

Brüstle, O., Jones, K. N., Learish, R. D., Karram, K., Choudhary, K., Wiestler, O. D., Duncan, I. D., and McKay, R. D. G. Embryonic stem cell-derived glial precursors: a source of myelinating transplants. Science, *285*:754–756, 1999.

Bruzzone, R., White, T. W., and Paul, D. L. Connections with connexins: the molecular basis of direct intercellular signaling. Eur. J. Biochem., *238*:1–27, 1996.

Caro, J. F., Jenquin, M., and Long, S. Effects of phorbol esters on insulin receptor function and insulin action in hepatocytes: evidence for heterogeneity. Mol. Cell. Biochem., *109*:115–118, 1992.

Celis, A., and Celis, J. E. General procedures for tissue culture. *In*: Cell Biology: A Laboratory Handbook, pp. 5–17. New York: Academic Press, 1994.

Chambard, M., Gabrion, J., and Mauchamp, J. Influence of collagen gel on the orientation of epithelial cell polarity: follicle formation from isolated thyroid cells and from preformed monolayers. J. Cell Biol., *91*:157–166, 1981.

Chan, G. L., and Little, J. B. Dissociated occurrence of single-gene mutation and oncogenic transformation in C3H 10T1/2 cells exposed to ultraviolet light and caffeine. J. Cell. Physiol., *111*:309–314, 1982.

Chatterjee, M., and Banerjee, M. R. Selenium mediated dose-inhibition of 7,12-dimethylbenz[*a*]anthracene-induced transformation of mammary cells in organ culture. Cancer Lett., *17*:187–195, 1982.

Chen, U., and Mok, H. Development of mouse embryonic stem (ES) cells: IV. Differentiation to mature T and B lymphocytes after implantation of embryoid bodies into nude mice. Dev. Immunol., *4*:79–84, 1995.

Chida, K., and Kuroki, T. Inhibition of DNA synthesis and sugar uptake and lack of induction of ornithine decarboxylase in human epidermal cells treated with mouse skin tumor promoters. Cancer Res., *44*:875–879, 1984.

Cho, H. Y., and Rhim, J. S. Cycloheximide-dependent reversion of human cells transformed by MSV and chemical carcinogen. Science, *205*:691–693, 1979.

Chouroulinkov, I., and Lasne, C. Two-stage (initiation-promotion) carcinogenesis *in vivo* and *in vitro*. Bull. Cancer, *65*:255–264, 1978.

Christman, J. K. DNA methylation in Friend erythroleukemia cells: the effects of chemically induced differentiation and of treatment with inhibitors of DNA methylation. Curr. Top. Microbiol. Immunol., *108*:49–76, 1984.

Colburn, N. H., Wendel, E., and Srinivas, L. Responses of preneoplastic epidermal cells to tumor promoters and growth factors: use of promoter-resistant variants for mechanism studies. J. Cell. Biochem., *18*:261–270, 1982.

Collins, S. J. The HL-60 promyelocytic leukemia cell line: proliferation, differentiation, and cellular oncogene expression. J. Am. Soc. Hematol., *70*:1233–1244, 1987.

Cooney, R. V., Pung, A., Harwood, P. J., Boynton, A. L., Zhang, L.-X., Hossain, M. Z., and Bertram, J. S. Inhibition of cellular transformation by triphenylmethane: a novel chemopreventive agent. Carcinogenesis, *13*:1107–1112, 1992.

Cowell, J. K., and Wigley, C. B. Chromosome changes associated with the progression of cell lines from preneoplastic to tumorigenic phenotype during transformation of mouse salivary gland epithelium in vitro. J. Natl. Cancer Inst., *69*:425–433, 1982.

Cram, L. S., Bartholdi, M. F., Ray, F. A., Travis, G. L., and Kraemer, P. M. Spontaneous neoplastic evolution of Chinese hamster cells in culture: multistep progression of karyotype. Cancer Res., *43*:4828–4837, 1983.

Croce, C. M., Aden, D., and Koprowski, H. Tumorigenicity of mouse-human diploid hybrids in nude mice. Science, *190*:1200–1202, 1975.

Decloitre, F., Lafarge-Frayssinet, C., Martin, M., and Frayssinet, C. Modifications of microfilaments and microtubules induced by two hepatic tumor promoters, phenobarbital and biliverdin in nontransformed and transformed hepatic cell lines. Cell Biol. Toxicol., *6*:23–34, 1990.

Dexter, D. L., Barbosa, J. A., and Calabresi, P. *N,N*-Dimethylformamide-induced alteration of cell culture characteristics and loss of tumorigenicity in cultured human colon carcinoma cells. Cancer Res., *39*:1020–1025, 1979.

Diamond, L., O'Brien, T. G., and Rovera, G. Tumor promoters: effects on proliferation and differentiation of cells in culture. Life Sci., *23*:1979–1988, 1978.

Dicker, P., and Rozengurt, E. Phorbol esters and vasopressin stimulate DNA synthesis by a common mechanism. Nature, *287*:607–612, 1980.

Dieterlen-Lièvre, F. Intraembryonic hematopoietic stem cells. Hematol./Oncol. Clin. North Am., *11*:1149–1170, 1997.

DiPaolo, J. A., Donovan, P. J., and Nelson, R. L. *In vitro* transformation of hamster cells by polycyclic hydrocarbons: factors influencing the number of cells transformed. Nature New Biol., *230*:240–243, 1971a.

DiPaolo, J. A., Donovan, P. J., and Nelson, R. L. Transformation of hamster cells *in vitro* by polycyclic hydrocarbons without cytotoxicity. Proc. Natl. Acad. Sci. U.S.A., *68*:2958–2961, 1971b.

DiPaolo, J. A., DeMarinis, A. J., Evans, C. H., and Doniger, J. Expression of initiated and promoted stages of irradiation carcinogenesis in vitro. Cancer Lett., *14*:243–249, 1981.

Dopp, E., Saedler, J., Stopper, H., Weiss, D. G., and Schiffmann, D. Mitotic disturbances and micronucleus induction in Syrian hamster embryo fibroblast cells caused by asbestos fibers. Environ. Health Perspect., *103*:268–271, 1995.

Doyle, L. A., Giangiulo, D., Hussain, A., Park, H.-J., Yen, R.-W. C., and Borges, M. Differentiation of human variant small cell lung cancer cell lines to a classic morphology by retinoic acid. Cancer Res., *49*:6745–6751, 1989.

Durkacz, B. W., Lunec, J., Grindley, H., Griffin, S., Horner, O., and Simm, A. Murine melanoma cell differentiation and melanogenesis induced by poly(ADP-ribose) polymerase inhibitors. Exp. Cell Res., *202*:287–291, 1992.

Earle, W. R., and Nettleship, A. Production of malignancy in vitro. V. Results of injections of cultures into mice. J. Natl. Cancer Inst., *4*:213–227, 1943.

Ellison, B. J., and Rubin, H. Individual transforming events in long-term cell culture of NIH 3T3 products of epigenetic induction. Cancer Res., *52*:667–673, 1992.

Elmore, E., Kakunaga, T., and Barrett, J. C. Comparison of spontaneous mutation rates of normal and chemically transformed human skin fibroblasts. Cancer Res., *43*:1650–1655, 1983.

Elson, A., and Leder, P. Identification of a cytoplasmic, phorbol ester-inducible isoform of protein tyrosine phosphatase e. Proc. Natl. Acad. Sci. U.S.A., *92*:12235–12239, 1995.

Embleton, M. J., and Noy, R. J. Inhibition of chemically induced neoplastic transformation in vitro by saturated fatty acids. Pathobiology, *59*:69–75, 1991.

Endo, S., Nettesheim, P., Oshimura, M., and Walker, C. Nonrandom chromosome alterations that correlate with progression to immortality in rat tracheal epithelial cells transformed with *N*-methyl-*N'*-nitro-*N*-nitrosoguanidine. Cancer Res., *50*:740–747, 1990.

Ephrussi, B. Hybridization of somatic cells and phenotypic expression. Nineteenth Annual Symposium on Fundamental Cancer Research, 1965.

Evans, C. H., and Boynton, A. L. Calcium dependence of chemical carcinogen induced morphological transformation of Syrian hamster embryo cells. Cancer Lett., *15*:271–279, 1982.

Evans, V. J., Price, F. M., Sanford, K. K., Kerr, H. A., and Handleman, S. L. Comparative effects of mare, stallion, gelding horse, and fetal bovine sera on neoplastic transformation *in vitro*. J. Natl. Cancer Inst., *49*:505–511, 1972.

Fibach, E., Gambari, R., Shaw, P. A., Maniatis, G., Reuben, R. C., Sassa, S., Rifkind, R. A., and Marks, P. A. Tumor promoter-mediated inhibition of cell differentiation: suppression of the expression of erythroid functions in murine erythroleukemia cells. Proc. Natl. Acad. Sci. U.S.A., *76*:1906–1910, 1979.

Flodström, S., Hemming, H., Wärngård, L., and Ahlborg, U. G. Promotion of altered hepatic foci development in rat liver, cytochrome P450 enzyme induction and inhibition of cell-cell communication by DDT and some structurally related organohalogen pesticides. Carcinogenesis, *11*:1413–1417, 1990.

Freed, L. E., and Vunjak-Novakovic, G. Culture of organized cell communities. Adv. Drug Delivery Rev., *33*:15–30, 1998.

Freedman, V. H., and Shin, S. Cellular tumorigenicity in *nude* mice: correlation with cell growth in semisolid medium. Cell, *3*:355–359, 1974.

Friedman, E., Gillin, S., and Lipkin, M. 12-*O*-tetradecanoylphorbol-13-acetate stimulation of DNA synthesis in cultured preneoplastic familial polyposis colonic epithelial cells but not in normal colonic epithelial cells. Cancer Res., *44*:4078–4086, 1984.

Friedman, S. J., and Skehan, P. Morphological differentiation of human choriocarcinoma cells induced by methotrexate. Cancer Res., *39*:1960–1967, 1979.

Fusenig, N. E., Breitkreutz, D., Dzarlieva, R. T., Boukamp, P., Herzmann, E., Bohnert, A., Pöhlman, J., Rausch, C., Schütz, S., and Hornung, J. Epidermal cell differentiation and malignant transformation in culture. Cancer Forum, *6*:209–240, 1982.

Fusenig, N. E., and Boukamp, P. Multiple stages and genetic alterations in immortalization, malignant transformation, and tumor progression of human skin keratinocytes. Mol. Carcinog., *23*:144–158, 1998.

Geiser, A. G., Der, C. J., Marshall, C. J., and Stanbridge, E. J. Suppression of tumorigenicity with continued expression of the c-Ha-*ras* oncogene in EJ bladder carcinoma-human fibroblast hybrid cells. Proc. Natl. Acad. Sci. U.S.A., *83*:5209–5213, 1986.

Gerharz, C. D., Gabbert, H. E., Engers, R., Ramp, U., Mayer, H., Biesalski, H. K., and Luley, C. Heterogeneous response to differentiation induction in different clonal subpopulations of a rat rhabdomyosarcoma cell line (BA-HAN-1). Cancer Res., *49*:7132–7140, 1989.

González-Espinosa, C., and García-Sáinz, J. A. Protein kinases and phosphatases modulate *c-fos* expression in rat hepatocytes. Effects of angiotensin II and phorbol myristate acetate. Life Sci., *56*:723–728, 1995.

Goodman, S. A., Esau, B., and Koontz, J. W. Insulin and phorbol myristic acetate induce ornithine decarboxylase in Reuber H35 rat hepatoma cells by different mechanisms. Arch. Biochem. Biophys., *266*:343–350, 1988.

Grafström, R. C. Carcinogenesis studies in human epithelial tissues and cells in vitro: emphasis on serumfree culture conditions and transformation studies. Acta Physiol. Scand., *140*:93–133, 1990.

Greiner, J. W., and Evans, C. H. Temporal dynamics of cortisol and dexamethasone prevention of benzo(*a*)pyrene-induced morphological transformation of Syrian hamster cells. Cancer Res., *42*:4014–4017, 1982.

Grisham, J. W., Greenberg, D. S., Smith, G. J., and Kaufman, D. G. Temporary culture in isoleucine-free medium enhances transformation of 10T½ cells by N-methyl-N′-nitro-N-nitrosoguanidine (MNNG). Biochem. Biophys. Res. Comm., *87*:969–975, 1979.

Grisham, J. W., Greenberg, D. S., Kaufman, D. G., and Smith, G. J. Cycle-related toxicity and transformation in 10T1/2 cells treated with *N*-methyl-*N*′-nitro-*N*-nitrosoguanidine. Proc. Natl. Acad. Sci. U.S.A., *77*:4813–4817, 1980.

Gruenert, D. C., Finkbeiner, W. E., and Widdicombe, J. H. Culture and transformation of human airway epithelial cells. Am. J. Physiol., *268*:L347–L360, 1995.

Guguen-Guillouzo, C., Clement, B., Baffet, G., Beaumont, C., Morel-Chany, E., Glaise, D., and Guillouzo, A. Maintenance and reversibility of active albumin secretion by adult rat hepatocytes co-cultured with another liver epithelial cell type. Exp. Cell Res., *143*:47–54, 1983.

Guillouzo, A. Use of isolated and cultured hepatocytes for xenobiotic metabolism and cytotoxicity studies. *In*: A. Guillouzo and C. Guguen-Guillouzo (Eds.), Research in Isolated and Culture Hepatocytes, pp. 313–332. London: John Libbey Eurotext, 1986.

Guillouzo, A., Guguen-Guillouzo, C., Boisnard, M., Bourel, M., and Benhamou, J.-P. Smooth endoplasmic reticulum proliferation and increased cell multiplication in cultured hepatocytes of the newborn rat in the presence of phenobarbital. Exp. Mol. Pathol., *28*:1–9, 1978.

Haber, D. A., and Thilly, W. G. Morphological transformation of C3H/10T1/2 cells subcultured at low cell densities. Life Sci., *2*:1663–1674, 1978.

Hahn, W. C., Counter, C. M., Lundberg, A. S., Beijersbergen, R. L., Brooks, M. W., and Weinberg, R. A. Creation of human tumour cells with defined genetic elements. Nature, *400*:464–468, 1999.

Hall, E. J., and Hei, T. K. Oncogenic transformation of cells in culture: pragmatic comparisons of oncogenicity, cellular and molecular mechanisms. Int. J. Radiat. Oncol. Biol. Phys., *12*:1909–1921, 1986.

Hamel, E., Katoh, F., Mueller, G., Birchmeier, W., and Yamasaki, H. Transforming growth factor β as a potent promoter in two-stage BALB/c 3T3 cell transformation. Cancer Res., *48*:2832–2836, 1988.

Han, A., and Elkind, M. M. Enhanced transformation of mouse 10T1/2 cells by 12-O-tetradecanoylphor-bol-13-acetate following exposure to x-rays or to fission-spectrum neutrons. Cancer Res., *42*:477–483, 1982.

Han, Z. T., Tong, Y. K., He, L. M., Zhang, Y., Sun, J. Z., Wang, T. Y., Zhang, H., Cui, Y. L., Newmark, H. L., Conney, A. H., and Chang, R. L. 12-O-Tetradecanoylphorbol-13-acetate (TPA)-induced increase in depressed white blood cell counts in patients treated with cytotoxic cancer chemotherapeutic drugs. Proc. Natl. Acad. Sci. U.S.A., *95*:5362–5365, 1998.

Hard, G. C., King, H., Borland, R., Stewart, B. W., and Dobrostanski, B. Length of in vivo exposure to a carcinogenic dose of dimethylnitrosamine necessary for subsequent expression of morphological transformation by rat kidney cells in vitro. Oncology, *34*:16–19, 1977.

Harris, H. Cell fusion and the analysis of malignancy. J. Natl. Cancer Inst., *48*:851–864, 1972.

Harris, H., and Bramwell, M. E. The suppression of malignancy by terminal differentiation: evidence from hybrids between tumour cells and keratinocytes. J. Cell Sci., *87*:383–388, 1987.

Hashimoto, Y., and Kitagawa, H. S. *In vitro* neoplastic transformation of epithelial cells of rat urinary bladder by nitrosamines. Nature, *252*:497–499, 1974.

Hasler, C. M., Bennink, M. R., and Trosko, J. E. Inhibition of gap junction-mediated intercellular communication by α-linolenate. Am. J. Physiol., *261*:C161–C168, 1991.

Hayashi, N., Hasegawa, K., Komine, A., Tanaka, Y., McLachlan, J. A., Barrett, J. C., and Tsutsui, T. Estrogen-induced cell transformation and DNA adduct formation in cultured Syrian hamster embryo cells. Mol. Carcinog., *16*:149–156, 1996.

Hayflick, L. The cellular basis for biological aging. *In*: Finch, C. E. and Hayflick, L. (Eds.), Handbook of the biology of aging, pp. 159–186. New York: Van Nostrand Reinhold, 1977.

Hayflick, L. Mortality and immortality at the cellular level. A review. Biochemistry, *62*:1180–1190, 1997.

Heidelberger, C. Chemical oncogenesis in culture. Adv. Cancer Res., *18*:317–366, 1973.

Hellman, K. B., and Hellman, A. Induction of type-C retrovirus by the tumor promoter TPA. Int. J. Cancer, *27*:95–99, 1981.

Himmelfarb, P., Thayer, P. S., and Martin, H. E. Spin filter culture: the propagation of mammalian cells in suspension. Science, *164*:555–557, 1969.

Hitotsumachi, S., Rabinowitz, Z., and Sachs, L. Chromosomal control of chemical carcinogenesis. Int. J. Cancer, *9*:305–315, 1972.

Hojo, M., Morimoto, T., Maluccio, M., Asano, T., Morimoto, K., Lagman, M., Shimbo, T., and Suthanthiran, M. Cyclosporine induces cancer progression by a cell-autonomous mechanism. Nature, *397*:530–534, 1999.

Hollands, P. Comparative stem cell biology. Int. J. Dev. Biol., *41*:245–254, 1997.

Holliday, R. Neoplastic transformation: the contrasting stability of human and mouse cells. Cancer Surv., *28*:103–115, 1996.

Honma, M., Mizusawa, H., Sasaki, K., Hayashi, M., Ohno, T., Tanaka, N., and Sofuni, T. Demonstration by DNA fingerprint analysis of genomic instability in mouse BALB 3T3 cells during cell transformation. Mutat. Res., *304*:167–179, 1994.

Howell, A. N., and Sager, R. Tumorigenicity and its suppression in cybrids of mouse and Chinese hamster cell lines. Proc. Natl. Acad. Sci. U.S.A., *75*:2358–2362, 1978.

Hozumi, M. Fundamentals of chemotherapy of myeloid leukemia by induction of leukemia cell differentiation. Adv. Cancer Res., *38*:121–169, 1983.

Hsu, S.-M., Zhao, X., Hsu, P.-L., and Lok, M. S. Extracellular matrix does not induce the proliferation, but promotes the differentiation, of Hodgkin's cell line HDLM-1. Am. J. Pathol., *127*:9–14, 1987.

Huband, J. C., Abernethy, D. J., and Boreiko, C. J. Potential role of treatment artifact in the effect of cell density upon frequencies of C3H/10T1/2 cell transformation. Cancer Res., *45*:6314–6321, 1985.

Huberman, E., and Sachs, L. Mutability of different genetic loci in mammalian cells by metabolically activated carcinogenic polycyclic hydrocarbons. Proc. Natl. Acad. Sci. U.S.A., *73*:188–192, 1976.

Ishii, D. N., Fibach, E., Yamasaki, H., and Weinstein, I. B. Tumor promoters inhibit morphological differentiation in cultured mouse neuroblastoma cells. Science, *200*:556–559, 1978.

Israel, B. A., and Schaeffer, W. I. Cytoplasmic mediation of malignancy. In Vitro Cell. Dev. Biol., *24*:487–490, 1988.

Iyer, A. P., and Banerjee, M. R. Sequential expression of preneoplastic and neoplastic characteristics of mouse mammary epithelial cells transformed in organ culture. J. Natl. Cancer Inst., 66:893–905, 1981.

Jackson, E. M. Review: A genealogy of tissue culture. J. Toxicol. Toxin Rev., 10:209–219, 1991.

Jansen, L. A. M., Mesnil, M., and Jongen, W. M. F. Inhibition of gap junctional intercellular communication and delocalization of the cell adhesion molecule E-cadherin by tumor promoters. Carcinogenesis, 17:1527–1531, 1996.

Johnson, G. S., Friedman, R. M., and Pastan, I. Restoration of several morphological characteristics of normal fibroblasts in sarcoma cells treated with adenosine-3′:5′-cyclic monophosphate and its derivatives. Proc. Natl. Acad. Sci. U.S.A., 68:425–429, 1971.

Jonasson, J., Povey, S., and Harris, H. The analysis of malignancy by cell fusion. VII. Cytogenetic analysis of hybrids between malignant and diploid cells and of tumours derived from them. J. Cell Sci., 24:217–254, 1977.

Jones, C. A., Callaham, M. F., and Huberman, E. Sodium fluoride promotes morphological transformation of Syrian hamster embryo cells. Carcinogenesis, 9:2279–2284, 1988.

Jones, P. A., Benedict, W. F., Baker, M. S., Mondal, S., Rapp, U., and Heidelberger, C. Oncogenic transformation of C3H/10T1/2 clone 8 mouse embryo cells by halogenated pyrimidine nucleosides. Cancer Res., 36:101–107, 1976.

Jones, P. A., Baker, M. S., Bertram, J. S., and Benedict, W. F. Cell cycle-specific oncogenic transformation of C3H/10T1/2 clone 8 mouse embryo cells by 1-β-D-arabinofuranosylcytosine. Cancer Res., 37:2214–2217, 1977.

Jones, P. H. Epithelial stem cells. Bioessays, 19:683–690, 1997.

Kaden, D., Gadi, I. K., Bardwell, L., Gelman, R., and Sager, R. Spontaneous mutation rates of tumorigenic and nontumorigenic Chinese hamster embryo fibroblast cell lines. Cancer Res., 49:3374–3379, 1989.

Kakunaga, T. The role of cell division in the malignant transformation of mouse cells treated with 3-methylcholanthrene. Cancer Res., 35:1637–1642, 1975.

Kam, E., and Pitts, J. D. Effects of the tumour promoter 12-O-tetradecanoylphorbol-13-acetate on junctional communication in intact mouse skin: persistence of homologous communication and increase of epidermal-dermal coupling. Carcinogenesis, 9:1389–1394, 1988.

Kanemitsu, M. Y., and Lau, A. F. Epidermal growth factor stimulates the disruption of gap junctional communication and connexin43 phosphorylation independent of 12-O-tetradecanoylphorbol 13-acetate-sensitive protein kinase C: the possible involvement of mitogen-activated protein kinase. Mol. Biol. Cell, 4:837–848, 1993.

Kaplan, P. L., and Ozanne, B. Cellular responsiveness to growth factors correlates with a cell's ability to express the transformed phenotypes. Cell, 33:931, 1983.

Katoh, F., Fitzgerald, D. J., Giroldi, L., Fujiki, H., Sugimura, T., and Yamasaki, H. Okadaic acid and phorbol esters: comparative effects of these tumor promoters on cell transformation, intercellular communication and differentiation in vitro. Jpn. J. Cancer Res., 81:590–597, 1990.

Katsuta, H., and Takaoka, T. Parameters for malignant transformation of mammalian cells treated with chemical carcinogens in tissue culture. In: W. Nakahara, S. Takayama, T. Sugimura, and S. Odashima (Eds.), Topics in Chemical Carcinogenesis, p. 389. Toyko: University of Tokyo Press, 1973.

Kaufmann, W. K., Ririe, D. G., and Kaufman, D. G. Phenobarbital-dependent proliferation of putative initiated rat hepatocytes. Carcinogenesis, 9:779–782, 1988.

Kayano, T., Nomura, K., Hino, O., and Kitagawa, T. Failure of phorbol ester TPA to promote growth of in vivo–initiated rat hepatocytes transferred into a culture system. Gann, 73:354–357, 1982.

Kennedy, A. R. The conditions for the modification of radiation transformation in vitro by a tumor promoter and protease inhibitors. Carcinogenesis, 6:1441–1446, 1985.

Kennedy, A. R., and Weichselbaum, R. R. Effects of dexamethasone and cortisone with X-ray irradiation on transformation of C3H 10T½ cells. Nature, 294:97–98, 1981.

Kerckaert, G. A., LeBoeuf, R. A., and Isfort, R. J. pH Effects on the lifespan and transformation frequency of Syrian hamster embryo (SHE) cells. Carcinogenesis, 17:1819–1824, 1996.

Kern, A., Bader, A., Pichlmayr, R., and Sewing, K.-F. Drug metabolism in hepatocyte sandwich cultures of rats and humans. Biochem. Pharmacol., *54*:761–772, 1997.

Kiguchi, K., Collart, F. R., Henning-Chubb, C., and Huberman, E. Induction of cell differentiation in melanoma cells by inhibitors of IMP dehydrogenase: altered patterns of IMP dehydrogenase expression and activity. Cell Growth Differ., *1*:259–270, 1990.

Kilkenny, A. E., Morgan, D., Spangler, E. F., and Yuspa, S. H. Correlation of initiating potency of skin carcinogens with potency to induce resistance to terminal differentiation in cultured mouse keratinocytes. Cancer Res., *45*:2219–2225, 1985.

Klaunig, J. E., Ruch, R. J., and Lin, E. L. C. Effects of trichloroethylene and its metabolites on rodent hepatocyte intercellular communication. Toxicol. Appl. Pharmacol., *99*:454–465, 1989.

Kleinman, H. K., Klebe, R. J., and Martin, G. R. Role of collagenous matrices in the adhesion and growth of cells. J. Cell Biol., *88*:473–485, 1981.

Köhler, G., and Milstein, C. Deviation of specific antibody-producing tissue culture and tumor lines by cell fusion. Eur. J. Immunol., *6*:511, 1976.

Koi, M., and Barrett, J. C. Loss of tumor-suppressive function during chemically induced neoplastic progression of Syrian hamster embryo cells. Proc. Natl. Acad. Sci. U.S.A., *83*:5992–5996, 1986.

Kokunai, T., Korosue, K., Tamaki, N., and Matsumoto, S. Promoting effect of 12-*O*-tetradecanoylphorbol-13-acetate on the *in vitro* malignant transformation of fetal rat brain cells exposed *in utero* to ethylnitrosourea. Cancer Res., *46*:1377–1381, 1986.

Komori, A., Yatsunami, J., Suganuma, M., Okabe, S., Abe, S., Sakai, A., Sasaki, K., and Fujiki, H. Tumor necrosis factor acts as a tumor promoter in BALB/3T3 cell transformation. Cancer Res., *53*:1982–1985, 1993.

Kopelovich, L. The use of a tumor promoter as a single parameter approach for the detection of individuals genetically predisposed to colorectal cancer. Cancer Lett., *12*:67–74, 1981.

Kopelovich, L., and Chou, T.-C. The proliferative response of low-density human cell cultures to tumor promoters and its relevance to carcinogenic mechanisms *in vitro*. Int. J. Cancer, *34*:781–788, 1984.

Korff, T., and Augustin, H. G. Integration of endothelial cells in multicellular spheroids prevents apoptosis and induces differentiation. J. Cell Biol., *143*:1341–1352, 1998.

Kraemer, P. M., Deaven, L. L., Crissman, H. A., and Van Dilla, M. A. DNA constancy despite variability in chromosome number. Adv. Cell Mol. Biol., *2*:47–106, 1972.

Krystosek, A., and Puck, T. T. The spatial distribution of exposed nuclear DNA in normal, cancer, and reverse-transformed cells. Proc. Natl. Acad. Sci. U.S.A., *87*:6560–6564, 1990.

Kumar, N. M., and Gilula, N. B. The gap junction communication channel. Cell, *84*:381–388, 1996.

Kuroki, T., and Huh, N.-h. Why are human cells resistant to malignant cell transformation *in vitro*? Jpn. J. Cancer Res., *84*:1091–1100, 1993.

Laerum, O. D., and Rajewsky, M. F. Neoplastic transformation of fetal rat brain cells in culture after exposure to ethylnitrosourea in vivo. J. Natl. Cancer Inst., *55*:1177–1187, 1975.

Landolph, J. R., and Heidelberger, C. Chemical carcinogens produce mutations to ouabain resistance in transformable C3H/10T1/2 Cl 8 mouse fibroblasts. Proc. Natl. Acad. Sci. U.S.A., *76*:930–934, 1979.

Lasne, C., Lu, Y.-P., Orfila, L., Ventura, L., and Chouroulinkov, I. Study of various transforming effects of the anabolic agents trenbolone and testosterone on Syrian hamster embryo cells. Carcinogenesis, *11*:541–547, 1990.

Lasnitzki, I. Growth pattern of the mouse prostate gland in organ culture and its response to sex hormones, vitamin A, and 3-methylcholanthrane. Natl. Cancer Inst. Monogr., *12*:381–403, 1963.

Lasnitzki, I. Reversal of methylcholanthrene-induced changes in mouse prostates *in vitro* by retinoic acids and its analogues. Br. J. Cancer, *34*:239–248, 1976.

Lau, A. F., Kanemitsu, M. Y., Kurata, W. E., Danesh, S., and Boynton, A. L. Epidermal growth factor disrupts gap-junctional communication and induces phosphorylation of connexin43 on serine. Mol. Biol. Cell, *3*:865–874, 1992.

Laws, J. O., and Flaks, A. Pulmonary adenomata induced by carcinogen treatment in organ culture. Br. J. Cancer, *20*:550–554, 1966.

Leeb-Lundberg, L. M. F., Cotecchia, S., Lomasney, J. W., DeBernardis, J. F., Lefkowitz, R. J., and Caron, M. G. Phorbol esters promote α_1-adrenergic receptor phosphorylation and receptor uncoupling from inositol phospholipid metabolism. Proc. Natl. Acad. Sci. U.S.A., *82*:5651–5655, 1985.

Lerman, M. I., Hegamyer, G. A., and Colburn, N. H. Cloning and characterization of putative genes that specify sensitivity to neoplastic transformation by tumor promoters. Int. J. Cancer, *37*:293–302, 1986.

Lerman, M. I., Sakai, A., Kai-Tai, Y., and Colburn, N. H. DNA sequences in human nasopharyngeal carcinoma cells that specify susceptibility to tumor promoter-induced neoplastic transformation. Carcinogenesis, *8*:121–127, 1987.

Levine, L. Tumour promoters and prostaglandin production. *In*: Nigam et al. (eds.), Eicosanoids, Lipid Peroxidation and Cancer, pp. 11–20. Heidelberg: Springer-Verlag Berlin, 1988.

Li, D., Noyes, I., Shuler, C., and Milo, G. E. Cloning and sequencing of *CATR1.3*, a human gene associated with tumorigenic conversion. Proc. Natl. Acad. Sci. U.S.A., *92*:6409–6413, 1995.

Li, R., Yerganian, G., Duesberg, P., Kraemer, A., Willer, A., Rausch, C., and Hehlmann, R. Aneuploidy correlated 100% with chemical transformation of Chinese hamster cells. Proc. Natl. Acad. Sci. U.S.A., *94*:14506–14511, 1997.

Lijian, Y., Nishino, H., and Iwashima, A. Stimulation of choline transport in cultured cells induced by 12-O-tetradecanoylphorbol-13-acetate: one of the earliest phenomena induced by the tumor promoter. Oncology, *45*:326–330, 1988.

Lillehaug, J. R., and Djurhuus, R. Effect of diethylstilbestrol on the transformable mouse embryo fibroblast C3H/10T1/2C18 cells. Tumor promotion, cell growth, DNA synthesis, and ornithine decarboxylase. Carcinogenesis, *3*:797–799, 1982.

Lin, J.-C., Smith, M. C., and Pagano, J. S. Activation of latent Epstein-Barr virus genomes: selective stimulation of synthesis of chromosomal proteins by a tumor promoter. J. Virol., *45*:985–991, 1983.

Lin, K. H., Maeda, S., Inagaki, H., and Saito, T. Long-term culture of primary rat hepatocytes on heparin- or lambda carrageenan-containing collagen gels. Biosci. Biotechnol. Biochem., *61*:971–974, 1997.

Lincoln, D. W. II, Kampcik, S. J., and Gierthy, J. F. 2,3,7,8-Tetrachlorodibenzo-*p*-dioxin (TCDD) does not inhibit intercellular communication in Chinese hamster V79 cells. Carcinogenesis, *8*:1817–1820, 1987.

Linge, C. Establishment and maintenance of normal human keratinocyte cultures. *In*: G. E. Jones (ed.), Methods in Molecular Medicine: Human Cell Culture Protocols, pp. 1–8. Totowa, NJ: Human Press, 1996.

Lotem, J., and Sachs, L. Regulation of normal differentiation in mouse and human myeloid leukemic cells by phorbol esters and the mechanism of tumor promotion. Proc. Natl. Acad. Sci. U.S.A., *76*:5158–5162, 1979.

Lyman, G. H., Papahadjopoulos, D., and Preisler, H. D. Phospholipid membrane stabilization by dimethylsulfoxide and other inducers of Friend leukemic cell differentiation. Biochim. Biophys. Acta, *448*:460–473, 1976.

Macieira-Coelho, A. Contributions made by the studies of cells in vitro for understanding of the mechanisms of aging. Exp. Gerontol., *28*:1–16, 1993.

Mamaeva, S. E. Karyotypic evolution of cells in culture: a new concept. Int. Rev. Cytol., *178*:1–40, 1998.

Manjeshwar, S., Rao, P. M., Rajalakshmi, S., and Sarma, D. S. R. Inhibition of DNA synthesis by phenobarbital in primary cultures of hepatocytes from normal rat liver and from hepatic nodules. Carcinogenesis, *13*:2287–2291, 1992.

Martin, S. J., Bradley, J. G., and Cotter, T. G. HL-60 cells induced to differentiate towards neutrophils subsequently die via apoptosis. Clin. Exp. Immunol., *79*:448–453, 1990.

Martinez-Valdez, H., and Cohen, A. Coordinate regulation of mRNAs encoding adenosine deaminase, purine nucleoside phosphorylase, and terminal deoxynucleotidyltransferase by phorbol esters in human thymocytes. Proc. Natl. Acad. Sci. U.S.A., *85*:6900–6903, 1988.

Matesic, D. F., Rupp, H. L., Bonney, W. J., Ruch, R. J., and Trosko, J. E. Changes in gap-junction permeability, phosphorylation, and number mediated by phorbol ester and non-phorbol-ester tumor promoters in rat liver epithelial cells. Mol. Carcinog., *10*:226–236, 1994.

McCormick, J. J., and Maher, V. M. Towards an understanding of the malignant transformation of diploid human fibroblasts. Mutat. Res., *199*:273–291, 1988.

McCormick, P. J., and Bertram, J. S. Differential cell cycle phase specificity for neoplastic transformation and mutation to ouabain resistance induced by *N*-methyl-*N'*-nitro-*N*-nitrosoguanidine in synchronized C3H10T1/2 CL8 cells. Proc. Natl. Acad. Sci. U.S.A., *79*:4342–4346, 1982.

Mehta, R. G., and Moon, R. C. Effects of 12-*O*-tetradecanoylphorbol-13-acetate on carcinogen-induced mouse mammary lesions in organ culture. Cancer Res., *46*:5832–5835, 1986.

Meyer, S. A., Gibbs, T. A., and Jirtle, R. L. Independent mechanisms for tumor promoters phenobarbital and 12-*O*-tetradecanoylphorbol-13-acetate in reduction of epidermal growth factor binding by rat hepatocytes. Cancer Res., *49*:5907–5912, 1989.

Michalopoulos, G., and Pitot, H. C. Primary culture of parenchymal liver cells on collagen membranes. Exp. Cell Res., *94*:70–78, 1975.

Miller, D. R., Istone, L., Burkart, W., Young, W., Blight, A. R., and Burns, F. J. Failure of the tumor promoter 12-*O*-tetradecanoylphorbol-13-acetate (TPA) to inhibit cell-cell coupling in newborn mouse epidermal cells and Chinese hamster V79 cells under non-standard culture conditions. Carcinogenesis, *8*:847–850, 1987.

Milo, G. E., Li, D., Casto, B. C., Theil, K., Shuler, C., Noyes, I., and Chen, J. Malignant conversion of chemically transformed normal human cells. Proc. Natl. Acad. Sci. U.S.A., *93*:5229–5234, 1996.

Minuth, W. W., Kloth, S., Aigner, J., Sittinger, M., and Rockl, W. Approach to an organo-typical environment for cultured cells and tissues. Biotechniques, *20*:498–501, 1996.

Mironescu, S., and Love, R. DNA synthesis and transformation induced in density-inhibited cultures of hamster embryo cells by the carcinogen benzo(*a*)pyrene. Cancer Res., *34*:2562–2570, 1974.

Miyamato, S., Guzman, R. C., Osborn, R. C., and Nandi, S. Neoplastic transformation of mouse mammary epithelial cells by *in vitro* exposure to *N*-methyl-*N*-nitrosourea. Proc. Natl. Acad. Sci. U.S.A., *85*:477–481, 1988.

Miyazaki, M., Bai, L., and Sato, J. Influence of liver tumor promoters and structurally related chemicals on survival of normal adult rat hepatocytes in primary culture. J. Cancer Res. Clin. Oncol., *116*:259–263, 1990.

Miyazaki, M., Mars, W. M., Runge, D., Kim, T. H., Bowen, W. C., and Michalopoulos, G. K. Phenobarbital suppresses growth and accelerates restoration of differentiation markers of primary culture rat hepatocytes in the chemically defined hepatocyte growth medium containing hepatocyte growth factor and epidermal growth factor. Exp. Cell Res., *241*:445–457, 1998.

Mondal, S., and Heidelberger, C. Transformation of C3H/10T1/2 CL8 mouse embryo fibroblasts by ultraviolet irradiation and a phorbol ester. Nature, *260*:710–711, 1976.

Montesano, R., Bannikov, G., Drevon, C., Kuroki, T., Saint Vincent, L., and Tomatis, L. Neoplastic transformation of rat liver epithelial cells in culture. Ann. N.Y. Acad. Sci., *349*:323–331, 1980.

Montesano, R., Mouron, P., Amherdt, M., and Orci, L. Collagen matrix promotes reorganization of pancreatic endocrine cell monolayers into islet-like organoids. J. Cell Biol., *97*:935–939, 1983.

Morel-Chany, E., Lafarge-Frayssinet, C., and Trincal, G. Progression of spontaneous malignant transformation of epithelial rat liver cell lines. Cell Biol. Toxicol., *1*:11–22, 1985.

Morrison, S. J., Shah, N. M., and Anderson, D. J. Regulatory mechanisms in stem cell biology. Cell, *88*:287–298, 1997.

Mosser, D. D., and Bols, N. C. Effect of saccharin on metabolic cooperation between human fibroblasts. Carcinogenesis, *4*:991–995, 1983.

Murray, A. W., and Fitzgerald, D. J. Tumor promoters inhibit metabolic cooperation in coculture of epidermal and 3T3 cells. Biochem. Biophys. Res. Commun., *91*:395–401, 1979.

Nakaya, K., Chou, S., Kaneko, M., and Nakamura, Y. Topoisomerase inhibitors have potent differentiation-inducing activity for human and mouse myeloid leukemia cells. Jpn. J. Cancer Res., *82*:184–191, 1991.

Nakano, S., and Ts'o, P. O. P. Cellular differentiation and neoplasia: characterization of subpopulations of cells that have neoplasia-related growth properties in Syrian hamster embryo cell cultures. Proc. Natl. Acad. Sci. U.S.A., *78*:4995–4999, 1981.

Namieno, T., Koito, K., Sato, N., Uchino, J., and Hosokawa, M. Co-cultured endothelial and Kupffer cells regulate hepatocyte replication. Int. J. Oncol., *9*:737–740, 1996.

Nardone, R. M. Cell culture methodology from donor to cell lines. Biotechniques, *5*:122–127, 1987.

Nettesheim, P., Klein-Szanto, A. J. P., Marchok, A. C., Steele, V. E., Terzaghi, M., and Topping, D. C. Studies of neoplastic development in respiratory tract epithelium. Arch. Pathol. Lab. Med., *105*:1–10, 1981.

Neveu, M. J., Hully, J. R., Paul, D. L., and Pitot, H. C. Reversible alteration in the expression of the gap junctional protein connexin 32 during tumor promotion in rat liver and its role during cell proliferation. Cancer Commun., *2*:21–31, 1990.

Noda, K., Umeda, M., and Ono, T. Effects of various chemicals including bile acids and chemical carcinogens on the inhibition of metabolic cooperation. Gann, *72*:772–776, 1981.

Oberleithner, H., Westphale, H.-J., and Gaßner, B. Alkaline stress transforms Madin-Darby canine kidney cells. Pflügers Arch, *419*:418–420, 1991.

O'Brien, R. M., Bonovich, M. T., Forest, C. D., and Granner, D. K. Signal transduction convergence: phorbol esters and insulin inhibit phospho*enol*pyruvate carboxykinase gene transcription through the same 10-base-pair sequence. Proc. Natl. Acad. Sci. U.S.A., *88*:6580–6584, 1991.

Oesch, F., Schäfer, A., and Wieser, R. J. 12-*O*-Tetradecanoylphorbol-13-acetate releases human diploid fibroblasts from contact-dependent inhibition of growth. Carcinogenesis, *9*:1319–1322, 1988.

Okada, F., Hosokawa, M., Hamada, J.-I., Hasegawa, J., Kato, M., Mizutani, M., Ren, J., Takeichi, N., and Kobayashi, H. Malignant progression of a mouse fibrosarcoma by host cells reactive to a foreign body (gelatin sponge). Br. J. Cancer, *66*:635–639, 1992.

Olsson, I., Bergh, G., Ehinger, M., and Gullberg, U. Cell differentiation in acute myeloid leukemia. Eur. J. Haematol., *57*:1–16, 1996.

O'Shea, K. S. Embryonic stem cell models of development. Anat. Rec. (New Anat.), *257*:32–41, 1999.

Oshimura, M., Hesterberg, T. W., Tsutsui, T., and Barrett, J. C. Correlation of asbestos-induced cytogenetic effects with cell transformation of Syrian hamster embryo cells in culture. Cancer Res., *44*:5017–5022, 1984.

Ozawa, N., Oshimura, M., McLachlan, J. A., and Barrett, J. C. Nonrandom karyotypic changes in immortal and tumorigenic Syrian hamster cells induced by diethylstilbestrol. Cancer Genet. Cytogenet., *38*:271–282, 1989.

Packard, B. S., Saxton, M. J., Bissell, M. J., and Klein, M. P. Plasma membrane reorganization induced by tumor promoters in an epithelial cell line. Proc. Natl. Acad. Sci. U.S.A., *81*:449–452, 1984.

Parfett, C. L. J., and Pilon, R. Tri-*n*-butyltin chloride promotes morphological transformation and induces proliferin expression in C3H10T1/2 cells. Cancer Lett., *71*:167–176, 1993.

Parodi, S., and Brambilla, G. Relationships between mutation and transformation frequencies in mammalian cells treated "in vitro" with chemical carcinogens. Mutat. Res., *47*:53–74, 1977.

Parsa, I., and Marsh, W. H. Long-term organ culture of embryonic rat pancreas in a chemically defined medium. Am. J. Pathol., *82*:119–128, 1976.

Patskan, G. J., and Baxter, C. S. Specific stimulation of histone H2B and H4 phosphorylation in mouse lymphocytes by 12-*O*-tetradecanoylphorbol 13-acetate. J. Biol. Chem., *260*:12899–12903, 1985.

Pedersen, R. A. Embryonic stem cells for medicine. Sci. Am., *280*:44–49, 1999.

Peehl, D. M., and Stanbridge, E. J. Anchorage-independent growth of normal human fibroblasts. Proc. Natl. Acad. Sci. U.S.A., *78*:3053–3057, 1981.

Peterson, A. R., Peterson, H., and Heidelberger, C. Oncogenesis, mutagenesis, DNA damage, and cytotoxicity in cultured mammalian cells treated with alkylating agents. Cancer Res., *39*:131–138, 1979.

Pitot, H. C. Criteria of neoplastic transformation. *In*: L. Golberg (Ed.), Carcinogenesis Testing of Chemicals, pp. 113–117. Cleveland, OH: CRC Press, 1974.

Poiley, J. A., Raineri, R., and Pienta, R. J. Two-stage malignant transformation in hamster embryo cells. Br. J. Cancer, *39*:8–14, 1979.

Poiley, J. A., Raineri, R., Cavanaugh, D. M., Ernst, M. K., and Pienta, R. J. Correlation between transformation potential and inducible enzyme levels of hamster embryo cells. Carcinogenesis, *1*:323–328, 1980.

Popescu, N. C., and DiPaolo, J. A. Chromosome alterations in Syrian hamster cells transformed *in vitro* by sodium bilsulfite, a nonclastogenic carcinogen. Cancer Res., *48*:7246–7251, 1988.

Potenberg, J., Schiffmann, D., Kahl, R., Hildebrandt, A. G., and Henschler, D. Modulation of benzo[*a*]pyrene-induced morphological transformation of Syrian hamster embryo cells by butylated hydroxytoluene and butylated hydroxyanisole. Cancer Lett., *33*:189–198, 1986.

Preston, G. A., Lang, J. E., Maronpot, R. R., and Barrett, J. C. Regulation of apoptosis by low serum in cells of different stages of neoplastic progression: enhanced susceptibility after loss of a senescence gene and decreased susceptibility after loss of a tumor suppressor gene. Cancer Res., *54*:4214–4223, 1994.

Pung, A., Rundhaug, J. E., Yoshizawa, C. N., and Bertram, J. S. β-Carotene and canthaxanthin inhibit chemically and physically induced neoplastic transformation in 10T1/2 cells. Carcinogenesis, 9:1533–1539, 1988.

Rabinowitz, Z., and Sachs, L. The formation of variants with a reversion of properties of transformed cells. V. Reversion to a limited life-span. Int. J. Cancer, *6*:388–398, 1970.

Radner, B. S., and Kennedy, A. R. Suppression of x-ray induced transformation by valium and aspirin in mouse C3H10T1/2 cells. Cancer Lett., *51*:49–57, 1990.

Ray, F. A., Peabody, D. S., Cooper, J. L., Cram, L. S., and Kraemer, P. M. SV40 T antigen *alone* drives karyotype instability that precedes neoplastic transformation of human diploid fibroblasts. J. Cell. Biochem., *42*:13–31, 1990.

Reid, L. M., and Jefferson, D. M. Cell culture studies using extracts of extracellular matrix to study growth and differentiation in mammalian cells. *In*: Mather, J. P. (Ed.), Mammalian Cell Culture, pp. 239–280. New York: Plenum Press, 1984.

Ren, P., and Ruch, R. J. Inhibition of gap junctional intercellular communication by barbiturates in long-term primary cultured rat hepatocytes is correlated with liver tumour promoting activity. Carcinogenesis, *17*:2119–2124, 1996.

Rifkin, D. B., Crowe, R. M., and Pollack, R. Tumor promoters induce changes in the chick embryo fibroblast cytoskeleton. Cell, *18*:361–368, 1979.

Rifkind, R. A., Marks, P. A., Bank, A., Terada, M., Reuben, R. C., Maniatis, G. M., Fibach, E., Nudel, U., Salmon, J. E., and Gazitt, Y. Regulation of differentiation in normal and transformed erythroid cells. In Vitro, *14*:155–161, 1978.

Rivedal, E. Reversal of the promotional effect of 12-O-tetradecanoylphorbol-13-acetate on morphological transformation of hamster embryo cells by glucocorticoids. Cancer Lett., *15*:105–113, 1982.

Rivedal, E., and Sanner, T. Metal salts as promoters of *in vitro* morphological transformation of hamster embryo cells initiated by benzo(*a*)pyrene. Cancer Res., *41*:2950–2953, 1981.

Rivedal, E., and Sanner, T. Promotional effect of different phorbol esters on morphological transformation of hamster embryo cells. Cancer Lett., *17*:1–8, 1982.

Rivedal, E., and Sanner, T. Caffeine and other phosphodiesterase inhibitors are potent inhibitors of the promotional effect of TPA on morphological transformation of hamster embryo cells. Cancer Lett., *28*:9–17, 1985.

Rivedal, E., Mikalsen, S.-O., and Sanner, T. The non-phorbol ester tumor promoter okadaic acid does not promote morphological transformation or inhibit junctional communication in hamster embryo cells. Biochem. Biophys. Res. Commun., *167*:1302–1308, 1990.

Rivera, E. M., Hill, S. D., and Taylor, M. Organ culture passage enhances the oncogenicity of carcinogen-induced hyperplastic mammary nodules. In Vitro, *17*:159–166, 1981.

Roesch, S. F., and Wiebel, F. J. Differential effects of 12-*O*-tetradecanoylphorbol 13-acetate on cytochrome *P*-450-dependent monooxygenase activities in rat hepatoma cells: induction of *P*-450I and suppression of *P*-450II. Toxicology, *61*:147–159, 1990.

Rojkind, M., Gatmaitan, Z., Mackensen, S., Giambrone, M.-A., Ponce, P., and Reid, L. M. Connective tissue biomatrix: its isolation and utilization for long-term cultures of normal rat hepatocytes. J. Cell Biol., *87*:255–263, 1980.

Rubin, A. L., Yao, A., and Rubin, H. Relation of spontaneous transformation in cell culture to adaptive growth and clonal heterogeneity. Proc. Natl. Acad. Sci. U.S.A., *87*:482–486, 1990.

Rubin, H., Vidair, C., and Sanui, H. Restoration of normal appearance, growth behavior, and calcium content to transformed 3T3 cells by magnesium deprivation. Proc. Natl. Acad. Sci. U.S.A., *78*:2350–2354, 1981.

Rubin, H., Yao, A., and Chow, M. Neoplastic development: paradoxical relation between impaired cell growth at low population density and excessive growth at high density. Proc. Natl. Acad. Sci. U.S.A., *92*:7734–7738, 1995.

Ruch, R. J., and Klaunig, J. E. Effects of tumor promoters, genotoxic carcinogens and hepatocytotoxins on mouse hepatocyte intercellular communication. Cell Biol. Toxicol., *2*:469–483, 1986.

Ruch, R. J., and Klaunig, J. E. Kinetics of phenobarbital inhibition of intercellular communication in mouse hepatocytes. Cancer Res., *48*:2519–2523, 1988.

Ruch, R. J., Klaunig, J. E., Kerckaert, G. A., and LeBoeuf, R. A. Modification of gap junctional intercellular communication by changes in extracellular pH in Syrian hamster embryo cells. Carcinogenesis, *11*:909–913, 1990.

Sachs, L. Regulation of membrane changes, differentiation, and malignancy in carcinogenesis. Harvey Lect., *68*:1–35, 1974.

Sachs, L. Regulators of normal development and tumor suppression. Int. J. Dev. Biol., *37*:51–59, 1993.

Sakai, R., Ikeda, I., Kitani, H., Fujiki, H., Takaku, F., Rapp, U., Sugimura, T., and Nagao, M. Flat reversion by okadaic acid of *raf* and *ret*-II transformants. Proc. Natl. Acad. Sci. U.S.A., *86*:9946–9950, 1989.

Sanchez, J. H., Abernethy, D. J., and Boreiko, C. J. Reversible expression of morphological transformation in C3H/10T1/2 mouse embryo cultures exposed to 12-*O*-tetradecanoylphorbol-13-acetate. Carcinogenesis, *7*:1793–1796, 1986.

Sanford, K. K., Barker, B. E., Parshad, R., Westfall, B. B., Woods, M. W., Jackson, J. L., King, D. R., and Peppers, E. V. Neoplastic conversion *in vitro* of mouse cells: cytologic, chromosomal, enzymatic, glycolytic, and growth properties. J. Natl. Cancer Inst., *45*:1071–1096, 1970.

Sanford, K. K., Boone, C. W., Merwin, R. M., Jones, G. M., and Garrison, C. U. The plate-implant as a bioassay for the neoplastic potential of cultured cells. Int. J. Cancer, *25*:509–516, 1980.

Sasabe, T., and Inana, G. Mechanism of suppression of malignancy in hybrids between Y79 retinoblastoma and NIH3T3 cells. Invest. Ophthalmol. Vis. Sci., *32*:2011–2019, 1991.

Sasaki, K., Chida, K., Hashiba, H., Kamata, N., Abe, E., Suda, T., and Kuroki, T. Enhancement by $1\alpha,25$-dihydroxyvitamin D_3 of chemically induced transformation of BALB 3T3 cells without induction of ornithine decarboxylase or activation of protein kinase C. Cancer Res., *46*:604–610, 1986.

Sastrodihardjo, S., Sasaki, Y., Shiba, Y., and Kanno, Y. Possible involvement of reorganization of actin filaments, induced by tumor-promoting phorbol esters, in changes in colony shape and enhancement of proliferation of cultured epithelial cells. J. Cell. Physiol., *132*:49–56, 1987.

Schaeffer, W. I. Terminology associated with cell, tissue and organ culture, molecular biology and molecular genetics. In Vitro Cell. Dev. Biol., *26*:97–101, 1990.

Schaeffer, W. I., and Heintz, N. H. A diploid rat liver cell culture. IV. Malignant transformation by aflatoxin B_1. In Vitro, *14*:418–427, 1978.

Schroy, P., Winawer, S., and Friedman, E. Effect on in vivo tumorigenicity of lengthy exposure of human colon cancer cells to the differentiation agent hexamethylene bisacetamide. Cancer Lett., *48*:53–58, 1989.

Semba, M., Honda, I., Shibagaki, M., and Nishi, Y. Antipromoting effects of 5-lipoxygenase inhibitors, 3-nitro-2,4,6-trihydroxybenzamide derivatives, on TPA-promoted transformation in BALB 3T3 cells. Cancer Lett., *71*:57–60, 1993.

Shamsuddin, A. K. M., Barrett, L. A., Autrup, H., Harris, C. C., and Trump, B. F. Long-term organ culture of adult rat colon. Pathol. Res. Pract., *163*:362–372, 1978.

Shimizu, T., Kato, M. V., Nikaido, O., and Suzuki, F. A specific chromosome change and distinctive transforming genes are necessary for malignant progression of spontaneous transformation in cultured Chinese hamster embryo cells. Jpn. J. Cancer Res., *86*:546–554, 1995.

Shive, W., and Matthews, K. S. Nutritional requirements for growth of human lymphocytes. Annu. Rev. Nutr., *8*:81–97, 1988.

Sidhu, J. S., and Omiecinski, C. J. Protein synthesis inhibitors exhibit a nonspecific effect on pheno-barbital-inducible cytochrome P450 gene expression in primary rat hepatocytes. J. Biol. Chem., *273*:4769–4775, 1998.

Široký, J., and Cervenka, J. Hybridization frequencies of different mammalian cell types by electrofusion. Gen. Physiol. Biophys., *9*:489–499, 1990.

Skouv, J., Christensen, B., and Autrup, H. Differential induction of transcription of c-*myc* and c-*fos* proto-oncogenes by 12-O-tetradecanoylphorbol-13-acetate in mortal and immortal human urothelial cells. J. Cell. Biochem., *34*:71–79, 1987.

Slaga, T. J., Viaje, A., Bracken, W. M., Buty, S. G., Miller, D. R., Fischer, S. M., Richter, C. K., and Dumont, J. N. *In vitro* transformation of epidermal cells from newborn mice. Cancer Res., *38*:2246–2252, 1978.

Smith, J. R., and Pereira-Smith, O. M. Replicative senescence: implications for in vivo aging and tumor suppression. Science, *273*:63–67, 1996.

Stampfer, M. R., and Bartley, J. C. Induction of transformation and continuous cell lines from normal human mammary epithelial cells after exposure to benzo[*a*]pyrene. Proc. Natl. Acad. Sci. U.S.A., *82*:2394–2398, 1985.

Stampfer, M. R., Bartholomew, J. C., Smith, H. S., and Bartley, J. C. Metabolism of benzo[*a*]pyrene by human mammary epithelial cells: toxicity and DNA adduct formation. Proc. Natl. Acad. Sci. U.S.A., *78*:6251–6255, 1981.

Stanbridge, E. J. Genetic analysis of tumorigenicity in human cell hybrids. Cancer Surv., *3*:335–350, 1984.

Steele, V. E., Beeman, D. K., and Nettesheim, P. Enhanced induction of the anchorage-independent pheno-type in initiated rat tracheal epithelial cell cultures by the tumor promoter 12-*O*-tetradecanoylphor-bol-13-acetate. Cancer Res., *44*:5068–5072, 1984.

Summerhayes, I. C., Cheng, Y.-S. E., Sun, T.-T., and Chen, L. B. Expression of keratin and vimentin inter-mediate filaments in rabbit bladder epithelial cells at different stages of benzo[*a*]pyrene-induced neoplastic progression. J. Cell Biol., *90*:63–69, 1981.

Szabo, E., Preis, L. H., Brown, P. H., and Birrer, M. J. The role of *jun* and *fos* gene family members in 12-*O*-tetradecanoylphorbol-13-acetate induced hemopoietic differentiation. Cell Growth Diff., *2*:475–482, 1991.

Tabib, A., and Bachrach, U. Polyamines induce malignant transformation in cultured NIH 3T3 fibroblasts. Int. J. Biochem. Cell Biol., *30*:135–146, 1998.

Tateno, C., Ito, S., Tanaka, M., Oyamada, M., and Yoshitake, A. Effect of DDT on hepatic gap junctional intercellular communication in rats. Carcinogenesis, *15*:517–521, 1994.

Taub, M. The use of defined media in cell and tissue culture. Toxicol. in Vitro, *4*:213–225, 1990.

Thomassen, D. G., and DeMars, R. Clonal analysis of the stepwise appearance of anchorage independence and tumorigenicity in CAK, a permanent line of mouse cells. Cancer Res., *42*:4054–4063, 1982.

Thomassen, D. G., Gray, T. E., Mass, M. J., and Barrett, J. C. High frequency of carcinogen-induced early, preneoplastic changes in rat tracheal epithelial cells in culture. Cancer Res., *43*:5956–5963, 1983.

Thomson, J. A., Itskovitz-Eldor, J., Shapiro, S. S., Waknitz, M. A., Swiergiel, J. J., Marshall, V. S., and Jones, J. M. Embryonic stem cell lines derived from human blastocysts. Science, *282*:1145–1147, 1998.

Tlsty, T. D., Margolin, B. H., and Lum, K. Differences in the rates of gene amplification in nontumorigenic and tumorigenic cell lines as measured by Luria-Delbrück fluctuation analysis. Proc. Natl. Acad. Sci. U.S.A., *86*:9441–9445, 1989.

Tomei, L. D., and Bertram, J. S. Restoration of growth control in malignantly transformed mouse fibro-blasts grown in a chemically defined medium. Cancer Res., *38*:444–451, 1978.

Tortora, G., Yokozaki, H., Pepe, S., Clair, T., and Cho-Chung, Y. S. Differentiation of HL-60 leukemia by type I regulatory subunit antisense oligodeoxynucleotide of cAMP-dependent protein kinase. Proc. Natl. Acad. Sci. U.S.A., *88*:2011–2015, 1991.

Trier, J. S. Organ-culture methods in the study of gastrointestinal-mucosal function and development. N. Engl. J. Med., *295*:150–155, 1976.

Trosko, J. E., Dawson, B., Yotti, L. P., and Chang, C. C. Saccharin may act as a tumor promoter by inhibit-ing metabolic cooperation between cells. Nature, *285*:109–110, 1980.

Trosko, J. E., Dawson, B., and Chang, C.-C. PBB Inhibits metabolic cooperation in Chinese hamster cells *in vitro*: its potential as a tumor promoter. Environ. Health Perspect., *37*:179–182, 1981.

Trott, D. A., Cuthbert, A. P., Overell, R. W., Russo, I., and Newbold, R. F. Mechanisms involved in the immortalization of mammalian cells by ionizing radiation and chemical carcinogens. Carcinogenesis, *16*:193–204, 1995.

Tsai, W.-H., Zarnegar, R., and Michalopoulos, G. K. Long-term treatment with hepatic tumor promoters inhibits mitogenic responses of hepatocytes to acidic fibroblast growth factor and hepatocyte growth factor. Cancer Lett., *59*:103–108, 1991.

Tsao, M. C., Walthall, B. J., and Ham, R. G. Clonal growth of normal human epidermal keratinocytes in a defined medium. J. Cell. Physiol., *110*:219–229, 1982.

Tsao, M.-S., and Zhang, X.-Y. The effects of continuous exposure to epidermal growth factor on the spontaneous transformation of cultured rat liver epithelial cells. Am. J. Pathol., *140*:85–94, 1992.

Tsuchiya, T., and Umeda, M. Relationship between exposure to TPA and appearance of transformed cells in MNNG-initiated transformation of BALB/c 3T3 cells. Int. J. Cancer, *73*:271–276, 1997.

Tsuda, H. Enhancing effect of tumor promoter 12-*O*-tetradecanoylphorbol-13-acetate on 8-azaguanine-resistant mutations induced by *N*-methyl-*N′*-nitro-*N*-nitrosoguanidine in cultured Chinese hamster cells. Jpn. J. Genet., *56*:9–18, 1981.

Tsutsui, T., Maizumi, H., McLachlan, J. A., and Barrett, J. C. Aneuploidy induction and cell transformation by diethylstilbestrol: a possible chromosomal mechanism in carcinogenesis. Cancer Res., *43*:3814–3821, 1983.

Tsutsui, T., Suzuki, N., and Ohmori, M. Sodium fluoride-induced morphological and neoplastic transformation, chromosome aberrations, sister chromatid exchanges, and unscheduled DNA synthesis in cultured Syrian hamster embryo cells. Cancer Res., *44*:938–941, 1984.

Tsutsui, T., Suzuki, N., Fukuda, S., Sato, M., Maizumi, H., McLachlan, J. A., and Barrett, J. C. 17β-Estradiol-induced cell transformation and aneuploidy of Syrian hamster embryo cells in culture. Carcinogenesis, *8*:1715–1719, 1987.

Tu, A. S., Tennant, R. W., and Spalding, J. W. Morphological transformation of Syrian hamster embryo cells by mezerein. Cancer Lett., *62*:159–165, 1992.

Ueo, H., Nakano, S., Ts'o, P. O. P., and Bruce, S. A. Tumor promoters retard the loss of a transient subpopulation of cells in low passage Syrian hamster cell cultures. J. Cell. Physiol., *142*:505–513, 1990.

Umans, R. S., and Kennedy, A. R. Effects of activators and inhibitors of protein kinase C on x-ray induced malignant transformation *in vitro*. Eur. J. Cancer, *28A*:732–735, 1992.

Vandenberghe, Y., Tee, L., Morel, F., Rogiers, V., Guillouzo, A., and Yeoh, G. Regulation of glutathione *S*-transferase gene expression by phenobarbital in cultured adult rat hepatocytes. Fed. Eur. Biochem. Soc., *284*:103–108, 1991.

Vizirianakis, I. S., and Tsiftsoglou, A. S. Induction of murine erythroleukemia cell differentiation is associated with methylation and differential stability of poly(A)$^+$ RNA transcripts. Biochim. Biophys. Acta, *1312*:8–20, 1996.

Warholm, M. Studies of the induction of ornithine decarboxylase activity in primary cultures of adult rat hepatocytes by the phorbol ester 12-*O*-tetradecanoyl-13-acetate and other substances. Toxicol. in Vitro, *6*:589–596, 1992.

Watt, F. M. Cell culture models of differentiation. FASEB J., *5*:287–294, 1991.

Weinstein, I. B., Wigler, M., and Stadler, U. Analysis of the mechanism of chemical carcinogenesis in epithelial cell cultures. *In*: R. Montesano, H. Bartsch, and L. Tomatis (Eds.), Screening Tests in Chemical Carcinogenesis, IARC Scientific Publications, No. 12, pp. 355–381. Lyon, France: International Agency for Research on Cancer, 1976.

Westerwoudt, R. J. Improved fusion methods. IV. Technical aspects. J. Immunol. Methods, *77*:181–196, 1985.

Whitesell, L., Mimnaugh, E. G., de Costa, B., Myers, C. E., and Neckers, L. M. Inhibition of heat shock protein HSP90-pp60[v-src] heteroprotein complex formation by benzoquinone ansamycins: essential role for stress proteins in oncogenic transformation. Proc. Natl. Acad. Sci. U.S.A., *91*:8324–8328, 1994.

Whong, W.-Z., Gao, H.-G., Zhou, G., and Ong, T. Genetic alterations of cancer-related genes in glass fiber-induced transformed cells. J. Toxicol. Environ. Health, 56:397–404, 1999.

Wiener, F., Klein, G., and Harris, H. The analysis of malignancy by cell fusion. VI. Hybrids between different tumour cells. J. Cell Sci., 16:189–198, 1974.

Wigley, C. B. TPA affects early and late stages of chemically-induced transformation in mouse submandibular salivary epithelial cells in vitro. Carcinogenesis, 4:101–106, 1983.

Willey, J. C., Saladino, A. J., Ozanne, C., Lechner, J. F., and Harris, C. C. Acute effects of 12-O-tetradecanoylphorbol-13-acetate, teleocidin B, or 2,3,7,8-tetrachlorodibenzo-p-dioxin on cultured normal human bronchial epithelial cells. Carcinogenesis, 5:209–215, 1984.

Williams, G. M., Elliott, J. M., and Weisburger, J. J. Carcinoma after malignant conversion in vitro of epithelial-like cells from rat liver following exposure to chemical carcinogens. Cancer Res., 33:606–612, 1973.

Wolffe, A. P., and Tata, J. R. Primary culture, cellular stress and differentiated function. FEBS Lett., 176:8–12, 1984.

Yamaguchi, N., and Weinstein, I. B. Temperature-sensitive mutants of chemically transformed epithelial cells. Proc. Natl. Acad. Sci. U.S.A., 72:214–218, 1975.

Yamanishi, K., Nishino, H., and Iwashima, A. Possible role of calmodulin in stimulation of hexose transport by 12-O-tetradecanoylphorbol-13-acetate, a tumor promoter. Experientia, 39:1036–1037, 1983.

Yamasaki, H. Gap junctional intercellular communication and carcinogenesis. Carcinogenesis, 11:1051–1058, 1990.

Yamasaki, H., and Fitzgerald, D. J. The role of selective junctional communication in cell transformation. In: R. Langenbach et al. (eds.), Tumor Promoters: Biological Approaches for Mechanistic Studies and Assay Systems, pp. 131–147. New York: Raven Press, 1988.

Yamasaki, H., Aguelon-Pegouries, A.-M., Enomoto, T., Martel, N., Furstenberger, G., and Marks, F. Comparative effects of a complete tumor promoter, TPA, and a second-stage tumor promoter, RPA, on intercellular communication, cell differentiation and cell transformation. Carcinogenesis, 6:1173–1179, 1985.

Yamasaki, H., Krutovskikh, V., Mesnil, M., Tanaka, T., Zaidan-Dagli, M. L., and Omori, Y. Role of connexin (gap junction) genes in cell growth control and carcinogenesis. Life Sci., 322:151–159, 1999.

Yang, J., Richards, J., Bowman, P., Guzman, R., Enami, J., McCormick, K., Hamamoto, S., Pitelka, D., and Nandi, S. Sustained growth and three-dimensional organization of primary mammary tumor epithelial cells embedded in collagen gels. Proc. Natl. Acad. Sci. U.S.A., 76:3401–3405, 1979.

Yang, J., Flynn, D., Larson, L., and Hamamoto, S. Growth in primary culture of mouse submandibular epithelial cells embedded in collagen gels. In Vitro, 18:435–442, 1982.

Yotti, L. P., Chang, C. C., and Trosko, J. E. Elimination of metabolic cooperation in Chinese hamster cells by a tumor promoter. Science, 206:1089–1091, 1979.

Yusof, Y. A. M., and Edwards, A. M. Stimulation of DNA synthesis in primary rat hepatocyte cultures by liver tumor promoters: interactions with other growth factors. Carcinogenesis, 11:761–770, 1990.

Yuspa, S. H., Hennings, H., and Lichti, U. Initiation and promoter induced specific changes in epidermal function and biological potential. J. Supramol. Struct. Cell. Biochem., 17:245–257, 1981.

Yuspa, S. H., Ben, T., and Lichti, U. Regulation of epidermal transglutaminase activity and terminal differentiation by retinoids and phorbol esters. Cancer Res., 43:5707–5712, 1983a.

Yuspa, S. H., Kulesz-Martin, M., Ben, T., and Hennings, H. Transformation of epidermal cells in culture. J. Invest. Dermatol., 81:162s–168s, 1983b.

Zhang, X., Wang, T., Batist, G., and Tsao, M.-S. Transforming growth factor β1 promotes spontaneous transformation of cultured rat liver epithelial cells. Cancer Res., 54:6122–6128, 1994.

15

The Cellular and Molecular Biology of Neoplasia in Vivo

The discoveries of chemical, physical, and biological carcinogenic agents and their actions have been among the most exciting and significant in our understanding of the causation of cancer and of many aspects of its prevention, but nothing has intrigued the biological scientist more than the molecular differences between cancer cells and normal cells. The first hint of this interest by biochemists in the cancer problem was shown during the first two decades of this century when the structures of nucleotides and sugar phosphates were just becoming known to biochemical scientists. In a review, Potter (1982) detailed much of the historical development of biochemical investigations into the cancer problem through 1975 (Table 15.1). Just as with the initial morphological and biological studies of the neoplastic process (see Chapter 1), the development of biochemistry and, more recently, cell and molecular biology has given rise to a series of hypotheses on the biochemical nature of neoplasia as well as the molecular mechanisms that result in the conversion of a normal cell to a neoplastic cell. This chapter considers, first, the historical development and bases for some of the better known theories of the biochemical nature and genesis of neoplasia in vivo. The evolution of such concepts into our more modern-day understanding of molecular lesions in neoplastic cells is then discussed.

BIOCHEMICAL THEORIES OF CARCINOGENESIS AND CANCER

Although some understanding of biochemical reactions occurring in living systems such as fermentation were known during the latter half of the nineteenth century, quantitative studies on such reactions were pioneered by the German chemist Otto Warburg. Warburg was recognized internationally for his investigations in photosynthesis; in addition, he made a very significant initial contribution to our understanding of biochemical reactions occurring in neoplastic cells.

Glycolysis of Cancer Cells: The Warburg Theory

During the 1920s, the predominant investigations of the biochemistry of cancer centered around the monumental studies of Otto Warburg. He observed that, in the absence of oxygen, tumor slices utilized glucose and produced lactic acid. Warburg termed this process *anaerobic glycolysis*. Generally, slices of cancer tissue were found to produce more lactic acid than did normal tissue slices. In addition, he observed that both normal and neoplastic tissue slices produced less lactic acid in the presence of oxygen (*aerobic glycolysis*) than in the presence of nitrogen. He called this latter phenomenon the *Pasteur effect* in reference to Pasteur's earlier observation that

Table 15.1 Historical Perspectives in Cancer Biochemistry

Period	Cancer Biochemistry	General Biochemistry
1913–23	Enzyme differences	1918, 3′RNtides[a] from RNA 1918, Fructose 6-P 1922, Glucose 6-P
1923–33	Aerobic glycolysis—respiratory defect (Warburg theory)	1924, Slice technique 1929, ATP 1930, Deoxyribose 1933, Glycolytic scheme
1933–43	Warburg theory	1934–1935, TPN, DPN (NADP, NAD) 1936, Homogenate technique 1937, Citric cycle 1939, Oxidative phosphorylation
1943–53	Convergence theory (Greenstein) Protein deletion theory (Miller and Miller)	1950, Alternative metabolic pathways 1951, 5′RNtides from RNA 1952, Pentose cycle 1952, Active transport across membranes
1953–63	Catabolic deletion theory (Potter) Morris hepatoma lines (Morris) Minimal deviation concept (Potter)	1953, DNA structure 1954, 5′RNtides in acid-soluble fraction 1956, Feedback 1957, Repression 1958, Cyclic AMP 1960, Cell hybridization 1961, Genetic code
1963–68	Altered feedback theory (does not imply presence or absence of somatic mutation) (Monod and Jacob; Pitot and Heidelberger; Potter) Molecular correlation concept (Weber) Altered mRNA template stability (Pitot) Metabolic activation of chemical carcinogens (Miller and Miller) Tumor promoters as reversible gene derepressors (Boutwell)	1964, Selection of cell hybrids 1964, Hormonal modulation of enzyme activity and synthesis in cell cultures 1967, Cell-free mRNA-directed enzyme synthesis 1967, Hormonal modulation of developmental enzyme formation
1968–75	Reconciling assumption: provirus as gene (Temin) Unbalanced retrodifferentiation (Uriel) Dysdifferentiation (Sugimura) Unbalanced blocked ontogeny (Potter) Altered gene expression (Weinhouse) Pleiotypic response (Tomkins) Pleiotropic controls (Weber)	1969, Regulated termination of gene transcription 1970, Reverse transcriptase 1971, Restriction endonucleases for specific sequences in DNA 1972, complementary DNA using reverse transcriptase on purified globin mRNA

[a]Ribonucleotides.
After Potter, 1982, with permission of the author and publisher.

yeast ceased fermentation when exposed to oxygen. In 1930, Warburg published his book on the metabolism of tumors, in which he demonstrated that in a wide variety of benign and malignant neoplasms investigated, tumors of both humans and lower animals exhibited a significant if not a very high rate of glycolysis (Warburg, 1930). Warburg's theory (based on his studies up to that time and reiterated in 1956) stated that cancer cells originate from normal cells as a result of an irreversible injury to their respiration, this injury to the normal cell being compensated for in the cancer cell by increased fermentation (glycolysis). Until 40 years ago, there were few if any exceptions to this generalization, although many normal tissues exhibited equally high and in some instances even higher rates of glycolysis than the vast majority of tumors studied; examples are embryonic tissue, the retina, and the renal papilla. In view of these findings, two questions arose that were never answered satisfactorily by proponents of the Warburg hypothesis. The first is the primary association of glycolysis with the growth rate of tumors rather than with the neoplastic transformation itself. A number of studies carried out in many laboratories demonstrated a reasonable degree of correlation of glycolytic rate with growth rate of tumors in many systems. Thus, glycolysis may be a secondary event as a result of the loss of control of cellular replication in most neoplasms. The second question concerns the validity of many comparisons of neoplastic tissues with their cells of origin. This problem recalls our original definition of relative autonomy, which was relative to the tissue from which the neoplasm arose. Normal tissues differ dramatically in their biochemistry as well as their cell and molecular biology, and neoplasms are found to do the same. This fact was not completely evident during the time of Warburg but now becomes a major factor in determining the significance of changes in neoplastic cells in relation to their normal counterparts.

Weinhouse (1976), in reviewing the Warburg theory on its fiftieth anniversary, summarized the experimental evidence pertaining to Warburg's hypothesis (Table 15.2). It was apparent that tumors do exhibit the Pasteur effect, although quantitatively not as efficiently as normal tissues. Weinhouse concluded, "There is no evidence either from Warburg's own observations or from those of his contemporaries that respiration in cancer is either quantitatively lower or fails to lower glycolysis." Warburg, and later Greenstein (see below), attempted to generalize their findings to include all neoplasms. Today it is clear that comparisons of normal liver with highly differentiated hepatocellular carcinomas reveal little if any difference in the glycolytic capacities of the two tissues, although, as these neoplasms continue to be transplanted, they tend to in-

Table 15.2 Condensed Tumor Metabolism Data of Warburg, Burk, and Others[a]

Tissue	QO_2	$Q^{N_2}_{CO_2}$	$A^{O_2}_{CO_2}$	Pasteur Effect
14 normal tissues of various animals	9.3 (3–21)	7.2 (2–19)	2.1 (0–10)	5.1 (1–16.5)
15 types of neoplasms of various animals	11.8 (5.3–19.8)	25.6 (14.0–34.8)	14.0 (4.7–24.6)	11.6 (6.3–17.8)
13 human neoplasms studied by Warburg	5.3 (2–6)	20.5 (13–29)	13.3 (5–19)	7.2 (3–11)
11 Flexner-Jobling carcinomas studied by Warburg	8.0 (3.5–13)	32.1 (27–37)	24.6 (19–28)	7.0 (3–9)

[a]Values are given in the Q notation, as µliters of gas absorbed or evolved/h/mg dry wt, with ranges given underneath in parentheses. The Q notation can be converted to µmol/min/g by multiplying the Q value by 0.15 on the assumption that 1 g fresh tissue is equivalent to 200 mg dry tissue.
After Weinhouse, 1976, with permission of the author and publisher.

crease their glycolytic activity. Investigations in the 1950s actually demonstrated the existence of primary hepatomas with little or no increased glycolytic rate compared with that of normal liver (cf. Greenstein, 1954). Malignant lymphoblasts glycolyze at essentially the same rate as their normal counterparts, and it is likely that malignant teratomas do not exhibit a degree of glycolysis in excess of that found in embryonic tissues. Thus, in support of Warburg's original hypothesis, most neoplasms do have relatively high rates of glycolysis, but, just as we saw normal karyotypes in early neoplasia, normal glycolytic rates do exist in many neoplasms, especially those that grow slowly and are well differentiated. Increased glycolysis may, therefore, be a characteristic of the stage of tumor progression, similar to the occurrence of many karyotypic changes in neoplasms.

Convergence Hypothesis of Greenstein

Some 45 years ago, the late Jesse Greenstein, author of *Biochemistry of Cancer* (1954) (the next major text after Warburg's work on the biochemical characterization of neoplasia), proposed that the biochemical constitution of neoplasms tended to converge to a relatively common enzymatic pattern. Several authors, including V. R. Potter (1964) of the McArdle Laboratory, pointed out that the Greenstein hypothesis had not challenged that of Warburg but actually extended it. Warburg's ideas of convergence were limited to the area of glycolysis and respiration, whereas those of Greenstein were extended to a number of enzymatic functions in the cell that could be analyzed in the 1940s. Greenstein understood and realized the importance of using valid tissue comparisons: he was among the first biochemists studying cancer to realize the importance of comparing liver with hepatomas, since they are relatively homogeneous cellular populations. In stating the hypothesis of convergence, Greenstein (1956) recognized the existence of exceptions to his theory, although perhaps not their importance for an understanding of the cancer problem in general. Since the enunciation of the convergence hypothesis, a number of exceptions have been reported on comparison of relatively highly differentiated neoplasms with their appropriate cells of origin (Morris, 1965; Mekhail-Ishak et al., 1989). However, like the Warburg hypothesis, the convergence hypothesis can be reconciled with our better understanding of the development of the stage of progression.

Deletion Hypothesis

Unlike the two hypotheses mentioned above, the deletion hypothesis, first advanced by the Millers (1947) more than 35 years ago, was not based on studies with many different neoplasms, but rather evolved from investigations on the production of hepatic cancer by the feeding of aminoazo dyes to experimental animals. The basic experimental observation was that the dye became bound in a covalent fashion to proteins of the liver of the dye-fed animal, whereas little or no dye binding occurred in the protein of the neoplasms ultimately produced (cf. Chapter 3). The Millers thus postulated that carcinogenesis resulted from "a permanent alteration or loss of protein essential for the control of growth . . . ." The reader should note that at this time the structure of DNA was not known and the concept of the gene was rather nebulous. Later studies by Sorof et al. (1958) and others indicated that the proteins to which the dyes were bound in greatest amounts constituted an electrophoretically slow-moving class termed the h_2 proteins. These proteins were found to be missing from the neoplasms that were produced by dye feeding. However, investigations with highly differentiated neoplasms have shown the presence of the h_2 protein(s), although little or no dye binding occurred in the h_2 fraction (Sorof et al., 1966).

It is now clear that, for the covalent linkage between amine carcinogens and liver macro-molecules to occur, aromatic amine carcinogens must be "activated" by N-hydroxylation and subsequent esterification, as described in Chapter 3. Lotlikar (1970) did demonstrate the capability for N-hydroxylation (Chapter 3) in several of the highly differentiated hepatomas. Thus, the absence of a portal blood supply and the generally lowered rate of blood perfusion through these neoplasms, as shown by Gullino and Grantham (1961), coupled with the low drug metabolism, may explain the lack of covalent interaction between the carcinogen and soluble proteins of the neoplasm. Elizabeth Miller (1951) and Heidelberger (1970) showed that a com-pletely analogous situation took place during skin carcinogenesis by hydrocarbons. A protein isolated from mouse skin binds hydrocarbons in a direct relationship to their carcinogenic activ-ity for the skin. Electrophoretically, this protein had many of the characteristics of the h_2 proteins of liver.

About 10 years after the original proposal of the deletion hypothesis, Potter (1958) sug-gested that the proteins deleted during carcinogenesis may be identical to or associated with en-zymes involved in catabolic reactions, a view compatible with the Greenstein hypothesis as well as with some of the biological aspects of neoplasia; for example, rapid growth. Furthermore, several experimental hepatomas demonstrated a complete lack of many catabolic reactions char-acteristic of liver, in support of the concept of "catabolic deletion." However, not long after the initial proposal of the catabolic deletion hypothesis, a series of hepatocellular carcinomas rang-ing from poorly differentiated to highly differentiated were produced in the laboratory of Harold Morris (Morris and Wagner, 1968), and their chemical characteristics were studied by numerous investigators. These studies demonstrated that the highly differentiated hepatocellular carcino-mas exhibited virtually all of the normal hepatic enzymatic functions investigated and, in several instances, lacked any abnormal glycolytic capacity, while the enzyme pattern of the poorly dif-ferentiated neoplasms was characteristic of the concept of "catabolic deletion."

The discovery of the Morris hepatomas and the investigation of their biochemical charac-teristics greatly altered the biochemical concepts of neoplasia that had developed up until 1961. Studies with these neoplasms demonstrated that simple qualitative measurements of enzymes and proteins of neoplasms were not sufficient to characterize the critical difference(s) between a normal and a neoplastic cell.

Minimal Deviation Concept

As a result of investigations with the first of the transplantable Morris hepatomas (no. 5123), Potter (1961) proposed the concept of the "minimal deviation" neoplasm, at the opposite end of the spectrum from those neoplasms conforming to the original Greenstein convergence hypo-thesis. Potter's concept was that some neoplasms were probably very closely related to or virtually identical with the initiated cell. An experimental program was proposed to examine a variety of transplantable hepatomas either to discover an essential alteration found in all examples or to disprove a generalization by finding exceptions. The phenotype of the highly differentiated hepatomas deviated only slightly from normal with respect to their growth charac-teristics and exhibited relatively few abnormalities except those necessary for the expression of neoplasia. As these cells progressed, their deviation from the cell(s) of origin increased to produce a moderately or maximally deviated neoplasm. The term *minimal deviation hepatoma* appeared to apply to a number of the Morris transplantable neoplasms. Although there has been some discussion of this concept in the literature, its correlation with both morphology and kary-otype appears to follow the distinction between neoplasms as to their degree of differentiation.

Molecular Correlation Concept

Shortly after the demonstration of the existence of a spectrum of transplantable hepatomas, Weber and associates (Weber, 1983) embarked on an extensive biochemical analysis of the enzymatic patterns of these neoplasms. These workers attempted to assemble the data into a modification of the idea of catabolic deletion, but in direct relation to cell replication and the growth rate of the neoplasm. Thus, by the molecular correlation concept, certain enzymatic abnormalities seen in a class of neoplasms compared with their cells of origin may be closely correlated with the growth rate of the neoplasm. Other functions, usually those more closely associated with the degree of differentiation of the organ, show little or no relation to the growth rate of the neoplasm. Weber's investigations were extended to include several different types of experimental neoplasms, numerous enzymatic functions, and specific metabolic pathways (Weber, 1983).

Biochemical Theories of Neoplasia Revisited

Although the four theories described above are not considered in most modern-day investigations of the cell and molecular biology of neoplasia, their influence on our basic knowledge of the biochemistry of neoplastic cells was very significant. Today, in retrospect, one may view the theories as related to studies of neoplastic cells in the stage of progression. Even those highly differentiated hepatocellular carcinomas forming the basis of the minimal deviation concept of Potter were almost all in the stage of progression as defined by karyotypic alterations (Nowell et al., 1967; Wolman et al., 1973). Thus, it is reasonable to suggest that the Warburg, Greenstein, and Weber concepts all involve studies of neoplasms in the stage of progression, while the deletion hypothesis may be more closely related to the stage of initiation, since the original theory, although ahead of its time, basically argued for the presence of a specific gene mutation as the seminal event in the conversion of a normal to a neoplastic cell. From all of these studies combined, however, it is reasonable to argue that there is as yet no evidence for a cellular pattern of metabolism specific to the neoplastic state, but there is evidence that in the natural history of neoplasia, there is a progression of neoplastic cells through morphological, karyotypic, and metabolic changes.

The reader should be aware that a number of other theories of carcinogenesis and of the neoplastic transformation have been proposed during the past half century. Several of these have been considered in earlier chapters, but it is not possible nor is it the function of this text to review all of the proposed theories of carcinogenesis. Rather, the rest of this chapter emphasizes several specific biochemical, cell, and molecular biological changes in preneoplastic and neoplastic cells, making appropriate comparisons wherever possible.

GENE EXPRESSION AND ITS REGULATION IN PRENEOPLASIA AND NEOPLASIA

Studies of the biochemistry of neoplasia during the first half of this century centered on qualitative and quantitative differences in enzyme levels reflecting gene expression. Approaches to an understanding of the most critical characteristic of neoplasia, that of relative autonomy, had to await methods for the investigation in the regulation of genetic expression in eukaryotic cells. Early investigations were concerned with changes in enzyme activities and, later, actual rates of enzyme synthesis and mRNA expression in neoplasms as compared with their appropriate tissue of origin in response to specific environmental agents including hormones, drugs, dietary factors, and other environmental changes.

The Regulatory Cybernetics of Preneoplasia and Neoplasia

Although the term *cybernetics* refers to the theoretical aspects of control processes in various systems, it is used here in a more general reference to the control of the variety of processes necessary for the viability of a cell. It is the regulation of these control processes, the regulation of genetic expression, whose alteration is likely the key to our ultimate understanding of the molecular nature of the neoplastic transformation. Here, a number of examples of the alteration of the regulation of genetic expression in neoplastic cells are considered; where possible, this discussion is extended to the cell and molecular mechanisms of such alteration, the basis of the relative autonomy of neoplasia (Chapter 2).

Preneoplasia

Compared with studies on neoplastic tissues, relatively few investigations have attempted to investigate the regulation of gene expression in preneoplastic tissues. In epidermal papillomas of mouse skin, overexpression of some genes occurs, including 12-lipoxygenase (Krieg et al., 1995), metallothionein (Hashiba et al., 1989), and mRNAs for which a function has not been defined (Krieg et al., 1993). In other instances, regulation of gene expression is abnormal or absent, such as with K14, a keratin protein (Roop et al., 1988), and enzymes of xenobiotic metabolism (Reiners et al., 1998).

Earlier studies by Kitagawa (1971) noted that partial hepatectomy did induce mitotic activity in preneoplastic nodules and hyperplasia of liver but less so in hepatomas in the rat. Studies of gene expression in altered hepatic foci have shown numerous differences in gene expression (Pitot, 1990) as well as altered responses to environmental agents compared with normal hepatocytes (Olsson et al., 1995). Removal of the inducing agent or promoting agent may cause not only a loss of cells through apoptosis, but also a reversal of the altered gene expression prior to cell death (Neveu et al., 1990; Li and Rozman, 1995). This latter point is indicative of the transient nature of cells in the stage of promotion as well as their altered gene expression.

Neoplasia

Studies on the cybernetics or regulation of gene expression in hepatocellular carcinoma cells in the stage of progression were initiated some four decades ago in studies on the hormonal and substrate regulation of several different enzymes of amino acid metabolism (Pitot, 1959; Pitot et al., 1961). Some of these earlier studies had been reviewed previously (cf. Goldfarb and Pitot, 1976; Sabine, 1975), but no generalization could be made. Table 15.3 gives examples of some of these earlier studies, which indicate both a normal response as well as an absence of response of gene expression to the administration of specific agents and under certain physiological conditions. While no specific regulatory mechanism is defective in all neoplastic cells when compared with these effects in their normal counterparts, even in most instances where an effect is noted in the neoplasm, this can be distinguished by differential sensitivity or other factors from that seen in the normal circumstance. An abnormality in control mechanisms that was thought to be characteristic of all hepatomas was that of the loss of the repressive control of cholesterol synthesis (Brown et al., 1973). However, in cell culture and in "preneoplastic" livers, the feedback both by dietary cholesterol in vivo and addition of the agent to cell culture resulted in some degree of repression of cholesterol biosynthesis (Sabine, 1976; Depass and Morris, 1982). The effect, which centers around the regulation of the synthesis of the key enzyme, hydroxymethylglutaryl-

Table 15.3 Some Alterations in Metabolic Regulation in Neoplasms

Function	Neoplasm	Regulatory Agent	Effect Control	Effect Neoplasm	Reference
Amino acid metabolism					
Urea cycle enzymes	Hepatoma (rat)	Dietary protein	+	+	Brebnor et al., 1981
Tryptophan oxygenase	Hepatoma (rat)	Tryptophan/cortisone	+	0	
Tyrosine aminotransferase (in B_6 deficiency)	Hepatoma (rat)	Hydrocortisone	+	0	Tryfiates et al., 1974
Cholesterol biosynthesis	Hepatoma (rat)	Cholesterol (diet)	–	0	Brown et al., 1973
HMG-CoA reductase	Hepatoma (rat)	Mevalonate (i.v.)	–	–	George and Goldfarb, 1980
DNA synthesis	Hepatomas (rat)	Liver regeneration	+	+/0	Kitagawa, 1971
	Hepatomas (rat)	Liver regeneration/ hydrocortisone	–	0	Jones and Irvin, 1972
Estrogen response					
Galactosyltransferase	Mammary cancer (rat)	Estradiol/prolactin	+	+/0	Ip and Dao, 1978
Glucose-6-phosphate dehydrogenase	Mammary cancer (rat)	Estradiol	+	+	Ringler and Hilf, 1975
Fatty acid synthesis	Hepatoma (rat)	Fasting	–	0	Halperin et al., 1975
	Pulmonary adenomas	Fast/refeed	+	+	Voelker et al., 1976
Xenobiotic metabolism					
Cytochrome P450	Hepatomas (mouse)	Phenobarbital	+	++	Becker and Stout, 1984
Benzphetamine met.	Hepatoma (rat)	Phenobarbital	+	+	Strobel et al., 1978
DAB	Hepatoma (rat)	Methylcholanthrene	+	+	Conney and Burns, 1963
γ-Glutamyltranspeptidase	Hepatomas (mouse)	Phenobarbital	0	+	Kitagawa et al., 1980
δ-Aminolevulinate synthetase	Hepatomas (rats)	Allylisopropylacetamide	+	0	Bonkowsky et al., 1973

Key: +, increase in function; –, decrease in function; 0, no change in function.

coenzyme A (HMG-CoA) reductase, a microsomal enzyme, has been described in both experimental and human neoplasms of the liver as well as leukemic cells. In view of the fact that hepatoma cells growing in vitro do exhibit cholesterol feedback of the expression of HMG-CoA reductase (Beirne and Watson, 1976), the original generalization developed in vivo was questioned as to its significance on the basis of the availability of the regulatory molecule(s) to the neoplastic cells because of differences in cholesterol accumulation and transport to the neoplasm itself (Harry et al., 1971). As with a number of other circumstances where enzyme regulation appears to be abnormal, the lack of effect of cholesterol on HMG-CoA reductase expression does not appear to be a result of structural alterations in the enzyme itself (e.g., Beirne et al., 1977).

In contrast to the attempted generalization of loss of cholesterol feedback in hepatomas, xenobiotic metabolism in such lesions is for the most part qualitatively not defective when neoplasms are compared with controlled tissues. Again, studies on the structure of the enzymes involved did not reveal significant differences (Ohmachi et al., 1985). The expression of several enzymes of amino acid metabolism in response to substrate and hormonal factors is abnormal (Tryfiates et al., 1974), while in other circumstances neoplasms appear to respond to the more general stimulus of dietary protein influx like normal tissues in liver (Brebnor et al., 1981). However, as noted in the table, the lack of response of hepatomas to the hydrocortisone induction of tyrosine aminotransferase seen in vivo in pyridoxine (B_6) deficiency is likely a result of the inability of the neoplasm to synthesize sufficient active forms of the vitamin in vivo (Thanassi et al., 1981). This is of note since the regulation of this specific gene has been extensively studied both in normal and neoplastic tissue in vivo and in vitro for a number of years as a model of the regulation of enzyme synthesis (Sorimachi et al., 1981; Thompson et al., 1966). Thyroid hormone is also capable of inducing mitochondrial α-glycerophosphate dehydrogenase in well-differentiated but not poorly differentiated hepatomas (Hunt et al., 1970). This finding, perhaps unexpected, indicates that as the stage of progression continues, regulation of specific genes will likely be further altered or lost altogether.

Thus, from these earlier studies it is not possible to draw any qualitative conclusions with respect to specific gene up- or downregulation. However, if one investigates quantitative differences in gene expression in different neoplasms, an interesting phenomenon occurs, at least in rat liver. This finding is seen in Figure 15.1, in which the activities of four different enzymes and the glycogen content of rat liver and of nine highly and well-differentiated hepatocellular carcinomas exhibiting chromosome numbers as shown is demonstrated. In each box there are three distinct points related to activities and content on a 12%, 30%, and 60% protein diet. The dark areas indicate the enzyme activity. While there are relatively few qualitative differences in normal and neoplastic tissue, the striking characteristic is that the set of data for each neoplasm is unique to that neoplasm and also distinguishes it from normal liver. Other studies have also indicated the heterogeneity of phenotypes of each neoplasm studied (Mehle et al., 1993; cf. Arvan, 1992). While this finding may be interpreted in many ways, one scenario is that the alterations reflect the beginning of karyotypic instability, which is the basic alteration in the stage of progression (Chapter 9). Interestingly, some degree of this has also been seen in preneoplastic lesions in the liver (see below).

This phenotypic heterogeneity of the regulation of gene expression in neoplasms, mostly hepatic in origin, is the complete opposite of the Warburg and Greenstein concepts of the biochemistry of neoplasia as described earlier in this chapter. The establishment of the Morris series of transplanted hepatocellular carcinomas as a major model system for the study of the biochemistry of neoplasia served to accelerate the search for critical biochemical differences between normal and neoplastic cells. Well-differentiated and, to a lesser extent, even poorly differentiated hepatic neoplasms (cf. Potter and Watanabe, 1968) exhibit phenotypic heterogeneity of altered regulation of genetic expression. Such diverse populations of neoplasms as mouse hepatomas

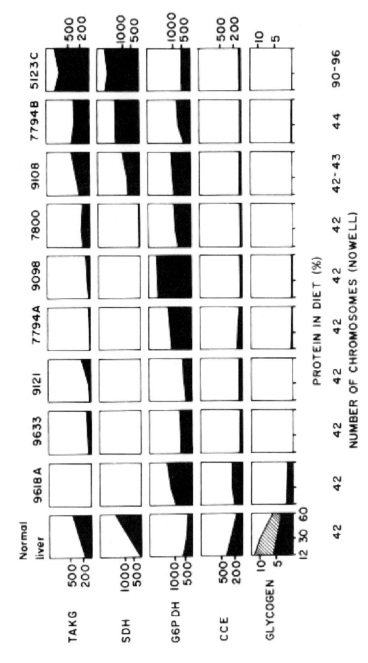

Figure 15.1 Activities of four enzymes and the glycogen content of rat liver and nine Morris hepatomas having the chromosome numbers shown in the bottom line. Each box indicates, by means of the darkened areas, the level of each of the four enzymes and the glycogen content of animals on a 12%, 30%, and 60% protein diet fed for at least 1 week. The abbreviations are as follows: TAKG, tyrosine aminotransferase; SDH, serine dehydratase; G6PDH, glucose 6-phosphate dehydrogenase; CCE, citrate cleavage enzyme. (From Potter et al., 1969, with permission of the authors and publisher.)

(Reynolds et al., 1971), myelomas (M. Potter, 1972), rat mammary adenocarcinomas (Hilf et al., 1970), human endometrial cancers (Siracky, 1979), human renal cell carcinomas (Mehle et al., 1993), and many others (Dexter and Calabresi, 1982) exhibit metabolic, genomic, and regulatory heterogeneity. The phenotypic heterogeneity shown in Figure 15.1 indicates the variation in quantitative enzyme levels under three different environmental conditions (dietary protein contents) in normal liver and in nine different, well-differentiated hepatocellular carcinomas. As the reader can appreciate, no vertical set of five boxes is identical with any other. On the other hand, there is no single enzyme abnormality or regulatory abnormality common to all neoplasms studied. Further investigations of the Morris tumors as well as other well-differentiated hepatic neoplasms have not uncovered any duplicate phenotypes. Unfortunately, with the possible exception of the regulation of cell replication or DNA synthesis, which may be considered to be abnormal in all neoplasms as the operational part of our definition (Chapter 2), no single regulatory mechanism has thus far been found to be abnormal in all neoplasms investigated. Thus, the search for a specific biochemical abnormality present in all neoplasms and directly related to the neoplastic transformation has not borne fruit, but all neoplasms exhibit one or more abnormalities in the regulation of genetic expression as might be expected from the definition of neoplasia (Chapter 2).

A somewhat analogous situation to the findings in Figure 15.1 may be implied by data on the phenotypic heterogeneity of preneoplastic enzyme-altered foci developing during the stage of promotion in rat hepatocarcinogenesis (Buchmann et al., 1992; Hendrich et al., 1987). While these data of phenotypic heterogeneity of preneoplastic lesions are not quantitative, the data are certainly compatible with the concept that preneoplastic cells and neoplastic cells during the early stages of progression show a degree of heterogeneity of gene expression that suggests that no single qualitative chemical defect common to all neoplasms will ever be discovered. However, such data do indicate that an understanding of the mechanism of this variability may be one key that helps to unlock the door to our understanding of the entire process of the neoplastic transformation.

Mechanisms of Regulatory Cybernetics and Its Abnormalities in Preneoplasia and Neoplasia

Although the listing in Table 15.3 and the data in Figure 15.1 describe a number of alterations in the regulation of metabolism or gene expression in several different neoplasms in rodents, the data do not give insight into the mechanisms involved in these alterations. This omission is not due to a lack of effort but rather to the paucity of information on such mechanisms at the time of these studies. Within the last two decades, considerable advances have been made in our understanding of the mechanisms of the regulation of genetic expression in mammalian systems. In this section, several major areas of these mechanisms and examples of their abnormalities both in preneoplasia and in neoplasia are considered.

Signal Transduction

The role of signal transduction as a means whereby environmental stimuli alter gene expression and cellular metabolism is now well established, as already discussed in previous chapters (Chapter 7 and 9). A reiteration of this material is not necessary or appropriate here, but some examples may clarify the subjects of this chapter.

Preneoplasia

As noted in Chapter 7, the principal if not sole function of promoting agents is the activation of signal transduction pathways mediated by specific receptors or indirectly through closely related pathways. The mechanisms of these effects involve reversible reactions between the promoting agent (ligand) and the receptor. Thus, the phenotype of cells in the stage of promotion (preneoplastic cells) is a function of the enhanced gene expression resulting from the induced signal transduction in the constant presence of the promoting agent. This is also true for the induction of reactive oxygen radicals, mostly indirectly, by promoting agents which cause oxidoreduction of glutathione, protein thiols (Dalton et al., 1999), and induced valence changes in heavy metals, especially iron (cf. Cimino et al., 1997; Chapter 3).

Although considerable effort has been directed toward an understanding of the mechanisms of action of promoting agents as signal transducers, the expression of genes involved in signal transduction pathways in preneoplastic lesions has not been a frequent topic of study. Table 15.4 shows a short list of alterations in growth factors and their receptors in preneoplastic lesions in several tissues induced by several different carcinogenic regimens. In mouse epidermis, there generally appears to be an increase in the expression of two different growth factors as well as their receptors. This in itself may lead to an enhancement of growth of such cells by an internal metabolic loop termed autocrine secretion in which the cell produces both a growth factor and the receptor mediating its signal transduction pathway (Chapter 16). In the mouse the more common basophilic preneoplastic foci exhibit little if any expression of transforming growth factor α, whereas the acidophilic foci almost all express this gene. In the rat, transforming growth factor α is rarely expressed in preneoplastic foci (Pitot et al., 1996). The more advanced lesion of nodular hyperplasia seen in the human liver in at least one study shows a majority of lesions expressing this growth factor. In contrast, in mouse liver foci, transforming growth factor β showed a significant decrease in all foci investigated (Moser et al., 1996). Growth factor receptors and G proteins for the most part showed some increase in almost all of the preneoplastic lesions listed in the table. Obviously, this table is not meant to be exhaustive, but rather to indicate that components of signal transduction pathways are altered, mostly with increases in various preneoplastic lesions. Since promoting agents in general induce the expression of signal transduction pathways (Chapter 7), the increases seen in this table might well be expected. However, it must be remembered that both the molecular and cellular phenomena of the stage of promotion are reversible upon removal of the promoting agent, and thus the changes seen in this table are in turn reversible. The molecular mechanisms of the changes listed in Table 15.4 were discussed in Chapter 7 and in detail with three commonly used promoting agents. Thus, such mechanisms would be underlying the changes seen in the table and are not reiterated here.

Neoplasia

As in preneoplasia, signal transduction pathways in neoplasia may also be expressed at higher levels than in their normal counterparts. In fact, true to the definition of neoplasia itself, at least one signal transduction pathway is defective in every neoplasm, although the defective pathway may not be the same in different neoplasms, as suggested by the phenotype heterogeneity noted earlier. As the stage of progression continues, the rule is to see more and more defective pathways regulating genetic expression. However, unlike the case in preneoplasia, these defects occur in the absence of any exogenous agent such as a promoting agent, although promoting agents may enhance the alterations seen in neoplasia. In neoplasia, unlike most preneoplasias, the defectiveness of the signal transduction pathways is, in a number of proven cases, the result of one or more mutations in the pathway, usually at critical points. Such mutations may be one or more of those listed in Table 6.1. In many other instances the mechanism of change is not known. While it is impossible to present a comprehensive listing of such defects seen in numerous neoplasms, a number of examples are given in Table 15.5. Although there have been some examples (Chapter 7) in which simple mutations (microlesions, Table 7.6) in key genes involved

Table 15.4 Alteration in Components of Signal Transduction Pathways in Preneoplasia

Growth factors	Tissue/Species	Lesion	% Altered	Change	Reference
Insulin-like growth factor-I	Epidermis/mouse	Papilloma	82	Increase	Rho et al., 1996
Transforming growth factor α	Epidermis/mouse	Papilloma	100	Increase	Rho et al., 1994
	Epidermis/human	Keratoacanthoma	0	—	Ho et al., 1991
	Esophagus/rat	Preneoplastic epithelium	0	—	Wang et al., 1996
	Liver/mouse	Basophilic foci	1.8	Increase	Moser et al., 1997
		Acidophilic foci	99	Increase	Moser et al., 1997
	Liver/human	Focal nodular hyperplasia	71	Increase	Schaff et al., 1994
	Renal cell/rat	Renal cell dysplasia	93	Increase	Everitt et al., 1997
Transforming growth factor β	Liver/mouse	Foci	100	Decrease	Moser et al., 1996
Growth Factor Receptors					
Epidermal growth factor receptor	Liver/mouse	Basophilic foci	3.0	Increase	Moser et al., 1997
		Acidophilic foci	55	Increase	Moser et al., 1997
	Esophagus/rat	Preneoplastic epithelium	0	—	Wang et al., 1996
	Epidermis/mouse	Papillomas	90	Increase	Rho et al., 1994
Insulin-like growth factor-I receptor	Epidermis/mouse	Papillomas	20	Increase	Rho et al., 1996
G Protein					
K-Ras	Pancreas/rat	Adenoma	33	Increase	Silverman et al., 1990

Table 15.5 Some Signal Transduction Pathway Alterations in Neoplasia in Vivo

Component	Tissue/Species	Change (No.)	Mechanism	Reference
Growth factors				
Epidermal growth factor	Pancreas, duct/hamster	0 (10)	—	Visser et al., 1996
Fibroblastic growth factor 1	Liver/human	↑ (6/31)	?	Chow et al., 1998
Insulin-like growth factor 1	Epidermis/mouse	↑ (13/21)	Enhanced transcription	Rho et al., 1996
Insulin growth factor 2	Stomach/human	↑ (5/6)	LOI	Wu et al., 1997
	Renal cell/human	↑ (7/7)	LOI	Oda et al., 1998
	Mammary/rat	↑ (10/10)	Enhanced transcription	Huynh et al., 1996
Fibroblastic growth factor-3 (int-2)	Breast/human	↑ (10/99)	Gene amplification	Donovan-Peluso et al., 1991
Transforming growth factor α	Breast/human	↑ (40/82)	?	Mizukami et al., 1990
	Renal cell/human	↑ (6/10)	Enhanced transcription	Gomella et al., 1989
Transforming growth factor β	Epidermis/mouse	↑ (10/10)	Enhanced transcription	Krieg et al., 1991
	Liver/human	↑ (10/10)	Enhanced transcription	Ito et al., 1990
	Renal cell/human	↑ (10/10)	Enhanced transcription	Gomella et al., 1989
Pleiotropin	Breast/human	↑ (16/27)	Enhanced transcription	Fang et al., 1992
Vascular endothelial growth factor	Breast/human	↑ (19/22)	Enhanced transcription	Brown et al., 1995
Growth factor receptors				
Epidermal growth factor receptor	Squamous cell carcinoma/human	↑ (8/21)	Gene amplification and enhanced transcription	Ishitoya et al., 1989
	Astrocytoma/human	↑ (3/10)	Gene amplification and rearrangement	Burgart et al., 1991
	Esophageal adenocarcinoma/human	↑ (5/13)	Gene amplification	Al-Kasspooles et al., 1993
ERBB2 (HER2-NEU)	Breast/human	↑ (~20%–25%)	Gene amplification	Schwab, 1998
		↑ (9%–39%)	Gene amplification	Tripathy and Benz, 1993
Hepatocyte growth factor receptor chain (c-met)	Stomach/human	↑ (15/64)	Gene amplification	Kuniyasu et al., 1992
Insulin-like growth factor-1 receptor	Epidermis/mouse	↑ (6/11)	Enhanced transcription	Rho et al., 1996

Gene/factor	Tissue/species	Change	Alteration	Reference
Insulin-like growth factor-2 receptor	Liver/rat and human	↓ (11/33)	Mutations (point) and deletions	Mills et al., 1998
Nerve growth factor (trk) receptor	Breast/human	↓ (70/80)	?	Natali et al., 1992
Transforming growth factor β receptor	Hereditary nonpolyposis colorectal cancer/human	↓ (~85%)	Various mutations, loss, rearrangement, truncation, etc.	cf. Reiss, 1997
G proteins and related factors				
H-Ras	Bladder/human	↑ (1/1)	Gene amplification	Hayashi et al., 1983
	Liver/mouse	↑ (25/50)	Point mutation	Bauer-Hofmann et al., 1992
	Breast/human	↑ (30/39)	?	Czerniak et al., 1989
K-Ras	Colon/human	↑ (?) (40%)	Point mutation	Bos, 1988
	Lung/human	↑ (?) (6/137)	Gene amplification	Shiraishi et al., 1989
	Ovary/human	↑ (5%–10%)	Gene amplification	Berchuck et al., 1992
N-Ras	Leukemia/human	↑ (67%)	Enhanced transcription	Gougopoulou et al., 1996
Protein kinases	Glioblastoma/human	? (1/1)	Gene rearrangement	Mitsunobu et al., 1989
c-Raf	Stomach/human	? (1/1)	Gene rearrangement	Nakatsu et al., 1986
Protein kinase C	Colon carcinoma/human	↓ (11/11)	?	Guillem et al., 1987
TRK	Papillary thyroid carcinoma/human	↑ (4/20)	Gene rearrangement	Bongarzone et al., 1989
Other signal transduction components				
β-catenin	Colon cancer/human	↑ (50%)	Point mutations	Munemitsu et al., 1995
	Liver/human	↑ (24/49)	Point mutations	de La Coste et al., 1998
				Koch et al., 1999

in signal transduction pathways may be found during the stage of promotion, it is likely that such mutations allow the preneoplastic cell the growth advantage necessary for its development as a readily identified lesion. Even with such mutations, however, preneoplastic cells in the absence of the promoting agent do not enjoy the growth advantage occurring with continued stimulus of the promoting agent.

Of the numerous studies on alterations in signal transduction pathways in neoplasms, only a relatively small number of the more commonly studied alterations are considered here. Some further detail, especially on growth factor components, are described in Chapter 16. Table 15.6 lists a number of alterations in specific components of signal transduction pathways, beginning with ligands, primarily growth factors, their receptors, and some of the better studied distal components of these pathways. The table consists of isolated examples that reflect the more general literature. In many instances the mechanism of the effect noted is not understood, but very likely reflects a change in gene expression. Whether this is due to amplification or some other major genetic alteration or simply a microlesional mutation that somehow affects expression is not clear at this time. However, where mechanisms are better understood, they are listed in the table. It is noteworthy that of the growth factors listed, only the example of epidermal growth factor production by pancreatic ductular carcinomas in the hamster shows no change in the expression of this gene. In virtually every other instance there is an increase in expression owing to enhanced transcription, loss of imprinting (LOI), or gene amplification.

In contrast to the growth factors themselves, the expression of growth factor receptors is increased in a number of instances; most of the examples given are due to gene amplification, but in other instances there is a marked decrease or even loss of expression of growth factor receptors such as the insulin-like growth factor-II receptor and the transforming growth factor β receptor. This appears to be the result of significant mutational alterations, both micro- and macrolesional. This raises the interesting possibility that the loss of growth factor receptors would make a neoplasm unresponsive to such growth factors, while their presence or even enhanced expression would give a distinct advantage to neoplasms having these characteristics. This is discussed more extensively in Chapter 16.

The G proteins of the *ras* family comprise an extremely large multigene family (Kaziro et al., 1991). The three examples in this table are those that have been best studied. It should be noted that both point mutations as well as gene amplification and enhanced transcription are mechanisms involved with the altered expression of these components, as well as their altered catalytic activity, as was discussed earlier (Chapter 7). The relatively high incidence of point mutation of the H-*ras* gene in mouse hepatomas is not seen in preneoplastic lesions in the liver of the mouse, where only 10% exhibit this mutation (Bauer-Hofmann et al., 1992). Enhanced expression of the protein kinase, c-*raf*, in the examples given is due to gene rearrangement. Similarly, the activation of the *abl* proto-oncogene is due to a gene rearrangement as described in Chapter 6. Many other such similar alterations in kinases as well as in transcription factors (see below) are listed in Table 6.8. Finally, in this table the signal transduction pathway involving the APC tumor suppressor gene (Chapter 5) has as a key component β-catenin (Figure 15.2). As noted in the figure, the APC gene, together with two other genes, GSK and AXIN, are required for proteolytic elimination of β-catenin by the proteasome. Mutations of APC prevent this effect, allowing the β-catenin concentration to build up and, together with other nuclear transcription factors, TCF and CPB, enhance transcription. It is of interest to note that this pathway is also linked to the pathways involved in cell-cell interactions through integrins (Chapter 10) and that mutations in β-catenin have been found in a large number of other neoplasms including those of the liver, melanomas, and ovarian neoplasms (cf. Morin, 1999).

Although it is very likely that abnormalities and signal transduction pathways play a major role in the abnormal growth and development of neoplastic tissue, other components of the cell's

Table 15.6 Alterations in Transcription Factors in Neoplasia in Vivo

Factor	Neoplasia/Species	Frequency	Mechanism	Result	Reference
c-Maf	Myeloma/human	25%	t(16q23)	Fusion protein	Chesi et al., 1998
c-Myb	Various/human	>50%	Gene amplification	Enhanced transcription	Oh and Reddy, 1999
c-Myc	Various/human	10%–20%	Gene amplification t(8:14)	Enhanced transcription	Garte, 1993
	Burkitt lymphoma/human	~80%	t(8:14)	Inappropriate expression	Neri et al., 1988
NF-kB	Cutaneous lymphoma/human	55%	Fusion gene	Enhanced transcription	Neri et al., 1996
REL	Diffuse large cell lymphoma/human	23%	Gene amplification	Enhanced transcription	Houldsworth et al., 1996
N-Myc	Neuroblastoma/human	35%	Gene amplification	Enhanced transcription	Cohn et al., 1990
p53	Various/human	~50%	Mutations	Reduced degradation of the protein	Hainaut and Hollstein, 2000
Retinoic acid receptor	Acute promyelocytic leukemia/human	~90%+	t(15:17)	Fusion protein	Warrell et al., 1993
WT1	Wilms tumor/human (stromal predominant)	60%	Deletion/mutation	Inactivation	Schumacher et al., 1997

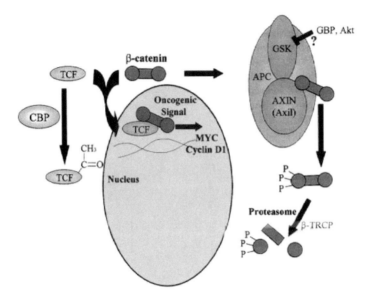

Figure 15.2   The APC/β-catenin pathway and its regulatory components. In a normal situation where no mutations occur in any of the proteins noted, β-catenin is actively targeted by the APC complex for proteasome degradation. However, mutations in β-catenin may stabilize the protein, preventing its proteasomal digestion and allowing it to activate the transcription factors noted including MYC and cyclin D_1. Other components may also control this pathway. (Modified from Morin, 1999, with permission of the author and publisher.)

metabolic machinery also play major roles in the molecular mechanisms of the "relative autonomy" and altered cell replication of neoplastic cells. The remainder of this chapter covers several of these cellular metabolic functions for which a reasonable amount of information is available on the mechanisms of the abnormalities seen in neoplastic tissue.

Transcription Factors

As seen from discussions in Chapter 7, the final common pathway of signal transduction is mediated by transcription factors interacting directly with specific sequences in DNA. Permanent alterations or mutations in transcription factors of a number of different types have been noted in neoplastic cells. These include dominant negative mutations in which an alteration in the structure of one allele of a transcription factor leads to the formation of a protein which interrupts the function of the normal allele (Sheppard, 1994). Also, amplification, deletion, and gene fusion following translocation resulting in the formation of new genes (Chapter 6) are seen with transcription factors in neoplasms.

Transcription factors and some of their functions have previously been cited in Chapters 6, 7, and 9, especially in relation to the action of tumor promoting agents and the transcriptional regulation of the cell cycle through the E2F family of transcription factors (Farnham et al., 1993; Bernards, 1997). However, the complexity of transcriptional activation of gene expression has become more apparent during the last few years. Not only are transcription factors themselves critical in this process, but also coactivators, accessory proteins, and other components are involved, some of which interact with other sequences in DNA while at the same time affecting the expression of the transcriptional factor through protein:protein interactions (cf. Martin,

1991). Figure 15.3 shows an artist's conception of the action of RNA polymerase in the presence and absence of the E2F/DP heterodimeric transcription factor, the latter in the presence of the activator Sp1 or the inhibitor Rb (Chapter 9). Several "basal factors" involved in RNA polymerase action are also noted. The diagram is a considerable oversimplification of this process, in analogy to other transcriptional activation processes.

Alteration in the expression of transcription factors in neoplasms is a relatively common event in neoplasia but relatively uncommon in preneoplasia. One example of the alteration of transcription factor expression, in particular c-*jun*, is seen in the expression of preneoplastic foci and even single hepatocytes in livers of mice administered diethylnitrosamine (Nakano et al., 1994). Its complexing partner, c-*fos*, has also seen increased expression in preneoplastic aberrant

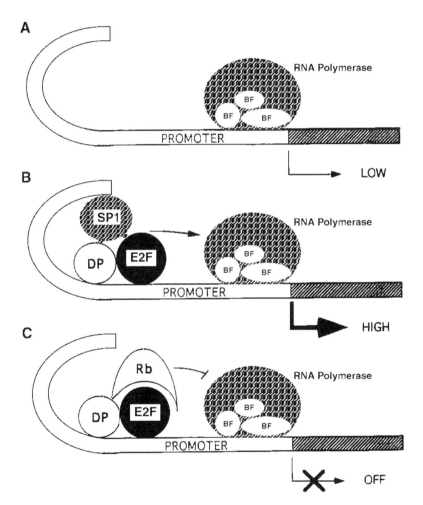

Figure 15.3 A scheme showing the action of a heterodimeric transcription complex of DP and E2F. A. When no transcription factor is bound, the rate of transcription by RNA polymerase is low. B. The heterodimeric transcription factor binds and is also associated with an enhancing factor, SP1, which in turn then interacts with RNA polymerase to stimulate transcription, resulting in a high rate of transcription of the gene. C. Unphosphorylated Rb binds to the DP/E2F complex and prevents its action with the RNA polymerase, thus suppressing the expression of the gene. BF, basal factors of the RNA polymerase complex (see text).

colonic crypts in rats (Stopera et al., 1992). In neoplastic lesions, alterations in several of the more commonly studied transcriptional factors are seen in Table 15.3. Only a few examples are given, but this does not mean that there are not other numerous examples, some of which are referred to in the reviews cited. Those factors that have been most extensively studied have also shown the greatest degree of alteration and types of alteration, as exemplified by the p53 tumor suppressor gene, the c-*myc* cellular oncogene, and the c-*myb* cellular oncogene. Numerous examples of fusion genes involving transcription factors have also been described (Chapter 6), and only a few of the more common examples are noted in the table. Interestingly, none of the E2F family members have been found to be mutated in human cancers. A similar finding has been reported with the transcription factor c-*jun*, a critical member of the important Ap-1 transcription heterodimer (cf. Rahmsdorf, 1996).

As noted in the table, several of the genes listed are amplified in a variety of different neoplasms, resulting in enhanced transcription. The fusion proteins involving c-*myc* and the retinoic acid receptor effect the expression of the former in cells where the protooncogene is normally not expressed, and of the retinoate receptor in an altered receptor/transcription factor that may inhibit the action of the normal factor such as in a dominant mutation (see above). The variety of mutations seen in the p53 gene involve both an alteration in the protein such that its normal turnover or degradation is reduced, allowing for an enhanced amount of protein present, and also in many instances interference with the function of the normal allele through a dominant mutation mechanism (Hainaut and Hollstein, 2000). The WT1 gene is found to be mutated in about 60% of a specific morphological type of Wilms tumor, that exhibiting a stromal-predominant pattern (Schumacher et al., 1997). Patients having neoplasms exhibiting different histologies have a lower apparent rate of mutation of the WT1 gene; as yet, it is not certain what gene is involved in a number of cases of Wilms tumor.

Although this table gives a very small representation of alterations in transcription factors in neoplasms, it is not unlikely that virtually every neoplasm exhibits some form of alteration in one or more transcription factors. Such changes, which are genetically determined as the stage of progression advances, then may interact with alterations in cell cycle components, leading to the altered growth patterns characteristic of neoplasms in general.

The Cell Cycle and Neoplasia

Alterations in the cell cycle and its components are generally considered to be found only in the stage of progression and not in promotion or preneoplasia. Studies of both mouse mammary tumor development (Said and Medina, 1995) and in human colorectal neoplasia (Polyak et al., 1996) support this statement, although cyclin A was found to be overexpressed in all hyperplasias in mouse mammary glands (Said and Medina, 1995). In addition, Robles and Conti (1995) have demonstrated that premalignant lesions in mouse skin carcinogenesis exhibited an increased level of cyclin D1 as investigated by an immunohistochemical technique. Interestingly, Balasubramanian et al. (1998) found dramatic increases in cyclin kinase inhibitors in skin papillomas, in contrast to the finding in most neoplasms (Table 15.7). On the other hand, there has been considerable work on the expression of cell cycle components in neoplasms (Draetta and Pagano, 1996); therefore this discussion focuses primarily on this topic.

As noted in Chapter 9, control mechanisms for the cell cycle involve both a cascade of protein phosphorylations that relay a cell from one stage to the next and a set of checkpoints that monitor the completion of critical events and may delay progression to the next stage of the cell cycle if required to maintain cell function (Collins et al., 1997). A diagram of the various regulators of the cell cycle is shown in Figure 15.4. In this figure, the crucial role of E2F is noted, as was discussed in Chapter 9 (Figure 9.5). Also noted in the figure by asterisks are those genes

Table 15.7 Alterations in Cell Cycle Regulators and Components in Neoplasia in Vivo

	Neoplasia/Species	Change	Mechanism	Reference
Cyclin-dependent kinases				
CDK1	Squamous cell carcinoma/mouse	↑	Enhanced transcription	Balasubramanian et al., 1998
CDK4	Sarcomas, gliomas/human	↑	Gene amplification	cf. Hall and Peters, 1996
Cyclin-dependent inhibitors				
p15	Squamous cell carcinoma/human	→	Mutation ?	cf. Michalides, 1999
p16	Various neoplasms/human	→	Deletions	cf. Hall and Peters, 1996
	Ovarian carcinoma/human		Aberrant transcription	Suh et al., 2000
p18	Various neoplasms/human	→	Mutations	cf. Millard and Koff, 1998
p27	Breast carcinoma/human	→	(Few mutations)	Tan et al., 1997
Cyclin-dependent phosphatases				
cdc25	Breast carcinoma/human	↑	?	cf. Orlowski and Furlanetto, 1996
Cyclins				
Cyclin A	Leukemias/human	↑	Enhanced transcription	Paterlini et al., 1993
	Squamous cell carcinoma/mouse	↑	Enhanced transcription	Balasubramanian et al., 1998
Cyclin D	Various neoplasms/human	↑	Gene amplification	cf. Hall and Peters, 1996
			Chromosomal rearrangement	cf. Peters, 1994
	Mammary carcinoma/rat	↑	Enhanced transcription	Sgambato et al., 1995
Cyclin E	Various neoplasms/human	↑	Gene amplification	cf. Donnellan and Chetty, 1999
Chromosomal function				
Bub1	Colon/human	→	Mutations (?)	Cahill et al., 1998

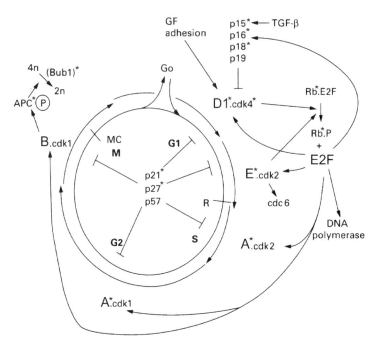

Figure 15.4 Positive ($\rightarrow$) and negative ($-|$) regulators of the cell cycle and the critical role of E2F in this process. Those symbols associated with an * indicate that that gene product is abnormally expressed in neoplasia, many of the abnormalities noted more particularly in Table 15.7. The designations for the components of the cell cycle, cyclins, phases, and cdks are the same as shown in Figure 9.5. Inhibitors of the cyclins are shown in two families, the INK4 family which encompasses p16, p15, p18, and p19, and the CIP/Kip family, including p21, p27, and p57 (cf. Michalides, 1999). Bub1, gene involved in chromosome segregation; GF, growth factors; adhesion, cell adhesion components and pathways; APC, tumor suppressor gene of familial adenomatous polyposis. (Modified from Michalides, 1999, with permission of the author and publisher.)

altered in one or more neoplasms by mutation of one or more mechanisms, e.g. amplification, base mutation, deletion, fusion, etc. In addition to the pathways noted in Figure 15.4, the role of E2F and its association with p53 in growth control, growth arrest, and apoptosis is noted in Figure 15.5. A more detailed listing of the functional abnormalities of these various components scored by an asterisk in Figures 15.4 and 15.5 is given in Table 15.7.

The central role of E2F when activated by release of Rb by phosphorylation is shown in this figure, as in Figure 9.5. In addition, the tempering effects of E2F on members of the INK4 family of cyclin inhibitors, while at the same time enhancing the expression of the cyclins and their kinases, indicate the delicate balance with which the cell cycle is regulated. The examples noted in Table 15.7 of alterations in several cell cycle regulators and components are by no means complete and are only given as examples. Again, it is quite likely that at least one and usually more than one of these components are abnormal through mutation, amplification, or enhanced transcription in virtually all neoplasms in the stage of progression. Furthermore, alterations in these components appear to become more severe as progression continues (Said and Medina, 1995). As noted from the table, gene amplification and mutations appear to be the more common changes seen in these various factors. In many instances, the nature of the mutation is unknown and may reflect other allelic changes, including deletion. Alterations in the p27 cyclin-

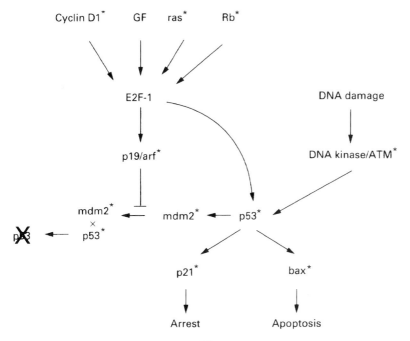

Figure 15.5 Diagram of the E2F-p19^{ARF}-p53 connection between growth control, growth arrest, and apoptosis. Those genes having an * indicate abnormalities in neoplastic cells, some of which are considered in Table 15.7 and others, e.g., p53, Rb, in the text previously. See text for discussions of mdm2, bax, ATM, and p19/arf. The figure emphasizes the critical roles of E2F-1 and p53. (Modified from Michalides, 1999, with permission of author and publishers.)

dependent inhibitor in which there is a decrease if not total elimination of expression appear not to result from mutations in most cases (cf. Millard and Koff, 1998). The changes in the cyclins that have been noted are largely due to gene amplification and chromosomal rearrangement, especially in the case of cyclin D1. A variety of neoplasms have exhibited such changes in the expression of this gene as well as in cyclin E, both of which play key roles in entrance into the cell cycle. Mutational inactivation of the Bub1, whose product is concerned with the proper segregation of chromosomes in cells, may play a significant role in the development of aneuploidy in neoplastic cells (Cahill et al., 1998).

Functional Consequences of Alterations in Cell Cycle Components

In general, as shown from studies in yeast (Hartwell and Kastan, 1994), significant alterations in the expression of any one of the components of the cell cycle may, over time, lead to derepression of the cycle, aneuploidy, and chromosomal abnormalities. However, in most instances one sees abnormalities in more than one component of the cell cycle within any neoplastic cell. Simple overexpression of cyclins D1 or E leads to accelerated transition through G1, reduced growth factor dependency. However, in the case of these two cyclins, simple overexpression does not appear to result in cell transformation in most instances (cf. Michalides, 1999), although association with alterations in p53 may do so. Amplification of cyclin D1 is a very common event in many human neoplasms (Hall and Peters, 1996).

Alterations in cyclin kinase, especially Cdk4, as well as cyclin-dependent kinase inhibitors, especially p16, have also been characterized in a number of human neoplasms (Hall and Peters, 1996). However, several of the cyclin kinase inhibitors such as p21 and p27 have rarely if at all been found in a mutation form in neoplasms. In human ovarian carcinoma, a lack of mutation of the p16 gene was found, although there was expression of aberrant p16 RNA transcripts (Suh et al., 2000). On the other hand, since p21 expression is regulated by p53 and mutations in p53 are found in a number of malignancies, loss of p53 function may result in loss of the normal functioning of p21 and other checkpoint control components (Orlowski and Furlanetto, 1996). Despite the lack of mutations in p27 found in human cancer, deletions of this gene have been seen in a number of aggressive carcinomas in the human (cf. Millard and Koff, 1998). Like p16, p18 is commonly mutated in a number of human neoplasms (cf. Millard and Koff, 1998).

As noted earlier (Chapter 6), a variety of "stress signals"—including DNA damage, hypoxia, etc.—lead to activation of the p53 tumor suppressor gene. This, in turn, can potentially lead to a variety of different functions, as noted in Figure 15.5. E2F-1 induces p53 expression which, like DNA damage via the DNA kinase, may cause arrest of the cell cycle in normal cells. The p19^{ARF} protein interacts with E2F-1 and is important in the transcriptional activation by E2F-1. Furthermore, p53 induces mdm-2, which subsequently binds and destabilizes p53 in the feedback loop noted in Figure 15.5. Although mdm-2 has been termed a proto-oncogene, it was originally discovered as one of several genes in a transformed cell line resulting from amplification of double minute particles, from which the terminology mouse double minute (mdm) was derived. The mdm-2 protein physically associates with the p53 tumor suppressor protein, blocking its transactivational effects. In addition, it seems to stimulate degradation of the protein (Haines, 1997). mdm gene amplification is quite common in a number of neoplasms (Haines, 1997; Flørenes et al., 1994). E2F-1 enhances the expression of p53 and also neutralizes mdm-2 through its stimulation of the expression of p19/arf (cf. Michalides, 1999). The ATM gene codes for a multifunctional enzyme having various kinase activities and involved in the response to DNA damage (Lavin and Shiloh, 1997). p53 also transactivates both the p21 cyclin-dependent inhibitor as well as BAX, which enhances apoptosis (cf. Brady and Gil-Gómez, 1998). Enhanced expression of BAX has been noted in prostatic neoplasia (Johnson et al., 1998), but low levels of BAX expression have been associated with a poor clinical outcome in breast cancer (Krajewski et al., 1995). Alternatively, p53 may induce apoptosis in cells. Mutations in this tumor suppressor gene thus lead to a lack of apoptotic response to DNA damage in neoplastic cells, which is quite commonly seen in many neoplasms.

Cell Cycle Checkpoints in Neoplasia

As noted in Figures 15.4 and 9.5, the checkpoints of the cycle occur at the G1/S interface, at the end of G2, and in M. Defects in each of these checkpoints have been noted in neoplasia. In addition, the restriction (R) point at which the decision is made whether to enter the mitotic cycle is another component that may be defective in neoplastic cells. The (R) and G1/S checkpoint defects may be in part due to the overexpression of D and E-type cyclins seen in so many neoplasms (Hunter and Pines, 1994). Defects in p53 also result in defective G1/S checkpoint function in neoplastic cells (cf. Sherr, 1996) as well as genetic instability (cf. Morgan and Kastan, 1997). Defects in the cyclin B-Cdk1 (Cdc2) phosphorylation, resulting in activation of the complex in neoplastic cells, allow the neoplastic cell to enter mitosis with damaged DNA (cf. Hunter and Pines, 1994). Mutations in the Bub1 gene (Figure 15.7), which controls the mitotic checkpoint and chromosome segregation, are seen in a variety of human neoplasms (Cahill et al., 1998). Alterations in this gene and related genes involved in the completion of normal mitosis can lead to aneuploidy, a hallmark characteristic of cells in the stage of progression (cf. Molinari, 2000).

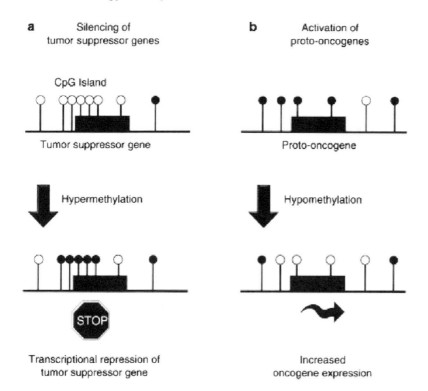

Figure 15.6 Mechanisms for potential roles of DNA methylation in neoplastic development. Unfilled circles denote unmethylated CpGs; filled circles indicate methylated CpGs. a. Aberrant hypermethylation of CpG islands could result in their transcriptional silencing or repression. In all examples, the gene is indicated by the filled rectangle. b. Hypomethylation of CpG dinucleotides in protooncogene promoter regions may facilitate an increased expression of the proto-oncogene. (Adapted from Laird, 1997, with permission of author and publisher.)

Thus, it may be noted that numerous defects occur in the cell cycle of neoplastic cells and contribute ultimately to the evolving karyotypic instability characteristic of the stage of progression (Chapter 9). Since, as noted earlier, enhanced mitotic activity may lay the foundation for enhanced aberrations in the cell cycle on the basis of mutation and/or selection, other mechanisms of regulating DNA expression may be found to be abnormal. Knowledge and understanding of such mechanisms may allow the elucidation of the transition of preneoplastic cells exhibiting few if any mutational alterations into neoplastic cells in the stage of progression that exhibit the profound mutational alterations discussed above. One such mechanism may be found in the alterations of DNA methylation, discussed below.

DNA Methylation in Preneoplasia and Neoplasia

As discussed in Chapter 3, the methylation of cytosine in DNA constitutes a mechanism not only of regulating the expression of DNA but also of maintaining the normal chromosomal integrity of the cell. These two mechanisms are quite interrelated, as more recent studies have indicated (cf. Jones and Laird, 1999; Gray et al., 1999). Methylation of cytosine residues in DNA occur primarily adjacent to guanine residues, forming CpG sequences in the DNA molecule. Where multiple CpG sequences are repeated up to about 1 kb in length, the region is termed a CpG island (cf. Laird, 1997). The methyl groups of the CpG sequence do not affect base pairing but do influence protein-DNA interaction by protruding into the major groove (Razin and Riggs, 1980). In general, DNA methylation in CpG islands within promoter regions of specific genes inhibits the transcription of the gene by interfering with transcription initiation through reducing the binding affinity of sequence-specific transcription factors (cf. Jones and Laird, 1999). Furthermore, methylation-dependent, sequence-specific DNA-binding proteins that have been described (cf. Hendrich and Bird, 1998) may act as transcriptional repressors. Particularly in relation to our consideration of the stage of progression, DNA hypomethylation of mammalian cells enhances mutation rates (Chen et al., 1998) and may lead to chromosome and genomic instability (cf. Jones and Gonzalgo, 1997; Xu et al., 1999).

Figure 15.6 is a simplistic diagram demonstrating the silencing of tumor suppressor genes and the activation of proto-oncogenes. In this diagram, tumor suppressor gene silencing involves hypermethylation of CpG islands, as has been documented in a number of instances (see below). Proto-oncogene activation, on the other hand, may occur as a result of decreased methylation of specific CpG dinucleotides rather than CpG islands. As discussed in Chapter 3, endogenous mutation of genes may result from oxidative deamination of 5-methylcytosine to thymine. The mismatch monitoring repair system reverses the effect of these mutations in the vast majority of instances where they occur in vivo (Chapter 3). Thus, alterations in DNA methylation may theoretically be involved in cancer causation by a variety of mechanisms, as indicated in Figure 15.6 and mentioned in the paragraph above.

Preneoplasia

There is substantial evidence that changes in DNA methylation occur during the stage of preneoplasia. This evidence comes from the demonstration both of global changes in DNA methylation as well as changes in CpG methylated sites in specific genes. At the moment there is little if any evidence for alterations in the methylation of CpG islands during the preneoplastic process. In addition, diets deficient in precursors of methyl groups have been shown to induce DNA hypomethylation quite effectively and rapidly (Wainfan and Poirier, 1992). Several such diets also induce neoplasia, especially in the liver, upon prolonged administration (cf. Poirier, 1994, Chapter 3). Some suggestions that alterations in DNA methylation alone are sufficient for initiation have also been made (Boehm and Drahovsky, 1983). However, other studies indicate that such is not the case (Sawada et al., 1990) but rather that diets deficient in methyl group precursors are effective promoting agents at least in the liver (Yokoyama et al., 1985). This may be expected, since alteration in DNA methylation results in alterations in gene expression (see above). Furthermore, the effects of methyl-deficient diets are completely reversible, both as to the lesions induced and the methylation status of the DNA in the liver (Christman et al., 1993). The latter process, involving global DNA methylation as well as methylation of specific genes, recovers more slowly than the restoration of the normal morphology of the liver. It is important to note, however, that these latter studies investigated only a relatively few CpG sites of specific genes by the technique of isoschizomer restriction enzyme analysis. Thus, the slower return to normal DNA methylation status with this technology may not reflect the methylation of many DNA CpG sites, since there is no substantial evidence that global DNA methylation is retarded upon return to normal dietary administration. The slow return to normal DNA methylation status of some sites may reflect cell turnover.

Table 15.8 shows examples of the relative global and specific gene alterations in DNA methylation in some putatively preneoplastic lesions. Global DNA methylation occurs quite early upon feeding severely methyl-deficient diets, as early as 1 week after initiation of the diet. Simultaneous with such global demethylation, increases in the levels of mRNAs were seen for

Table 15.8 Alterations in DNA Methylation in Preneoplasia

DNA Region of Methylation	Carcinogen or Process	Tissue/Species	Alteration[a]	Reference
Global	Methyl-deficient diets	Liver/rat	Hypomethylation	Wainfan and Poirier, 1992 Christman et al., 1993
Global	Dichloro- or tri-chloroacetic acid	Liver/mouse	Hypomethylation (transient)	Tao et al., 1998
c-*myc*	1,2-Dimethyl-hydrazine	Liver nodules/rat	Hypomethylation*	Rao et al., 1989
	N-nitrosomor-pholine	Liver nodules/rat	Hypomethylation*	Münzel et al., 1991
c-Ha-*ras*, c-*fos*	Methyl-deficient, amino acid-defined diet	Liver/rat	Hypomethylation*	Zapisek et al., 1992
CDKN2/p16	Spontaneous	Esophageal dysplasia/human	Hypermethylation**	Klump et al., 1998
	NNK[b]	Squamous metaplasia in lung/rat	Hypermethylation**	Belinsky et al., 1998
β-hydroxy-β-methylglutaryl coenzyme A reductase	1,2-Dimethylhydra-zine or aristo-cholic acid	Liver nodules/rat	Hypomethylation*	Rossiello et al., 1994
Growth hormone	Spontaneous	Colon polyps/human	Hypomethylation*	Goelz et al., 1985
Glutathione S-transferase π	Methyl-deficient diet	Liver/rat	Hypomethylation**	Steinmetz et al., 1998

[a]In most studies of global hypomethylation, total 5-methylcytosine amounts in the DNA were determined. However, in those studies having an * by the alteration, the isoschizomer technique was utilized; in those with **, the bisulfite, with DNA sequencing, was used to analyze and determine the presence or absence of DNA methylation.
[b]NNK = 4-(Methylnitrosamino)-1-(3-pyridyl)-1-butanone.

several oncogenes and decreases in other genes such as epidermal growth factor receptors (Wainfan and Poirier, 1992). Even administration of a specific hepatocarcinogen, such as dichloroacetic or trichloroacetic acid, causes transient decreases in the level of 5-methylcytosine in DNA in the liver. Interestingly, determination of exposure to dichloroacetic, but not trichloroacetic acid, resulted in an increase of 5-methylcytosine in adenomas to the level found in noninvolved liver, suggesting different mechanisms for the two carcinogens (Tao et al., 1998). The majority of the studies on alterations in CpG methylation in specific sites with the isoschizomer restriction enzyme technique could be related to alterations in the expression of the gene. Interesting exceptions were noted in a specific gene, CDKN2/p16, an inhibitor of the cell cycle in which bisulfite conversion of unmethylated cytosines to uracil results in DNA sequence changes, which can be analyzed and the specific methylcytosine sites determined. This technique is more accurate than the isoschizomer technology, which looks at only several specific sequences but not at many other regions containing methylated cytosines (Saluz and Jost, 1993). Similar findings were seen with the glutathione S-transferase pi gene, specifically in the promoter region of animals placed on a methyl-deficient diet (Steinmetz et al., 1998). In this instance, specific sites in the promoter region of the gene, several involving transcription factors that might otherwise not have been noted with the isoschizomer technique were found to be hypomethylated. This is in congruence with the high expression of the gene both in the livers of animals fed the methyl-deficient diet and in preneoplastic and neoplastic lesions in the livers of these animals. The presence of hypomethylation of specific genes in benign neoplasms of the liver in the rodent and in the colon in the human (Table 15.8) further suggests that some changes in methylation of specific CpGs may be important in the early development of neoplasia during the stage of promotion and extending into the stage of progression.

Neoplasia

It is becoming increasingly clear that alterations in DNA methylation in one or more genes in neoplasia are likely without exception (cf. Liang et al., 1998; Baylin et al., 1998). The examples of global hypomethylation in neoplastic cells are numerous and most definitive in rapidly growing, less differentiated neoplasms (Gama-Sosa et al., 1983; Kim et al., 1994). A few examples of altered methylation of specific genes in neoplasms may be noted in Table 15.9. In many of the references given, the newer and more definitive technology of bisulfite treatment with subsequent PCR and sequencing is utilized. Both hypo- and hypermethylation of CpG dinucleotides are seen in components of the various genes listed. In most instances, the methylation occurs in the regulatory region of the gene and in general this may be correlated with an enhanced expression of the gene in the case of DNA hypomethylation or a repression of expression with DNA hypermethylation. In the case of glutathione S-transferase, π hypermethylation occurs in two different types of neoplasms in the human, whereas hypomethylation occurs in hepatomas in the

Table 15.9 Altered Methylation of Specific Genes in Neoplasia

Gene	Change[a]	Tissue/Species	Reference
Albumin	Hypermethylation*	Hepatoma/rat	Vedel et al., 1983
α-Fetoprotein	Hypomethylation*	Hepatoma/human	Peng et al., 1993
Glutathione S-transferase π (1)	Hypermethylation**	Hepatoma/human	Tchou et al., 2000
	Hypermethylation*	Prostate carcinoma/human	Lee et al., 1994
	Hypomethylation**	Hepatoma/rat	Steinmetz et al., 1998
E-cadherin	Hypermethylation*	Hepatoma/human	Kanai et al., 1997
	Hypermethylation**	Gastric carcinoma/human	Tamura et al., 2000
Methylguanine-DNA methyltransferase	Hypermethylation**	Many types/human	Esteller et al., 1999
Oncogenes and tumor suppressor genes			
bcr-abl fusion gene	Hypermethylation**	Chronic myelogenous leukemia/human	Zion et al., 1994
DNA mismatch repair gene – hMLH1	Hypermethylation**	Gastric cancer/human	Fleisher et al., 1999
BRCA1 gene	Hypermethylation**	Sporadic breast and ovarian cancer/human	Esteller et al., 2000
p16 tumor suppressor gene	Hypermethylation**	Lung adenocarcinoma/rat	Belinsky et al., 1998
c-myc	Hypomethylation*	Hepatoma/human	Nambu et al., 1987

[a]The indication of methodology used is the same as that in Table 15.8.

rat. In all of these instances, the correlation with expression of the gene is quite close. Hypermethylation of the repair enzyme methylguanine-DNA methyltransferase, with resultant repression, may be associated with alteration in response to specific drugs or carcinogens (Esteller et al., 1999). Hypermethylation has been consistently associated with the repression of tumor suppressor genes, several examples of which are noted in the table. In the case of proto-oncogenes, one might suppose that hypomethylation would be the rule, as is noted in the case of c-*myc* in human hepatomas, where increased expression is associated with hypomethylation (Nambu et al., 1987). However, an interesting exception to this generalization is noted in the progressive de novo DNA methylation at the *bcr-abl* cellular oncogene locus during the progression of chronic myelogenous leukemia (Zion et al., 1994). In this instance, patients with this condition who exhibit dramatic hypomethylation of this gene at the time of diagnosis invariably demonstrate increased methylation of the fusion gene as the disease progresses. Thus, the great majority of the information available in this field demonstrates that alterations in DNA methylation occur early during the natural history of the development of neoplasia and progressively become more deviant as the cell enters and continues in the stage of progression. As already noted, such changes in DNA methylation lead to dramatic alterations in the expression of specific genes as well as in genomic stability. While it is tempting to speculate that such alterations in DNA methylation may be the basis for the evolving karyotypic instability seen in the stage of progression, such a conclusion is clearly premature at this time.

Alterations in Genomic Imprinting

In Chapter 5 the phenomenon of genomic imprinting was discussed (Figure 5.7), and several neoplasms having a genetic basis to their etiology were discussed in relation to the potential importance of genomic imprinting in their neoplastic expression (Table 5.7). In neoplasms not having a genetic basis, the loss of imprinting (LOI) or alteration in the normal imprinting pattern of a specific gene may be seen in a variety of neoplasms (Table 15.10). Although the table indicates only five genes that have been relatively well studied in neoplasms as compared with their normal counterparts, some 20 or more imprinted genes have been described in the mouse (Kelsey and Reik, 1998), involving at least seven different chromosomes. Many of these genes

Table 15.10 Some Imprinted Genes in Rat (r), Mouse (m), and Human (h) and Their Alterations in Neoplasia

Imprinted Gene/Function	Expressed Allele in Normal Tissue	Alteration in Neoplasia	Neoplasm/ Syndrome	Reference
Igf2/growth factor	Paternal (m, h)	LOI	Glioma (h)	Uyeno et al., 1996
		LOI	Ewing's sarcoma (h)	Zhan et al., 1995
		LOI	Gastric cancer (h)	Wu et al., 1997
		LOI	Renal cell cancer (h)	Oda et al., 1998
H19/RNA, function unknown	Maternal (m, h)	LOI	Numerous types (h) of neoplasms	Looijenga et al., 1997
Igf2R/Igf2 clearance receptor/mannose 6 PO$_4$ receptor	Maternal (r, m)	LOI?	Liver, mammary gland (r, m)	de Souza et al., 1997
p57^{KIP2}/cyclin-cdk inhibitor	Maternal (m, h)	LOI	Wilms tumor (h)	Taniguchi et al., 1997
p73/homologous to *p53*	Maternal (h)	LOI	Renal cell cancer (h)	Mai et al., 1998

have counterparts in the human and rat, in which imprinting has also been demonstrated, although occasionally the imprinting pattern between species differs (Bartolomei and Tilghman, 1997). As noted in the table, the imprinted genes most extensively investigated in neoplasia are the *Igf2* (insulin growth factor-2) and *H19* genes. LOI of *Igf2* has been seen in a variety of neoplasms, as noted in the table; in hepatic neoplasms in the human, however, biallelic expression of the gene in this tissue occurs after birth (cf. Aihara et al., 1998). But in the rodent, the imprinting of this gene is maintained during adult life (cf. Bartolomei and Tilghman, 1997). While this species differential may be related to imprinting of specific promoter regions in this gene (Wutz and Barlow, 1998), the *Igf2* gene lies immediately adjacent to the *H19* gene in rodents and the human. Note that the *H19* gene expresses the maternal allele, while *Igf2*, the paternal allele (Table 15.10). Thus, the expression of the two genes is closely linked, and the differential imprinting has led to a number of theories related to the mechanism of this effect (Tilghman et al., 1993; Banerjee and Smallwood, 1995). The abnormal expression of these two genes is felt to be an important factor in the phenotype of patients with the Beckwith-Wiedemann syndrome (Table 5.1), which is characterized by extensive overgrowth postnatally and neoplasms such as Wilms tumor of the kidney (Reik and Maher, 1997). A couple of recent investigations have suggested that CTCF, a specific DNA binding protein that binds in the region intermediate between the two genes, may play a major role in this mechanism (Bell and Felsenfeld, 2000; Hark et al., 2000).

While the *Igf2* receptor gene (mannose 6-phosphate receptor) is paternally imprinted, most of the alterations that have been described involve major mutations and deletions of the gene rather than specifically LOI. Such lack of or uncontrolled expression of the gene is felt to play a role in both the early and late stages of hepatic neoplasia (de Souza et al., 1997). The $p57^{KIP2}$ cdk inhibitor is also found in the same region as the *Igf2/H19* complex in mouse, human, and rat; thus one might expect to see the effects noted in the table in Wilms tumors. The actual function of p73 is not clear as yet, and thus it is difficult to relate the LOI of this gene to specific functions in neoplasia. However, it is apparent from even these few studies that LOI can play an important role in the alteration of genetic expression so characteristically seen in neoplasms in the stage of progression.

Altered Mechanisms of Apoptosis in Neoplasia

As discussed in Chapter 7, one of the characteristics of promoting agents is their effectiveness in inhibiting the process of apoptosis in preneoplastic cells. Just as with many other mechanisms that are transiently altered in preneoplastic cells by the presence of the promoting agent, alterations in mechanisms of apoptosis, as in cell replication, likely are altered in some way in virtually every malignant neoplasm (cf. Laderoute, 1994). Furthermore, an extensive study by Staunton and Gaffney (1995) suggested that the apoptotic index was characteristic of each histogenetic type of neoplasm. The apoptotic index generally was greater than or similar to the mitotic index for the individual type of neoplasm under study. Already discussed is the importance of the increased expression of the *bcl-2* proto-oncogene, the apoptotic inhibitor, in follicular lymphomas (Figure 6.8).

While a variety of pathways have been shown to be involved in the induction of apoptosis (Figure 7.14), central themes are now becoming obvious in relation to the development of apoptosis in normal and neoplastic cells. Figure 15.7 is a simplified diagram of potential mechanisms for the effects of DNA damage- as well as oncogene-induced apoptosis. Already discussed is the importance of the *p53* tumor suppressor gene in activating apoptosis in normal cells as a result of DNA damage, the effect apparently mediated through the ATM gene (Figure 15.5). In this figure, it is noted that the p53 protein enhances the expression of the proapoptic gene, *bax*,

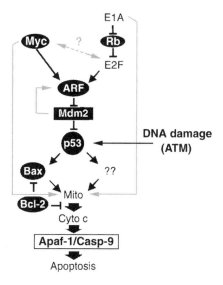

Figure 15.7   Diagram of DNA damage- and oncogene-induced apoptosis. Oncogenes and proto-onco-genes such as E1A and c-*myc* respectively induce apoptosis through both p53-dependent and -independent pathways as noted in the figure. Both pathways may facilitate cytochrome c release from mitochondria which in turn effects the activation of the caspase cascade. Components of this pathway that have been shown to be mutated in neoplasms are shown in black. Mito, mitochondria; Cyto c, cytochrome c; Apaf-1, caspase adapter; Casp-9, caspase-9 and caspase cascade. (Modified from Lowe and Lin, 2000, with permission of the authors and publisher.)

which effects alterations in mitochondrial permeability, resulting ultimately in activation of the caspase pathway to apoptosis. Similarly, the proto-oncogene c-*Myc*, as well as the viral onco-gene E1A, inhibits the effect of the specific p53 inhibitor Mdm2 mediated through ARF. By this mechanism *p53* is activated and the same situation as noted with DNA damage occurs. Muta-tions of genes, as noted in the figure, can result in alteration of the apoptotic pathway either through the *p53* tumor suppressor gene or by bypassing it and acting directly on the *bax/bcl-2* pathway or other pathways not completely understood (Lowe and Lin, 2000).

   A variety of other methods for the induction of apoptosis through specific ligand/receptor mechanisms are also present in many cells throughout the organism. Several of these are dis-cussed later in the text (Chapter 17). However, as noted in the figure, the extensive potential for alteration in genes required for the basic apoptotic mechanism seen in Figure 15.7 is indicative of the statement that most if not all neoplasms exhibit one or more abnormalities in these steps in this critical process governing the ultimate growth of neoplasms in the host.

Telomerase and Its Alteration in Neoplasia

Telomeres are repeat sequences found at the distal ends of chromosomes, forming a cap or end to the chromosome and preventing interactions between chromosomes that may threaten their structure and/or stability (Greider and Blackburn, 1996). While the repeated sequence occurring in telomeres may vary in length from 5 to 15 kb, the maintenance of telomere length presents a problem in cell replication because lagging-strand synthesis is not able to fully replicate the te-lomere end (Figure 15.8). From the figure, it becomes obvious that cells must possess one or more mechanisms to solve the problem noted in the figure—i.e., to prevent telomeres from be-

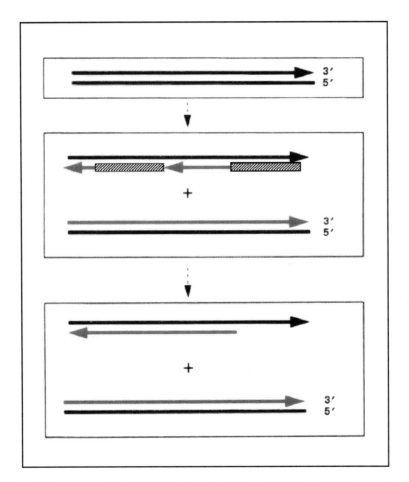

Figure 15.8 The telomere end-replication problem seen diagrammatically. During DNA replication, synthesis of the lagging strand requires an RNA primer (lined box). The primers that are extended by DNA polymerase are subsequently removed, leaving gaps which the polymerase can repair as long as they do not occur at the end of the telomere because there is the absence of a primer 5′. As a result, one daughter strand will lack the DNA previously encoded by the terminal sequence. If no correction is made, then the DNA sequence will decrease in length each time cell replication occurs. (Adapted from Hamilton and Corey, 1996, with permission of the authors and publisher.)

coming progressively shorter during successive cell divisions, as such a process ultimately leads to a loss of viability. The solution of this problem by the cell was reported by Blackburn and associates (Greider and Blackburn, 1985) in the discovery of telomerase, an enzyme that has the function of extending telomeres.

Telomerase is actually an RNA-dependent DNA polymerase of specialized function. Figure 15.9 presents a model for telomerase action in which the enzyme possesses an RNA having sequences complementary to the telomeric DNA of the region. As shown in the figure, telomerase may extend the DNA sequences by the telomeric repeats for the appropriate number of species and tissue. In this way, telomeres would not decrease in size, as shown in the problem diagrammed in Figure 15.8. Recent studies by Griffith and associates (1999) indicate that proteins binding to telomeres may also be involved in the formation of a large duplex loop of the telomere, which may be concerned with the protection and replication of telomeres. There is also evidence that cells may use other mechanisms besides polymerase to solve the end-replication problem, specifically mechanisms involved in the repair of double-strand DNA breaks (cf. Colgin and Reddel, 1999). Mice whose telomerase gene has been eliminated by gene targeting (Chapter 5) did not appear to show any significant phenotypic differences from normal animals when first reported (Blasco et al., 1997), but later investigations of a similar strain of telomerase-negative mice indicated that these animals exhibited a somewhat shortened life span and increased incidence of spontaneous neoplasia (Rudolph et al., 1999).

Following Blackburn's discovery, a number of observations noted that chromosome ends became shorter in cells during aging, both in vivo and in vitro (cf. Shay, 1995). In addition, telomerase activity in the majority of somatic tissues in adult animals was found to be essentially nonexistent. Exceptions were in the germ cells and also in some stem cell populations (cf. Bacchetti, 1996). Investigation of neoplastic cells demonstrated that, in contrast to normal cells, most neoplastic cells do possess telomerase activity, although they usually have relatively short telomeres (cf. Ishikawa, 1997). More detailed studies, however, have not shown a consistent absence of telomerase in normal tissues and an increased activity in the neoplastic tissues (e.g., King et al., 1999; Kojima et al., 1997). An example of one study of a variety of human neoplasms and the activity of telomerase in these tissues is seen in Table 15.11. Note that many normal tissues do not exhibit activity of the enzyme, while others do. In some instances, such as large cell carcinoma of the lung, the telomerase activity is essentially equal to that of normal tissue. Preneoplastic lesions of liver (Kitamoto and Ide, 1999; Tsujiuchi et al., 1996), prostate (Zhang et al., 1998), lung (Yashima et al., 1997), and ovary (Wan et al., 1997) did exhibit telomerase activity, but usually at a lesser level than that seen in neoplastic tissues. Other studies, however, have indicated that there may be no general tendency toward telomere reduction in malignant tissues (Schmitt et al., 1994) and that telomerase activity may well be a biomarker of cell proliferation rather than malignant transformation (Belair et al., 1997). In some studies, progressive telomere shortening and telomerase reactivation are associated with tumor progression (Miura et al., 1997; Sawyer et al., 1996) and the cell cycle (Harley and Sherwood, 1997). Thus, while many neoplasms exhibit increased telomerase activity and some degree of telomeric presence in their cells, it does not appear that all neoplasms exhibit this interesting change in vivo. The next chapter takes up telomerase loss and reactivation during cell culture as a characteristic of the neoplastic transformation in vitro.

Isozymes, Mutant or "Unique" Proteins, and Fetal Gene Expression in Neoplasia

One of the anticipated results of biochemical studies of neoplasia was the discovery of an enzyme or protein unique to the neoplastic cell. However, an apparently unique protein species could be the result of the derepression of a normally quiescent segment of the genome expressed in fetal but not in adult tissue of the same lineage, or it could be genuinely unique, as the result of one or more mutations in a gene for an enzyme or protein of the normal cell of origin. The presence in tumor tissue of "new" proteins not found in their cell of origin but resulting from expression of genetic information normally repressed in the cell of origin has been described repeatedly. This latter mechanism is directly related to the "relative autonomy" of the neoplastic cell in the sense of its inability to regulate the expression of its own genetic material, as is done by its cell of origin.

In 1959, Markert and Moller coined the term *isozyme*, which was generally defined as a member of a family of multiple, separable forms of enzymes occurring within the same organism and having the same or very similar catalytic activity. Examination of such isozyme families

in neoplasms, especially those of rodent liver, demonstrated that several isozymic forms of enzymes occurred in experimental hepatomas but were either absent or at very low levels in normal
liver. In 1982, Weinhouse reviewed much of the literature to date on this subject in relation to
murine hepatic lesions, demonstrating that the new and unique isozymic forms seen in neoplasms, as compared with their cell of origin, could almost always be found in other normal
tissues in the adult or in the cell of origin of the neoplasm during fetal life. A "unique" aldehyde
dehydrogenase was found in rat hepatomas by Lindahl (1979) but was later found to be induced
in normal adult tissues by some carcinogenic agents, especially 2,3,7,8-tetrachlorodibenzo-*p*-
dioxin (Hempel et al., 1989). Some enzymes and proteins in tumors were found to differ in the
nonprotein portion of the molecule, thus leading to an apparent new "isozyme," as reported with
γ-glutamyltranspeptidase (Tsuchida et al., 1979), and also with the iron storage protein ferritin
(Linder et al., 1975).

The altered isozyme composition of neoplasms is not ubiquitous but appears to be more
characteristic of the poorly differentiated, rapidly growing tumors than of the highly differentiated, slowly growing neoplasms. Thus, the appearance of fetal or other isozymes in neoplasms
may be related to tumor progression, as suggested by Weinhouse (1973). On the other hand, the
appearance of fetal forms of proteins in neoplastic cells is not unique to isozymes. In fact, the
expression of fetal genes in neoplasms in the adult is the rule rather than the exception. As with
other biochemical characteristics of neoplasms, however, this expression also appears to be quite

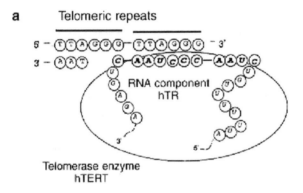

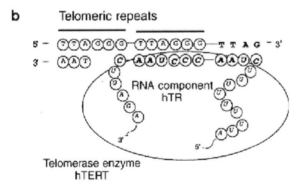

Figure 15.9   Model for telomerase action. a. Binding of telomerase to the end of telomeric DNA via the
RNA component of the enzyme. b. The RNA component of telomerase serves as a template for the extension of the telomere 3′ end. c. Translocation of telomerase along the newly synthesized strand. d. Further
extension of the telomere 3′ end occurs, and the process continues with subsequent translocation-extension

variable and heterogeneous. Furthermore, expression of a fetal gene is not unique to the neoplastic state but may occur in vivo in certain pathological conditions such as inflammation and regeneration. Cultured cells may also express fetal genes in vitro, as exemplified by the investigations of Sirica and associates (1979).

While these earlier studies laid the foundation for identifying and understanding differences in phenotypes of various neoplasms, it was not until the advent of the "explosion" in molecular biological techniques and knowledge in the last two decades that structural differences in a variety of proteins in neoplasms resulting from mutational alterations in the genes for such proteins became well documented. Unlike the situation 25 years ago, when few if any documented alterations in protein structure could not be accounted for by altered gene expression in neoplasms, today there is considerable evidence for the presence of mutant proteins and their genes within neoplastic cells. The majority of such examples occur within cellular oncogenes, which by definition are mutated cellular genes, and in tumor suppressor genes. Many of these

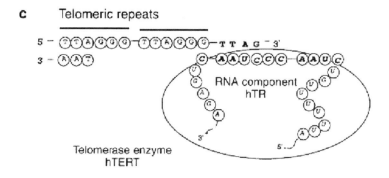

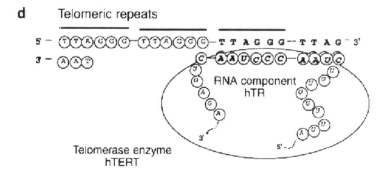

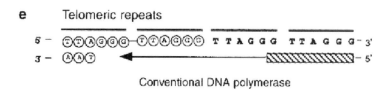

steps. e. Synthesis of the complementary strand (C-rich) then occurs by extension of an RNA primer by a conventional DNA polymerase. Removal of the RNA primer leaves a 3′ overhang at the telomeric end. hTR, human telomerase RNA component; hTERT, human telomerase reverse transcriptase. (Adapted from Urquidi et al., 1998, with permission of the authors and publisher.)

Table 15.11 Expression of Normalized Telomerase in Tumors and Corresponding Healthy Tissues

Cell or Tissue Type	Tissue	Normalized Telomerase[a]	Tumor in Sample, %[b]
Pancreas	Healthy tissue	0.00	
	Healthy tissue	0.00	
	Healthy tissue	0.00	
	Adenocarcinoma	0.36	30
	Adenocarcinoma	6.11	70
	Neuroendocrine tumor	2.77	90
Lung	Healthy tissue	0.54	
	Healthy tissue	0.51	
	Healthy tissue	0.34	
	Large cell carcinoma	0.53	40
	Adenocarcinoma	20.1	40
	Adenocarcinoma	2.41	60
	Adenocarcinoma	6.57	60
	Nondifferentiated carcinoma	5.84	40
Colon	Healthy tissue	6.54	
	Healthy tissue	7.44	
	Adenocarcinoma	1.95	60
	Adenocarcinoma	3.49	20
	Adenocarcinoma	19.8	80
	Adenocarcinoma	3.43	40
	Adenocarcinoma	0.00	40
Esophagus	Healthy squamous epithelium	0.50	
	Healthy squamous epithelium	4.94	
	Healthy squamous epithelium	1.26	
	Adenocarcinoma	3.40	20
	Adenocarcinoma	8.54	50
	Adenocarcinoma	5.94	30
	Adenocarcinoma	7.35	15
	Adenocarcinoma	6.47	10
	Adenocarcinoma	10.57	10
Bladder	Healthy epithelium	0.00	
	Healthy epithelium	0.00	
	Healthy epithelium	0.00	
	Carcinoma	1.37	80
	Carcinoma	14.80	50
	Carcinoma	1.80	70
	Carcinoma	10.17	70
	Carcinoma	25.25	75
	Carcinoma	7.41	50

[a]Normalized telomerase = $100 \times$ (telomerase/*rRNA*).
[b]Percentage of tumor cells in frozen tumor sections stained with hematoxylin and eosin was scored by a pathologist.
Adapted from de Kok et al., 2000, with permission of the authors and publisher.

alterations have been discussed in this chapter and earlier chapters, but by way of review some of the better-documented structural alterations in such genes are listed in Table 15.12. Although the p53 tumor suppressor gene has been discussed earlier, it is important to emphasize the extremely high rate of mutations seen in this gene in human neoplasia (cf. Hainaut and Hollstein, 2000). In Figure 15.10 may be noted the percentage and relationship of transitional and transversional mutations in this gene in a variety of different human neoplasms.

The importance of p53 function has been previously noted in Figure 15.9 in a highly simplified diagram. The role of p53 as "guardian of the genome" is implied from that figure in that, in the presence of DNA, damage with subsequent activation of p53 by the ATM kinase mediated by a checkpoint kinase (Hirao et al., 2000; Morgan and Kastan, 1997) can lead to arrest of the cell cycle by transactivation of the cyclin inhibitor p21, allowing repair to occur. This is paralleled by activation of an apoptotic pathway which, if the cell damage is not repaired in a timely fashion or cannot be repaired, leads to death of the cell. Mutations in p53 to a great extent alter its transactivation capabilities, thus interrupting its guardian function and allowing the cell to survive and replicate with major DNA damage. Although mutation of the p53 gene may be considered an initiation event, most studies both in humans (e.g., Navone et al., 1993; Tanaka et al., 1993; Kuwabara et al., 1998) and animals (Miller, 1999) indicate that such mutations are identified predominantly during the stage of progression. Furthermore, during the stage of progression there is ample evidence that elimination of wild-type p53 activity leads to gene amplification (Livingstone et al., 1992), chromosome instability (Shao et al., 2000), and genomic instability due to alteration in checkpoint function (cf. Smith and Fornace, 1995). Thus, loss of p53 function may contribute in a major way to the evolving karyotypic instability characteristic of the stage of progression.

The PTEN tumor suppressor gene appears to be a regulator of specific kinases involved in signal transduction (Sun et al., 1999). Somatic mutations of the PTEN gene have been seen in acute myeloid leukemia (Liu et al., 2000) and hepatocellular carcinomas (Kawamura et al., 1999). The PTEN gene appears to function in neoplasms of the endometrium as a "gatekeeper," as does the p53 gene for a number of other tissues as well (Ali, 2000). Genes having "caretaker" functions may be those such as the mismatch repair genes found defective in hereditary non-polyposis colorectal carcinoma (Chapter 5). The concept of gatekeeper and caretaker has been proposed and discussed by Kinzler and Vogelstein (1997). Allelic imbalances and somatic mutations of the p16 tumor suppressor gene, an inhibitor of CDK4 (Table 15.7), were seen in soft tissue sarcomas (Schneider-Stock et al., 1998).

Mutations in cellular adhesion molecules involved in invasion and metastasis have also been described, as indicated previously in Chapter 10. In particular, genes of the cadherin family, which are considered tumor suppressor genes, are mutated in a fairly high percentage of breast cancers (Berx et al., 1996) and very likely in a variety of other human neoplasms (cf. Semb and Christofori, 1998). Mutations in the catenin gene, which is involved in the function of

Table 15.12 Genes and Gene Families Commonly Exhibiting Mutations in Neoplasia

---

p53
PTEN
Cell cycle inhibitors, e.g., p16
Cadherins, catenins, and other genes involved in cell-cell interactions
Receptors
G proteins
Transcription factors

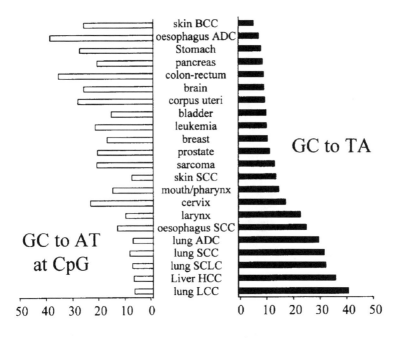

Percentage of Mutations

Figure 15.10 Relationship between CpG transitions and GC to TA transversions in the p53 cDNA. Neoplasms have been listed according to the frequency of GC to TA transversions (increasing from top to bottom). Note that those neoplasms exhibiting a low frequency of GC to TA transversions show a high frequency of CpG transitions and vice versa. Generally it is considered that neoplasms exhibiting a low level of p53 CpG transitional mutations and high GC to TA transversion mutations are associated with or caused by exogenous risk factors. (Adapted from Hainut and Hollstein, 2000, with permission of the authors and publisher.)

the APC tumor suppressor gene (Chapter 5), have been noted in both human neoplasms (Koch et al., 1999) and those induced in animals (Ogawa et al., 1999). Other proteins involved in such cell adhesion function include integrins and the CD44 glycoprotein family. In both of these instances, neoplasms express isoforms that their cells of origin frequently do not (cf. Rudzki and Jothy, 1997; Schapira, 1981). The other three types of protein listed in the table have been discussed rather extensively in this chapter and will not be discussed again here. It is sufficient to say that mutations in proto-oncogenes, resulting in their conversion to cellular oncogenes, and in tumor suppressor genes are undoubtedly ubiquitous in neoplasia although it is not yet clear in exactly which stage of neoplastic development the predominant mutations occur, nor, with the exception of specific hereditary conditions involving single tumor suppressor genes (Chapter 5), what the actual initiation mutation is.

Secondary Biochemical Changes Resulting from Alteration of Genetic Expression

It appears that the principal mechanisms resulting in the alteration of genetic expression in neoplastic cells concern themselves with the processes of transcription or translation or both, but changes in the concentration and/or presence of specific enzymes have distinct ramifications in the ultimate phenotype of the neoplastic cell. Such changes are seen in structural lipids, especially the glycolipids, and in their presence or absence on the surface membrane of the cell. Hakomori and Kannagi (1983) have summarized many of the data concerning changes in the expression of these molecules that result from alterations in levels of enzymes responsible for their synthesis in a variety of different neoplasms. Such surface changes may affect the antigenicity of the neoplastic cell (Chapter 15) or its metastatic potential. The appearance or disappearance of specific glycolipid structures on the surface of the cell may also express a fetal phenotype.

In addition to glycolipids, the lipid composition of neoplasms, especially hepatomas, differs from that of normal liver (cf. Ruggieri and Fallani, 1979), as does the fatty acid composition of phosphatides of normal and malignant epidermis (Carruthers, 1967). Such changes would be expected because of the altered regulation of enzymes synthesizing sterols as well as fatty acids (Sabine, 1975). In particular, Van Hoeven and his associates (1975) demonstrated in a study of several different mouse and rat hepatomas that the plasma membranes of such cells exhibited increased cholesterol content and a decrease in the degree of unsaturation in the fatty acids of most lipid classes in the neoplasms.

Illustrating further ramifications of such structural alterations resulting from changes in the regulation of genetic expression, a number of studies have indicated both altered and decreased interaction of hormones with their receptors and the activation of adenylate cyclase in neoplasms of both the human and lower animals (cf. Hunt and Martin, 1979). Pezzino et al. (1979) have shown that five malignant hepatomas of varying growth rates have lowered capacities for binding insulin and glucagon to membrane receptors; this may be due to a decrease in receptor number, lowered affinity, or site-site interactions of the hormones, receptors, and plasma membrane structures. These findings further demonstrate the ramifications of altered genetic expression, which can, in turn, lead to alterations in the ability of environmental factors to initiate intracellular mechanisms leading to the control of gene expression.

The importance of structural alterations in proteins resulting from changes in the regulation of genetic expression is probably not completely appreciated at the present time. The pioneering studies of Hakomori and associates pointed out the importance of glycolipid and other structural component changes which in turn alter the function of the cell. Olden (1993) has emphasized that the expression of aberrant oligosaccharide moieties of glycoproteins and glycolipids is a typical characteristic of essentially all animal and human neoplasms regardless of their causative mechanisms. Thus, it is obviously not necessary to have mutations in specific proteins in order to alter functional characteristics of cells; rather, alterations and the regulation of genetic expression may be of equal or greater importance than mutational alterations in specific proteins and groups of proteins.

THE CELL AND MOLECULAR BIOLOGY OF PRENEOPLASIA AND NEOPLASIA—ITS ROLE IN OUR UNDERSTANDING OF THE NEOPLASTIC PROCESS

As noted in this chapter, the development of our understanding of the cell and molecular biology of the neoplastic process has closely paralleled advances in our understanding of the cell and molecular biology of normal cells. In retrospect, initially naïve concepts of the biochemistry of neoplasia were based on the assumption that a single biochemical abnormality could explain the neoplastic phenotype. As knowledge of the natural history of neoplastic development and of cellular and molecular biology advanced, such a concept was no longer tenable. However, today the pendulum has swung entirely in the opposite direction, in that the complexity of the cell and the molecular biology of the neoplasia are becoming more obvious, and there is no evidence of a ubiquitous, single defect resulting in this disease. Rather, it is apparent that the vast majority of the phenotypic and genotypic alterations seen in neoplasia—i.e., cells in the stage of progression—are a direct result of the primary characteristic of this stage, evolving karyotypic instability (Chapter 9).

In Table 15.13 may be seen a summary of our knowledge to date of a number of processes and functions in the cell and molecular biology of preneoplasia and neoplasia. Although the table indicates that in virtually every instance of neoplasia the cell and molecular process stated is defective, it is important to note that there is no single component of any of these processes that is ubiquitously abnormal in all neoplasms. However, the majority of neoplasms exhibit at least one defective process in each of those listed. This is indicated by ++++. In all other instances, there are examples of neoplasms that do not exhibit abnormalities in the process listed. In viewing the listing in preneoplasia, it is noted that the majority show either no or a few examples of abnormalities in the process listed. Furthermore, such as in signal transduction, the processes occurring in the preneoplastic cell are essentially normal but hyperexpressed as a result of the chronic administration of the promoting agent. Removal of the promoting agent will, of course, result in loss of cell viability (Chapter 7). The three exceptions to this generalization are seen with DNA methylation, apoptosis mechanisms, and the expression of mutant proteins. In this last instance, by our definition of initiation, one should expect that every initiated cell will have mutations in various genes and thus express mutant proteins, although examples of this are not nearly so extensive as that in neoplasia. Abnormalities in apoptosis—i.e., inhibition of this process—are characteristic of the action of promoting agents, but such an effect is lost in the absence of these agents in preneoplastic tissue. The increase or changes in DNA methylation in preneoplasia are likely ubiquitous to all preneoplastic cells, although only certain examples have been tendered (Table 15.8), but in virtually every carefully studied case such abnormalities are noted. Alterations in DNA methylation may be the basis for the transition from promotion to progression and, at least initially, for the development of karyotypic instability in progression. However, at our present state of knowledge, this is clearly a tenuous statement, and it may be that further information will bring a variety of other mechanisms to the fore as candidates for the basis of the cellular and molecular biology of neoplasia. A comparison of the cellular and mo-

Table 15.13 The Cell and Molecular Biology of Preneoplasia and Neoplasia—Summary

Cell and Molecular Process	Preneoplasia	Neoplasia
Glycolysis	+/−	+++
Regulation of gene expression	0/+	++++
Signal transduction	0/++	++++
Transcription factors	+/−	++++
Cell cycle	+	++++
DNA methylation	+++	++++
Apoptosis mechanisms	+++	++++
Telomerase	+/−	+++
Unique protein expression	0 (?)	++++
Mutant protein expression	++ (?)	++++
Unique lipid and carbohydrates	0 (?)	+++

Key: 0, no change from normal; +/−, variable or no change; + to ++++, little to substantial and consistent change from normal.

lecular biology of preneoplasia with that of neoplasia does, however, emphasize the importance of an understanding of the molecular transition between these two stages as critical to our understanding of the ultimate formation of the cancer cell.

It should be noted here, however, that alterations in a number of the cell and molecular processes that are seen in neoplasia—i.e. the stage of progression—contribute significantly to the evolving karyotypic instability characteristic of this stage. This includes alterations in components of the transcription mechanism, cell cycle, DNA methylation, telomerase, and the altered or eliminated function of specific tumor suppressor genes such as p53. This would suggest that the basis for the karyotypic instability in neoplastic cells develops from a large number of molecular alterations in the cell. The natural history of the stage of progression is thus likely to result from the successive alteration of individual mechanisms, each of which by itself could lead to genomic instability. Such a scenario may make it very difficult to design therapeutic modalities that are able to correct or interdict the evolution of karyotypic instability of the neoplastic cell.

REFERENCES

Aihara, T., Noguchi, S., Miyoshi, Y., Nakano, H., Sasaki, Y., Nakamura, Y., Monden, M., and Imaoka, S. Allelic imbalance of insulin-like growth factor II gene expression in cancerous and precancerous lesions of the liver. Hepatology, *28*:86–89, 1998.

Ali, I. U. Gatekeeper for endometrium: the PTEN tumor suppressor gene. J. Natl. Cancer Inst., *92*:861–863, 2000.

Al-Kasspooles, M., Moore, J. H., Orringer, M. B., and Beer, D. G. Amplification and over-expression of the *EGF*R and *erb*B-2 genes in human esophageal adenocarcinomas. Int. J. Cancer, *54*:213–219, 1993.

Arvan, D. A. Tumor cell heterogeneity: an overview. Clin. Chim. Acta, *206*:3–7, 1992.

Bacchetti, S. Telomere dynamics and telomerase activity in cell senescence and cancer. Semin. Cell Dev. Biol., *7*:31–39, 1996.

Balasubramanian, S., Ahmad, N., Jeedigunta, S., and Mukhtar, H. Alterations in cell cycle regulation in mouse skin tumors. Biochem. Biophys. Res. Commun., *243*:744–748, 1998.

Banerjee, S., and Smallwood, A. A chromatin model of *IGF2/H19* imprinting. Nature Genet., *11*:237–238, 1995.

Bartolomei, M. S., and Tilghman, S. M. Genomic imprinting in mammals. Annu. Rev. Genet., *31*:493–525, 1997.

Bauer-Hofmann, R., Klimek, F., Buchmann, A., Müller, O., Bannasch, P., and Schwarz, M. Role of mutations at codon 61 of the c-Ha-*ras* gene during diethylnitrosamine-induced hepatocarcinogenesis in C3H/He mice. Mol. Carcinog., *6*:60–67, 1992.

Baylin, S. B., Herman, J. G., Graff, J. R., Vertino, P. M., and Issa, J. P. Alterations in DNA methylation—A fundamental aspect of neoplasia. Adv. Cancer Res., *72*:141–196, 1998.

Becker, F. F., and Stout, D. L. A constitutive deficiency in the monooxygenase system of spontaneous mouse liver tumors. Carcinogenesis, *5*:785–788, 1984.

Beirne, O. R., and Watson, J. A. Comparison of regulation of 3-hydroxy-3-methylglutaryl coenzyme A reductase in hepatoma cells grown *in vivo* and *in vitro*. Proc. Natl. Acad. Sci. U.S.A., *73*:2735–2739, 1976.

Beirne, O. R., Heller, R., and Watson, J. A. Regulation of 3-hydroxy-3-methylglutaryl coenzyme A reductase in minimal deviation hepatoma 7288C. J. Biol. Chem., *252*:950–954, 1977.

Belair, C. D., Yeager, T. R., Lopez, P. M., and Reznikoff, C. A. Telomerase activity: a biomarker of cell proliferation, not malignant transformation. Proc. Natl. Acad. Sci. U.S.A., *94*:13677–13682, 1997.

Belinsky, S. A., Nikula, K. J., Palmisano, W. A., Michels, R., Saccomanno, G., Gabrielson, E., Baylin, S. B., and Herman, J. G. Aberrant methylation of *p16*[INK4a] is an early event in lung cancer and a potential biomarker for early diagnosis. Proc. Natl. Acad. Sci. U.S.A., *95*:11891–11896, 1998.

Bell, A. C., and Felsenfeld, G. Methylation of a CTCF-dependent boundary controls imprinted expression of the *Igf2* gene. Nature, *405*:482–485, 2000.

Berchuck, A., Kohler, M. F., and Bast, R. C. Jr. Oncogenes in ovarian cancer. Hematol. Oncol. Clin. North Am., *6*:813–827, 1992.

Bernards, R. E2F: a nodal point in cell cycle regulation. Biochim. Biophys. Acta, *1333*:M33–M40, 1997.

Berx, G., Cleton-Jansen, A.-M., Strumane, K., de Leeuw, W. JF, Nollet, F., van Roy, F., and Cornelisse, C. E-cahderin is inactivated in a majority of invasive human lobular breast cancers by truncation mutations throughout its extracellular domain. Oncogene, *13*:1919–1925, 1996.

Blasco, M. A., Lee, H.-W., Hande, M. P., Samper, E., Lansdorp, P. M., DePinho, R. A., and Greider, C. W. Telomere shortening and tumor formation by mouse cells lacking telomerase RNA. Cell, *91*:25–34, 1997.

Boehm, T. L. J., and Drahovsky, D. Alteration of enzymatic methylation of DNA cytosines by chemical carcinogens: a mechanism involved in the initiation of carcinogenesis. J. Natl. Cancer Inst., *71*:429–432, 1983.

Bongarzone, I., Pierotti, M. A., Monzini, N., Mondellini, P., Manenti, G., Donghi, R., Pilotti, S., Grieco, M., Santoro, M., Fusco, A., Vecchio, G., and Della Porta, G. High frequency of activation of tyrosine kinase oncogenes in human papillary thyroid carcinoma. Oncogene, *4*:1457–1462, 1989.

Bonkowsky, H. L., Tschudy, D. P., Collins, A., and Doherty, J. M. Control of δ-aminolevulinic acid synthetase and tyrosine aminotransferase in tumors and livers of tumor-bearing rats. J. Natl. Cancer Inst., *50*:1215–1225, 1973.

Bos, J. L. The *ras* gene family and human carcinogenesis. Mutat. Res., *195*:255–271, 1988.

Boyd, K. E., and Farnham, P. J. Identification of target genes of oncogenic transcription factors. Proc. Soc. Exp. Biol. Med., *222*:9–28, 1999.

Brady, H. J. M., and Gil-Gómez, G. Molecules in focus. Bax. The pro-apoptotic Bcl-2 family member, Bax. Int. J. Biochem. Cell Biol., *30*:647–650, 1998.

Brebnor, L. D., Grimm, J., and Balinsky, J. B. Regulation of urea cycle enzymes in transplantable hepatomas and in the livers of tumor-bearing rats and humans. Cancer Res., *41*:2692–2699, 1981.

Brown, L. F., Berse, B., Jackman, R. W., Tognazzi, K., Guidi, A. J., Dvorak, H. F., Senger, D. R., Connolly, J. L., and Schnitt, S. J. Expression of vascular permeability factor (vascular endothelial growth factor) and its receptors in breast cancer. Hum. Pathol., *26*:86–91, 1995.

Brown, M. S., Goldstein, J. L., and Siperstein, M. D. Regulation of cholesterol synthesis in normal and malignant tissue. Fed. Proc., *32*:2168–2173, 1973.

Buchmann, A., Bock, K. W., and Schwarz, M. Enzyme and immunohistochemical phenotyping of diethylnitrosamine-induced liver lesions of male C3H/He, B6C3F1 and C57BL/6J mice. Carcinogenesis, *13*:691–697, 1992.

Burgart, L. J., Robinson, R. A., Haddad, S. F., and Moore, S. A. Oncogene abnormalities in astrocytomas: *EGF-R* gene alone appears to be more frequently amplified and rearranged compared with other protooncogenes. Mod. Pathol., *4*:183–186, 1991.

Cahill, D. P., Lengauer, C., Yu, J., Riggins, G. J., Willson, J. K. V., Markowitz, S. D., Kinzler, K. W., and Vogelstein, B. Mutations of mitotic checkpoint genes in human cancers. Nature, *392*:300–303, 1998.

Carruthers, C. The fatty acid composition of the phosphatides of normal and malignant epidermis. Cancer Res., *27*:1–6, 1967.

Chen, R. Z., Pettersson, U., Beard, C., Jackson-Grusby, L., and Jaenisch, R. DNA hypomethylation leads to elevated mutation rates. Nature, *395*:89–92, 1998.

Chesi, M., Bergsagel, P. L., Shonukan, O. O., Martelli, M. L., Brents, L. A., Chen, T., Schrock, E., Ried, T., and Kuehl, W. M. Frequent dysregulation of the c-*maf* proto-oncogene at 16q23 by translocation to an Ig locus in multiple myeloma. Blood, *91*:4457–4463, 1998.

Chow, N.-H., Cheng, K.-S., Lin, P.-W., Chan, S.-H., Su, W.-C., Sun, Y.-N., and Lin, X.-Z. Expression of fibroblast growth factor-1 and fibroblast growth factor-2 in normal liver and hepatocellular carcinoma. Dig. Dis. Sci., *43*:2261–2266, 1998.

Christman, J. K., Chen, M.-L., Sheikhnejad, G., Dizik, M., Abileah, S., and Wainfan, E. Methyl deficiency, DNA methylation, and cancer: studies on the reversibility of the effects of a lipotrope-deficient diet. J. Nutr. Biochem., *4*:672–680, 1993.

Cimino, F., Esposito, F., Ammendola, R., and Russo, T. Gene regulation by reactive oxygen species. Curr. Topics Cell. Regul., 35:123–148, 1997.

Cohn, S. L., Rademaker, A. W., Salwen, H. R., Franklin, W. A., Gonzales-Crussi, F., Rosen, S. T., and Bauer, K. D. Analysis of DNA ploidy and proliferative activity in relation to histology and *N-myc* amplification in neuroblastoma. Am. J. Pathol., 136:1043–1052, 1990.

Colgin, L. M., and Reddel, R. R. Telomere maintenance mechanisms and cellular immortalization. Curr. Opin. Genet. Dev., 9:97–103, 1999.

Collins, K., Jacks, T., and Pavletich, N. P. The cell cycle and cancer. Proc. Natl. Acad. Sci. U.S.A., 94:2776–2778, 1997.

Conney, A. H., and Burns, J. J. Induced synthesis of oxidative enzymes in liver microsomes by polycyclic hydrocarbons and drugs. *In*: G. Weber (Ed.), Advances in Enzyme Regulation, Vol. 1, pp. 189–214. Oxford, UK: Pergamon Press, 1963.

Czerniak, B., Chen, R., Tuziak, T., Markiewski, M., Kram, A., Gorczyca, W., Deitch, D., Herz, F., and Koss, L. G. Expression of *ras* oncogene p21 protein in relation to regional spread of human breast carcinomas. Cancer, 63:2008–2013, 1989.

Dalton, T. P., Shertzer, H. G., and Puga, A. Regulation of gene expression by reactive oxygen. Annu. Rev. Pharmacol. Toxicol., 39:67–101, 1999.

de Kok, J. B., Ruers, T. J. M., van Muijen, G. N. P., van Bokhoven, A., Willems, H. L., and Swinkels, D. W. Real-time quantification of human telomerase reverse transcriptase mRNA in tumors and healthy tissues. Clin. Chem., 46:313–318, 2000.

de La Coste, A., Romagnolo, B., Billuart, P., Renard, C.-A., Buendia, M.-A., Soubrane, O., Fabre, M., Chelly, J., Beldjord, C., Kahn, A., and Perret, C. Somatic mutations of the β-catenin gene are frequent in mouse and human hepatocellular carcinomas. Proc. Natl. Acad. Sci. U.S.A., 95:8847–8851, 1998.

Depass, L. R., and Morris, M. D. Feedback control of cholesterol biosynthesis in mice fed the liver carcinogens benzidine and 2-acetylaminofluorene. Cancer Biochem. Biophys., 6:47–51, 1982.

de Souza, A. T., Yamada, T., Mills, J. J., and Jirtle, R. L. Imprinted genes in liver carcinogenesis. FASEB J., 11:60–67, 1997.

Dexter, D. L., and Calabresi, P. Intraneoplastic diversity. Biochim. Biophys. Acta, 695:97–112, 1982.

Donnellan, R., and Chetty, R. Cyclin E in human cancers. FASEB J., 13:773–780, 1999.

Donovan-Peluso, M., Contento, A. M., Tobon, H., Ripepi, B., and Locker, J. Oncogene amplification in breast cancer. Am. J. Pathol., 138:835–845, 1991.

Draetta, G., and Pagano, M. Cell cycle control and cancer. Ann. Rep. Med. Chem., 31:241–248, 1996.

Esteller, M., Hamilton, S. R., Burger, P. C., Baylin, S. B., and Herman, J. G. Inactivation of the DNA repair gene *O6-methylguanine-DNA methyltransferase* by promoter hypermethylation is a common event in primary human neoplasia. Cancer Res., 59:793–797, 1999.

Esteller, M., Silva, J. M., Dominguez, G., Bonilla, F., Matias-Guiu, X., Lerma, E., Bussaglia, E., Prat, J., Harkes, I. C., Repasky, E. A., Gabrielson, E., Schutte, M., Baylin, S. B., and Herman, J. G. Promoter hypermethylation and BRCA1 inactivation in sporadic breast and ovarian tumors. J. Natl. Cancer Inst., 92:564–569, 2000.

Everitt, J. I., Walker, C. L., Goldsworthy, T. W., and Wolf, D. C. Altered expression of transforming growth factor-α: an early event in renal cell carcinoma development. Mol. Carcinog., 19:213–219, 1997.

Fang, W., Hartmann, N., Chow, D. T., Riegel, A. T., and Wellstein, A. Pleiotrophin stimulates fibroblasts and endothelial and epithelial cells and is expressed in human cancer. J. Biol. Chem., 267:25889–25897, 1992.

Farnham, P. J., Slansky, J. E., and Kollmar, R. The role of E2F in the mammalian cell cycle. Biochim. Biophys. Acta, 1155:125–131, 1993.

Fleisher, A. S., Esteller, M., Wang, S., Tamura, G., Suzuki, H., Yin, J., Zou, T.-T., Abraham, J. M., Kong, D., Smolinski, K. N., Shi, Y.-Q., Rhyu, M.-G., Powell, S. M., James, S. P., Wilson, K. T., Herman, J. G., and Meltzer, S. J. Hypermethylation of the *hMLH1* gene promoter in human gastric cancers with microsatellite instability. Cancer Res., 59:1090–1095, 1999.

Flørenes, V. A., Mælandsmo, G. M., Forus, A., Andreassen, Å., Myklebost, O., and Fodstad, Ø. MDM2 gene amplification and transcript levels in human sarcomas: relationship to TP53 gene status. J. Natl. Cancer Inst., 86:1297–1302, 1994.

Gama-Sosa, M. A., Slagel, V. A., de Bustros, A., Trewyn, R. W., Oxenhandler, R., Kuo, K. C., Gehrke, C. W., and Ehrlich, M. The 5-methylcytosine content of DNA from human tumors. Nucleic Acids Res., *11*:6883–6894, 1983.

Garte, S. J. The c-*myc* oncogene in tumor progression. Crit. Rev. Oncog., *4*:435–449, 1993.

George, R., and Goldfarb, S. Inhibition of 3-hydroxy-3-methylglutaryl coenzyme A reductase activity in Morris hepatoma 7800 after intravenous injection of mevalonic acid. Cancer Res., *40*:4717–4721, 1980.

Goelz, S. E., Vogelstein, B., Hamilton, S. R., and Feinberg, A. P. Hypomethylation of DNA from benign and malignant human colon neoplasms. Science, *228*:187–190, 1985.

Goldfarb, S., and Pitot, H. C. Enzymology of highly differentiated hepatocellular carcinomas. *In*: L. van der Reis (Ed.), Frontiers of Gastrointestinal Research, Vol. II, pp. 194–242. Basel: Karger, 1976.

Gomella, L. G., Sargent, E. R., Wade, T. P., Anglard, P., Linehan, W. M., and Kasid, A. Expression of transforming growth factor α in normal human adult kidney and enhanced expression of transforming growth factors α and β1 in renal cell carcinoma. Cancer Res., *49*:6972–6975, 1989.

Gougopoulou, D., Kiaris, H., Ergazaki, M., Anagnostopoulos, N., Grigoraki, V., and Spandidos, D. Mutations and expression of the Ras family genes in leukaemias. Stem Cells, *14*:725–729, 1996.

Gray, S. G., Eriksson, T., and Ekström, T. J. Methylation, gene expression and the chromatin connection in cancer. Int. J. Mol. Med., *4*:333–350, 1999.

Greenstein, J. P. Biochemistry of Cancer, 2nd ed., New York: Academic Press, 1954.

Greider, C. W., and Blackburn, E. H. Identification of a specific telomere transferase activity in *Tetrahymena* extracts. Cell, *43*:405–413, 1985.

Greider, C. W., and Blackburn, E. H. Telomeres, telomerase and cancer. Sci. Am., *276*:92–97, 1996.

Griffith, J. D., Comeau, L., Rosenfield, S., Stansel, R. M., Bianchi, A., Moss, H., and de Lange, T. Mammalian telomeres end in a large duplex loop. Cell, *97*:503–514, 1999.

Guerrero, I., Villasante, A., Mayer, A., and Pellicer, A. Carcinogen- and Radiation-Induced Mouse Lymphomas Contain an Activated c-*ras* Oncogene. Cold Spring Harbor, NY: Cold Spring Harbor Laboratory Press, 1984.

Guillem, J. G., O'Brian, C. A., Fitzer, C. J., Forde, K. A., LoGerfo, P., Treat, M., and Weinstein, I. B. Altered levels of protein kinase C and Ca^{2+}-dependent protein kinases in human colon carcinomas. Cancer Res., *47*:2036–2039, 1987.

Gullino, P. M., and Grantham, F. H. Studies on the exchange of fluids between host and tumor. II. The blood flow of hepatomas and other tumors in rats and mice. J. Natl. Cancer Inst., *27*:1465–1491, 1961.

Hainaut, P., and Hollstein, M. p53 and human cancer: the first ten thousand mutations. Adv. Cancer Res., *77*:81–137, 2000.

Haines, D. S. The mdm2 proto-oncogene. Leuk. Lymph., *26*:227–238, 1997.

Hakomori, S.-I., and Kannagi, R. Guest editorial. Glycosphingolipids as tumor-associated and differentiation markers. J. Natl. Cancer Inst., *71*:231–251, 1983.

Hall, M., and Peters, G. Genetic alterations of cyclins, cyclin-dependent kinases, and Cdk inhibitors in human cancer. Adv. Cancer Res., *68*:67–108, 1996.

Halperin, M. L., Taylor, W. M., Cheema-Dhadli, S., Morris, H. P., and Fritz, I. B. Effects of fasting on the control of fatty-acid synthesis in hepatoma 7777 and host liver. Eur. J. Biochem., *50*:517–522, 1975.

Hamilton, S. E., and Corey, D. R. Telomerase: anti-cancer target or just a fascinating enzyme? Chem. Biol., *3*:863–867, 1996.

Hark, A. T., Schoenherr, C. J., Katz, D. J., Ingram, R. S., Levorse, J. M., and Tilghman, S. M. CTCF mediates methylation-sensitive enhancer-blocking activity at the *H19/Igf2* locus. Nature, *405*:486–489, 2000.

Harley, C. B., and Sherwood, S. W. Telomerase, checkpoints and cancer. Cancer Surv., *29*:263–284, 1997.

Harry, D. S., Morris, H. P., and McIntyre, N. Cholesterol biosynthesis in transplantable hepatomas: evidence for impairment of uptake and storage of dietary cholesterol. J. Lipid Res., *12*:313–317, 1971.

Hartwell, L. H., and Kastan, M. B. Cell cycle control and cancer. Science, *266*:1821–1828, 1994.

Hashiba, H., Hosoi, J., Karasawa, M., Yamada, S., Nose, K., and Kuroki, T. Induction of metallothionein mRNA by tumor promoters in mouse skin and its constitutive expression in papillomas. Mol. Carcinog., *2*:95–100, 1989.

Hayashi, K., Kakizoe, T., and Sugimura, T. *In vivo* amplification and rearrangement of the c-Ha-*ras*-1 sequence in a human bladder carcinoma. Gann, *74*:798–801, 1983.

Heidelberger, C. Chemical carcinogenesis, chemotherapy: cancer's continuing core challenges. G.H.A. Clowes Memorial Lecture. Cancer Res., *30*:1549–1569, 1970.

Hempel, J., Harper, K., and Lindahl, R. Inducible (class 3) aldehyde dehydrogenase from rat hepatocellular carcinoma and 2,3,7,8-tetrachlorodibenzo-*p*-dioxin-treated liver: distant relationship to the class 1 and 2 enzymes from mammalian liver cytosol/mitochondria. Biochemistry, *28*:1160–1167, 1989.

Hendrich, B., and Bird, A. Identification and characterization of a family of mammalian methyl-CpG binding proteins. Mol. Cell. Biol., *18*:6538–6547, 1998.

Hendrich, S., Campbell, H. A., and Pitot, H. C. Quantitative stereological evaluation of four histochemical markers of altered foci in multistage hepatocarcinogenesis in the rat. Carcinogenesis, 8:1245–1250, 1987.

Hilf, R., Goldenberg, H., Gruenstein, M., Meranze, D. R., and Shimkin, M. B. Lack of correlation between morphological and biochemical parameters in mammary adenocarcinomas of rats induced with 7,12-dimethylbenz(a)-anthracene. Cancer Res., *30*:1223–1230, 1970.

Hirao, A., Kong, Y.-Y., Matsuoka, S., Wakeham, A., Ruland, J., Yoshida, H., Liu, D., Elledge, S. J., and Mak, T. W. DNA damage-induced activation of p53 by the checkpoint kinase Chk2. Science, *287*:1824–1827, 2000.

Ho, T., Horn, T., and Finzi, E. Transforming growth factor α expression helps to distinguish keratoacanthomas from squamous cell carcinomas. Arch. Dermatol., *127*:1167–1171, 1991.

Houldsworth, J., Mathew, S., Rao, P. H., Dyomina, K., Louie, D. C., Parsa, N., Offit, K., and Chaganti, R. S. K. *REL* proto-oncogene is frequently amplified in extranodal diffuse large cell lymphoma. Blood, *87*:25–29, 1996.

Huang, G.-T., Lee, H.-S., Chen, C.-H., Chiou, L.-L., Lin, Y.-W., Lee, C.-Z., Chen, D.-S., and Sheu, J.-C. Telomerase activity and telomere length in human hepatocellular carcinoma. Eur. J. Cancer, *34*:1946–1949, 1998.

Hunt, N. H., and Martin, T. J. Cyclic nucleotide metabolism in tumours. Aust. N.Z. J. Med., *9*:584–599, 1979.

Hunt, S. M., Osnos, M., and Rivlin, R. S. Thyroid hormone regulation of mitochondrial α-glycerophosphate dehydrogenase in liver and hepatoma. Cancer Res., *30*:1764–1768, 1970.

Hunter, T., and Pines, J. Cyclins and cancer II: cyclin D and CDK inhibitors come of age. Cell, *79*:573–582, 1994.

Huynh, H., Alpert, L., and Pollak, M. Pregnancy-dependent growth of mammary tumors is associated with overexpression of insulin-like growth factor II. Cancer Res., *56*:3651–3654, 1996.

Ip, C., and Dao, T. L. Effect of estradiol and prolactin on galactosyltransferase and α-lactalbumin activities in rat mammary gland and mammary tumor. Cancer Res., *38*:2077–2083, 1978.

Ishikawa, F. Telomere crisis, the driving force in cancer cell evolution. Biochem. Biophys. Res. Commun., *230*:1–6, 1997.

Ishitoya, J., Toriyama, M., Oguchi, N., Kitamura, K., Ohshima, M., Asano, K., and Yamamoto, T. Gene amplification and overexpression of EGF receptor in squamous cell carcinomas of the head and neck. Br. J. Cancer, *59*:559–562, 1989.

Ito, N., Kawata, S., Tamura, S., Takaishi, K., Yabuuchi, I., Matsuda, Y., Nishioka, M., and Tarui, S. Expression of transforming growth factor-β1 mRNA in human hepatocellular carcinoma. Jpn. J. Cancer Res., *81*:1202–1205, 1990.

Johnson, M. I., Robinson, M. C., Marsh, C., Robson, C. N., Neal, D. E., and Hamdy, F. C. Expression of Bcl-2, Bax, and p53 in high-grade prostatic intraepithelial neoplasia and localized prostate cancer: relationship with apoptosis and proliferation. Prostate, *37*:223–229, 1998.

Jones, P. A., and Gonzalgo, M. L. Altered DNA methylation and genome instability: a new pathway to cancer? Proc. Natl. Acad. Sci. U.S.A., *94*:2103–2105, 1997.

Jones, P. A., and Laird, P. W. Cancer epigenetics comes of age. Nature Genet., *21*:163–167, 1999.

Jones, R. B., and Irvin, J. L. Effect of hydrocortisone on the synthesis of DNA and histones and the acetylation of histones in regenerating liver. Arch. Biochem. Biophys., *152*:828–838, 1972.

Kanai, Y., Ushijima, S., Hui, A.-M., Ochiai, A., Tsuda, H., Sakamoto, M., and Hirohashi, S. The E-cadherin gene is silenced by CpG methylation in human hepatocellular carcinomas. Int. J. Cancer, *71*:355–359, 1997.

Kawamura, N., Nagai, H., Bando, K., Koyama, M., Matsumoto, S., Tajiri, T., Onda, M., Fujimoto, J., Ueki, T., Konishi, N., Shiba, T., and Emi, M. *PTEN/MMAC1* mutations in hepatocellular carcinomas: somatic inactivation of both alleles in tumors. Jpn. J. Cancer Res., *90*:413–418, 1999.

Kaziro, Y., Itoh, H., Kozasa, T., Nakafuku, M., and Satoh, T. Structure and function of signal-transducing GTP-binding proteins. Annu. Rev. Biochem., *60*:349–400, 1991.

Kelsey, G., and Reik, W. Analysis and identification of imprinted genes. Methods, *14*:211–234, 1998.

Kim, Y.-I., Giuliano, A., Hatch, K. D., Schneider, A., Nour, M. A., Dallal, G. E., Selhub, J., and Mason, J. B. Global DNA hypomethylation increases progressively in cervical dysplasia and carcinoma. Cancer, *74*:893–899, 1994.

King, L. M., Song, J., Wojcinski, Z. W., Baker, K. W., and Walker, R. M. Absence of correlation between telomerase activity and hepatic neoplasia in B6C3F1 mice. Toxicol. Lett., *106*:247–254, 1999.

Kitagawa, T. Responsiveness of hyperplastic lesions and hepatomas to partial hepatectomy. Gann, *62*:217–224, 1971.

Kitagawa, T., Watanabe, R., and Sugano, H. Induction of γ-glutamyl transpeptidase activity by dietary phenobarbital in "spontaneous" hepatic tumors of C3H mice. Gann, *71*:536–542, 1980.

Kitamoto, M., and Ide, T. Telomerase activity in precancerous hepatic nodules. Cancer, *85*:245–246, 1999.

Klump, B., Hsieh, C.-J., Holzmann, K., Gregor, M., and Porschen, R. Hypermethylation of the CDKN2/p16 promoter during neoplastic progression in Barrett's esophagus. Gastroenterology, *115*:1381–1386, 1998.

Koch, A., Denkhaus, D., Albrecht, S., Leuschner, I., von Schweinitz, D., and Pietsch, T. Childhood hepatoblastomas frequently carry a mutated degradation targeting box of the β-catenin gene. Cancer Res., *59*:269–273, 1999.

Kojima, H., Yokosuka, O., Imazeki, F., Saisho, H., and Omata, M. Telomerase activity and telomere length in hepatocellular carcinoma and chronic liver disease. Gastroenterology, *112*:493–500, 1997.

Krajewski, S., Blomquist, C., Franssila, K., Krajewska, M., Wasenius, V. M., Niskanen, E., Nordling, S., and Reed, J. C. Reduced expression of the proapoptotic gene BAX is associated with poor response rates to combination chemotherapy and shorter survival in women with metastatic breast adenocarcinoma. Cancer Res., *55*:4471–4478, 1995.

Krieg, P., Schnapke, R., Fürstenberger, G., Vogt, I., and Marks, F. TGF-β1 and skin carcinogenesis: antiproliferative effect in vitro and TGF-β1 mRNA expression during epidermal hyperproliferation and multistage tumorigenesis. Mol. Carcinog., *4*:129–137, 1991.

Krieg, P., Feil, S., Fürstenberger, G., and Bowden, G. T. Tumor-specific overexpression of a novel keratinocyte lipid-binding protein. J. Biol. Chem., *268*:17362–17369, 1993.

Krieg, P., Kinzig, A., Ress-Löschke, M., Vogel, S., Vanlandingham, B., Stephan, M., Lehmann, W.-D., Marks, F., and Fürstenberger, G. 12-Lipoxygenase isoenzymes in mouse skin tumor development. Mol. Carcinog., *14*:118–129, 1995.

Kuniyasu, H., Yasui, W., Kitadai, Y., Yokozaki, H., Ito, H., and Tahara, E. Frequent amplification of the c-*met* gene in scirrhous type stomach cancer. Biochem. Biophys. Res. Commun., *189*:227–232, 1992.

Kuwabara, A., Watanabe, H., Ajioka, Y., Yasuda, K., Saito, H., Matsuda, K., Kijima, H., and Hatakeyama, K. Alteration of *p53* clonality accompanying colorectal cancer progression. Jpn. J. Cancer Res., *89*:40–46, 1998.

Laderoute, M. P. A new perspective on the nature of the cancer problem: anti-cellular senescence. Mol. Carcinog., *10*:125–133, 1994.

Laird, P. W. Oncogenic mechanisms mediated by DNA methylation. Mol. Med. Today, *3*:223–229, 1997.

Lavin, M. F., and Shiloh, Y. The genetic defect in ataxia-telangiectasia. Annu. Rev. Immunol., *15*:177–202, 1997.

Lee, W.-H., Morton, R. A., Epstein, J. I., Brooks, J. D., Campbell, P. A., Bova, G. S., Hsieh, W.-S., Isaacs, W. B., and Nelson, W. G. Cytidine methylation of regulatory sequences near the π-class glutathione S-transferase gene accompanies human prostatic carcinogenesis. Proc. Natl. Acad. Sci. U.S.A., *91*:11733–11737, 1994.

Li, X., and Rozman, K. K. Subchronic effects of 2,3,7,8-tetrachlorodibenzo-*p*-dioxin (TCDD) and their reversibility in male Sprague-Dawley rats. Toxicology, *97*:133–140, 1995.

Liang, G., Salem, C. E., Yu, M. C., Nguyen, H. D., Gonzales, F. A., Nguyen, T. T., Nichols, P. W., and Jones, P. A. DNA methylation differences associated with tumor tissues identified by genome scanning analysis. Genomics, *53*:260–268, 1998.

Lindahl, R. Subcellular distribution and properties of aldehyde dehydrogenase from 2-acetylaminofluorene-induced rat hepatomas. Biochem. J., *183*:55–64, 1979.

Linder, M. C., Moor, J. R., Munro, H. N., and Morris, H. P. Structural differences in ferritins from normal and malignant rat tissues. Biochim. Biophys. Acta, *386*:409–421, 1975.

Liu, T.-C., Lin, P.-M., Chang, J.-G., Lee, J.-P., Chen, T.-P., and Lin, S.-F. Mutation analysis of PTEN/MMAC1 in acute myeloid leukemia. Am. J. Hematol., *63*:170–175, 2000.

Livingstone, L. R., White, A., Sprouse, J., Livanos, E., Jacks, T., and Tlsty, T. D. Altered cell cycle arrest and gene amplification potential accompany loss of wild-type p53. Cell, *70*:923–935, 1992.

Looijenga, L. H. J., Verkerk, A. J. M. H., de Groot, N., Hochberg, A. A., and Oosterhuis, J. W. H19 in normal development and neoplasia. Mol. Reprod. Dev., *46*:419–439, 1997.

Lotlikar, P. D. Effects of 3-methylcholanthrene pretreatment on microsomal hydroxylation of 2-acetamidofluorene by various rat hepatomas. Biochem. J., *118*:513–518, 1970.

Lowe, S. W., and Lin, A. W. Apoptosis in cancer. Carcinogenesis, *21*:485–495, 2000.

Mai, M., Qian, C., Yokomizo, A., Tindall, D. J., Bostwick, D., Polychronakos, C., Smith, D. I., and Liu, W. Loss of imprinting and allele switching of p73 in renal cell carcinoma. Oncogene, *17*:1739–1741, 1998.

Markert, C. L., and Moller, F. Multiple forms of enzymes: tissue, ontogenetic, and species specific patterns. Proc. Natl. Acad. Sci. U.S.A., *45*:753–763, 1959.

Martin, K. J. The interactions of transcription factors and their adaptors, coactivators and accessory proteins. Bioessays, *13*:499–503, 1991.

Mehle, C., Ljungberg, B., Stenling, R., and Roos, G. DNA fingerprinting of renal cell carcinoma with special reference to tumor heterogeneity. Genes Chromosom. Cancer, *6*:86–91, 1993.

Mekhail-Ishak, K., Medina, D., and Batist, G. Biochemical characteristics of mouse mammary tissues, preneoplastic lesions and tumors. Carcinogenesis, *10*:2363–2366, 1989.

Michalides, R. J. A. M. Cell cycle regulators: mechanisms and their role in aetiology, prognosis, and treatment of cancer. J. Clin. Pathol., *52*:555–568, 1999.

Millard, S. S., and Koff, A. Cyclin-dependent kinase inhibitors in restriction point control, genomic stability, and tumorigenesis. J. Cell. Biochem. Suppl., *30/31*:37–42, 1998.

Miller, E. C. Studies on the formation of protein-bound derivatives of 3,4-benzpyrene in the epidermal fraction of mouse skin. Cancer Res., *11*:100–108, 1951.

Miller, E. C., and Miller, J. A. The presence and significance of bound aminoazo dyes in the livers of rats fed *p*-dimethylaminoazobenzene. Cancer Res., *7*:468–480, 1947.

Miller, M. S. Tumor suppressor genes in rodent lung carcinogenesis—mutation pf *p53* does not appear to be an early lesion in lung tumor pathogenesis. Toxicol. Appl. Pharmacol., *156*:70–77, 1999.

Mills, J. J., Falls, J. G., De Souza, A. T., and Jirtle, R. L. Imprinted *M6p/Igf2 receptor* is mutated in rat liver tumors. Oncogene, *16*:2797–2802, 1998.

Mitsunobu, F., Fukui, M., Oda, T., Yamamoto, T., and Toyoshima, K. A mechanism of c-*raf*-1 activation: fusion of the lipocortin II amino-terminal sequence with the c-*raf*-1 kinase domain. Oncogene, *4*:437–442, 1989.

Miura, N., Horikawa, I., Nishimoto, A., Ohmura, H., Ito, H., Hirohashi, S., Shay, J. W., and Oshimura, M. Progressive telomere shortening and telomerase reactivation during hepatocellular carcinogenesis. Cancer Genet. Cytogenet., *93*:56–62, 1997.

Mizukami, Y., Nonomura, A., Yamada, T., Kurumaya, H., Hayashi, M., Koyasaki, N., Taniya, T., Noguchi, M., Nakamura, S., and Matsubara, F. Immunohistochemical demonstration of growth factors, TGF-α, TGF-β, IGF-I and *neu* oncogene product in benign and malignant human breast tissues. Anticancer Res., *10*:1115–1126, 1990.

Molinari, M. Cell cycle checkpoints and their inactivation in human cancer. Cell Prolif., *33*:261–274, 2000.

Morgan, S. E., and Kastan, M. B. p53 and ATM: cell cycle, cell death, and cancer. Adv. Cancer Res., *71*:1–25, 1997.

Morin, P. J. β-Catenin signaling and cancer. Bioessays, *21*:1021–1030, 1999.

Morris, H. P. Studies on the development, biochemistry, and biology of experimental hepatomas. Adv. Cancer Res., *9*:227–302, 1965.

Morris, H. P., and Wagner, B. P. Induction and transplantation of rat hepatomas with different growth rate (including "minimal deviation" hepatomas). Methods Cancer Res., *4*:125–152, 1968.

Moser, G. J., Wolf, D. C., Harden, R., Standeven, A. M., Mills, J., Jirtle, R. L., and Goldsworthy, T. L. Cell proliferation and regulation of negative growth factors in mouse liver foci. Carcinogenesis, *17*:1835–1840, 1996.

Moser, G. J., Wolf, D. C., and Goldsworthy, T. L. Quantitative relationship between transforming growth factor-alpha and hepatic focal phenotype and progression in female mouse liver. Toxicol. Pathol., *25*:275–283, 1997.

Munemitsu, S., Albert, I., Souza, B., Rubinfeld, B., and Polakis, P. Regulation of intracellular β-catenin levels by the adenomatous polyposis coli (APC) tumor-suppressor protein. Proc. Natl. Acad. Sci. U.S.A., *92*:3046–3050, 1995.

Münzel, P. A., Pfohl-Leszkowicz, A., Röhrdanz, E., Keith, G., Dirheimer, G., and Bock, K. W. Site-specific hypomethylation of c-*myc* protooncogene in liver nodules and inhibition of DNA methylation by N-nitrosomorpholine. Biochem. Pharmacol., *42*:365–371, 1991.

Nakano, H., Hatayama, I., Satoh, K., Suzuki, S., Sato, K., and Tsuchida, S. c-Jun expression in single cells and preneoplastic foci induced by diethylnitrosamine in B6C3F1 mice: comparison with the expression of pi-class glutathione *S*-transferase. Carcinogenesis, *15*:1853–1857, 1994.

Nakatsu, Y., Nomoto, S., Oh-Uchida, M., Shimizu, K., and Sekiguchi, M. Structure of the activated c-*raf-1* gene from human stomach cancer. Cold Spring Harbor Symp. Quant. Biol., *51*:1001–1008, 1986.

Nambu, S., Inoue, K., and Sasaki, H. Site-specific hypomethylation of the c-*myc* oncogene in human hepatocellular carcinoma. Jpn. J. Cancer Res. (Gann), *78*:695–704, 1987.

Natali, P. G., Nicotra, M. R., Sures, I., Mottolese, M., Botti, C., and Ullrich, A. Breast cancer is associated with loss of the c-*kit* oncogene product. Int. J. Cancer, *52*:713–717, 1992.

Navone, N. M., Troncoso, P., Pisters, L. L., Goodrow, T. L., Palmer, J. L., Nichols, W. E., von Eschenbach, A. C., and Conti, C. J. p53 protein accumulation and gene mutation in the progression of human prostate carcinoma. J. Natl. Cancer Inst., *85*:1657–1669, 1993.

Neri, A., Barriga, F., Knowles, D. M., Magrath, I. T., and Dalla-Favera, R. Different regions of the immunoglobulin heavy-chain locus are involved in chromosomal translocations in distinct pathogenetic forms of Burkitt lymphoma. Proc. Natl. Acad. Sci. U.S.A., *85*:2748–2752, 1988.

Neri, A., Fracchiolla, N. S., Migliazza, A., Trecca, D., and Lombardi, L. The involvement of the candidate proto-oncogene NFKB2/lyt-10 in lymphoid malignancies. Leuk. Lymph., *23*:43–48, 1996.

Neveu, M. J., Hully, J. R., Paul, D. L., and Pitot, H. C. Reversible alteration in the expression of the gap junctional protein connexin 32 during tumor promotion in rat liver and its role during cell proliferation. Cancer Commun., *2*:21–31, 1990.

Nowell, P. C., Morris, H. P., and Potter, V. R. Chromosomes of "minimal deviation" hepatomas and some other transplantable rat tumors. Cancer Res., *27*:1565–1579, 1967.

Oda, H., Kume, H., Shimizu, Y., Inoue, T., and Ishikawa, T. Loss of imprinting of *igf2* in renal-cell carcinomas. Int. J. Cancer, *75*:343–346, 1998.

Ogawa, K., Yamada, Y., Kishibe, K., Ishizaki, K., and Tokusashi, Y. β-catenin mutations are frequent in hepatocellular carcinomas but absent in adenomas induced by diethylnitrosamine in B6C3F1 mice. Cancer Res., *59*:1830–1833, 1999.

Oh, I.-H., and Reddy, E. P. The *myb* gene family in cell growth, differentiation and apoptosis. Oncogene, *18*:3017–3033, 1999.

Ohmachi, T., Sagami, I., Fujii, H., and Watanabe, M. Microsomal monooxygenase system in Morris hepatoma: purification and characterization of cytochromes P-450 from Morris hepatoma 5123D of 3-methylcholanthrene-treated rats. Arch. Biochem. Biophys., *236*:176–184, 1985.

Olden, K. Adhesion molecules and inhibitors of glycosylation in cancer. Semin. Cancer Biol., *4*:269–276, 1993.

Olsson, J. M., Schedin, S., Teclebrhan, H., Eriksson, L. C., and Dallner, G. Enzymes of mevalonate pathway in rat liver nodules induced by 2-acetylaminofluorene treatment. Carcinogenesis, 16:599–605, 1995.

Orlowski, C. C., and Furlanetto, R. W. The mammalian cell cycle in normal and abnormal growth. Endocrinol. Metab. Clin. North Am., 25:491–502, 1996.

Paterlini, P., Suberville, A. M., Zindy, F., Melle, J., Sonnier, M., Marie, J. P., Dreyfus, F., and Bréchot, C. Cyclin A expression in human hematological malignancies: a new marker of cell proliferation. Cancer Res., 53:235–238, 1993.

Peng, S.-Y., Lai, P.-L., Chu, J.-S., Lee, P.-H., Tsung, P.-T., Chen, D.-S., and Hsu, H.-C. Expression and hypomethylation of α-fetoprotein gene in unicentric and multicentric human hepatocellular carcinomas. Hepatology, 17:35–41, 1993.

Peters, G. The D-type cyclins and their role in tumorigenesis. J. Cell Sci., 18:89–96, 1994.

Pezzino, V., Vigneri, R., Siperstein, M. D., and Goldfine, I. D. Insulin and glucagon receptors in Morris hepatomas of varying growth rates. Cancer Res., 39:1443–1446, 1979.

Pitot, H. C. Metabolic adaptations and the neoplastic cell. Bull. Tulane Univ. Med. Fac., 19:17, 1959.

Pitot, H. C. Altered hepatic foci: their role in murine hepatocarcinogenesis. Annu. Rev. Pharmacol. Toxicol., 30:465–500, 1990.

Pitot, H. C., Potter, V. R., and Morris, H. P. Metabolic adaptations in rat hepatomas. I. The effect of dietary protein on some inducible enzymes in liver and hepatoma 5123. Cancer Res., 21:1001–1008, 1961.

Pitot, H. C., Dragan, Y. P., Teeguarden, J., Hsia, S., and Campbell, H. Quantitation of multistage carcinogenesis in rat liver. Toxicol. Pathol., 24:119–128, 1996.

Poirier, L. A. Methyl group deficiency in hepatocarcinogenesis. Drug Metab. Rev., 26:185–199, 1994.

Polyak, K., Hamilton, S. R., Vogelstein, B., and Kinzler, K. W. Early alteration of cell-cycle-regulated gene expression in colorectal neoplasia. Am. J. Pathol., 149:381–387, 1996.

Potter, M. Immunoglobulin-producing tumors and myeloma proteins of mice. Physiol. Rev., 52:631–719, 1972.

Potter, V. R. The biochemical approach to the cancer problem. Fed. Proc., 17:691–697, 1958.

Potter, V. R. Transplantable animal cancer, the primary standard. Guest editorial. Cancer Res., 21:1331–1333, 1961.

Potter, V. R. Biochemical perspectives in cancer research. Cancer Res., 24:1085–1098, 1964.

Potter, V. R. Recent trends in cancer biochemistry: the importance of studies on fetal tissue. Can. Cancer Conf., 8:9–30, 1969.

Potter, V. R. Biochemistry of cancer. In: J. F. Holland and E. Frei III (Eds.), Cancer Medicine, 2nd ed., pp. 133–148. Philadelphia: Lea & Febiger, 1982.

Potter, V. R., and Watanabe, M. Some biochemical essentials of malignancy: the challenge of diversity. In: C. J. D. Zarafonetis (Ed.), Proceedings of the International Conference on Leukemia-Lymphoma, pp. 33–46. Philadelphia: Lea & Febiger, 1968.

Potter, V. R., Watanabe, M., Pitot, H. C., and Morris, H. P. Systematic oscillations in metabolic activity in rat liver and hepatomas. Survey of normal diploid and other hepatoma lines. Cancer Res., 29:55–78, 1969.

Rahmsdorf, H. J. Jun: transcription factor and oncoprotein. J. Mol. Med., 74:725–747, 1996.

Rao, P. M., Antony, A., Rajalakshmi, S., and Sarma, D. S. R. Studies on hypomethylation of liver DNA during early stages of chemical carcinogenesis in rat liver. Carcinogenesis, 10:933–937, 1989.

Razin, A., and Riggs, A. D. DNA methylation and gene function. Science, 210:604–616, 1980.

Reik, W., and Maher, E. R. Imprinting in clusters: lessons from Beckwith-Wiedemann syndrome. Trends Genet., 13:330–334, 1997.

Reiners, J. J. Jr., Jones, C. L., Hong, N., and Myrand, S. P. Differential induction of Cyp1a1, Cyp1b1, Ahd4, and Nmo1 in murine skin tumors and adjacent normal epidermis by ligands of the aryl hydrocarbon receptor. Mol. Carcinog., 21:135–146, 1998.

Reiss, M. Transforming growth factor-β and cancer: a love-hate relationship? Oncol. Res., 9:447–457, 1997.

Reynolds, R. D., Potter, V. R., Pitot, H. C., and Reuber, M. D. Survey of some enzyme patterns in transplantable Reuber mouse hepatomas. Cancer Res., 31:808–812, 1971.

Rho, O., Beltrán, L. M., Gimenez-Conti, I. B., and DiGiovanni, J. Altered expression of the epidermal growth factor receptor and transforming growth factor-α during multistage skin carcinogenesis in SENCAR mice. Mol. Carcinog., *11*:19–28, 1994.

Rho, O., Bol, D. K., You, J., Beltrán, L., Rupp, T., and DiGiovanni, J. Altered expression of insulin-like growth factor I and its receptor during multistage carcinogenesis in mouse skin. Mol. Carcinog., *17*:62–69, 1996.

Ringler, M. B., and Hilf, R. Effect of estrogen on synthesis of glucose-6-phosphate dehydrogenase in R3230AC mammary tumors and uteri. Biochim. Biophys. Acta, *411*:50–62, 1975.

Robles, A. I., and Conti, C. J. Early overexpression of cyclin D1 protein in mouse skin carcinogenesis. Carcinogenesis, *16*:781–786, 1995.

Roop, D. R., Krieg, T. M., Mehrel, T., Cheng, C. K., and Yuspa, S. H. Transcriptional control of high molecular weight keratin gene expression in multistage mouse skin carcinogenesis. Cancer Res., *48*:3245–3252, 1988.

Rossiello, M. R., Rao, P. M., Rajalakshmi, S., and Sarma, D. S. R. Similar patterns of hypomethylation in the β-hydroxy-β-methylglutaryl coenzyme A reductase gene in hepatic nodules induced by different carcinogens. Mol. Carcinog., *10*:237–245, 1994.

Rudolph, K. L., Chang, S., Lee, H.-W., Blasco, M., Gottlieb, G. J., Greider, and DePinho, R. A. Longevity, stress response, and cancer in aging telomerase-deficient mice. Cell, *96*:701–712, 1999.

Rudzki, Z., and Jothy, S. CD44 and the adhesion of neoplastic cells. J. Clin. Pathol. Mol. Pathol., *50*:57–71, 1997.

Ruggieri, S., and Fallani, A. Lipid composition of Morris hepatoma 5123c, and of livers and blood plasma from host and normal rats. Lipids, *14*:781–788, 1979.

Sabine, J. R. Defective control of lipid biosynthesis in cancerous and precancerous liver. Progr. Biochem. Pharmacol., *10*:269–307, 1975.

Sabine, J. R. Metabolic controls in precancerous liver—VII. Time course of loss of dietary feedback control of cholesterol synthesis during carcinogen treatment. Eur. J. Cancer, *12*:299–303, 1976.

Said, T. K., and Medina, D. Cell cyclins and cyclin-dependent kinase activities in mouse mammary tumor development. Carcinogenesis, *16*:823–830, 1995.

Saluz, H., and Jost, J.-P. Major techniques to study DNA methylation. *In*: J. P. Jost and H. P. Saluz (Eds.), DNA Methylation: Molecular Biology and Biological Significance, pp. 11–26. Basel, Switzerland: Birkhäuser Verlag, 1993.

Sawada, N., Poirier, L., Moran, S., Xu, Y.-H., and Pitot, H. C. The effect of choline and methionine deficiency on the number and volume percentage of altered hepatic foci in the presence and absence of diethylnitrosamine initiation in rat liver. Carcinogenesis, *11*:273–281, 1990.

Sawyer, J. R., Roloson, G. J., Bell, J. M., Thomas, J. R., Teo, C., and Chadduck, W. M. Telomeric associations in the progression of chromosome aberrations in pediatric solid tumors. Cancer Genet. Cytogenet., *90*:1–13, 1996.

Schaff, Z., Hsia, C. C., Sarosi, I., and Tabor, E. Overexpression of transforming growth factor-α in hepatocellular carcinoma and focal nodular hyperplasia from European patients. Hum. Pathol., *25*:644–651, 1994.

Schapira, F. Resurgence of fetal isozymes in cancer: study of aldolase, pyruvate kinase, lactic dehydrogenase, and β-hexosaminidase. Isozymes: Curr. Top. Biol. Med. Res., *5*:27–75, 1981.

Schmitt, H., Blin, N., Zankl, H., and Scherthan, H. Telomere length variation in normal and malignant human tissues. Genes Chromosom. Cancer, *11*:171–177, 1994.

Schneider-Stock, R., Walter, H., Haeckel, C., Radig, K., Rys, J., and Roessner, A. Gene alterations at the CDKN2A (p16/MTS1) locus in soft tissue tumors. Int. J. Oncol., *13*:325–329, 1998.

Schumacher, V., Schneider, S., Figge, A., Wildhardt, G., Harms, D., Schmidt, D., Weirich, A., Ludwig, R., and Royer-Pokora, B. Correlation of germ-line mutations and two-hit inactivation of the *WT1* gene with Wilms tumors of stromal-predominant histology. Proc. Natl. Acad. Sci. U.S.A., *94*:3972–3977, 1997.

Schwab, M. Amplification of oncogenes in human cancer cells. Bioessays, *20*:473–479, 1998.

Semb, H., and Christofori, G. Insights from model systems. The tumor-suppressor function of E-cadherin. Am. J. Hum. Genet., *63*:1588–1593, 1998.

Sgambato, A., Han, E. K.-H., Zhang, Y.-J., Moon, R. C., Santella, R. M., and Weinstein, I. B. Deregulated expression of cyclin D1 and other cell cycle-related genes in carcinogen-induced rat mammary tumors. Carcinogenesis, *16*:2193–2198, 1995.

Shao, C., Deng, L., Henegariu, O., Liang, L., Stambrook, P. J., and Tischfield, J. A. Chromosome instability contributes to loss of heterozygosity in mice lacking p53. Proc. Natl. Acad. Sci. U.S.A., *97*:7405–7410, 2000.

Shay, J. W. Aging and cancer: are telomeres and telomerase the connection? Mol. Med. Today, *1*:378–384, 1995.

Sheppard, D. Dominant negative mutants: tools for the study of protein function *in vitro* and *in vivo*. Am. J. Respir. Cell Mol. Biol., *11*:1–6, 1994.

Sherr, C. J. Cancer cell cycles. Science, *274*:1672–1677, 1996.

Shiraishi, M., Noguchi, M., Shimosato, Y., and Sekiya, T. Amplification of protooncogenes in surgical specimens of human lung carcinomas. Cancer Res., *49*:6474–6479, 1989.

Silverman, J. A., Kuhlmann, E. T., Zurlo, J., Yager, J. D., and Longnecker, D. S. Expression of c-*myc*, c-*raf*-1, and c-Ki-*ras* in azaserine-induced pancreatic carcinomas and growing pancreas in rats. Mol. Carcinog., *3*:379–386, 1990.

Siracky, J. An approach to the problem of heterogeneity of human tumour-cell populations. Br. J. Cancer, *39*:570–577, 1979.

Sirica, A. E., Richards, W., Tsukada, Y., Sattler, C. A., and Pitot, H. C. Fetal phenotypic expression by adult rat hepatocytes on collagen gel/nylon meshes. Proc. Natl. Acad. Sci. U.S.A., *76*:283–287, 1979.

Smith, M. L., and Fornace, A. J. Jr. Genomic instability and the role of p53 mutations in cancer cells. Curr. Opin. Oncol., *7*:69–75, 1995.

Sorimachi, K., Niwa, A., and Yasumura, Y. Hormonal regulation of tyrosine aminotransferase and phenylalanine hydroxylase in rat hepatoma cells continuously cultured in a serum-free medium. Effect of serum, dexamethasone and insulin. Cell Struct. Funct., *6*:61–68, 1981.

Sorof, S., Young, E. M., and Ott, M. G. Soluble liver h proteins during hepatocarcinogenesis by aminoazo dyes and 2-acetylaminofluorene in the rat. Cancer Res., *18*:33–46, 1958.

Sorof, S., Young, E. M., Coffey, C. B., and Morris, H. P. On protein binding of fluorenyl carcinogens by minimal deviation hepatomas. Cancer Res., *26*:81–88, 1966.

Staunton, M. J., and Gaffney, E. F. Tumor type is a determinant of susceptibility to apoptosis. Am. J. Clin. Pathol., *103*:300–307, 1995.

Steinmetz, K. L., Pogribny, I. P., James, S. J., and Pitot, H. C. Hypomethylation of the rat *glutathione S-transferase π (GSTP)* promoter region isolated from methyl-deficient livers and GSTP-positive liver neoplasms. Carcinogenesis, *19*:1487–1494, 1998.

Stopera, S. A., Davie, J. R., and Bird, R. P. Colonic aberrant crypt foci are associated with increased expression of c-*fos*: the possible role of modified c-*fos* expression in preneoplastic lesions in colon cancer. Carcinogenesis, *13*:573–578, 1992.

Strobel, H. W., Dignam, J. D., Saine, S. E., Fang, W.-F., and Fennell, P. M. The drug metabolism systems of liver and liver tumors: a comparison of activities and characteristics. Mol. Cell. Biochem., *22*:79–90, 1978.

Suh, S.-I., Cho, J.-W., Baek, W.-K., Suh, M.-H., and Carson, D. A. Lack of mutation at p16INK4A gene but expression of aberrant p16INK4A RNA transcripts in human ovarian carcinoma. Cancer Lett., *153*:175–182, 2000.

Sun, H., Lesche, R., Li, D.-M., Liliental, J., Zhang, H., Gao, J., Gavrilova, N., Mueller, B., Liu, X., and Wu, H. PTEN modulates cell cycle progression and cell survival by regulating phosphatidylinositol 3,4,5-trisphosphate and Akt/protein kinase B signaling pathway. Proc. Natl. Acad. Sci. USA, *96*:6199–6204, 1999.

Tamura, G., Yin, J., Wang, S., Fleisher, A. S., Zou, T., Abraham, J. M., Kong, D., Smolinski, K. N., Wilson, K. T., James, S. P., Silverberg, S. G., Nishizuka, S., Terashima, M., Motoyama, T., and Meltzer, S. J. E-Cadherin gene promoter hypermethylation in primary human gastric carcinomas. J. Natl. Cancer Inst., *92*:569–573, 2000.

Tan, P., Cady, B., Wanner, M., Worland, P., Cukor, B., Magi-Galluzzi, C., Lavin, P., Draetta, G., Pagano, M., and Loda, M. The cell cycle inhibitor p27 is an independent prognostic marker in small ($T_{1a,b}$) invasive breast carcinomas. Cancer Res., *57*:1259–1263, 1997.

Tanaka, S., Toh, Y., Adachi, E., Matsumata, T., Mori, R., and Sugimachi, K. Tumor progression in hepatocellular carcinoma may be mediated by *p53* mutation. Cancer Res., *53*:2884–2887, 1993.

Taniguchi, T., Okamoto, K., and Reeve, A. E. Human p57(KIP2) defines a new imprinted domain on chromosome 11p but is not a tumour suppressor gene in Wilms tumour. Oncogene, *14*:1201–1206, 1997.

Tao, L., Kramer, P. M., Ge, R., and Pereira, M. A. Effect of dichloroacetic acid and trichloroacetic acid on DNA methylation in liver and tumors of female B6C3F1 mice. Toxicol. Sci., *43*:139–144, 1998.

Tchou, J. C., Lin, X., Freije, D., Isaacs, W. B., Brooks, J. D., Rashid, A., De Marzo, A. M., Kanai, Y., Hirohashi, S., and Nelson, W. G. *GSTP1* CpG island DNA hypermethylation in hepatocellular carcinomas. Int. J. Oncol., *16*:663–676, 2000.

Thanassi, J. W., Nutter, L. M., Meisler, N. T., Commers, P., and Chiu, J.-F. Vitamin B_6 metabolism in Morris hepatomas. J. Biol. Chem., *256*:3370–3375, 1981.

Thompson, E. B., Tomkins, G. M., and Curran, J. F. Induction of tyrosine α-ketoglutarate transaminase by steroid hormones in a newly established tissue culture cell line. Proc. Natl. Acad. Sci. U.S.A., *56*:296–303, 1966.

Tilghman, S. M., Bartolomei, M. S., Webber, A. L., Brunkow, M. E., Saam, J., Leighton, P. A., Pfeifer, K., and Zemel, S. Parental imprinting of the *H19* and *Igf2* genes in the mouse. Cold Spring Harbor Symp. Quant. Biol., *58*:287–295, 1993.

Tripathy, D., and Benz, C. C. Activated oncogenes and putative tumor suppressor genes involved in human breast cancers. *In*: C. C. Benz and E. T. Liu (Eds.), Oncogenes and Tumor Suppressor Genes in Human Malignancies, pp. 15–60. Boston: Kluwer, 1993.

Tryfiates, G. P., Shuler, J. K., Hefner, M. H., and Morris, H. P. Effect of B_6 deficiency on hepatoma 7794A growth rate: activities of tyrosine transaminase and serine dehydratase before and after induction by hydrocortisone. Eur. J. Cancer, *10*:147–154, 1974.

Tsuchida, S., Hoshino, K., Sato, T., Ito, N., and Sato, K. Purification of γ-glutamyltransferases from rat hepatomas and hyperplastic hepatic nodules, and comparison with the enzyme from rat kidney. Cancer Res., *39*:4200–4205, 1979.

Tsujiuchi, T., Tsutsumi, M., Kido, A., Kobitsu, K., Takahama, M., Majima, T., Denda, A., Nakae, D., and Konishi, Y. Increased telomerase activity in hyperplastic nodules and hepatocellular carcinomas induced by a choline-deficient L-amino acid-defined diet in rats. Jpn. J. Cancer Res., *87*:1111–1115, 1996.

Urquidi, V., Tarin, D., and Goodison, S. Telomerase in cancer: clinical applications. Ann. Med., *30*:419–430, 1998.

Uyeno, S., Aoki, Y., Nata, M., Sagisaka, K., Kayama, T., Yoshimoto, T., and Ono, T. *IGF2* but not *H19* shows loss of imprinting in human glioma. Cancer Res., *56*:5356–5359, 1996.

Van Hoeven, R. P., Emmelot, P., Krol, J. H., and Oomen-Meulemans, E. P. M. Studies on plasma membranes. XXII. Fatty acid profiles of lipid classes in plasma membranes of rat and mouse livers and hepatomas. Biochim. Biophys. Acta, *380*:1–11, 1975.

Vedel, M., Gomez-Garcia, M., Sala, M., and Sala-Trepat, J. M. Changes in methylation pattern of albumin and α-fetoprotein genes in developing rat liver and neoplasia. Nucleic Acids Res., *11*:4335–4354, 1983.

Visser, C. J. T., Bruggink, A. H., Korc, M., Kobrin, M. S., de Weger, R. A., Seifert-Bock, I., van Blokland, W. T. M., van Garderen-Hoetmer, A., and Woutersen, R. A. Overexpression of transforming growth factor-α and epidermal growth factor receptor, but not epidermal growth factor, in exocrine pancreatic tumours in hamsters. Carcinogenesis, *17*:779–785, 1996.

Voelker, D. R., Lee, T.-C., and Snyder, F. Fatty acid biosynthesis and dietary regulation in pulmonary adenomas. Arch. Biochem. Biophys., *176*:753–756, 1976.

Wainfan, E., and Poirier, L. A. Methyl groups in carcinogenesis: effects on DNA methylation and gene expression. Cancer Res., *52*:2071s–2077s, 1992.

Wan, M., Li, W.-Z., Duggan, B. D., Felix, J. C., Zhao, Y., and Dubeau, L. Telomerase activity in benign and malignant epithelial ovarian tumors. J. Natl. Cancer Inst., *89*:437–441, 1997.

Wang, Q.-S., Sabourin, C. L. K., Bijur, G. N., Robertson, F. M., and Stoner, G. D. Alterations in transform-
    ing growth factor-α and epidermal growth factor receptor expression during rat esophageal tumori-
    genesis. Mol. Carcinog., *15*:144–153, 1996.

Warburg, O. Metabolism of Tumors, translated by F. Dickens. London: Constable, 1930.

Warburg, O. On the origin of cancer cells. Science, *123*:309–314, 1956.

Warrell, R. P. Jr., de Thé, H., Wang, Z.-Y., and Degos, L. Acute promyelocytic leukemia. N. Engl. J. Med.,
    329:177–189, 1993.

Weber, G. Biochemical strategy of cancer cells and the design of chemotherapy. G. H. A. Clowes Memorial
    Lecture. Cancer Res., *43*:3466–3492, 1983.

Weinhouse, S. Isozyme patterns of hepatomas and tumour progression. Neoplasma, *20*:559–562, 1973.

Weinhouse, S. The Warburg hypothesis fifty years later. Z. Krebsforsch. Klin. Onkol., *87*:115–126, 1976.

Weinhouse, S. What are isozymes telling us about gene regulation in cancer? J. Natl. Cancer Inst.,
    68:343–348, 1982.

Wolman, S. R., Horland, A. A., and Becker, F. F. Altered karyotypes of transplantable "diploid" tumors. J.
    Natl. Cancer Inst., *51*:1909–1914, 1973.

Wu, M.-S., Wang, H.-P., Lin, C.-C., Sheu, J.-C., Shun, C.-T., Lee, W.-J., and Lin, J.-T. Loss of imprinting
    and overexpression of IGF2 gene in gastric adenocarcinoma. Cancer Lett., *120*:9–14, 1997.

Wutz, A., and Barlow, D. P. Imprinting of the mouse *Igf 2r* gene depends on an intronic CpG island. Mol.
    Cell. Endocrinol., *140*:9–14, 1998.

Xu, G.-L., Bestor, T. H., Bourc'his, D., Hsieh, C.-L., Tommerup, N., Bugge, M., Hulten, M., Qu, X.,
    Russo, J. J., and Viegas-Péquignot, E. Chromosome instability and immunodeficiency syndrome
    caused by mutations in a DNA methyltransferase gene. Nature, *402*:187–191, 1999.

Yashima, K., Litzky, L. A., Kaiser, L., Rogers, T., Lam, S., Wistuba, I. I., Milchgrub, S., Srivastava, S.,
    Piatyszek, M. A., Shay, J. W., and Gazdar, A. F. Telomerase expression in respiratory epithelium
    during the multistage pathogenesis of lung carcinomas. Cancer Res., *57*:2373–2377, 1997.

Yokoyama, S., Sells, M. A., Reddy, T. V., and Lombardi, B. Hepatocarcinogenic and promoting action of a
    choline-devoid diet in the rat. Cancer Res., *45*:2834–2842, 1985.

Zapisek, W. F., Cronin, G. M., Lyn-Cook, B. D., and Poirier, L. A. The onset of oncogene hypomethylation
    in the livers of rats fed methyl-deficient, amino acid-defined diets. Carcinogenesis, *13*:1869–1872,
    1992.

Zhan, S., Shapiro, D. N., and Helman, L. J. Loss of imprinting of IGF2 in Ewing's sarcoma. Oncogene,
    11:2503–2507, 1995.

Zhang, W., Kapusta, L. R., Slingerland, J. M., and Klotz, L. H. Telomerase activity in prostate cancer, pro-
    static intraepithelial neoplasia, and benign prostatic epithelium. Cancer Res., *58*:619–621, 1998.

Zion, M., Ben-Yehuda, D., Avraham, A., Cohen, O., Wetzler, M., Melloul, D., and Ben-Neriah, Y. Progres-
    sive *de novo* DNA methylation at the *bcr-abl* locus in the course of chronic myelogenous leukemia.
    Proc. Natl. Acad. Sci. U.S.A., *91*:10722–10726, 1994.

16

Cellular and Molecular Biology of Neoplastic Transformation in Vitro

Although the study of the biochemistry and the cell and molecular biology of neoplasia in vivo has elucidated many significant and important characteristics of neoplasia, the ability to transform cells in vitro with various carcinogenic agents has been a very popular and useful tool. This is particularly true in systems of cultured cells exhibiting a normal phenotype and genotype that may be transformed to neoplasia by viruses, chemicals, or radiation and where direct comparisons with the parent culture may be made. While "pure" cultures of normal tissues, ideally developing as clones, may not always be completely feasible, cultures of fibroblasts, keratinocytes, T cells (lymphocytes), and some other cell types do fit this criterion and have been used in comparison with their transformed counterparts. However, the majority of studies attempting to identify critical differences between normal and neoplastic cells have not followed these rigorous criteria. Despite this fact, considerable valuable information about the cell and molecular biology of neoplastic transformation in vitro has been obtained.

One of the first systems studied was that of normal embryonic chick fibroblasts compared with cells from cultures of the same tissue that had been transformed by the Rous sarcoma virus in vitro. This system and most others that have been studied are of mesenchymal origin; thus broad extrapolation of such findings to the in vivo situation may be somewhat limited. Biological transformation of cells in vitro has several distinct advantages over chemical- and radiation-induced transformation, the most important of which is the use of mutants of the oncogenes involved in the transformation. On the other hand, chemical- and radiation-induction of transformation in vitro may have greater general application, especially in relation to transformation of epithelial cells such as keratinocytes and hepatocytes.

MEMBRANE TRANSPORT IN NORMAL AND TRANSFORMED CELLS

Some of the earliest investigations of the biochemical changes accompanying transformation in vitro involve the study of glycolysis as well as the transport of small molecules across plasma membranes, especially sugars. In 1968, Temin reported that the glycolysis of chick embryo fibroblasts infected with a strain of the Rous sarcoma virus exhibited a considerably higher rate than uninfected cultures (Figure 16.1). Studies by others confirmed these findings, but the actual mechanism was not clear—i.e., transport, phosphorylation, or both (Temin, 1974), until later studies demonstrated that infection by the virus actually induced expression of the glucose transporter gene in the infected cells (Birnbaum et al., 1987; White and Weber, 1988). In addition, the rate of uptake of glucose analogs was also dramatically enhanced in Rous sarcoma virus–trans-

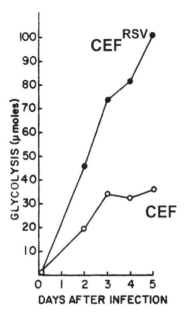

Figure 16.1 Glycolysis of cultures of uninfected chick embryo fibroblasts (CEF) and Rous sarcoma virus (RSV) infected CEF in media containing limiting amounts of serum. For infection, RSV (Fujinami strain) was added to the culture 40 minutes before zero time. Cultures were harvested at each of the days indicated, and the lactate in the medium determined as a measure of glycolysis. (Modified from Temin, 1968, with permission of the author and publisher.)

formed chick embryo fibroblasts (Table 16.1), but the apparent rate of uptake of a variety of other nutrients and substrates was not significantly different from that of normal growing chick embryo fibroblasts (Weber et al., 1984). In these earlier studies, it was demonstrated that glucose uptake was concomitant with the first appearance of morphological changes in the virus-infected cells (cf. Hatanaka, 1974) and that hexokinase activity did not change at the time of transformation with the RNA oncogenic virus. Perhaps the most conclusive evidence that the alteration in

Table 16.1   Rates of Nutrient Uptake by Chicken Embryo Fibroblasts

	Uptake Rate		
Nutrient	Density-Inhibited	Normal Growing	Rous Sarcoma Virus–Transformed
2-Deoxyglucose	1.0	6.8	23.9
3-O-Methylglucose	1.0	6.5	32.8
Uridine	1.0	4.0	3.4
Adenosine	1.0	2.1	—
Thymidine	1.0	9.0	8.9
α-Aminoisobutyric acid	1.0	4.5	4.5
Phosphate	1.0	1.9	1.8
Potassium	1.0	1.8	1.6

From Weber et al., 1984, with permission of the author and publisher.

glucose uptake was a function of the viral infection was through the use of temperature-sensitive mutants of the virus. Cells infected with a temperature-sensitive mutant of the Rous sarcoma virus were morphologically and biologically transformed in vitro at 35°C but not at 39.5°C. In experiments demonstrating the induction of expression of the glucose transporter gene after infection with the Rous sarcoma virus, both wild-type virus and temperature-sensitive mutants produced the morphological and biochemical changes at the permissive temperature of 36°C; but when the temperature was raised to 41.5°C, only the cells infected by the wild-type virus exhibited the enhancement of glucose transporter expression (White and Weber, 1988). The use of such temperature-sensitive viral mutants in demonstrating the importance of a variety of other functions in the transformation of chick embryo fibroblasts has also been reported, including the membrane association of actin (see below) (Wickus et al., 1975), the synthesis of several membrane polypeptides (Isaka et al., 1975), and the synthesis of glycosaminoglycan in chick embryo chondroblasts (Shanley et al., 1983). At the time many of these experiments were carried out, the existence and function of oncogenes was still not completely understood, and thus the use of such mutants was very helpful in determining functions of the cell that were directly related to the function of the gene responsible for the oncogenic transformation.

Relatively early studies with mammalian cells transformed by RNA sarcoma viruses suggested that enhanced phosphorylation, not enhanced transport of hexoses, was the mechanism for differences seen in hexose metabolism (Bissell et al., 1973; Jullien et al., 1982). However, both the studies by White and Weber (1988) and those by Birnbaum et al. (1987) clearly demonstrated, by using temperature-sensitive mutants, that infection with RNA sarcoma viruses induced a dramatic increase in glucose transporter gene expression. Unlike cells transformed by RNA oncogenic viruses, transformation by small DNA viruses of mouse cells does not specifically enhance sugar transport (cf. Hatanaka, 1974). The transport of amino acids studied with the use of nonmetabolized α-aminoisobutyrate in cells transformed by the SV40 virus gave varied results. Human cells (Patterson et al., 1976) transformed by this virus showed no difference in transport of α-aminoisobutyrate as compared with nontransformed cells, whereas mouse cells infected by the same virus showed an increase in the sodium ion gradient–dependent transport of α-aminoisobutyrate (Lever, 1976). While transport mechanisms after chemical carcinogenesis in vitro have not as yet been studied in detail, the cellular and molecular changes that occur after infection with oncogenic viruses depend on both the virus and the species of recipient cells.

CHARACTERISTICS OF THE SURFACE MEMBRANE OF NORMAL AND TRANSFORMED CELLS IN VITRO

In Chapters 10 and 14, the importance of the structure of the external plasma membrane in relation to tumor invasion, tumor metastases, and the phenomenon of contact inhibition of both cell movement and cell replication were discussed. Thus it was appropriate that one of the earliest investigations of the biochemistry and cell biology of transformed cells was related to the surface membrane. In 1969 Burger (cf. Burger, 1973) demonstrated that the addition of certain plant proteins, loosely termed *agglutinins*, would cause the agglutination of virally transformed cells in culture. In contrast, the parent cells from which the transformed cells were derived did not agglutinate when specific plant materials were added to the medium. The purified material responsible for the agglutination was found to be a glycoprotein with a molecular weight of approximately 18,000. This material reacted in a similar manner with a number of neoplastic cell types obtained from neoplasms growing in vivo as well as cells transformed in culture by chemicals, ionizing radiation, viruses, or "spontaneously." In many instances, cells that had reverted or lost their transformed phenotype also lost their capacity for agglutination in the presence of the plant agglutinin.

Several other plant agglutinins or lectins, as they are known, have been found to affect neoplastic cells in a similar manner. In addition, some nontransformed cells also exhibit agglutinability, thus making the original generalization invalid. Furthermore, Burger and others (cf. Sharon, 1977) demonstrated that treatment of normal cells with trypsin for very short periods of time rendered them agglutinable. This last experiment indicated that normal cells contained receptor sites for the plant agglutinins but that these sites were normally "protected" by some peptide components of the surface membrane. Furthermore, it was shown by Sachs (1974) that some variants of polyoma-transformed cells showed varying degrees of agglutination by concanavalin A, another plant lectin. Sachs' laboratory also demonstrated that normal fibroblasts in mitosis are agglutinated by concanavalin A as well as by the wheat germ lectin, whereas transformed fibroblasts in mitosis are not agglutinated by these lectins.

As can be seen from Table 16.2, lectins from both plant and animal sources interact rather specifically with certain sugars and their derivatives. Those from plant sources react primarily with specific sugar moieties, while lectins or selectins from mammalian sources (Chapter 10) react with more complex oligosaccharide structures. As noted from the table, lectins are proteins with a selective affinity for simple or complex sugars. Their specificity is dependent not only on the presence of the sugar in the terminal position but also on its anomeric confirmation, the attachment site to and nature of the subterminal sugar, the number of receptor sites, and the degree of steric hindrance caused by surrounding structures. In the mammal, as exemplified in the human, lectins are involved in the interaction of specific cells with other specific cell types (Chapter 10). Their functions in plants is not entirely clear.

The binding of lectins to the carbohydrate moieties listed in Table 16.2 is not by means of covalent linkages but rather through weak molecular interactions such as van der Waals forces. Other studies (cf. Nicolson, 1976) have demonstrated that whether cells were agglutinated by a

Table 16.2 Some Examples of Specific Lectins in Plants and Animals

Source (trivial name)	Predominant Chemical Specificity	Reference
Canavalia ensiformis (concanavalin A from jack bean)	D-mannose	cf. Rapin and Burger, 1974
Glycine max (soybean agglutinin)	N-acetyl-D-galactosamine	cf. Rapin and Burger, 1974
Triticum vulgaris (wheat germ agglutinin)	N-acetylglucosamine	cf. Rapin and Burger, 1974
Phaseolus vulgaris (phytohemagglutinin of red kidney bean)	N-acetyl-D-galactosamine	cf. Rapin and Burger, 1974
Ricinus communis (castor bean agglutinin)	D-galactose	cf. Rapin and Burger, 1974
Lotus tetragonolobus (lotus agglutinin)	L-fucose	cf. Rapin and Burger, 1974
Limulus polyphemus (hemolymph agglutinin of the horseshoe crab)	Sialic acid	cf. Rapin and Burger, 1974
Homo sapiens (galectin-3)	β-galactosides	Ochieng et al., 1998
Homo sapiens [P-selectin (GNP-140)]	Galβ1-4 (Fucα1-3) GlcNAcβ1-3Galβ1-4Glc	Brandley et al., 1990
Homo sapiens [E-selectin (ELAM-1)]	NeuNAcα2-3Galβ1-4(Fucα1-3) GlcNAc	Brandley et al., 1990

Taken in part from data of Rapin and Burger, 1974, with permission of the authors and publisher.

lectin or not, the total number of lectin molecules bound to the surface was usually the same for both normal and neoplastic cells. The answer to this puzzle became apparent when lectin molecules labeled with fluorescent dyes were used to interact with normal and neoplastic cells. Such experiments demonstrated a difference in the surface distribution of lectins bound to normal cells compared with lectins bound to tumor cells. On normal cells, the lectin molecules were distributed randomly, whereas they appeared to be aggregated into clusters on the surface of tumor cells. This is shown in Figure 16.2. Furthermore, lectins in their polyvalent form are capable of inducing a redistribution of lectin-binding sites on the plasma membrane of the cell, which then becomes agglutinated. This latter process may extend to the clustering of such sites to form a large mass on one portion of the cell surface, which has been termed a cap. Capping occurs more rapidly on transformed fibroblast cell lines than on untransformed cells under identical circumstances (cf. Nicolson and Poste, 1976) and occurs commonly on normal lymphocytes (see below). Capping involves an interaction of the surface receptor molecules (such as lectin receptors as well as a variety of other receptors including those for hormones, growth factors, and so on) with elements of the cytoskeleton, discussed later in this chapter (Bourguignon and Bourguignon, 1984). The effectiveness and rapidity of capping, as well as agglutination, which results from cluster formation of lectin-binding sites, is dependent on these and several other factors including the cell density of the culture (Inbar et al., 1977) and the ATP content of the cells (Vlodavsky et al., 1973) but not the ploidy of the cell (Sivak and Wolman, 1972). In addition, the fatty acid and cholesterol composition of the cell membrane also affects the effectiveness and

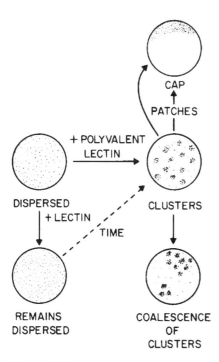

Figure 16.2 Pathways of ligand (concanavalin A)-induced receptor redistribution on cells. After ligand binding, initially dispersed receptors may remain dispersed or undergo clustering. The clustered receptor-ligand complexes may coalesce or form patches and eventually caps. (After Nicolson and Poste, 1976, with permission of the authors and publisher.)

speed of agglutination of cells (Hill and Borysenko, 1979). This latter characteristic may be related in part to the microviscosity (fluidity-rigidity behavior) of the cell membrane. However, a
number of studies using fibroblast-like cells in culture reported various results from increased
fluidity of the plasma membrane of transformed fibroblasts to a lowered fluidity of the membrane of these cells compared with that of normal or untransformed fibroblasts (cf. Nicolson,
1976; Shinitzky and Inbar, 1976). Normal lymphocytes exhibited a greater microviscosity
(lesser fluidity) than malignant lymphocytes grown in suspension (Shinitzky and Inbar, 1976).
This phenomenon may be related to the cholesterol content of these cells in that normal lymphocytes contain about twice the amount of this molecular species as lymphoma cells (Shinitzky
and Inbar, 1974). Lectin and antibody-induced capping of receptor sites is readily seen in normal
lymphocytes, but may not occur under the same circumstances with neoplastic lymphocytes (Inbar et al., 1973). Furthermore, redistribution of surface receptors may occur on lymphocytes in
hypertonic medium even in the absence of any ligands (Yahara and Kakimoto-Sameshima,
1977). Thus, the mobility of receptors and related molecules on the surface of various cell types
is dependent on a variety of factors, including the valency of the ligand, microviscosity of the
membrane, and interaction of the plasma membrane molecule, receptor or otherwise, with intracellular components, including elements of the cytoskeleton and other members of the signal
transduction pathway (e.g., Graziadei et al., 1990).

After these extensive studies on differential lectin agglutination of normal and transformed
cells in culture, some investigators extended these studies into the in vivo situation. Becker
(1974) demonstrated a differential lectin agglutination of fetal and malignant hepatocytes compared with adult hepatocytes. The latter cells, even after treatment with protease, cannot be agglutinated by concanavalin A, whereas fetal liver cells and hepatoma cells are agglutinated by
this lectin. Weiser (1972) also demonstrated that intestinal epithelial cells of the human fetus,
but not of the adult, can be agglutinated by concanavalin A. These studies suggest that in at least
some cell populations the property of agglutination by lectins is another example of the expression of fetal characteristics by neoplastic cells. In both normal and neoplastic keratinocytes, both
in vivo and in vitro, the expression of lectin binding by using a variety of different lectins exhibited significant differentiation-dependent expression. Normal keratinocytes in culture bound
those lectins that neoplastic keratinocytes also bound with the exception of the *Ulex europaeus*
agglutinin I (peanut agglutinin), which was bound to neoplastic keratinocytes but not to normal
cells (Suter et al., 1991).

In accord with the changes in lectin-binding sites described above, biochemical studies of
the surface membrane of normal and transformed cells in vitro have shown differences. Surface
glycoproteins and gangliosides of cells transformed by viruses, chemicals, and x-rays in vitro
show significant but not necessarily common differences when compared with nontransformed
cells cultured in vitro (Baker et al., 1980; Srinivas and Colburn, 1984; Glick, 1979). Smets et al.
(1978) demonstrated that alterations in membrane glycopeptides of transformed cells did not
always correlate with anchorage-independent growth in vitro, although tumors derived from cell
lines showed a correlation of the two characteristics. Furthermore, the addition of retinoic acid
to transformed mouse fibroblasts greatly increases their adhesive properties, which appear to be
related to the effect of this vitamin A derivative on the biosynthesis of cell-surface glycoproteins
(Sasak et al., 1980). In agreement with these findings is the demonstration by several investigators of lowered levels in transformed cells of a glycosyltransferase involved in the synthesis of glycoproteins and gangliosides on the surface membrane (Roth et al., 1974; Patt and
Grimes, 1974).

A frequent finding in transformed cells in culture was the absence or marked decrease of a
cell surface glycoprotein of molecular weight of about 250,000 (Chen et al., 1976). This protein

had been designated as LETS (large external transformation-sensitive protein). The protein was shown to be absent from the surface of cells transformed by some oncogenic DNA viruses. Interestingly, when cells were transformed by a temperature-sensitive mutant of the SV40 virus, the LETS protein did not disappear from the surface of infected cells cultured at the nonpermissive temperature (Shopsis and Sheinin, 1976). Another cell surface protein that is greatly reduced in many transformed cells in culture is fibronectin, a large, adhesive protein found in many cells, in connective tissue, and in plasma (Chapter 10). This protein is involved in the maintenance of the cellular cytoskeleton and the interaction of cells with collagen and with other intercellular molecular matrices. It is now apparent that the LETS protein and fibronectin are quite likely one and the same molecular species (cf. McDonagh, 1981). Several secretory glycoprotein species, one having a molecular weight of 35,000 (Gottesman and Cabral, 1981) and another protein family of molecular weight 60,000 to 62,000 (Senger et al., 1980, 1983) were identified and correlated with transformation of both fibroblastic and epithelial cells in culture. While these early findings posed many more questions than they answered, knowledge of characteristics of the surface membrane of the cells in culture in part laid the foundation for our understanding of cell-cell interaction, which has become so important in our understanding of the processes of invasion and metastases during the stage of progression in vivo.

ARCHITECTURE OF TRANSFORMED CELLS IN VITRO

Although early histologists suggested that the cytoplasm of cells possessed a characteristic architecture, the full impact of these observations did not become clear until the demonstration of cytoskeletal components, microtubules, contractile microfilaments, and intermediate (10-nm) filaments in cells. The most common method of demonstration of these structures has been by fluorescent antibody techniques.

Microtubules are ultramicroscopic tubular structures found in virtually all cells. They comprise a family of proteins called tubulins α, β, and γ (cf. Burns, 1991). The α- and β-tubulins form heterodimers and assemble into microtubules. γ-Tubulin is primarily associated with the poles of the microtubule structure. Originally, microtubules were felt to be primarily involved in mitosis, where they make up a major portion of the mitotic spindle. However, it is now apparent that microtubules have definitive patterns of organization within cells, depending on the cell type, and are associated with a variety of other proteins that are important in a number of cellular functions. A listing of some of the structure/function relationships of microtubules in cells is given in Table 16.3. A number of proteins have been associated with microtubules and are essen-

Table 16.3 Structure/Function Relationships of Microtubules in Cells

Structure	Function
Mitotic spindle	Chromosome segregation
Interphase microtubule network	Intracellular organization, organelle movements, and coordination of membrane traffic, including secretion
Dendrites	Neural morphogenesis, postsynaptic densities
Axon	Neural morphogenesis, presynaptic densities, axonal transport
Cilia, flagella	Cell motility

tial for several of the functions noted in Table 16.3. As expected, different cells express different protein families for such microtubule expression (cf. Lane and Allan, 1998; Avila, 1992). Microfilaments are the smallest of the components of the cytoskeleton and consist of one or more of several contractile proteins and their associated molecular species related to actin and myosin (cf. Goldman et al., 1979).

Intermediate filaments are a more diverse group of cytoskeletal elements, which have been divided into a number of groupings including keratins, vimentin, desmin, and neurofilament proteins (Table 16.4; Weber and Osborn, 1982). These cytoskeletal elements are members of a large multigene family, many of which are differentially expressed in different tissues (Fuchs and Hanukoglu, 1983; Moll et al., 1982). Such variation in the expression of components of the multigene family of intermediate filaments has also been seen in neoplastic cells, both in vivo and in vitro (Wada et al., 1992; Skalli et al., 1988; Caulín et al., 1993), and this finding has been used diagnostically to distinguish general classes of neoplasms (cf. Miettinen et al., 1983). Summerhayes et al. (1981) demonstrated that rat bladder epithelium in culture as well as nontumorigenic foci altered by exposure to benzo[a]pyrene demonstrated no detectable vimentin filaments. However, tumorigenic cell lines from this tissue did express this protein. In mouse epidermal keratinocytes, both viral and chemical transformation resulted in abnormalities in the expression of keratins (cf. Caulín et al., 1993). Specifically, keratin K8 was upregulated in transformed epidermal cell lines and in neoplasms resulting from injection of the cells back into appropriate mouse hosts.

One of the most striking changes exhibited in the cytoskeleton of transformed cells is exemplified by Figure 16.3. The upper figure is an artist's conception of the patterns of microfilaments forming networks of "actin cables" extending in a parallel fashion throughout the cytoplasm of the cultured cell resting on a surface. Below this is shown the microfilament pattern in a transformed cell. Here the filaments display very little parallel arrangement, and there is diffuse fluorescence to indicate depolymerization of microfilaments into their constitutive molecules, which react to give the diffuse pattern. The normal patterns of microtubule (Brinkley and Fuller, 1978) and intermediate filaments (Ben-Ze'ev, 1984) lose the organization seen in nontransformed cells when they become transformed.

Both microfilaments and microtubules interact directly with the surface membrane of the cell. Thus, both the morphology of a cell and the mobility of its lectin-binding sites are in all likelihood directly related to microtubule and microfilament organization. This probability has been demonstrated by a direct relationship between concanavalin A capping and a redistribution of microtubules as well as the changes induced by a temperature-sensitive Rous sarcoma virus (cf. Nicolson and Poste, 1976). In the latter instance, both cell morphology and surface topography are altered concomitantly with changes in the organization and assembly of microfilaments. Therefore, it is quite likely that the mobility of lectin-binding sites in neoplastic cells is more directly related to changes in the microfilament-microtubule system governing cell architecture than to membrane microviscosity. In transformed fibroblasts exhibiting this disruption of microfilaments, receptor proteins that are normally associated with a relatively rigid organization of the structures would become more mobile, allowing for the lectin induction of clustering and capping (Wang and Goldberg, 1976). In the case of the lymphocyte, capping induced by lectins and by antibodies to specific surface receptors may be directly related to the interaction of microfilaments with surface membrane receptors and other proteins (Bourguignon and Bourguignon, 1984). Ultimately in the normal lymphocyte, as discussed in Chapter 20, interaction with lectins or antibodies stimulates cell replication, but such stimulation may not always be effective in neoplastic lymphocytes.

Table 16.4 Expression of Different Intermediate Filament (IF) Proteins in Cells, Tissues, and Tumors[a]

IF type	No. of Polypeptides	Molecular Mass (kDa)	Cell Types Positive	Tumor Types Positive
Keratins	19	40–68	Keratinizing and nonkeratinizing epithelia	Carcinomas
Vimentin	1	54	"Mesenchymal cells," e.g., fibroblasts, chondrocytes, endothelial cells, etc.	Nonmuscle sarcomas Most lymphomas Melanoma
Desmin	1	53	Sarcomeric muscle Visceral smooth muscle Some vascular smooth muscle cells	Muscle sarcomas, i.e., rhabdomyosarcoma leiomyosarcoma
Glial fibrillary acidic protein (GFAP)	1	51	Astrocytes Bergmann glia	Gliomas
Neurofilament proteins	3	NF-L 63 NF-M 160 NF-H 200	Neurons of central and peripheral nerves	Neuroblastoma Ganglioneuroblastoma Pheochromocytoma

[a] IF contents of only a few selected major cell types are listed. Certain cells and tumors show characteristic coexpression of more than one IF protein. For example, some vascular smooth muscle cells coexpress vimentin and desmin, some glial cells coexpress vimentin and GFAP. This coexpression can also be useful in differential diagnosis. Thus, mesothelial cells, mesotheliomas, pleomorphic adenomas, and some but not all carcinomas of the kidney and thyroid coexpress keratin and vimentin, while some Merkel cell carcinomas and neuroendocrine tumors seem to coexpress neurofilaments and keratin. A few tumors express different IF proteins in different tumor parts; for example, teratomas and biphasic synovial sarcomas.
Adapted from Osborn and Weber, 1986, with permission of the authors and publisher.

NORMAL

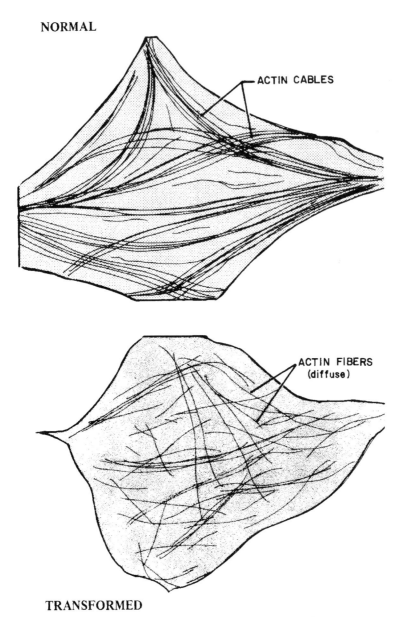

TRANSFORMED

Figure 16.3 Patterns of microfilaments (actin cables or fibers) in normal and transformed fibroblasts growing in vitro. The regular pattern of parallel microfilaments in the normal cell can be contrasted with the disarray and diffuseness of the cables and fibers in the transformed cell.

PROTEINS AND mRNA IN TRANSFORMED CELLS

Because of the relative homogeneity of transformed cell populations in vitro, it has been possible to make direct comparisons between both messenger RNA and protein populations of transformed cells with those of their nontransformed counterparts. In these instances, it becomes extremely important to be rigorous in the populations being compared, as noted above.

Messenger RNAs in Normal and Transformed Cells in Culture

Comparative studies of different RNA populations in normal and transformed cells have been somewhat cyclic with respect to methodologies. As an example, in 1980, Moyzis and associates compared nuclear RNA and polysomal poly(adenylic acid) messenger RNA in normal SHE cells and a cell line that had originally been treated with benzo[a]pyrene. Utilizing the liquid hybridization techniques popular at that time, they were able to demonstrate relatively few changes in the qualitative pattern of gene expression in these two cell populations. However, when specific messenger RNAs were investigated after transformation by a variety of methods, distinct quantitative changes could be found between normal and transformed cells in culture. Some examples of such instances are seen in Table 16.5. While many more examples might be given, many of them do not satisfy the criteria discussed at the beginning of this chapter. However, the examples given do indicate dramatic differences in the messenger RNA levels of the specific genes indicated. Most of the examples are matrix or cytoskeletal proteins, with one oncogene-related example. There are obviously numerous other examples that could be given in the oncogene area, but that would only further emphasize the point made in the table.

Within the last few years, a variety of technologies have been developed for examining large numbers of messenger RNAs in cells, both in vivo and in vitro. Because of the ease and "purity" of the use of cells in culture, many of the examples of these technologies are in cultured cells. Table 16.6 lists some of the more modern technologies that have been utilized, with appropriate references. The student is urged to examine the references for details of the methods themselves. Of the methods listed, the differential display method is relatively simple and

Table 16.5 Expression of Some Specific mRNAs in Transformed Compared with Their Nontransformed Controls

Gene	Cell Type	Carcinogen	Relative Change (t/nt)	Reference
Actin	Rat fibroblast	CMV	$\downarrow$ (0/1)	Leavitt et al., 1985
Collagen precursor	CEF	RSV	$\downarrow$ (1/10)	Adams et al., 1977
Fibronectin	CEF	Avian sarcoma virus	$\downarrow$ (1/10)	Fagan et al., 1981
fms-related	Rat tracheal epithelial cells	MNNG or γ radiation	$\uparrow$ (5–19/1)	Walker et al., 1987
Keratins (3)	Mouse epidermal cells	Spontaneous	$\downarrow$ (~0/1)	Roop et al., 1983
Pro α1 collagen	SHE cells	4-nitroquinoline-1-oxide	$\downarrow$ (0/1)	Majmudar et al., 1988

Key: t/nt, transformed/nontransformed; CEF, chick embryo fibroblasts; SHE, Syrian hamster embryo; CMV, cytomegalovirus; RSV, Rous sarcoma virus; MNNG, N-methyl-N-nitro-N-nitrosoguanidine.

Table 16.6 Methods for Screening the Expression of Large Populations of Messenger
RNAs in Cells

Method	Basis	Reference
Differential display	Use of synthetic DNA "tags" to probe and display differentially expressed mRNAs	Martin et al., 1998
DNA microarray and "gene screens"	Individual gene sequences "fixed" to a "chip," screen, or other frame for subsequent hybridization to mRNA populations	Ramsay, 1998; Iyer et al., 1999
Subtractive hybridization	Liquid hybridization of two related mRNA and cDNA populations, with subsequent isolation of cDNAs not hybridizing	Lee et al., 1991

inexpensive but exhibits difficulties from false positives and negatives. Subtractive hybridization
is an elegant technology that requires some experience to obtain appropriate results. The DNA
microarray methods presently in use allow for the examination of the expression of 10^4 or more
genes but are extremely expensive. The less expensive "gene screens" usually have fewer than
10^3 genes with which to examine differential expression from different mRNA populations. As an
example, the subtractive hybridization method has been utilized to compare a normal strain of human mammary cells with an aneuploid neoplastic cell line obtained from a pleural effusion (Lee et
al., 1991). Although the comparison here does not conform to the criteria indicated at the beginning of this chapter, it does demonstrate that the method allows for the identification of differential
expression of specific genes in two populations as well as the identification of genes not yet
described.

Differential Protein Expression in Normal and Transformed Cells

Studies of differential protein contents in transformed cells related to those in normal cells were
initially concerned with the investigation of specific proteins or related groups of proteins. One
such protein species that was intensively studied was related to earlier investigations, more than
half a century ago, of certain neoplastic cells grown in vitro that have the ability to lyse plasma
clots rapidly. This observation was further investigated by Reich and associates (cf. Unkeless et
al., 1973), who demonstrated that many cells transformed in vitro release a proteolytic factor
into the culture medium that has the ability to activate plasminogen, an inactive precursor of the
proteolytic enzyme plasmin. The plasminogen activator of SV40-transformed hamster cells
growing in vitro was characterized as a protein with a molecular weight of 50,000. The production of this activator can be correlated in many transformed cells with the other characteristics of
transformation (Table 14.1). Again, however, we are faced with the fact that the plasminogen
activator is not produced by all cells transformed in vitro or in vivo (San et al., 1977). Furthermore, the production of plasminogen activator does not correlate with certain biochemical characteristics of transformed cells, such as the increased rate of hexose transport in Rous sarcoma
virus–transformed fibroblasts (Wolf and Goldberg, 1976). Thus, although plasminogen activator
production may be an important characteristic of specific transformed cells, it is not an ubiquitous characteristic of the neoplastic transformation. On the other hand, its obvious relationship
to proteases involved in neoplastic invasion and metastases (Chapter 10) strongly suggests that
this characteristic in vitro has its counterparts in vivo (Duffy and O'Grady, 1984).

In analogy to the search for specific and ubiquitous biochemical changes characteristic of the neoplastic state, the production of a variety of different proteins and enzymes were investigated in transformed cells in culture. Some examples in systems involving reasonable comparative studies, as discussed at the beginning of this chapter, are seen in Table 16.7. As with the messenger RNAs noted in Table 16.5, the functions of the proteins in this table are concerned with intercellular and intracellular proteins as well as components of the cell cycle. As expected, a variety of other differences in cell cycle function between normal and transformed cells have also been described (e.g., Crissman et al., 1991; Xiong et al., 1993), but a more extensive consideration is beyond the boundaries of this text.

Ornithine decarboxylase catalyzing the initial step of polyamine biosynthesis has been implicated as a major rate-limiting step early in the stage of promotion in mouse epidermis, particularly its response to TPA (O'Brien, 1976). As noted in the table, infection of mouse 3T3 cells with murine sarcoma virus (MSV) produces a dramatic increase in the protein content in such cells within 4 days after infection (Gazdar et al., 1976). Some of this increase may be due to stabilization of the protein rather than new synthesis and expression (Bachrach, 1976). In an interesting contrast, spontaneously transformed mouse epidermal cells for the most part exhibit a basal level less than that seen in the nontransformed cells and for the most part are induced to higher levels by the addition of TPA (Yuspa et al., 1980). Transfection of ornithine decarboxylase constructs into mouse 3T3 cells induces transformation (Moshier et al., 1993). Thus, while polyamine synthesis is critical for cell growth and normal maintenance, these somewhat disparate findings again indicate that there is no ubiquitous change in polyamine metabolism in neoplasia as evidenced by this single important key enzyme.

Another protein not listed in the table but having critical functions in the neoplastic transformation both in vivo and in vitro is p53, as already discussed elsewhere (Chapters 6 and 15). This protein, having a molecular weight of 53,000 (from which it derives its name), was first described in association with the large T antigen of SV40-transformed cells (cf. Crawford, 1983). The relative levels of this protein in normal and transformed mouse cells are listed in Table 16.8. As shown by many, the presence of this protein is not characteristic of all transformed or neoplastic cells in animals, but it clearly plays a major role in cell replication, response of the cell to injury, and neoplastic transformation (Chapter 15). The level of p53 messenger RNA in many nontransformed mouse cells was found to be the same as that in their SV40-transformed progeny. The marked difference in the levels of p53 was largely the result of

Table 16.7 Altered Levels of Specific Proteins in Transformed Cells

Protein	Cell Type	Carcinogen	Relative Change (t/nt)	Reference
Actin	CEF	RSV	↓ (0.3–0.5/1)	Wickus et al., 1975
Calmodulin	Mouse 3T3	SV40	↑ (2/1)	Chafouleas et al., 1981
cdc2 (p34)	Human keratinocytes	Spontaneous	↑ (7/1)	Rice et al., 1993
Collagen polypeptides	CEF	RSV	↓ (1/10)	Levinson et al., 1975
Cyclins A and B	Human keratinocytes	Spontaneous	↑ (~6/1)	Rice et al., 1993
Integrin $\alpha_5\beta_1$	Rat fibroblasts	RSV	↓ (0.5/1)	Plantefaber and Hynes, 1989
Ornithine decarboxylase	Mouse 3T3	MSV	↑ (20–25/1)	Gazdar et al., 1976
	Mouse epidermis	Spontaneous	↑ (~0.5/1)	Yuspa et al., 1980

Key: CEF, chick embryo fibroblasts; RSV, Rous sarcoma virus; SV40, simian virus 40; MSV, murine sarcoma virus.

Table 16.8   Relative Levels of p53 in Mouse Cells

Cell	Description	Amount of p53[a] (%)
SVA31E7	SV40-transformed BALB/c 3T3	100
MCA	Methylcholanthrene-induced C56BL/6 fibrosarcoma	31
CQ15	Spontaneously transformed C3H.Q embryo fibroblast	19
3T6	Mouse embryo fibroblast Swiss	16
Py A31C2	Polyoma-transformed BALB/c 3T3	16
PYS	Parietal yolk sac carcinoma	3
PCC4	Embryonal carcinoma	2
F9	Embryonal carcinoma	2
F9 AC C19	Differentiated carcinoma	2
WME 10	Whole mouse embryo, 10 days gestation	≤1
WME 12	Whole mouse embryo, 12 days gestation	≤1
WME 14	Whole mouse embryo, 14 days gestation	≤1
WME 15	Whole mouse embryo, 15 days gestation	≤1
BMK	Baby mouse kidney, strain TO	≤1
3T12	Mouse embryo fibroblast, BALB/c	2
3T3.A31	Mouse embryo fibroblast, BALB/c	≤1
3T3K	Mouse embryo fibroblast, Swiss	≤1
L929	Methylcholanthrene-induced tumor	≤1
NS1	Mouse myeloma	≤1
Thymocytes	Baby mouse thymus, strain TO	≤1

[a] All the values, corrected for the total protein content of the extract, are given relative to SVA31E7 as 100%.
From Crawford, 1983, with permission of the author and publisher.

sequestration and inactivation of the p53 by the SV40 large T antigen (cf. Herzig et al., 1999). Although p53 is a tumor suppressor gene, it has been shown to have transforming activity both in human (Slingerland and Benchimol, 1991) and rat (Rovinski and Benchimol, 1988) cells. The phosphorylation of p53 plays a major role in its intracellular function, although discrepancies have been found with respect to its phosphorylation and the effect of this change on transformation in vitro (cf. Milczarek et al., 1997). However, transformation in vitro is associated with phosphorylation of a number of other proteins (Arrigo et al., 1983; Kobayashi et al., 1981; Cooper et al., 1983). In contrast, sulfation of proteins on their tyrosine residues was dramatically decreased in embryonic rat fibroblasts infected with the Rous sarcoma virus (Liu and Lipmann, 1984).

Two-Dimensional Electrophoresis of Proteins in Normal and Transformed Cells

In analogy to the techniques noted in Table 16.6 but developed somewhat earlier, the two-dimensional electrophoretic separation of proteins in cells was seen as a method to examine the synthesis of many proteins simultaneously (Anderson and Anderson, 1979; O'Farrell, 1975). With this technique, a number of investigations have found quantitative differences in the protein populations of normal as compared with transformed cells. Bravo and Celis (1982) separated about 1300 polypeptides from normal and SV40-transformed human fibroblasts and from normal and spontaneously transformed human amnion cells. These investigators were unable to detect any new major polypeptide in the transformed cells, although perhaps as many as 10% of the peptides varied quantitatively between normal and transformed cells. Croy and Pardee (1983) resolved approximately 1000 polypeptides in normal and benzo[a]pyrene-transformed mouse 3T3 cells and identified a protein exhibiting a greater rate of synthesis and of stability in transformed as compared with nontransformed cells. Garrels and Franza (1989) compared protein maps containing about 1600 distinct polypeptides in nontransformed rat embryo fibroblasts and these cells transformed by the SV40-, adenovirus, or Kirsten murine sarcoma virus. No overall correlation between growth-regulated changes and transformation-induced changes was seen, although some 26 coregulated proteins were found overexpressed in the transformed cells. Figure 16.4 shows a computer interpretation of a two-dimensional gel electrophoresis of normal human fibroblasts (Celis et al., 1987). In this study, comparing the nontransformed cells with those transformed by the SV40 virus, a striking decrease in the levels of many proteins was seen in the transformed cells as well as the appearance (or increased synthesis) of some 47 polypeptides that were either absent or present in very low amounts in normal cells. These are noted as black spots on the computer printout. Although this study did not attempt to identify the polypeptides exhibiting such differences, the technology to do so rapidly became available. From other studies (e.g., Leavitt et al., 1982), the use of this technology allowed the identification of mutations in the β-actin gene of transformed human fibroblasts. However, isolation and characterization of such mutants is extremely difficult with two-dimensional gel electrophoresis; with the advent of the technologies indicated in Table 16.6, the nucleic acid methodologies have largely supplanted those involving the electrophoresis of proteins.

CYCLIC NUCLEOTIDES, CALCIUM, BASE ANALOGS, AND TRANSFORMATION IN VITRO

In Chapter 14, modulation of cell transformation in vitro was discussed. The effects of a variety of structurally dissimilar chemicals in modulating the transformation process were listed in Table 14.9. However, several such chemical modulators of the transformation phenotype in vitro were purposely omitted to be discussed in this chapter, primarily because their effects can be closely related to other mechanisms, and in some instances a fair amount of knowledge exists as to the mechanism of the effects themselves. Each of these three factors is considered separately.

Cyclic Nucleotides and Cell Transformation

A possible role for cyclic nucleotides in cell transformation in vitro was suggested some three decades ago when studies by Pastan and associates (cf. Johnson et al., 1971) demonstrated that the addition of cyclic AMP to CEF cultures transformed by the Rous sarcoma virus (RSV) resulted in an alteration in their morphology to that of normal, contact-inhibited cells with a lower growth rate. However, further investigation demonstrated that not all transformed cells responded in this manner upon the addition of cyclic AMP to the medium (Roth et al., 1982). The concentration of cyclic AMP in cells transformed in vitro was significantly less than that in corresponding nontransformed cells, especially during conditions of little or no cell replication (cf. Pastan, 1975). However, at least in cell lines transformed by temperature-sensitive SV40 mutants, a change in temperature from the restrictive to the permissive temperature or vice versa did not alter the cyclic AMP levels of these cells (Burstin et al., 1974). Otten et al. (1971) demonstrated an inverse correlation between growth rate and cyclic AMP levels when many cell lines were compared during logarithmic growth. Furthermore, in RSV-transformed chick embryo fibroblasts, plasma membrane adenylate cyclase activity was reduced, and its K_m for ATP was

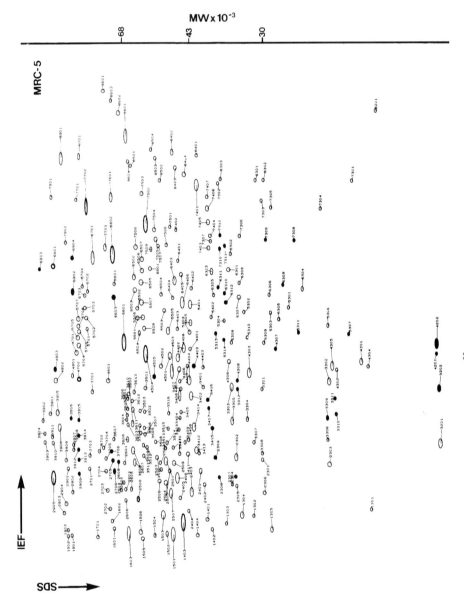

Figure 16.4 Computer interpretation of the [^{35}S]-methionine-labeled proteins (IEF) secreted by normal human fibroblasts (MRC-5). Polypeptides present preferentially in the media from SV40-transformed fibroblasts have been included in the map and are indicated in black. (Adapted from Celis et al., 1987, with permission of the authors and publisher.)

significantly lower in normal cells than in the transformed cells. Anderson et al. (1973) suggested that these changes may be mediated through some modification of the plasma membrane by viral transformation. Other studies by Sharma and associates (1977) as well as by Simantov and Sachs (1975) demonstrated apparent structural changes in cyclic AMP–binding proteins in an adrenocortical carcinoma and neuroblastoma, respectively.

Alterations in the cyclic AMP levels in normal and transformed cells have also been correlated with changes associated with the plasma membrane. Willingham and Pastan (1974) demonstrated that, in cultured mouse 3T3 cells, low levels of intracellular cyclic AMP may be correlated with increased agglutinability by concanavalin A, whereas high levels of the cyclic nucleotide are seen in those cells exhibiting decreased agglutinability. Cyclic AMP also appears to affect the glycopeptide composition of the surface membranes of cultured cells (Roberts et al., 1973), and the morphological changes seen in cultured neoplastic cells after the addition of cyclic nucleotides are also associated with a reappearance of contact inhibition of growth in these cells (cf. Pastan, 1975).

Another cyclic nucleotide, cyclic GMP, was shown by Goldberg and associates (see Hadden et al., 1972) to vary with cell replication in a manner opposite to that seen with cyclic AMP—that is, cyclic GMP levels increase when lymphocytes are stimulated to replicate, whereas the levels of this cyclic nucleotide are decreased in starved cells, in which cyclic AMP levels increase. In embryonic hamster kidney fibroblasts in culture, the addition of serum, insulin, or other growth factors caused a decrease in cyclic AMP levels but had no effect on cyclic GMP levels. However, when these cells were transformed by polyomavirus, the cyclic GMP concentration increased sixfold (Richman et al., 1981). The inverse relation between cyclic AMP levels in cells and their rate of replication has led to applications both in experimental and clinical situations. Bang et al. (1994) has shown the induction of terminal differentiation by externally added cAMP to a line of cells derived from adenocarcinoma of the prostate in the human. The addition induced terminal differentiation of these cells in vitro. In addition, Cho-Chung and associates (cf. Tagliaferri et al., 1988), using analogs of cAMP, induced both growth inhibition and phenotypic reversion of murine sarcoma virus–transformed mouse 3T3 cells. A more extensive review by these investigators laid the foundation for potential clinical uses of such chemicals in the therapy of neoplasia (Cho-Chung et al., 1991).

Calcium Ions and the Neoplastic Transformation in Vitro

Already discussed is the importance of calcium ions in activating protein kinase C, an enzyme that appears to be important in the mediation of some tumor promoters (Chapters 7 and 15). Calcium ions were shown to be very important in mediating the action of cyclic AMP in a variety of functions (cf. Rasmussen, 1974; Whitfield et al., 1979). It is now apparent that a large number of intracellular Ca^{2+}-binding proteins are involved in signaling mechanisms (cf. Niki et al., 1996). One of the most important of these proteins is calmodulin, which is involved in the regulation of protein phosphorylation–dependent cascades as well as in interaction with cytoskeletal elements (cf. Veigl et al., 1984). Generally speaking, the calmodulin levels of transformed cells of mesenchymal origin are higher than those present in nontransformed cells (cf. Veigl et al., 1984). Early studies showed that both mouse and chicken fibroblasts transformed by oncogenic viruses, as compared with their normal counterparts, required a markedly decreased concentration of Ca^{2+} in the medium to sustain cell replication in culture (Boynton and Whitfield, 1976; Balk et al., 1979). This was also found to be true for keratinocytes, in which high concentrations of calcium induce differentiation and ultimately apoptosis, but low concentrations of the ion favor keratinocyte replication. Transformed keratinocytes could not be induced to differentiate in high concentrations of calcium ions and, in fact, replicated quite well in low concentrations (cf. Whitfield, 1992). Although the mechanisms of many of these differences are not absolutely clear, it is now apparent that cells not only have specific Ca^{2+} channels for entrance but also Ca^{2+}-sensing receptors. This is diagrammed in Figure 16.5, which also indicates the importance of the endoplasmic reticulum as a transporter and storehouse for calcium within cells (cf. Hebert and Brown, 1995). Thus, it is likely that transformed cells that do not respond to calcium in normal ways have defects in one or more of the pathways shown in Figure 16.5 as well as in the regulation of the expression of various calcium-binding proteins, especially calmodulin.

Effects of Nucleic Acid Analogs on Transformed Cells

In Chapter 13, the use of the thymine analog 5-bromodeoxyuridine was discussed in relation to the demonstration of sister chromatid exchanges (Figures 13.5 and 13.6). Almost 30 years ago, Silagi (1971) demonstrated an interesting effect of the incorporation of 5-bromodeoxyuridine into the DNA of mouse melanoma cells. Growth of these cells in media containing the analog caused a suppression of growth, loss of pigment formation, and a lost or markedly decreased ability to grow as tumors when inoculated into appropriate hosts. These effects were completely

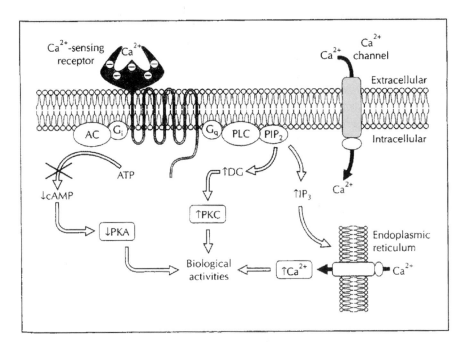

Figure 16.5 Diagram illustrating the manner in which Ca^{2+} acts as an extracellular messenger. Activation of the Ca^{2+}-sensing receptor (by binding of Ca^{2+} to negatively charged regions) activates phospholipase C (PLC; possibly via a G_q protein), leading to increased intracellular levels of diacylglycerol (DG) and inositol 1,4,5-trisphosphate (IP_3), and concomitant release of Ca^{2+} from internal stores (e.g., the endoplasmic reticulum). The rise in Ca^{2+} is sustained by influx of Ca^{2+} through channels in the plasma membrane. The Ca^{2+}-sensing receptor can also reduce receptor-mediated increases in cAMP levels (possibly via a G_i protein). The Ca^{2+}-induced changes in the activities of these second messenger systems leads to changes in the activities of a series of kinases (e.g., PKC and PKA), which in turn alter the biological activities of the cell. AC, adenylate cyclase; PIP_2, phosphatidylinositol bisphosphate. (From Hebert and Brown, 1995, with permission of the authors and publisher.)

reversed by growing the cells in thymine without 5-bromodeoxyuridine. This was of great interest, since—in addition to the induction of sister chromatid exchange—5-bromodeoxyuridine also induces specific-locus mutations and the expression of fragile sites in cultured cells (Morris, 1991). More recently, Anisimov and associates (1993) demonstrated the carcinogenicity of this analog in association with other agents when administered in vivo for chronic periods. Other effects of addition of this analog to the medium of cultured cells include the induction of endogenous oncogenic viruses, especially RNA viruses (cf. Goz, 1978). In a sense, it would appear that the analog tends to enhance "differentiation" of the expression of the viral genome.

In addition to 5-bromodeoxyuridine, 5-azacytidine, an analog of cytidine, also has the capacity to "activate" retroviral genomes within a variety of cells in vitro (Jaenisch et al., 1985). In addition, in other systems the analog induces the appearance of differentiated characteristics in a variety of different cell types (Jones, 1985). It is presumed that the effects of this analog are due to its effects on DNA methyltransferase responsible for the methylation of cytosines in DNA (Jüttermann et al., 1994). However, exactly how the 5-bromodeoxyuridine exerts its effect on reversing neoplasia and altering differentiation is not clear at the present time.

GROWTH FACTORS AND THE NEOPLASTIC TRANSFORMATION

Biologists have long recognized the presence and critical importance of factors, both exogenous and endogenous, capable of regulating either positively or negatively the growth, development, and cell replication of cell populations within an organism. Paramount among these factors are the trophic hormones of endocrine origin, such as those from the anterior pituitary, pancreatic islets, and gonads. However, the importance of trophic factors in regulating cell growth and replication was not entirely appreciated until the advent of tissue culture methodology. The critical importance of serum in the maintenance, growth, and replication of mammalian cells in culture was obvious with the very earliest experiments of Carrel and others (cf. Carrel and Lindbergh, 1938).

Serum and the Nutrition of Transformed Cells

One of the earliest studies showing distinctive differential serum requirements for transformed cells was that of Temin (1966), who demonstrated a lowered requirement for serum by cells transformed by the RSV compared with nontransformed chick embryo fibroblasts. Similarly, SV40-transformed human lung fibroblasts exhibited a lowered requirement for a number of serum factors including some ions (McKeehan et al., 1981). Chemically transformed 3T3 mouse cells also had a much lower serum requirement than normal cells, although these cells exhibited "normal" growth controls at low serum concentrations (Holley et al., 1976).

In contrast to the lowered serum requirement of transformed cells, a number of publications have indicated that neoplastic cells in culture exhibit an increased requirement for the essential amino acid methionine (Halpern et al., 1974; Hoffman, 1982; Breillout et al., 1990). Studies discussed in Chapter 17 also indicate that certain neoplasms have specific requirements for other individual amino acids. With this knowledge, it has also been possible to develop serum-free cell culture media for both normal and neoplastic cells (cf. Taub, 1990; Bjare, 1992). However, the development of such serum-free media initially required the isolation and characterization of factors—virtually all polypeptide in nature—occurring in serum and having both trophic and inhibitory effects on cells in culture. A number of these growth factors and related agents are discussed below.

Growth-Enhancing and -Inhibitory Factors in Cell Transformation

In his original experiments, Temin (1966) proposed that the lowered requirement for serum was related to growth factors within this medium. At that time, only one or two such growth factors had been isolated and characterized, although there had been many experiments in a variety of systems with crude serum or tissue extracts, demonstrating both the enhancement and inhibition of the replication of cells in culture (cf. Keski-Oja et al., 1988; Siegfried, 1992). Furthermore, as pointed out by Siegfried (1992), there is some difficulty in the precise definition of a growth factor, because some molecules may have quite different effects on different tissues within the organism. An example of such overlapping functions may be seen in Figure 16.6, wherein a polypeptide may act as a growth factor in one tissue, as a hormone-controlling secretion in another tissue, and as a neurotransmitter in the brain (cf. Siegfried, 1992). Thus, one may consider an operational definition for a growth factor as a peptide that produces a biological signal via a specific high-affinity receptor that results in altered growth or differentiation (Siegfried, 1992). A listing of such growth factors exhibiting either growth enhancement, growth inhibition, or both, is seen in Table 16.9.

The rather extensive listing in Table 16.9 is by no means complete. For example, it omits the trophic hormones, growth hormone, and insulin, and some of the families are incomplete, such as the transforming growth factor-β family (Lawrence, 1996). Most of the factors listed in Table 16.9 are of a molecular weight below 20 kDa and with no known modifications of the polypeptide, such as carbohydrate or lipid. The exceptions are the platelet-derived growth factor family, whose members in their dimeric forms are in excess of 30 kDa, and transforming growth factor-β whose dimers are 25 kDa. Erythropoietin, a circulating hormone produced by kidney and liver and acting as a growth factor for the erythroid progenitor population, is a complex, glycosylated protein of molecular weight 46 kDa. Transforming growth factor-β, the tumor necrosis factor, and the interferon families are generally considered to be inhibitors of cell growth (Keski-Oja et al., 1988). Some 50 years ago, investigators proposed that cell replication in vivo may be controlled by a negative feedback mechanism through endogenous inhibitors of replication. Such inhibitors were termed *chalones* and thought to be cell type–specific (cf. Patt and Houck, 1980). Other cell growth inhibitors have been partially characterized (Miyazaki and Horio, 1989), but the three families noted are perhaps the best characterized of the "chalones" at present.

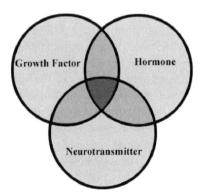

Figure 16.6 Overlapping functions of polypeptides exerting distinctive effects in biological systems. (Adapted from Siegfried, 1992, with permission of the author and publisher.)

Table 16.9 Families of Growth-Enhancing and -Inhibiting Factors

Family	Source	Target Cells	Major Effect
Epidermal growth factor family			
Epidermal growth factor (EGF)	Epithelial cells	Epithelial, mesenchymal cells	Mitogen
Transforming growth factor-α (TGFα)	Tumor-derived, transformed cell lines	Epithelial, mesenchymal cells	Mitogen, transforming for fibroblasts
Amphiregulin (AP)	Carcinoma cell lines	Epithelial, mesenchymal cells	Mitogen for fibroblasts, inhibits breast carcinoma cell growth
Schwannoma-derived growth factor (SDGF)	Schwann cells	Astrocytes, fibroblasts, Schwann cells	Mitogen
gp30	Breast carcinoma cells	*c-erb*B2-positive cells	Mitogen
Heparin-binding growth factor family			
Acidic-fibroblast growth factor (aFGF)	Ubiquitous	Ubiquitous	Mitogen, angiogenesis, neurotrophic
Basic fibroblast growth factor (bFGF)	Ubiquitous	Ubiquitous	Mitogen, motility factor
int-2 oncoprotein (FGF-3)	Embryonic cells	Fibroblasts	Mitogen
hst oncoprotein (FGF-4)	Embryonic cells	Fibroblasts	Mitogen
Fibroblast growth factor-5 (FGF-5)	Fibroblasts	Fibroblasts	Mitogen
Keratinocyte growth factor (KGF)	Stromal cells	Keratinocytes	Mitogen, angiogenesis
Vascular endothelial cell growth factor (VEGF)	Monocytes/macrophages	Vascular endothelial cells	Mitogen, angiogenesis, vascular permeability factor
Platelet-derived growth factor family			
Platelet-derived growth factor (PDGF)	Mesenchymal cells, platelets	Mesenchymal cells	Mitogen
αα			
ββ			
αβ			
Insulin-like growth factor family			
Insulin-like growth factor-I (IGF-I)	Ubiquitous	Ubiquitous	Mediates growth hormone activity, insulin-like effects
Insulin-like growth factor-II (IGF-II)	Ubiquitous	Ubiquitous	Insulin-like effects
Nerve growth factor family			
Nerve growth factor (NGF)	Schwann cells, neurons	Peripheral neurons, melanocytes, cholinergic neurons in brain	Neurotrophic, increases ACh synthesis

(table continues)

Table 16.9 (continued)

Family	Source	Target Cells	Major Effect
Nerve growth factor family (continued)			
Brain-derived neurotrophic factor (BDNF)	Neurons, glial cells	Dopaminergic neurons in brain	Neurotrophic
Neurotrophin-3 (NT-3)	Many cell types	Peripheral proprioceptive neurons	Neurotrophic
Transforming growth factor-β family			
Transforming growth factor (TGF)			
-β₁	Ubiquitous	Ubiquitous	Mitogen for fibroblasts, inhibits proliferation of many cell types, angiogenesis
-β₂			
-β₃			
-β₄			
Growth factors not classified into the above families			
Hepatocyte growth factor (HGF)	Many cell types	Hepatocytes, epithelial cells	Mitogen
Platelet-derived endothelial growth factor (PDEGF)	Platelets	Endothelial cells	Angiogenesis, mitogen
Endothelin-1	Many cell types	Endothelial, mesenchymal cells	Vasoconstriction, mitogen
Gro (melanocyte growth factor)	Many cell types	Melanocytes, inflammatory cells	Mitogen, proinflammatory
Hematopoietic growth factors			
Erythropoietin (Epo)	Kidney, liver	Erythroid progenitors	Mitogen and red cell maturation
Granulocyte colony-stimulating factor (G-CSF)	Macrophages, endothelial cells, fibroblasts	Stem cells, neutrophil precursors	Mitogen and enhancement of function
Granulocyte-macrophage colony-stimulating factor (GM-CSF)	T lymphocytes, macrophages, endothelial cells, fibroblasts	Progenitors for neutrophils, eosinophils, monocytes	Mitogen and enhancement of function
CSF-1 (M-CSF)	Many cell types	Mononuclear phagocytes	Mitogen
Lymphocyte-activating factor (IL-1β)	Endothelial cells	T cells and others	Mitogen and enhanced function
T cell growth factor (IL-2)	T lymphocytes	T cells, B cells, macrophages	Mitogen
Multi-CSF (IL-3)	T lymphocytes	Precursors of neutrophils, platelets, monocytes, eosinophils, basophils, stem cells	Mitogen, maturation, and enhanced function
B cell stimulatory factor I(IL-4)	T lymphocytes	B cells, mast cells	Mitogen

B cell growth factor II (IL-5)	T lymphocytes	B cells, eosinophils	Mitogen and enhanced eosinophil differentiation
Eosinophil differentiation factor			
Inteferon β2 (IL-6)	T lymphocytes, macrophages	Stem cells, B cells	Mitogen
Hybridoma growth factor			
Hepatocytic growth factor			
Tumor necrosis factor (TNF) family			
TNF-α (cachectin)	Primarily monocytes, but many other cell types may secrete	Ubiquitous	Functional activation, apoptosis
TNF-β (lymphotoxin)	Lymphocytes	Lymphocytes	Decreased proliferation and apoptosis
Interferons (IFN)			
IFNα	Ubiquitous	Virus-infected cell	Resistance to virus infections
IFNβ	Ubiquitous	Virus-infected cell	Resistance to virus infections
IFNγ	T lymphocytes and natural killer cells	Lymphocytes and other cells of the immune system	Activation of the immune system to eradicate infections and neoplasms in cells

Modified and extended from Pusztai et al., 1993, with permission of the authors and publisher.

Growth Factor Receptors

In order for growth factors to exert their trophic effects, it is necessary for such polypeptides to interact with specific receptors on the surface of the target cell. We have already noted this in previous chapters (3, 7, and 15). However, in the case of growth factors, their receptors are predominantly of the type involving a single polypeptide chain or its dimeric or trimeric forms, having both external and cytoplasmic domains with a single transmembrane domain. Examples of a number of diagrammatic structures for the receptors for growth factors may be seen in Figure 16.7. Virtually all of these receptors are glycoproteins having a high affinity for their specific growth factor, with their molecular weights being considerably in excess of those of the ligand growth factors themselves, usually in the range of 50 kDa to 150 kDa. As noted in the figure, many but not all growth factor receptors exhibit tyrosine protein kinase activity in the cytoplasmic domain, such activity being activated by interaction with the ligand, as was previously discussed in Chapter 7. In virtually all instances, interaction of the receptor with its ligand involves a dimerization or in some instances a trimerization of the receptor molecules in the cell membrane (cf. Weiss and Schlessinger, 1998).

Signaling mechanisms that are initiated and result in transduction to the nucleus have already been discussed in relation to receptors containing an intrinsic tyrosine kinase (Chapter 7; Fantl et al., 1993). However, as noted from Figure 16.7, receptors involved in hematopoietic and lymphoid cells do not contain tyrosine kinase in their cytoplasmic domain. In this instance, the signal transduction pathway must involve tyrosine kinases that are separate molecules within the cytoplasm of the cell. A considerable amount of work has elucidated many of the details of this pathway (Silvennoinen et al., 1997; McCubrey et al., 2000). A diagram of the pathway that involves a family of tyrosine kinases known as JAK kinases (Janus kinases) and STAT transcription factors (signal transducers and activators of transcription) is seen in Figure 16.8. As noted in the figure, the JAKs phosphorylate the cytokine receptor and at the same time phosphorylate members of signal transduction pathways, not only the STAT pathway but, as noted in the figure, other pathways involved in signal transduction of receptors having inherent tyrosine kinase within their cytoplasmic domains. This "cross-talk" between the JAK-STAT pathways and other signaling pathways allows such cells to activate a variety of transcription factors and subsequently genetic expression. Such cross-talk also exists between peptide growth factor transduction pathways and steroid hormone receptor signaling pathways (cf. Ignar-Trowbridge et al., 1995). As discussed in the next chapter, tumor necrosis factors utilize a different signaling pathway, which in many instances directs the cell into apoptosis (Chapter 17).

Transforming Growth Factors

Following the characterization of epidermal growth factor (cf. Carpenter and Cohen, 1990) and nerve cell growth factor (Levi-Montalcini, 1987), the search for other growth factors and their characterization became a popular area of research in the 1970's. During this time, Todaro and associates reported the striking observation that media from murine sarcoma virus–transformed cells possessed growth factor properties when added to normal or some other neoplastic cells (De Larco and Todaro, 1978). Most striking was the fact that these "growth factors" actually induced the morphological transformation of normal cells and anchorage-independent growth, one property in cell culture that correlates quite well with tumorigenicity in vivo (Table 14.1). This striking effect may be noted microscopically in Figure 16.9. Untreated normal rat cells shown in A exhibit a single monolayer of growth and a quite regular pattern. Treatment with media from murine sarcoma–transformed rat cells induced the normal cells to growth in the pattern seen in B, in which cells become quite crowded and pile up on one another as characterized

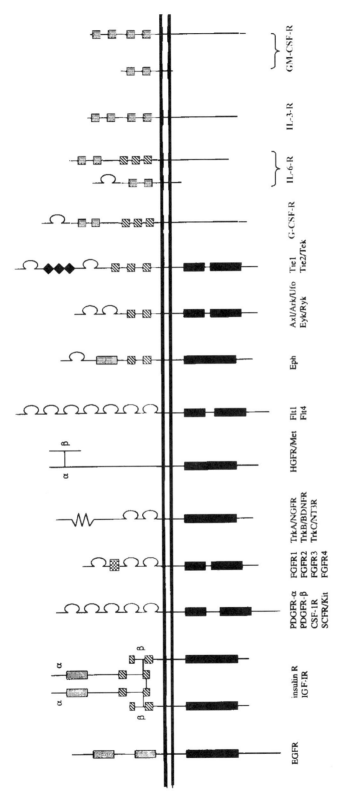

Figure 16.7 Diagrammatic structures of members of growth factor receptor families. The solid closed rectangles indicate cytoplasmic tyrosine kinase domains; the heavy double line indicates the plasma membrane. Dotted rectangles, cysteine-rich domains; hatched boxes, fibronectin domains; vertical lines box, acid box consisting of eight consecutive acidic residues; closed diamonds, EGF-like domains; half-circles, immunoglobulin domains; zig-zag line, leucine-rich domain; EGF, epidermal growth factor; IGF, insulin growth factor receptor; PDGF, platelet-derived growth factor; FGF, fibroblast growth factor; NGF, nerve growth factor; HGF, hepatocyte growth factor; Flt, vascular endothelial growth factor receptor. The reader is referred to the original article for definition of other acronyms used in this figure. The last four growth factors are listed in Table 16.9. (Modified and extended from Heldin, 1996, with the permission of the author and publisher.)

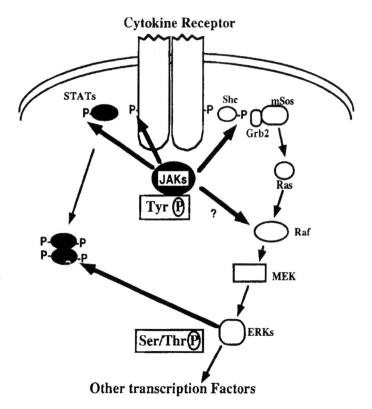

Figure 16.8 Diagram of interaction between the JAK-STAT and Ras pathways in signaling in hemato-poietic and lymphoid cells. The arrows indicate action of components toward others. (Adapted from Leaman et al., 1996, with permission of the authors and publisher.)

by the transformed phenotype. Even more striking is the absence of anchorage-dependent growth of the normal rat cells in C but the growth in single colonies of more than 500 cells each in the soft agar, as noted in D (Todaro et al., 1981). Subsequent to these studies, Todaro and associates (Marquardt et al., 1984) isolated and determined the amino acid sequence of the "sarcoma growth factor," which was subsequently termed *transforming growth factor-α* (TGF-α). The structural similarity of TGF-α to epidermal growth factor is seen in Figure 16.10. Although not shown in the figure, both growth factors are originally synthesized as a large transmembrane precursor, and the active growth factor as seen in Figure 16.10 is cleaved from the cell surface and released into the surrounding environment (cf. Kumar et al., 1995). Interestingly, the "normal" epidermal growth factor (EGF) may also induce transformed properties in cells in vitro by addition to the medium (Liboi et al., 1986). Other studies have indicated that many cells in culture may respond to a variety of growth factors by exhibiting properties of the transformed phenotype (Kaplan and Ozanne, 1983; van Zoelen et al., 1988). Furthermore, as might be expected, both TGF-α and EGF interact with the EGF receptor, and both are produced by a variety of normal tissues (Rall et al., 1985; Salomon et al., 1990).

A second transforming growth factor, TGF-β, was independently discovered by two laboratories (Moses et al., 1981; Roberts et al., 1981). TGF-β was later shown to be a component of the crude "sarcoma growth factor" present in the media of retrovirus-transformed cells (cf. Lawrence, 1996). Subsequent studies have demonstrated that this growth factor is one of a very

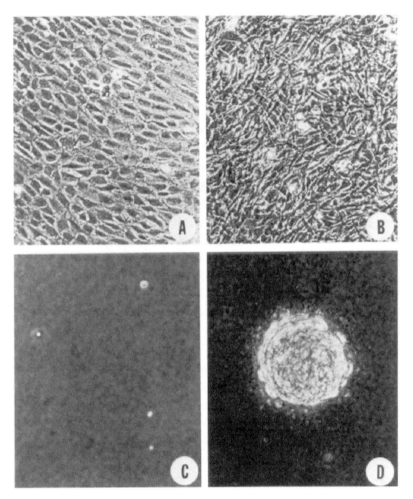

Figure 16.9 A. Untreated normal rat kidney cells. B. Normal rat kidney cells treated with crude "sarcoma growth factor" for 6 days. C. Untreated normal rat kidney cells plated in 0.3% soft agar. D. Colony of normal rat kidney cells plated in 0.3% soft agar, treated with "sarcoma growth factor," and photographed two weeks after treatment. See text for details. (Adapted from Todaro et al., 1981, with permission of the authors and publisher.)

large family of growth factors occurring normally in a variety of species with quite divergent functionalities. TGF-β itself occurs in three different forms, TGF-β1, -β2, and -β3, which are produced from a large precursor form nearly three times the size of the active growth factor monomer (Figure 16.11). As seen from the figure, there is considerable sequence conservation in the active TGF-β component, but the pro and pre components exhibit much less conservation. The extended polypeptide containing the pro- and active TGF-β are combined within the cell as dimers, which are proteolytically cleaved, and a binding protein [latent TGF-β-binding protein (LTPB)] is linked by a disulfide bond to the pro region. Secretion of these latent complexes of TGF-β are secreted into the cellular environment, as noted in Figure 16.12. The active dimeric form of TGF-β is freed from the complex by one or more of the components seen in the figure, and this dimeric active form may then interact with receptors with subsequent cell signaling

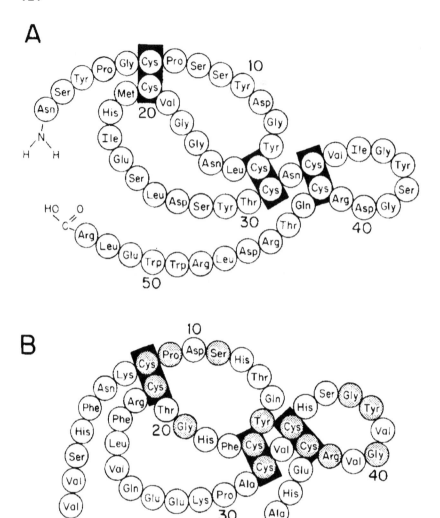

Figure 16.10   Structures of epidermal growth factor (A) and transforming growth factor α (B) in the mouse and rat, respectively. The extreme similarity of the positions of the disulfide (CYS-CYS) bridges and the lengths and sequence similarities of the intervening chains are readily noted. Invariant amino acid residues present in all known epidermal growth factor-like structures are depicted with shaded circles in the transforming growth factor structure.

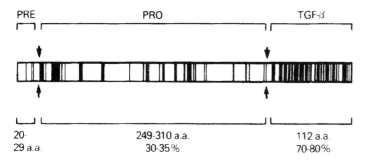

Figure 16.11 Regions of homology and overall structure of mammalian TGF-β isoforms. The three mammalian TGF-βs are highly homologous to one another in the C-terminal region of 112 amino acids (a.a.) but show much more sequence divergence in the precursor (pre) and pro regions. The black bars indicate regions of sequence identity between TGF-β1, -β2, and -β3. The percentage identity in each domain is given below the numbers of a.a. Other members of the TGF-β family show virtually no homology in the pro region but still are quite homologous in the C-terminal 112 a.a. (Adapted from Wakefield et al., 1991, with permission of the authors and publisher.)

(Roberts and Sporn, 1996). In contrast to the predominantly growth-stimulatory activity of TGF-α and other growth factors listed in Table 16.9, TGF-β and members of its family have a number of other functions. In fact, TGF-β acts as a growth-stimulatory agent for only a few cell types of mesenchymal origin (cf. Wakefield et al., 1991). TGF-βs are strongly growth-inhibitory for most epithelial cells, as well as cells of the hematopoietic system. TGF-β may also serve to enhance or inhibit the expression of the differentiated phenotype of a number of cells.

TGF-β Signaling Mechanisms

The TGF-β receptor complex differs from those depicted in Figure 16.9 in that, while having a cytoplasmic protein kinase domain, the specificity for this protein kinase is not tyrosine but serine/threonine. Furthermore, there are two types of TGF-β receptors, and interaction with the ligand requires an interaction with each of the two types, type 1 and type 2. Since type 2 receptors may bind ligand directly from the medium while type 1 receptors cannot, it is likely that the final complex involves a heterotetramer in which the type 1 receptor may differ depending on the member of the TGF-β family involved (cf. Ruscetti et al., 1998). A diagram indicating the interaction with TGF-β and the two forms of the receptor as a heterotetramer with activation of the kinase domain is seen in Figure 16.13. For this signal transduction pathway, a different series of downstream signaling molecules known as Smad proteins are involved, with a series of phosphorylations, as noted in the figure, ultimately resulting in an activated complex of Smad proteins that may associate with transcription factors and activate DNA transcription of specific genes (Visser and Themmen, 1998).

Influences of Growth Factors on Cell Transformation

Prior to the discovery of transforming growth factors, there was a general belief that cells producing hormones or growth factors did not possess receptors for the hormone or growth factor produced by the cell itself. The secretion by such cells of endocrine glands was termed *endocrine secretion*. Alternatively, cells producing a hormone or growth-enhancing or -inhibitory factor might be in close association with target cells containing the receptor for such ligands, with the endocrine cell itself still not possessing such receptors. The demonstration by Todaro

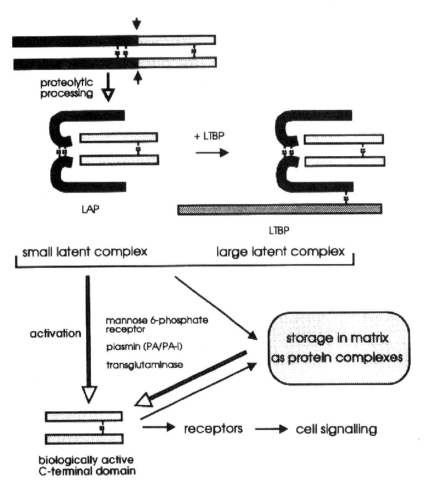

Figure 16.12 Diagram of the formation and activation of latent complexes of TGF-β. Latent TGF-β consists of a noncovalent complex between the LAP form and the mature TGF-β. In the large latent complex, LAP is covalently bound to a protein called the latent TGF-β–binding protein (LTBP) by a disulfide linkage. These complexes may be either sequestered by extracellular matrix or activated by a cooperative proteolytic process involving the mannose-6-phosphate receptor and a surface-bound protease after secretion from the cell. Only the mature, biologically active, C-terminal domain of TGF-β binds to its signaling receptors. (Adapted from Roberts and Sporn, 1996, with permission of the authors and publisher.)

and his associates of the production of a transforming growth factor, TGF-α, soon led to the demonstration that cells producing this factor also possess the EGF receptor, thus allowing both the production and the stimulation by the growth factor product all within a single cell. This was termed *autocrine* secretion, and these three types of secretion are diagrammed in Figure 16.14. At first, this phenomenon was felt to be unique to neoplastic cells and to possibly explain their enormous growth advantage over their normal counterparts (cf. Todaro et al., 1981). During the past two decades, however, examples of both paracrine and autocrine secretion in normal cells have been reported (cf. Wysolmerski and Stewart, 1998; Tsao et al., 1993).

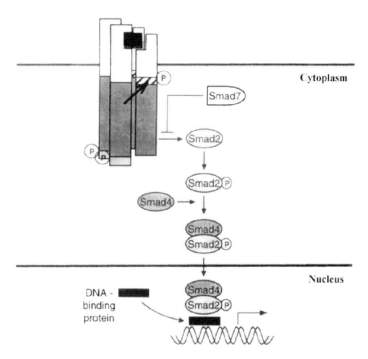

Figure 16.13 Diagram of the TGF-β heterotetramer receptor and its signaling pathway. Upon activation of the serine/threonine receptor kinase by interaction with its ligand, pathway-specific Smads are phosphorylated leading to heterodimerization with Smad4, the complex then translocating to the nucleus where it binds directly, or in a complex with other factors, to DNA. The inhibitory Smads (Smad7) bind to the type 1 receptor and prevent phosphorylation of the pathway-specific Smads. (Adapted from Visser and Themmen, 1998, with permission of the authors and publisher.)

Transforming Growth Factors and Multistage Carcinogenesis

Since TGF-α as well as EGF itself may induce phenotypic transformation in normal cells in vitro, it is reasonable to suggest that these agents may act as promoters in vivo. Furthermore, there is now ample evidence that TGF-α is expressed in a variety of malignant neoplasms, and many of these neoplasms exhibit an enhanced level of the EGF receptor, many times owing to gene rearrangements or amplification of the EGF receptor gene as a component of the stage of tumor progression (cf. Salomon et al., 1990).

Various types of "dysregulation" of growth factor–receptor pathways in transformed cells have been described (cf. Hatakeyama and Taniguchi, 1988). A number of examples of changes in the epidermal growth factor–receptor pathway in transformed cells have been described (Todaro et al., 1976; Cherington et al., 1979; Hollenberg et al., 1979). Several of these reports (e.g., Hollenberg et al., 1979; Cherington et al., 1979) have demonstrated a decreased requirement for epidermal growth factor in transformed cells. The role that autocrine stimulation of such cells played in these findings was not clear at that time. In addition, in Syrian hamster embryo cells transformed in vitro, alterations and the responsiveness of these cells to epidermal growth factor, platelet-derived growth factor, and transforming growth factor β were significantly altered (Isfort et al., 1994).

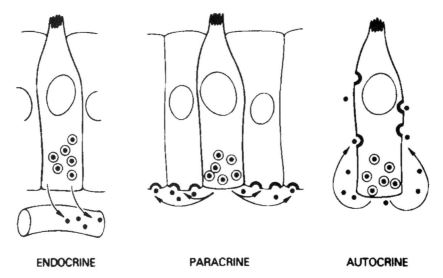

ENDOCRINE   PARACRINE   AUTOCRINE

Figure 16.14 Diagram of the types of cellular secretion. The black dots represent the secretory product or ligand and the heavy black half circles on the cell membrane the specific receptor for the secreted ligand. (Adapted from Todaro et al., 1981, with permission of the authors and publisher.)

The response of transformed and neoplastic cells to TGF-β tends to be lost, primarily during the stage of progression. Since TGF-β acts primarily to inhibit the growth of epithelial and many mesenchymal cells, such a loss of receptor activity and function is perhaps to be expected. There is now substantial evidence that much of this TGF-β resistance is the consequence of inactivating mutations either in the type 1 or type 2 TGF-β receptors or one of the several Smad proteins (Reiss, 1997). In fact, Smad2 has been implicated as a tumor suppressor gene involved in the control of cell invasion (Prunier et al., 1999). In contrast, Oft and associates (1998) have argued that TGF-β signaling may be rather important for the invasiveness and metastasis of certain carcinoma cells both in vivo and in vitro. Krieg et al. (1991) reported that constitutive overexpression of TGF-β1 mRNA was observed in malignant carcinomas but not in benign premalignant lesions. Furthermore, 100% of pancreatic and 83% of colonic neoplasms have a mutation affecting at least one component of the TGF-β pathway (cf. Blobe et al., 2000). However, the activity of the entire pathway was not investigated. An autocrine type of secretion for TGF-β has been described in transformed fibroblasts, and in many instances this is associated with aberrant EGF receptor regulation (Newman, 1993). Repression or inactivation of TGF-β receptors has also been described in the genetically based retinoblastoma and in hereditary nonpolyposis colorectal cancer (cf. Ruscetti et al., 1998).

Thus, it appears that growth factor signaling pathways are largely aberrant in transformed cells in vivo as they are in many neoplastic cells in vitro. Furthermore, a number of pathways in other growth factors are also abnormal in transformed cells, as noted in Table 16.10. The EGF/TGF-α autocrine pathway is not functional in all neoplasms, although all cells transformed by chemicals appear to exhibit an enhancement in TGF-α expression (cf. Lee et al., 1993). It is likely that such increased expression of these growth factors makes up the basis for the decreased requirement for EGF in chemically transformed mouse cells (Cherington et al., 1979). Furthermore, some neoplastic cells may begin to express growth factor receptors and thus respond to growth factors to which their normal counterparts would not (cf. Descamps et al.,

Table 16.10 Defective Growth Factor Pathways in Transformed Cells

Growth Factor System	Cell System	Change Related to Transformation	Reference
Epidermal growth factor/transforming growth factor α	Cells transformed in vitro by chemicals	Increased expression with or without enhanced receptor expression	Cf. Lee et al., 1993
Fibroblast growth factor	Mouse 3T3 cell lines	Mutant and normal forms of these genes induce transformation	Cf. Hatakeyama and Taniguchi, 1988
Hepatocyte growth factor	Hepatocellular carcinoma cell lines	Growth inhibition	Shiota et al., 1992
	Spontaneous transformation of 3T3 cells	Increase in HGF receptor due to gene amplification	Cooper et al., 1986
Insulin growth factor-1	SV40 transformed 3T3 cells	Increased expression	Porcu et al., 1992
Interleukin-2	HTLV-transformed cell lines	Increased expression of IL-2 receptor	Hatakeyama and Taniguchi, 1988
Platelet-derived growth factor (PDGF)	Syrian hamster embryo cell transformation	Decreased responsiveness in half of transformed cell lines tested	Isfort et al., 1994
Transforming growth factor β	Retinoblastoma cell lines	Absence of TGF-β receptors	Kimchi et al., 1988

1998). A similar effect had earlier been reported with the platelet-derived growth factor and its receptor (Bowen-Pope et al., 1984). Insulin-like growth factors I and II may also be expressed at higher levels in a variety of neoplasms in vivo and in vitro, often with their receptor exhibiting expression as well, leading to autocrine growth potential (Werner and LeRoith, 1996). Mutations in the IGF-II/mannose-6-phosphate receptor, which prevent such autocrine effects or growth factor effects on the neoplastic cells themselves, have been reported, as discussed in Chapter 15. Interestingly, hepatocyte growth factor may actually inhibit proliferative activity of a variety of neoplastic cell lines (Tajima et al., 1991). In another cell culture system, Seslar et al. (1995) demonstrated an interaction between TGF-β production and hepatocyte growth factor expression, with a clear interaction between various cell types in the culture.

Since the responses to growth factors in the neoplastic cell may be altered as a result of the development of autocrine stimulation, mutations in signaling pathways, interactions between growth factors and adjacent cell types (paracrine secretion), or altered imprinting, it is very likely that growth factors do play a role in the enhanced cell replication during the stage of progression. It is very likely that many of the characteristics described in this section are the result of evolving karyotypic instability in this stage, and thus, while many interesting different patterns of responses may be seen in transformed and neoplastic cells, no single alteration may be seen ubiquitously in all transformed and neoplastic cells.

DNA METHYLATION, TELOMERASE, CELL SENESCENCE, AND TRANSFORMATION

In Chapter 15 the importance of alterations in DNA methylation was discussed, as well as telomerase activity and telomere length as common alterations in neoplasia. In cultured cells, these functions appear to play a quite significant role, especially in the phenomenon of cell senescence, which was briefly described in Chapter 14. In short, essentially all cells that are placed in culture have a finite period or finite number of doublings during which they remain structurally and genetically normal cells (Hayflick, 1997). At the end of this time, the cells either die or some of them become "transformed" to an immortal phenotype that is accompanied by an altered karyotype, which usually expresses instability subsequently as the cells are continued in culture. In recent years, the association of DNA methylation and telomerase and telomeres has been a subject of intense investigation. These are considered separately here, although in fact they are closely related functions.

DNA Methylation and Transformation

When cells are first placed into culture, there is usually a rapid general loss of DNA methylation; but as immortal cells emerge, the methylated DNA content of such cell lines appears to increase (cf. Razin and Cedar, 1991). Recall that in neoplastic cells in vivo there is a general hypomethylation of DNA, although there are clearly areas of hypermethylation within the DNA of a variety of human neoplasms (cf. Laird and Jaenisch, 1994). Baylin and associates (1997) have reviewed some of the changes that may be seen in the DNA methylation capability of cells in culture as a function of the level of the DNA-methyltransferase activity. Figure 16.15 summarizes much of the experimental data for the relations between DNA methyltransferase activity to fibroblast aging and senescence as well as infection with the SV40 oncogenic virus. The changes in methylation seen on initial explantation are not appreciated from the graph, although the relative DNA methyltransferase of young fibroblasts may be considered as reflecting the initial loss of DNA methyl groups and, presumably, the activity of the enzyme, especially in epithelial cell cultures. The further loss of methyltransferase as the fibroblasts are continued in culture is reflective of a further loss in DNA methylation as well. At the time of senescence there is a reversal of this effect, occurring over a shorter time period; at the time of crisis—i.e., in this case transformation by SV40 virus—DNA methyltransferase is subsequently enhanced and then stabilizes. This was further investigated by Slack et al. (1999), who showed that T-antigen expression in transformed cells is accompanied by an elevation in DNA methyltransferase mRNA and protein as well as global genomic DNA methylation. These results and others (e.g., Kautiainen and Jones, 1986) suggest that transformed cells in cell culture may actually have enhanced levels of DNA methylation, which is an interesting contrast to the global demethylation seen in neoplasms in vivo.

Telomeres, Telomerase, and Cell Senescence and Transformation

As suggested in Chapter 15, the normal adult mammal tends to have extremely short or virtually absent telomeres in many of the highly differentiated cell types within the organism. When cells are initially placed in culture, especially mesenchymal cells, they initially have telomeres as well as exhibit telomerase activity. As mesenchymal cells are maintained in culture, their telomeres decrease in length until they become extremely short; the cells then stop replicating and subsequently die or go through a crisis (see above), at which time immortal cells develop. These immortal cells now exhibit telomerase activity and have telomeres, although usually shorter than those in the original cell population at explantation. Transformation by oncogenic viruses or

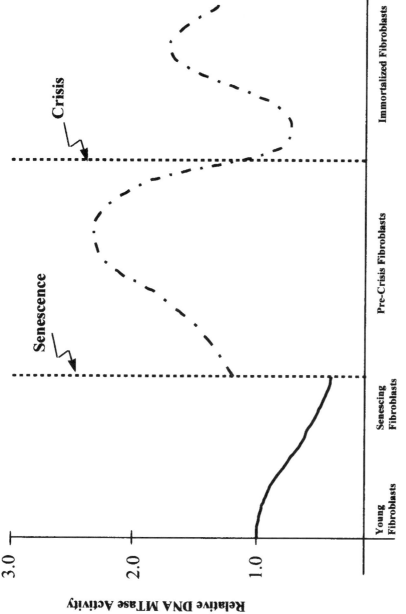

Figure 16.15 Graphical summary of experimental data for the relations of DNA-methyltransferase (MTase) activity to fibroblast aging and infection with SV40 virus in vitro. The graph depicts the full changes in DNA-MTase activity relative to 1.0 as the level seen in normal cells between passages 0 and 25. The three components of the graph are (1) as a function of young human fibroblasts from about passage 25 to when they are senescing (passage 50); (2) cells in the precrisis stage from about passage 50 to 70 after infection with SV40 at about passage 30; and (3) crisis phase cells from about passage 70 to 90, finally immortalized at passages 130 to 200. (Adapted from Baylin et al., 1998, with permission of the authors and publisher.)

chemicals will also reactivate telomerase and in many instances allow for the immortality of such transformed cells, as noted in Chapter 14 (Table 14.1). A diagram of this process is given in Figure 16.16.

It should be noted from the figure that germ cells and stem cells have a constant and relatively high level of telomerase activity and possess telomeres of substantial size. Induced differentiation of immortal cells causes a pronounced downregulation of telomerase activity in a wide variety of transformed cells (Sharma et al., 1995) but a lack of effect in some other cell lines (Bestilny et al., 1996). There is also evidence that the p53 gene is involved in the entrance of cells into the senescent period (Wynford-Thomas, 1996). The decrease in telomerase activity as

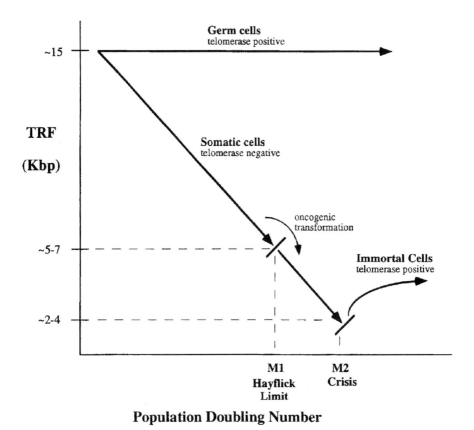

Figure 16.16 The telomere hypothesis of cell aging. TRF is the terminal restriction fragment length made up of the terminal TTAGGG repeats in human cells plus a small, variable length, proximal fragment. Germ cells maintain telomerase activity as well as their telomere length upon cell division. Somatic cells in general are telomerase negative and, as a consequence, their telomeres shorten with each cell division by approximately 50 bp (cf. Krupp et al., 2000). When somatic cell telomeres shorten sufficiently, cell cycle arrest occurs, with the activation of a senescent phenotype (M1 or Hayflick limit). If cells are transformed, they may bypass M1, but their telomeres continue to shorten, since telomerase has not been activated. When telomeres shorten to the point where chromosome function is impaired, cells enter a crisis period (Figure 16.15 or M2). In the absence of transforming virus infection, a few cells emerge from crisis that have activated the telomere maintenance machinery and telomerase. It is these cells that are immortal and maintain stable telomere lengths during culture. (Adapted from Morin, 1997, with permission of the author and publisher.)

cells in vitro approach senescence does not appear to be a direct function of DNA methylation, although this process can contribute to the repression of telomerase in some cells (Dessain et al., 2000). The marked shortening of telomeres as cells approach senescence is associated with increasing chromosome instability in mammals (Pommier et al., 1995) as well as in lower forms, where inhibition of telomerase induces chromosomal destabilization (Izbicka et al., 1999). In fact, Reddel (2000) has emphasized that many of the more common genetic changes seen in neoplasia may play a key role in the immortalization process of cells transformed in vitro.

Thus, while there is reasonable evidence to argue that telomerase activity as well as telomere length is associated with aging and senescence in vitro and in many instances in vivo (Krupp et al., 2000), the presence of the enzyme and of telomeres, even shortened, has not been universal in neoplasia (Krupp et al., 2000). Still, inhibition of telomerase may be an appropriate method with which to induce death in appropriate neoplasms (Herbert et al., 1999).

THE MOLECULAR AND CELL BIOLOGY OF CELL TRANSFORMATION IN VITRO—ITS CONTRIBUTION TO OUR UNDERSTANDING OF THE NEOPLASTIC PROCESS

As noted in Chapter 14 as well as in this chapter, cells in culture have many but not all of the characteristics of neoplastic cells in vivo. In particular, the cell and molecular alterations in transformed cells sometimes appear to be relatively unique to the situation. However, with careful comparison between normal and transformed cells in vitro, some characteristics seen in transformed cells may be directly applied to the in vivo situation. This was certainly the case with telomerase and its disappearance in senescence and reappearance during transformation, thus making it a potential therapeutic target in the management of neoplastic disease. Although the multistage nature of neoplasia has not been extensively studied in cell culture, probably because of the lack of good model systems, the SHE cell system has shown that there are considerable similarities in the biology and quite likely the cell and molecular changes occurring during the three stages of carcinogenesis in this in vitro system. Cell culture offers an exciting tool with which to study the neoplastic transformation and a variety of other processes that impinge on our knowledge and ultimate control of the neoplastic process.

REFERENCES

Adams, S. L., Sobel, M. E., Howard, B. H., Olden, K., Yamada, K. M., de Crombrugghe, B., and Pastan, I. Levels of translatable mRNAs for cell surface protein, collagen precursors, and two membrane proteins are altered in Rous sarcoma virus-transformed chick embryo fibroblasts. Proc. Natl. Acad. Sci. U.S.A., *74*:3399–3403, 1977.

Anderson, N. G., and Anderson, N. L. Molecular anatomy. Behring Inst. Mitt., *63*:169–210, 1979.

Anderson, W. B., Russell, T. R., Carchman, R. A., and Pastan, I. Interrelationship between adenylate cyclase activity, adenosine 3′:5′ cyclic monophosphate phosphodiesterase activity, adenosine 3′:5′ cyclic monophosphate levels, and growth of cells in culture. Proc. Natl. Acad. Sci. U.S.A., *70*:3802–3805, 1973.

Anisimov, V. N., and Osipova, G. Y. Carcinogenesis induced by combined neonatal exposure to 5-bromo-2′-deoxyuridine and subsequent total-body x-ray irradiation in rats. Cancer Lett., *70*:81–90, 1993.

Arrigo, A.-P., Darlix, J.-L., and Spahr, P.-F. A cellular protein phosphorylated by the avian sarcoma virus transforming gene product is associated with ribonucleoprotein particles. EMBO J., *2*:309–315, 1983.

Avila, J. Microtubule functions. Life Sci., *50*:327–334, 1992.

Bachrach, U. Polyamines and neoplastic growth: stabilization of ornithine decarboxylase during transformation. Biochem. Biophys. Res. Commun., *72*:1008–1013, 1976.

Baker, S. R., Blithe, D. L., Buck, C. A., and Warren, L. Glycosaminoglycans and other carbohydrate groups bound to proteins of control and transformed cells. J. Biol. Chem., *255*:8719–8728, 1980.

Balk, S. D., Polimeni, P. I., Hoon, B. S., LeStourgeon, D. N., and Mitchell, R. S. Proliferation of Rous sarcoma virus-infected, but not of normal, chicken fibroblasts in a medium of reduced calcium and magnesium concentration. Proc. Natl. Acad. Sci. U.S.A., *76*:3913–3916, 1979.

Bang, Y.-J., Pirnia, F., Fang, W.-G., Kang, W. K., Sartor, O., Whitesell, L., Ha, M. J., Tsokos, M., Sheahan, M. D., Nguyen, P., Niklinski, W. T., Myers, C. E., and Trepel, J. B. Terminal neuroendocrine differentiation of human prostate carcinoma cells in response to increased intracellular cyclic AMP. Proc. Natl. Acad. Sci. U.S.A., *91*:5330–5334, 1994.

Baylin, S. B., Herman, J. G., Graff, J. R., Vertino, P. M., and Issa, J.-P. Alterations in DNA methylation: a fundamental aspect of neoplasia. Adv. Cancer Res., *72*:141–196, 1998.

Becker, F. F. Differential lectin agglutination of fetal, dividing-postnatal, and malignant hepatocytes. Proc. Natl. Acad. Sci. U.S.A., *71*:4307–4311, 1974.

Ben-Ze'ev, A. Inhibition of vimentin synthesis and disruption of intermediate filaments in simian virus 40–infected monkey kidney cells. Mol. Cell. Biol., *4*:1880–1889, 1984.

Bestilny, L. J., Brown, C. B., Miura, Y., Robertson, L. D., and Riabowol, K. T. Selective inhibition of telomerase activity during terminal differentiation of immortal cell lines. Cancer Res., *56*:3796–3802, 1996.

Birnbaum, M. J., Haspel, H. C., and Rosen, O. M. Transformation of rat fibroblasts by FSV rapidly increases glucose transporter gene transcription. Science, *235*:1495–1497, 1987.

Bissell, M. J., White, R. C., Hatie, C., and Bassham, J. A. Dynamics of metabolism of normal and virus-transformed chick cells in culture. Proc. Natl. Acad. Sci. U.S.A., *70*:2951–2955, 1973.

Bjare, U. Serum-free cell culture. Pharmacol. Ther., *53*:355–374, 1992.

Blobe, G. C., Schiemann, W. P., and Lodish, H. F. Role of transforming growth factor β in human disease. N. Engl. J. Med., *342*:1350–1358, 2000.

Bourguignon, L. Y. W., and Bourguignon, G. J. Capping and the cytoskeleton. Int. Rev. Cytol., *87*:195–224, 1984.

Bowen-Pope, D. F., Vogel, A., and Ross, R. Production of platelet-derived growth factor-like molecules and reduced expression of platelet-derived growth factor receptors accompany transformation by a wide spectrum of agents. Proc. Natl. Acad. Sci. U.S.A., *81*:2396–2400, 1984.

Boynton, A. L., and Whitfield, J. F. Different calcium requirements for proliferation of conditionally and unconditionally tumorigenic mouse cells. Proc. Natl. Acad. Sci. U.S.A., *73*:1651–1654, 1976.

Brandley, B. K., Swiedler, S. J., and Robbins, P. W. Carbohydrate ligands of the LEC cell adhesion molecules. Cell, *63*:861–863, 1990.

Bravo, R., and Celis, J. E. Human proteins sensitive to neoplastic transformation in cultured epithelial and fibroblast cells. Clin. Chem., *28*:949–954, 1982.

Breillout, F., Antoine, E., and Poupon, M. F. Methionine dependency of malignant tumors: a possible approach for therapy. J. Natl. Cancer Inst., *82*:1628–1632, 1990.

Brinkley, B. R., and Fuller, G. M. Tubulin and actin immunofluorescence as an aid in detecting cell transformation *in vitro*. Texas Rep. Biol. Med., *37*:26–42, 1978.

Burger, M. M. Surface changes in transformed cells detected by lectins. Fed. Proc., *32*:91–101, 1973.

Burns, R. G. α-, β-, and γ-Tubulins: sequence comparisons and structural constraints. Cell Motil. Cytoskeleton, *20*:181–189, 1991.

Burstin, S. J., Renger, H. C., and Basilico, C. Cyclic AMP levels in temperature sensitive SV40 transformed cell lines. J. Cell. Physiol., *84*:69–74, 1974.

Carpenter, G., and Cohen, S. Epidermal growth factor. J. Biol. Chem., *265*:7709–7712, 1990.

Carrel, A., and Lindbergh, C. A. The Culture of Organs. London: Hamish Hamilton, 1938.

Caulín, C., Bauluz, C., Gandarillas, A., Cano, A., and Quintanilla, M. Changes in keratin expression during malignant progression of transformed mouse epidermal keratinocytes. Exp. Cell Res., *204*:11–21, 1993.

Celis, J. E., Ratz, G. P., and Celis, A. Secreted proteins from normal and SV40 transformed human MRC-5 fibroblasts: toward establishing a database of human secreted proteins. Leukemia, *1*:707–717, 1987.

Chafouleas, J. G., Pardue, R. L., Brinkley, B. R., Dedman, J. R., and Means, A. R. Regulation of intracellular levels of calmodulin and tubulin in normal and transformed cells. Proc. Natl. Acad. Sci. U.S.A., *78*:996–1000, 1981.

Chen, L. B., Gallimore, P. H., and McDougall, J. K. Correlation between tumor induction and the large external transformation sensitive protein on the cell surface. Proc. Natl. Acad. Sci. U.S.A., *73*:3570–3574, 1976.

Cherington, P. V., Smith, B. L., and Pardee, A. B. Loss of epidermal growth factor requirement and malignant transformation. Proc. Natl. Acad. Sci. U.S.A., *76*:3937–3941, 1979.

Cho-Chung, Y. S., Clair, T., Tortora, G., and Yokozaki, H. Role of site-selective cAMP analogs in the control and reversal of malignancy. Pharmacol. Ther., *50*:1–33, 1991.

Cooper, C. S., Tempest, P. R., Beckman, M. P., Heldin, C.-H., and Brookes, P. Amplification and overexpression of the *met* gene in spontaneously transformed NIH3T3 mouse fibroblasts. EMBO J., *5*:2623–2628, 1986.

Cooper, J. A., Reiss, N. A., Schwartz, R. J., and Hunter, T. Three glycolytic enzymes are phosphorylated at tyrosine in cells transformed by Rous sarcoma virus. Nature, *302*:218–223, 1983.

Crawford, L. The 53,000-dalton cellular protein and its role in transformation. Int. Rev. Exp. Pathol., *25*:1–50, 1983.

Crissman, H. A., Gadbois, D. M., Tobey, R. A., and Bradbury, E. M. Transformed mammalian cells are deficient in kinase-mediated control of progression through the G_1 phase of the cell cycle. Proc. Natl. Acad. Sci. U.S.A., *88*:7580–7584, 1991.

Croy, R. G., and Pardee, A. B. Enhanced synthesis and stabilization of M_r 68,000 protein in transformed BALB/c-3T3 cells: candidate for restriction point control of cell growth. Proc. Natl. Acad. Sci. U.S.A., *80*:4699–4703, 1983.

De Larco, J. E., and Todaro, G. J. Growth factors from murine sarcoma virus-transformed cells. Proc. Natl. Acad. Sci. U.S.A., *75*:4001–4005, 1978.

Descamps, S., Lebourhis, X., Delehedde, M., Boilly, B., and Hondermarck, H. Nerve growth factor is mitogenic for cancerous but not normal human breast epithelial cells. J. Biol. Chem., *273*:16659–16662, 1998.

Dessain, S. K., Yu, H.-y., Reddel, R. R., Beijersbergen, R. L., and Weinberg, R. A. Methylation of the human telomerase gene CpG island. Cancer Res., *60*:537–541, 2000.

Duffy, M. J., and O'Grady, P. Plasminogen activator and cancer. Eur. J. Cancer Clin. Oncol., *20*:577–582, 1984.

Fagan, J. B., Sobel, M. E., Yamada, K. M., de Crombrugghe, B., and Pastan, I. Effects of transformation on fibronectin gene expression using cloned fibronectin cDNA. J. Biol. Chem., *256*:520–525, 1981.

Fantl, W. J., Johnson, D. E., and Williams, L. T. Signalling by receptor tyrosine kinases. Annu. Rev. Biochem., *62*:453–481, 1993.

Fuchs, E., and Hanukoglu, I. Unraveling the structure of the intermediate filaments. Cell, *34*:332–334, 1983.

Garrels, J. I., and Franza, B. R. Jr. Transformation-sensitive and growth-related changes of protein synthesis in REF52 cells. J. Biol. Chem., *264*:5299–5312, 1989.

Gazdar, A. F., Stull, H. B., Kilton, L. J., and Bachrach, U. Increased ornithine decarboxylase activity in murine sarcoma virus infected cells. Nature, *262*:696–698, 1976.

Glick, M. C. Membrane glycopeptides from virus-transformed hamster fibroblasts and the normal counterpart. Biochemistry, *18*:2525–2532, 1979.

Goldman, R. D., Milsted, A., Schloss, J. A., Starger, J., and Yerna, M.-J. Cytoplasmic fibers in mammalian cells: cytoskeletal and contractile elements. Annu. Rev. Physiol., *41*:703–722, 1979.

Gottesman, M. M., and Cabral, F. Purification and characterization of a transformation-dependent protein secreted by cultured murine fibroblasts. Biochemistry, *20*:1659–1665, 1981.

Goz, B. The effects of incorporation of 5-halogenated deoxyuridines into the DNA of eukaryotic cells. Pharmacol. Rev., *29*:249–272, 1978.

Graziadei, L., Riabowol, K., and Bar-Sagi, D. Co-capping of *ras* proteins with surface immunoglobulins in B lymphocytes. Nature, *347*:396–400, 1990.

Hadden, J. W., Hadden, E. M., Haddox, M. K., and Goldberg, N. D. Guanosine 3':5'-cyclic monophosphate: a possible intracellular mediator of mitogenic influences in lymphocytes. Proc. Natl. Acad. Sci. U.S.A., *69*:3024–3027, 1972.

Halpern, B. C., Clark, B. R., Hardy, D. N., Halpern, R. M., and Smith, R. A. The effect of replacement of methionine by homocysteine on survival of malignant and normal adult mammalian cells in culture. Proc. Natl. Acad. Sci. U.S.A., *71*:1133–1136, 1974.

Hatakeyama, M., and Taniguchi, T. Dysregulation of growth factor-receptor system in cellular transformation. Jpn. J. Cancer Res., *79*:885–901, 1988.

Hatanaka, M. Transport of sugars in tumor cell membranes. Biochim. Biophys. Acta, *355*:77–104, 1974.

Hayflick, L. Mortality and immortality at the cellular level. A review. Biochemistry, *62*:1180–1190, 1997.

Hebert, S. C., and Brown, E. M. The extracellular calcium receptor. Curr. Opin. Cell Biol., *7*:484–492, 1995.

Heldin, C.-H. Protein tyrosine kinase receptors. Cancer Surv., *27*:7–24, 1996.

Herbert, B.-S., Pitts, A. E., Baker, S. I., Hamilton, S. E., Wright, W. E., Shay, J. W., and Corey, D. R. Inhibition of human telomerase in immortal human cells leads to progressive telomere shortening and cell death. Proc. Natl. Acad. Sci. U.S.A., *96*:14276–14281, 1999.

Herzig, M., Novatchkova, M., and Christofori, G. An unexpected role for p53 in augmenting SV40 large T antigen-mediated tumorigenesis. Biol. Chem., *380*:203–211, 1999.

Hill, D. J., and Borysenko, J. Z. Restriction of patching of bound concanavalin A after incorporation of arachidonic acid into the plasma membrane of virally transformed fibroblasts. J. Cell Biol., *83*:218–230, 1979.

Hoffman, R. M. Methionine dependence in cancer cells—a review. In Vitro, *18*:421–428, 1982.

Hollenberg, M. D., Barrett, J. C., Ts'o, P. O. P., and Berhanu, P. Selective reduction in receptors for epidermal growth factor-urogastrone in chemically transformed tumorigenic Syrian hamster embryo fibroblasts. Cancer Res., *39*:4166–4169, 1979.

Holley, R. W., Baldwin, J. H., Kiernan, J. A., and Messmer, T. O. Control of growth of benzo[*a*]pyrene-transformed 3T3 cells. Proc. Natl. Acad. Sci. U.S.A., *73*:3229–3232, 1976.

Ignar-Trowbridge, D. M., Pimentel, M., Teng, C. T., Korach, K. S., and McLachlan, J. A. Cross talk between peptide growth factor and estrogen receptor signaling systems. Environ. Health Perspect., *103*:35–38, 1995.

Inbar, M., Ben-Bassat, H., and Sachs, L. Difference in the mobility of lectin sites on the surface membrane of normal lymphocytes and malignant lymphoma cells. Int. J. Cancer, *12*:93–99, 1973.

Inbar, M., Yuli, I., and Raz, A. Contact-mediated changes in the fluidity of membrane lipids in normal and malignant transformed mammalian fibroblasts. Exp. Cell Res., *105*:325–335, 1977.

Isaka, T., Yoshida, M., Owada, M., and Toyoshima, K. Alterations in membrane polypeptides of chick embryo fibroblasts induced by transformation with Avian sarcoma viruses. Virology, *65*:226–237, 1975.

Isfort, R. J., Cody, D. B., Kerckaert, G. A., and LeBoeuf, R. A. Growth factor responsiveness and alterations in growth factor homeostasis in Syrian hamster embryo cells during *in vitro* transformation. Carcinogenesis, *15*:1203–1209, 1994.

Iyer, V. R., Eisen, M. B., Ross, D. T., Schuler, G., Moore, T., Lee, J. C. F., Trent, J. M., Staudt, L. M., Hudson, J. Jr., Boguski, M. S., Lashkari, D., Shalon, D., Botstein, D., and Brown, P. O. The transcriptional program in the response of human fibroblasts to serum. Science, *283*:83–86, 1999.

Izbicka, E., Nishioka, D., Marcell, V., Raymond, E., Davidson, K. K., Lawrence, R. A., Wheelhouse, R. T., Hurley, L. H., Wu, R. S., and Von Hoff, D. D. Telomere-interactive agents affect proliferation rates and induce chromosomal destabilization in sea urchin embryos. Anticancer Drug Des., *14*:355–365, 1999.

Jaenisch, R., Schnieke, A., and Harbers, K. Treatment of mice with 5-azacytidine efficiently activates silent retroviral genomes in different tissues. Proc. Natl. Acad. Sci. U.S.A., *82*:1451–1455, 1985.

Johnson, G. S., Friedman, R. M., and Pastan, I. Cyclic AMP-treated sarcoma cells acquire several morphological characteristics of normal fibroblasts. Ann. N.Y. Acad. Sci., *185*:413–416, 1971.

Jones, P. A. Effects of 5-azacytidine and its 2′-deoxyderivative on cell differentiation and DNA methylation. Pharmacol. Ther., *28*:17–27, 1985.

Jullien, M., Blat, C., and Harel, L. Early effect of the expression of SRC gene on phosphate metabolism in mammalian cells. Biol. Cell (Paris), *44*:93–100, 1982.

Jüttermann, R., Li, E., and Jaenisch, R. Toxicity of 5-aza-2′-deoxycytidine to mammalian cells is mediated primarily by covalent trapping of DNA methyltransferase rather than DNA demethylation. Proc. Natl. Acad. Sci. U.S.A., *91*:11797–11801, 1994.

Kaplan, P. L., and Ozanne, B. Cellular responsiveness to growth factors correlates with a cell's ability to express the transformed phenotype. Cell, *33*:931–938, 1983.

Kautiainen, T. L., and Jones, P. A. DNA methyltransferase levels in tumorigenic and nontumorigenic cells in culture. J. Biol. Chem., *261*:1594–1598, 1986.

Keski-Oja, J., Postlethwaite, A. E., and Moses, H. L. Transforming growth factors in the regulation of malignant cell growth and invasion. Cancer Invest., *6*:705–724, 1988.

Kimchi, A., Wang, X.-F., Weinberg, R. A., Cheifetz, S., and Massagué, J. Absence of TGF-β receptors and growth inhibitory responses in retinoblastoma cells. Science, *240*:196–198, 1988.

Kobayashi, N., Tanaka, A., and Kaji, A. *In vitro* phosphorylation of the 36K protein in extract from Rous sarcoma virus–transformed chicken fibroblasts. J. Biol. Chem., *256*:3053–3058, 1981.

Krieg, P., Schnapke, R., Fürstenberger, G., Vogt, I., and Marks, F. TGF-β1 and skin carcinogenesis: antiproliferative effect in vitro and TGF-β1 and mRNA expression during epidermal hyperproliferation and multistage tumorigenesis. Mol. Carcinog., *4*:129–137, 1991.

Krupp, G., Klapper, W., and Parwaresch, R. Cell proliferation, carcinogenesis and diverse mechanisms of telomerase regulation. Cell. Mol. Life Sci., *57*:464–486, 2000.

Kumar, V., Bustin, S. A., and McKay, I. A. Transforming growth factor alpha. Cell Biol. Int., *19*:373–388, 1995.

Laird, P. W., and Jaenisch, R. DNA methylation and cancer. Hum. Mol. Genet., *3*:1487–1495, 1994.

Lane, J., and Allan, V. Microtubule-based membrane movement. Biochim. Biophys. Acta, *1376*:27–55, 1998.

Lawrence, D. A. Transforming growth factor-β: a general review. Eur. Cytokine Netw., *7*:363–374, 1996.

Leaman, D. W., Leung, S., Li, X., and Stark, G. R. Regulation of STAT-dependent pathways by growth factors and cytokines. FASEB J., *10*:1578–1588, 1996.

Leavitt, J., Goldman, D., Merril, C., and Kakunaga, T. Actin mutations in a human fibroblast model for carcinogenesis. Clin. Chem., *28*:850–860, 1982.

Leavitt, J., Gunning, P., Kedes, L., and Jariwalla, R. Smooth muscle α-actin is a transformation-sensitive marker for mouse NIH 3T3 and Rat-2 cells. Nature, *316*:840–842, 1985.

Lee, D. C., Luetteke, N. C., and Petch, L. A. Transforming growth factor-alpha and its role in neoplastic progression. *In*: C. C. Benz and E. T. Liu (Eds.), Oncogenes and Tumor Suppressor Genes in Human Malignancies, pp. 233–254. Boston: Kluwer, 1993.

Lee, S. W., Tomasetto, C., and Sager, R. Positive selection of candidate tumor-suppressor genes by subtractive hybridization. Proc. Natl. Acad. Sci. U.S.A., *88*:2825–2829, 1991.

Lever, J. E. Regulation of amino acid and glucose transport activity expressed in isolated membranes from untransformed and SV 40-transformed mouse fibroblasts. J. Cell. Physiol., *89*:779–788, 1976.

Levi-Montalcini, R. The nerve growth factor 35 years later. Science, *237*:1154–1162, 1987.

Levinson, W., Bhatnagar, R. S., and Liu, T.-Z. Loss of ability to synthesize collagen in fibroblasts transformed by Rous sarcoma virus. J. Natl. Cancer Inst., *55*:807–810, 1975.

Liboi, E., Pelosi, E., Testa, U., Peschle, C., and Rossi, G. B. Proliferative response and oncogene expression induced by epidermal growth factor in EL2 rat fibroblasts. Mol. Cell. Biol., *6*:2275–2278, 1986.

Liu, M.-C., and Lipmann, F. Decrease of tyrosine-*O*-sulfate-containing proteins found in rat fibroblasts infected with Rous sarcoma virus or Fujinami sarcoma virus. Proc. Natl. Acad. Sci. U.S.A., *81*:3695–3698, 1984.

Majmudar, G., Schalk, E., Bateman, J., and Peterkofsky, B. Uncoupled expression of mRNAs for α1(I) and α2(I) procollagen chains in chemically transformed Syrian hamster fibroblasts. J. Biol. Chem., *263*:5555–5559, 1988.

Marquardt, H., Hunkapiller, M. W., Hood, L. E., and Todaro, G. J. Rat transforming growth factor type 1: structure and relation to epidermal growth factor. Science, *223*:1079–1082, 1984.

Martin, K. J., Kwan, C.-P., O'Hare, M. J., Pardee, A. B., and Sager, R. Identification and verification of differential display cDNAs using gene-specific primers and hybridization arrays. Biotechniques, *24*:1018–1026, 1998.

McCubrey, J. A., May, W. S., Duronio, V., and Mufson, A. Serine/threonine phosphorylation in cytokine signal transduction. Leukemia, *14*:9–21, 2000.

McDonagh, J. Fibronectin. Arch. Pathol. Lab. Med., *105*:393–396, 1981.

McKeehan, W. L., McKeehan, K. A., and Calkins, D. Extracellular regulation of fibroblast multiplication. J. Biol. Chem., *256*:2973–2981, 1981.

Miettinen, M., Lehto, V.-P., and Virtanen, I. Monophasic synovial sarcoma of spindle-cell type. Virchows Arch. B Cell Pathol., *44*:187–199, 1983.

Milczarek, G. J., Martinez, J., and Bowden, G. T. p53 phosphorylation: biochemical and functional consequences. Life Sci., *60*:1–11, 1997.

Miyazaki, K., and Horio, T. Growth inhibitors: molecular diversity and roles in cell proliferation. In Vitro Cell. Dev. Biol., *25*:866–871, 1989.

Moll, R., Franke, W. W., Schiller, D. L., Geiger, B., and Krepler, R. The catalog of human cytokeratins: patterns of expression in normal epithelia, tumors and cultured cells. Cell, *31*:11–24, 1982.

Morin, G. B. Telomere control of replicative lifespan. Exp. Gerontol., *32*:375–382, 1997.

Morris, S. M. The genetic toxicology of 5-bromodeoxyuridine in mammalian cells. Mutat. Res., *258*:161–188, 1991.

Moses, H. L., Branum, E. L., Proper, J. A., and Robinson, R. A. Transforming growth factor production by chemically transformed cells. Cancer Res., *41*:2842–2848, 1981.

Moshier, J. A., Dosescu, J., Skunca, M., and Luk, G. D. Transformation of NIH/3T3 cells by ornithine decarboxylase overexpression. Cancer Res., *53*:2618–2622, 1993.

Moyzis, R. K., Grady, D. L., Li, D. W., Mirvis, S. E., and Ts'o, P. O. P. Extensive homology of nuclear ribonucleic acid and polysomal poly(adenylic acid) messenger ribonucleic acid between normal and neoplastically transformed cells. Biochemistry, *19*:821–832, 1980.

Newman, M. J. Transforming growth factor beta and the cell surface in tumor progression. Cancer Metast. Rev., *12*:239–254, 1993.

Nicolson, G. L. Trans-membrane control of the receptors on normal and tumor cells. II. Surface changes associated with transformation and malignancy. Biochim. Biophys. Acta, *458*:1–72, 1976.

Nicolson, G. L., and Poste, G. The cancer cell: dynamic aspects and modifications in cell-surface organization. N. Engl. J. Med., *295*:197–203, 1976.

Niki, I., Yokokura, H., Sudo, T., Kato, M., and Hidaka, H. Ca^{2+} signaling and intracellular Ca^{2+} binding proteins. J. Biochem., *120*:685–698, 1996.

O'Brien, T. G. The induction of ornithine decarboxylase as an early, possibly obligatory, event in mouse skin carcinogenesis. Cancer Res., *36*:2644–2653, 1976.

Ochieng, J., Leite-Browning, M. L., and Warfield, P. Regulation of cellular adhesion to extracellular matrix proteins by galectin-3. Biochem. Biophys. Res. Commun., *246*:788–791, 1998.

O'Farrell, P. H. High resolution two-dimensional electrophoresis of proteins. J. Biol. Chem., *250*:4007–4021, 1975.

Oft, M., Heider, K.-H., and Beug, H. TGFβ signaling is necessary for carcinoma cell invasiveness and metastasis. Curr. Biol., *8*:1243–1252, 1998.

Osborn, M., and Weber, K. Intermediate filament proteins: a multigene family distinguishing major cell lineages. Trends Biochem. Sci., *11*:469–472, 1986.

Otten, J., Johnson, G. S., and Pastan, I. Cyclic AMP levels in fibroblasts: relationship to growth rate and contact inhibition of growth. Biochem. Biophys. Res. Commun., *44*:1192–1198, 1971.

Pastan, I. The role of cyclic AMP in malignant transformation. Am. J. Clin. Pathol., *63*:669–670, 1975.

Patt, L. M., and Grimes, W. J. Cell surface glycolipid and glycoprotein glycosyltransferases of normal and transformed cells. J. Biol. Chem., *249*:4157–4165, 1974.

Patt, L. M., and Houck, J. C. The incredible shrinking chalones. FEBS Lett., *120*:163–168, 1980.

Patterson, M. K. Jr., Birckbichler, P. J., Conway, E., and Orr, G. R. Amino acid and hexose transport of normal and simian virus 40-transformed human cells. Cancer Res., *36*:394–397, 1976.

Plantefaber, L. C., and Hynes, R. O. Changes in integrin receptors on oncogenically transformed cells. Cell, *56*:281–290, 1989.

Pommier, J. P., Lebeau, J., Ducray, C., and Sabatier, L. Chromosomal instability and alteration of telomere repeat sequences. Biochimie, *77*:817–825, 1995.

Porcu, P., Ferber, A., Pietrzkowski, Z., Roberts, C. T., Adamo, M., LeRoith, D., and Baserga, R. The growth-stimulatory effect of simian virus 40 T antigen requires the interaction of insulinlike growth factor I with its receptor. Mol. Cell. Biol., *12*:3883–3889, 1992.

Prunier, C., Mazars, A., Noë, V., Bruyneel, E., Mareel, M., Gespach, C., and Atfi, A. Evidence that Smad2 is a tumor suppressor implicated in the control of cellular invasion. J. Biol. Chem., *274*:22919–22922, 1999.

Pusztai, L., Lewis, C. E., Lorenzen, J., and McGee, J. O. D. Growth factors: regulation of normal and neoplastic growth. J. Pathol., *169*:191–201, 1993.

Rall, L. B., Scott, J., Bell, G. I., Crawford, R. J., Penschow, J. D., Niall, H. D., and Coghlan, J. P. Mouse prepro-epidermal growth factor synthesis by the kidney and other tissues. Nature, *313*:228–231, 1985.

Ramsay, G. DNA chips: state-of-the art. Nat. Biotechnol., *16*:40–44, 1998.

Rapin, A. M. C., and Burger, M. M. Tumor cell surfaces: general alterations detected by agglutinins. Adv. Cancer Res., *20*:1–91, 1974.

Rasmussen, H. Ions as "second messengers." Hosp. Pract., *9*:99–107, 1974.

Razin, A., and Cedar, H. DNA methylation and gene expression. Microbiol. Rev., *55*:451–458, 1991.

Reddel, R. R. The role of senescence and immortalization in carcinogenesis. Carcinogenesis, *21*:477–484, 2000.

Reiss, M. Transforming growth factor-β and cancer: a love-hate relationship? Oncology Res., *9*:447–457, 1997.

Rice, R. H., Steinmann, K. E., deGraffenried, L. A., Qin, Q., Taylor, N., Schlegel, R. Elevation of cell cycle control proteins during spontaneous immortalization of human keratinocytes. Mol. Biol. Cell, *4*:185–194, 1993.

Richman, R. A., Johnson, R. A., and Friedman, D. L. Cyclic nucleotides and growth regulation in BHK cells (41259). Proc. Soc. Exp. Biol. Med., *168*:196–203, 1981.

Roberts, A. B., and Sporn, M. B. Transforming growth factor-β. *In*: R. A. F. Clark (Ed.), The Molecular and Cellular Biology of Wound Repair, 2nd ed., pp. 275–308. New York: Plenum Press, 1996.

Roberts, A. B., Anzano, M. A., Lamb, L. C., Smith, J. M., and Sporn, M. B. New class of transforming growth factors potentiated by epidermal growth factor: isolation from non neoplastic tissues. Proc. Natl. Acad. Sci. U.S.A., *78*:5339–5343, 1981.

Roberts, R. M., Walker, A., and Cetorelli, J. J. Fucose-containing glycopeptides from the cell surface of Chinese hamster ovary cells grown in the presence or absence of cyclic AMP. Nat. New Biol., *244*:86–89, 1973.

Roop, D. R., Hawley-Nelson, P., Cheng, C. K., and Yuspa, S. H. Expression of keratin genes in mouse epidermis and normal and malignantly transformed epidermal cells in culture. J. Invest. Dermatol., *81*:144s–149s, 1983.

Roth, C. W., Singh, T., Pastan, I., and Gottesman, M. M. Rous sarcoma virus transformed cells are resistant to cyclic AMP. J. Cell. Physiol., *111*:42–48, 1982.

Roth, S., Patteson, A., and White, D. Surface glycosyltransferases on cultured mouse fibroblasts. J. Supramol. Struct., *2*:1–6, 1974.

Rovinski, B., and Benchimol, S. Immortalization of rat embryo fibroblasts by the cellular p53 oncogene. Oncogene, *2*:445–452, 1988.

Ruscetti, F. W., Birchenall-Roberts, M. C., McPherson, J. M., and Wiltrout, R. H. Transforming Growth Factor β1. pp. 415–432. New York: Academic Press, 1998.

Sachs, L. Regulation of membrane changes, differentiation, and malignancy in carcinogenesis. Harvey Lect. (1972–73), *68*:1–35, 1974.

Salomon, D. S., Kim, N., Saeki, T., and Ciardiello, F. Transforming growth factor-α: an oncodevelopmental growth factor. Cancer Cells, 2:389–397, 1990.

San, R. H. C., Rice, J. M., and Williams, G. M. Lack of correlation between plasminogen activating factor production and tumorigenicity in rat liver epithelial cells. Cancer Lett., 3:243–246, 1977.

Sasak, W., De Luca, L. M., Dion, L. D., and Silverman-Jones, C. S. Effect of retinoic acid on cell surface glycopeptides of cultured spontaneously transformed mouse fibroblasts (BALB/c 3T12-3 cells). Cancer Res., 40:1944–1949, 1980.

Senger, D. R., Wirth, D. F., and Hynes, R. O. Transformation-specific secreted phosphoproteins. Nature, 286:619–621, 1980.

Senger, D. R., Asch, B. B., Smith, B. D., Perruzzi, C. A., Dvorak, H. F. A secreted phosphoprotein marker for neoplastic transformation of both epithelial and fibroblastic cells. Nature, 302:714–715, 1983.

Seslar, S., Nakamura, T., and Byers, S. Tumor-stroma interactions and stromal cell density regulate hepatocyte growth factor protein levels: a role for transforming growth factor-β activation. Endocrinology, 136:1945–1953, 1995.

Shanley, D. J., Cossu, G., Boettiger, D., Holtzer, H., and Pacifici, M. Transformation by Rous sarcoma virus induces similar patterns of glycosaminoglycan synthesis in chick embryo skin fibroblasts and vertebral chondroblasts. J. Biol. Chem., 258:810–816, 1983.

Sharma, H. W., Sokoloski, J. A., Perez, J. R., Maltese, J. Y., Sartorelli, A. C., Stein, C. A., Nichols, G., Khaled, Z., Telang, N. T., and Narayanan, R. Differentiation of immortal cells inhibits telomerase activity. Proc. Natl. Acad. Sci. U.S.A., 92:12343–12346, 1995.

Sharma, R. K., Shanker, G., Ahrens, H., and Ahmed, N. K. Partial purification and characterization of the defective cyclic adenosine 3′:5′-monophosphate binding protein kinase from adrenocortical carcinoma. Cancer Res., 37:3297–3300, 1977.

Sharon, N. Lectins. Sci. Am., 236:108–116, 118–119, 1977.

Shinitzky, M., and Inbar, M. Difference in microviscosity induced by different cholesterol levels in the surface membrane lipid layer of normal lymphocytes and malignant lymphoma cells. J. Mol. Biol., 85:603–615, 1974.

Shinitzky, M., and Inbar, M. Microviscosity parameters and protein mobility in biological membranes. Biochim. Biophys. Acta, 433:133–149, 1976.

Shiota, G., Rhoads, D. B., Wang, T. C., Nakamura, T., and Schmidt, E. V. Hepatocyte growth factor inhibits growth of hepatocellular carcinoma cells. Proc. Natl. Acad. Sci. U.S.A., 89:373–377, 1992.

Shopsis, C., and Sheinin, R. Biosynthesis of plasma membrane components by SV40-virus–transformed 3T3 mouse cells temperature sensitive for expression of some transformed cell properties. Biochim. Biophys. Acta, 433:101–117, 1976.

Siegfried, J. M. Strategies for identification of peptide growth factors. Pharmacol. Ther., 56:233–245, 1992.

Silagi, S. Modification of malignancy by 5-bromodeoxyuridine. Studies of reversibility and immunological effects. In Vitro, 7:105–114, 1971.

Silvennoinen, O., Saharinen, P., Paukku, K., Takaluoma, K., and Kovanen, P. Cytokine receptor signal transduction through Jak tyrosine kinases and Stat transcription factors. APMIS, 105:497–509, 1997.

Simantov, R., and Sachs, L. Temperature sensitivity of cyclic adenosine 3′:5′-monophosphate–binding proteins and the regulation of growth and differentiation in neuroblastoma cells. J. Biol. Chem., 250:3236–3242, 1975.

Sivak, A., and Wolman, S. R. Classification of cell types: agglutination and chromosomal properties. In Vitro, 8:1–6, 1972.

Skalli, O., Gabbiani, G., Babai, F., Seemayer, T. A., Pizzolato, G., and Schürch, W. Intermediate filament proteins and actin isoforms as markers for soft tissue tumour differentiation and origin. J. Pathol., 130:515–531, 1988.

Slack, A., Cervoni, N., Pinard, M., and Szyf, M. DNA methyltransferase is a downstream effector of cellular transformation triggered by simian virus 40 large T antigen. J. Biol. Chem., 274:10105–10112, 1999.

Slingerland, J. M., and Benchimol, S. Transforming activity of mutant human p53 alleles. J. Cell. Physiol., *148*:391–395, 1991.

Smets, L. A., Van Beek, W. P., Van Rooy, H., and Homburg, Ch. The relationship between membrane glycoprotein alterations and anchorage-independent growth in neoplastic transformation. Cancer Biochem. Biophys., *2*:203–207, 1978.

Srinivas, L., and Colburn, N. H. Reduced trisialoganglioside synthesis in chemically but not *mos*-transformed mouse epidermal cells. Cancer Res., *44*:1510–1514, 1984.

Summerhayes, I. C., Cheng, Y.-S. E., Sun, T.-T., and Chen, L. B. Expression of keratin and vimentin intermediate filaments in rabbit bladder epithelial cells at different stages of benzo[a]pyrene-induced neoplastic progression. J. Cell Biol., *90*:63–69, 1981.

Suter, M. M., Augustin-Voss, H. G., Pantano, D. M., Flanders, J. A., and Varvayanis, M. Differentiation-dependent expression of lectin binding sites on normal and neoplastic keratinocytes in vivo and in vitro. J. Histochem. Cytochem., *39*:1103–1112, 1991.

Tagliaferri, P., Katsaros, D., Clair, T., Neckers, L., Robins, R. K., and Cho-Chung, Y. S. Reverse transformation of Harvey murine sarcoma virus-transformed NIH/3T3 cells by site-selective cyclic AMP analogs. J. Biol. Chem., *263*:409–416, 1988.

Tajima, H., Matsumoto, K., and Nakamura, T. Hepatocyte growth factor has potent anti-proliferative activity in various tumor cell lines. FEBS Lett., *291*:229–232, 1991.

Taub, M. The use of defined media in cell and tissue culture. Toxicol. in Vitro, *4*:213–225, 1990.

Temin, H. M. Studies on carcinogenesis by avian sarcoma viruses. III. The differential effect of serum and polyanions on multiplication of uninfected and converted cells. J. Natl. Cancer Inst., *37*:167–175, 1966.

Temin, H. M. Studies on carcinogenesis by avian sarcoma viruses: VIII. Glycolysis and cell multiplication. Int. J. Cancer, *3*:273–282, 1968.

Temin, H. M. The cellular and molecular biology of RNA tumor viruses, especially avian leukosis-sarcoma viruses, and their relatives. Adv. Cancer Res., *19*:47–104, 1974.

Todaro, G. J., and De Larco, J. E. Transformation by murine and feline sarcoma viruses specifically blocks binding of epidermal growth factor to cells. Nature, *264*:26–31, 1976.

Todaro, G. J., De Larco, J. E., Fryling, C., Johnson, P. A., and Sporn, M. B. Transforming growth factors (TGFs): properties and possible mechanisms of action. J. Supramol. Struct. Cell. Biochem., *15*:287–301, 1981.

Tsao, M.-S., Zhu, H., Giaid, A., Viallet, J., Nakamura, T., and Park, M. Hepatocyte growth factor/scatter factor is an autocrine factor for human normal bronchial epithelial and lung carcinoma cells. Cell Growth Differ., *4*:571–579, 1993.

Unkeless, J. C., Tobia, A., Ossowski, L., Quigley, J. P., Rifkin, D. B., and Reich, E. An enzymatic function associated with transformation of fibroblasts by oncogenic viruses. I. Chick embryo fibroblast cultures transformed by Avian RNA tumor viruses. J. Exp. Med., *137*:85–111, 1973.

van Zoelen, E. J. J., van Oostwaard, T. M. J., and de Laat, S. W. The role of polypeptide growth factors in phenotypic transformation of normal rat kidney cells. J. Biol. Chem., *263*:64–68, 1988.

Veigl, M. L., Vanaman, T. C., and Sedwick, W. D. Calcium and calmodulin in cell growth and transformation. Biochim. Biophys. Acta, *738*:21–48, 1984.

Visser, J. A., and Themmen, A. P. N. Downstream factors in transforming growth factor-β family signaling. Mol. Cell. Endocrinol., *146*:7–17, 1998.

Vlodavsky, I., Inbar, M., and Sachs, L. Membrane changes and adenosine triphosphate content in normal and malignant transformed cells. Proc. Natl. Acad. Sci., USA, *70*:1780–1784, 1973.

Wada, T., Yasutomi, M., Hashmura, K., Kunikata, M., Tanaka, T., and Mori, M. Vimentin expression in benign and malignant lesions in the human mammary gland. Anticancer Res., *12*:1973–1982, 1992.

Wakefield, L. M., Colletta, A. A., McCune, B. K., and Sporn, M. B. Roles for transforming growth factors-β in the genesis, prevention, and treatment of breast cancer. *In*: R. B. Dickson and M. E. Lippman (Eds.), Genes, Oncogenes, and Hormones: Advances in Cellular and Molecular Biology of Breast Cancer, pp. 97–136. Boston: Kluwer, 1991.

Walker, C., Nettesheim, P., Barrett, J. C., and Gilmer, T. M. Expression of a *fms*-related oncogene in carcinogen-induced neoplastic epithelial cells. Proc. Natl. Acad. Sci. U.S.A., *84*:1804–1808, 1987.

Wang, E., and Goldberg, A. R. Changes in microfilament organization and surface topography upon transformation of chick embryo fibroblasts with Rous sarcoma virus. Proc. Natl. Acad. Sci. U.S.A., *73*:4065–4069, 1976.

Weber, K., and Osborn, M. Cytoskeleton: definition, structure, and gene regulation. Pathol. Res. Pract., *175*:128–145, 1982.

Weber, M. J., Evans, P. K., Johnson, M. A., McNair, T. F., Nakamura, K. D., and Salter, D. W. Transport of potassium, amino acids, and glucose in cells transformed by Rous sarcoma virus. Fed. Proc., *43*:107–112, 1984.

Weiser, M. M. Concanavalin A agglutination of intestinal cells from the human fetus. Science, *177*:525–526, 1972.

Weiss, A., and Schlessinger, J. Switching signals on or off by receptor dimerization. Cell, *94*:277–280, 1998.

Werner, H., and LeRoith, D. The role of the insulin-like growth factor system in human cancer. Adv. Cancer Res., *68*:183–223, 1996.

White, M. K., and Weber, M. J. Transformation by the *src* oncogene alters glucose transport into rat and chicken cells by different mechanisms. Mol. Cell. Biol., *8*:138–144, 1988.

Whitfield, J. F. Calcium signals and cancer. Crit. Rev. Oncog., *3*:55–90, 1992.

Whitfield, J. F., Boynton, A. L., Macmanus, J. P., Sikorska, M., and Tsang, B. K. The regulation of cell proliferation by calcium and cyclic AMP. Mol. Cell. Biochem., *27*:155–179, 1979.

Wickus, G., Gruenstein, E., Robbins, P. W., and Rich, A. Decrease in membrane-associated actin of fibroblasts after transformation by Rous sarcoma virus. Proc. Natl. Acad. Sci. U.S.A., *72*:746–749, 1975.

Willingham, M. C., and Pastan, I. Cyclic AMP mediates the concanavalin A agglutinability of mouse fibroblasts. J. Cell Biol., *63*:288–294, 1974.

Wolf, B. A., and Goldberg, A. R. Rous-sarcoma-virus-transformed fibroblasts having low levels of plasminogen activator. Proc. Natl. Acad. Sci. U.S.A., *73*:3613–3617, 1976.

Wynford-Thomas, D. Telomeres, p53 and cellular senescence. Oncology Res., *8*:387–398, 1996.

Wysolmerski, J. J., and Stewart, A. F. The physiology of parathyroid hormone-related protein: an emerging role as a developmental factor. Annu. Rev. Physiol., *60*:431–460, 1998.

Xiong, Y., Zhang, H., and Beach, D. Subunit rearrangement of the cyclin-dependent kinases is associated with cellular transformation. Genes Dev., *7*:1572–1583, 1993.

Yahara, I., and Kakimoto-Sameshima, F. Ligand-independent cap formation: redistribution of surface receptors on mouse lymphocytes and thymocytes in hypertonic medium. Proc. Natl. Acad. Sci. U.S.A., *74*:4511–4515, 1977.

Yuspa, S. H., Hawley-Nelson, P., Koehler, B., and Stanley, J. R. A survey of transformation markers in differentiating epidermal cell lines in culture. Cancer Res., *40*:4694–4703, 1980.

17

The Host–Tumor Relationship—
Nutritional Factors and Biomarkers

It is important to remember, in considering neoplasia as defined in this book, that *two* entities are involved, the host and the neoplasm. Each is independent yet in many ways dependent on the other. The neoplasm is dependent on the host for its blood supply and other supporting tissues, and the host responds to the viability and the nutritional requirements of the neoplasm in the maintenance of the internal milieu of the organism. Weiss (1976) pointed out that the host-tumor relation is quite analogous to the host-parasite relation, which is usually considered in infectious diseases. The tumor-bearing host is confronted with a population of living cells sufficiently independent of the host (relative autonomy) and sufficiently different at the molecular level to warrant designation as parasitic. Yet the analogy of the neoplastic cell to an exogenous parasite is not altogether correct, because in this case the relation to the host is much more subtle, in that the parasitic element is derived from the host's own tissues.

This relation between host and tumor is perhaps the major factor in the clinical symptomatology seen in patients with cancer. According to the late Jesse Greenstein (1958), "The host-tumor relationship is the key to the cancer problem." With the rapid advances in our knowledge of mechanisms in pathobiology, however, the problem of the host-tumor relation has been somewhat deemphasized; yet it is as significant today as it has ever been.

CANCER CACHEXIA

It is not unusual for humans and lower animals with advanced cancer to lose weight and to become emaciated even to the point that the host appears to die of starvation rather than as a result of any localized effects of the neoplasm. In the initial growth phase, the neoplasm may give evidence of host restraints. However, after the neoplasm reaches a substantial size within the host, it often continues to grow, regardless of the nutritional and hormonal needs of the host. A neoplasm transplanted to mice that were fasted for 48 or 60 hours with interval 24-hour access to food showed a significant decrease in growth (Pavelić, 1982). In some experimental animals, body growth ceases when the neoplasm becomes grossly demonstrable; thereafter, the body weight may remain essentially constant or decrease somewhat, while the neoplasm continues to increase in size and cell number. In animals this latter phase may be correlated with the involution of the thymus (Ertl, 1972).

The sum of the changes noted above has been termed *cachexia*, which may also be seen as a similar symptomatology in a number of disease states other than cancer, such as the acquired immunodeficiency syndrome (AIDS), major trauma, extensive surgery, malabsorption syndromes, and severe sepsis (Tisdale, 1997). Cachexia differs from starvation, either self-induced (anorexia nervosa) or as the result of circumstances, in that in the latter situations, especially during continued starvation, there is a much greater loss of adipose tissue than other components, while in cancer cachexia there is equal loss of both fat and muscle (Moley et al., 1987). Furthermore, in contrast to simple starvation, the changes in body composition seen in patients with cancer cachexia cannot be reversed by the provision of extra calories.

Cachexia has been defined by Costa (1963) as "the sum of those effects produced by neoplasms in the host, which are not the immediate result of mechanical interference with recognizable structures." About 50% of all cancer patients exhibit the syndrome of cancer cachexia, characterized by loss of adipose tissue and skeletal muscle mass, weakness, anorexia (loss of appetite), depletion of host components such as lipid and protein, electrolyte and water abnormalities, and a progressive fading of vital functions (cf. Tisdale, 1997, Table 17.1). Accompanying asthenia is a prevalence of fatigue, which may, in turn, be related to anemia, pain, nutritional deficiency, infection with fever, or depression (Groopman, 1998). In cancer patients receiving chemotherapy (Chapter 20), the prevalence of fatigue has been reported to range from 75 to 96% (cf. Stone et al., 1998). The degree of cachexia, however, is not correlated in any simple manner with caloric intake, tumor burden, tumor cell type, or anatomical site of involvement. Some individuals with widespread neoplasms exhibit no clinically recognizable cachexia, whereas others with extremely small neoplasms may show characteristics of this syndrome (cf. Costa and Donaldson, 1980). For example, cachexia is relatively uncommon in patients with adenocarcinoma of the breast, while it is very common in other forms of adenocarcinoma, as of the lung or pancreas (MacDonald et al., 1995).

Nutrition and Cancer Cachexia—Anorexia

The mechanisms of the development of cancer cachexia are complex and not completely understood. Costa (1977) likened the cachectic state to the diseases of protein-calorie malnutrition, kwashiorkor, and marasmus, which are more commonly seen in relatively undeveloped areas of the world. In fact, patients with advanced cancer may lose significant amounts of nitrogen and fat and exhibit protein-calorie malnutrition (Nixon et al., 1980). As with malnutrition, some of the characteristics of cachexia may be overcome by forced feeding programs involving either total parenteral nutrition, that is, intravenous feeding, or hyperalimentation by means of stomach intubation or similar methods. However, such methods do not appear to prolong survival or affect many of the complications of advanced neoplasia (Balducci and Hardy, 1985; Vigano et al., 1994). In view of this lack of effectiveness of such nutritional modalities, various pharmacological approaches to the treatment of cachexia in advanced cancer patients have been utilized (Loprinzi et al., 1992; Vigano et al., 1994). The drug therapy utilized involves either hormones

Table 17.1 Manifestations of Cancer Cachexia

1. Anorexia
2. Weight loss
3. Asthenia (weakness)
4. Changing body image
5. Chronic nausea
6. Negative energy balance
7. Anemia, metabolic alterations (protein, lipid, carbohydrate)

such as corticosteroids, progestational drugs, and anabolic steroids administered in an attempt to change the altered hormonal milieu of the tumor-bearing host or mood-altering drugs such as cannabinoids to alter the psychology of the host. In the final analysis, however, cancer cachexia cannot be completely reversed without the elimination of the neoplasm (van Eys, 1982).

Warnold and associates (1978) demonstrated that the development of cachexia may be accompanied by an increase in the resting metabolic rate and the daily energy expenditure in cancer patients, even in the absence of significant physical activity. In comparing cancer patients with healthy subjects, these authors found that while energy intake was not significantly different between the two groups, the daily energy expenditure and resting metabolic rate were significantly greater in cancer patients than in controls (Table 17.2). Shortly thereafter, Bozzetti and colleagues (1980) reported that resting metabolic rates were increased by 60% in a heterogeneous group of 65 patients with advanced cancer. These investigators found a significant correlation between resting metabolic expenditure and percentage of body weight loss. Furthermore, a number of investigations have found that weight loss in cancer patients, especially that found at initial diagnosis, had a dramatic effect on survival (Table 17.3). This table shows that weight loss is quite common in patients with cancer, and it may be stated that nearly every patient who dies from cancer will develop weight loss at some time during the course of the disease (Langstein and Norton, 1991).

Anorexia, Weight Loss, and Cancer Cachexia

Despite the relatively low plasma glucose levels in many cachectic patients, a factor that usually stimulates appetite, a typical characteristic of cachexia is anorexia or loss of appetite. This symptom is an extremely important characteristic of the syndrome of cachexia, as anorexia may aggravate weight loss, weakness, hormonal changes, and progressive alterations in a number of vital functions. Grosvenor and colleagues (1989) determined that anorexia occurs in approximately 50% of newly diagnosed cancer patients. Even in the 1930s, it was recognized that at least 20% of all cancer deaths were due solely to malnutrition (Warren, 1932). It is not clear that any single cause is primary in the anorexia of cancer, but a number of possible factors have been described over the past two decades (Table 17.4). However, since the publication of Table 17.4, substantial evidence has developed to indicate that humoral factors, many affecting the central nervous system, may be very important in the development of anorexia in cancer patients and can be directly related to several of the factors listed in Table 17.4. In addition, recent studies in animals have demonstrated that spontaneous physical exercise may modify the cachectic state, particularly in slowing the muscle wasting, although, toward the end of the experiments, the energy costs of exercise accelerated the catabolic state (Deuster et al., 1985; Daneryd et al., 1990).

Within the last decade, studies on the mechanism of anorexia have been oriented toward the effects of circulating hormones and metabolic constituents. In a rat hepatoma experimental model, Chance and associates (1991) demonstrated a correlation between increases in ammonia

Table 17.2   Energy Relationships in Cancer Patients

	Controls	Cancer Patients
Energy intake	1470 kcal/day	1270 kcal/day
Energy expenditure	1420 kcal/day	2020 kcal/day
Basal metabolic rate	1170 kcal/day	1630 kcal/day

Table 17.3   Weight Loss in Cancer Patients at Initial Diagnosis: Its Effect on Survival
Following Cancer Treatment

Diagnosis	No. Patients	Percent with Weight Loss at Diagnosis	Survival (Weeks)	
			Weight Loss	No Weight Loss
Breast	289	36	45	70[a]
Sarcoma	189	39	25	46[a]
Colon	307	54	21	43[a]
Prostate	78	56	24	46[a]
Small cell lung	436	60	27	34[a]
Lung	590	61	14	20[a]
Pancreas	111	83	12	14
Gastric	179	83	27	41[a]

[a]Significantly different from weight loss patients.
Adapted from Langstein and Norton, 1991, with permission of the authors and publisher.

concentration in the blood and the development of cancer-induced anorexia. A number of investigations, some of which are considered later in this chapter, have demonstrated that specific hormones in the general class of cytokines (Chapter 19; Matthys and Billiau, 1997) may also be important in the development of anorexia. Perhaps primary among these is tumor necrosis factor α (TNF-α; see below), but other cytokines such as interleukin-1 (IL-1; Laviano et al., 1996), and even endogenous opioids that are involved in the regulation of food intake may also play a role in the mechanism of the anorexia of cancer (Yim and Lowy, 1984). Several investigations have implicated the amine hormones serotonin and dopamine as playing significant roles in the mechanism of the anorexia of cancer. Initial studies by Chance et al. (1983) demonstrated increased concentrations of tryptophan, the precursor of serotonin, as well as the amine itself and 5-hydroxyindoleacetic acid, one of its metabolites, in specific regions of the brain related to the control of food intake and appetite in tumor-bearing rats. These studies were extended by Rossi-Fanelli and associates (Muscaritoli et al., 1996; Cangiano et al., 1996; Laviano et al., 1996). In particular, these authors demonstrated a correlation between the ratio of free tryptophan to neutral amino acids (valine, leucine, isoleucine, tyrosine, and phenylalanine) and the content of se-

Table 17.4   Possible Causes of Anorexia in Individuals with Cancer

1. Nonspecific manifestation of disease
2. Mechanical interference with the gastrointestinal tract
3. Alterations of taste and/or smell perception
4. Learned food aversions
5. Production of lactate
6. Production of ketones
7. Hypothetical tumor toxins
8. Direct effect on appetite center
9. Psychological factors
10. Treatment (chemotherapy, radiation therapy)

Modified from Costa and Donaldson, 1980, with permission of the authors and publisher.

rotonin in brain. This led to a hypothesis depicted in Figure 17.1, in which tumor growth resulted in increased plasma tryptophan concentrations, which, in turn, successively competed with neutral amino acids for access to the central nervous system across the blood-brain barrier. From this, the hypothalamus metabolized tryptophan to serotonin, in turn resulting in anorexia by a direct effect of this amine hormone on centers controlling food intake. However, as pointed out by these authors, the simple concentration of serotonin in the hypothalamus is not the only factor involved, but its metabolism and release by neurons in the hypothalamus and the effect of cytokines acting directly on cells of the central nervous system are involved in the development of anorexia (Laviano et al., 1996). Later studies by Varma et al. (1999), using elaborate surgical techniques with cannulation of the hypothalamic area and ventromedial nucleus concerned with the regulation of food intake, came to similar conclusions as those noted in Figure 17.1.

While it is likely that serotonin and perhaps dopamine are involved in the mechanism of anorexia in cancer patients, it is also clear that a number of other polypeptide factors, some of which have been mentioned above, play significant roles in the anorexia of cancer. These, particularly tumor necrosis factor, are discussed later in this chapter.

Protein Metabolism and Neoplastic Growth

As noted above, the weight loss associated with malignant disease involves a reduction of both body fat and body protein. In the normal adult mammal, proteins are continuously synthesized and degraded. This dynamic process, termed *protein turnover*, is regulated by a variety of hormonal as well as nutritional factors. In the healthy adult, a state of nitrogen balance occurs, with protein synthesis equal to protein degradation. In the tumor-bearing host, this relationship is dis-

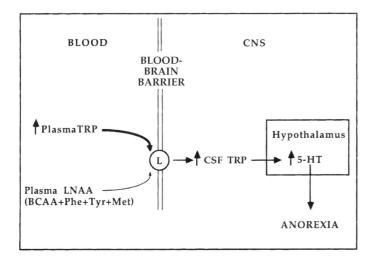

Figure 17.1 Postulated pathogenic mechanism involved in the development of cancer anorexia. In the tumor-bearing animal, plasma tryptophan (TRP) concentrations increase, facilitating the competition with other large neutral amino acids (LNAA) in crossing the blood-brain barrier via the specific L-transport system. BCAA, branched-chain amino acids; Phe, phenylalanine; Tyr, tyrosine; Met, methionine; CSF, cerebrospinal fluid. As a consequence of the successful competition of TRP across the blood-brain barrier, TRP concentrations in the central nervous system (CNS) increase, leading to enhanced serotonin (5-HT) synthesis in the hypothalamus, ultimately leading to anorexia. (Adapted from Laviano et al., 1996, with permission of the authors and publisher.)

turbed, so that there is usually a net loss of nitrogen from nonmalignant tissues as protein degradation exceeds synthesis. The relationship of the host to the neoplasm with respect to protein and amino acid metabolism is depicted diagrammatically in Figure 17.2.

As depicted in the figure and noted in numerous studies, protein degradation in the cancer-bearing host occurs to the greatest extent in the musculature of the organism. In experimental systems, protein synthesis in muscle decreases (Paxton et al., 1987) while protein degradation in this same tissue increases dramatically, as measured by several different methods (Tessitore et al., 1987; Lazarus et al., 1999). In a mouse model, this enhanced protein degradation in muscle was associated with a rise in PGE_2, one of the prostaglandins, (Smith and Tisdale, 1993). In turn, the protein degradation in muscle could be inhibited by administration of the ω-3 polyunsaturated fatty acid, eicosapentaenoic acid (Beck et al., 1991). These factors may be considered as a direct or indirect effect of the neoplasm on the host via known and unknown humoral influences (Figure 17.2). In the human, Emery et al. (1984) reported that protein synthesis in muscle could account for only about 8% of total body protein synthesis in cancer patients, as compared with

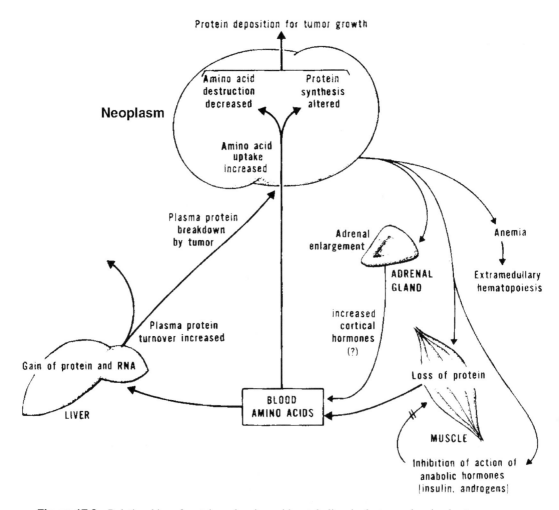

Figure 17.2   Relationships of protein and amino acid metabolism in the tumor-bearing host.

53% in normal control subjects. In contrast to skeletal muscle, protein synthesis in liver increased during cachexia (Paxton et al., 1987), although—in one experimental system—as tumor growth continued, protein degradation became predominant in that organ (Tessitore et al., 1987). Unlike these other tissues, the adrenals in experimental systems become enlarged and remain so during the entire experimental period (Tessitore et al., 1993). This is probably due to a generalized stress response, both psychologically and physically, which in turn results in increased levels of gluconeogenic hormones such as glucagon and cortisol (cf. Hulsewé et al., 1997). Although overall protein synthesis in livers of cancer-bearing animals increased, there was no change in the synthesis of serum albumin, the major protein component of serum, in either humans (Lundholm et al., 1980) or experimental animals (Ove et al., 1972); however, in tumor-bearing rats, albumin catabolism was increased, an effect abolished by adrenalectomy (Jewell and Hunter, 1971). But in patients with hepatocellular carcinoma, O'Keefe et al. (1990) demonstrated that amino acid incorporation into serum albumin and other serum proteins was higher than that in controls or in patients with hepatic metastasis.

As noted in Figure 17.2, the intermediary between muscle and liver and, in turn, the neoplasm is the blood amino acid concentrations. In general, as noted earlier in this chapter, patients exhibit decreases in the concentrations of gluconeogenic amino acids, including the branched-chain neutral amino acids (Figure 17.1). This is in contrast to individuals exhibiting severe malnutrition, in whom the concentration of these amino acids is usually normal or increased (cf. Tisdale, 1997). As might be expected of a rapidly growing tissue, neoplastic cells under both in vitro and in vivo conditions have a high capacity for concentrating amino acids. Furthermore, tumor-bearing animals fed a protein-containing diet were actually observed to excrete less nitrogen and consequently appeared to be in a more positive nitrogen balance than controls without neoplasms (cf. Goodlad, 1964). This is also true of human patients with advanced cancer (Brennan and Burt, 1981). In animal experiments, analysis of the tumors showed them to contain more nitrogen than was retained during the experimental period. Thus, part of the tumor protein must have been obtained at the expense of the tissues of the host. This ability of the tumor to draw directly on its host tissue proteins is also illustrated by the observation that tumor growth in animals maintained on a protein-free diet was still about three-quarters of the rate observed in protein-fed animals. Observations such as these in both humans and animals have led investigators, originally Mider et al. (1948), to describe the growing tumor as a *nitrogen trap*.

Although the original studies leading to the concept of the nitrogen trap were carried out with only a few neoplasms, there is substantial reason to believe that the concept is applicable to many forms of cancer. Some neoplasms appear to have special types of nitrogen traps in the form of enzymatic capacities for the selective degradation of essential amino acids (Pitot et al., 1961). When such a circumstance is present, the host becomes deficient in an essential amino acid (e.g., threonine) while the neoplasm retains its ability to synthesize protein and to grow. Another specific amino acid "trap" has been shown for the nonessential amino acid glutamine in experimental systems (cf. de Blaauw et al., 1997). While glutamine is the most abundant free amino acid in the organism, because of the increased protein synthesis and need for this amino acid as well as its concomitant breakdown by neoplasms, glutamine may become a "conditionally" essential amino acid because the capacity for the endogenous biosynthesis of this amino acid is exceeded by tissue utilization (cf. de Blaauw et al., 1997). Stein (1978) has suggested that the progressive weight loss, abnormal gluconeogenesis, and lactate recycling seen in cachexia may be the result of an imbalance of essential amino acids within the host that results from selective uptake of essential amino acids. This imbalance may prevent the host from effectively decreasing gluconeogenesis as long as the tumor persists in causing an amino acid imbalance. The capacity of a neoplasm to act as a selective nitrogen trap is undoubtedly associated with the characteristic of relative autonomy of the tumor cell, but other factors may also play a role. Sidransky and Verney (1979) demonstrated that the livers of hepatoma-bearing rats do not respond to several nutritional stresses, such as a protein-free diet or tryptophan administration, as do the livers of non-tumor-bearing animals. Thus the neoplasm, directly or indirectly, may alter the regulatory mechanisms of normal tissues. On the other hand, it would appear that the breakdown of protein in muscle is not necessarily due to an enhancement of protein degradation but rather to an inhibition of protein synthesis, leading to a greater net degradation of muscle protein (Svaninger et al., 1983).

Many neoplasms, especially those exhibiting relatively rapid growth during the process of cachexia, have a decidedly greater ability to concentrate many if not most amino acids within their cells (cf. Goodlad, 1964). Shortly after the administration of a labeled amino acid, the "pools" of amino acids within various normal tissues are labeled to a much greater extent than those in neoplastic tissue. Some years ago, Busch and associates (1961) showed that when labeled amino acids were administered to animals in the form of proteins such as albumin, tumor proteins were found to have a much greater specific activity than proteins in nonneoplastic tissue. This suggests that the amino acids in the form of proteins are better substrates for protein synthesis in neoplasms and that tumors perhaps have a selective advantage in extracting whole proteins from the bloodstream. Furthermore, humans and animals with large or rapidly growing neoplasms usually exhibit hypoalbuminemia.

The amino acid requirements of tumors do not appear to differ significantly from those of normal tissues except with regard to nutritional requirements apparently associated with growth and possible specific abnormalities seen in certain neoplasms. A peculiarity of tumor nutrition has been exploited therapeutically by the use of the enzyme asparaginase to treat certain leukemias and lymphomas in which the tumor cells themselves require the amino acid asparagine for growth and survival (Uren and Handschumacher, 1977). The use of this enzyme to deplete the host of a specific amino acid that apparently does not significantly compromise normal tissue metabolism differs from other studies, in which diets missing certain amino acids were fed in an attempt to determine the effect of nutritional deficiencies on tumor growth. Other attempts have also been carried out with enzymes that selectively degrade other amino acids, such as phenylalanine and methionine, in experimental systems. However, unlike the asparaginase system, the amino acids degraded by these enzymes are essential for normal cells in general and, although inhibition of tumor growth was demonstrated, such preparations have not come into clinical use. Because of the metabolic importance of glutamine (see above), glutaminase prepared from bacterial sources has been used in both experimental and human systems with some success (Roberts et al., 1971; Spiers and Wade, 1976), but it has not found general use, possibly because of its toxicity. Furthermore, comparable experiments have been attempted with amino acid–deficient or –limited diets, again with variable results (Lorincz et al., 1969). On the other hand, the use of vitamin-deficient diets has received some attention, especially since at least one vitamin analog, methotrexate (an analog of folic acid), is used routinely in clinical chemotherapy (Jolivet et al., 1983). In this instance it has been demonstrated that, in experimental animals, the drug is more effective when folic acid–deficient diets are fed (Rosen et al., 1964). Patients receiving methotrexate for prolonged periods must also be carefully monitored to ensure that the drug therapy, while combating neoplastic growth, does not produce a folic acid deficiency.

Many patients with advanced cancer also exhibit significant anemia. Although the exact mechanism for this anemia is not clear at present, there is substantial evidence that humoral factors produced by the neoplasm (Zucker et al., 1980) or by the host in response to the neoplasm (Ludwig and Fritz, 1998) result in a decreased production of the hormone erythropoietin. The decrease in the production of this hormone appears to be the general common denominator seen in cancer-related anemia (cf. Spivak, 1994) and is likely due to the effect of cytokines produced as a result of neoplastic interaction with the host. A diagram of the proposed pathophysiology of the anemia of cancer is seen in Figure 17.3. The nomenclature of the various cytokines indicated in the figure is discussed further in Chapter 19. Besides the general mechanism, there are other causes of anemia in cancer patients, such as direct blood loss, autoimmune hemolysis, cachexia, nutritional deficiencies, and the therapy of the neoplasm itself (Ludwig and Fritz, 1998).

Carbohydrate Metabolism and Gluconeogenesis in the Cancer-Bearing Organism

One of the earliest metabolic abnormalities described in cancer patients was that of glucose intolerance (Rohdenberg et al., 1919). Glucose intolerance is evidenced by increased concentrations and delayed clearance of blood glucose following oral or intravenous glucose administration (Holroyde and Reichard, 1981). Such an effect may be due, at least in part, to tissue insensitivity to insulin as well as a defective response of β cells of the pancreas to insulin secretion following hyperglycemia. Despite this fact, in experimental systems, insulin may actually modify or even reverse the cachexia of neoplasia (Moley et al., 1985; Beck and Tisdale, 1989a).

Another abnormality commonly seen in cancer patients with advanced disease is an increase in glucose turnover as measured by isotopic techniques (cf. Chlebowski and Heber, 1986). Although few difference in the rates of glucose production and oxidation have been observed in patients with cancer, there is substantial evidence for differential cycling of the molecule. Although glucose is converted to a variety of metabolites, a major metabolite that may be recycled is lactate. This recycling through the process of gluconeogenesis, which is predominantly a function of liver and kidney, is diagrammatically represented in Figure 17.4. Under normal conditions, lactate produced in peripheral tissues would provide the individual with maximum energy available from glucose oxidation (cf. Holroyde and Reichard, 1981). In patients with neoplasia, especially those exhibiting weight loss, measurements of the Cori cycle have demonstrated dramatic increases in this process (Table 17.5). This is particularly true in patients who have increased basal metabolic rates (BMR), where the Cori cycle contributes a

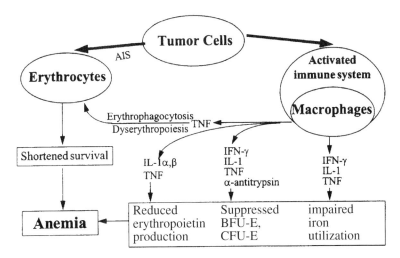

Figure 17.3 Diagram of the pathophysiology of anemia in cancer patients. AIS, anemia-inducing substance; BFU-E and CFU-E, precursors of red blood cells; IFN, interferon; IL, interleukin; TNF, tumor necrosis factor. (Reproduced from Nowrousian et al., 1996, with permission of the authors and publisher.)

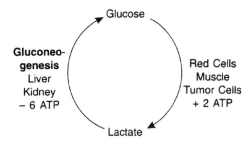

Figure 17.4 Diagram of the Cori cycle, in which peripheral tissues, including neoplastic cells, metabolize glucose to lactate. The lactate is circulated by the bloodstream to the liver and kidneys, where it is converted back to glucose; but in the process, a substantial amount of energy is required.

little less than two-thirds of the total glucose turnover, requiring considerable energy expenditure by the host.

Part of the assumed mechanism for this phenomenon is the high rate of glycolysis that is characteristic of malignant neoplasms (Chapter 15). Glucose uptake and lactate release has been found to be dramatically increased in neoplastic cells, possibly in part a consequence of the predominant form of hexokinase seen in neoplasms, which is essentially unresponsive to hormonal and external stimuli (Mathupala et al., 1995). Thus, in a sense, the neoplasm may also be considered a glucose trap, which is further evidenced by some human (Marks et al., 1974) and experimental (McDevitt and Tisdale, 1992) studies showing that hypoglycemia is found in cancer-bearing hosts. The exact mechanism of this phenomenon is not clear but may be related not simply to the "glucose trap" effect of the neoplasm but also to humoral factors induced by the cancer itself (Chapter 18).

As noted in Figure 17.4, a major component of the Cori cycle is the phenomenon of gluconeogenesis or the conversion of lactate and other related molecules to glucose. These other molecules include amino acids such as leucine, alanine, and those whose metabolism gives rise to potentially gluconeogenic substrates. As indicated earlier, gluconeogenesis is further enhanced by hormones within the organism, especially corticosteroids and glucagon, the former being a product of the stress response contributing to the altered protein metabolism in the tumor-bearing host (Figure 17.2). Metabolically, it is possible to reverse, at least transiently, the gluconeogenesis of the tumor-bearing host, as noted in Figure 17.5. In this experiment, ^{14}C-alanine

Table 17.5 Total Glucose Turnover and Cori Cycle Measurements in Cancer Patients and Normal Subjects

	Total Glucose Turnover	Cori Cycle
	g/1.73m²/24 h	
Normal, overnight fast	200	36
Normal, 7-day fast	144	36
Cancer, stable weight	187	33
Cancer, progressive weight loss	268	115
Cancer, progressive weight loss with increased basal metabolic rate	370	212

Modified from Holroyde and Reichard, 1981, with permission of the authors and publisher.

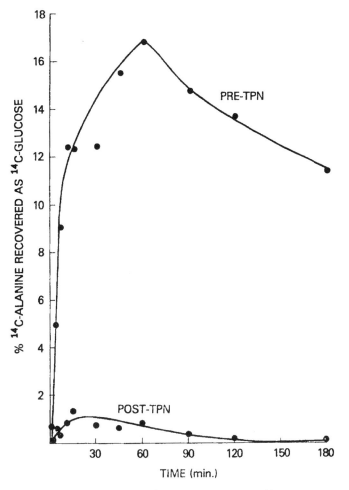

Figure 17.5   Percentage of ^{14}C-alanine recovered as ^{14}C-glucose after a single injection of ^{14}C-alanine to a cancer-bearing patient before and 2 weeks after total parenteral nutrition (TPN). (Adapted from Brennan and Burt, 1981.)

was administered to a cancer-bearing patient, and the glucose was isolated from the blood before (pre) and after (post) total parenteral nutrition (TPN). By forcing the metabolism of the host through administration of carbohydrate, lipid, and amino acids intravenously, one may suppress the gluconeogenesis in the cancer patient, showing that responses in normal tissues still appear to be functional. However, the tumor burden, the metabolism of the neoplasm, and the altered hormonal milieu of the host lead ultimately to the abnormalities in carbohydrate metabolism noted.

Lipid Metabolism in the Tumor-Bearing Host

During prolonged starvation, the organism gradually converts its metabolism from that dependent on glucose and amino acids to one dependent on lipids and their breakdown products—

ketone bodies. This change results in a decrease in oxygen consumption and a sparing of protein breakdown (cf. McAndrew, 1986). In patients with cancer cachexia, these metabolic adaptations normally seen during starvation do not occur. As noted earlier, there is a recycling of lactate (Figure 17.4) as well as pyruvate and an increase in the use of acetoacetate (ketone body) by neoplastic tissue (cf. McAndrew, 1986).

Alterations in fat metabolism in the entire tumor-bearing organism have been seen both in experimental animals and in patients. These alterations include increases in circulating triglycerides, free fatty acids (FFA), and glycerol (Noguchi et al., 1988; Legaspi et al., 1987). Body fat constitutes 90% of energy reserves in the adult organism, and loss of whole-body fat is a consistent feature of cancer cachexia (cf. Tisdale, 1997). While normal individuals suppress lipid mobilization after administration of glucose, this process is impaired in patients with neoplastic disease, in whom the oxidation of fatty acids continues throughout the stage of progression. The hypertriglyceridemia seen in animals bearing neoplasms may also be due in part to the fact that lipoprotein lipase expression and activity in both fat and muscle decline from the normal level, possibly owing to some humoral factor produced by or as a result of the neoplastic growth (Noguchi et al., 1991). The effect of neoplastic growth on adipose tissue extends even to apoptosis of adipocytes in most of the cancer-bearing patients studied (Prins et al., 1994). It has been speculated that the liver exhibits a demand for the utilization of free fatty acid to supply the energy for increased gluconeogenesis in cancer patients (Levin and Gevers, 1981). In this vein, the feeding of a diet in which up to 80% of the calories was supplied as medium-chain triglycerides resulted in a reduction in weight loss as well as in the percentage contribution of the neoplasm to the final body weight (Tisdale et al., 1987). Furthermore, this regimen restored the nitrogen balance to that seen in non-tumor-bearing controls (Beck and Tisdale, 1989b). More recently, Pariza et al. (1999) have demonstrated that conjugated isomers of the fatty acid linoleic acid have effects in experimental animals that may inhibit carcinogenesis at each of the major stages. In relation to this discussion, dietary conjugated linoleic acid (CLA) was found to protect against cachexia induced in mice by the administration of tumor necrosis factor. The suggested mechanism for this effect is an alteration or inhibition of the signal transduction pathway induced by this cytokine (Pariza et al., 1999). In concert with the increases in triglycerides, there is an elevation in the low-density lipoproteins in the plasma. It is these lipoproteins that are synthesized in the liver and carry triglycerides to peripheral tissues and to a great extent to the neoplasm (Clark and Crain, 1986). Thus, the lack of glucose inhibition of fat mobilization from the fat depots, the continued oxidation of fatty acids, and the absence of increased dietary fat intake lead to a depletion of fat stores with concomitant increase in metabolic rate from fatty acid oxidation required for gluconeogenesis. Maintenance of the Cori cycle combines with alterations in fat metabolism to contribute to a net loss of body weight in the cancer-bearing patient.

HUMORAL FACTORS IN CANCER CACHEXIA

As indicated earlier in this chapter, a variety of humoral or circulating factors influence the development of cancer cachexia and many nutritional aspects of the host-tumor relationship. Furthermore, the interactions and interrelations of many of these factors add to the complexity of the mechanisms of cachexia seen in the tumor-bearing host. No single amino acid, cytokine, steroid, or polypeptide hormone can account for the syndrome of cancer cachexia. A list of some of the major humoral factors and their interrelationships are seen in Table 17.6.

Table 17.6 Humoral Factors and Their Interrelations in Cancer Cachexia

Factor	Interrelating Factors	Some Major Effects
Corticosteroids	Catecholamines, insulin	Gluconeogenesis, insulin resistance
Glucagon	Corticosteroids	Gluconeogenesis, hyperglycemia
Insulin	Glucagon, corticosteroids	Hypoglycemia and glucose utilization by Cori cycle
Interleukin-1	Serotonin, tumor necrosis factor-α	Anorexia, weight loss, hypoalbuminemia
Interleukin-6	Interferon-γ, tumor necrosis factor-α	Muscle atrophy
Leptin	Tumor necrosis factor-α, interleukin-1	Regulation of food intake
Prostaglandins	Interleukin-6, interferon-γ, tumor necrosis factor α	Lipolysis, protein degradation, fever and immune suppression
Serotonin	Interleukin-1	Appetite suppression
Tumor necrosis factor-α	Interleukin-1, interleukin-6, leptin	Anorexia, lipolysis, apoptosis

Table 17.6 is not meant to be exhaustive, as may be noted later in the chapter, but rather indicates the complexity of the various hormones, cytokines, and amines that contribute to the clinical picture of cachexia in the cancer patient. The reader is referred to various reviews on the effects of other factors noted in the table (Tisdale, 1997; Inui, 1999; Laviano et al., 1995; Matthys and Billiau, 1997; Roubenoff, 1997). The cytokines interleukin-1, interleukin-6, interferon-γ, and tumor necrosis factor-α all appear to have some degree of effectiveness in inducing some aspects of the syndrome of cancer cachexia (Tisdale, 1997). However, in some instances little or no change is seen in the serum levels of one or the other of these cytokines, again suggesting that no single factor is effective in inducing the syndrome of cancer cachexia. Of these cytokines, the best studied, which may serve to model the others as well as many other components of the syndrome of cancer cachexia, is tumor necrosis-α (TNF-α). Prostaglandins are produced both by host cells and in some cases by neoplastic cells. Thus, administration of inhibitors of prostaglandin synthesis will have variable effects. However, in mice in which several cytokines were eliminated by gene targeting, inhibition of prostaglandin production by the neoplasm and host resulted in improvement of the cachectic state (Cahlin et al., 2000).

Tumor Necrosis Factor-α and Related Cytokines in Cancer Cachexia

The effects of TNF were first observed in the latter part of the nineteenth century by Coley (1893) based on the observation that patients with streptococcal infections might also exhibit a partial remission of some neoplasms. Subsequent investigations demonstrated that injection of bacterial products, specifically a lipopolysaccharide, could induce hemorrhagic necrosis of transplantable neoplasms in mice. Subsequently, a serum factor associated with administration of the bacterial product was isolated and named *tumor necrosis factor* (Carswell et al., 1975). Since that time, there has been a dramatic increase in our knowledge of TNF-α, its genetics, and its function. TNF-α is a member of a superfamily of genes of which more than 10 are presently known, along with their respective receptors (cf. Gruss, 1996). Neoplasms engineered to express high levels of TNF when grown in mice rapidly induce a syndrome of cancer cachexia (Oliff et al., 1987). An interesting comparison of the clinical and metabolic alterations seen in cancer cachexia with those of the in vivo effects of TNF-α are listed in Table 17.7. As noted, there are relatively few differences in the syndrome and the effects of the cytokine, at least in those parameters listed. However, in some model systems it was possible to dissociate some of the effects of TNF-α from the cachectic syndrome. In particular, a number of studies have failed to detect elevated circulating levels of TNF-α in cachectic cancer patients or to associate an elevation of this cytokine with the development of cachexia (cf. Tisdale, 1997). Still, the effects of the cytokine serve as an excellent model with which to consider the mechanisms whereby such humoral substances may exert effects leading to cachexia in the cancer patient.

TNF-α is produced predominantly by tissue macrophages, but other cell types—including endothelial cells, fibroblasts, and epithelium—synthesize significant amounts of this polypeptide when subjected to appropriate stimuli (cf. Luster et al., 1999). A closely related member of the TNF-α family, lymphotoxin-α, is produced exclusively by lymphocytes, but its functions are not as well known as those of TNF-α, although both ligands interact with the same receptors (see below). TNF-α is synthesized as a large transmembrane molecule (Figure 17.6). It may be activated by a proteolytic cleavage at the surface of the cell membrane, releasing the 17-kDa active ligand, which may circulate in an endocrine manner or interact with adjacent cells in a paracrine manner.

Mechanisms of TNF-α Action—Signaling Pathways

As noted above, TNF-α is a member of a superfamily of ligands each having its own receptor, although TNF-α may interact with either of two different receptors. This is shown schematically

Table 17.7 Some Clinical and Metabolic Alterations in Cancer Cachexia: Comparison with the In Vivo Effects of Tumor Necrosis Factor

Parameter	Cachexia	Tumor Necrosis Factor
Anorexia	Yes	Yes
Weight loss	Yes	Yes
Anemia	Yes	Yes
Skeletal muscle		
catabolism	↑	↑
synthesis	↓	↑
Hepatic protein		
synthesis	↑	↑
gluconeogenesis	↑	NA[a]
Serum glucose	±/↓	↑ then ↓
Lactate recycling	↑	↑
Total body water	↑	↑
Serum lipid/triglyceride	↑	↑
Lipoprotein lipase activity	↓	↓
Lipid stores	↓	↓
Lipogenesis	↑	↑

[a]NA = not available
Reproduced from Alexander and Norton (1993) with permission of the authors and publisher.

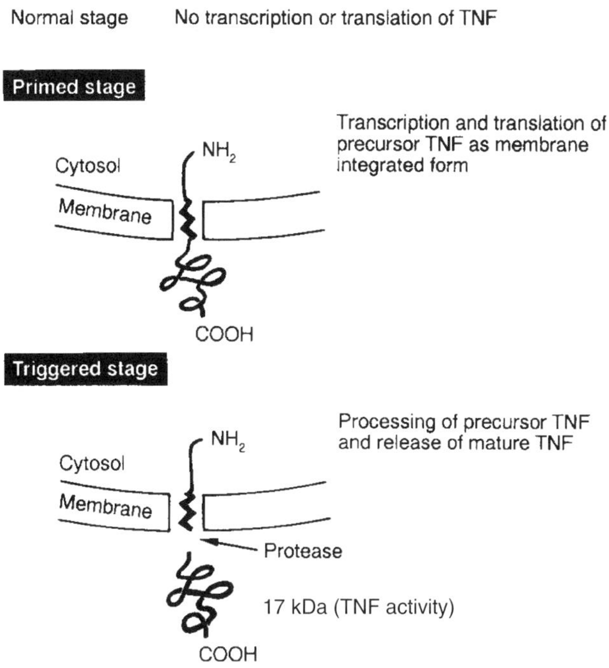

Figure 17.6 Proposed mechanism for priming and activation of TNF production from the macrophage. (Reproduced from Mizuno, 1992, with permission of the author and publisher.)

in Figure 17.7, which indicates that most cells of the organism possess receptors for TNF-α. As noted in the figure, interaction with the 55-kDa receptor (now known as CD120a) involves significantly more functions than interaction with the 75-kDa receptor. In the latter case, it appears that activation is preferentially by the cell-bound form of TNF, and it is likely that many of its functions are as yet unknown (cf. Wallach et al., 1999). As with many other receptors, the active form is the dimer, and the predominant form of the soluble TNF-α ligand is a homotrimer, which likely has as one of its functions the induction of dimerization and subsequent signal transduction from the receptor.

A schematic representation of the 55- and 75-kDa (CD1206) receptors for TNF and lymphotoxin-α is seen in Figure 17.8. In addition, another receptor, *Fas*, is shown because of its similarity to the 55-kDa TNF receptor. It has a separate ligand and associates with a kinase that is involved in the induction of apoptosis by the interaction of *Fas* with its ligand (cf. Baker and Reddy, 1996). The interesting characteristic of the *Fas* and 55-kDa TNF-α receptor are domains in the intracellular portion of the molecule known as *death domains*. These domains interact with proteins as shown, having the names of TRADD and FADD. While the exact molecular mechanisms of these proteins is unknown, it is likely that they recruit other proteins, possibly activating such to ultimately result in apoptosis or, in the case of the 55-kDa TNF-α receptor, activation of the nuclear transcription factor NF-κB (Beyaert and Fiers, 1998). The 75-kDa receptor, on the other hand, associates with different proteins known as TRAFs, which apparently have specific regions involved in the ultimate signaling pathway to NF-κB activation as shown (cf. Wallach et al., 1999). Not shown in this diagram but appar-

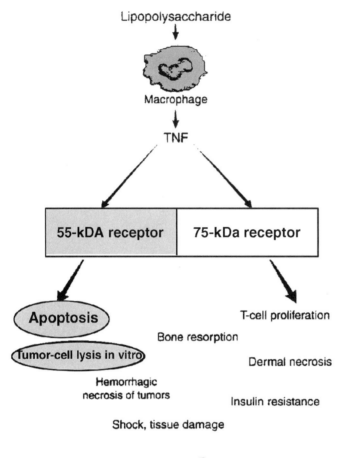

Figure 17.7   Diagram of TNF-α-receptor interactions leading to various effects within the organism. The receptors occur on virtually all cells throughout the organism, thus accounting for the generalized organismal response resulting from circulating levels of TNF. (Adapted from Bazzoni and Beutler, 1996, with permission of the authors and publisher.)

ently involved in TNF-α induction of apoptosis is the sphingomyelin signaling pathway, which involves lipid intermediates, notably ceramide, and NF-κB translocation to the nucleus (Yang et al., 1993).

Thus, TNF-α has effects that induce both cell replication, presumably through signal transduction pathways to activation of nuclear transcription factors, and apoptosis, via the death domains of the receptor and associated proteins, leading to activation of the apoptotic pathway. It is of interest that in the mouse skin, TNF-α acts as a tumor promoter (Fujiki and Suganuma, 1994) and may also serve as an autocrine growth factor for human B lymphocytes (Boussiotis et al., 1994). All of this illustrates the complexity with which these humoral factors exert their effects at a mechanistic level, leading to their part in the induction of cancer cachexia in the whole organism.

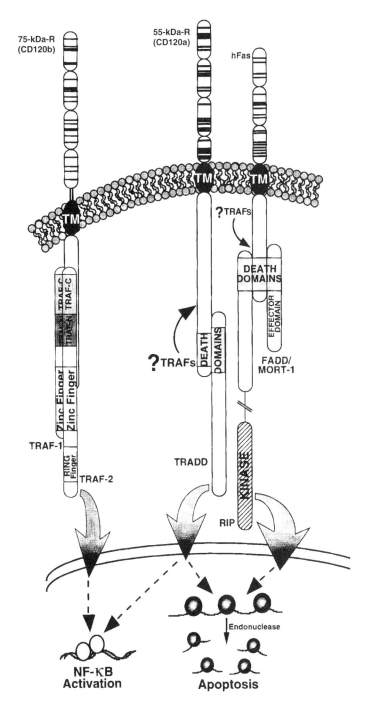

Figure 17.8 Diagrammatic representation of the proposed interaction between three members of the TNF receptor superfamily and their associated proteins. Both CD120a (55 kDa) and *Fas* transduce apoptotic signals via a C-terminal death domain following activation by the ligand. The death domain region, in addition to its function as an effector in apoptosis, also appears to mediate protein-protein interactions resulting in nuclear events including NF-κB activation. In contrast, the other TNF receptor, CD120b (75 kDa), recruits a different set of proteins, the TRAF protein, resulting in signal transmission. This in turn transduces nuclear events that may result in the modulation of cellular responses and gene expression. The figure depicts the receptors as monomers for clarity, but it should be remembered that it is their dimeric form that is active. (Modified from Baker and Reddy, 1996, with permission of the authors and publisher.)

THE COMPLEXITY OF CANCER CACHEXIA

As indicated at the beginning of this chapter, the syndrome of cancer cachexia resembles several nutritional syndromes such as starvation or protein-calorie malnutrition. It is clear, however, that this aspect of the host-tumor relationship is extremely complex, involving not only nutritional factors but also a wide variety of humoral and hormonal components, many of which are known and a number of which are undoubtedly unknown. The idea that humoral factors or hormones may be critical in the causation of cachexia was actually first suggested more than four decades ago by Nakahara and Fukuoka (1958), who proposed that a hormone-like substance that they termed *toxohormone* was responsible for significant changes in the tumor-bearing host, particularly a depression of the level of the enzyme catalase in the liver. Although the concept of toxohormone is generally not considered as significant in the cachectic syndrome today, this original work pointed the way to the present-day understanding that numerous hormones and humoral factors are involved in the cancer cachexia syndrome.

Cancer cachexia is among the most devastating syndromes associated with advanced cancer and may account directly for between 10% and 22% of all cancer deaths (cf. Tisdale, 1997). The ideal therapy of cancer cachexia is obviously complete removal of the offending neoplasm. Since this is usually not possible because of metastatic spread, various modes of therapy have been employed to relieve symptomatology when treatment of the neoplasm has been relatively unsuccessful. These include the use of several different steroid hormones, both natural and synthetic, and more recently eicosapentaenoic acid which may be able to prevent the muscle wasting (Beck et al., 1991). The use of anabolic steroids as well as corticosteroids may produce transient effects on appetite but have not been generally successful. As with many other aspects of the cancer problem, it is apparent that only when a complete understanding of the variety of factors contributing to the syndrome of cancer cachexia is achieved will it be possible to develop effective treatment modalities for this complex interaction between the neoplasm and the host.

CALCIUM HOMEOSTASIS IN THE HOST-TUMOR RELATIONSHIP

Our discussion thus far of the nutritional aspects of the host-tumor relationship has included only organic nutrients as well as humoral factors of an organic nature. However, studies have demonstrated the inhibition of neoplastic growth by the depletion of essential inorganic constituents such as zinc (Mills et al., 1984a) and magnesium (Mills et al., 1984b). While such parameters are of undoubted importance in the nutrition of the tumor-bearing host, a far more significant inorganic constituent is calcium. A diagram of normal adult calcium homeostasis is seen in Figure 17.9. Since calcium, unlike organic nutritional components, is not "degraded" by the organism, a balance, just as with nitrogen, is established by the organism. In the adult, where bone growth has essentially ceased, calcium balance is neutral, as shown in the figure. However, in the young, growing individual, there is a positive calcium balance with greater retention of ingested calcium than excretion, while individuals critically ill from a variety of different diseases as well as those with renal insufficiency sometimes occurring as a complication of chemotherapy will be in a negative calcium balance (Abramson et al., 1990). Hypercalcemia, an increase in serum calcium concentration, is probably the most common metabolic complication of malignant disease (Ralston, 1994). This condition occurs in about one-third of patients with multiple myeloma and in five or more percent of all patients with solid neoplasms (Glover and Glick, 1987). Of patients with breast cancer, 30% to 40% exhibit this complication (Muggia, 1990). In fact, the most frequent metabolic oncological emergency is hypercalcemia (Glover and

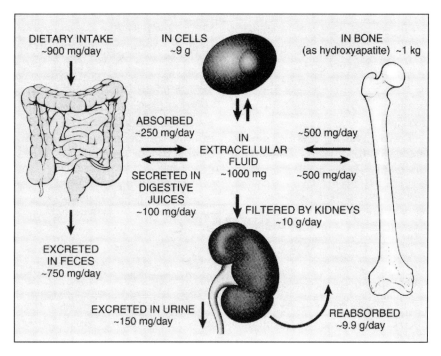

Figure 17.9 Pathways leading to calcium homeostasis in the adult organism. (Modified from Seymour, 1995, with permission of the author and publisher.)

Glick, 1987). From the pathways noted in Figure 17.9, one may note that hypercalcemia can result from at least one of three mechanisms acting alone or in combination. These are increased calcium absorption from the gut, decreased excretion of calcium in the kidney, and accelerated calcium resorption into the serum from bone (Warrell, 1992). In cancer patients exhibiting hypercalcemia, calcium absorption from the gut is generally suppressed and contributes relatively little calcium to the systemic circulation (Coombes et al., 1976). An interesting exception to this generalization is seen with some lymphomas in which the neoplasm itself synthesizes the vitamin 1,25-dihydroxyvitamin D, which regulates the absorption of calcium from the gut (Davies et al., 1994).

During the first two-thirds of the twentieth century and earlier, hypercalcemia due to malignant disease was thought to be primarily a function of the effects of metastases in bone, causing resorption of the skeleton and increase in serum calcium. The three most common neoplasms in humans—breast, prostate, and lung cancer—frequently affect the skeleton with metastases to bone. Since these three types of neoplasms are diagnosed in almost three-quarters of a million new individuals each year, the 5% suffering from hypercalcemia becomes a very significant figure. However, it was not until some 15 years ago that a better understanding of the mechanism of hypercalcemia became apparent. The major internal hormone that regulates calcium metabolism is secreted by the parathyroid gland, parathyroid hormone. Neoplasms of the parathyroid gland in many cases secrete excessive amounts of this hormone, as discussed in Chapter 18. This leads to hypercalcemia but may be considered a special case, although occasionally neoplasms of other tissues may secrete parathyroid hormone ectopically and result in hypercalcemia (Nussbaum et al., 1990). However, in 1987, several laboratories reported the isolation of a polypeptide significantly larger than the parathyroid hormone but having at least some of the sequences of this hormone at its amino terminal end (cf. Broadus et al., 1988). Figure 17.10 shows the organization of the human parathyroid hormone (PTH) gene and that of the parathyroid hormone-related protein (PTHRP) gene. While at first PTHRP and its product were felt to be exclusively produced in neoplasms, it was rapidly shown that PTHRP is a normal hormone essential both for normal development of the mammal as well as for normal homeostasis in the adult. Figure 17.11 lists tissues in the fetus and the adult in which PTHRP is produced and exerts its hormonal effect. Interestingly, the parathyroid glands of both the fetus and the adult produce PTHRP. Furthermore, many of the tissues noted produce the hormone, and it has a paracrine effect on adjacent tissues as well as endocrine effects on distant tissues. Furthermore, as noted from Figure 17.10, there are two promoters for the PTHRP gene, resulting in several forms produced in different tissues (Burtis, 1992). PTH is a polypeptide of 84 amino acids in the human, whereas the various forms of PTHRP range from 139 to 173 amino acids in length (Seymour, 1995). The first 34 amino acids beginning from the N-terminal are structurally similar and functionally equivalent in PTH and the forms of PTHRP. However, the remainder of the polypeptides are different, and in PTHRP there is a region involved in calcium transport in the middle of the polypeptide, whereas the C-terminal domains are involved in osteoclast metabolism in bone (Seymour, 1995; Strewler, 2000). Figure 17.12 gives the plasma levels of PTHRP in normal individuals as well as in those exhibiting the humoral hypercalcemia of malignancy (HHM), several different types of neoplasms, as well as two non-neoplastic conditions. Essentially, it is only neoplasms that exhibit higher than normal levels of PTHRP in the plasma (Martin and Grill, 1992).

As already noted, the secretion of PTHRP, while accounting for the vast majority of hypercalcemia of malignancy, is not the only hormone that can trigger or affect this parameter of the host-tumor relationship. In Table 17.8 is a short list of other factors that induce hypercalcemia, primarily through their action on bone. Notably in this list are the growth factors TGF-α and

HUMAN PTH GENE:

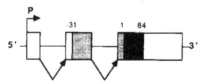

HUMAN PTHRP GENE:

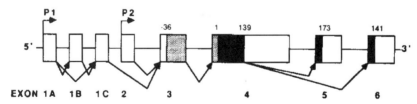

Figure 17.10 Diagram of organization of human parathyroid hormone (PTH) and parathyroid hormone–related protein (PTHRP) genes. The PTH gene has three exons that encode a pre-pro region (light shading) and the mature protein (dark shading). A more complex PTHRP gene possesses two promoters (P1, P2), either of which can initiate transcription. The distal three of its eight exons can be alternatively spliced (arrows) to yield at least three different mRNA transcripts, encoding different lengths of the mature protein. (Reproduced from Burtis, 1992, with permission of the author and publisher.)

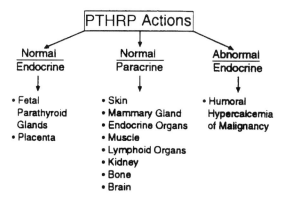

Figure 17.11   Diagrammatic summary of the sites of parathyroid hormone–related protein (PTHRP) production and action. PTHRP can function either in an endocrine or paracrine manner in normal adult and fetal tissues depending on whether it acts locally or is secreted into the circulation. Neoplasms which produce this hormone primarily do so in an endocrine manner. (Reproduced from Rosol and Capen, 1992, with permission of the authors and publisher.)

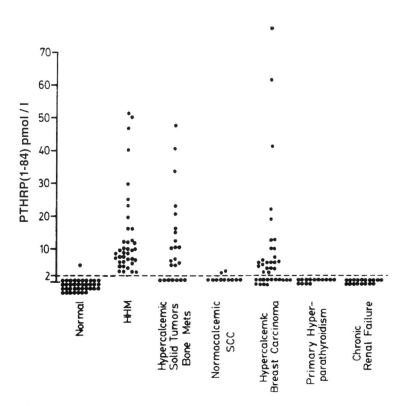

Figure 17.12   Plasma levels of PTHRP in patients with neoplasms and other disease states as well as normal controls. HHM, humoral hypercalcemia of malignancy; SCC, squamous cell carcinoma. (Reproduced from Martin and Grill, 1992, with permission of the authors and publisher.)

Table 17.8 Other Factors Contributing to the Hypercalcemia of Malignancy

Transforming growth factor-α
Transforming growth factor-β
Interleukin-1
Tumor necrosis factor-α
Lymphotoxin
Prostaglandins
Colony-stimulating factors

TGF-β, which act on osteoblasts and osteoclasts, two cell types critical in bone formation and resorption (Mundy, 1989). Not surprisingly, IL-1 and TNF-α, as well as lymphotoxin, also cause hypercalcemia and probably play a significant role in hypercalcemia seen with multiple myeloma and various lymphomas. One of the earlier fashionable theories for the pathogenesis of hypercalcemia was the production of prostaglandins of the E series, which were shown to stimulate osteoclastic bone resorption (cf. Gutierrez et al., 1990).

While all of these factors may be important in certain types of neoplasms, such as those of the immune system and some epithelial neoplasms, all of the evidence argues that PTHRP is the primary stimulator of the hypercalcemia in the majority of neoplasms.

BIOMARKERS OF THE HOST-TUMOR RELATIONSHIP

In addition to explaining the basis for the majority of cases of hypercalcemia of malignancy, the presence of high levels of PTHRP in the plasma indicates the presence of a neoplasm in the host, although not specifically defining the histogenetic type of neoplasm (Figure 17.12). Thus, PTHRP is one of a large number of substances that are secreted, are present on or within the neoplastic cell, or may be produced by normal cells in response to the presence of or factors in or released by the neoplasm. This large group of such substances are termed *tumor markers*, since they indicate the presence or specific characteristics of one or more neoplasms. Generally speaking, tumor markers may be characterized at virtually all levels of genetic expression. This is seen diagrammatically in Figure 17.13. Markers at the genomic level include cytogenetic markers, loss of heterozygosity (LOH), and specific mutations. Messenger RNAs produced specifically in neoplastic cells may be used as markers in tissue sections, while proteins within and secreted by neoplastic cells can be used as markers in tissue sections as well as in body fluids. Products of metabolism and/or specific enzymic function, such as polyamines, lactate, etc., may also be considered as tumor markers. As seen in Chapters 15 and 16, intracellular tumor markers are very useful in our understanding of the critical alterations that give rise to the neoplastic cell. However, a number of these changes have found usefulness in cytological and histological diagnoses, and materials secreted or released from neoplastic cells have been measured in blood, urine, cerebrospinal fluid, etc. It is the diagnostic, prognostic, and screening usefulness of tumor markers that are considered here.

Tumor Markers in Clinical Studies

Tumor markers useful in the diagnosis of specific neoplasms date back to the middle of the nineteenth century with the description of Bence-Jones urinary proteins as markers for multiple myeloma (cf. Virji et al., 1988). Since that time, a large number of markers have been developed

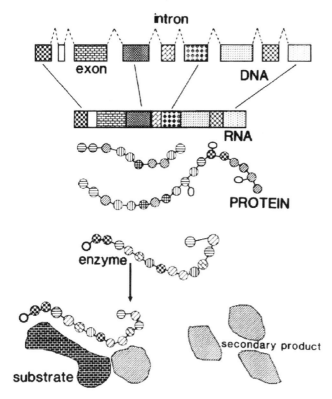

Figure 17.13   Tumor markers occur in or are produced from neoplastic cells at several levels of genetic expression. DNA-based markers may be the result of specific nucleotide alterations, sequence alterations, as well as cytogenetic changes. When transcribed, many such genomic alterations will be reflected both at the mRNA and protein level (transcription and translation). Markers at the protein and enzyme level may be detected within the cell on sample sections or within body fluids, having been released from normal or dying neoplastic cells. Low-molecular-weight products include abnormal nucleic acid bases, polyamines, amine hormones, and others. (Modified from Lehto and Pontén, 1989, with permission of the authors and publisher.)

both from experimental studies and studies directly in the human. However, only a relative few tumor markers in body fluids are generally useful for screening, diagnostic, therapeutic, and prognostic studies. Tissue markers may be more successful in the future, particularly with the advances of methodologies allowing for the identification of mutational, cytogenetic, mRNA, and protein markers within tissue sections.

The important criteria for the usefulness of a tumor marker are its sensitivity and specificity with respect to identifying the neoplastic cell in which or from which the marker arose. A sensitive marker detects a high percentage of patients with the disease, while a specific marker is present only in cancer patients and not in those without cancer (Magdelénat, 1992). Table 17.9 shows an outline and definition of sensitivity and specificity as predictive values in neoplasia. The values in Table 17.9 are linked to both sensitivity and specificity, but also to the prevalence (P) or incidence of the disease in the population studied. Knowing this latter parameter and calculating sensitivity and specificity, one may obtain a "positive predictive value" as shown in the following equation:

Table 17.9   Sensitivity and Specificity as Values Predictive of Neoplasia

		Cancer	No Cancer	
Marker	Positive	TP	FP	Positive predictive value
	Negative	FN	TN	Negative predictive value
	Sensitivity = TP/TP + FN	Specificity = TN/TN + FP		

Key: TP, true positive or patients having cancer; FP, false positive or patients expressing the marker but not having cancer; FN, false negative or patients not expressing the marker but having cancer; TN, true negative, patients not expressing the marker and not having cancer.
Adapted from Magdelénat, 1992, with permission of the author and publisher.

$$\text{Positive predictive value} = \frac{(S) \times (P)}{(S)(P) + (1 - Sp)(1 - P)}$$

where S equals sensitivity, Sp equals specificity and P equals prevalence. The positive predictive value is extremely useful in screening large groups of patients for the purpose of monitoring the presence of neoplasia at an early time point when the disease is most treatable (cf. Nielsen and Lang, 1999). An example of using this information to determine the predictive value in screening for ovarian cancer with a specific tumor marker, CA 125, a serum protein, may be seen in Table 17.10. As noted in the table, screening in the general population gives a very high predictive value far in excess of the actual prevalence. However, by screening only women with pelvic masses, the number of false positives can be dramatically reduced.

In order to screen large populations effectively for a neoplasm, a very high degree of specificity (greater than 95%) and good sensitivity would be required considering the relatively low

Table 17.10   Results of Screening for Ovarian Cancer with the Tumor Marker CA 125 in Several Different Populations of Women

Screening in the general population (20 to 40 cases of ovarian cancer/100,000 persons)
Sensitivity = 80%
Specificity = 99% in a healthy population
Prevalence = 30/100,000 = 0.0003

$$\text{Positive predictive value} = \frac{(0.80)(0.0003)}{(0.80)(0.0003) + (1 - 0.99)(1 - 0.0003)} = 0.023 \, (2.3\%)$$

Screening in American women with pelvic masses
Sensitivity = 80%
Specificity = 78%
Prevalence = 18/182 = 0.0989

$$\text{Positive predictive value} = \frac{(0.80)(0.0989)}{(0.80)(0.0989) + (1 - 0.78)(1 - 0.0989)} = 0.285 \, (28.5\%)$$

Screening in Scandinavian women with pelvic masses
Sensitivity = 87%
Specificity = 88%
Prevalence = 91/184 = 0.5

$$\text{Positive predictive value} = \frac{(0.87)(0.5)}{(0.87)(0.5) + (1 - 0.88)(1 - 0.5)} = 0.88 \, (88\%)$$

Adapted from Bates, 1991, with permission of the author and publisher.

prevalence of the neoplasm in the general population, as noted above. In fact, a simple calculation shows that in ideal conditions (1% incidence of the disease, 99% sensitivity and specificity), the frequency of false positives would be in the neighborhood of 50% (Magdelénat, 1992). Perhaps the best example where screening for a specific tumor marker has had a major impact in mortality reduction is the assay of human chorionic gonadotropin (HCG) in choriocarcinoma. The relatively high incidence of the neoplasm (5% to 10%) in women who have had an hydatiform mole, together with the excellent sensitivity and specificity of the assay and the high chemosensitivity of the neoplasm, has resulted in the combination of these factors leading to excellent detection and care of patients with this neoplasm.

One may also look at this problem in another way, as seen in Figure 17.14. In this instance, if one assumes a bell-shaped curve of the distribution of marker values for diseased and nondiseased individuals with a slight overlap as shown in the figure, one may calculate a "cutoff" value beyond which one considers marker values under the curve (3,4) as positive. However, in selecting such a value, one must take into account a number of other factors such as (1) the risk of complications associated with the screening test, (2) the dollar cost of the screening test and subsequent cost for further testing, (3) the subject's anxiety as well as anticipated medical and economic burdens, and (4) the social and public health impact of either missing positive cases or identifying truly nondiseased patients as being diseased (Makuch and Muenz, 1987). These are questions involving the "risk/benefit" ratio, discussed in Chapter 13 but in a different context.

A major use of several tumor markers is in following the course of the disease after therapy. As long as the neoplasm is present in substantial amount in the organism, the marker will also, of course, be present in the tissue but also in secreted markers or those released by the neoplasm into body fluids. On removal of the neoplasm, if almost all or all of the neoplastic tissue has been surgically excised, the level of the marker will fall to near normal or normal levels. If there is regrowth of the primary or metastatic lesions of the neoplasm, in almost all instances the level of the marker itself will also increase and indicate to the clinician that significant neoplastic growth is occurring. A diagram of what might be expected in the circumstance of primary therapy with remission following recurrence in relation both to tumor burden and expression of the tumor marker is seen in Figure 17.15. As noted from the figure, the appearance of the marker in most instances usually occurs after significant growth of the neoplasm has oc-

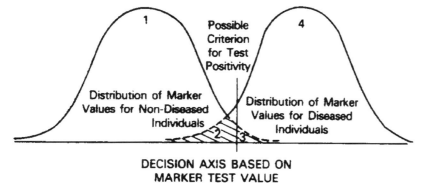

Figure 17.14 Potential outcomes in classifying patients into one group or another based on the true distribution of tumor marker values in two distinct populations: (1) true negatives; (2) false negatives; (3) false positives; (4) true positives. (Adapted from Makuch and Muenz, 1987, with permission of the authors and publisher.)

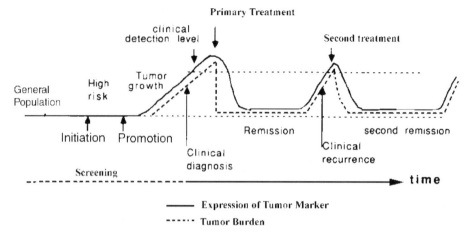

Figure 17.15 Graphical relationships of marker expression in the serum and tumor growth or burden. Note that there is a direct parallel between the level of expression of the marker and the tumor burden, although in primary treatment, which many times is surgical, there is a very abrupt drop in tumor burden because of removal of the neoplasm, whereas secondary treatment may be chemotherapy and/or radiation leading to a somewhat slower loss of tumor burden. Regrowth of the neoplasm a second time usually causes demise of the patient. (Adapted from Magdelénat, 1992, with permission of the author and publisher.)

curred. Following primary therapy with excision and/or destruction of the vast majority of neoplastic cells, the level of the marker decreases in accord with the loss of the tumor burden. Serum markers decrease dramatically following the removal of the neoplasm, usually with half-lives of less than 1 week (cf. Duffy, 1996; Takashi et al., 1989). If the neoplasm is not completely removed, some low level of the marker will remain in body fluids and then increase again as the residual neoplasm grows, as noted in the figure. In this way, the clinician may monitor the effectiveness of therapy as well as recurrence of the neoplasm.

As Virji et al. (1988) have pointed out, to date no tumor marker has been shown to be specific or sufficiently sensitive to be used in the detection and screening of neoplasms in the general population. However, some years ago, Weber (1982) proposed a list of characteristics for detecting and utilizing biological markers in monitoring human neoplastic disease (Table 17.11). The table includes not only screening and diagnosis but also the following therapy by using a tumor marker, as discussed below. With the ready availability of biopsy material from a variety of neoplasms, which in the past could not be had, an additional requirement would be its detection in tissue sections and samples of the neoplasm itself. The rather arbitrary upper limit of 200 million cells for detection does not indicate a lower limit. Utilizing tissue sections and modern methodologies (see below), it is now possible to detect markers in only a few cells or in extremely low concentrations in body fluids. Recently, Hayes et al. (1996) have proposed a tumor marker utility grading system (TMUGS) for the evaluation of the clinical utility of tumor markers and the establishment of an investigational program for evaluation of new tumor markers.

Tumor Markers of Carcinogenesis and Carcinogen Exposure

In addition to the use of markers for the detection, diagnosis, therapeutic efficacy, and prognosis of neoplasms within organisms, markers have also been utilized to monitor both experimental

Table 17.11 Requirements for Biological Markers for the Detection and Monitoring of Human Neoplastic Disease

1. Specificity for neoplasia
2. Specificity for tumor type
3. Should indicate cancer cells in patient before they are clinically evident
4. Should indicate extent of tumor burden
5. Should be a sensitive indicator of success of anticancer treatment
6. Should signal presence of micrometastatic lesions
7. Should indicate recurrence of neoplasia
8. Should be detectable in blood, urine, and tissues
9. Simplicity and low cost of test
10. Assay should be sensitive to detect less than 200 million cells

animals and human populations for their exposure to a variety of environmental carcinogens. This general field, when applied to humans, has come to be known as *molecular epidemiology*. In some publications, this terminology has been relatively global, including not only markers resulting from environmental exposures but also markers of genetic predisposition to neoplasia, some of which were considered in Chapter 5 (Perera, 1996). Some of the markers that have been utilized, as well as an indication of their sensitivity and specificity, may be seen in Table 17.12. The determination of urinary 8-hydroxy-2′-deoxyguanosine is utilized as a biological marker of in vivo oxidative DNA damage (Shigenaga et al., 1989). Metabolites of carcinogens, particularly aflatoxin, have also been useful in monitoring exposure of patients to this carcinogen (cf.

Table 17.12 Some Commonly Utilized Molecular Epidemiology Markers[a]

Marker	Methodology	Sensitivity	Specificity	T. Comp.
Urinary aflatoxin metabolites	HPLC/fluorescence Immunoaffinity chromatography	+	+++	+
Urinary 3-methyladenine	GCMS	+	++	++
Urinary nitrosoproline	HPLC	+	++	+
Urinary 8-hydroxyguanosine	HPLC	++	−	+
Hemoglobin alkylation	GCMS	+	++	++
DNA adducts	HPLC/GCMS	++	+++	+++
	ELISA	+	+	+
	[32]P postlabeling	+++	−	+++
Protein adducts	HPLC/GCMS	++	+++	+++
HPRT mutation	In vitro cell viability	−	−	+
Glycophorin-A mutation	flow cytometry	−	−	+
Oncogene mutations	PCR	+++	+	+++
Tumor suppressor gene mutations	PCR	+++	−	+++

Key: −, low; +, medium; ++, high; +++, very high. T. Comp., technical complexity; HPLC, high-pressure liquid chromatography; GCMS, gas chromatography—mass spectroscopy; PCR, polymerase chain reaction.
[a]*Sensitivity* refers to the level of exposure inducing the biomarker modification (low sensitivity, high exposure needed). *Specificity* attests to the rate of false positives and principally the ability of the test to indicate the involvement of specific carcinogens.
Adapted from Izzotti et al., 1997.

Wogan, 1992). Adducts of hemoglobin by several different chemical carcinogens, including aflatoxin and polycyclic hydrocarbons as well as aromatic amine carcinogens in smokers, have also been used as a form of molecular dosimetry to chemical carcinogens in humans (Skipper and Tannenbaum, 1990). Measurement of the levels of DNA adducts by the techniques described by a number of workers includes studies both in experimental animals and in humans (La and Swenberg, 1996; Poirier and Weston, 1996). Such measurements may be used not only as dosimetry studies of exposure but also studies on the effects of preventive environmental factors on the presence of such adducts in blood cells in vivo (Peluso et al., 2000). Bhatnagar and Talaska (1999) have presented a provocative model of expected cancer rate, exposure history, and biomarker levels in workers exposed to a specific carcinogen during this century (Figure 17.16). In the model, one can see the potential "latent" period followed by an increase in risk, which then tapers off after cessation of exposure. Such a model could certainly explain a variety of different exposures, especially in the nineteenth century, to various chemical carcinogens. Recently, Bartsch (2000) reviewed studies on biomarkers in cancer etiology and prevention over the last two decades, indicating the potential usefulness of such markers in programs and trials of cancer prevention.

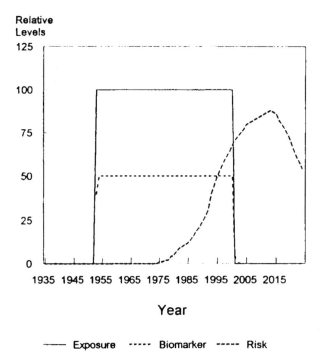

Figure 17.16 A model of expected cancer rate, exposure history, and biomarker levels of workers born in 1935 and beginning work with exposure to a carcinogen at age 18. The biomarker levels shown would be consistent with a steady 8 hours per day, 5 days per week exposure and a biomarker with a 120-day half-life. In this model the risk or cancer rate is based on recent age-specific lung cancer rates in the United States. Note that the biomarker for exposure is present basically only during the period that the worker is exposed because of the relatively brief half-life. (Adapted from Bhatnagar and Talaska, 1999, with permission of the authors and publisher.)

Tumor Markers in Human Neoplastic Disease

The number of tumor markers that could be utilized in some experimental or human situation is extremely large, but to date only a relatively small number have been used in screening, detection, and diagnosis, prognosis, and follow-up of human neoplastic disease. Table 17.13 provides a listing of a variety of markers that are utilized for any one of these parameters in specific human neoplasms. One of the first generally accepted markers was originally recognized by Gold and Freedman (1965) as a glycoprotein, which they termed carcinoembryonic antigen (CEA). They found that it was produced in large quantities in the large bowel and initially was felt to be relatively specific for that lesion (cf. Moertel et al., 1993). Even some patients with colonic polyps had elevated CEA levels (Doos et al., 1975). It is now apparent that a large number of neoplasms and even normal tissues produce varying amounts of CEA. Furthermore, CEA is a family of proteins that are normally found at high levels in fetal gut and appear to be involved in intercellular adhesion (Benchimol et al., 1989) as well as signal transduction (Dráber and Skubitz, 1998). Another glycoprotein is CA 125, which has been used as a marker of ovarian neoplasms, but is even more generally found in normal tissues as well as other neoplasms (cf. Jacobs and Bast, 1989).

Notice from the table that a number of markers are still in the experimental stage, and actually only those so indicated are approved by the U.S. Food and Drug Administration for use in the United States. In mesenchymal neoplasms as well as lymphomas and leukemias, it is apparent that the cytogenetic markers are primarily for diagnostic purposes. Similarly, but not shown in the table, is the use of cytoskeletal proteins as tissue markers for a variety of different types of neoplasms that aid the pathologist in specific diagnoses (Virtanen et al., 1984; Table 16.4). If one analyzes the tumor markers associated with any specific type of neoplasm, a wide variety of different markers, both in tissue and body fluid, may be seen. Table 17.14 presents a short list of markers found in two different types of lung cancer at two different stages (Chapter 10). However, this is only a small part of the total number of markers that have been described in human bronchogenic carcinoma (e.g., Coombes et al., 1976).

As discussed in Chapter 10 (Table 10.7), a variety of tissue markers in the form of changes in expression and mutation in proto-oncogenes and tumor suppressor genes have been utilized to make predictions about the natural history of neoplastic growth in specific individuals—i.e., the prognosis of the disease in such persons. Within the last few years, it has also been possible to detect mutations of tumor suppressor genes and proto-oncogenes in plasma DNA of cancer patients (e.g., Silva et al., 1999; Kopreski et al., 2000). In addition, antibodies to the p53 tumor suppressor protein have been found in human cancer patients with a specificity of 96% but sensitivity of 30% (Soussi, 2000). Whether such markers will be a useful adjunct to prognosis, detection, or therapy still remains to be seen.

One of the most frequently utilized tumor markers at the present time is the prostate-specific antigen (PSA). This protein is a glycoprotein with a molecular mass of 33 to 34 kDa existing in at least five isomers. It is a serine protease capable of catalyzing the hydrolysis of a variety of proteins. PSA is not synthesized exclusively by the prostate, since both normal tissues (breast and endometrium) as well as nonprostatic neoplasms (breast, and salivary glands) also secrete this material into the serum (cf. Duffy, 1996). In men, the normal serum PSA values increase with age (DeAntoni, 1997). PSA concentrations in black men are significantly higher than those in whites (Morgan et al., 1996), leading to a differential discrimination in prostate cancer diagnosis between these two races based on PSA concentrations. Recently, it has been noted that PSA in the serum is predominantly bound to α-1-antichymotrypsin (PSA-ACT) with a smaller percentage bound to a macroglobulin. Recent studies have suggested that measurement

Table 17.13 The Use of Tumor Markers in Monitoring Parameters in Human Neoplasia

Disease	Marker	Screening	Detection and Diagnosis	Staging and Prognosis	Follow-Up	Marker Still at Experimental Stage
Colon cancer	Carcinoembryonic antigen		(X)[a]	X[a]		
Breast cancer	Estrogen receptor			X[a]		X
	CA15.3			X	X	X
	CA27.29					X
	Her-2/neu			X		X
Hepatocellular carcinoma	α Fetoprotein		X[a]		X[a]	
Prostate cancer	Prostate specific antigen	(X)[a]			X[a]	
	Prostatic acid phosphatase			X[a]	X[a]	
Ovarian cancer	CA125		X		X	
	CA19.9 (CA74.2)					X
Thyroid cancer	Thyroglobulin		X		X	
	Calcitonin		X		X	
Testicular cancer	Human chorionic gonadotropin		X[a]		X[a]	
	α Fetoprotein		X[a]		X[a]	
Sarcoma:						
Synovial sarcoma	t(X;18)		X		X	
Ewing sarcoma	t(11;22)		X			
Alveolar rhabdomyo-sarcoma	t(2;13)		X			

Tumor/Disease	Marker		
Granulocytic sarcoma	t(9;11)	X	X
Myxoid liposarcoma	t(12;16)	X	X
Round cell liposarcoma	t(12;16)	X	X
Congenital fibrosarcoma	t(2;15)	X	X
Clear cell sarcoma	t(12;22)	X	X
Dermatofibrosarcoma protuberans	t(17;22)	X	X
Melanoma	Tyrosinase	X	
Adrenal carcinoma	Steroids	X	
	Catecholamines	X	
Lymphoma	t(8;14)	X	X
	t(11;14)	X	X
	t(2;5)	X	X
	t(3;14)	X	X
	sCD25		X
	sCD44		X
Leukemia	Numerous cytogenetic alterations	X	X
	Terminal transferase	X[a]	X[a]

[a]Approved for use in the United States.
Modified from Lindblom and Liljegren, 2000, with permission of the authors and publisher.

Table 17.14 Serum Biomarkers in Lung Cancer

Marker	Non-Small-Cell Lung Cancer (Approximate % Elevated)		Small-Cell Lung Cancer (Approximate % Elevated)		Comment
	Local-Regional	Metastatic	Limited	Extensive	
CEA	20–45	30–65	0–38	40–65	Marked elevations usually associated with metastatic disease in SCLC and NSCLC
CA-125	15–35	35–75	20–30	60	May help predict resectability in NSCLC
SCC Ag	15–35	15–35	5–10	5–10	Frequency of elevation not significantly higher in disseminated than in localized disease
TPA	20–35	50–75	40–50	40–50	Abnormal pretreatment TPA value heralds an adverse prognosis within all stage groupings
AGP	NR	NR	80–90	80–90	Elevated in vast majority of SCLC independent of stage
NSE	0–10	10–20	30–40	70–85	Powerful prognostic variable in SCLC
CK BB	NR	NR	Rare	25–35	Marked elevation in SCLC predicts poor response to chemotherapy
ChrA	0–10	10–20	50	70	Elevations in SCLC predict response to chemotherapy
CA 19–9	50–55	45–55	35–50	45–55	Limited data available in lung cancer

CEA, carcinoembryonic antigen; CA-125, cancer antigen 125; SCC Ag, squamous cell carcinoma antigen; TPA, tissue polypeptide antigen; AGP, alpha-1-acid glycoprotein; NSE, neuron-specific enolase; CK BB, BB isoenzyme of creatine kinase; ChrA, chromogranin A; CA 19-9, cancer antigen 19-9.
Adapted from Strauss and Skarin, 1994.

of PSA not bound to protein may increase the sensitivity of the test (Potter et al., 1999). While the sensitivity of the assay, especially if free PSA is taken into account, may reach 100%, the specificity of the assay ranges from 20% to 95% in a variety of series (Potter et al., 1999). In Figure 17.17 may be noted serum PSA levels in healthy controls as well as a variety of conditions in which one might expect to see an increase in the marker. While patients with prostate cancer exhibit a very high median level, the overlap with patients having the benign condition, benign prostatic hyperplasia (BPH)—as well as with other genitourinary cancers or diseases in patients who had undergone prostatectomy—is still exhibiting some overlap. It is possible that the analysis of free PSA may tighten these numbers so there will be much less overlap, increasing the sensitivity of the assay. Despite these shortcomings, this tumor marker is being utilized for screening and monitoring of men over 50 years of age together with a measurement of other clinical parameters.

Thus, it is apparent that tumor markers have some usefulness in certain neoplasms, especially in the diagnosis of mesenchymal neoplasms and the usefulness of PSA in monitoring the presence of prostatic carcinoma. Like so much in cancer research, the potential for

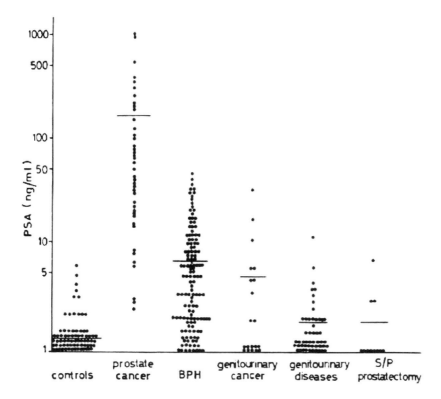

Figure 17.17   Serum PSA levels in healthy male controls, patients with prostate cancer, patients with benign prostatic hyperplasia (BPH), patients with other genitourinary cancers or diseases, and patients who had undergone prostatectomy. The individual dots each represent a single patient and the horizontal line show the mean PSA levels for each group. (Adapted from Barak et al., 1989, with permission of the authors and publisher.)

the usefulness of these markers, many of which contribute to the host-tumor relationship, is as yet unfulfilled.

REFERENCES

Abramson, E. C., Garjardo, H., and Kukreja, S. C. Hypocalcemia in cancer. Bone Miner., *10*:161–169, 1990.

Alexander, H. R., and Norton, J. A. Pathophysiology of cancer cachexia. *In*: D. Doyle, G. Hanks, and M. MacDonald (Eds.), Oxford Textbook of Palliative Medicine, Chap. 4.3.5, pp. 316–329. Oxford, UK: Oxford University Press, 1993.

Baker, S. J., and Reddy, E. P. Transducers of life and death: TNF receptor superfamily and associated proteins. Oncogene, *12*:1–9, 1996.

Balducci, L., and Hardy, C. Cancer and malnutrition—a critical interaction. Am. J. Hematol., *18*:91–103, 1985.

Barak, M., Mecz, Y., Lurie, A., and Gruener, N. Evaluation of prostate-specific antigen as a marker for adenocarcinoma of the prostate. J. Lab. Clin. Med., *113*:598–603, 1989.

Bartsch, H. Studies on biomarkers in cancer etiology and prevention: a summary and challenge of 20 years of interdisciplinary research. Mutat. Res., *462*:255–279, 2000.

Bates, S. E. Clinical applications of serum tumor markers. Ann. Intern. Med., *115*:623–638, 1991.

Bazzoni, F., and Beutler, B. The tumor necrosis factor ligand and receptor families. N. Engl. J. Med., *334*:1717–1725, 1996.

Beck, S. A., and Tisdale, M. J. Effect of insulin on weight loss and tumour growth in a cachexia model. Br. J. Cancer, *59*:677–681, 1989a.

Beck, S. A., and Tisdale, M. J. Nitrogen excretion in cancer cachexia and its modification by a high fat diet in mice. Cancer Res., *49*:3800–3804, 1989b.

Beck, S. A., Smith, K. L., and Tisdale, M. J. Anticachectic and antitumor effect of eicosapentaenoic acid and its effect on protein turnover. Cancer Res., *51*:6089–6093, 1991.

Benchimol, S., Fuks, A., Jothy, S., Beauchemin, N., Shirota, K., and Stanners, C. P. Carcinoembryonic antigen, a human tumor marker, functions as an intercellular adhesion molecule. Cell, *57*:327–334, 1989.

Beyaert, R., and Fiers, W. Tumor necrosis factor and lymphotoxin. *In*: A. Mire-Sluis and R. Thorpe (Eds.), Cytokines, pp. 335–360. San Diego, CA: Academic Press, 1998.

Bhatnagar, V. K., and Talaska, G. Carcinogen exposure and effect biomarkers. Toxicol. Lett., *108*:107–116, 1999.

Boussiotis, V. A., Nadler, L. M., Strominger, J. L., and Goldfeld, A. E. Tumor necrosis factor α is an autocrine growth factor for normal human B cells. Proc. Natl. Acad. Sci. U.S.A., *91*:7007–7011, 1994.

Bozzetti, F., Pagnoni, A. M., and DelVecchia, M. Excessive caloric expenditure as a cause of malnutrition in patients with cancer. Surg. Gynecol. Obstet, *150*:229–234, 1980.

Brennan, M. F., and Burt, M. E. Nitrogen metabolism in cancer patients. Cancer Treat. Rep., *65*(Suppl. 5):67–78, 1981.

Broadus, A. E., Mangin, M., Ikeda, K., Insogna, K. L., Weir, E. C., Burtis, W. J., and Stewart, A. F. Humoral hypercalcemia of cancer. Identification of a novel parathyroid hormone-like peptide. N. Engl. J. Med., *319*:556–563, 1988.

Burtis, W. J. Parathyroid hormone-related protein: structure, function, and measurement. Clin. Chem., *38*:2171, 1992.

Busch, H., Fujiwara, E., and Firszt, D. C. Studies on the metabolism of radioactive albumin in tumor-bearing rats. Cancer Res., *21*:371–377, 1961.

Cahlin, C., Körner, A., Axelsson, H., Wang, W., Lundholm, K., and Svanberg, E. Experimental cancer cachexia: the role of host-derived cytokines interleukin (IL)-6, IL-12, interferon-γ, and tumor necrosis factor α evaluated in gene knockout, tumor-bearing mice on C57 Bl background and eicosanoid-dependent cachexia. Cancer Res., *60*:5488–5493, 2000.

Cangiano, C., Laviano, A., Muscaritoli, M., Meguid, M. M., Cascino, A., and Fanelli, F. R. Cancer anorexia: new pathogenic and therapeutic insights. Nutrition, *12*:S48–S51, 1996.

Carswell, E. A., Old, L. J., Kassel, R. L., Green, S., Fiore, N., and Williamson, B. An endotoxin-induced serum factor that causes necrosis of tumors. Proc. Natl. Acad. Sci. USA, *72*:3666–3670, 1975.

Chance, W. T., von Meyenfeldt, M. F., and Fischer, J. E. Changes in brain amines associated with cancer anorexia. Neurosci. Biobehav. Rev., *7*:471–479, 1983.

Chance, W. T., Zhang, F.-S., Foley-Nelson, T., and Fischer, J. E. Hyperammonemia and anorexia in Morris hepatoma-bearing rats. Physiol. Behav., *50*:397–401, 1991.

Chlebowski, R. T., and Heber, D. Metabolic abnormalities in cancer patients: carbohydrate metabolism. Surg. Clin. North Am., *66*:957–968, 1986.

Clark, R. W., and Crain, R. C. Characterization of alterations in plasma lipoprotein lipid and apoprotein profiles accompanying hepatoma-induced hyperlipidemia in rats. Cancer Res., *46*:1894–1903, 1986.

Coley, W. B. The treatment of malignant tumors by repeated inoculations of erysipelas; with a report of ten original cases. Am. J. Med. Sci., *105*:487–490, 1893.

Coombes, R. C., Ward, W. K., Greenberg, P. B., et al. Calcium metabolism in cancer: studies using calcium isotopes and immunoassay for parathyroid hormone and calcitonin. Cancer, *38*:2111–2120, 1976.

Costa, G. Cachexia, the metabolic component of neoplastic diseases. Prog. Exp. Tumor Res., *3*:321–369, 1963.

Costa, G. Cachexia, the metabolic component of neoplastic diseases. Cancer Res., *37*:2327–2335, 1977.

Costa, G., and Donaldson, S. The nutritional effects of cancer and its therapy. Nutr. Cancer, *2*:22–29, 1980.

Daneryd, P. L.-E., Hafström, L. R., and Karlberg, I. H. Effects of spontaneous physical exercise on experimental cancer anorexia and cachexia. Eur. J. Cancer, 26:1083–1088, 1990.

Davies, M., Hayes, M. E., Yin, J. A. L., Berry, J. L., and Mawer, E. B. Abnormal synthesis of 1,25-dihydroxyvitamin D in patients with malignant lymphoma. J. Clin. Endocrinol. Metab., 78:1202–1207, 1994.

DeAntoni, E. P. Age-specific reference ranges for PSA in the detection of prostate cancer. Oncology, 11:475–489, 1997.

de Blaauw, I., Deutz, N. E. P., and von Meyenfeldt, M. F. Metabolic changes in cancer cachexia—first of two parts. Clin. Nutr., 16:169–176, 1997.

Deuster, P. A., Morrison, S. D., and Ahrens, R. A. Endurance exercise modifies cachexia of tumor growth in rats. Med. Sci. Sports Exerc., 17:385–392, 1985.

Doos, W. G., Wolff, W. I., Shinya, H., DeChabon, A., Stenger, R. J., Gottlieb, L. S., and Zamcheck, N. CEA levels in patients with colorectal polyps. Cancer, 36:1996–2003, 1975.

Dráber, P., and Skubitz, K. M. Signal transduction mediated by the CEA family. In: C. P. Stanners (Ed.), Cell Adhesion and Communication Mediated by the CEA Family: Basic and Clinical Perspectives, pp. 121–140. Amsterdam: Harwood, 1998.

Duffy, M. J. PSA as a marker for prostate cancer: a critical review. Ann. Clin. Biochem., 33:511–519, 1996.

Emery, P. W., Edwards, R. H., Rennie, M. J., Souhami, R. L., and Halliday, D. Protein synthesis in muscle measured in vivo in cachectic patients with cancer. Br. Med. J. Clin. Res., 289:584–586, 1984.

Ertl, H. A contribution to the clarification of the relation between tumor cachexia and thymus involution. Oncology, 26:329–334, 1972.

Fujiki, H., and Suganuma, M. Tumor necrosis factor-α, a new tumor promoter, engendered by biochemical studies of okadaic acid. J. Biochem., 115:1–5, 1994.

Glover, D. J., and Glick, J. H. Metabolic oncologic emergencies. CA, 37:302–320, 1987.

Gold, P., and Freedman, S. O. Demonstrations of tumor specific antigens in human colonic carcinomata by immunologic tolerance and absorption techniques. J. Exp. Med., 121:439–462, 1965.

Goodlad, G. A. J. Protein metabolism and tumor growth. In: H. N. Munro and J. B. Allison (Eds.), Mammalian Protein Metabolism, Vol. 2, pp. 415–444. New York: Academic Press, 1964.

Greenstein, J. P. Biochemistry of Cancer. New York: Academic Press, 1958.

Groopman, J. E. Fatigue in cancer and HIV/AIDS. Oncology, 12:335–351, 1998.

Grosvenor, M., Bulcavage, L., and Chlebowski, R. T. Symptoms potentially influencing weight loss in a cancer population. Cancer, 63:330–334, 1989.

Gruss, H.-J. Molecular, structural, and biological characteristics of the tumor necrosis factor ligand superfamily. Int. J. Clin. Lab. Res., 26:143–159, 1996.

Gutierrez, G. E., Poser, J. W., Katz, M. S., Yates, A. J. P., Henry, H. L., and Mundy, G. R. Mechanisms of hypercalcaemia of malignancy. Baillière's Clin. Endocrinol. Metab., 4:119–138, 1990.

Hayes, D. F., Bast, R. C., Desch, C. E., Fritsche, H., Jr., Kemeny, N. E., Jessup, J. M., Locker, G. Y., Macdonald, J. S., Mennel, R. G., Norton, L., Ravdin, P., Taube, S., and Winn, R. J. Tumor marker utility grading system: a framework to evaluate clinical utility of tumor markers. J. Natl. Cancer Inst., 88:1456–1466, 1996.

Holroyde, C. P., and Reichard, G. A. Carbohydrate metabolism in cancer cachexia. Cancer Treat. Rep., 65(Suppl. 5):55–59, 1981.

Hulsewé, K. W. E., Deutz, N. E. P., de Blaauw, I., van der Hulst, R. R. W. J., von Meyenfeldt, M. M. F., and Soeters, P. B. Liver protein and glutamine metabolism during cachexia. Proc. Nutr. Soc., 56:801–806, 1997.

Inui, A. Cancer anorexia-cachexia syndrome: are neuropeptides the key? Cancer Res., 59:4493–4501, 1999.

Izzotti, A., Neri, M., Vecchio, D., and Puntoni, R. Molecular epidemiology in cancer research. Int. J. Oncol., 11:1053–1069, 1997.

Jacobs, I., and Bast, R. C., Jr. The CA 125 tumour-associated antigen: a review of the literature. Hum. Reprod., 4:1–12, 1989.

Jewell, W. R., and Hunter, L. The effect of adrenalectomy and high-protein diet on tumor-altered albumin metabolism. Cancer Res., 31:257–259, 1971.

Jolivet, J., Cowan, K. H., Curt, G. A., Clendeninn, N. J., and Chabner, B. A. The pharmacology and clinical use of methotrexate. N. Engl. J. Med., *309*:1094–1104, 1983.

Kopreski, M. S., Benko, F. A., Borys, D. J., Khan, A., McGarrity, T. J., and Gocke, C. D. Somatic mutation screening: identification of individuals harboring K-ras mutations with the use of plasma DNA. J. Natl. Cancer Inst., *92*:918–923, 2000.

La, D. K., and Swenberg, J. A. DNA adducts: biological markers of exposure and potential applications to risk assessment. Mutat. Res., *365*:129–146, 1996.

Langstein, H. N., and Norton, J. A. Mechanisms of cancer cachexia. Nutr. Cancer, 5:103–123, 1991.

Laviano, A., Renvyle, T., Meguid, M. M., Yang, Z.-J., Cangiano, C., and Fanelli, F. R. Relationship between interleukin-1 and cancer anorexia. Nutrition, *11*:680–683, 1995.

Laviano, A., Meguid, M. M., Yang, Z.-J., Gleason, J. R., Cangiano, C., and Fanelli, F. R. Cracking the riddle of cancer anorexia. Nutrition, *12*:706–710, 1996.

Lazarus, D. D., Destree, A. T., Mazzola, L. M., McCormack, T. A., Dick, L. R., Xu, B., Huang, J. Q., Pierce, J. W., Read, M. A., Coggins, M. B., Solomon, V., Goldberg, A. L., Brand, S. J., and Elliott, P. J. A new model of cancer cachexia: contribution of the ubiquitin-proteasome pathway. Am. J. Physiol., *277*:E332–E341, 1999.

Legaspi, A., Jeevanandam, M., Starnes, H. F. Jr., and Brenna, M. F. Whole body lipid metabolism in the cancer patient. Metabolism, *36*:958–963, 1987.

Lehto, V.-P., and Pontén, J. Tumor markers in human biopsy material. Rev. Oncol., 2:743–762, 1989.

Levin, L., and Gevers, W. Metabolic alterations in cancer. Part II. Protein and fat metabolism. S. Afr. Med. J., *59*:553–556, 1981.

Lindblom, A., and Liljegren, A. Tumour markers in malignancies. Br. Med. J., *320*:424–427, 2000.

Loprinzi, C. L., Goldberg, R. M., and Burnham, N. L. Cancer-associated anorexia and cachexia. Implications for drug therapy. Drugs, *43*:499–506, 1992.

Lorincz, A. B., Kuttner, R. E., and Brandt, M. B. Tumor response to phenylalanine-tyrosine-limited diets. J. Am. Diet. Assoc., *54*:198–205, 1969.

Ludwig, H., and Fritz, E. Anemia in cancer patients. Semin. Oncol., *25*(Suppl. 7):2–6, 1998.

Lundholm, K., Karlberg, I., and Scherstén, T. Albumin and hepatic protein synthesis in patients with early cancer. Cancer, *46*:71–76, 1980.

Luster, M. I., Simeonova, P. P., Gallucci, R., and Matheson, J. Tumor necrosis factor α and toxicology. Crit. Rev. Toxicol., *29*:491–511, 1999.

MacDonald, N., Alexander, H. R., and Bruera, E. Cachexia-anorexia-asthenia. J. Pain Symptom Management, *10*:151–155, 1995.

Magdelénat, H. Tumour markers in oncology: past, present and future. J. Immunol. Meth., *150*:133–143, 1992.

Makuch, R. W., and Muenz, L. R. Evaluating the adequacy of tumor markers to discriminate among distinct populations. Semin. Oncol., *14*:89–101, 1987.

Marks, L. J., Steinke, J., Podolsky, S., and Egdahl, R. H. Hypoglycemia associated with neoplasia. Ann. N.Y. Acad. Sci., *230*:147–160, 1974.

Martin, T. J., and Grill, V. Hypercalcemia in cancer. J. Steroid Biochem. Mol. Biol., *43*:123–129, 1992.

Mathupala, S. P., Rempel, A., and Pedersen, P. L. Glucose metabolism in cancer cells. Isolation, sequence, and activity of the promoter for type II hexokinase. J. Biol. Chem., *270*:16918–16925, 1995.

Matthys, P., and Billiau, A. Cytokines and cachexia. Nutrition, *13*:763–770, 1997.

McAndrew, P. F. Fat metabolism and cancer. Surg. Clin. North Am., *66*:1003–1012, 1986.

McDevitt, T. M., and Tisdale, M. J. Tumour-associated hypoglycaemia in a murine cachexia model. Br. J. Cancer, *66*:815–820, 1992.

Mider, G. B., Tesluk, J., and Morton, J. J. Effects of Walker carcinoma 256 on food intake, body weight, and nitrogen metabolism of growing rats. Acta Unio Int. Contra Cancrum., *6*:409–415, 1948.

Mills, B. J., Broghamer, W. L., Higgins, P. J., and Lindeman, R. D. Inhibition of tumor growth by zinc depletion of rats. J. Nutr., *114*:746–752, 1984a.

Mills, B. J., Broghamer, W. L., Higgins, P. J., and Lindeman, R. D. Inhibition of tumor growth by magnesium depletion of rats. J. Nutr., *114*:739–745, 1984b.

Mizuno, D. Significance of endogenous production of TNF. *In*: T. Osawa and B. Bonavida (Eds.), Tumor Necrosis Factor: Structure-Function Relationship and Clinical Application, pp. 1–24. Basel: Karger, 1992.

Moertel, C. G., Fleming, T. R., Macdonald, J. S., Haller, D. G., Laurie, J. A., and Tangen, C. An evaluation of the carcinoembryonic antigen (CEA) test for monitoring patients with resected colon cancer. J.A.M.A., *270*:943–947, 1993.

Moley, J. F., Morrison, S. D., and Norton, J. A. Insulin reversal of cancer cachexia in rats. Cancer Res., *45*:4925–4931, 1985.

Moley, J. F., Aamodt, R., Rumble, W., Kaye, W., and Norton, J. A. Body cell mass in cancer bearing and anorexia patients. J. Parenter. Enter. Nutr., *11*:219–222, 1987.

Morgan, T. O., Jacobsen, S. J., McCarthy, W. F., Jacobson, D. J., McLeod, D. G., and Moul, J. W. Age-specific reference ranges for serum prostate-specific antigen in black men. N. Engl. J. Med., *335*:304–310, 1996.

Muggia, F. M. Overview of cancer-related hypercalcemia: epidemiology and etiology. Semin. Oncol., *17*:3–9, 1990.

Mundy, G. R. Hypercalcemic factors other than parathyroid hormone-related protein. Endocrinol. Metab. Clin. North Am., *18*:795–806, 1989.

Muscaritoli, M., Meguid, M. M., Beverly, J. L., Yang, Z.-J., Cangiano, C., and Rossi-Fanelli, F. Mechanism of early tumor anorexia. J. Surg. Res., *60*:389–397, 1996.

Nakahara, W., and Fukuoka, F. A. The newer concept of cancer toxin. Adv. Cancer Res., *5*:157–177, 1958.

Nielsen, C., and Lang, R. S. Principles of screening. Med. Clin. North Am., *6*:1323–1337, 1999.

Nixon, D. W., Heymsfield, S. B., Cohen, A. E., Kutner, M. H., Ansley, J., Lawson, D. H., and Rudman, D. Protein-calorie undernutrition in hospitalized cancer patients. Am. J. Med., *68*:683–690, 1980.

Noguchi, Y., Vydelingum, N. A., Conlon, K. C., and Brenna, M. F. Hypertriglyceridemia in the tumor bearing state is associated with decreased hepatic malic enzyme activity. Surg. Forum, *39*:462–463, 1988.

Noguchi, Y., Vydelingum, N. A., Younes, R. N., Fried, S. K., and Brennan, M. F. Tumor-induced alterations in tissue lipoprotein lipase activity and mRNA levels. Cancer Res., *51*:863–869, 1991.

Nowrousian, M. R., Kasper, C., Oberhoff, C., et al. Pathophysiology of cancer-related anemia. *In*: J. F. Smyth, M. A. Boogaerts, and B.R.-M. Ehmer (Eds.), Erythropoietin in Cancer Supportive Treatment, pp. 13–34. New York: Marcel Dekker, 1996.

Nussbaum, S. R., Gaz, R. D., and Arnold, A. Hypercalcemia and ectopic secretion of parathyroid hormone by an ovarian carcinoma with rearrangement of the gene for parathyroid hormone. N. Engl. J. Med., *323*:1324–1329, 1990.

O'Keefe, S. J. D., Ogden, J., Ramjee, G., and Rund, J. Contribution of elevated protein turnover and anorexia to cachexia in patients with hepatocellular carcinoma. Cancer Res., *50*:1226–1230, 1990.

Oliff, A., Defeo-Jones, D., Boyer, M., Martinez, D., Kiefer, D., Vuocolo, G., Wolfe, A., and Socher, S. H. Tumors secreting human TNF/cachectin induce cachexia in mice. Cell, *50*:555–563, 1987.

Ove, P., Coetzee, M. L., Chen, J., and Morris, H. P. Differences in synthesis and degradation of serum proteins in normal and hepatoma-bearing animals. Cancer Res., *32*:2510–2518, 1972.

Pariza, M. W., Park, Y., and Cook, M. E. Conjugated linoleic acid and the control of cancer and obesity. Toxicol. Sci., *52*(Suppl.):107–110, 1999.

Pavelić, J. Influence of fasting on tumor growth. IRCS Med. Sci., *10*:881, 1982.

Paxton, K., Ward, L. C., and Wilce, P. A. Protein synthesis in the tumour-bearing rat. Biochem. Int., *14*:1055–1063, 1987.

Peluso, M., Airoldi, L., Magagnotti, C., Fiorini, L., Munnia, A., Hautefeuille, A., Malaveille, C., and Vineis, P. White blood cell DNA adducts and fruit and vegetable consumption in bladder cancer. Carcinogenesis, *21*:183–187, 2000.

Perera, F. P. Molecular epidemiology: insights into cancer susceptibility, risk assessment, and prevention. J. Natl. Cancer Inst., *88*:496–509, 1996.

Pitot, H. C., Potter, V. R., and Morris, H. P. Metabolic adaptations in rat hepatomas. I. The effect of dietary protein on some inducible enzymes in liver and hepatoma 5123. Cancer Res., *21*:1001–1008, 1961.

Poirier, M. C., and Weston, A. Human DNA adduct measurements: state of the art. Environ. Health Perspect., *104*:883–893, 1996.

Potter, S. R., Reckwitz, T., and Partin, A. W. The use of percent free PSA for early detection of prostate cancer. J. Androl., *20*:449–453, 1999.

Prins, J. B., Walker, N. I., Winterford, C. M., and Cameron, D. P. Human adipocyte apoptosis occurs in malignancy. Biochem. Biophys. Res. Commun., *205*:625–630, 1994.

Ralston, S. H. Pathogenesis and management of cancer-associated hypercalcaemia. Cancer Surv., *21*:179–196, 1994.

Roberts, J., Holcenberg, J. S., and Dolowy, W. C. Glutaminase induced prolonged regression of established Ehrlich carcinoma. Life Sci., *10*:251–255, 1971.

Rohdenberg, G. L., Bernhard, A., and Krehbiel, O. Sugar tolerance in cancer. J.A.M.A., *72*:1528–1529, 1919.

Rosen, F., Sotobayashi, H., and Nicol, C. A. Different effects of folic acid deficiency and treatment with amethopterin on the growth of several rat tumors (abstr.). Proc. Am. Assoc. Cancer Res., *5*:54, 1964.

Rosol, T. J., and Capen, C. C. Mechanisms of cancer-induced hypercalcemia. Lab. Invest., *67*:680–702, 1992.

Roubenoff, R. Inflammatory and hormonal mediators of cachexia. J. Nutr., *127*:1014S–1016S, 1997.

Seymour, J. F. Malignancy-associated hypercalcemia. Sci. Am., *2*:48–57, 1995.

Shigenaga, M. K., Gimeno, C. J., and Ames, B. N. Urinary 8-hydroxy-2'-deoxyguanosine as a biological marker of *in vivo* oxidative DNA damage. Proc. Natl. Acad. Sci. U.S.A., *86*:9697–9701, 1989.

Sidransky, H., and Verney, E. Effect of nutritional alterations on protein synthesis in transplantable hepatomas and host livers of rats. Cancer Res., *39*:1995–2000, 1979.

Silva, J. M., Gonzalez, R., Dominguez, G., Garcia, J. M., España, P., and Bonilla, F. *TP53* gene mutations in plasma DNA of cancer patients. Genes, Chromosom. Cancer, *24*:160–161, 1999.

Skipper, P. L., and Tannenbaum, S. R. Protein adducts in the molecular dosimetry of chemical carcinogens. Carcinogenesis, *11*:507–518, 1990.

Smith, K. L., and Tisdale, M. J. Mechanism of muscle protein degradation in cancer cachexia. Br. J. Cancer, *68*:314–318, 1993.

Soussi, T. p53 antibodies in the sera of patients with various types of cancer: a review. Cancer Res., *60*:1777–1788, 2000.

Spiers, A. S. D., and Wade, H. E. Bacterial glutaminase in treatment of acute leukaemia. Br. Med. J., *1*:1317–1319, 1976.

Spivak, J. L. Cancer-related anemia: its causes and characteristics. Semin. Oncol., *21*:3–8, 1994.

Stein, T. P. Cachexia, gluconeogenesis and progressive weight loss in cancer patients. J. Theor. Biol., *73*:51–59, 1978.

Stone, P., Richards, M., and Hardy, J. Fatigue in patients with cancer. Eur. J. Cancer, *34*:1670–1676, 1998.

Strauss, G. M., and Skarin, A. T. Use of tumor markers in lung cancer. Hematol. Oncol. Clin. North Am., *8*:507–532, 1994.

Strewler, G. J. The physiology of parathyroid hormone-related protein. N. Engl. J. Med., *342*:177–185, 2000.

Svaninger, G., Bennegard, K., Ekman, L., Ternell, M., and Lundholm, K. Lack of evidence for elevated breakdown rate of skeletal muscles in weight-losing, tumor-bearing mice. J. Natl. Cancer Inst., *71*:341–346, 1983.

Takashi, M., Haimoto, H., Tanaka, J., Murase, T., and Kato, K. Evaluation of gamma-enolase as a tumor marker for renal cell carcinoma. J. Urol., *141*:830–834, 1989.

Tessitore, L., Bonelli, G., and Baccino, F. M. Early development of protein metabolic perturbations in the liver and skeletal muscle of tumour-bearing rats. Biochem. J., *241*:153–159, 1987.

Tessitore, L., Costelli, P., Bonetti, G., and Baccino, F. M. Cancer cachexia, malnutrition, and tissue protein turnover in experimental animals. Arch. Biochem. Biophys., *306*:52–58, 1993.

Tisdale, M. J. Biology of cachexia. J. Natl. Cancer Inst., *89*:1763–1773, 1997.

Tisdale, M. J., Brennan, R. A., and Fearon, K. C. Reduction of weight loss and tumour size in a cachexia model by a high fat diet. Br. J. Cancer, *56*:39–43, 1987.

Uren, J. R., and Handschumacher, R. E. Enzyme therapy. *In*: F. F. Becker (Ed.), Cancer—A Comprehensive Treatise, Vol. 5, Chap. 16, pp. 457–488. New York: Plenum Press, 1977.

van Eys, J. Nutrition and neoplasia. Nutr. Rev., *40*:353–359, 1982.

Varma, M., Torelli, G. F., Meguid, M. M., Chai, J.-K., Blaha, V., Laviano, A., and Kim, H.-J. Potential strategies for ameliorating early cancer anorexia. J. Surg. Res., *81*:69–76, 1999.

Vigano, A., Watanabe, S., and Bruera, E. Anorexia and cachexia in advanced cancer patients. Cancer Surv., *21*:99–115, 1994.

Virji, M. A., Mercer, D. W., and Herberman, R. B. Tumor markers in cancer diagnosis and prognosis. CA, *38*:104–126, 1988.

Virtanen, I., Miettinen, M., and Lehto, V.-P. Cytoskeletal proteins as tissue markers for cancer. Cancer Bull., *36*:174–178, 1984.

Wallach, D., Varfolomeev, E. E., Malinin, N. L., Goltsev, Y. V., Kovalenko, A. V., and Boldin, M. P. Tumor necrosis factor receptor and Fas signaling mechanisms. Annu. Rev. Immunol., *17*:331–367, 1999.

Warnold, I., Lundholm, K., and Schersten, T. Energy balance and body composition in cancer patients. Cancer Res., *38*:1801–1807, 1978.

Warrell, R. P. Jr. Etiology and current management of cancer-related hypercalcemia. Oncology, *6*:37–50, 1992.

Warren, S. The immediate cause of death in cancer. Am. J. Med. Sci., *184*:610, 1932.

Weber, G. Markers of malignancy in cancer cells. Proceedings of the Sixth Meeting of the European Association for Cancer Research, Budapest, October 12–15, 1981, pp. 335–341. Amsterdam: Kugler, 1982.

Weiss, D. W. Neoplastic disease and tumor immunology from the perspective of host-parasite relationships. Natl. Cancer Inst. Monogr., *44*:115–122, 1976.

Wogan, G. N. Molecular epidemiology in cancer risk assessment and prevention: recent progress and avenues for future research. Environ. Health Perspect., *98*:167–178, 1992.

Yang, Z., Costanzo, M., Golde, D. W., and Kolesnick, R. N. Tumor necrosis factor activation of the sphingomyelin pathway signals nuclear factor κB translocation in intact HL-60 cells. J. Biol. Chem., *268*:20520–20523, 1993.

Yim, G. K. W., and Lowy, M. T. Opioids, feeding, and anorexias. Fed. Proc., *43*:2893–2897, 1984.

Zucker, S., Lysik, R. M., and DiStefano, J. F. Cancer cell inhibition of erythropoiesis. J. Lab. Clin. Med., *96*:770–782, 1980.

18

The Host–Tumor Relationship—
Endocrine Factors and Stromal Reaction

As noted in the last chapter, neoplastic growth significantly alters the homeostasis of the host. The presence of the neoplasm may alter the host's nutritional status to the point of starvation, termed *cachexia* in the tumor-bearing host. The complexity of the mechanisms of tumor cachexia was emphasized, but clearly the effects of the neoplasm on the host and the relatively autonomous growth of the neoplasms are the key factors in the development of the cachexia of cancer.

Normal homeostasis is controlled in the organism by a delicate balance of multiple intercellular regulatory molecules generally known as *hormones*. This is not to say that small molecules such as glucose, nonesterified fatty acids, amino acids, and other small molecule substrates are not important in the homeostasis of the organism. However, generally speaking, the functional, trophic (replicative), and tissue-specific controlling factors that maintain organismal homeostasis are hormones. Hormones may be polypeptide in character, such as growth hormone and insulin, or of low molecular weight, such as prostaglandins and steroid hormones. Some groups of hormones have distinctive designations dependent on their function, such as cytokines (Chapter 19), interleukins (Chapter 19), growth factors (Chapter 16), and others. Still, in the general sense, these chemicals produced by specific cells and acting in an autocrine, paracrine, or endocrine manner may be considered as hormones. In previous chapters we have discussed a number of such hormones, including growth factors (Chapter 16), tumor necrosis factor alpha (Chapter 17), and the parathyroid hormone-related protein (PTHRP) (Chapter 17). Many of these and other components designated, in the general sense, as hormones are produced by a variety of cell types, whereas other polypeptides, steroids, and small molecules are produced primarily by specific cell types and have largely an endocrine function, such as growth hormone, steroid hormones, and insulin. This chapter considers the latter class both from the standpoint of the effect of such hormone production by the host on the neoplasm and the effect of the production of such hormones by neoplasms on the host.

Effects of the Endocrinology of the Host on the Neoplasm

As emphasized at the beginning of the last chapter, neoplasia must always be taken in the context of the neoplasm and the host. Since neoplastic cells must exist within the environment of the host, factors produced by the host that directly affect the neoplastic cell will obviously alter the neoplasm's growth and function. In Chapter 3 (Figure 3.19), the cybernetic relationship of endocrine glands within the mammalian organism was depicted in relation to the demonstration of the carcinogenicity of endogenous hormones (Figure 3.20). Earlier studies by Furth and associates (cf. Furth, 1961) demonstrated the inhibition of the development of mammary neoplasms in rats induced with 3-methylcholanthrene by ovariectomy and hypophysectomy shortly after administration of the carcinogen. These authors demonstrated that administration of mammotrophic pituitary polypeptide hormones for several months after surgery would allow the development of mammary neoplasms, indicating their growth responsiveness to the effects of these pituitary trophic hormones. Briand et al. (1982) carried out similar experiments but induced mammary adenocarcinomas by treatment of ovariectomized mice with progesterone or estrone. Continued treatment with the hormone resulted in mammary neoplasms, but absence of such treatment resulted in the development of very few neoplasms. However, if the animals were kept for extended periods of time (a year or more), then some neoplasms developed. Similar findings have been demonstrated experimentally with other types of neoplasms that grow only in animals possessing very high levels of circulating hormones of the type to which the cell of origin is normally responsive (cf. Clifton and Sridharan, 1975).

In a more detailed experiment, Furth and colleagues (cf. Furth, 1961) performed a variation of the experiment depicted in Figure 3.20, utilizing, as a source of hormone, functional pituitary neoplasms that could be transplanted into the host. In this instance, as outlined in Figure 18.1, a functional pituitary thyrotropin-producing neoplasm was transplanted into a rat, and the thyroid gland was sampled at various periods. Initially lesions histologically indistinguishable from neoplasms of the thyroid developed in the gland, but—as noted in the figure—surgical removal of the functional pituitary transplant resulted in complete regression of these "neoplasms." Furthermore, transplantation of these lesions into animals of the same inbred strain but with no functional pituitary thyrotropic neoplasm transplant (FPTNT) allowed for no growth. However, if the FPTNT was maintained in the host for longer periods, some neoplasms developed which on removal of the transplant did not entirely regress, although substantial regression occurred (Figure 18.1). Finally, if the thyrotropin-producing transplant was maintained sufficiently long in the host, neoplasms would develop which even in the absence of the transplant and the thyrotropic stimulus grew, could be transplanted into other animals, and metastasized. Furth termed these three "stages" in the development of completely autonomous neoplasms as *dependent*, *responsive*, and *autonomous* (Figure 18.1). The reader will immediately see the complete analogy to the stages of promotion and progression in neoplastic development. The fully dependent neoplasm is a preneoplastic lesion arising from a spontaneously initiated cell but still completely dependent on the promoter (thyrotropin). The responsive neoplasm is one with a cel-

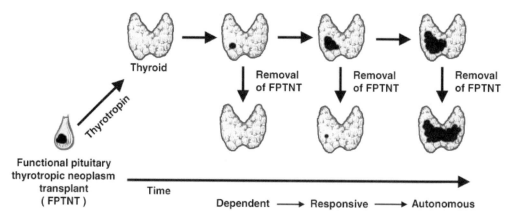

Figure 18.1 Diagram of the development of dependent, responsive, and autonomous neoplasia following chronic exposure of the thyroid in vivo to thyrotropin from a functional pituitary thyrotropic neoplasm transplant.

lular population that can survive and exist in the absence of the hormone but grows relatively slowly in the stage of progression. The completely autonomous lesion is that of the usual malignant neoplasm in the stage of progression. Theoretically, a neoplasm of any of the tissues depicted in Figure 3.19 may undergo a similar series of "stages" in the development to neoplasia. In the human there are no unequivocal examples of *dependent* neoplasms, although in one respect the placenta may be considered a dependent tumor, its maintenance dependent entirely on the "abnormal" hormonal environment of the pregnant female.

Continued proliferation of such "dependent" cells can lead to a gradual progression in proliferative vigor as a result either of environmental stimuli, of host-induced modification of cells, or of a natural selection of a more aggressive cell type, in a manner analogous to tumor progression (Chapter 9). Such neoplasms may exist in the host even in the absence of the trophic hormone or environmental stimulus, although at relatively low growth rates in many instances. Such neoplasms are termed *hormonally responsive* tumors and are exemplified by such neoplasms as carcinoma of the prostate or of the breast in the human, since castration or treatment with hormones substantially reduces the growth rate of many of these neoplasms. Less often, hormone-responsive neoplasms give rise to nonresponsive or *reversely responsive* variants—the original inhibitor becoming a stimulant of the tumor cell in the latter case (Clifton and Sridharan, 1975). Although the latter situation is rare, it may be brought about by therapy in humans and has also been shown to develop in experimental situations. This may be related to the demonstration of the development of mutations or variants in the steroid hormone receptors present within the neoplastic cell (cf. Sluyser, 1994; see below). Finally, responsive tumors may progress to an *autonomous* neoplasm, in which hormones have little if any effect on its growth rate. The natural history in humans of neoplasms of endocrine tissue is a progression from responsive to the autonomous stage.

Host Effects on Human Neoplasia

Although Furth, Clifton, and their colleagues discovered an experimental basis for hormone dependency and responsiveness of endocrine neoplasms, their work was actually anticipated by the demonstration by Beatson (1896) that surgical removal of the ovaries in patients with advanced cancer of the breast caused a slowing of growth and even regression in some cases. In 1941 Huggins and his associates (Huggins et al., 1941a,b) applied some of the principles suggested by Beatson's study to the treatment of cancer of the prostate in human males. They noted that castration and estrogen administration caused a prolongation of life in patients with prostate cancer, as well as changes and regression in the neoplastic gland itself. This led to a major area of clinical investigation involving the predictability of the hormone responsiveness of several neoplasms in the human and in animals, especially that of mammary carcinoma. The methodology involved in these studies concerns the measurement of receptor proteins in cells that interact with steroid hormones (Figures 3.23 and 3.24). A somewhat more detailed diagram of the components and action of this hormone-receptor complex may be seen in Figure 18.2. As noted in the figure, the estrogen receptor, a transcription factor (Figure 3.24) occurs in the cytoplasm in association with heat-shock proteins (hsp90) (Ylikomi et al., 1998) and immunophilin chaperones (Pratt and Toft, 1997). Binding of estrogen leads to dissociation of the heat-shock proteins, receptor dimerization with an enhancement of phosphorylation of serine 167 in the estrogen receptor protein (Castaño et al., 1998). The phosphorylated receptor dimer-ligand then enters the nucleus and, in association with several coactivators (Freedman, 1999), activates transcription of specific genes within the cell.

Those breast cancers in the human that exhibit moderate to elevated levels of the estrogen-receptor protein are usually found in more highly differentiated (lower-grade) carcinomas exhib-

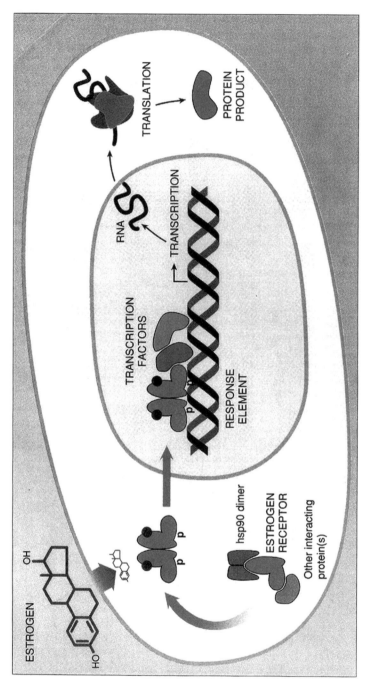

Figure 18.2 Model of estrogen action mediated by the estrogen receptor. Estrogens enter cells by simple or facilitated diffusion and then bind to specific estrogen receptors. The estrogen receptor protein exists in an inactive state in the cytoplasm in association with heat shock protein 90 immunophilins and other proteins (Pratt and Toft, 1997). Upon estrogen binding to the receptor, the receptor is freed from the other protein and undergoes phosphorylation (p) and dimerization (Castaño et al., 1998). This complex enters the nucleus and, in association with other proteins termed coactivators (Freedman, 1999), binds to specific estrogen response elements in target gene promoter regions. Transcription of the estrogen-responsive gene then occurs with subsequent translation and formation of the protein product. (Modified from Kuiper et al., 1998, with permission of the authors and publisher.)

iting a relatively slow rate of cellular replication (Martin et al., 1979). Furthermore, patients with estrogen receptor–positive breast cancers usually experience longer survival after treatment than do patients with estrogen receptor–negative neoplasms (Furmanski et al., 1980). Metastatic lesions from primary breast cancers usually exhibit a lower level of estrogen-receptor proteins than the primary lesions (Görlich and Jandrig, 1997). Interestingly, those carcinomas exhibiting Barr bodies (Chapter 10) in more than 10% of the tumor cells examined were much more likely to have high levels of the estrogen-receptor protein than those neoplasms exhibiting a lower proportion of Barr body–containing cells (Rosen et al., 1977).

Measurement of the estrogen-receptor content of mammary neoplasms has demonstrated that the absence of such receptors usually predicts a lack of response to hormone therapy, that is, a lack of hormone responsiveness (Osborne and McGuire, 1978). Unfortunately, the presence of the receptor does not assure that the neoplasm will be hormone-responsive but it does increase the chances of such an occurrence to about 1 in 2. Several studies in animals (King et al., 1976; Vignon and Rochefort, 1978) have also shown that the presence of estrogen-receptor proteins in mammary tumors does not necessarily confer an estrogen responsiveness to the growth of these neoplasms. However, the analysis of a second steroid hormone receptor, the progesterone receptor, has indicated that neoplasms exhibiting both estrogen and progesterone receptors have a relatively high degree of responsiveness, usually 70% to 80% of the cases (cf. McGuire et al., 1978). Responsiveness to endocrine therapy may occur in a variety of ways, including modification of the internal hormonal milieu of the host by surgical adrenalectomy or hypophysectomy, the administration of androgens or large doses of estrogens or, during the last two decades, administration of antiestrogens (cf. Jensen, 1981). Responsiveness to these various types of endocrine therapy as a function of the presence or absence of the estrogen and progesterone receptors is shown in Table 18.1. Interestingly, estrogen receptor–negative neoplasms are usually more responsive to cytotoxic chemotherapy in metastatic breast cancer than are neoplasms that are estrogen receptor–positive (Lippman et al., 1978). In contrast, the presence of the estrogen receptor may impart a poorer prognosis for young women with breast cancer (Aebi et al., 2000). As noted above, estrogen receptor–positive breast cancers are more often diploid than are their negative counterparts, and their proliferative activity is inversely related to the estrogen receptor content, as noted above (Raber et al., 1982). As an additional variable, estrogen receptor–negative breast cancers that do not express the epidermal growth factor receptor (EGFR) are usually more responsive to primary endocrine therapy than those expressing EGFR (cf. Robertson, 1996). Thus, in general, one may conclude that estrogen receptor–negative breast cancers are further along in the stage of progression than are estrogen receptor–positive breast cancers. While most of the epidemiological risk factors for estrogen receptor–positive and estrogen receptor–negative or –deficient breast cancers were similar, one striking difference was that the

Table 18.1 Response to Endocrine Therapy in Patients as a Function of the Presence (+) or Absence (–) of the Estrogen Receptor (ER) and Progesterone Receptor (PR)

Hormone Status	Number of Patients	Percent Responding (number)
ER+/PR+	319	68 (217)
ER–/PR+	26	42 (11)
ER+/PR–	223	32 (72)
ER–/PR–	197	9 (18)

Adapted from Sunderland and McGuire, 1991, with permission of the authors and publisher.

late age at first full-term pregnancy was a risk factor for estrogen receptor–rich breast cancer but not for estrogen receptor–poor breast cancer (McTiernan et al., 1986).

Resistance to Endocrine Therapy in Breast Cancer

While the lack of estrogen receptors would be the obvious cause for resistance to endocrine therapy, another potential mechanism is the mutational alteration in the estrogen-receptor gene that prevents the normal interaction of the hormone with its receptor. Interestingly, genetic variants in estrogen receptors have been found in normal breast tissue (Leygue et al., 1996). Many of these variants appear to be the result of various splicing differences in the formation of the messenger RNA for the receptor protein (cf. Miksicek, 1994). Although there has never been a clear association with altered estrogen receptors and the responsiveness to endocrine therapy, some preliminary data suggest that this might be true (Raam et al., 1988). There are, however, other potential changes in the cell that may lead to the resistance of the neoplastic cell to endocrine therapy, as noted in Figure 18.3. It is quite likely that the development of hormone resistance as the stage of progression continues is multifactorial, involving changes in more than one of the various potential alterations seen in Figure 18.3.

Steroid Receptors in Neoplasms Other Than Those of Mammary Origin

Steroid-receptor proteins have also been studied and found in other neoplasms (Stedman et al., 1980). A number of such examples are seen in Table 18.2. Although this table is by no means complete, it does give the reader an indication that these various receptor proteins are expressed in a wide variety of neoplasms in the human as well as some in the animals that have been studied. In the case of hepatocellular adenomas and renal neoplasms in the rat, both associated with

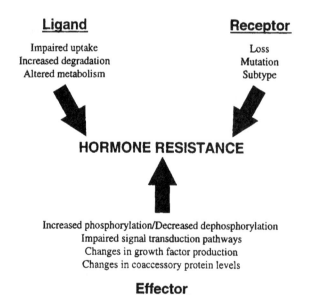

Figure 18.3 Potential multifactorial resistance to hormones of breast neoplasms. Resistance to the hormone may occur by changes at the level of the ligand, receptor, or a variety of other effectors. (Adapted from Hansen and Fuqua, 1999, with permission of the authors and publisher.)

Table 18.2   Steroid Receptor Proteins in Extramammary Neoplasms

Neoplasm	Receptor	Incidence	Reference
Human			
Chronic lymphocytic leukemia	ER	8/11	Rosen et al., 1983
Endometrial carcinoma	ER	132/154	Ingram et al., 1989
	PR	144/154	Ingram et al., 1989
Glioma	ER	3/20	Fujimoto et al., 1984
Hepatocellular carcinoma	ER	12/30	Nagasue et al., 1986
Lung cancer	ER	6/15	Beattie et al., 1985
	PR	2/15	Beattie et al., 1985
	GR	31/43	Beattie et al., 1985
	AR	21/30	Beattie et al., 1985
Melanoma	ER	61/141	Walker et al., 1987
	AR	10%–35%	cf. Walker, 1988
	GR	28%–86%	cf. Walker, 1988
Meningioma	ER	18/36	Fujimoto et al., 1984
Prostate cancer	AR	8/10	Habib et al., 1986
	ER	11%–62%	Bonkhoff et al., 1999
Renal cell carcinoma	ER	17%–31%	Karr et al., 1983
	PR	17%–29%	Karr et al., 1983
	AR	20%	Karr et al., 1983
Thyroid carcinoma	ER	32/76	Diaz et al., 1991
Animal			
Pituitary neoplasms (rat)	ER	100%	Winneker et al., 1981
Renal neoplasms (rat)	ER	100%	Anderson et al., 1979

Key: AR, androgen receptor; ER, estrogen receptor; GR, glucocorticoid receptor; PR, progesterone receptor.

estrogen administration, virtually all of these neoplasms, as might be expected, contain estrogen-receptor proteins (cf. Schmid et al., 1985; Anderson et al., 1979).

With this knowledge, it was logical to try to determine whether or not those neoplasms possessing steroid receptors might be responsive to the effects of doses of the steroid or antisteroid. There have been several attempts to treat specific neoplasms containing estrogen receptors, such as hepatocellular carcinomas and melanomas, with antiestrogens; the most successful of these have been attempts relating steroid receptor protein content with responses to antiandrogens or estrogens in prostate cancer (Sadi and Barrack, 1994) and glucocorticoid receptors to corticosteroid responses in lymphatic leukemias (cf. Homo-Delarche, 1984). However, in neither of these conditions has the determination of steroid-binding proteins been successfully related to the effectiveness of therapy to the same degree that estrogen- and progesterone-receptor content has been related to the therapy of breast cancer.

Hormonal Effects of Neoplasms on the Host

The concept that neoplasms may produce hormones and/or hormone-like substances has already been introduced. The parathyroid hormone–related protein (PTHRP, Chapter 17) that regulates calcium metabolism in peripheral tissues is an example. A number of neoplasms derived from tissues that, in the adult, normally produce this hormone have been described (Chapter 17). In addition, as pointed out below, neoplasms produce a number of as yet unidentified materials that exert significant effects on host tissues. However, the best-understood aspect of hormonal effects of neoplasms on the host involves functional neoplasms of endocrine tissues.

Effects of Functioning Neoplasms of the Endocrine System on the Host-Tumor Relationship

It has been known since the nineteenth century that neoplasms derived from endocrine tissues can retain the function of their cell of origin. However, the extent of this phenomenon was not appreciated until the last four decades. Table 18.3 is a partial list of functional neoplasms of endocrine tissues in the human. These neoplasms elaborate the hormones normally produced by their cell of origin. However, the regulation of the production of one or more hormones normally produced by that tissue is clearly aberrant in all cases, many times to such a degree that the pathophysiological changes that result from the excess hormone give rise to specific clinical findings. Therefore such neoplasms reflect the relative autonomy characteristic of all neoplasia, but this aberrant regulation is manifest not so much in growth control as in the regulation of the elaboration of their secretory products. In most instances the production of the hormone shows little or no environmental regulation by the host. On the other hand, there are now specific in-

Table 18.3   Some Functional Neoplasms of Endocrine Tissue

Neoplastic Classification	Hormones Elaborated by Tumors	Clinical Findings
Interstitial cell tumor of testis	Androgens	Masculinization
Arrhenoblastoma	Androgens	Masculinization
Granulosa-theca cell tumor of ovary	Estrogens	Feminization
Acidophilic adenoma of pituitary	Somatotrophic hormone	Pituitary gigantism or acromegaly
Chromophobe adenoma of pituitary	Thyrotropin	Hyperthyroidism
"Prolactin-cell" adenoma of pituitary	Prolactin	Amenorrhea-galactorrhea syndrome, hypogonadism
Adrenocortical adenoma	Aldosterone	Conn syndrome
Adrenocortical adenoma	Cortisone	Cushing syndrome
Pheochromocytoma	Adrenalin and/or noradrenalin	Paroxysmal hypertension
Medullary carcinoma of thyroid	Calcitonin, etc.	Dysphagia, diarrhea
Thyroid carcinoma	Thyroxine, T_3	Graves' disease (thyrotoxicosis)
Parathyroid adenoma	Parathormone	Hyperparathyroidism
Islet cell adenoma (see Figure 18.4)	Insulin	Paroxysmal hypoglycemia
	Glucagon	Migratory erythema, diabetes
	Gastrin	Zollinger-Ellison syndrome, peptic ulceration
	Somatostatin	Mild diabetes, hypochlorhydria
Renal cell carcinoma (Wilms tumor)	Erythropoietin	Polycythemia
Carcinoid	Serotonin, substance P, histamine, kallikrein	Carcinoid syndrome
Hodgkin disease	Various cytokines and growth factors	Lymphoid hyperplasia, immunosuppression, and fibrosis

stances in which such regulation still occurs to some extent, as in the production of calcitonin by medullary carcinoma of the thyroid (Deftos et al., 1971). In this example, calcitonin secretion by the tumor can be regulated by the administration of calcium, glucagon, or hypocalcemic agents. This may be the reflection of the presence of receptors in the neoplastic cell. In support of this is the fact that the responsiveness of carcinoid neoplasms to the administration of the somatostatin analog, octreotide is dependent on the presence of somatostatin receptors in the neoplasm (Kvols and Reubi, 1993).

Just as with the pancreatic islet, the anterior pituitary consists of a variety of different hormone-secreting cell populations and thus gives rise to a variety of different functional neoplasms, each producing primarily but not exclusively one of the polypeptide hormones of the pituitary. The three listed in Table 18.2 comprise the more common lesions, but in addition neoplasms producing excessive amounts of adrenocorticotropic hormones as well as various gonadotropins have been described (cf. Thapar et al., 1995). Thyrotropin-secreting pituitary adenomas have rarely been seen; the vast majority are not associated with hypersecretion of other anterior pituitary hormones (Beck-Peccoz et al., 1996). Similarly, in the adrenal cortex one finds cells producing either aldosterone, a hormone regulating potassium metabolism and blood pressure, or cortisone, the steroid hormone affecting sodium metabolism as well as gluconeogenesis (Chapter 17). Conn syndrome resulting from hyperaldosteronism is associated with hypertension and hypokalemia; Cushing syndrome is associated with hypertension, sodium retention, and a peculiar form of truncal obesity and rounded facies as well as abdominal stria. Neoplasms of the adrenal medulla are mostly pheochromocytomas that secrete excessive amounts of catecholamines, primarily adrenalin (epinephrine), noradrenalin (norepinephrine), and dopamine, resulting in frequent severe bouts of hypertension. In the thyroid, medullary carcinoma of the "C" cells (which normally produce calcitonin) results in diarrhea and dysphagia (difficulty in swallowing) when these cells produce excessive amounts of calcitonin (Cohen and Modigliani, 1993). The normal function of this hormone is to decrease levels of calcium in the blood. In contrast, as discussed in Chapter 17, parathormone, the product of the parathyroid gland, when produced in excess by parathyroid adenomas, produces excessive hypercalcemia, loss of bone, and renal kidney pathology. Carcinoid neoplasms may occur in a variety of tissues of the gastrointestinal tract and lungs developing from neuroendocrine cells in these tissues (see below). These neoplasms in their differentiated state produce excessive amounts of serotonin and other hormones, as noted, producing among other effects vasoactive changes that appear to be associated with episodic flushing, diarrhea, abdominal pain, and eventually right-sided valvular heart disease (Kulke and Mayer, 1999). An interesting functional process of neoplastic cells in Hodgkin lymphomas is their production of a variety of cytokines (Chapter 19). These hormone-like substances have a variety of effects on immune cells and, together with growth factors produced by these malignant lymphocytes, apparently produce the changes seen in this disease as noted in the table (Gruss et al., 1994; Hsu et al., 1993; Teruya-Feldstein et al., 2000).

In endocrine tissues with multiple cellular populations—such as the pituitary, adrenal, thyroid, and islets of Langerhans—separate and distinct clinical syndromes are produced, the specific kind depending on which of the cell types of the gland becomes neoplastic. The spectrum of hormones produced by the various cell types of neoplasms of the islets of Langerhans is shown in Figure 18.4 (cf. review by Friesen, 1982). The β cell classically produces insulin and presumably is the neoplastic element found in insulinomas. The δ or α_1 cell of the islet produces gastrin, and neoplasms derived from this cell are responsible for the peptic ulceration of the stomach and duodenum found in the Zollinger-Ellison syndrome. In addition, other cellular species of the islets have been found to be producers of amines and the hormone secretin. Neoplasms of the α cells may produce glucagon, giving rise to hyperglycemia. As a result, these individuals express clinical diabetes as well as a peculiar necrolytic migratory erythema appear-

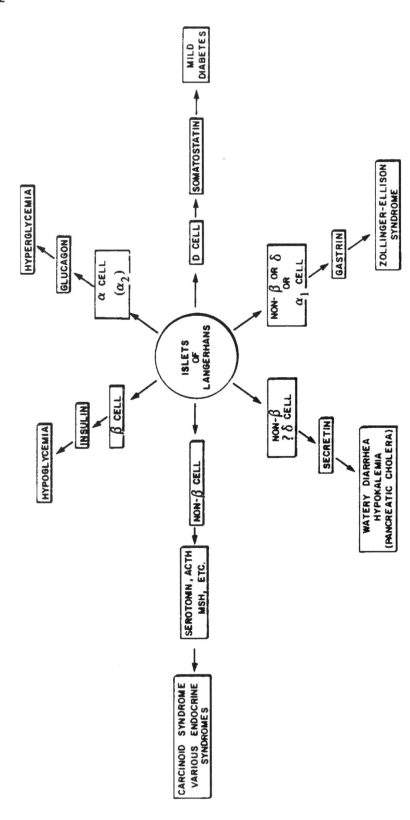

Figure 18.4 Spectrum of neoplasms derived from the islets of Langherans of the pancreas. The hormones produced by each of the neoplasms are noted, together with the syndromes resulting from excessive production of these hormones. (Modified from Schein, 1973, with permission of the author and publisher.)

ing as a skin rash–like phenomenon, with healing and reappearance (Wermers et al., 1996). Several neoplasms producing the hormone somatostatin, a polypeptide also produced in the hypothalamus (Pimstone et al., 1979), have been reported (Vinik et al., 1987). As this hormone regulates the secretion of a number of other hormones including insulin, glucagon, gastrin, and pituitary polypeptides, neoplasms of the D cell appear to result in a syndrome indistinguishable from mild diabetes. Such interrelationships of hormones have been known for some time and play a role in the pathophysiology of syndromes resulting in the excessive production of other hormones of endocrine neoplasms. Furthermore, a number of these hormones are produced in precursor forms, such as those noted in Figure 18.5. Of the pre-pro forms, only those shaded in the diagram actually are the functional components, although a number of neoplasms secrete the pro hormones, whereas their tissues of origin seldom secrete significant amounts of such structures (cf. Rehfeld et al., 1996). Since processing of the pre-pro forms of these proteins is post-translational, their secretion is a further indication of the altered regulatory mechanisms present in such neoplasms.

Another group of neoplasms of endocrine tissues that appear to be related are those of the amine precursor uptake and decarboxylation (APUD) system (cf. Baylin, 1975; Pearse, 1968). Cells of the APUD system include pancreatic islet cells, pituitary cells producing adreno-corticotropic hormone (ACTH) and melanotropin, C cells of the thyroid, gastrointestinal argentaffin cells, and adrenal medullary cells. This concept, which was first proposed by Pearse (1968), relates functional cell types to their synthesis and storage of polypeptide and amine hormones. Such cell types are thought to arise from the neural crest. A diagram of the APUD system is seen in Figure 18.6. This concept not only links various neoplasms by their embryological origin, but also accounts for the production of amine and polypeptide hormones by some neoplasms that arise in tissues where APUD cells were thought to be absent or in the minority, such as in the lung, thymus, and urogenital tract. Today the term "neuroendocrine" is used more frequently than "APUD" to characterize neoplasms that produce polypeptide hormones as well as amines in which identical or similar forms are secreted by cells of the nervous system (Capella et al., 1994). A number of members of this group produce more than a single hormone (cf. Weil, 1985).

Mechanisms of Altered Hormone Gene Expression in Endocrine Neoplasms

The mechanism of the excessive production of hormones by many endocrine neoplasms is not completely understood in most instances. Obviously, alterations in the levels of transcription factors, receptors, or perturbations in signal transduction pathways might explain a number of the examples. It is unlikely that the evolving karyotypic instability of the stage of progression is directly involved in most examples, since the most common examples of functioning endocrine neoplasms are in adenomas and in highly differentiated carcinomas that are likely to be very early in the stage of progression. However, several investigations have demonstrated specific mutational alterations in receptors and components of signal transduction pathways that are probably responsible for the excessive specific hormone production in the individual cases described.

In 1990 Lyons and associates (Lyons et al., 1990) described a putative cellular oncogene termed *gsp*. The wild-type protooncogene of *gsp* is the α-subunit of the G protein involved in the response of pituitary cells to growth hormone–releasing hormone (GHRH). A diagram of the effect of the mutations that have been found in this proto-oncogene is seen in Figure 18.7. The amino acid substitutions noted result in constitutive activation of adenyl cyclase (AC) and subsequent cyclic AMP formation, which, in turn, activates a signal transduction pathway leading to both hyperplasia and hyperfunction (cf. Spada et al., 1994, 1998).

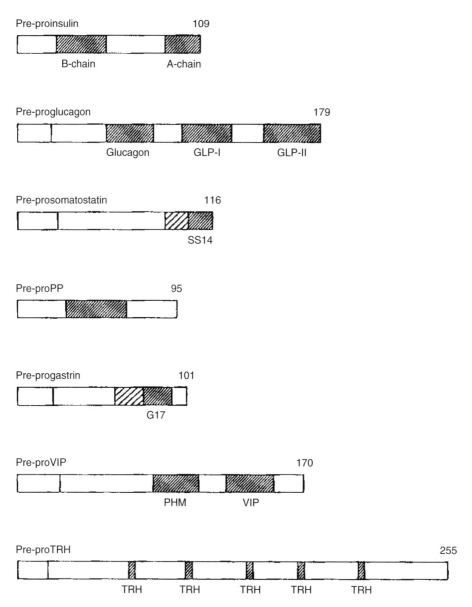

Figure 18.5 Structure and organization of different pre-pro hormones expressed in the pancreas. The numbers at the upper right of each structure indicate the number of amino acid residues. Pre-pro insulin is an example of a precursor from which the entire sequence is used for synthesis of one bioactive peptide. Pre-pro glucagon and pre-pro VIP (vasoactive intestinal peptide) are polyprotein precursors containing several homologous but not identical bioactive peptides. Pre-pro TRH (thyrotropin releasing hormone) is an example of a polyprotein precursor containing five identical copies of the bioactive peptide. (Adapted from Rehfeld et al., 1996, with permission of the authors and publisher.)

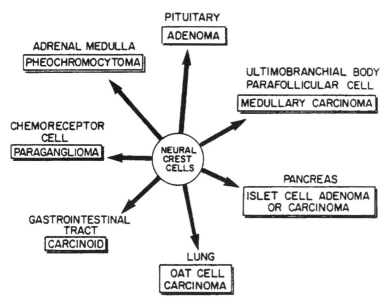

Figure 18.6 Distribution of some peptide hormone-producing tissues arising from the neural crest and belonging to the APUD system. The associated neoplasms of these tissues are designated by boxes. (After Schein, 1973, with permission of the author and publisher.)

At least one of these mutations has been found in about 40% of growth hormone–secreting pituitary neoplasms in several series (Johnson et al., 1999; cf. Spada et al., 1998). However, another series from Australia (Boothroyd et al., 1995) found a much lower incidence of such mutations in pituitary and other neoplasms. A second cellular oncogene, *gip2*, has mutations in similar regions of an α subunit of a different G protein whose function results in decreased cyclic AMP levels and decreased calcium ion mobilization (cf. Spada et al., 1992). The *gip2* cellular oncogene has been identified in about 10% of nonfunctioning pituitary adenomas as well as in neoplasms of the ovary and adrenal cortex. However, the exact functional alteration contributing to the neoplastic process or alterations in function in these neoplasms is not absolutely clear (cf. Spada et al., 1998).

Another example of mutations in a proto-oncogene leading to the formation of a cellular oncogene is seen with the thyrotropin receptor in adenomas of the thyroid gland. In this instance, the multimembrane domain receptor has been shown to be mutated in from 50% (Krohn et al., 1998) to 80% (Parma et al., 1995) of hyperfunctioning thyroid adenomas. Figure 18.8 gives a diagram of the thyrotropin receptor, indicating in black the amino acids where mutations were demonstrated (Parma et al., 1995). Mutation in the receptor appears to cause hyperfunction and proliferation of the adenomatous thyroid epithelium by constitutively elevating cyclic AMP (Krohn et al., 1998; Parma et al., 1995). About 30% of hyperfunctioning thyroid adenomas also exhibit the presence of the *gsp* cellular oncogene (O'Sullivan et al., 1991; Suarez et al., 1991).

In contrast to mutations in the G proteins in endocrine neoplasms noted above, mutations in N-*ras*, H-*ras*, and K-*ras* are relatively infrequent in thyroid and adrenal neoplasms in the human (Moley et al., 1991; Moul et al., 1993). Only about a quarter of adenomas and carcinomas of the thyroid exhibit *ras* gene mutations (Namba et al., 1990). Interestingly, Shi et al. (1991) reported that a 50% to 80% rate of *ras* codon 61 mutations occurred in thyroid tumors developing in an iodide-deficient area. While adrenocortical neoplasms exhibited low levels of G-pro-

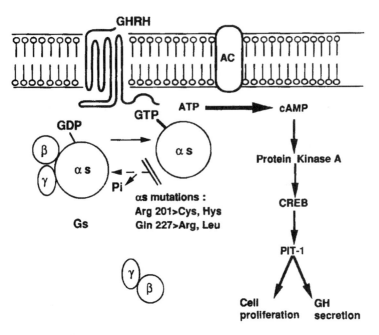

Figure 18.7 Diagram of the effect of single amino acid substitutions replacing Arg 201 with either Cys or His, or Gln 227 with either Arg or Leu in the protooncogene α-subunit of Gs, a G protein. The substitutions lead to the constitutive activation of adenyl cyclase (AC) and cyclic AMP formation by inhibiting GTPase activity. Increased cyclic AMP levels activate protein kinase A, which in turn phosphorylates CREB, initiating gene transcription. (Adapted from Spada et al., 1994, with permission of the authors and publisher.)

tein mutations, they were found to overexpress insulin growth factor-II in more than 80% of carcinomas studied (Gicquel et al., 1995).

One may speculate that the mutations seen in the G proteins and receptors in pituitary and thyroid adenomas reflect initiating mutations, since they appear to function in a dominant manner and would likely produce effects in the cell even if only one allele were mutated. However, considerable further studies will be required before such questions can be answered.

Effects on the Host-Tumor Relationship Produced by Hormones Elaborated by Neoplasms of "Nonendocrine Tissues"

Ectopic hormone production, a term coined by Liddle and associates (1962), refers to the production of hormones by neoplasms of nonendocrine origin or the production of hormones by endocrine neoplasms not associated with the normal gland of origin (cf. Smith, 1975). It is also possible that the "ectopic" production of a hormone by a neoplasm is the result of a relatively small number of cells in the tumor that are derived from normal endocrine tissue and produce the hormone in question. Under these circumstances, such hormone production by the neoplastic tissue cannot be considered as truly ectopic. In fact, a number of criteria have been delineated, one or more of which must be satisfied in order to demonstrate that the neoplasm is producing the hormone inappropriately or ectopically (cf. Wajchenberg et al., 1994; Baylin and Mendelsohn, 1980). These characteristics, which confirm that a given neoplasm is the source of ectopic hormone production, are listed below. There have been suggestions that all neoplasms produce

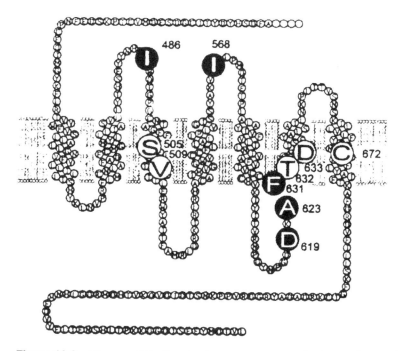

Figure 18.8 Diagram of the thyrotropin receptor structure in the membrane of thyroid epithelial cells. The circles with letters indicate the amino acids in which mutations have been found. The black symbols refer to mutations found in a series of adenomas for which the entire exon 10 of the protein was sequenced (Parma et al., 1995), while the white circles refer to other mutations found in toxic adenomas of the thyroid. (Reproduced from Parma et al., 1995, with permission of the authors and publisher.)

at least one hormonally active substance ectopically (Odell et al., 1977). On this basis as well as other studies, it is likely that many of the unexplained changes seen in the tumor-bearing host may be the result of one or more known or unknown hormones being elaborated by neoplasms.

1. Abnormal endocrine function
2. Disappearance of endocrine abnormalities following removal of neoplasms
3. Persistence of elevated levels of hormone following removal of gland normally producing the hormone
4. Increased concentrations of the hormone in the neoplasm compared with surrounding tissues
5. Molecular evidence for the synthesis of the hormone by the neoplastic cells

The first recognition that hormones elaborated by neoplasms arose from cells not considered to elaborate such hormones was described by Brown in 1928. More than 30 years later, Liddle et al. (1969) recognized that lung cancers were associated with Cushing syndrome, normally seen with hyperadrenocorticism, and demonstrated that the neoplasms contained large amounts of biologically active adrenocorticotropic hormone (ACTH). While originally considered relatively rare, Cushing syndrome resulting from ectopic production of ACTH-like polypeptides by lung and other neoplasms is increasingly being recognized such that a wide variety of neoplasms may be associated with "ectopic" Cushing syndrome (cf. Odell, 1997). Some of these neoplasms produce a hormone that is biologically, physically, chemically, and immunologically indistinguishable from human pituitary adrenocorticotropic hormone. Others produce variously modified forms of the hormone, as discussed below. Through its action on the adrenal glands, this ectopically produced hormone may cause all of the symptomatology of Cushing syndrome, a clinical picture of moon face, enlarged abdomen with linear streaking of the skin of the lower trunk, hypertension, and salt retention. The production of such a hormone is not suppressible by the administration of corticosteroid hormones, natural or synthetic.

Table 18.4 lists a variety of neoplasms derived from nonendocrine tissues that elaborate one or more hormone-like substances resulting in specific clinical findings. As noted in the table, several neoplasms—e.g., small-cell carcinoma of lung, renal cell carcinoma, adrenal neoplasms—may give rise to more than one hormone produced ectopically. In fact, lung cancers may elaborate more than 20 different hormones, most of which are not elaborated by pulmonary tissue in the normal state (Keffer, 1996). While ectopic hormone production is relatively common in some neoplasms, such as small-cell carcinoma of the lung, and contributes to the majority of the clinical symptomatology seen in general regardless of the source of the hormone, some ectopic hormone production is relatively rare, such as prolactin and rennin (cf. Odell, 1997).

Table 18.4   Some Ectopic Hormone–Producing Neoplasms and Their Effects[a]

Neoplasm	Hormone-like Substances Elaborated by Neoplasm	Clinical Findings
Small-cell carcinoma of the lung, carcinoids, thymoma, carcinoma of colon	ACTH, corticotropin-releasing factor	Cushing syndrome
Small-cell carcinoma of lung, carcinoma of pancreas	Antidiuretic hormone	Hyponatremia (low serum sodium)
Hepatoblastoma	Luteinizing hormone	Precocious puberty
Bronchogenic carcinoma, adrenocortical carcinoma, renal cell carcinoma	Chorionic gonadotropin	Gynecomastia
Hydatidiform mole, choriocarcinoma, embryonal carcinoma of testis	Thyroid-stimulating hormone	Hyperthyroidism
Cerebellar hemangioblastoma, adrenal adenoma, uterine fibroma, hepatoma	Erythropoietin	Erythrocytosis
Squamous cell carcinoma, acute myeloblastic leukemia	Parathormone	Hypercalcemia (increased serum calcium)
Pulmonary carcinoma	Growth hormone	Acromegaly Hypertrophic pulmonary osteo-arthropathy
Fibrosarcoma, mesothelioma, adrenocortical carcinomas	Insulin-like growth factor-II	Hypoglycemia
Small-cell carcinoma of lung	Antidiuretic hormone (ADH), arginine vasopressin (AVP)	Hyponatremia, renal sodium loss
Renal cell carcinoma, bronchogenic carcinoma, breast cancer, and others	Prolactin	Generally negligible
Lung cancer, ovarian cancer	Renin	Hypokalemia (low serum potassium)

[a]Further information on ectopic hormone-producing neoplasms may be obtained from the following references: Keffer, 1996; Odell, 1997; Macaulay and Smith, 1995.

Mechanisms Involved in Ectopic Hormone Production by Nonendocrine Neoplasms

In most of the examples given in Table 18.4, one might suggest that such a change in gene expression is the result of defect(s) at the gene, transcription, or posttranscriptional level. Many of the mechanisms discussed in Chapter 15 would thus be applicable. However, another potential mechanism is that related to posttranslational processing of polypeptides such as depicted in Figure 18.5 with reference to the production of pancreatic hormones. Such appears to be the case for the production of ACTH, where a 31-kDa peptide is the initial translation product, then leading to a variety of different products including ACTH, lipotropin, and β-endorphin, as well as melanocyte-stimulating hormone (MSH). A diagram of the posttranslational processing of the precursor peptide proopiomelanocortin (POMC) is seen in Figure 18.9. It will be noted from this that ACTH is only one of many peptides produced by this posttranslational processing mechanism. Wajchenberg and associates (1994) have presented evidence that probably all tissues synthesize at least small amounts of POMC-derived peptides, but only in neoplasms where it is produced in substantial amounts does one see significant clinical findings. Thus, one might argue that the "ectopic" production of ACTH by small-cell lung cancers and a variety of other tissues is not truly ectopic, since such tissues appear to have the capability of producing the precursor. In other neoplasms, however, there is evidence for differential splicing of the POMC transcript, giving rise to different mRNA species, some of which may be associated with the ectopic ACTH syndrome and others not (cf. Wajchenberg et al., 1994).

Overexpression of insulin-like growth factor-II (IGF-II) in mesenchymal and adrenal neoplasms may be related to the loss of imprinting of the gene, as discussed in Chapter 15 (Gicquel et al., 1995). The high level of IGF-II may induce hypoglycemia by inhibiting the output of glucose from the liver (cf. Fradkin et al., 1989). However, these mechanisms may not comprise the majority of alterations leading to the elaboration of hormone-like substances by nonendocrine neoplasms. It is tempting to speculate that in a number of instances the aberrant hormone production may be the result of evolving karyotypic instability with its associated gene amplification and gene translocations.

Paraneoplastic Syndromes Unassociated with Increased Production of Known Hormones

The term *paraneoplastic syndrome* has been used to denote clinical signs and symptoms that are not directly related to the neoplasm or its metastases (cf. Eckhardt, 1994). This rather broad classification would then include almost any determinant of the host-tumor relationship, including cachexia, anorexia, hormones elaborated by endocrine neoplasms, as well as hormones secreted by neoplasms developing from nonendocrine tissues and the production of nonhormonal elements leading to host responses resulting in specific syndromes. The clinical effects resulting in these syndromes are thus not dependent on the bulk of the neoplastic tissue but on its functioning within the organism (Eckhardt, 1994). In this broad definition, one could perhaps include almost all neoplasms, since all produce some remote effect not dependent on the bulk or the invasive or metastatic characteristics of the neoplasm itself. Thus, as others have done (cf. Agarwala, 1996; Zimmermann and Greenberg, 1996; Macaulay and Smith, 1995), the term *paraneoplastic syndromes* is here restricted to those resulting from hormones elaborated by neoplasms of nonendocrine tissues, nonhormonal components elaborated by neoplasms but directly or indirectly inducing specific signs and symptoms in the organism, and physical effects resulting from overproduction of products of the neoplasm. Already discussed are paraneoplastic syndromes resulting from hormone production by neoplasms of nonendocrine tissues (see above); considered below are the effects of nonhormonal components elaborated by neoplasms on the host.

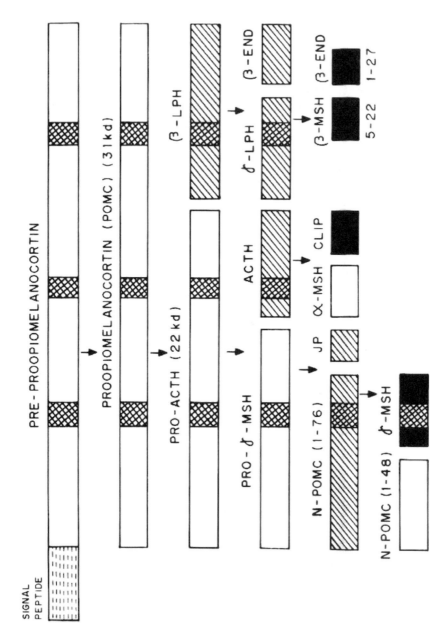

Figure 18.9 Posttranslational processing of proopiomelanocortin (POMC) in normal pituitary and in neoplasms of the anterior pituitary and in ectopic ACTH-secreting neoplasms. The hatched areas indicate peptides that are more abundant in the pituitary, while the cross-hatched areas indicate melanocyte-stimulating hormone (MSH) sequences, and the black areas represent "abnormal" polypeptide fragments seen in the ectopic ACTH syndrome. (From Wajchenberg et al., 1995, with permission of the authors and publisher.)

Paraneoplastic Syndromes Associated with Production of Nonhormonal Factors by the Neoplasm

By the definition indicated above, one could include cancer cachexia as a paraneoplastic syndrome; but generally this has not been done, since it is such a complex, little understood phenomenon that occurs to one degree or another in organisms bearing any malignant neoplasm. Table 18.5 shows a listing of a number of clinical syndromes associated with neoplasms but for which there is no known *hormonal* cause. Acanthosis nigrans—a lesion of the skin that is usually symmetrical, elevated, rough-surfaced, and hyperpigmented—is usually associated with carcinomas of the gastrointestinal tract, especially the stomach, but it may also be seen with malignancies of the breast, prostate, lung, breast, and ovary (cf. Poole and Fenske, 1993). There has been some suggestion that this lesion may be related to the production of melanocyte-stimulating hormone (see above), but other suggestions implicate some as yet unknown epidermal growth substance (cf. Poole and Fenske, 1993). Mucocutaneous pigmentation is seen with the inherited Peutz-Jeghers syndrome. This syndrome is associated with benign tumorous malformations of the gastrointestinal tract known as hamartomas, which are probably not neoplastic (cf. Utsunomiya et al., 1975). Other mucocutaneous manifestations of paraneoplastic effects of neoplasms have also been described but are not included in the table (cf. Poole and Fenske, 1993; Herzberg, 1998; Kurzrock and Cohen, 1995). Arthralgia and hypertrophic pulmonary osteoarthropathy (forms of arthritis) have long been known to be associated with neoplasms affecting the lung and pleura (cf. Naschitz et al., 1995). Hypertrophic pulmonary osteoarthropathy is basically an overgrowth of soft tissue in the distal phalanges (fingers and toes) leading to a phenomenon known as "clubbing." One of the first hematological paraneoplastic disorders described was that of Trousseau syndrome, the association of thrombosis with malignancy. Deep vein thrombosis of the lower extremities and pulmonary embolism result from a hypercoagulable state induced by the neoplasm, most commonly a mucin-producing neoplasm of the gastrointestinal tract or of the lung and pelvic organs (cf. Staszewski, 1997). Multiple myeloma, a neoplasm of antibody-producing plasma cells, in most instances produces excessive amounts of circulating immunoglobulins, which can deposit in various organs leading to renal failure, where there is actual blockage of the renal tubular system, and to amyloidosis, a disease characterized by extracellular deposition of complex proteins causing dysfunction of the organ by the presence of large amounts of amyloid (cf. Barlogie et al., 1992; Dhodapkar et al., 1997; Tan and Pepys, 1994). However, the most common paraneoplastic syndromes associated with neoplastic elaboration of nonhormonal substances are those related to autoimmune reactions to proteins produced by the neoplasms themselves. Autoimmunity is discussed more extensively in Chapter 19, but it is basically the immune reaction of the host to products of its own genetic makeup, so-called self-antigens.

Table 18.5 Paraneoplastic Syndromes Resulting from Excessive Production of Nonhormonal Components by Neoplasms

Neoplasm	Clinical Findings
Adenocarcinoma of stomach, breast, lung	Acanthosis nigricans
Peutz-Jeghers syndrome (hamartomas of gastro-intestinal tract)	Mucocutaneous pigmentation (lips, mucous membranes, skin)
Pulmonary and pleural neoplasms	Hypertrophic pulmonary osteoarthropathy
Gastrointestinal and pulmonary neoplasms	Deep vein thrombosis
Multiple myeloma	Renal failure and amyloidosis
Multiple different histogenetic types of neoplasms	Autoimmunity to various tissues (see Table 18.6)

Paraneoplastic Neurological Syndromes

Paraneoplastic syndromes affecting the central and peripheral nervous systems may make up a substantial part of host-tumor effects, especially when certain neoplasms are considered (Dalmau and Posner, 1997). For example, it has been estimated that 75% of patients with lung neoplasms suffer from a paraneoplastic myopathy (cf. Müller-Felber and Pongratz, 1998). A large number of other syndromes are associated with the production of autoantibodies and the effects of their reaction with antigens within and on cells in both the central and the peripheral nervous system, as delineated in Table 18.6. As noted in the table, a number of autoantibodies are induced by antigens in neoplasms that without exception are not neural in origin. In addition to the paraneoplastic neurological syndromes, there are a number of other paraneoplastic myopathies which likely are related to autoantibodies, including a dermatopolymyositis involving inflammation of skeletal muscle (Müller-Felber and Pongratz, 1998), an autoimmune mucocutaneous disease, paraneoplastic pemphigus associated with lymphomas (Fullerton et al., 1992), and paraneoplastic autoimmune hemolytic anemias and thrombocytopenias also associated with leukemias and lymphomas (Staszewski, 1997).

The significant characteristic of these types of paraneoplastic syndromes is the production of proteins whose genes are not normally expressed in the tissue of origin of the neoplasm. This is quite comparable to the elaboration of hormones from nonendocrine tissues. Darnell (1996) has suggested that the antigens produced by the neoplasms are normally not exposed to the immune system in the adult because of the protected nature of the central nervous system. The immune response, in the form of cells or antibodies, may then somehow traverse the blood-brain barrier and react with the antigens normally produced in cells of the nervous system, as postulated in Figure 18.10. This mechanism, however, does not completely explain the other autoimmune phenomena such as those directed to muscle tissue, red cells, and platelets.

Potential Mechanisms for the Production of Paraneoplastic Syndromes in the Host-tumor Relationship

Most cells within the mammalian organism with the exception of the egg, sperm, and certain cells of the immune system (Chapter 19) contain the same genetic information in one form or another. Differentiation results from a selective suppression and expression of the genetic information available in the cell. There is significant evidence that neoplasia may be a disease of differentiation (Chapter 6). The paraneoplastic syndromes, on the other hand, appear to involve almost exclusively the production of proteins expressed from a single gene, although several such proteins may be expressed within the same neoplasm. It would appear more likely, although not proven, that a reasonable mechanism is a direct relation of this altered "differentiation" to the evolving karyotypic instability characteristic of the stage of progression. Virtually all of the neoplasms involved in paraneoplastic syndromes as well as the production of hormones by neoplasms of nonendocrine tissue are in the stage of progression. In view of the multiple potential alterations that can occur in the genome during the evolution of the unstable karyotype (Chapter 9), it is not unreasonable to consider that the "ectopic" production of hormones, a variety of other proteins, and the excessive amount of proteins leading to the syndromes described in this chapter are the result of the instability of the genome of the neoplastic cell.

Stromal Reaction of the Host to Neoplasms

In our discussion of benign neoplasms (Chapter 2), it was demonstrated that the host may form a fibrous capsule around the neoplasm, apparently in an attempt to separate this growth from the

Table 18.6 Autoantibodies, Antigen Site and Function, Associated Neoplasms, and Clinical Findings in Paraneoplastic Neurological Syndromes

Antibody	Neural Site	Function	Syndrome/Clinical Findings	Associated Neoplasm
Anti-Hu	Neuronal nuclei	RNA binding	Sensory neuronopathy, encephalomyelitis	Small-cell lung carcinoma, neuroblastoma, prostate
Anti-Yo	Purkinje cells of cerebellum	Transcription factor	Cerebellar degeneration	Breast, ovary
Anti-Ri	Neuronal nuclei of central nervous system	RNA binding protein	Truncal ataxia, myoclonus, opsoclonus	Breast, small-cell carcinoma of lung
Anti-recoverin	Photoreceptor	Rhodopsin recovery (calcium binding)	Photophobia and retinal degeneration	Hodgkin disease
Anti-VGCC (P/Q type)[a]	Nerve terminal	Transmembrane calcium channel	Myasthenia (muscle weakness)	Small-cell carcinoma of lung
Antiamphiphysin	Synaptic vesicles	Synaptic vesicle release	Stiff-man syndrome (painful muscle contractions, hypertension, tachycardia)	Carcinoma of breast
Anti-AchR[b]	Cholinergic synapse (postsynaptic)	Transmitter receptor	Weakness of oculobulbar and respiratory muscles	Thymoma

[a]VGCC, voltage-gated calcium channel.
[b]AchR, acetylcholine receptor.
This table was developed from the following references: Posner and Dalmau, 1997; Inuzuka, 2000; Anhalt and Nousari, 1998; Hildebrand, 1989.

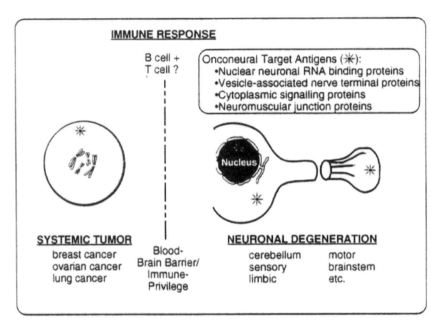

Figure 18.10   Model for the pathogenesis of paraneoplastic neurological disorders. Proteins normally made only in neurons are expressed in the systemic neoplasm with concomitant reaction of the immune system to the neural protein as foreign, since it is not normally presented to the immune system because of the immunologically privileged state of neurons. The antibodies and/or immunocytes (T cells, Chapter 19) cross the blood-brain barrier and react with sites of the protein production in normal neurons and related cells. (Adapted from Darnell, 1996, with permission of the author and publisher.)

remainder of the organism. Although the exact mechanism that stimulates the production of this capsule is not yet clear, a number of potential mechanisms are now becoming apparent. In some cases a portion of the capsule is probably the result of collapse and degeneration of neoplastic as well as normal tissue in the area. A very important factor in this situation as well as in the growth of all neoplasms is the fact that the host supplies the blood—vascular system—for the nutrition of the neoplasm. Denekamp and Hobson (1982) demonstrated almost two decades ago that in a large number of experimental neoplasms, the rate of proliferation of vascular endothelium within the neoplasm is much greater than the vascular endothelial proliferation in nonneoplastic tissues of the host. Even more striking is the demonstration by several authors (cf. van den Hooff, 1988) that fibroblasts in the stroma (the nonneoplastic supporting host tissue of the neoplasm) exhibit some features usually considered characteristic of neoplastic cells, including chromosomal alterations and several interesting characteristics seen by transformed cells in vitro, such as disorganized growth patterns, differential agglutinability by lectins, and extended life span. It should be kept in mind that all cells in a neoplasm other than the neoplastic cells themselves are derived from normal host tissues. These include blood and lymphatic vessels, fibrous tissue, and other normal tissues that support the neoplasm or become trapped by its growth. In rare instances, the host stromal tissue, especially blood vessels, appears to undergo malignant transformation in vivo. The mechanism of this change is unknown, but may be seen in certain neoplasms of the central nervous system (cf. McMenemey, 1966).

In certain neoplasms the host may react to the growth of the tumor by the production of extensive amounts of fibrous tissue. Such a reaction has been termed a *scirrhous* reaction and the neoplasm a *scirrhous tumor* (Figure 18.11). This type of reaction may be seen in some carcinomas of the breast, pancreas, colon, and others, as well as in their metastases. In the past, neoplasms inducing a scirrhous reaction in the host were considered limited to epithelial tumors that secrete glycoproteins and mucopolysaccharides. In some instances, as seen in carcinoma of the breast that metastasizes to the liver, the scirrhous reaction in the metastatic lesions may be so severe as to compromise or even virtually destroy liver function. More than 50 years ago, investigators pointed out a spatial relationship often seen between peripheral lung cancer and collagenous scars, usually in the vicinity of the pleura. A number of instances of neoplasms arising in or near the scar, usually adenocarcinomas and many in association with old tuberculosis, made some investigators suggest that the scar itself was a major factor in the pathogenesis of these neoplasms (cf. van den Hooff, 1988). As yet, however, there is no mechanistic relationship between pulmonary neoplasia and pulmonary scarring other than this interesting statistical and histological association between the two. Neoplasms that possess relatively little scirrhous reaction have been termed medullary tumors when they are soft and easily dissected from the host (Figure 18.11). In some such medullary neoplasms, there is a substantial lymphoid infiltrate which in many instances leads to a very favorable prognosis with few if any metastases (Rapin et al., 1988).

A different type of reaction, that of production of amyloid, an amorphous mixture of glycoproteins resulting from a combination of cellular secretion and proteolysis (cf. Hawkins, 1988), occurs in association with several types of neoplasms, including those of the APUD system (Pearse, 1980), as well as both carcinomas and mesenchymal neoplasms (Husby et al., 1982). The production of amyloid is quite common in myelomas, where its source is the excessive amount of immunoglobulins produced by the neoplasm (Isobe and Osserman, 1974).

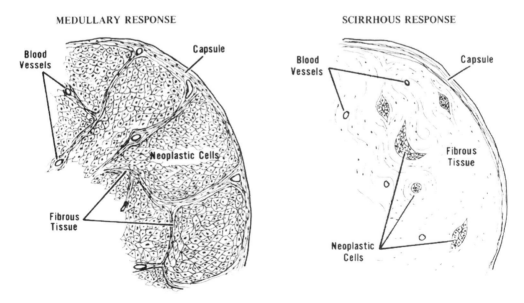

Figure 18.11 Diagram of the stromal reaction of the host to epithelial neoplasms, showing the extensive fibrous reaction in the scirrhous response compared with the relatively small fibrous reaction in the medullary response.

Potential Mechanisms Controlling Stromal Reaction of the Host to the Neoplasm

It is very likely that a major mechanism whereby neoplasms induce a stromal response of the host is through their secretion of various growth factors, which, in turn, can regulate the development of the extracellular matrix, angiogenesis, and fibrous tissue. Transforming growth factor-β has been implicated in several of these reactions such as an effect on regulating the expression and structure of extracellular matrix chondroitin/dermatan sulfate proteoglycans (Bassols and Massagué, 1988; Taipale et al., 1998) as well as specific proteoglycan gene expression (Iozzo and Cohen, 1993). Transforming growth factor-β plays a major role in tissue fibrosis (Border and Noble, 1994) and thus, together with other growth factors such as basic fibroblast growth factor (Table 16.9), may be important in the scirrhous reaction developing in relation to certain epithelial neoplasms (Figure 18.11). In addition to the apparent changes seen in stromal fibroblasts noted above, Scanlan et al. (1994) have described the induction of a protein on stromal fibroblasts, termed the fibroblast activation protein, possessing serine protease activity, which could mimic some of the cellular-extracellular matrix interactions discussed in Chapter 10 in tumor invasion. Wernert (1997) has pointed out that the stroma of neoplasms in fact has a variety of different functions, including the production of growth factors and a variety of other proteins that may transduce signals capable of modification of proliferation of neoplastic cells. However, the most important aspect of the stromal host-tumor relationship may be the development of a blood supply supporting neoplastic growth.

Angiogenesis

Although the vasculature or blood supply of neoplasms has been investigated since the nineteenth century, it is only in the past few decades that the morphology and mechanisms of blood vessel formation in neoplasms have been studied extensively. Blood vessels in neoplastic tissue appear to differ from blood vessels in normal tissues with respect to their growth and neogenesis, especially at the areas of greatest growth of the neoplasm along its borders with normal tissue (cf. Beckner, 1999). In 1971 Folkman proposed a theory that neoplasms lie dormant yet viable and unable to grow beyond 2 to 3 mm^3 in size in the absence of vascularization from the host. He proposed that neoplasms produced a diffusible product that stimulated angiogenesis by host vessels to supply the vasculature for the neoplasm. Another term, *vasculogenesis*, refers to the formation of a primary vascular network during embryonic development of the vascular system (cf. Malonne et al., 1999). Angiogenesis, on the other hand, develops from preexisting vessels from which capillary sprouts migrate to produce new vessels.

Angiogenesis may occur in the organism as a result of a number of different stimuli. A simplified diagram of the "angiogenic cascade" is seen in Figure 18.12. As noted, the phase of initiation of angiogenesis may be stimulated by vascular injury, wounds, neoplastic growth, and/or local inflammation. Proliferation of the new vascular sprout with "invasion" into the extracellular matrix (ECM, Chapter 10) occurs with many of the characteristics seen with neoplastic invasion. Finally, maturation with lumen formation and differentiation of the new vessel occurs. As noted in the figure, the initiation phase of angiogenesis as well as to some extent the proliferation phase depend on the presence of growth factors and other hormones, while the maturation phase in normal tissues depends to a great extent on various inhibitors of angiogenesis, allowing for differentiation and normal vascular formation in the healing sequence. A list of various angiogenic stimulators and inhibitors is seen in Table 18.7.

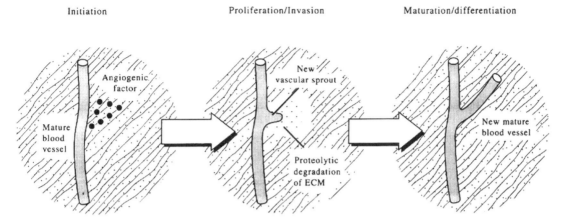

Figure 18.12   The angiogenic cascade. Angiogenesis is depicted as a continuum of three phases or stages as shown. Initiation of angiogenesis may occur from vascular injury, neoplastic growth, or activation by a variety of cytokines. The proliferative/invasive stage is characterized by an increased release of proteolytic enzymes, differential regulation of cell adhesion molecules, endothelial cell migration, proliferation, and invasion of adjacent tissues. The maturation/differentiation phase occurs on the basis of cell-cell and cell-ECM interactions, as well as the release of various angiogenesis inhibitors and maturation components resulting in differentiation into mature blood vessels. (Adapted from Brooks, 1996, with permission of the author and publisher.)

Growth Factors and Angiogenesis

Of all of the growth factors listed in Table 18.7 as angiogenesis stimulators, only two, vascular endothelial growth factor (VEGF) and placental growth factor (PlGF), influence the behavior and replication of endothelial cells directly (cf. Norrby, 1997). Many of the other stimulators appear to act indirectly, possibly by stimulating other cells such as macrophages and mast cells as well as endothelial cells themselves to produce VEGF (Norrby, 1997). VEGF itself is a highly specific mitogen for vascular endothelial cells, and at least five isoforms have been described, generated as a result of alternative splicing from a single VEGF gene (cf. Neufeld et al., 1999). At least three VEGF receptors have been identified, each showing some specificity for VEGF and PlGF. A diagram of the receptors and their ligand specificities in seen in Figure 18.13. Note that the VEGFR-3 is also involved in lymphangiogenesis as well as angiogenesis. The lymphatics are extremely important in the overall circulation of any tissue and in neoplasms as well, offering another pathway for the release of neoplastic cells into the lymphatic circulation. VEGF-mediated angiogenesis is very important in the developing embryo but is relatively rare in the normal adult, the exceptions being the female reproductive system (in the ovary) as well as wound healing and tissue repair (cf. Klagsbrun and Moses, 1999). Some of the other angiogenesis stimulators, such as the angiopoietins, appear to play a major role in angiogenesis in the developing embryo (cf. Klagsbrun and Moses, 1999).

Just as in neoplastic invasion, VEGF induces significant increases in specific integrins (Senger et al., 1997), and others have identified integrin $\alpha_v\beta_3$ as a marker of angiogenic and proliferating vessels (Brooks et al., 1994a). Antagonists to this integrin actually induce apoptosis in angiogenic blood vessels (Brooks et al., 1994b). Another very important factor regulating the expression of VEGF is hypoxia (Shweiki et al., 1992). This phenomenon may actually mediate

Table 18.7 Factors Modulating the Angiogenic Cascade

Angiogenesis Stimulators	Angiogenesis Inhibitors
Basic fibroblast growth factor (bFGF)	Platelet factor 4 (fragment)
Acidic fibroblast growth factor (aFGF)	Thrombospondin-1
Transforming growth factor-α (TGF-α)	Interferon-alpha/beta
Transforming growth factor-β (TGF-β)	Prolactin fragment
Platelet-derived growth factor (PDGF)	Angiostatin (fragment of plasminogen)
Insulin-like growth factor (IGF)	Tissue inhibitors of metalloproteinases
Vascular endothelial growth factor (VEGF)	TIMP-1
Platelet-derived endothelial cell growth factor	TIMP-2
Hepatocyte growth factor (HGF)/SF	bFGF soluble receptor
Angiopoietin-1	Placental proliferin-related protein
Angiogenin	Endostatin (fragment of type XVIII collagen)
Placental growth factor (PlGF)	Vasostatin (fragment of calreticulin)
Interleukin-8	Angiopoietin-2 (in absence of VEGF)
Prostaglandins E_1 and E_2	
Androgens	
Proliferin	
Estrogens	
Angiopoietin-2 (in presence of VEGF)	

hypoxia-initiated angiogenesis through the induction of hypoxia-inducible factor (HIF)-1α, a transcription factor regulating specific genes involved in cell cycle control and other important cell functions (Carmeliet et al., 1998).

Angiogenesis in Neoplastic Growth

In accord with Folkman's (1971) prediction that neoplasms produce factors stimulating angiogenesis by the host, Denekamp and Hobson (1982) demonstrated that endothelium in neoplasms had an extremely high proliferative index, in marked contrast to the reportedly low DNA labeling of normal tissue endothelium. On the basis of the large number of angiogenesis stimulators listed in Table 18.7, as well as the fact that all neoplasms produce at least one or more such factors ectopically or as a result of the differentiation program of their tissue of origin, the result of Denekamp and Hobson can be readily explained. While a number of normal tissues— especially heart, skeletal muscle, ovary, and intestine—produce significant amounts of one or more of the isoforms of VEGF, one or more isoforms of this growth factor are likely produced by virtually every malignant neoplasm (Nicosia, 1998). Furthermore, there is now ample evidence that several cellular oncogenes may modulate angiogenesis via indirect effects on VEGF production by neoplastic cells (Bouck, 1993; Rak et al., 1995; Schlessinger, 2000).

The Angiogenic Switch During Carcinogenesis

Folkman and his colleagues (Folkman et al., 1989) were among the first to report that angiogenic activity as assayed in an in vitro system first appeared in "hyperplastic" islet cells of the pancreas in transgenic mice expressing the SV40 large T antigen in these cells prior to the onset of formation of neoplasms. They extended this observation to other transgenic models and have applied it to the development of human neoplasms, as noted in Figure 18.14. In this figure, the

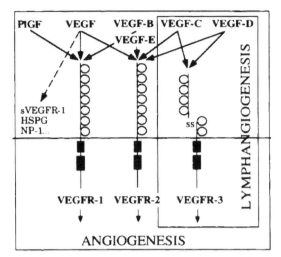

MIGRATION, GROWTH, SURVIVAL, PERMEABILITY

Figure 18.13 The three known VEGF receptors, VEGFR-1, VEGFR-2, and VEGFR-3, and their inter-action with specific VEGF isoforms. Ligand binding induces receptor signal transduction leading to vari-ous responses, some of which are listed below the figure. While all ligands are capable of mediating signals for angiogenesis, at least VEGF-C induces lymphangiogenesis. sVEGFR-1, soluble VEGFR-1, encoded by alternatively spliced mRNA; HSPG, heparan sulfate proteoglycan; NP-1, neuropilin-1, a cell surface glyco-protein involved in the central nervous system. (Adapted from Veikkola and Alitalo, 1999, with permission of the authors and publisher.)

early expression during carcinogenesis of genes whose products are involved in angiogenesis, such as VEGF, occurs at the morphological stage of dysplasia or carcinoma in situ (CIS). Fol-lowing that, angiogenesis itself occurs with ultimate invasive malignancy. This model is com-pletely in accord with the stages of initiation, promotion, and progression, as indicated in the figure. The preneoplastic lesion is the hyperplastic ductular proliferation, while progression be-gins with carcinoma in situ, extending to invasive carcinoma. Thus, in this model, one of the critical genetic alterations occurring in the transition from the reversible stage of promotion to the irreversible stage of progression is activation of angiogenesis. As expected, overproduction of VEGF by neoplastic cells contributes to malignant progression in model systems (Aonuma et al., 1999). Recently, another accompanying genetic change in the angiogenic switch is the acti-vation of a metalloproteinase also involved early in the stage of progression (Fang et al., 2000).

Thus, it becomes apparent that angiogenesis is not only critical for the growth of malig-nant neoplasms but also may well be an important marker in the critical transition from the stage of promotion to that of progression in epithelial and probably other neoplasms. Mechanisms in-volved in the exact activation of these genes—such as altered methylation, gene amplification, translocation, or direct enhanced transcription—are not apparent as yet.

As discussed in Chapter 20, antiangiogenesis has now developed into a field with potential chemotherapeutic effectiveness in the treatment of solid neoplasms. Although, as with any such therapeutic modality, there are difficulties (Westphal et al., 2000), there is also considerable promise, since the therapy is not related to the neoplasm directly, with its unstable karyotype, allowing for a variety of mechanisms of drug resistance (Chapter 20), but rather the therapy is directed at a normal tissue with a stable karyotype, namely the endothelium. While studies have

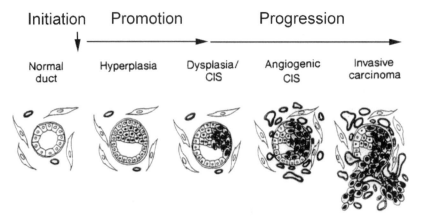

Figure 18.14   The angiogenic switch in neoplasia: reference to the stages of initiation, promotion, and progression. The diagram is of the carcinogenesis of ductal epithelium of the mammary gland going through the various morphological stages noted. The appearance of darkened cells at the dysplasia/carcinoma in situ (CIS) phase is the transition from the stage of promotion to that of progression. (Adapted from Hanahan and Folkman, 1996, with permission of the authors and publisher.)

demonstrated the effectiveness of antiangiogenesis factors (Kim et al., 1993; Kerbel, 2000), it will be only after extensive studies in the human that the effectiveness of this form of therapy for the treatment of neoplasia will be realized.

REFERENCES

Aebi, S., Gelber, S., Castiglione-Gertsch, M., Gelber, R. D., Collins, J., Thurlimann, B., Rudenstam, C. M., Lindtner, J., Crivellari, D., Cortes-Funes, H., Simoncini, E., Werner, I.D., Coates, A. S., and Goldhirsch, A. Presence of estrogen receptor imparts a poorer prognosis for young women with breast cancer. Lancet, *355*:1869–1874, 2000.

Agarwala, S. S. Paraneoplastic syndromes. Med. Clin. North Am., *80*:173–184, 1996.

Anderson, N. S., III, David, Y., and Fanestil, D. D. Estrogen receptor in hamster kidney during estrogen-induced renal tumorigenesis. J. Steroid Biochem., *10*:123–128, 1979.

Anhalt, G. J., and Nousari, H. C. Paraneoplastic autoimmune syndromes. *In*: The Autoimmune Diseases, 3rd ed., pp. 795–804. New York, Academic Press, 1998.

Aonuma, M., Saeki, Y., Akimoto, T., Nakayama, Y., Hattori, C., Yoshitake, Y., Nishikawa, K., Shibuya, M., and Tanaka, N. G. Vascular endothelial growth factor overproduced by tumour cells acts predominantly as a potent angiogenic factor contributing to malignant progression. Int. J. Exp. Pathol., *80*:271–281, 1999.

Barlogie, B., Alexanian, R., and Jagannath, S. Plasma cell dyscrasias. J.A.M.A., *268*:2946–2951, 1992.

Bassols, A., and Massagué, J. Transforming growth factor β regulates the expression and structure of extracellular matrix chondroitin/dermatan sulfate proteoglycans. J. Biol. Chem., *263*:3039–3045, 1988.

Baylin, S. B. Ectopic production of hormones and other proteins by tumors. Hosp. Pract., *10*:117, 1975.

Baylin, S. B., and Mendelsohn, G. Ectopic (inappropriate) hormone production by tumors: mechanisms involved and the biological and clinical implications. Endocr. Rev., *1*:45–77, 1980.

Beatson, G. T. On the treatment of inoperable cases of carcinoma of the mamma. Suggestions for a new method of treatment with illustrative cases. Lancet, *2*:104–107, 1896.

Beattie, C. W., Hansen, N. W., and Thomas, P. A. Steroid receptors in human lung cancer. Cancer Res., *45*:4206–4214, 1985.

Beck-Peccoz, P., Brucker-Davis, F., Persani, L., Smallridge, R. C., and Weintraub, B. D. Thyrotropin-secreting pituitary tumors. Endocr. Rev., *17*:610–638, 1996.

Beckner, M. E. Factors promoting tumor angiogenesis. Cancer Invest., *17*:594–623, 1999.

Bonkhoff, H., Fixemer, T., Hunsicker, I., and Remberger, K. Estrogen receptor expression in prostate cancer and premalignant prostatic lesions. Am. J. Pathol., *155*:641–647, 1999.

Boothroyd, C. V., Grimmond, S. M., Cameron, D. P., and Hayward, N. K. G protein mutations in tumours of the pituitary, parathyroid and endocrine pancreas. Biochem. Biophys. Res. Commun., *211*:1063–1070, 1995.

Border, W. A., and Noble, N. A. Transforming growth factor β in tissue fibrosis. N. Engl. J. Med., *331*:1286–1292, 1994.

Bouck, N. Angiogenesis: a mechanism by which oncogenes and tumor suppressor genes regulate tumorigenesis. *In*: C. C. Benz and E. T. Liu (Eds.), Oncogenes and Tumor Suppressor Genes in Human Malignancies, pp. 359–370. Boston: Kluwer Academic Publishers, 1993.

Briand, P., Rose, C., and Thorpe, S. M. Spontaneous regrowth of regressed hormone-dependent tumours after long periods of time. Eur. J. Cancer Clin. Oncol., *18*:1391–1393, 1982.

Brooks, P. C. Role of integrins in angiogenesis. Eur. J. Cancer, *32A*:2423–2429, 1996.

Brooks, P. C., Clark, R. A. F., and Cheresh, D. A. Requirement of vascular integrin $\alpha_v\beta_3$ for angiogenesis. Science, *264*:569–571, 1994a.

Brooks, P. C., Montgomery, A. M. P., Rosenfeld, M., Reisfeld, R. A., Hu, T., Klier, G., and Cheresh, D. A. Integrin $\alpha_v\beta_3$ antagonists promote tumor regression by inducing apoptosis of angiogenic blood vessels. Cell, *79*:1157–1164, 1994b.

Brown, W. H. A case of pluriglandular syndrome: diabetes of bearded women. Lancet, *2*:1022–1023, 1928.

Capella, C., Heitz, P. U., Höfler, H., Solcia, E., and Klöppel, G. Revised classification of neuroendocrine tumors of the lung, pancreas and gut. Digestion, *55*(Suppl 3):11–23, 1994.

Carmeliet, P., Dor, Y., Herbert, J.-M., Fukumura, D., Brusselmans, K., Dewerchin, M., Neeman, M., Bono, F., Abramovitch, R., Maxwell, P., Koch, C. J., Ratcliffe, P., Moons, L., Jain, R. K., Collen, D., and Keshet, E. Role of HIF-1α in hypoxia-mediated apoptosis, cell proliferation and tumour angiogenesis. Nature, *394*:485–490, 1998.

Castaño, E., Chen, C. W., Vorojeikina, D. P., and Notides, A. C. The role of phosphorylation in human estrogen receptor function. J. Steroid Biochem. Mol. Biol., *65*:101–110, 1998.

Clifton, K. H., and Sridharan, B. N. Endocrine factors and tumor growth. *In*: F. F. Becker (Ed.), Cancer—A Comprehensive Treatise, Vol. 3, Chap. 10, pp. 249–285. New York: Plenum Press, 1975.

Cohen, R., and Modigliana, E. Medullary thyroid carcinoma: 25 years on. Cancer J., *6*:59–64, 1993.

Dalmau, J. O., and Posner, J. B. Paraneoplastic syndromes affecting the nervous system. Semin. Oncol., *24*:318–328, 1997.

Darnell, R. B. Onconeural antigens and the paraneoplastic neurologic disorders: at the intersection of cancer, immunity, and the brain. Proc. Natl. Acad. Sci. USA, *93*:4529–4536, 1996.

Deftos, L. J., Goodman, A. D., Engleman, K., and Potts, J. T. Jr. Suppression and stimulation of calcitonin secretion in medullary thyroid carcinoma. Metabolism, *20*:428–431, 1971.

Denekamp, J., and Hobson, B. Endothelial-cell proliferation in experimental tumours. Br. J. Cancer, *46*:711–720, 1982.

Dhodapkar, M. V., Merlini, G., and Solomon, A. Biology and therapy of immunoglobulin deposition diseases. Hematol./Oncol. Clin. North Am., *11*:89–110, 1997.

Diaz, N. M., Mazoujian, G., and Wick, M. R. Estrogen-receptor protein in thyroid neoplasms. Arch. Pathol. Lab. Med., *115*:1203–1207, 1991.

Eckhardt, S. J. Paraneoplastic syndromes. Cancer Surv., *21*:197–209, 1994.

Fang, J., Shing, Y., Wiederschain, D., Yan, L., Butterfield, C., Jackson, G., Harper, J., Tamvakopoulos, G., and Moses, M. A. Matrix metalloproteinase-2 is required for the switch to the angiogenic phenotype in a tumor model. Proc. Natl. Acad. Sci. U.S.A., *97*:3884–3889, 2000.

Folkman, J. Tumor angiogenesis: therapeutic implications. N. Engl. J. Med., *285*:1182–1186, 1971.

Folkman, J., Watson, K., Ingber, D., and Hanahan, D. Induction of angiogenesis during the transition from hyperplasia to neoplasia. Nature, *339*:58–61, 1989.

Fradkin, J. E., Eastman, R. C., Lesniak, M. A., and Roth, J. Specificity spillover at the hormone receptor—exploring its role in human disease. N. Engl. J. Med., *320*:640–645, 1989.

Freedman, L. P. Increasing the complexity of coactivation in nuclear receptor signaling. Cell, *97*:5–8, 1999.

Friesen, S. R. Tumors of the endocrine pancreas. N. Engl. J. Med., *306*:580–590, 1982.

Fujimoto, M., Yoshino, E., Hirakawa, K., Fujimoto, J., and Tamaya, T. Estrogen receptors in brain tumors. Clin. Neuropharmacol., *7*:357–362, 1984.

Fullerton, S. H., Woodley, D. T., Smoller, B. R., and Anhalt, G. J. Paraneoplastic pemphigus with autoantibody deposition in bronchial epithelium after autologous bone marrow transplantation. J.A.M.A., *267*:1500–1502, 1992.

Furmanski, P., Saunders, D. E., Brooks, S. C., Rich, M. A., and the Breast Cancer Prognostic Study Clinical and Pathology Associates. The prognostic value of estrogen receptor determinations in patients with primary breast cancer: an update. Cancer, *46*:2794–2796, 1980.

Furth, J. Vistas in the etiology and pathogenesis of tumors. Fed. Proc., *20*:865–873, 1961.

Gicquel, C., Bertagna, X., and Le Bouc, Y. Recent advances in the pathogenesis of adrenocortical tumours. Eur. J. Endocrinol., *133*:133–144, 1995.

Görlich, M., and Jandrig, B. Steroid hormone receptors related to parameters characterizing the biology of human breast cancer. Tumori, *83*:930–397, 1997.

Gruss, H.-J., Herrmann, F., and Drexler, H. G. Hodgkin's disease: a cytokine-producing tumor—a review. Crit. Rev. Oncogen., *5*:473–538, 1994.

Habib, F. K., Odoma, S., Busuttil, A., and Chisholm, G. D. Androgen receptors in cancer of the prostate. Correlation with the stage and grade of the tumor. Cancer, *57*:2351–2356, 1986.

Hanahan, D., and Folkman, J. Patterns and emerging mechanisms of the angiogenic switch during tumorigenesis. Cell, *86*:353–364, 1996.

Hansen, R. K., and Fuqua, S. A. W. The estrogen receptor and breast cancer. *In*: A. M. Bowcock (Ed.), Breast Cancer: Molecular Genetics, Pathogenesis, and Therapeutics. Totowa, NJ: Humana Press, 1999.

Hawkins, P. N. Amyloidosis. Blood Rev., *2*:270–280, 1988.

Herzberg, J. J. Cutaneous markers of internal malignancy: paraneoplastic dermatoses. *In*: U. Rüther, C. Nunnensiek, and C. Bokemeyer (Eds.), Paraneoplastic Syndromes, Vol. 52, pp. 201–231. Basel: Karger, 1998.

Hildebrand, J. Signs, symptoms, and significance of paraneoplastic neurological syndromes. Oncology, *3*:57–61, 1989.

Homo-Delarche, F. Glucocorticoid receptors and steroid sensitivity in normal and neoplastic human lymphoid tissues: a review. Cancer Res., *44*:431–437, 1984.

Hsu, S.-M., Waldron, J. W. Jr., Hsu, P.-L., and Hough, A. J. Jr. Cytokines in malignant lymphomas: review and prospective evaluation. Hum. Pathol., *24*:1040–1057, 1993.

Huggins, C., and Hodges, C. L. Studies on prostatic cancer. I. The effect of castration, of estrogen and of androgen injection on serum phosphatase in metastatic carcinoma of the prostate. Cancer Res., *1*:293, 1941a.

Huggins, C., Stevens, R. E., and Hodges, C. L. Studies on prostatic cancer. II. The effect of castration on clinical patients with carcinoma of the prostate. Arch. Surg., *43*:209, 1941b.

Husby, G., Marhaug, G., and Sletten, K. Amyloid A in systemic amyloidosis associated with cancer. Cancer Res., *42*:1600–1603, 1982.

Ingram, S. S., Rosenman, J., Heath, R., Morgan, T. M., Moore, D., and Varia, M. The predictive value of progesterone receptor levels in endometrial cancer. Int. J. Rad. Oncol. Biol. Phys., *17*:21–27, 1989.

Inuzuka, T. Autoantibodies in paraneoplastic neurological syndrome. Am. J. Med. Sci., *319*:217–226, 2000.

Iozzo, R. V., and Cohen, I. Altered proteoglycan gene expression and the tumor stroma. Experientia, *49*:447–455, 1993.

Isobe, T., and Osserman, E. F. Patterns of amyloidosis and their association with plasma-cell dyscrasia, monoclonal immunoglobulins and Bence-Jones proteins. N. Engl. J. Med., *290*:473–477, 1974.

Jensen, E. V. Hormone dependency of breast cancer. Cancer, *47*:2319–2326, 1981.

Johnson, M. C., Codner, E., Eggers, M., Mosso, L., Rodriguez, J. A., and Cassorla, F. *gps* Mutations in Chilean patients harboring growth hormone-secreting pituitary tumors. J. Pediatr. Endocrinol. Metab., *12*:381–387, 1999.

Karr, J. P., Pontes, J. E., Schneider, S., Sandberg, A. A., and Murphy, G. P. Clinical aspects of steroid hormone receptors in human renal cell carcinoma. J. Surg. Oncol., *23*:117–124, 1983.

Keffer, J. H. Endocrinopathy and ectopic hormones in malignancy. Hematol./Oncol. Clin. North Am., *10*:811–823, 1996.

Kerbel, R. S. Tumor angiogenesis: past, present and the near future. Carcinogenesis, *21*:505–515, 2000.

Kim, K. J., Li, B., Winer, J., Armanini, M., Gillett, N., Phillips, H. S., and Ferrara, N. Inhibition of vascular endothelial growth factor-induced angiogenesis suppresses tumour growth *in vivo*. Nature, *362*:841–844, 1993.

King, R. J. B., Cambray, G. J., and Robinson, J. H. The role of receptors in the steroidal regulation of tumour cell proliferation. J. Steroid Biochem., *7*:869–873, 1976.

Klagsbrun, M., and Moses, M. A. Molecular angiogenesis. Chem. Biol., *6*:R217–R224, 1999.

Krohn, K., Führer, D., Holzapfel, H.-P., and Paschke, R. Clonal origin of toxic thyroid nodules with constitutively activating thyrotropin receptor mutations. J. Clin. Endocrinol. Metab., *83*:130–134, 1998.

Kuiper, G. G. J. M., Carlquist, M., and Gustafsson, J.-Å. Estrogen is a male and female hormone. Sci. Med., *5*:36–45, July/August 1998.

Kulke, M. H., and Mayer, R. J. Carcinoid tumors. N. Engl. J. Med., *340*:858–868, 1999.

Kurzrock, R., and Cohen, P. R. Mucocutaneous paraneoplastic manifestations of hematologic malignancies. Am. J. Med., *99*:207–216, 1995.

Kvols, L. K., and Reubi, J. C. Metastatic carcinoid tumors and the malignant carcinoid syndrome. Acta Oncol., *32*:197–201, 1993.

Leygue, E. R., Watson, P. H., and Murphy, L. C. Estrogen receptor variants in normal human mammary tissue. J. Natl. Cancer Inst., *88*:284–290, 1996.

Liddle, G. W., Island, D., and Meador, C. K. Normal and abnormal regulation of corticotropin secretion in man. Recent Prog. Horm. Res., *18*:125, 1962.

Liddle, G. W., Nicholson, W. E., Island, D. P., Orth, D. N., Abe, K., and Lowder, S. C. Clinical and laboratory studies of ectopic humoral syndromes. Recent Prog. Horm. Res., *25*:283–324, 1969.

Lippman, M. E., Allegra, J. C., Thompson, E. B., Simon, R., Barlock, A., Green, L., Huff, K. K., Do, H. M. T., Aitken, S. C., and Warren, R. The relation between estrogen receptors and response rate to cytotoxic chemotherapy in metastatic breast cancer. N. Engl. J. Med., *298*:1223–1228, 1978.

Lyons, J., Landis, C. A., Harsh, G., Vallar, L., Grünewald, K., Feichtinger, H., Duh, Q.-Y., Clark, O. H., Kawasaki, E., Bourne, H. R., and McCormick, F. Two G protein oncogenes in human endocrine tumors. Science, *249*:655–658, 1990.

Macaulay, V. M., and Smith, I. E. Paraneoplastic syndromes. *In*: M. Peckham, H. Pinedo, and U. Veronesi (Eds.). Oxford Textbook of Oncology, Vol. 2, pp. 2228–2253. New York: Oxford University Press, 1995.

Malonne, H., Langer, I., Kiss, R., and Atassi, G. Mechanisms of tumor angiogenesis and therapeutic implications: angiogenesis inhibitors. Clin. Exp. Metast., *17*:1–14, 1999.

Martin, P. M., Rolland, P. H., Jacquemier, J., Rolland, A. M., and Toga, M. Multiple steroid receptors in human breast cancer. III. Relationships between steroid receptors and the state of differentiation and the activity of carcinomas throughout the pathologic features. Cancer Chemother. Pharmacol., *2*:115–120, 1979.

McGuire, W. L., Horwitz, K. B., Zava, D. T., Garola, R. E., and Chamness, G. C. Hormones in breast cancer: update 1978. Metabolism, *27*:487–501, 1978.

McMenemey, W. H. The central nervous system. *In*: G. P. Wright and W. St. C. Symmers (Eds.), Systemic Pathology, Vol. II, Chap. 34, pp. 1137B–1298B. New York: American Elsevier, 1966.

McTiernan, A., Thomas, D. B., Johnson, L. K., and Roseman, D. Risk factors for estrogen receptor-rich and estrogen receptor-poor breast cancers. J. Natl. Cancer Inst., *77*:849–854, 1986.

Miksicek, R. J. Steroid receptor variants and their potential role in cancer. Semin. Cancer Biol., *5*:369–379, 1994.

Moley, J. F., Brother, M. B., Wells, S. A., Spengler, B. A., Biedler, J. L., and Brodeur, G. M. Low frequency of *ras* gene mutations in neuroblastomas, pheochromocytomas, and medullary thyroid cancers. Cancer Res., *51*:1596–1599, 1991.

Moul, J. W., Bishoff, J. T., Theune, S. M., and Chang, E. H. Absent ras gene mutations in human adrenal cortical neoplasms and pheochromocytomas. J. Urol., *149*:1389–1394, 1993.

Müller-Felber, W., and Pongratz, D. E. Paraneoplastic myopathies. *In*: U. Rüther, C. Nunnensiek, and C. Bokemeyer (Eds.), Paraneoplastic Syndromes, Vol. 52, pp. 187–200. Basel: Karger, 1998.

Nagasue, N., Ito, A., Yukaya, H., and Ogawa, Y. Estrogen receptors in hepatocellular carcinoma. Cancer, *57*:87–91, 1986.

Namba, H., Rubin, S. A., and Fagin, J. A. Point mutations of *ras* oncogenes are an early event in thyroid tumorigenesis. Mol. Endocrinol., *4*:1474–1479, 1990.

Naschitz, J. E., Yeshurun, D., and Rosner, I. Rheumatic manifestations of occult cancer. Cancer, *75*:2954–2958, 1995.

Neufeld, G., Cohen, T., Gengrinovitch, S., and Poltorak, Z. Vascular endothelial growth factor (VEGF) and its receptors. FASEB J., *13*:9–22, 1999.

Nicosia, R. F. What is the role of vascular endothelial growth factor-related molecules in tumor angiogenesis? Am. J. Pathol., *153*:11–16, 1998.

Norrby, K. Angiogenesis: new aspects relating to its initiation and control. APMIS, *105*:417–437, 1997.

Odell, W. D. Endocrine/metabolic syndromes of cancer. Semin. Oncol., *24*:299–317, 1997.

Odell, W., Wolfsen, A., Yoshimoto, Y., Weitzman, R., Fisher, D., and Hirose, F. Ectopic peptide synthesis: a universal concomitant of neoplasia. Trans. Assoc. Am. Physicians, *90*:204–227, 1977.

Osborne, C. K., and McGuire, W. L. Current use of steroid hormone receptor assays in the treatment of breast cancer. Surg. Clin. North Am., *58*:777–788, 1978.

O'Sullivan, C., Barton, C. M., Staddon, S. L., Brown, C. L., and Lemoine, N. R. Activating point mutations of the gsp oncogene in human thyroid adenomas. Mol. Carcinog., *4*:345–349, 1991.

Parma, J., Van Sande, J., Swillens, S., Tonacchera, M., Dumont, J., and Vassart, G. Somatic mutations causing constitutive activity of the thyrotropin receptor are the major cause of hyperfunctioning thyroid adenomas: identification of additional mutations activating both the cyclic adenosine 3′,5′-monophosphate and inositol phosphate-Ca^{2+} cascades. Mol. Endocrinol., *9*:725–733, 1995.

Pearse, A. G. E. Common cytochemical and ultrastructural characteristics of cells producing polypeptide hormones (the AUPD series) and their relevance to thyroid and ultimobranchial 'C' cells and calcitonin. Proc. R. Soc. Lond. Ser. B, *170*:71, 1968.

Pearse, A. G. E. APUD: concept, tumours, molecular markers and amyloid. Mikroskopie (Wien), *36*:257–269, 1980.

Pimstone, B. L., Sheppard, M., Shapiro, B., Kronheim, S., Hudson, A., Hendricks, S., and Waligora, K. Localization in and release of somatostatin from brain and gut. Fed. Proc., *38*:2330–2332, 1979.

Poole, S., and Fenske, N. A. Cutaneous markers of internal malignancy. II. Paraneoplastic dermatoses and environmental carcinogens. J. Am. Acad. Dermatol., *28*:147–164, 1993.

Posner, J. B., and Dalmau, J. Paraneoplastic syndromes. Curr. Opin. Immunol., *9*:723–729, 1997.

Pratt, W. B., and Toft, D. O. Steroid receptor interactions with heat shock protein and immunophilin chaperones. Endocr. Rev., *18*:306–360, 1997.

Raam, S., Robert, N., Pappas, C. A., and Tamura, H. Defective estrogen receptors in human mammary cancers: their significance in defining hormone dependence. J. Natl. Cancer Inst., *80*:756–761, 1988.

Raber, M. N., Barlogie, B., Latreille, J., Bedrossian, C., Fritsche, H., and Blumenschein, G. Ploidy, proliferative activity and estrogen receptor content in human breast cancer. Cytometry, *3*:36–41, 1982.

Rak, J., Filmus, J., Finkenzeller, G., Grugel, S., Marmé, D., and Kerbel, R. S. Oncogenes as inducers of tumor angiogenesis. Cancer Metast. Rev., *14*:263–277, 1995.

Rapin, V., Contesso, G., Mouriesse, H., Bertin, F., Lacombe, M. J., Piekarski, J. D., Travagli, J. P., Gadenne, C., and Friedman, S. Medullary breast carcinoma. A reevaluation of 95 cases of breast cancer with inflammatory stroma. Cancer, *61*:2503–2510, 1988.

Rehfeld, J. F., Bardram, L., and Hilsted, L. Gastroenteropancreatic tumours and prohormones. Scand. J. Gastroenterol., *31* (Suppl. 216):39–45, 1996.

Robertson, J. F. R. Oestrogen receptor: a stable phenotype in breast cancer. Br. J. Cancer, *73*:5–12, 1996.

Rosen, P. P., Savino, A., Menendez-Botet, C., Urban, J. A., Mike, V., Schwartz, M. K., and Melamed, M. R. Barr body distribution and estrogen receptor protein in mammary carcinoma. Ann. Clin. Lab. Sci., 7:491–499, 1977.

Rosen, S. T., Maciorowski, Z., Wittlin, F., Epstein, A. L., Gordon, L. I., Kies, M. S., Kucuk, O., Kwaan, H. C., Vriesendorp, H., Winter, J. N., Fors, E., and Molteni, A. Estrogen receptor analysis in chronic lymphocytic leukemia. Blood, 62:996–999, 1983.

Sadi, M. V., and Barrack, E. R. Androgen receptors in human prostate cancer. Biochem. Mol. Asp. Selected Cancers, 2:239–265, 1994.

Scanlan, M. J., Raj, B. K. M., Calvo, B., Garin-Chesa, P., Sanz-Moncasi, M. P., Healey, J. H., Old, L. J., and Rettig, W. J. Molecular cloning of fibroblast activation protein α, a member of the serine protease family selectively expressed in stromal fibroblasts of epithelial cancers. Proc. Natl. Acad. Sci. U.S.A., 91:5657–5661, 1994.

Schein, P. S. Islet cell tumors: current concepts and management. Ann. Intern. Med., 79:239–257, 1973.

Schlessinger, J. New roles for Src kinases in control of cell survival and angiogenesis. Cell, 100:293–296, 2000.

Schmid, M., Pirovino, M., Arrenbrecht, S., and Altorfer, J. Sex steroid receptors and liver tumors. In: H. Brunner and H. Thaler (Eds.), Hepatology: A Festschrift for Hans Popper, pp. 79–83. New York: Raven Press, 1985.

Senger, D. R., Claffey, K. P., Benes, J. E., Perruzzi, C. A., Sergiou, A. P., and Detmar, M. Angiogenesis promoted by vascular endothelial growth factor: regulation through $\alpha_1\beta_1$ and $\alpha_2\beta_1$ integrins. Proc. Natl. Acad. Sci. U.S.A., 94:13612–13617, 1997.

Shi, Y., Zou, M., Schmidt, H., Juhasz, F., Stensky, V., Robb, D., and Farid, N. R. High rates of ras codon 61 mutation in thyroid tumors in an iodide-deficient area. Cancer Res., 51:2690–2693, 1991.

Shweiki, D., Itin, A., Soffer, D., and Keshet, E. Vascular endothelial growth factor induced by hypoxia may mediate hypoxia-initiated angiogenesis. Nature, 359:843–848, 1992.

Sluyser, M. Hormone resistance in cancer: the role of abnormal steroid receptors. Crit. Rev. Oncog., 5:539–554, 1994.

Smith, L. H. Ectopic hormone production. Surg. Gynecol. Obstet., 141:443–453, 1975.

Spada, A., Vallar, L., and Faglia, G. G protein oncogenes in pituitary tumors. Trends Endocrinol. Metab., 3:355–360, 1992.

Spada, A., Vallar, L., and Faglia, G. Cellular alterations in pituitary tumors. Eur. J. Endocrinol., 130:43–52, 1994.

Spada, A., Lania, A., and Ballarè, E. At the cutting edge. G protein abnormalities in pituitary adenomas. Mol. Cell. Endocrinol., 142:1–14, 1998.

Staszewski, H. Hematological paraneoplastic syndromes. Semin. Oncol., 24:329–333, 1997.

Stedman, K. E., Moore, G. E., and Morgan, R. T. Estrogen receptor proteins in diverse human tumors. Arch. Surg., 115:244–248, 1980.

Suarez, H. G., du Villard, J. A., Caillou, B., Schlumberger, M., Parmentier, C., and Monier, R. gsp Mutations in human thyroid tumours. Oncogene, 6:677–679, 1991.

Sunderland, M. C., and McGuire, W. L. Hormones and breast cancer. Trends Endocrinol. Metab., 2:72–76, 1991.

Taipale, J., Saharinen, J., and Keski-Oja, J. Extracellular matrix-associated transforming growth factor-β: role in cancer cell growth and invasion. Adv. Cancer Res., 75:87–134, 1998.

Tan, S. Y., and Pepys, M. B. Amyloidosis. Histopathology, 25:403–414, 1994.

Teruya-Feldstein, J., Tosato, G., and Jaffe, E. S. The role of chemokines in Hodgkin's disease. Leuk. Lymph., 38:363–371, 2000.

Thapar, K., Kovacs, K., and Laws, E. R. The classification and molecular biology of pituitary adenomas. In: L. Symon et al. (Eds.), Advances and Technical Standards in Neurosurgery, Vol. 22:3–53. Vienna: Springer-Verlag, 1995.

Utsunomiya, J., Gocho, H., Miyanaga, T., Hamaguchi, E., Kashimure, A., Aoki, N., and Komatsu, I. Peutz-Jeghers syndrome: its natural course and management. Johns Hopkins Med. J., 136:71–82, 1975.

van den Hooff, A. Stromal involvement in malignant growth. Adv. Cancer Res., 50:159–196, 1988.

Veikkola, T., and Alitalo, K. VEGFs, receptors and angiogenesis. Semin. Cancer Biol., 9:211–220, 1999.

Vignon, F., and Rochefort, H. Nuclear translocation of the estrogen receptor in autonomous C3H mouse mammary tumors. Cancer Res., *38*:1808–1814, 1978.

Vinik, A. I., Strodel, W. E., Eckhauser, F. E., Moattari, A. R., and Lloyd, R. Somatostatinomas, PPomas, neurotensinomas. Semin. Oncol., *14*:263–281, 1987.

Wajchenberg, B. L., Mendonca, B. B., Liberman, B., Pereira, M. A. A., Carneiro, P. C., Wakamatsu, A., and Kirschner, M. A. Ectopic adrenocorticotropic hormone syndrome. Endocr. Rev., *15*:752–787, 1994.

Wajchenberg, B. L., Mendonça, B. B., Liberman, B., Pereira, M. A. A., and Kirschner, M. A. Ectopic ACTH syndrome. J. Steroid Biochem. Mol Biol., *53*:139–151, 1995.

Walker, M. J. Role of hormones and growth factors in melanomas. Semin. Oncol., *15*:512–523, 1988.

Walker, M. J., Beattie, C. W., Patel, M. K., Ronan, S. M., and Das Gupta, T. K. Estrogen receptor in malignant melanoma. J. Clin. Oncol., *5*:1256–1261, 1987.

Weil, C. Gastroenteropancreatic endocrine tumors. Kliwo, *63*:433–459, 1985.

Wermers, R. A., Fatourechi, V., Wynne, A. G., Kvols, L. K., and Lloyd, R. V. The glucagonoma syndrome. Clinical and pathologic features in 21 patients. Medicine, *75*:53–63, 1996.

Wernert, N. The multiple roles of tumour stroma. Virchows Arch., *430*:433–443, 1997.

Westphal, J. R., Ruiter, D. J., and De Waal, R. M. W. Anti-angiogenic treatment of human cancer: pitfalls and promises. Int. J. Cancer, *86*:870–873, 2000.

Winneker, R. C., Welshons, W. V., and Parsons, J. A. Estrogen receptor-like macromolecule in MtTW15 rat pituitary tumors: effects of antiestrogens. Mol. Cell. Endocrinol., *23*:333–344, 1981.

Ylikomi, T., Wurtz, J.-M., Syvälä, H., Passinen, S., Pekki, A., Haverinen, M., Bläuer, M., Tuohimaa, P., and Gronemeyer, H. Reappraisal of the role of heat shock proteins as regulators of steroid receptor activity. Crit. Rev. Biochem. Mol. Biol., *33*:437–466, 1998.

Zimmermann, C. W., and Greenberg, H. S. Paraneoplastic syndromes. *In*: Neurological Disorders: Course and Treatment, Chap. 56, pp. 627–635. New York: Academic Press, 1996.

19

Immunobiology of the Host–Tumor Relationship

For more than a century it has been evident that the various tissues of an organism are structurally different at both the morphological and molecular levels. In terms of immunobiology, this is reflected in the fact that tissues are antigenically distinct—that is, each tissue possesses unique macromolecules capable of stimulating a specific immune response within a foreign host. This fact has certainly been obvious to the biochemist, as each tissue has a relatively unique enzymatic content and thus would be expected to be antigenically distinct. An *antigen* may be defined as a substance capable of eliciting an immune response when the immune system of the organism is exposed to the antigen. An *antibody* is a circulating globulin specifically reactive with the antigen responsible for its production or with a comparable (cross-reactive) antigenic species. Antigens that are relatively specific to the tissue in which they are found have been termed *tissue-specific* antigens (Milgrom, 1966) or, in another context, *differentiation antigens*. A differentiation antigen is operationally defined as a determinant, detected in immunological tests (usually specific antibody-containing sera), that is limited in its pattern of expression to specific tissues (cf. Old et al., 1962; Old and Stockert, 1977). Lymphocyte populations express particular differentiation antigens on their surfaces. When a number of monoclonal antibodies (Chapter 14) recognize or react with the same differentiation antigen, these antibodies define *clusters of differentiation*, or CD. The nomenclature for some of these CD antigens is considered below.

ONTOGENY AND PHYLOGENY OF THE IMMUNE RESPONSE

Many invertebrates exhibit cellular recognition and aggressive reaction against foreign cells and antigenic structures. Such organisms also exhibit innate constitutive mechanisms, such as cellular engulfment or phagocytosis of foreign materials and the formation of bactericidal substances. Some relatively primitive vertebrates such as sharks have circulating serum immunoglobulins that have considerable structural similarity to the same types of molecules in mammals (Marchalonis and Schluter, 1994). The evolution of the vertebrate immune system has been in the direction of greater diversity and complexity in relation to the recognition of "non-self," the specificity of the immune response, and the structures of the molecules involved (Du Pasquier, 1992). The immune response of vertebrates exhibits the highest degree of specificity in that all vertebrates are capable of generating an immunological response upon stimulation by an antigen (cf. Roitt, 1977). The immune response in vertebrates initially involves *innate* immunity, which is a rapid and nonspecific, more primitive response usually occurring on the initial exposure of the immune system to foreign substances. Adaptive or anticipatory immunity (Klein, 1997),

which is characteristic of higher vertebrates, involves specificity in the response by the formation of specific immune globulins (antibodies) and cells that react specifically with certain antigens. Innate or nonanticipatory immunity is more characteristic of invertebrates (see above),
many of which have little if any adaptive immunity. However, vertebrates also possess innate
immunity, which depends on proteins directly encoded in the germline that identify potentially
noxious substances such as bacterial surface proteins, lipopolysaccharides, and protozoan as
well as multicellular parasitic organisms (Fearon and Locksley, 1996; Hoffmann et al., 1999).
Innate immunity is mediated by several cell types including macrophages and natural killer
cells, circulating proteins such as the complement system, and a number of antimicrobial peptides produced by secretory cells, especially of the gut (cf. Abbas and Janeway, 2000). It is also
apparent that unmethylated DNA of such parasitic organisms may play a significant role in innate immunity (Krieg, 2000). However, it is the adaptive immune response that primarily concerns us in this chapter.

The cellular interrelations of the immune system during embryonic development in the
vertebrate follow similar pathways in a number of vertebrate species. The first systematic study
of the developmental biology of the immune system was undertaken in the chicken. Stem cells
from the yolk sac of the early embryo and the primitive bone marrow appeared to develop in this
species along two general lines, one of which populated the thymus and the other a structure in
the intestine of the bird known as the *bursa*. From this schema, cells that populated the thymus
came to be known as T cells, while cells developing from the bursa were termed B cell. In mammals, that do not possess the anatomical structure known as the bursa, it has become apparent
that several other tissues, predominantly the bone marrow, appear to be the equivalent of the
bursa. Figure 19.1 shows a scheme for the development and migration of lymphocytes in fetal
life and to some extent continuing into adult life. Stem cells derived from the yolk sac in the

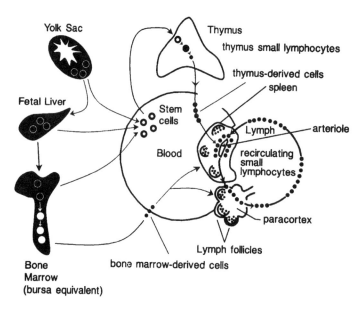

Figure 19.1 Development and migration of lymphocytes. Stem cells originating in the yolk sac, fetal
liver, or bone marrow are disseminated in the bloodstream, where some migrate to the thymus, ultimately
differentiating into T lymphocytes, while others differentiate within the bone marrow to produce B cells.
Such T and B cells eventually circulate in blood and lymph and colonize the appropriate areas of lymphoid
tissues. (From Miller, 1992, with permission of the author and publishers.)

embryo, as well as fetal liver and bone marrow—the latter in both the embryo and the adult—circulate and populate the thymus in the case of T cells and the follicles and medullary cords of the lymphocyte in the case of B cells (Miller, 1992). Within the thymus, T cells further differentiate into several varieties expressing CD (see above) antigens, specifically CD4 and CD8, each having specific functions, as discussed below (Weissman, 1994). In addition, later in life, T cell differentiation occurs extensively in extrathymic tissues such as liver, intestine, and omentum, as the thymus itself tends to atrophy with age (Abo, 1993).

MEDIATION OF THE IMMUNE RESPONSE

Differentiation of the lymphocyte population also results in the differentiation of function. T cells generally are involved in the mediation of responses that directly involve the interaction of the T cell with cells bearing antigenic components. B cells, in contrast, when activated directly or indirectly by a specific antigen, produce antibodies, which in turn circulate in the organism, reacting with antigen occurring at a distance from the cell and producing the antibody. This latter response, characteristic of B cells, is termed the *humoral immune response*. Each is considered separately below.

The Humoral Immune Response

Humoral immunity is the result of the formation of specific antibodies reactive with specific antigens and the ultimate consequences of such a reaction either by eliminating foreign antigens or in producing abnormal reactions within the host itself (autoantibodies). In order to consider the humoral immune response, however, it becomes necessary to understand the principal molecular species involved in this response.

Structure and Function of Antibodies

Antibodies are the proteins that form the basis for the humoral response to foreign antigens. Their structure has been known for some years and may be seen in schematic form in Figure 19.2. The upper portion of the figure gives a schematic structure of the basic immunoglobulin monomer (IgG). Each such structure consists of two identical heavy (H) chains and two identical light (L) chains. Segments of each of the molecules contain intrachain disulfide bonds within *domains* and *homology regions*. The domains marked V_H and V_L exhibit great variation in their amino acid sequence, especially in the hypervariable (HV) regions. Interspersed between the hypervariable regions are the less variable framework (FW) residues. The peptide chains are connected to each other by disulfide bonds as shown. The "hinge" region is characterized by a sequence of three prolines, which serve to give the molecule a specific confirmation in that region (Putnam, 1969). The constant (C) regions of the heavy and light chains are shaded with diagonal lines. There are three domains, 1, 2, and 3, for the constant region of the heavy chain. The structures of the constant regions of the heavy chain differ among the five different types of immunoglobulins as discussed below. The F_{ab} and F_c fragments may be produced by treatment of the molecule with the enzyme, papain, which cleaves the structures near the hinge region, leaving two F_{ab} molecules and a single F_c fragment. The F_c region contains carbohydrate as well as functional regions as shown in the figure.

The light chains consist of two classes or isotypes, κ and λ, for all immunoglobulin classes. The immunoglobulin classes are shown in schematic form as units or multiples of the basic immunoglobulin monomer in the figure. The class is determined by the type of the con-

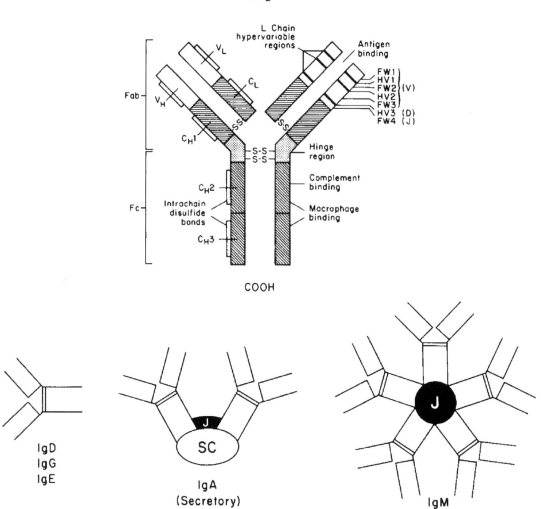

Figure 19.2 The structure of immunoglobulins. The upper portion of the figure details the structure of an individual antibody molecule. The different parts of the heavy chain *V* region are indicated on the right, and the segments of the gene that code for these nucleotides are shown in parentheses. The interchain disulfide bonds are shown as –S-S–, whereas the amino (NH$_2$) and carboxyl (COOH) ends of the molecule are as designated. (Adapted and modified from Teillaud et al., 1983, with permission of the authors and publisher.)

The diagrams in the lower portion of the figure are the comparative structures of the several immunoglobulins. IgG is the most commonly found immunoglobulin, while IgM is the immunoglobulin characteristically formed as an immediate response to the administration of a new foreign antigen. The overall structure of the IgD, IgG, and IgE is comparable to the upper figure, with the individual peptide chains and interchain disulfides shown as single lines. The IgA and IgM molecules are polymers of this monomeric structure held together by a joining piece (J) and, in the case of IgA, an additional piece, the secretory component (SC), which seems to be necessary to allow IgA entrance into mucosal secretions. (Lower portion of the figure modified from Goldman and Goldman, 1984, with permission of the authors and publisher.)

stant regions (C) of the heavy chains (μ, δ, γ, α, and ε) corresponding respectively to IgM, IgD, IgG, IgA, and IgE. Any individual immunoglobulin molecule possesses only one type of heavy chain and one type of light chain.

In the case of the multimeric IgA and IgM immunoglobulins, the individual monomers are covalently interactive through a separate polypeptide, termed the *J chain*, whose synthesis occurs within B cells (cf. Mestecky et al., 1974). In addition, IgA molecules may be secreted into saliva, milk, sweat, and other body secretions. The secreted dimeric IgA molecule contains a separate glycoprotein termed the *secretory component* (SC), which it obtains during the transcytosis of the IgA from the basal to the luminal surface of the secretory cell through which it passes. Figure 19.3 is a schematic representation of the uptake of both IgA and IgM by secretory mucosal cells following the interaction of these immunoglobulins secreted by plasma cells in the immediate adjacent tissue, termed the *lamina propria*. SC is synthesized as an inherent plasma

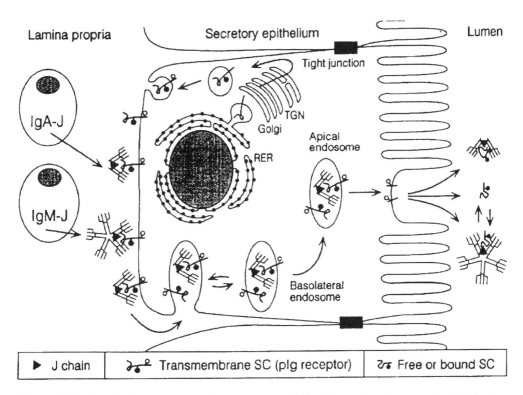

Figure 19.3 Steps in the production of human secretory IgA (right, top) and secretory IgM (right, bottom) via SC-mediated epithelial transport of J chain–containing polymeric IgA (IgA-J) and pentameric IgM (IgM-J) secreted by local plasma cells (left). Transmembrane SC is synthesized in the rough endoplasmic reticulum (RER) of secretory epithelial cell and matures by terminal glycosylation (●) in the Golgi complex. After sorting through the trans-Golgi network (TGN), SC is phosphorylated (○) and expressed as polymeric Ig (pIg) receptor at the basolateral plasma membrane. Endocytosis of noncovalently ligand-complexed and unoccupied pIg receptor is followed by transcytosis to apical endosomes and finally by cleavage and release of secrtory Ig molecules with bound SC as well as excess of free SC at the luminal cell face. During the external translocation, covalent stabilization of the IgA-SC complexes regularly occurs (two disulphide bridges indicated in secretory IgA), whereas free SC in the secretion apparently serves to stabilize the noncovalent IgM-SC complexes (dynamic equilibrium indicated for secretory IgM). (From Brandtzaeg, 1995, with permission of the author and publisher.)

membrane protein, which also acts as a receptor for these immunoglobulins. Following interaction, the IgA or IgM complexed with the plasma membrane receptor FC is transcytosed through the cytoplasm of the cell to be secreted through its luminal surface. Either prior to or at the time of secretion, the SC molecule loses its membrane interactive component (Solari and Kraehenbuhl, 1985). In this way the secretory component has been termed the *sacrificial receptor*, since the molecule is utilized only once, partially cleaved, and secreted in association with the immunoglobulin. The association of the glycoprotein SC with the immunoglobulin protects the molecules against proteolytic attack (Brandtzaeg, 1985). These mucosal immunoglobulins are considered the first line of defense against infectious agents coming in contact with various mucous membranes (Mestecky, 1987).

Regulation of Antibody Formation

Exposure of the immune system to certain antigens results in the production of antibody reactive with antigen. Later in this chapter the interaction of T and B cells in the regulation of antibody production is discussed. After the administration of an antigen, there is a relatively abundant production of IgM antibody, which continues and then falls off, while the production of IgG increases beginning shortly after that of IgM and does not fall as rapidly after peaking (Figure 19.4). Administration of a second dose of the antigen some 4 weeks later results in a relatively rapid increase in the level of IgG with some IgA and IgE but with much less increase in IgM. This is continued even after a third injection. The IgG that is produced following the second and third injections usually has a much greater affinity for the antigen, while that of IgM increases only slightly (Janeway and Travers, 1996).

The production of antibody is also regulated in a feedback manner. Administration of specific antibody to an animal immunized against the antigen specific to the antibody results in an inhibition of the formation of the specific antibody. This result has been clinically useful in the prevention of Rh incompatibility in pregnant women after the initial sensitizing pregnancy

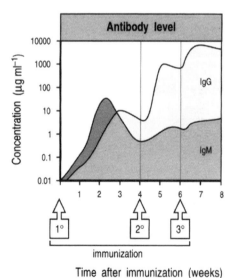

Figure 19.4 Synthesis of antibody types during the primary and secondary and later responses to the administration of an antigen at the periods shown by the numerical boxes and arrows on the X axis. (Adapted from Janeway and Travers, 1996, with permission of the authors and publisher.)

(Clarke, 1973). While the suppression by IgG molecules is antigen-specific, such antibodies binding to one epitope of a complex antigen may suppress the antibody response to all epitopes of this antigen. An *epitope* is the simplest antigenic determinant specifically reactive with an antibody molecule, as depicted in Figure 19.5. Although the exact mechanism of this regulation is not understood, it appears that intact F_c regions of the molecules are required for the effect (cf. Heyman, 1990).

Another as yet largely theoretical but potentially very important mechanism of the regulation of antibody formation is the proposed network theory of the immune system in which idiotypic determinants are primarily involved in the recognition and regulation of other immune response products and mechanisms (Jerne, 1974). An idiotype, as noted in Figure 19.5, consists of epitopes found in or near the antigen-combining sites of immunoglobulins and, as discussed below, in the T cell receptor. Since the variable regions possess an extremely wide variety of idiotopes (see below), the opportunity for the immune system to produce antibodies to such idiotopes is always present. While as yet there is not substantial evidence that anti-idiotype antibodies play a major role in the regulation of antibody formation or the immune system in general, there is evidence that anti-idiotypic antibodies are formed within the organism and possibly play a significant role in regulating the formation of autoantibodies, i.e., antibodies to the proteins of the organism or "self" antigens (Dwyer, 1992; Rodey, 1992).

A variety of other factors also regulate antibody response—including drugs, hormones, and dietary factors—but a detailed discussion of these topics is beyond the scope of this text.

B Lymphocytes and the Antibody Response

For the production of circulating antibodies, B cells must mature into secretory plasma cells. However, the immune response is highly specific, and thus only certain B cells will respond to certain antigens. For many years it had been argued that such a response was the result of a

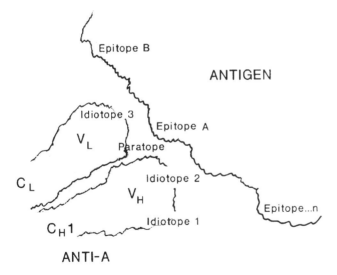

Figure 19.5 Terminology of the immunoglobulin-antigen interaction. A paratope is the antigen-combining site formed by the combined variable region segments of the heavy and light chains of immunoglobulins or the appropriate chains of the T-cell receptor. Idiotopes are epitope conformations in or around the antigen combining site, the paratope. The region labeled as paratope may also serve as an idiotope. (Reproduced from Rodey, 1992, with permission of the author and publisher.)

direct specific interaction of the antigen with an immunoglobulin-like molecule on the surface of the B cell, such an antibody being specific for the epitope of the antigen. During the last decade, the general structure of such a receptor on B cells has been described, as shown in Figure 19.6. In this figure, the antigen receptor complex is composed of two heavy chains that are transmembrane and two light chains that are extracellular. Associated in the membrane with this immunoglobulin are two other components termed Ig-α and Ig-β. These molecules are known to bind several different protein-tyrosine kinases which in turn are capable of activating signal transduction pathways, which ultimately result in an increase in replication and differentiation of the B cell interacting with the specific antigen (DeFranco, 1992; Justement, 1994).

In the uncommitted B cell that has developed from the stem cells of the bone marrow or other sites of lymphopoiesis, the receptor immunoglobulin is the monomeric transmembrane form of IgM or IgD. The further differentiation of the uncommitted B cell and the production of IgG, IgA, and IgE involve complex genetic rearrangements, as discussed below.

B-Cell Differentiation and the Genetics of Antibody Production

As noted above, millions of B lymphocytes mature, having on their surface millions of different IgM and IgD receptor molecules complementary to what many feel are billions of antigen species. An understanding of the mechanism of this highly complicated biological phenomenon has evolved rapidly over the last several decades, since the determination of the structure of immunoglobulin molecules. Contributory to such an understanding was the "clonal selection theory" proposed initially by Burnet (1970) and refined by many others. Major support for this theory came from the finding that myelomas in different patients each secreted a single molecular species of immunoglobulin and thus were clonal for that species. The receptor concept developed above was in part based on such findings. The remaining dilemma, however, was the mechanism for the production of the extreme diversity of antibodies to respond to an even greater diversity of antigens. Two general theories to explain this were entertained. The first, the germline theory, argued that immunoglobulin genes are expressed in exactly the same way as those for any other protein. This model required an enormous number of genes simply coding for the millions of immunoglobulin molecules. A second theory argued that there were only a limited number of immunoglobulin genes, which somehow diversified as the antibody-forming B lymphocytes developed from their stem cells. However, at the time, the theory demanded a completely original

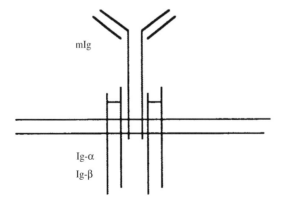

Figure 19.6   Model for the major portion of the antigen-receptor complex of B lymphocytes. mIg is composed of two heavy chains of the types depicted in Figure 19.2 that are transmembrane and two light chains (κ or λ) as shown. (Reproduced from DeFranco, 1992, with permission of the author and publisher.)

mechanism for such diversification. An answer to this dilemma came from the studies of Tone-gawa and associates (cf. Brack et al., 1978), who demonstrated that DNA of the embryo contained a number of λ gene sequences, only one of which could be found in plasma cell DNA. Tonegawa and associates argued that the most likely explanation of these data was that somatic recombination had occurred during the development of plasma cell DNA coding for a single molecular species of the λ chain, suggesting that embryonic DNA contained a number of possible λ chains. Subsequent studies by numerous investigators (Goldman and Goldman, 1984; Leder, 1983; Early et al., 1980) confirmed and extended these findings. In the genome, immunoglobulin genes occur in various places throughout the karyotype (cf. Matsuda and Honjo, 1996). Within each immunoglobulin genomic region there are multiple exon segments coding for different portions of the heavy or light chain. As a B cell matures and becomes committed to the production of a specific antibody, rearrangements, recombinations, and deletions of the vast majority of genes coded for the portions of the peptide chains occur. The result is that the mature B cell possesses a single pair of genes coding for a functional specific antibody. A diagram of the generation of a specific κ chain resulting from gene rearrangement and RNA processing may be seen in Figure 19.7. For the light chain, some species may have as many as 200 variable region genes in the embryo as well as in most non–antibody-producing cells in the adult. Each of the V

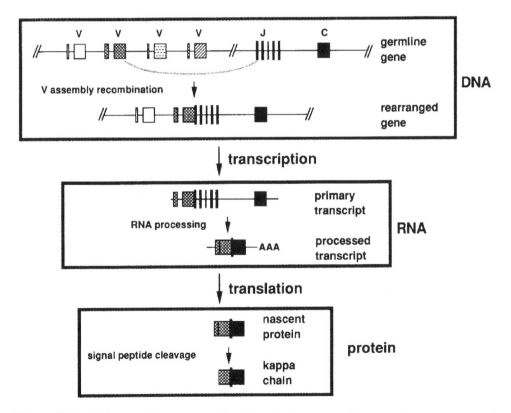

Figure 19.7   A diagram of κ gene expression. Note that the pathway from germline κ genes to proteins that are secreted involves alterations in the structure of DNA, RNA, and protein. The critical and unique component is the extensive DNA recombination which joins one of many germline Vκ regions to one of several J gene segments, resulting in a rearranged gene which is then transcribed, processed, secreted by cleavage of the signal peptide, finally resulting in a κ chain to be associated with the heavy chain. (After Max, 1993, with permission of the author and publisher.)

genes, whether of the κ or λ type, retains certain structural features, including a "leader" sequence coding for a hydrophobic sequence of amino acids involved in the secretion of the antibody molecule through the cell membrane. As noted in Figure 19.7, there are also a series of small sequences termed the J or joining sequences for the human κ chain. Five J sequences are present, each capable of joining with variations of the V gene (Figure 19.7). In the human λ chain system there are six C genes, each one linked to its own J sequence, while in the mouse there are four such combinations. During lymphocyte development, one V gene with its leader sequence is recombined with one of the J sequences along with a single C gene to form an active light chain. During RNA processing, intervening sequences and extra J genes in the transcript are spliced out to yield a coherent messenger RNA, which is then translated into a protein. If the protein is secreted, the leader sequence is first cleaved off.

The formation of the heavy-chain variable region is similar to that of the light chain except that the V genes are situated at a much greater distance from the C genes in the DNA of the embryo, and a second region, the D or diversity gene, is also present between the V and J genes. The D genes are segments from 12 to 15 base pairs in length, which in the human comprise about 30 different sequences. In Table 19.1 may be seen an estimate of the number of the light and heavy chain combinations. The table is taken from data in Janeway and Travers (1996) and is of the human. Similar numbers in the mouse vary somewhat from those of the human but are generally similar overall. Such values for other species have not been established as yet. In addition, as other factors enter into the diversity so that the total number of potential antibody structures is many orders of magnitude more than the final number in Table 19.1 (see below).

The formation of the heavy-chain constant region is considerably more complex than that of the light chain, since there are at least five classes of heavy chains, as shown diagrammatically in Figure 19.8. The final formation of the C genes in the plasma cell DNA results from "isotype switching," in which various segments of the DNA in the C gene region are deleted with subsequent recombination. By a similar technique, the V-D-J combination may be moved to other immunoglobulin genes. In the figure, 5′ of the C genes are long stretches of repeated noncoding sequences. In noncommitted B cells expressing IgM or IgD, the gene structure retains two C genes, those for the μ and the δ constant region. In this case one of the sequences is excised during RNA processing so that only a single heavy chain is produced (cf. Janeway and Travers, 1996).

It should be noted that in any single B cell, only one of the pair of genes coding for an immunoglobulin molecule is expressed. This phenomenon, termed *allelic exclusion*, indicates that if, for a given immunoglobulin gene in a single B lymphocyte, the alleles, one from each parent, are different, the lymphocyte will express only one of the alleles. The mechanism for this phenomenon is not known, although recent studies suggest a role for DNA methylation in allelic exclusion (Mostoslavsky et al., 1999; Bergman, 1999). A further factor in antibody diversity is the fact that antibody genes exhibit somatic hypermutation, especially in domains around the rearranged V region of the molecule (Neuberger and Milstein, 1995). The mutation rates in these regions have been estimated to be as high as one point mutation per 1000 bp per cell generation,

Table 19.1 Numbers in the Antibody Repertoire of the Human

Gene Segment	Ig_H	$Ig_{L(k \text{ and } d)}$
Variable segments	51	69
Diversity segments	30	—
Joining segments	5	5
Combinatorial joining	4650	350
Combinatorial association	1.6×10^6	

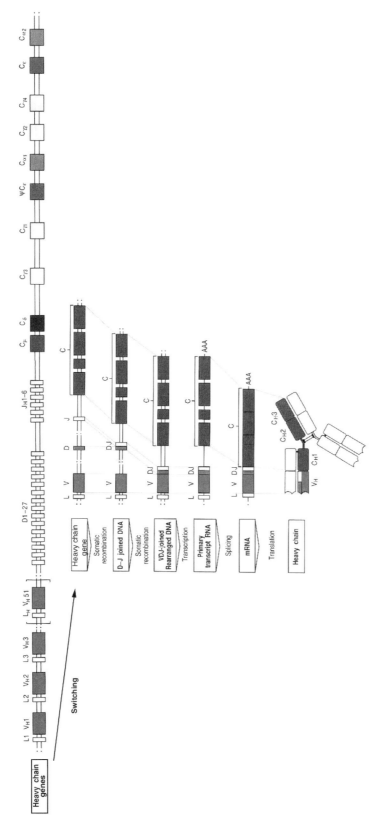

Figure 19.8 Diagrammatic representation of the heavy-chain genes and formation of the mRNA and protein products. The coding segments of the variable regions, diversity (D) and junctional (J), are comparable to those in Figure 19.17. The multiple constant region genes occurring in the germline DNA are removed by isotype switching that involves recombination between specific DNA sequences 5' to each of the constant region genes. After establishment of a specific constant region gene together with individual variable, D and J segments, somatic recombinations occur, leading to a single V(D)J-joined rearranged DNA from which is transcribed the nuclear RNA that matures to the mRNA from which the heavy chain gene is translated and subsequently associated with light chains as shown in the figure. The figure as shown is the general case with the constant region (C) following isotype switching, representing any of the various constant regions shown in genomic DNA with individual exons separated by introns. (Adapted and modified from Janeway and Travers, 1996.)

which is many orders of magnitude higher than the spontaneous mutation rate (cf. Storb, 1996). This hypermutation occurs during a narrow period of B-cell differentiation in germinal centers of lymphoid tissues, involves primarily transitions and transversions, especially the former (Neuberger and Milstein, 1995); and is not a result of defective DNA repair mechanisms (cf. Jacobs et al., 1998). A recent study (Muramatsu et al., 2000) suggested that RNA editing may be involved in this process, which increases the diversity potential and also generates antibodies of a higher affinity, with subsequent selection for the expression of those antibodies producing a more effective immune response (French et al., 1989).

Mechanisms of V(D)J Recombination

The rearrangements and deletions leading to mature immunoglobulin genes and their products (Figures 19.7 and 19.8), as well as the formation of T cell receptor genes (see below), are mediated by a common type of recombination signal sequence (RSS) that flanks virtually all recombinationally competent genes segments within the gene families of immunoglobulins and the T-cell receptor (cf. Oettinger, 1999). A diagram of the steps in V(D)J recombination is seen in Figure 19.9. Two genes specific for lymphoid tissue, RAG1 and RAG2 (recombination activat-

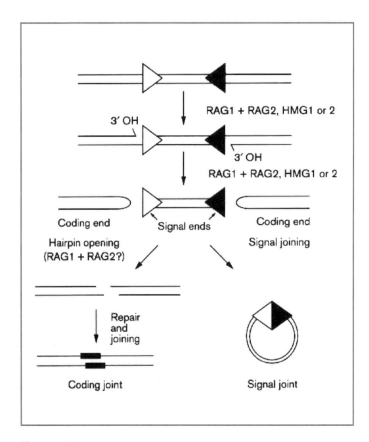

Figure 19.9 Diagram of V(D)J recombination. In the first stage of the reaction, the RAG1 and RAG2 proteins aided by HMG1 or HMG2 bind to a pair of recombination signal sequences (RSS) and introduce a double-strand break in a two-step reaction. In the second stage the hairpinned coding ends and blunt "signal" ends are resolved to form the coding and signal junctions as noted. The two RSS are indicated as white and shaded triangles. (Adapted from Oettinger, 1999, with permission of the author and publisher.)

ing gene), together make up the V(D)J recombinase and collaborate with one or the other of two high-mobility-group (HMG) proteins to form the V(D)J recombinase, recognize the RSS, and cleave between the latter and the coding sequence. Subsequent rejoining to form the mature coding segment as well as the signal joint involves a number of other proteins including terminal deoxytransferase and DNA-dependent protein kinase (Fugmann et al., 2000). The signal joint or complex that contains the RAG and HMG proteins appears to function in the downregulation of RAG gene expression, consistent with the need to remove RAG proteins from the signal end complex before joining occurs to produce the coding sequence (cf. Fugmann et al., 2000). This general mechanism appears to be applicable to many if not all of the recombinatorial events occurring in immunoglobulin and T-cell-receptor diversity.

The Cellular Immune Response

While the discovery of antibodies and an understanding of some of the characteristics of humoral immunity began during the turn of this century, an understanding of the cell-mediated immunity took much longer and appears to be considerably more complicated. T cells do not produce antibody but exert most of their immunological effects through direct interaction with a variety of cells. Considered below are, first, the characteristics of the T cell and how it responds to foreign antigens and second, the interaction of the T- and B-cell populations.

The T-Cell Receptor

T cells, just like B cells, must have a mechanism for recognizing and interacting with foreign antigens in a specific manner, namely, through a receptor mechanism (see above). Initial evidence identifying T-cell receptors came from the use of monoclonal antibodies (Chapter 14) specific for individual T cells, indicating a unique molecular species on the surface of such cells. Refinement of these experiments led to the conclusion that each T cell bears about 30,000 T-cell receptor molecules on its surface. Subsequent studies by numerous investigators have demonstrated that the T-cell receptor consists of two different polypeptide chains originally termed the α and β chains bound to each other by a disulfide bond. The entire structure is quite homologous to the Fab fragment of IgG (Figure 19.2). Such $\alpha{:}\beta$ heterodimers appear to account for antigen recognition by more than 90% of the various functional classes of T cells (cf. Janeway and Travers, 1996).

The two T-cell receptor proteins are anchored to the cell membrane through a transmembrane region that extends into the cytoplasm (Figure 19.10). Just as with the B-cell receptor, several proteins are associated with the T-cell receptor to serve in the mediation of signals resulting from the interaction of the T cell receptor with an antigen. These proteins are known collectively as CD3 and consist of a γ, δ, and ϵ forms which have sequence homologies to immunoglobulins. In addition, two other proteins, either ζ and η, also are part of this complex either as homo- or heterodimers. Finally, adjacent to the T cell receptor complex are molecules known as coreceptors, the CD4 and CD8 molecules, which are involved in the functional interaction of specific T cells, which may express either CD4 or CD8, with antigen presenting cells (see below). It is through the cytoplasmic portion of the ζ/η protein dimer of the T cell receptor:CD3 complex and the cytoplasmic domain of the CD4 or CD8 molecule that signal transduction is mediated (Figure 19.10).

The Genes of the T Cell Receptor

Just as with immunoglobulins, both membrane and soluble forms, one might conclude that a great degree of diversity must be inherent in the expression of the genes, since T cells react with

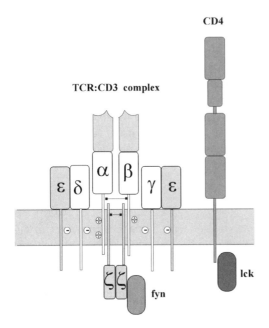

Figure 19.10 Diagram of the T-cell receptor:CD3 complex in association with a CD4 molecule and potential protein tyrosine kinases. A similar structure would be seen for CD8 T-cells where the CD8 molecule replaces the CD4 molecule. Similarly, some TCR:CD3 complexes have η molecules in place of one of the ζ species. The positions of the various proteins indicate interactions. (Modified from Janeway and Travers, 1996, with permission of the authors and publisher.)

so many different molecular species of antigens, many of which do not induce B cell responses (see below). A diagram of the T-cell receptor gene complexes that are presently known is seen in Figure 19.11. The α and β gene complexes are those primarily expressed in T lymphocytes, as noted above. In contrast, human γ/δ T lymphocytes recognize unconventional antigens via their heterodimeric T cell receptor in a non-MHC-restricted fashion (see below) (Kabelitz et al., 2000). Only a small percentage (1% to 5%) of mature T lymphocytes express the γ/δ T cell receptor heterodimer (Kabelitz et al., 2000). γ/δ T cells are distributed in different anatomical sites—such as the epidermis, intestines, and reproductive organs—as compared with the α/β T cells (Yoshikai, 1991). Despite the relatively small representation of these cells in the organism in general, the predominant T-cell type found in murine epidermis and epithelium is largely γ/δ cells. Still, the exact differential function of the γ/δ T cells is not known, and it is assumed that the predominant T-cell response is through the α/β T cell.

As noted from Figure 19.11, T-cell receptor genes express variable (V), constant (C), joining (J), and diversity (D) regions with the exception of the γ gene complex, which has no D regions. Interestingly, the δ gene complex is a component within the α gene complex and thus, during maturation of a T cell to an α/β form, the δ gene is eliminated (cf. Breit and van Dongen, 1994). The maturation of T cells occurs through the elimination by recombination and deletion of gene segments just as with immunoglobulins (see above). The potential total diversity of immunoglobulins and T cell receptors of the α/β type is seen in Table 19.2. As noted in the table, while T cell receptor genes have many fewer D segments than immunoglobulins, there is a greater diversity, where the D segments can be read in three different frames, thus dramatically increasing the total actual D segments and J segments. This leads to an increase by two orders of

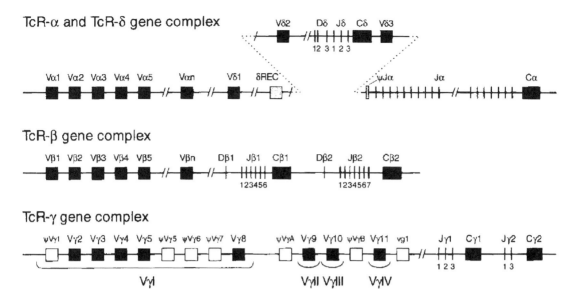

Figure 19.11 Schematic diagram of the germline configuration of the four human T-cell receptor (TcR) gene complexes. The TcR-α gene complex consists of more than 50 V_α gene segments, a long stretch of J gene segments, and 1 C_α gene segment. The TcR-δ locus is located within the TCR-α gene complex as shown and consists of many fewer V_δ (about 6), D_δ (3), J_δ (3), and 1C_δ gene segment. The TcR-β gene complex contains about 51 V_β gene segments grouped in 24 families and two C_β gene segments that are preceded by one D_β and six or seven J_β gene segments. The TcR-γ gene complex consists of two C_γ gene segments preceded by two or three J_γ gene segments and a restricted number of V_γ gene segments, which are grouped into four families as shown. (After Breit and van Dongen, 1994, with permission of the authors and publisher.)

magnitude in junctional diversity, resulting in approximate equal numbers of epitopes that can be recognized by immunoglobulins or the T cell α/β receptor (cf. Janeway and Travers, 1996). The γ/δ T-cell receptor diversity is very similar, but T-cell receptor genes appear to undergo no somatic hypermutations (cf. Raulet, 1989; Zheng et al., 1994), and they are usually not associated with CD4 and CD8 molecules (Pardoll et al., 1987; Raulet, 1989). Hypermutation of immunoglobulin genes also contributes to the diversity of immunoglobulin genes. This process increases with age and with reentry of memory B cells into the hypermutation process (cf. Neuberger and Milstein, 1995).

Cellular Interactions in the Immune Response

As already noted, the immune response involves several different types of cells (T and B lymphocytes), each of which has various forms as noted both by morphology and surface antigens. However, it is clear that the immune response involves many more different types of cells, their subtle interactions, and numerous protein signals termed *cytokines* or *lymphokines*, which regulate both the expression of specific genes as well as cell proliferation in the target cell. The relations of some of these cell types may be seen in Figure 19.12. In the figure, the developmental origin of T and B cells as well as macrophages from the bone marrow is depicted. The macrophage or antigen-presenting cell—which takes on various forms in tissues such as "dendritic" cells, monocytes, and sinusoidal-lining cells—plays a key role in cellular interactions in the im-

Table 19.2 Comparison of the Total Diversity of Immunoglobulins and of T Cell α/β Receptors in the Human

Element	Immunoglobulin		αβ Receptors	
	H	κ	α	β
Variable segments (V)	51	69	~70	52
Diversity segments (D)	~30	0	0	2
D segments read in three frames	rarely	–	–	often
Joining segments (J)	5	5	61	13
Joints with N and P nucleotides[a]	2	(1)	1	2
Number of V gene pairs	3519		640	
Junctional diversity	~10^{13}		~10^{13}	
Total diversity	~10^{16}		~10^{16}	

[a]During the recombination events leading to the ultimate immunoglobulin molecule, there occurs loss or addition of nucleotides at the recombination junctions. Additions of nucleotides at this junction fall into two categories: template-dependent (P nucleotides) and template-independent (N regions) (cf. Komori et al., 1993). N region addition may be effected by the enzyme, terminal deoxytransferase, in B cells (Desiderio et al., 1984).
From Janeway and Travers, 1996, with permission of the authors and publisher.

mune response. The mechanism of antigen processing and presentation will be considered below. Although antigens may interact directly with B cells to evoke or accelerate subsequent immune responses (see below), most foreign antigens, including tumor antigens, are first processed by one of several pathways. In the sequence of events that follow the presentation of the processed antigen by the macrophage to unstimulated T and B cells, the T cells play a major role. Some T cells, termed *helper* cells, interact with B cells in the presence of the antigen to stimulate the further differentiation of the B cell to the effector plasma cell that produces antibodies specifically reactive with the antigen (cf. Janeway and Travers, 1996). Such an inter-

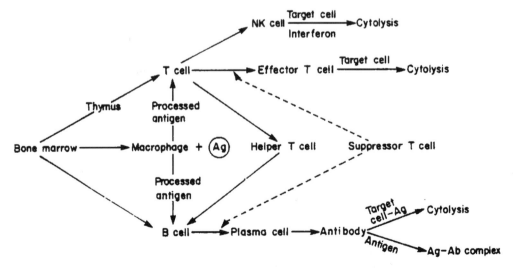

Figure 19.12 Pathways of cellular responses to a foreign antigen (Ag). The figure indicates the various cell types and their interactions with various other cell types as noted by the arrows.

action results in the elaboration by the helper T cell of a number of lymphokines which in turn stimulate the B or T recipient cell to proliferate, thus enhancing and accelerating the clonal expansion of the effector T or B cells. The effector or killer T cell has on its surface, along with the T-cell receptor, the CD8 coreceptor, as noted in Figure 19.13. The helper T cell has a similar structure but with the CD4 coreceptor in place of the CD8 molecule.

In addition to the coreceptors seen in Figure 19.13, it is now apparent that there are several different costimulatory receptors that interact between the antigen-presenting cell and the T lymphocyte. CD28 is a major costimulatory receptor on T cells, and B7 its costimulatory ligand on antigen-presenting cells (cf. Robey and Allison, 1995). Another regulatory molecule, CTLA-4, also occurring on the surface of T cells when interacting with B7, causes a block in the production of cytokines, cell cycle progression, and cell differentiation (cf. Lee et al., 1998).

Subgroups of T-Helper Cells

As we have noted above, a class of T cells appears to exist, the T suppressor cell population, whose function is to inhibit specific immune responses. In opposition to this, helper T cells enhance the immune response, both cell-mediated and humoral. However, it is now apparent that there are at least two different types of T-helper cells, known as Th1 and Th2, which are committed before antigenic stimulation (cf. Abbas et al., 1996). But the most potent differentiation-inducing stimuli are specific cytokines or lymphoid growth factors. Interleukin-12 (IL-12), produced by activated macrophages and dendritic cells, is the principal Th1-inducing cytokine, while IL-4 induces the development of Th2 cells. In turn, each of these classes of T-helper cells produces a variety of cytokines and exhibits functions as shown in Table 19.3.

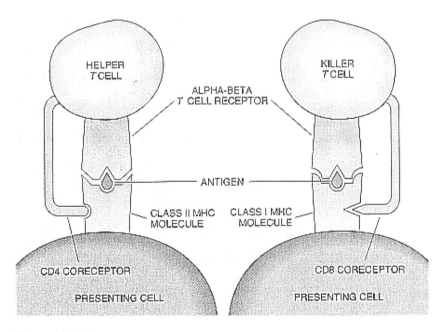

Figure 19.13   Diagram of the interaction of helper and killer (effector) T cells with presenting cells. The interaction involves the association of the T cell receptor and its coreceptor (CD4 or CD8) with the presentation of antigen in association with appropriate MHC (major histocompatibility complex) molecules (see below). (After von Boehmer and Kisielow, 1991, with permission of the authors and publisher.)

Table 19.3   Principal Features of Human CD4 T Cell Subsets

	T_H1	T_H2
Cytokines Produced		
Interferon-γ	+++	–
Tumor necrosis factor-β	+++	–
Interleukin-2	+++	– or +
Tumor necrosis factor-α	+++	+
Granulocyte-macrophage CSF	++	++
Interleukin-3	++	+++
Interleukin-10	– or +	+++
Interleukin-13	+	++
Interleukin-4	–	+++
Interleukin-5	–	+++
Functions		
B-cell help (total Ig)	+	+++
Help for IgE and IgG$_4$	–	+++
Eosinophil and mast cell differentiation and activation	–	+++
Macrophage activation	+++	–
Delayed-type hypersensitivity	+++	–
Cytolytic activity	+++	–

Adapted from Romagnani, 1994, with permission of the author and publisher.

T Cell–Independent B-Cell Response

As noted above, there is a subset of B lymphocytes, termed B1, that do not interact with T cells in order to produce antibodies. Such cells respond directly to antigens by their interaction with the B-cell receptor. B1 cells are usually not found in the bone marrow but rather home predominantly in the peritoneal and pleural cavities. Such cells recognize common bacterial antigens as well as self-antigens (cf. Fagarasan and Honjo, 2000). They appear to contribute to the mucosal immune response (Figure 19.3) and also in the production of autoantibodies.

Suppressor T Cells

Another population of T cells that is central to the regulation of the immune response is that of suppressor T cells. These cells modulate both T and B cell–effected immunity by suppressing the replication, maturation, and/or function of potential effector cells (Kapp et al., 1984). There has been some controversy with respect to their actual existence (Arnon and Teitelbaum, 1993). A number of suppressor T cells are antigen-specific, while others may suppress pathways by nonspecific cellular interactions (Kapp et al., 1984). Earlier studies have suggested that suppressor T cells are restricted—i.e., require an interaction by a specific gene product, that of the I-J gene in the mouse, which is involved in macrophage–T cell interactions (Dorf and Benacerraf, 1985; Hayes and Klyczek, 1985; Asano and Tada, 1989). The development of suppressor T cells involves many fewer antigen-presenting cells (macrophages) for their induction than T-helper cells (Dorf et al., 1992). In addition, there is substantial evidence that T-suppressor cells mediate the suppressor action via factors comparable to lymphokines (Dorf et al., 1992). These factors may include transforming growth factor-β (Chapter 16) and interleukin-10 (Mason and Powrie, 1998).

γδ T Cells

While the majority of T-cell receptors are made up of the α and β chains (greater than 90%), a small percentage (1% to 10%) of T cells express the heterodimer T-cell receptor consisting of γ and δ chains (Figure 19.11). While the function of these cells is not absolutely clear, it is noted that they do have distinct properties. They are relatively small cells that express almost no CD4 and considerably less CD8 than αβ T cells (cf. Kabelitz et al., 1999). Furthermore, the interaction of the γδ T cell with an antigen-presenting cell does not require the MHC molecules as do the αβ T cells, as noted in Figure 19.13. While their function is not clear at present, they do appear to express reactivity towards a variety of foreign, self, and neoplastic antigens.

Natural Killer Cells

Another subset of lymphocytes is the natural killer (NK) cells, which are shown in Figure 19.12 as derived from T cells. Other evidence suggests that these lymphocytes are unique and different in their origin from either T or B cells and thus likely derived in the bone marrow, like all other major players in the immune response (Lotzová, 1993). NK cells appear to function in graft rejection, tumor immunity, and the regulation of hematopoiesis (Robertson and Ritz, 1990). NK cells spontaneously react with cells exhibiting foreign antigens on their surface, but may also interact with specific carbohydrates on the cell surface (Brennan et al., 1995) as well as a variety of other surface targets (Storkus and Dawson, 1991). However, in contrast to cytotoxic T cells, NK cells not only do not require the presence of proteins of the MHC locus (see below) in order to exert their lytic effect but such proteins actually inhibit NK cells from interacting with cells containing such proteins. Such inhibition appears to be mediated by specific membrane receptors expressed on NK cells (cf. Lanier, 1998). In this way, NK cells complement the T- and B-cell repertoire of the cell-mediated and humoral responses that are restricted by the presence of such histocompatibility antigens (Gumperz and Parham, 1995; Reyburn et al., 1997). The production of NK cells in the host may also be enhanced by immunostimulatory agents such as interferon and lymphokines, especially interleukin-2 (Robertson and Ritz, 1990). Newborn humans are deficient in NK cell activity—a factor that may be involved in the peculiar immunological reactivity of neonates (Kaplan et al., 1982).

REGULATION OF THE IMMUNE RESPONSE

As noted in Figure 19.12, the development of the immune response is extremely complex but also must be highly regulated if the host is to mount an appropriate response to one or more specific antigens. The mechanisms of the regulation of the immune response involve the presence of specific surface gene products as well as the production of stimulatory and inhibitory signals both within the immunocyte and via signals secreted and received by cells in the immune response. These regulatory factors are considered below under several different headings.

Genetics in the Regulation of the Immune Response

While it is obvious that specific genes control the amino acid sequence of the immunoglobulins and T cell–receptor components involved in the immune response, the elucidation of the genetics involved in cellular interactions that mediate the immune response has also been a major topic of immunobiology. Many of the genes coding for products involved in the regulation of the immune response of the organism are located in regions of the genome designated as the major histocompatibility complex (MHC), located in the human on chromosome 6 (the HLA complex) and in the mouse on chromosome 17 (H-2 complex). A diagram of the major components of these two MHC regions is seen in Figure 19.14, along with a diagram of the protein structures of the major histocompatibility complex antigens. Class I antigens are ubiquitous and found on most cells within the organism. Class I molecules have a single integral membrane unit consisting of three domains—α1, α2, and α3—as shown in Figure 19.14. This molecule is in association noncovalently with β2 microglobulin, a 12 kDa soluble protein. This latter protein is, in the mouse, found on the H-3 minor histocompatibility locus present on chromosome 2 (Rammensee and Klein, 1983). The class II MHC antigen is a heterodimer of two transmembrane units, α (33 kDa) and β (29 kDa), both encoded in the MHC. Class II antigens are expressed primarily on B cells, macrophages, and all antigen-presenting cells as well as endothelium (cf. Germain, 1994). Recently, another set of MHC-like genes, termed the CD1 family, have been described. These genes appear to be involved in antigen presentation to a subset of phenotypically identifiable CD1-restricted T cells (cf. Park et al., 1998). In general, the antigens presented by this system involve glycolipid structures and related molecules (e.g., Prigozy et al., 2001).

Antigen Processing and Presentation in the Immune Response

As indicated earlier (Figure 19.5), a specific antibody reacts with a specific epitope or confirmation of a relatively small peptide unit or comparable structure within an antigen. While the struc-

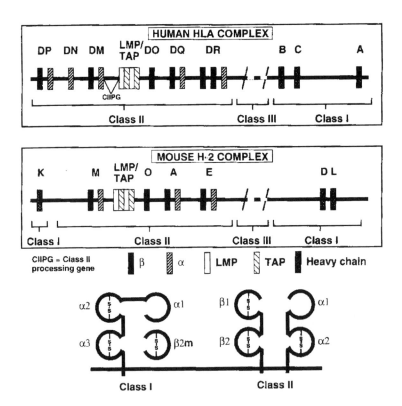

Figure 19.14 Schematic representations of the gene organization of the human HLA and mouse H-2 major histocompatibility complexes as well as cartoons of the class I and class II MHC antigen molecules with their domain organizations. Details of the class III regions of the MHC are not shown. It is in this region that other genes, especially those for complement, occur (cf. Claman, 1992). (After Germain, 1994, with permission of the author and publisher.)

ture of the antibody-combining region dictated a relatively small molecular size for the epitope, the mechanism for selection of the epitope by the antibody-producing cell as well as the T-cell receptor of the T lymphocyte was not clear. It is now apparent that this is dictated by the processing of antigens by antigen-presenting cells. In addition, antigen processing is required for the T-cell receptor to engage molecules of the MHC that are associated with a small polypeptide chain bearing the epitope. The receptor does not engage the antigen unless the antigen forms part of the complex involving the MHC molecule. This requirement of the interaction of the T-cell receptor with MHC molecules is termed *MHC restriction*. Such restriction then requires that for a T cell to become activated by processed antigens, there must be an interaction between the T-cell receptor and the peptide carried in the cleft of the MHC antigen. As noted earlier, exceptions to this restriction are δγ T cells and NK cells.

Since at least two sets of MHC molecules, class I and class II, are required for the recognition of protein antigens, other factors in such association and recognition are the CD8 and CD4 molecules on the surface of cytolytic and helper T lymphocytes respectively. In addition to CD8 and CD4 molecules, several other "costimulatory" molecules have been described that enhance the stimulation of the T cell interacting through its receptor with the polypeptide fragment carried by the MHC class 1 or class 2 antigen (cf. Jenkins, 1994; Yoshinaga et al., 1999).

While the processing and presentation of antigens are clearly effective in adult and developed tissues, there is evidence that neonatal macrophages are deficient in their ability to present antigen and express cell-surface MHC antigens (Lu and Unanue, 1985). Although T-cell differentiation in the thymus is presumably complete by 18 to 20 weeks of fetal life in the human, T cells of the newborn show a decreased potential to provide help and suppression for antibody production by B lymphocytes, and they do not develop into cytotoxic T lymphocytes (Hanson et al., 1997).

Mechanisms of Antigen Processing and Presentation

During the past several years it has become apparent that antigens from different locations vis-à-vis the cell are processed by somewhat different routes. A diagram of this is seen in Figure 19.15. As noted in the figure, peptides produced from endogenous cytosolic proteins that enter

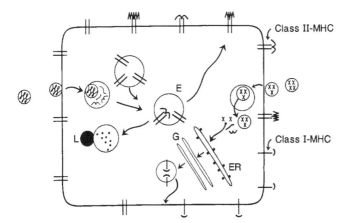

Figure 19.15 Pathways of antigen presentation by MHC class I and class II molecules. Antigens taken up into the cell are internalized into endosomes (E), where they are partially degraded and subsequently bind to class II MHC molecules and are thence transported to the cell surface. Proteins that either occur in the cytosol or migrate there from external sources (X) are processed by the proteasome, transported into the cisternae of the endoplasmic reticulum through the Golgi and subsequently to the surface. (Adapted from Unanue and Cerottini, 1989, with permission of the authors and publisher.)

the cytosol either endogenously or from exogenous sources, as noted, are processed probably through a structure known as the *proteasome*, which results in relatively short peptides of 10 to 20 amino acids length. These are transported through the membrane of the endoplasmic reticulum by a "transporter associated with antigen processing" (TAP). From thence the peptide associates with an MHC class I molecule occurring in the endoplasmic reticulum, the complex that is subsequently passed through the Golgi and ultimately expressed on the surface of the plasma membrane (Germain, 1994; Unanue and Cerottini, 1989). Within the proteosome are components, LMP proteins, which appear to alter the substrate specificity of the protein degradation occurring in the proteosome, favoring cleavage near residues suitable for binding of the peptide within the "pocket" or "cleft" of class I MHC molecules. Proteins to be processed for presentation in MHC class II molecules are those internalized from the exterior into endosomes, where they are partially degraded and subsequently bound to the "cleft" of class II MHC molecules and then exteriorized by fusion of the endosome to the plasma membrane. A diagram of the peptide-binding clefts of class I and class II MHC molecules is seen in Figure 19.16. The overall structure of the MHC class I and class II molecules as shown in Figure 19.16 is strikingly similar to the antibody-reactive site of immunoglobulins (Figures 19.2 and 19.5). However, the molecular diversity of the MHC molecules is much less than that of the immunoglobulins, numbering only in the hundreds (Le Bouteiller, 1994).

Regulation of the Expression of MHC Genes

Just as with the expression of immunoglobulin genes (see above), the expression of MHC genes can also be modified by a variety of different factors. Several endogenous materials—most notably some of the interferons and the tumor necrosis factor-α (TNF-α), previously discussed in Chapter 15—induce MHC class I gene expression in a variety of cell types (cf. David-Watine et al., 1990) including brain cells (Wong et al., 1984). Chemical inducers of differentiation such as sodium butyrate or hexamethylene bisacetamide may also amplify the expression of MHC class I antigens (Fenig et al., 1993).

Among the principal exogenous factors regulating the expression of MHC antigens are viruses, both oncogenic and nononcogenic (cf. Maudsley and Pound, 1991). In the majority of instances, especially of oncogenic viruses, the effects are to downregulate the expression of both

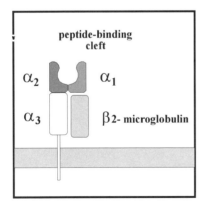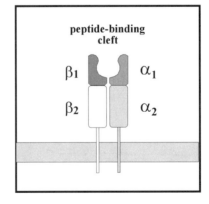

Figure 19.16 Diagrams of the class I (left) and class II (right) molecules of the MHC showing the peptide-binding cleft and the subunit association thereof. (Adapted from Janeway and Travers, 1996, with permission of the authors and publisher.)

class I and class II MHC antigens. Some viruses, even including HIV, actually upregulate the expression of MHC class II antigens. The importance of this effect in the interaction of the host immune system with neoplastic cells is outlined later in this chapter.

Signaling Pathways and Lymphocyte Activation

As noted earlier, the interaction of T-helper and -suppressor lymphocytes with both T cells and B cells results in the secretion and release of a variety of factors, most of which are components of the cytokine system, some of whose members are indicated in Table 19.4. The table is not meant

Table 19.4 Some Examples of Specific Cytokines—Their Sources and Activities

Cytokine	Cellular Sources	Major Activities
Interleukin-1	Macrophages	Activation of T cells and macrophages; promotion of inflammation
Interleukin-2	Type 1 (Th1) helper T cells	Activation of lymphocytes, natural killer cells, and macrophages
Interleukin-4	Type 2 (Th2) helper T cells, mast cells, basophils, and eosinophils	Activation of lymphocytes, monocytes, and IgE class switching
Interleukin-5	Type 2 (Th2) helper T cells, mast cells, and eosinophils	Differentiation of eosinophils
Interleukin-6	Type 2 (Th2) helper T cells and macrophages	Activation of lymphocytes; differentiation of B cells; stimulation of the production of acute-phase proteins
Interleukin-8	T cells and macrophages	Chemotaxis of neutrophils, basophils, and T cells
Interleukin-11	Bone marrow stromal cells	Stimulation of the production of acute-phase proteins
Interleukin-12	Macrophages and B cells	Stimulation of the production of interferon-γ by type 1 (Th1) helper T cells and by natural killer cells; induction of type 1 (Th1) helper T cells
Tumor necrosis factor-α	Macrophages, natural killer cells, T cells, B cells, and mast cells	Promotion of inflammation
Lymphotoxin (tumor necrosis factor β)	Type 1 (Th1) helper T cells and B cells	Promotion of inflammation
Transforming growth factor β	T cells, macrophages, B cells, and mast cells	Immunosuppression
Granulocyte-macrophage colony-stimulating factor	T cells, macrophages, natural killer cells, and B cells	Promotion of the growth of granulocytes and monocytes
Interferon-α	Virally infected cells	Induction of resistance of cells to viral infection
Interferon-β	Virally infected cells	Induction of resistance of cells to viral infection
Interferon-γ	Type 1 (Th1) helper T cells and natural killer cells	Activation of macrophages; inhibition of type 2 (Th2) helper T cells

Adapted from Delves and Roitt, 2000, with permission of the authors and publisher.

to be exhaustive, since other cytokines—including other interleukins, hematopoietic factors, thymus hormones, and somatic growth factors—could be included (Borecký, 1993). Most of the cytokines have specific receptors, and thus their interaction with such molecules on a cell surface can result in the initiation of signal pathways and alteration of gene expression involving a variety of genes including the MHC class I and II antigens, protein kinases, guanylate-binding proteins, and even tumor-associated antigens (Borecký, 1993).

Another major consequence of cytokine release and interaction with specific receptors is cell proliferation. Interleukin-2 or the T-cell growth factor is one of the major cytokines released during T-cell interactions involving MHC molecules and the T-cell receptor. As with other interactions of ligands with their receptors, a series of reactions is initiated involving signal transduction mechanisms very similar to those described in Chapters 7 and 15. In Table 19.5 are listed the major events involved in T-lymphocyte activation from the time that cell-cell interaction occurs until proliferation of the T lymphocyte ensues. A similar sort of pathway is involved in the activation of B lymphocytes (DeFranco, 1993).

A diagram of signal transduction pathways in T lymphocytes may be seen in Figure 19.17. In the figure the function of the costimulatory protein, CD28, as well as the CD4/CD8 interaction is shown. Obviously, all of these factors are involved in the signal transduction pathway leading to the activation of transcription factors in the nucleus, altered gene expression, and ultimately cell proliferation. As noted above, the activation of T cells as well as that of D cells by mechanisms shown in Figure 19.17 and Table 19.5, leads to the production of various cytokines such as those listed in Table 19.4. Many of these cytokines, especially the interleukins and interferons, interact with specific receptors on target cells such as other T cells and B cells to further stimulate gene transcription and cell replication. As indicated earlier with TNF-α and TGF-β, signal transduction pathways differ in their effector molecules. In the case of interferons and interleukins, the signal transduction pathway involves protein kinases termed JAKs as well as

Table 19.5   Major Events Involved in T-Lymphocyte Activation

Event	Example
Cell–cell interaction	T-cell—APC
	T cell—target cell
Receptor–ligand binding	TCR-antigen/MHC
Transmembrane signal transduction	Activation of protein tyrosine kinase
Tyrosine phosphorylation	Phospholipase C γ1
Generation of second messengers	1,4,5-IP$_3$ and DG
Second messenger effects	Ca^{2+} mobilization
	Protein kinase C activation
Biochemical pathways	Raf-1 kinase activation, MAP kinase cascade
	Intracellular alkalinization
Cellular events	Cytoskeletal reorganization
	Secretion of cytolytic granules
Early transcriptional factor gene activation	c-*myc*, c-*fos*
Intermediate gene activation	Lymphokines, lymphokine receptors, nutrient receptors
Late gene activation	Genes involved in cell proliferation

Adapted from Weiss, 1993, with permission of the author and publishers.

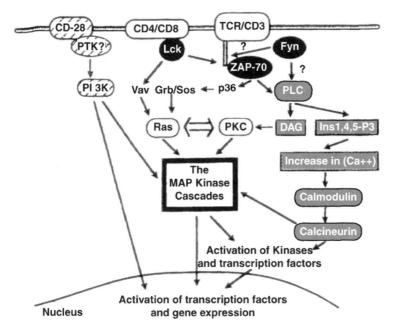

Figure 19.17 Signal transduction pathways in T lymphocytes. Not all known interactions with various costimulatory molecules and other cellular components are shown in the figure for simplicity. The principal events involved are ultimately the activation of transcription factors through the MAP kinase cascades (Chapter 7). As seen in this figure, the costimulatory molecule CD28 signals via a protein tyrosine kinase (PTK) and phosphoinositide kinase. Activation of the T cell receptor (TCR) is also mediated through tyrosine and MAP kinases. The CD4 or CD8 molecule is bound to the tyrosine kinase Lck, which phosphorylates TCR enabling another tyrosine kinase, Zap-70, to bind to the T-cell receptor complex and become localized to the membrane. Zap-70 activates phospholipase C, resulting in increased diacylglycerol and inositol 1,4,5-P$_3$ levels. These latter changes result in a calcium-activated pathway which together with the other pathways shown can activate the MAP kinase cascade. The different pathways are also indicated by the different shading of their components as noted. (Adapted from Hardy and Chaudhri, 1997, with permission of the authors and publisher.)

STAT proteins which are phosphorylated, bind to each other and translocate directly to the nucleus in a fashion somewhat similar to that of the Smads seen in signal transduction with TGF-β (Figure 16.8; Heim, 1999).

Effecting the Immune Response

As noted from Figure 19.12, the effective response of the humoral immune system involves either interaction of antibodies with cells or antigens, the antigen-antibody complex being then effectively phagocytosed by appropriate scavenger cells such as macrophages in the instance of nonviable particles—or the reaction of the antibody with an antigen on the cell surface to which proteins of the complement system adhere—with subsequent formation of pores through the action of a component of complement, C9, also termed perforin (Lowin et al., 1992).

Cytotoxic T cells when interacting with target cells exhibiting the specific epitope to which they are sensitive and the presence of the MHC class I antigen result in a series of reactions depicted in Figure 19.18, which include the formation of pores as with antigen-antibody-complement reactions noted above, as well as other mechanisms involving the direct induction of apoptosis by specific surface molecules. In addition, cytolytic T cells on interaction with the MHC-antigen epitope via the T-cell receptor produce granules filled with various lytic enzymes, which pass through the pores and further serve to cause apoptosis in the target cell (Figure 19.18).

For some years the exception to this mechanism was the NK cell which did not require MHC complex antigens for its action in causing apoptosis in target cells. NK cells do not express the T-cell receptor on their surface, although they may express other surface molecules involved in the T-cell antigen receptor complex such as components of CD3 and the Fc receptor. Furthermore, NK cells do not require expression of MHC class I molecules on the surface of their targets; rather, they are inhibited from killing cells expressing such molecules (see above). NK cells use a cytolytic machinery somewhat similar to that of specific cytolytic T cells (Figure 19.18), especially the perforin pathway (van den Broek et al., 1998). Investigations by Yokoyama (1995) do suggest that recognition of MHC class I molecules by NK cells may be involved in their cytolytic effects since the initial responses of NK cells to the target cell occur in the presence of MHC class I molecules on the target cell surface. It is likely that other molecules, some of which have yet to be defined, may allow the cytolytic effect of the NK cell to reach certain targets while protecting others.

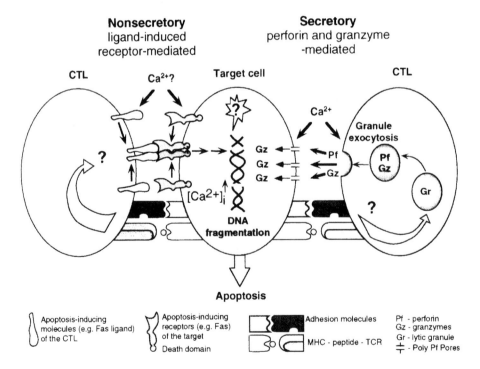

Figure 19.18 Mechanisms of lymphocyte-mediated cytolysis. The figure is a schematic diagram of the nonsecretory receptor (left) and the secretory, perforin/granzyme-mediated (right) mechanisms of lymphocytotoxicity. (After Berke, 1995, with permission of the author and publisher.)

IMMUNOBIOLOGY OF NEOPLASIA

The experimental and theoretical basis for the field of immunobiology of neoplasia did not become reasonably established until after 1950, despite studies on tumor transplantation as discussed below. The observation by Foley in 1953 that mouse neoplasms may be immunogenic for their host as well as a reformulation by Thomas in 1959 of the theory of immune surveillance first proposed by Ehrlich in 1909 formed major aspects of the beginnings of an understanding of the immunobiology of the host-tumor relationship (cf. Brodt, 1983). Although, over the last half century, there has been considerable clinical promise of the utilization of the immunobiology of the host–tumor relationship in the control and therapy of neoplasia (cf. Scott and Cebon, 1997), such promise has never been effectively realized. In fact, some investigators questioned the significance of any major role that tumor immunology may play in ultimate therapeutic ventures (cf. Chigira et al., 1993). Despite these conflicting ideas and approaches to this problem, there is no question but that the host immune system does interact with malignant neoplasms in a variety of ways. However, as shown further on, in most instances the neoplasm effectively escapes from any definitive resistance of the host to the presence of the neoplasm, despite the fact that neoplasms clearly express antigens recognized by the host immune system and that definitive responses are produced.

Tumor Antigens

Ever since the early reports by Nowinsky (1876) and Hanau (1889) of the transplantation of cancer tissue in dogs and rats, respectively (in contrast to the failure of many others to achieve such results at that time), the antigenicity of neoplastic cells has been recognized. Since then numerous examples of tumor transplantation both within individuals and even between species have been reported. In considering the antigenicity of tissue transplantation, certain terms should be defined (Roitt, 1977). An *autograft* is tissue grafted from one site to another in the same individual. *Isograft* designates transplantation between *syngeneic* individuals (that is, of identical genetic constitution), such as identical twins or animals of the same pure inbred line. *Allografts* are transplants between *allogeneic* individuals (that is, members of the same species having different genetic constitutions), for example, transplants between unrelated humans or from one animal strain to another of the same species. A *xenograft* is a transplant (graft) between *xenogeneic* individuals (that is, of different species), for example, pig to human.

When considering the antigenic structure of neoplasms, the critical question is whether the antigenicity of neoplasms is different in any way from that of their cells of origin. Early investigations in this field with inbred mice and hydrocarbon-induced sarcomas showed that immunological resistance of the host to the syngeneic neoplasm could be established, although no immunological response could be obtained to certain spontaneously arising neoplasms (Klein and Klein, 1977; Ritts and Neel, 1974). As a result of these studies, Prehn (1973) and Klein (1973), utilizing whole-animal experiments, were able to demonstrate that chemically induced and transplanted neoplasms evoke specific reactions of the cellularly mediated type (T cell) in recipient or host animals. A diagram of the methodology utilized to demonstrate the biological effect of such antigens is given in Figure 19.19. The antigens evoking such reactions were termed tumor-specific transplantation antigens (TSTA) and, more recently, tumor-associated transplantation antigens (TATA) (cf. Brodt, 1983; Herberman, 1977). For the demonstration of such antigens, it was important to utilize neoplasms of recent origin, since serial passage through many generations caused neoplasms to undergo antigenic changes by mechanisms not totally understood but quite possibly related to the phenomenon of tumor progression with karyotypic

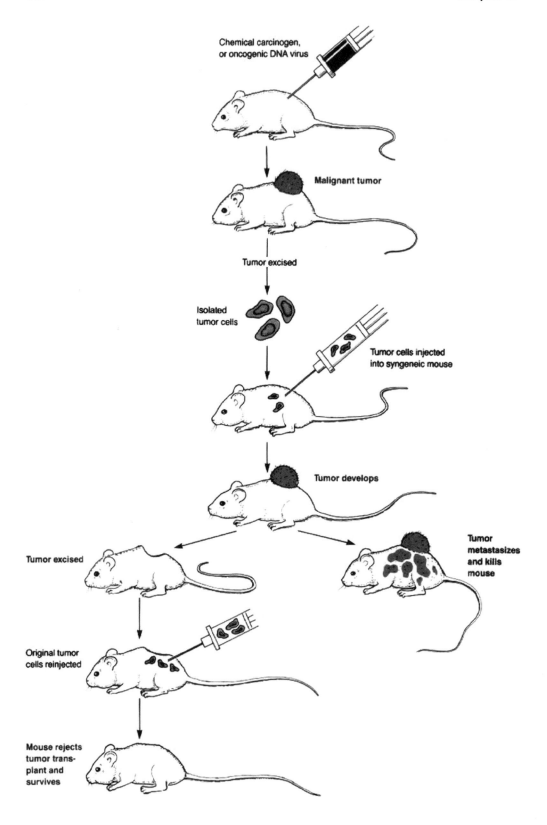

alterations (Chapter 8). The TSTAs appeared to be complex surface antigens, which are lost upon destruction of the surface membrane of the cell. Klein (1973) also made the interesting observation that TSTAs of chemically induced neoplasms were essentially unique to each neoplasm, whereas those of virally induced neoplasms were identical for each virus. Furthermore, it is clear that the TSTAs of virus-induced cancers are quite distinct from the S and T antigens mentioned earlier in the discussion on viral oncology (Chapter 4). Each neoplasm produced by radiation also appears to have its own unique tumor-specific transplantation antigen. The TSTAs of chemically or radiation-induced neoplasms are in no way related to the specific chemical agent or type of radiation causing the neoplasm, because a single chemical or the same wavelength of radiation can be shown to induce numerous primary neoplasms in one animal, each neoplasm having a different TSTA. Since the original findings of Prehn, Klein, and their associates, there have been reports of chemically induced tumors that do contain common TSTAs (or TATAs) on the basis that immunization of a host with one neoplasm led to some protection against challenge by other neoplasms (cf. Herberman, 1977). Some of these findings might be explained by more recent results, as discussed below.

Neoplasms arising spontaneously in animals fail to elicit a specific immunological resistance in the transplantation tests in syngeneic animals (cf. Brodt, 1983). Occasionally a resistance reaction is found, but it is invariably weak, and some investigators argue that, because of this finding, spontaneous tumors do have TSTAs but that, for practical purposes, they are not sufficiently antigenic to stimulate specific immunologic resistance in the host.

Little is actually known about the chemical nature of TSTAs; however, they may represent the cumulative antigenicity of a number of surface components of the cell, and this allows the host to recognize such a structure as foreign. MHC antigens, while required for the T-cell response, do not appear to be significant components of the TSTAs, and the expression of "alien antigens" on neoplastic cells does not appear to constitute a significant biological phenomenon (Parham, 1989).

Following the discovery of tumor-specific transplantation antigens, T-cell immunity has been recognized as the predominant immune response with the potential to significantly influence the outcome of neoplastic disease and probably other diseases as well (Shu et al., 1997). A number of antigens produced by neoplasms that may induce the T cell responses are listed in Table 19.6. As would be expected, viral gene products that are foreign to the host's immune system can stimulate T-cell responses, as noted in the table; most T-cell responses to viral gene products would utilize the MHC class I pathway (Figure 19.15). The SV40 T antigen, which occurs primarily in the nucleus, does in fact induce T-cell responses, and there is evidence that T antigen also occurs on the cell surface (Mora, 1982). This finding, together with the evidence for T cell–mediated responses to some of the early gene products of the SV40 virus, has been suggested as composing the TSTA of neoplasms induced by this virus (Dalianis, 1990). Cellular oncogenes, specifically the *ras* mutant proteins, can induce MHC class II–restricted T cells capable of recognizing the mutations (Peace et al., 1993). Presumably this occurs as a result of apoptosis of neoplastic cells bearing the mutated protein, which are then engulfed by antigen-

Figure 19.19 Diagram of methodology utilized to determine the presence and, by subsequent experiments, the specificity of a tumor-specific transplantation antigen. The neoplastic cells under study are injected into a syngeneic mouse with subsequent development of the neoplasm that may metastasize and kill the animal. Excision of the neoplasm before it has metastasized (lower left) allows the rejection of a second implant of the same neoplasm, presumably as a consequence of the immunity acquired from exposure to the original transplant. (Adapted from Rubin and Farber, 1988, with permission of the authors and publisher.)

Table 19.6 Antigens of Neoplasms That May Induce T-Cell Responses

Tumor Antigen	Examples of Occurrence
Tumor-specific transplantation antigens (TSTA)	Carcinogen and radiation-induced neoplasms (unique to neoplasm)
Viral gene products	Viral-induced neoplasms (unique to virus species inducing the neoplasm); EBNA of EBV, papilloma virus E6 and E7 gene products, SV40 T antigen
Cellular oncogene products	p21 *ras* mutations, *bcr/abl* fusion gene
Tumor suppressor gene mutant products	p53, β catenin
Overexpressed normal gene products	HER-2/neu protein in ovarian/breast cancer
Fetal antigens/testis	MAGE-1 in melanoma, GAGE
Tissue differentiation antigens	Tyrosinase and MART-1/MELANA in melanoma, thyroid peroxidase in thyroid neoplasia

presenting cells, and the peptide is presented to T cells. The BCR-ABL fusion cellular oncogene may likewise be induced to cause MHC class II–restricted T cells responsive to specific peptides of the chimeric protein (Chen et al., 1992). Both cellular and humoral immune responses to the mutated (Houbiers et al., 1993) and wild-type (Röpke et al., 1996) p53 gene product have been demonstrated in mice and humans. Although β catenin may be more properly considered a proto-oncogene, its association with the APC tumor suppressor gene (Figure 15.2) that regulates its degradation in association with other proteins (Kawahara et al., 2000) may place it in the suppressor gene category. Melanomas have been described having β catenin mutations that result in the stabilization of the mutated protein, thus favoring the transcriptional pathway seen in Figure 15.2 (Van den Eynde and van der Bruggen, 1997). Even normal gene products that are overexpressed in neoplastic cells may induce a T cell–mediated response. One of the best examples is the HER-2/neu gene, which codes for an epidermal growth factor–like receptor (see below).

During the last decade, with the realization of the processing of antigens and their presentation to T cells, investigations have attempted to isolate and characterize the peptides of antigens on neoplastic cells that are presented to the T-cell antigen receptor. A family of such genes whose products are expressed in a variety of neoplasms is seen in Table 19.7. The gene products recognized are specific peptides from the entire protein antigen. The only normal tissues expressing these genes appear to be the testis and placenta (cf. Van den Eynde and Boon, 1997). These genes appear to be methylated in most normal cells, and their expression in neoplastic cells may be the result of a genome-wide demethylation seen in neoplastic cells (Chapter 16). A number of differentiation antigens occurring in specific neoplastic cell types as well as their cell of origin have also been found to induce T-cell responses, several of which occur in melanomas but also in other tissues as noted in the table. In fact, several other melanoma differentiation antigens have been described that induce T cell–mediated responses (cf. Rosenberg, 1996; Van den Eynde and van der Bruggen, 1997). Some of these may be responsible for the relative efficacy of immunotherapy with this particular type of neoplasm (see below).

It should be noted that, within the last several years, the methods developed allow the identification of antigenic peptides presented by MHC class I molecules to tumor-specific cytolytic T cells. Both genetic and peptide purification methodologies have been utilized; the reader is referred to specific references for the techniques involved (De Plaen et al., 1997; Cox et al., 1994). With such techniques and others that will undoubtedly be developed in the future, it is becoming increasingly likely that T cell–mediated immunity to specific antigens in specific neoplasms may be enhanced on a rational basis.

Table 19.7 Expression of Genes MAGE-1, -3, BAGE, GAGE, and RAGE in Samples of Human Neoplasms[a]

Histological Type	Percentage of Tumors Positive for				
	MAGE-1	MAGE-3	BAGE	GAGE-1, 2	RAGE-1
Melanomas					
Primary lesions	16	36	8	13	2
Metastases	48	76	26	28	5
Non-small-cell lung carcinomas	49	47	4	19	0
Head and neck tumors	28	49	8	19	2
Bladder carcinomas	22	36	15	12	5
Sarcomas	14	24	6	25	14
Mammary carcinomas	18	11	10	9	1
Prostatic carcinomas	15	15	0	10	0
Colorectal carcinomas	2	17	0	0	0
Renal carcinomas	0	0	0	0	2
Leukemias and lymphomas	0	0	0	1	0
Testicular seminomas	4/6	3/6	1/6	5/6	0/3

[a]Expression was measured by reverse transcriptase-polymerase chain reaction on total RNA using primers specific for each gene.
Adapted from Van den Eynde and Boon, 1997, with permission of the authors and publisher.

Antigens of Neoplastic Cells Inducing Humoral Responses

Although, as indicated above, the most effective immune response to neoplasms in the host appears to be that of cellular immunity dependent on T-cell responses, a variety of antigens of neoplasms have been described that either induce the formation of antibodies within the host or can be used as antigens to produce antibodies, usually in xenogeneic hosts, which then may be used as reagents in attempts to kill specific neoplastic cells in vivo. In Table 19.8 is a listing of a number of antigens associated with neoplastic cells that are reactive with specific antibodies or induce B-cell humoral immune responses. As noted in the table, a number of differentiation an-

Table 19.8 Antigens of Neoplastic Cells That Induce B-Cell Humoral Responses

Tumor Antigen	Examples of Occurrence
Differentiation antigens (e.g., CD10, CD19, CD20, CD33, CD45, thyroid peroxidase, smooth muscle antigen)	Leukemias/lymphomas; thyroid carcinoma, sarcomas
Glycoproteins (e.g., CEA, TAG-72, Eplam, A33, MUC1, G250)	Colon cancer and other adenocarcinomas
Glycolipids (e.g., gangliosides, GD2 and GD3, etc.)	Melanoma, neuroblastoma and astrocytoma
Glycoprotein carbohydrate chains (e.g., Lewis monosaccharide antigens)	Gastric and colon cancers
Growth-factor receptors (e.g., EGFR, HER2/neu)	Breast and ovarian cancer
Embryonal antigens	SOX genes expressed in small-cell lung cancer

tigens from the *clusters of differentiation* (CD) that normally occur on lymphoid cells and other immunocytes may be expressed at high levels in individual neoplasms. Such antigens can induce an antibody response as well as the formation of monoclonal antibodies (Chapter 14). Of the CD antigens seen on the surface of leukemias and lymphomas, one that was extensively studied more than a decade ago, CD10 or the CALLA (common acute lymphoblastic leukemia antigen), is perhaps the best known. This antigen, which actually is a membrane-associated neutral metal-loendopeptidase (Shipp et al., 1989), was the target of immunotherapy with specific antibodies (cf. LeBien and McCormack, 1989). Thyroid peroxidase, a major differentiation antigen of thyroid carcinomas, as noted in Table 19.6, also induces the formation of circulating antibodies in 25% to 50% of patients with thyroid carcinoma (cf. Baker and Fosso, 1993). Earlier studies (Moore and Hughes, 1973) demonstrated circulating antibodies to a smooth muscle protein in 45% of patients with sarcomas. Interestingly, about one-third of normal human adult sera tested (Ollert et al., 1996) contain a natural IgM antibody cytotoxic for human neuroblastoma cells. The antigen appears to be a 260-kDa antigen expressed on neuroblastoma cells in vivo. This natural humoral immunological host tumor relationship may be associated with the in vivo phenomenon of spontaneous neuroblastoma regression (Carlsen, 1990; Evans et al., 1976). The variety of glycoproteins that occur on the surface7 of cells have also been utilized for the development of both cell-mediated and antibody responses. We have discussed the carcinoembryonic antigen (CEA) gene expression as a marker for gastrointestinal neoplasia (Chapter 17). Another interesting potential for immunotherapy is the fact that many epithelial cells lining ducts and glands express MUC1, a cell-associated mucin. In the normal cells this protein is fully glycosylated, usually on a specific region of the cell as shown in Figure 19.20. In contrast, as briefly discussed in Chapter 16, glycosylation of proteins on neoplastic surfaces many times is incomplete and/or abnormal. This is shown in the figure on the right as a neoplastic cell expressing MUC1 as well as the MHC class I molecule, but with the MUC1 markedly underglycosylated. In this way, components of the protein that are normally not seen by the immune system because of glycosylation now become apparent, and the immune system responds with the formation of antibodies as well as cell-mediated immunity. Also, as briefly discussed in Chapter 16, glycolipids may appear as unique structures on the surface of neoplastic cells because of the abnormalities in the expression of genes coding for enzymes that normally produce the structure of the glycolipid, especially gangliosides (Lloyd, 1993). Alteration in the structure of mucins may also play other roles in host–tumor relationships as well as in neoplastic progression (cf. Irimura et al., 1999). Specific carbohydrate structures as components of glycoproteins on the surface of cells have also been shown to induce antibodies. The Lewis monosaccharide antigens are among these, and just as with the mucoproteins (Figure 19.20), alterations in the level of enzymes catalyzing the specific formation of terminal carbohydrate structures result in alteration in antigenicity and the potential for such an immune response (Feizi and Childs, 1985). The Her-2/neu protein on mammary and ovarian cancer cells induces not only T cell–mediated immunity (Table 19.6) but also B-cell humoral immunity (Disis and Cheever, 1997). The expression of this gene product is extremely high in the majority of mammary lesions, and thus specific or monoclonal antibodies are now being used clinically as a therapy for this type of neoplasm (see below). Similarly, melanoma antigens induce antibodies within patients as well as those immunized with genetically modified autologous neoplastic cells (Cai and Garen, 1995). A tumor-specific antigen in human glioblastoma multiforme as defined by monoclonal antibodies has also been described (de Tribolet and Carrel, 1980). A series of embryonic neural proteins expressed from the 50 K genes that are highly immunogenic have also been described in small-cell lung cancers in humans which induce B cell-mediated responses in vivo (Güre et al., 2000).

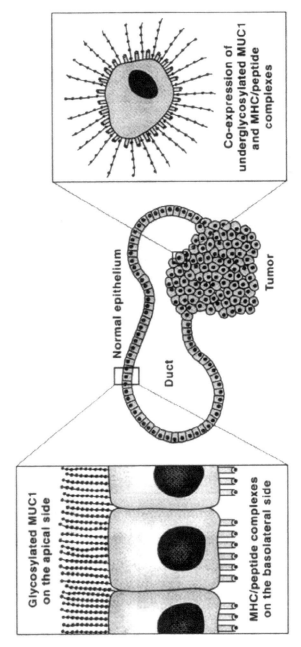

Figure 19.20 Changes in the level of expression, distribution, and glycosylation of MUC1 occurring in neoplastic as compared with normal ductular epithelium. (Adapted from Finn and Gendler, 1998, with permission of the authors and publisher.)

Table 19.9 Integrated Immune Response to Human Tumor Antigens

Antigen	CD8+ T cell	CD4+ T cell	B cell
gp75[a]	+		+
Tyrosinase	+	+	+
MART-1/MELAN A	+		
MAGE family	+		+
GAGE family	+		
BAGE	+		
Her2/neu	+	+	+
p53	+		+
Mutant Ras	+	+	+
E6/E7	+		+
MUC-I	+		+

[a]gp75 is another differentiation antigen of melanomas (cf. Van den Eynde and van der Bruggen, 1997). Adapted from Sahin et al., 1997, with permission of the author and publisher.

Even circulating antibodies to the p53 protein have frequently been found in the serum of some patients with ovarian carcinoma (Angelopoulou et al., 1996).

In the past, several of the antigens listed in Table 19.8 were considered as tumor-specific antigens (TSA) that were unique to the histogenetic type or class of neoplasm. In the table, this would include thyroid peroxidase and smooth muscle antigen as well as several of the melanoma antigens. While it was felt that these TSAs were relatively unique to the neoplasm expressing such antigens and that primarily humoral responses were evoked by their presence, today this distinction has become less clear, as noted below (Table 19.9).

From this brief discussion of tumor antigens and the responses they induce, it is apparent that neoplastic cells can and do stimulate immune responses within the host. Furthermore, although separated for the sake of convenience, the reader will note that many antigens induce both T- and B-cell responses, as seen in Table 19.9. It is thus likely that the immune system is quite capable and effective in producing both T- and B-cell responses to specific antigens of neoplastic cells. As noted above, apoptosis of neoplastic cells enhances such reactions by the engulfment of internal antigens of neoplastic cells with subsequent processing and presentation through the MHC class II pathway. However, given the considerable antigenicity of neoplastic cells and the effectiveness of the host immune system until the terminal stages of the disease (see below), how is it that the immunobiology of the host-tumor relationship predominantly favors the neoplasm?

FAILURE OF THE IMMUNOBIOLOGIC HOST–TUMOR RELATIONSHIP

Since it is in the stage of progression that most of our knowledge of the immunobiology of the host–tumor relationship has been gained, it is perhaps not surprising that neoplasms have exhibited a variety of methodologies with which to escape the host immune response. As we shall see, it is not unlikely that evolving karyotypic instability, the hallmark of the stage of progression, may be the basis for many of the mechanisms of the failure of the immunobiological host–tumor relation. In a very real sense, as has been so aptly stated, "The tumor fakes out the host." The variety of modes and mechanisms whereby the neoplasm escapes the host immune response is exemplified in Table 19.10.

Table 19.10 Mechanisms of Evasion of the Immune System by Neoplasms

---

1. Host may not express appropriate or sufficient MHC molecules to bind and present antigen
2. MHC expression may be downregulated or ineffective
    Virus infections
    Cellular oncogenes
3. Neoplasms may express antigens in a tolerable form
    Neonatal tolerance (like self)
    Lack of proper costimulators, B7-1 and/or B7-2 leading to anergy
    Clonal deletion
4. Antigen modulation
    "Hiding" of the antigen from antibodies that then do not destroy the cell
5. Antigen masking
    Glycosylated molecules that are produced at high levels in tumor cells and/or α globulins produced
        by host. These molecules can surround the tumor antigen so that it is inaccessible to the immune
        cells. Neoplasms can shield themselves in a fibrin "cocoon" by activating a coagulating system.
    "Blocking" antibodies
    Complement resistance
6. Antigens shed by neoplasm can interact with other immune responses (mechanism unknown)
7. Induction by suppressor cells that downregulate T_{helper} cells. Th2 cells > Th1 cells
    "Sneaking through" by small neoplasms—insufficient antigen to trigger cytolytic immune response,
        but may trigger $T_{suppressor}$ cells
8. Immunosuppression may be induced by products of the neoplasm or other chemical, physical, or viral
    agents
    TGFβ is secreted by many neoplasms and inhibits many lymphocyte and macrophage functions
    Fas ligand production by neoplastic cells
    Prostaglandin production by neoplastic cells

Alterations in MHC Expression and Structure in Neoplasia

As briefly discussed above, some workers had reported the occurrence of "alien" MHC molecules on the surface of neoplastic cells. While this concept is open for discussion, there are several concrete examples of altered expression and structure of MHC molecules on neoplastic
cells. Mutations within both HLA class I genes (Koopman et al., 1999) as well as class II determinants (cf. Möller and Hämmerling, 1992) have been described. In addition, alterations in
chromatin structure of the MHC genes in neoplasms of mice have been described (Maschek et
al., 1989). A somewhat unique mechanism for neoplastic cells to escape MHC restricted toxicity
is the expression of HLA antigens that normally are expressed only on the placenta, specifically
HLA-G. This MHC form apparently does not function well in antigen presentation for the remainder of the cell types in the organism, but does prevent the action of natural killer (NK) lymphocytes in effecting the destruction of neoplastic cells that do not express other HLA forms
(see below; Paul et al., 1998). In some instances, neoplastic cells express very low levels of
MHC class I determinants in amounts that are insufficient to trigger a normal T-cell response
(Cohen and Kim, 1994). Furthermore, in experimental situations prostaglandins downregulate
the expression of specific MHC antigens in neoplastic cells (Arvind et al., 1995).

   Far more common than the few examples given above is the fact that the majority of neoplasms do not express or downregulate MHC class I and class II antigens. One of the earliest
recognitions of this fact was the finding that cells transformed by adenovirus type 12 have a
markedly reduced or almost absent expression of MHC class I antigens after infection (Bernards
et al., 1983). As a result, such cells were not recognized by the immune system because of the

failure to present antigenic peptides in the MHC molecules to the T-cell receptor. Following this finding, a variety of other viral infections have been shown to produce similar effects by a variety of different mechanisms (cf. Rinaldo, 1994). A sample of the frequency of MHC downregulation in human neoplasms may be noted in Table 19.11, which depicts a large number of neoplasms from a variety of different histogenetic origins (Algarra et al., 1997). The loss of expression of MHC antigens is also associated with the natural history of neoplastic development. Marx et al. (1996) demonstrated that the majority of adrenocortical adenomas still express MHC class II antigens, whereas such expression is abrogated in all of the carcinomas of this tissue that were examined. Similarly, metastases from primary melanotic lesions exhibited a greater downregulation of HLA class I antigen expression, as well as molecules necessary in the pathway of antigen presentation (Kageshita et al., 1999). This loss of MHC antigen expression in the stage of progression is seen diagrammatically in Figure 19.21, as evidenced from immunohistochemical studies of the development of lesions from the stage of promotion to that of progression (Garrido et al., 1993).

Mechanisms of Altered MHC Expression

Because of the considerable complexity of the expression of HLA antigens and their immunogenic peptides, one might conclude that a variety of different mechanisms will lead to the loss of MHC expression in neoplastic cells. Figure 19.22 presents a brief diagram of potential alterations that can lead to the lack of cytotoxic T-cell recognition of antigens presented on the surface of neoplastic cells. As noted, alterations in the digestion of the antigen by the proteasome because of the lack of the LMP-2 and LMP-7 subunits of the complex (cf. Figure 19.14) or the elimination of the transporter proteins, TAP-1 and TAP-2 or defects in any of these proteins lead to little or no expression of the MHC antigen with its appropriate immunogenic peptide. Furthermore, alterations in the transcription of MHC genes can occur as the result of mutational or excessive expression of protooncogenes including *ras* (Weijzen et al., 1999), *myc* (Schrier and Peltenburg, 1993), and NF-κB–binding activity to the promoter region of class I genes (Blanchet et al., 1992). Another mechanism of altered MHC expression is the loss of β2-microglobulin synthesis and expression. As we have previously noted (Figure 19.16), this molecule is an essential component of MHC class I antigens, and in its absence there may be either a lack of expression of the major MHC class I molecule or the expression of the latter may produce an abnormal MHC class I molecule. In either event, the T-cell receptor does not recognize the abnormal protein (cf. Ljunggren, 1992).

Table 19.11 Frequency (%) of HLA Class I Altered Phenotypes in Invasive Neoplasms

HLA Loss	Breast	Cervix	Colon	Larynx	Melanoma	Pancreas	Prostate
Total losses	52	18	21	9	16	12	34
HLA-A locus losses	4	3	8	19		19	ND
HLA-B locus losses	8	19	5	16	10	8	ND
HLA-A+B loci losses	9	2	5	9			ND
HLA allelic losses	15	21	26	26	25	ND[a]	51
Total	88	63	65	79	51	39	85

[a]ND, not determined.
Adapted from Algarra et al., 1997, with permission of the authors and publisher.

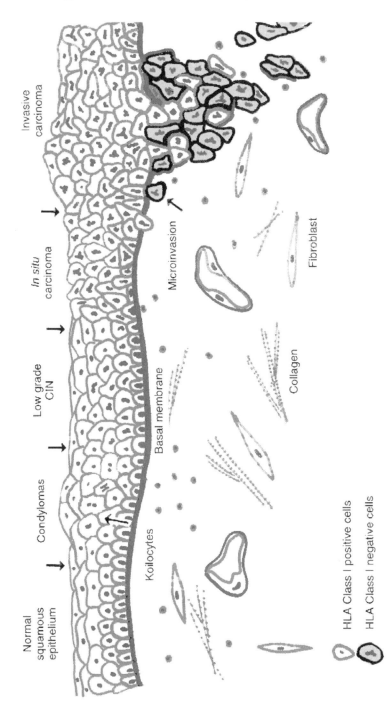

Figure 19.21 Diagram of changes seen in the development of cervical carcinoma illustrating alterations in HLA class I expression in normal, preneoplastic, and neoplastic epithelium. Note that the HLA class I losses occur when the "in situ" carcinoma becomes invasive and from this may ultimately produce metastases. Similar patterns have been observed in colon, breast, and laryngeal carcinomas. (Adapted from Garrido et al., 1993, with permission of the authors and publisher.)

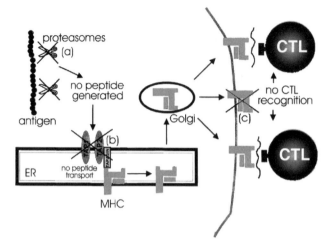

Figure 19.22 Diagram of defects in MHC class I-restricted antigen processing in neoplastic cells. The defects noted inclu*de (a) downregulation of LMP2 and LMP7 expression and; (b) downregulation of TAP-1 and TAP-2 and/or alteration in the expression of MHC class I antigen proteins. As noted earlier (Figure 19.14), loss of LMP2 and LMP7 expression blocks the generation of specific peptide epitopes. Loss of TAP-1 and TAP-2 blocks or prevents the transport of peptide epitopes from the cytoplasmic compartment into the endoplasmic reticulum, where it comes into association with the MHC protein. Any one or all of these defects may result in the lack of expression of MHC molecules carrying appropriate peptide epitopes, thus preventing an interaction with cytotoxic T cells. (Modified from Khanna, 1998, with permission of the author and publisher.)

Perhaps paramount among such alterations is the basic process of the stage of progression, that of evolving karyotypic instability. Such has been argued as the critical mechanism for the alterations in MHC expression seen in neoplastic cells, allowing their evasion from the host immune system (Ellem et al., 1998).

Host Tolerance to Antigens of Neoplastic Cells

Any consideration of tolerance of the immune system to specific antigens must take into account the distinction between "self" antigens and "non-self" antigens. In the normal condition, the host immune system is tolerant to *self* antigens, which consist of MHC antigens with their peptide ligands derived from normal tissues that are available to the immune system during fetal and early neonatal life. *Non-self* antigens are those originating in the external environment as well as those in immune privileged sites such as the testis or anterior chamber of the eye. These latter sites constitutively express Fas ligand, which interacts with any T cells contacting such tissues, resulting in the death of the interloping T cell (cf. Sotomayor et al., 1996). While the mechanism of the development of tolerance of T cells to self antigens is not entirely clear (Antonia et al., 1998; Basten, 1998; Sakaguchi, 2000), the immune system of the adult does not normally react to self antigens. As we shall see below, however, the phenomenon of autoimmunity may result from a failure of one or more of the mechanisms of self tolerance, with the resultant production of various disease states.

Since neoplastic cells for the most part express self antigens, the presentation and processing of such antigens would not be expected to induce alterations in the immunobiology of the host–tumor relationship. However, tolerance to some fetal antigens such as CEA or α-fetoprotein occurs in the host during neonatal life, thus abrogating a T-cell response to such antigens when they are expressed in neoplasms in the adult. Tolerance to specific antigens on neoplastic cells that might be considered non-self by the immune system may also occur by several other mechanisms. Clonal deletion of small numbers of T cells when confronted with an excess of antigen occurs presumably via apoptosis (cf. Starzl and Zinkernagel, 1998). T-cell deletion may also result from reactions with "superantigens," which may occur on some viruses such as the mouse mammary tumor virus (see below).

Peripheral tolerance of T cells to specific antigens may also occur through the induction of anergy, i.e., the nonresponsiveness of T cells to an antigenic signal. This phenomenon has been reported in several instances when cytotoxic T cells may interact with neoplasms expressing a non-self antigen through the MHC protein but lacking costimulatory molecules needed for the complete interaction of the cytotoxic T cell with the target tumor cell (Kabelitz, 1997). One such family of costimulatory molecules, the B7 family, is upregulated on B cells and antigen-presenting cells shortly after activation of such cells. These molecules interact with specific receptors, CD28, for members of the B7 family, found on the vast majority of T cells. Neoplastic cells frequently lack such costimulatory molecules and are thus unable to elicit substantial T-cell responses, even when sufficient amounts of relevant MHC molecules are present (Kabelitz, 1997). Thus, the lack of such costimulatory molecules can lead to T-cell anergy, i.e., failure of T-cell response even with appropriate MHC antigens and peptide presentation. In at least one study, the development of antigen-specific T-cell anergy appears to be an early event during tumor progression (Staveley-O'Carroll et al., 1998).

Clonal deletion of T cells as a result of interaction with neoplastic cells may occur by at least two mechanisms. The first, described above, is the formation on the neoplasm of a superantigen that is capable of stimulation of T cells but circumventing the requirement for strict MHC restriction. Furthermore, processing of superantigens by the antigen-presenting cell is not required. A diagram of the interaction of a superantigen with the T-cell receptor and MHC complex on an antigen-presenting cell is seen in Figure 19.23. Presentation of superantigens requires MHC class II antigens on the presenting cell, but there is less specificity than is seen with usual

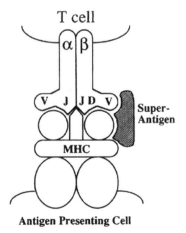

Figure 19.23   Schematic representation of the complex between a superantigen, the T-cell receptor, and an MHC class II protein on an antigen-presenting cell. As noted, the superantigen does not present itself within the cleft of the MHC but rather binds to the β chain of the T-cell receptor and components of the MHC class II protein. (Adapted from Herman et al., 1991, with permission of the authors and publisher.)

MHC-restricted responses (cf. Herman et al., 1991). While superantigens activate T cells, they also are capable of eliminating T cells with specific components of the T-cell receptor, particularly the β chain (Figure 19.23). Expression of the superantigen on cells with the integrated mouse mammary tumor virus genome resulted in the deletion of specific T-cell clones; this is thought to be critical in the productive infection by the virus and the ultimate formation of malignant neoplasms (Ross, 1997).

Another mechanism for deletion of T-cell clones reactive against specific antigens on neoplasms is the production of the Fas ligand by the neoplasm. Interaction of such neoplastic cells with T cells can result in the release of the Fas ligand, which interacts with the Fas receptor on the surface of all T cells, leading to their apoptosis (Chapter 17). Increased expression of the Fas ligand on neoplastic cells has been reported with several different neoplasms in both animals and humans (cf. Sotomayor et al., 1996; Shiraki et al., 1997; Strand and Galle, 1998).

Antigenic Modulation and Masking

In 1968, Old and associates (1968) described the phenomenon of "antigenic modulation" as the antibody-induced resistance to the cytotoxic action of antibody plus complement. This phenomenon appears to be associated with the redistribution of antigen-antibody complexes on the cell surface. In the original experiments by Old et al. (1968), neoplastic cells expressing a specific thymocyte antigen (TL) incubated in the presence of the antibody to the antigen lost the expression of the TL antigen. Simultaneously, there was an increased expression of H-2-D antigens. This modulation was temperature-dependent and inhibited by actinomycin D, suggesting that RNA synthesis is required for the process. Later studies showed that complete clearance of the antigen-antibody complex from the surface of the cell was not required, even in the presence of both specific antibody and complement (Gordon and Stevenson, 1981). It was clear from these studies, however, that neoplastic cells may escape from the antibody-complement reaction by the elimination of most or all of the complexes formed with specific antigens on the surface of the neoplastic cell, thus abrogating the humoral response to the neoplasm. This phenomenon was reportedly a factor in the failure of treatment of lymphocytic leukemia with anti-idiotypic antibody (Gordon et al., 1984). In addition, some neoplastic B cells retain their capability for hypermutations (see above) and may change the expression of the idiotype on the surface of the B cell, thus becoming unresponsive to anti-idiotype antibody therapy (Raffeld et al., 1985).

Another method of interference of the interaction with antigens on neoplasms and antibodies or cytolytic T cells is that of "masking" of the antigen on the neoplastic cell, so that it is not "seen" by the immune system. Earlier studies (cf. Apffel and Peters, 1969) found that a group of glycoproteins found in the slow-moving α_2-globulin electrophoretic class became associated with the surface of neoplastic cells, thereby affecting the antigenicity of the neoplastic cell as well as the entire immunologic response of the host to the neoplasm. These authors termed such proteins *symbodies*. Such proteins appear in the plasma in response to wound repair as well as regeneration. Their synthesis is mediated by hormones from the adrenal cortex and thus is likely to be related to the "stress" response of the host to the neoplasm, as seen in cachexia (Chapter 17). Since then, a number of other materials found circulating in the plasma, mostly proteins, appear to have similar direct inhibitory effects between the immune system and surface antigens of the neoplastic cell. The Hellströms and their associates (Hellström and Hellström, 1979) demonstrated factors in the serum of patients that are protein in nature and possibly contain antibody structures. These factors appear to prevent the action of sensitized T lymphocytes on neoplastic cells. They term such proteins *blocking factors*, which serve to coat the surface of neoplastic cells, thus preventing the reaction of cellular and humoral immunity from occurring in response to antigens on the neoplastic cell. The molecular nature of such "blocking factors" appears to be more complex than simple excess immune globulins, possessing both specific and nonspecific components, including tumor antigens (Rao and Bonavida, 1977), antigen-antibody complexes (cf. Robins and Baldwin, 1978), and other as yet unidentified components (cf. Hellström and Hellström, 1979). Furthermore, some of these and other plasma components as well as materials produced by the neoplastic cells themselves (cf. Sedlacek, 1994) lead to a resistance of neoplastic cells to the effect of complement, which is necessary for the effectiveness of antibody-induced cytotoxicity (Jurianz et al., 1999).

In addition to antigen modulation and antigen masking, neoplasms, both through apoptosis and possibly normal rapid cell replication, shed molecular components of the neoplastic cell into the circulation. While the phenomenon has been best documented in experimental situations (cf. Raz et al., 1978; Viñuela et al., 1991), a potentially similar finding has been described in both animals and humans—i.e., the formation of immune complexes between antibodies and circulating antigens of neoplastic cells (cf. Salinas et al., 1983). Such circulating complexes appear to have immunosuppressive effects and may produce significant physical changes in the organism, especially in leukemia (Sutherland and Mardiney, 1973) and myelomas (cf. Dhodapkar et al., 1997). The binding of the extracellular matrix protein laminin to neoplastic cells inhibits not only cytotoxic T cells but also the effects of NK cells (Hiserodt et al., 1985). Perhaps the most overlooked factor unique to neoplasms is a persistent antigen overload to the host. This includes many of the factors mentioned above as well as the number of individual neoplastic cells or clusters occurring in veins draining various neoplasms such as those of the colon, ovary, stomach, breast, and others, sometimes on the order of 5 to 50 cells or more per milliliter of blood (cf. Smith, 1994).

Suppressor Cells and Factors Downregulating the Host Immune Response to Neoplasia

While there still may be some question as to the exact actual existence of suppressor T cells (cf. Arnon and Teitelbaum, 1993), there is also ample evidence arguing for the existence of such cells and their importance in the immune response, as cited by these authors and others (Dorf et al., 1992; North, 1985; Hoover et al., 1990), as well as the existence of macrophages exhibiting suppressor effects on the immune response (Walker et al., 1993). The effect of such suppressor T cells can be readily seen in the growth of some transplanted neoplasms following the initial inoculum. A diagram of this is seen in Figure 19.24. Other studies (e.g., Hoover et al., 1990) utilized the alkylating agent cyclophosphamide to inhibit the generation of suppressor T cells when used at very low doses.

Almost four decades ago, a number of authors (cf. Prehn, 1977) noted that a transplant of an antigenic neoplasm may fail to produce effective immunity against its own growth if the inoculum is sufficiently small. A diagram of such an experiment with a variety of different sizes of cell inocula of a transplanted neoplasm in mice is seen in Figure 19.25A. With relatively small inocula, 100 to 500 cells, a substantial number of animals develop neoplastic growths, significantly more than animals receiving only 5- or 10-cell inocula. However, the surprising effect was that at doses of 1000 or 10,000 cells, relatively few animals developed neoplasms—in fact, a number quite comparable to those receiving only 5 or 10 cells. At doses of 100,000 or 1 million cells, almost 100% of the animals developed neoplasms, presumably because this large number overcame any immunological host resistance. This "sneaking-through" effect was completely abrogated by pretreatment of the animals with low doses of cyclophosphamide, as seen in Figure 19.25B. As noted in the latter figure, the alkylating agent also appeared to depress to some extent the overall immune response of the host to the transplanted neoplasm.

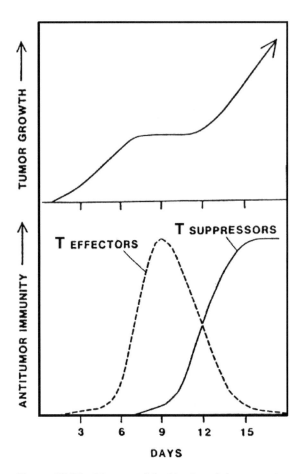

Figure 19.24　Diagram of the kinetics of the generation of effector and suppressor T cells during the growth of an immunogenic neoplasm following transplantation. In this experiment, after day 9 of neoplastic growth, there is a progressive increase in the ratio of suppressor to effector T cells. (Adapted from North, 1985, with permission of the author and publisher.)

Contributory to this suppressive effect, although not entirely explained, is the potential that neoplastic cells, especially small inocula, induce a far greater Th2 than Th1 cell response (Table 19.3). Since the Th2 response is directed primarily toward humoral immunity, which has distinctly less efficacy in eliminating neoplastic cells than the cell-mediated immunity of the Th1 response, a similar phenotypic response might be the result of variable Th2 and Th1 responses to the various-sized inocula. In any event, different subsets of lymphocytes and probably macrophages are involved in the neoplastic cell-induced abrogation of a potential immune response to antigens within the neoplasm.

Immunosuppressive Factors in the Immunobiology of the Host-Tumor Relationship

In addition to all of the various methods whereby neoplasms evade the immune system, there is a rather large area generally classified as immunosuppression by products of neoplasms or the

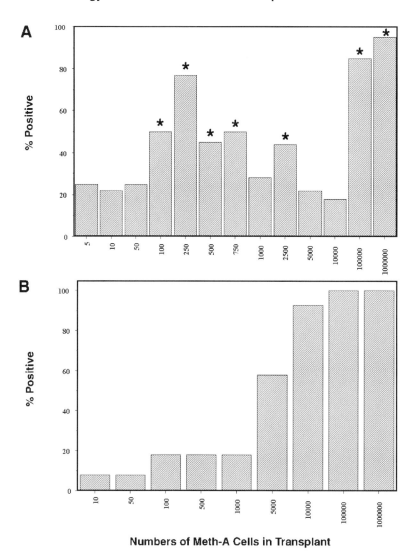

Figure 19.25 A. Incidence (% positive) of neoplasms following varying doses of Meth-A, a transplanted ascites neoplasm, in intact female BALB/c mice. The * bars are significantly greater than the number of neoplasms resulting from an inoculum of 10^4 cells. B. Incidence of neoplasms as in A after transplantation of Meth-A cells in BALB/c female mice that had received cyclophosphamide 24 hours prior to tumor inoculum. No evidence of "sneaking through" was demonstrated, and the number of tumor takes was lower at the lowest doses than in A, suggesting some generalized effect on the resistance to neoplastic growth. (Adapted from Gatenby et al., 1981, with permission of the authors and publisher.)

host, the latter resulting from the host–tumor relationship. Several cytokines and growth factors produced both by the host and the neoplasm, although primarily the latter, have immunosuppressive effects on the host response to the neoplasm. Several such prominent factors are listed in Table 19.12. As noted in the table, several of these cytokines and growth factors augment the effects we have already discussed, such as T-cell anergy, shift of T-helper cells toward the Th2 population, and downregulation of costimulatory molecules.

Table 19.12 Immunosuppressive Effects of IL-10, TGF-β, and VEGF on the Immune Response of the Host to the Neoplasm

Effect	TGF-β	IL-10	VEGF
Inhibition of T-cell growth	+	−	+
Inhibition of CTL differentiation	+	+	+
Inhibition of cytokine production	+	+	−
Induction of T-cell anergy	+	−	−
Downregulation of cytotoxic potential	+	+	−
Inhibition of antigen presentation	+	+	−
Shift in the Th1-Th2 balance toward Th2	+	+	−
Downregulation of adhesion/costimulatory molecules	+	+	−
Resistance to CTL-mediated lysis	−	+	−

Key: CTL, cytotoxic T lymphocyte; IL, interleukin; TGF-β, transforming growth factor β; Th, T helper; VEGF, vascular endothelial growth factor.
Adapted from Chouaib et al., 1997.

In addition to these cytokines, several other molecular species serve to suppress the immune response of the host to the neoplasm. These include prostaglandins (Bankhurst, 1982; cf. Wojtowicz-Praga, 1997), gangliosides shed from neoplastic cells (Heitger and Ladisch, 1996; McKallip et al., 1999), and micromolecular degradation products of fibrinogen (Girmann et al., 1976). The effect of prostaglandins may be related to the chemopreventive effect of prostaglandin synthetase inhibitors on the development of neoplasms (Chapter 8). Interestingly, Ladisch et al. (1994) suggested that gangliosides with shorter fatty acyl chains are most immunosuppressive and are known to be preferentially shed by neoplastic cells. Other immunosuppressive factors have also been described, both well and partially characterized (cf. Sulitzeanu, 1985). An interesting immunosuppressive effect as yet not totally characterized is an apparent defect in macrophage chemotaxis seen in patients with neoplastic disease, presumably mediated by a serum-borne molecule (Walter et al., 1986).

SUCCESSES OF THE IMMUNOBIOLOGICAL HOST–TUMOR RELATIONSHIP

Although, as evidenced from Table 19.10 and discussed above, there are a variety of mechanisms for the neoplastic cell to evade the immune response of the host, there are also a number of examples of successful immunological responses of the host to the neoplasm. Several of the more important of these are considered below.

Immunosurveillance

More than 40 years ago, Thomas (1959) suggested that the host possessed a normal homeostatic cellular mechanism active in eliminating non-self antigenic components such as parasites, mutated cells, and neoplastic cells. This concept predicted that patients with immunodeficiency not only would be more susceptible to parasitic infections but should be expected to be quite susceptible to the development of malignant disease. Later studies by Good (1971) and associates demonstrated that this was so in that genetic defects of the immune system usually rendered such patients highly prone to the development of neoplasms, although these neoplasms were almost always of cells from the immune system. Application of this concept to neoplasms was articulated by Burnet (1970), who predicted the occurrence of tumor-specific antigens and T cell–dependent elimination of neoplastic cells. Further substantiation of this concept came from the widespread therapeutic use of organ transplantation with associated chemical and radiological immunosuppression in order to obtain reasonably functioning transplants in the face of the host immune defenses. As a result of a survey, it has been shown that the incidence of lymphomas in such transplant patients is approximately 25 times higher than in the normal population (Fraumeni and Hoover, 1977). In one specific instance, that of reticulum cell sarcoma, the incidence of this neoplasm in patients who had been immunosuppressed for organ transplants was 350 times higher than in the normal population (Hoover and Fraumeni, 1973). The dramatic increase in neoplasia, especially lymphomas and particular Kaposi sarcoma in AIDS patients (Spina et al., 1999), who are immunosuppressed as a result of the action of the HIV virus (Chapter 12), is further evidence for the existence of an immunosurveillance mechanism in the tumor-bearing host. In addition to these types of neoplasms, an increase in epithelial neoplasms also occurs in immunosuppressed patients, usually for transplantation (Penn, 1993). While in the case of lymphomas and Kaposi sarcoma one can make a case that these are primarily virus-induced neoplasms with immunosuppression of the host allowing the infection to proceed, it is difficult to make such a case for many epithelial neoplasms whose incidence is increased following active immunosuppression.

The discovery that a recessive mutation, the so-called nude mouse, results in a virtually complete absence of thymic development has offered another system in which to study neoplastic growth in the absence of cell-mediated immunity. The T cell–mediated response of such mutant animals is essentially nonexistent, yet the incidence of spontaneous carcinomas and neoplasms other than those of the immune system is actually no different from that of nonmutant controls and laboratory mice in general (cf. Stutman, 1979). On the other hand, if newborn nude mice are inoculated with polyomavirus, they develop more neoplasms faster than would a mouse with an intact immune system under the same circumstances (cf. Vandeputte, 1982). These findings in this mutant mouse are similar to those seen in the immunodepressed human with the exception of the lack of spontaneous carcinomas. However, it must be remembered that the NK-cell response of the nude mouse is perfectly normal. This fact may be very important in the lack of spontaneous carcinogenesis, as we shall note below. Immunosurveillance in the host may also be mediated by NK cells, macrophages, and antibodies occurring naturally within the plasma of the host (cf. Wheelock and Robinson, 1983). Furthermore, immunosurveillance is a likely mechanism for the dormancy seen with a number of neoplasms (Chapter 10). The fact that some neoplasms, such as those of the breast or melanoma, may recur many, many years after apparent successful treatment of the primary growth may be, at least in part, owing to immunosurveillance. Experimental studies have suggested that the dormant state is mediated predominantly by cytolytic T cells, although long-term maintenance of this situation likely requires the additional presence of macrophages (cf. Stevenson, 1991).

Cell Populations Potentially Active in Immunosurveillance Toward Neoplasia

Although the host fails to respond in many instances to the neoplasm by the usual T- and B-cell mechanisms as outlined in Table 19.10, several cell populations appear to be effective in recognizing and eliminating neoplastic cells.

Natural Killer Cells

As discussed earlier in this chapter, NK cells are likely derived in the bone marrow from a common precursor with T cells. NK cells have clearly distinctive characteristics, both morphologically and biochemically. While T cells carrying the T-cell receptor recognize and respond to MHC antigens bearing peptide epitopes, NK cells are inhibited in their activity and replication by such MHC complexes. This inhibition is mediated by receptors of somewhat limited diversity, that recognize distinct MHC class I antigen epitopes and are shared by a large number of MHC alleles (Seebach and Waneck, 1997; Raulet, 1999). Therefore many have argued that NK cells are the basis of host immunosurveillance, since the NK cell can play a major role in the host immunity to many neoplasms as well as certain virus infections. In these instances, the downregulation of the MHC class I and class II antigen would eliminate the inhibitory effect of these antigens on NK-cell activity toward such cells, thus allowing for the destruction of these cells. Studies have strongly suggested that such destruction occurs through the perforin pathway (Figure 19.19) (van den Broek et al., 1995). However, NK cells do produce cytokines including TNF-α and interferon-γ, the latter also involved in the activation of NK cells in the presence of other cytokines such as interleukin-2 (Naume and Espevik, 1994).

As might be expected, neoplastic cells with the greatest downregulation of MHC antigens—namely, metastatic lesions well into the stage of progression—are more susceptible to the effects of NK cells. This has been shown in genetic systems in mice that are deficient in NK cells (Talmadge et al., 1980), where metastases of transplanted neoplasms normally sensitive to natural killer activity were much more extensive than in wild-type mice. Other studies showed similar effects in in vitro and in vivo systems, even with human cells (Hanna, 1985). Thus, in a heterogeneous population of neoplastic cells in vivo, it would be those cells that are least differentiated, exhibiting the greatest downregulation of MHC antigens, that would be susceptible to NK cell–mediated lysis (cf. Uchida, 1986). However, animals with a large tumor burden exhibit impaired NK-cell cytotoxicity (Boom et al., 1988); in another model system, NK cells apparently play a significant role early in the growth of the neoplasm, fostering the generation of antineoplastic cytotoxic T cells (Kurosawa et al., 1995).

Macrophages, Dendritic Cells, and Antigen-Presenting Cells

Of the monocyte-macrophage-dendritic cell group, it is the dendritic cell that is most efficient at presenting antigen to naïve T cells and stimulating their proliferation in response to specific MHC-bound peptide epitopes. It is only in the last two decades that the dendritic cell has been distinguished from the monocyte found in the circulation and from the macrophage, a primarily phagocytic cell. While the latter two cell types presumably may act as antigen-presenting cells, they are 1% to 10% as effective as dendritic cells in antigen presentation. Dendritic cells are characterized morphologically by the presence of numerous membrane processes that can extend for hundreds of micrometers from the cell. Such cells are far more effective at pinocytosis of soluble antigen than macrophages or monocytes, while the latter are more efficient at phagocytosis of large particles such as cellular debris and bacteria (cf. Fong and Engleman, 2000). Dendritic cells also occur from a variety of hematopoietic lineages, including monocytes, granulocytes, T cells, B cells, and others. They are found in a variety of tissues including the skin, intestinal mucosa, lymph nodes, and spleen. As expected, dendritic cells from different precursor lineages exhibit different populations of antigens and receptors on their surfaces (Björck, 1999). Thus, the principal role of the dendritic cell in the immunological host–tumor relationship is the processing of antigens and presentation to various T-cell populations, which would then interact with appropriate neoplastic cells provided they carry the MHC class I or class II protein antigens. However, there is substantial evidence that the less efficient antigen-presenting cells, particularly macrophages, have the ability to recognize neoplastic cells selectively and either destroy them or impede their growth (McBride, 1986; Fauve, 1993). Activation of macrophages occurs through their interaction with cytokines, particularly interferon γ (cf. Killion and Fidler, 1998).

Macrophages occur within neoplasms in both animals and humans. Normann (1985), from a number of different published reports, suggested that intratumoral macrophage density was related to tumor growth, as seen diagrammatically in Figure 19.26. It appears that macrophage killing of neoplastic cells involves a process that can discriminate between neoplastic and normal cells by a process independent of MHC antigens, tumor-specific antigens, the cell cycle, or the histogenetic phenotype of the transformed cell (cf. Whitworth et al., 1990). Neoplasms that are regressing, possibly through some degree of apoptosis, usually exhibit macrophages throughout the neoplastic tissue; however, in those neoplasms that are proliferating and continuing in the stage of progression, especially sarcomas, macrophages are confined to the periphery of the neoplasm (cf. Killion and Fidler, 1998). Normann (1985) reported that the induction time of neoplasms in rodents varies with their macrophage content; the more rapidly growing neoplasms are those containing fewer infiltrating macrophages. However, the accumulation of macrophages in neoplasms does not necessarily correlate with the metastatic properties or the immunogenicity of the neoplasms. In some instances, the presence in the neoplasm of nonactivated (noncytotoxic) macrophages may actually enhance the growth of the neoplasm (cf. Killion and Fidler, 1998).

While the mechanism of this antineoplastic effect of macrophages is not understood, some evidence suggests that macrophage recognition of plasma membrane phosphatidylserine is at least correlated with an increased binding of macrophages to neoplastic cells. Since the mechanism for the specific recognition by activated macrophages of neoplastic cells is nonimmunological and requires cell-to-cell contact, it would appear that some membrane recognition

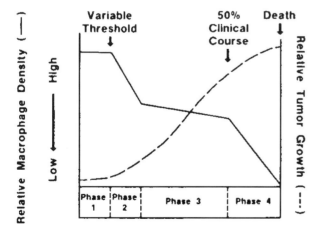

Figure 19.26 Diagrammatic representation of macrophage density within neoplasms during growth. Of the four phases indicated, phases I and II have been demonstrated for micrometastases and might be presumed to exist for carcinoma in situ as well as early invasive neoplasms. Phases III and IV have been demonstrated for autochthonous and transplanted neoplasms and phase IV for metastases. (Adapted from Normann, 1985, with permission of the author and publisher.)

phenomenon of activated macrophages towards neoplastic cells is related to this immunological host–tumor relationship.

There have also been relationships between dendritic cells in human neoplasms and the prognosis of the lesion. Zeid and Muller (1993) demonstrated that well-differentiated squamous cell carcinomas of the lung contained a much higher density of a specific type of dendritic cell, the Langerhans cell, than did poorly differentiated lesions. Another interesting neoplasm in the human in which the immunocytic infiltrate is directly related to the prognosis is breast carcinoma displaying a considerable infiltration by lymphocytes and monocytes. Such neoplasms are termed *medullary carcinomas* (Figure 18.11). While the infiltrate contains a variety of T cells, both suppressor and cytotoxic, macrophages and NK cells are also seen in the intraneoplastic cell population (Naukkarinen and Syrjänen, 1990). In line with the relatively favorable prognosis of such lesions, significant apoptosis of neoplastic cells was also demonstrated in medullary carcinomas of the breast (Grekou et al., 1996).

Dendritic Cells, Suppressors, and Ultraviolet Epidermal Carcinogenesis

As discussed in Chapter 13, ultraviolet radiation is a known carcinogen for both humans and animals. More than six decades ago, Roffo (1933) and Rusch et al. (1941) demonstrated that ultraviolet radiation, particularly UVB lying within the range of 275 to 315 nm, was carcinogenic for the epidermis of both mice and rats. Later studies by Kripke (1974) demonstrated the interesting phenomenon that in syngeneic mice, epidermoid carcinomas induced by UVB were quite immunogenic and could not be readily transplanted into nonirradiated syngeneic hosts. However, transplants into UV-irradiated hosts readily grew, even after relatively short exposure to UV radiation (Figure 19.27). Not shown in the figure is the fact that epidermal neoplasms developing after UV irradiation do not grow when transplanted into nonirradiated hosts (see above). This fact indicates that the host-immune response is quite effective against this particular neoplasm in this species. Other studies have also demonstrated that chronic UV irradiation enhances carcinogenesis by benzo[a]pyrene-induced (Gensler, 1988) and N-methyl-N′-nitro-N-nitrosoguanidine–induced skin cancers in similarly irradiated mice (Gensler, 1992). The latter experiment indicates that the chronic UV irradiation effect is not mediated through activation of the chemical carcinogen. Furthermore, UV radiation does not suppress the normal or inducible NK-cell activity in association with the appearance of the epidermal carcinomas in mice (Steerenberg et al., 1997).

Cutaneous Immunity and Ultraviolet B Radiation

As expected, because of the strategic location of the skin as an interface with the environment, this organ has its own components of the immune system, as outlined diagrammatically in Figure 19.28. Langerhans cells are virtually eliminated or markedly reduced from skin exposed to UVB radiation (Streilein et al., 1994; Thiers et al., 1984; Meunier, 1999). The inhibition of antigen-presenting activity of dendritic cells resulting from UV radiation in the skin appears to be dependent on UV-induced DNA damage in the cutaneous antigen-presenting cell population (Vink et al., 1997). Contact hypersensitivity to various antigens is lost from the area of skin that is subjected to the UV radiation (cf. Streilein et al., 1994). Such cells appear to have lost the ability to present antigens to T cells, resulting in the failure of the induction of Th1 responses but still allowing Th2 responses to occur (Simon et al., 1990; Cruz, 1992; cf. Meunier, 1999). A direct test of this conclusion is seen in Table 19.13. These studies then underline the importance of the role of Langerhans cells in the skin in presenting antigen, including tumor antigens, from

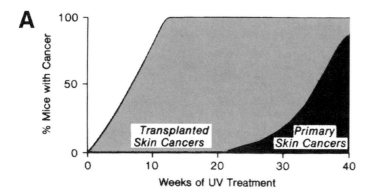

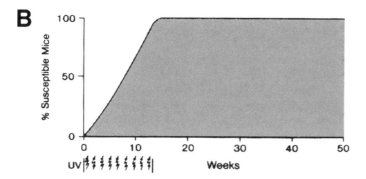

Figure 19.27 A. Time course for development of primary skin cancers and the susceptibility to the growth of transplanted skin cancers in C3H mice continuously exposed three times per week to UVB radiation. B. The percentage susceptibility of mice treated for 12 weeks (3 times per week) with UVB radiation to the growth of transplants of UV-induced neoplasms of the skin. (Adapted from Kripke, 1986, with permission of the author and publisher.)

epidermoid carcinomas to the immune system, with subsequent rejection of the transplant in the case of the UV-induced carcinomas.

Ultraviolet-Mediated Immunosuppression

Since the transplantation of UV-induced epidermal carcinomas in mice could be accomplished virtually anywhere in the organism, it was clear that the effects of UVB irradiation were not simply local, as suggested by the failure of contact hypersensitivity only in regions of UV radiation. It now appears that there are several mechanisms for such generalized immunosuppression by UV radiation. The first of these is the fact that suppressor T cells that are specific for the UV radiation–induced neoplasms (Trial and McIntyre, 1990) have been induced in the organism as a result of UV radiation. This may be because a different population of antigen-presenting cells in the skin, relatively nonsusceptible to UVB irradiation, can act as antigen-presenting cells for suppressor T lymphocytes that likely express the $\gamma\delta$ T cell receptor (see below) (cf. Meunier, 1999). In addition, there is evidence that immunosuppression by UV radiation of the skin is mediated by the UV-induced formation of the abnormal *cis* isomer of urocanic acid from the product of the action of histidine ammonia-lyase in the skin, which is the *trans* isomer. A diagram of

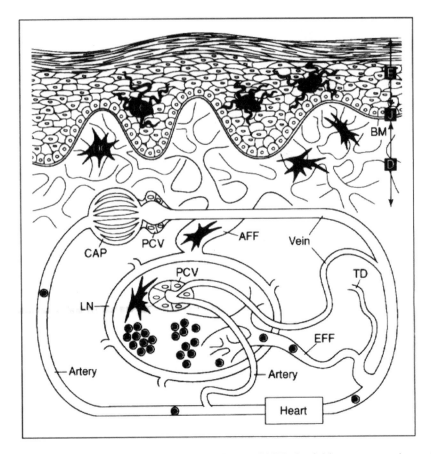

Figure 19.28 Skin-associated lymphoid tissues (SALT) that initiate cutaneous immunity are located in the epidermis (E) and dermis (D) and are separated by the dermal-epidermal junction (J) and the basement membrane (BM). Dendritic cells in the dermis (DC) and Langerhans cells (LC) residing in the epidermis are the antigen-presenting cells of the skin. The dermis contains blood vessels [capillaries (CAP) and post-capillary venules (PCV)] and lymphatic channels. Afferent lymphatic ducts (AFF) carry lymph contents to lymph nodes (LN) containing lymphoreticular cells and postcapillary venules. Lymphocytes exit the LN via efferent lymphatics (EFF) into the thoracic duct (TD) and eventually into the bloodstream. (Adapted from Streilein et al., 1994, with permission of the authors and publisher.)

the reaction is seen in Figure 19.29 depicting primary metabolic products in the metabolism of histidine in skin and the effect of UV radiation. Evidence for this hypothesis was seen in animals having a mutant histidine-ammonia lyase gene with less than 10% of the wild-type levels of skin urocanic acid. Such animals did not exhibit the marked UV-induced immune suppression seen in wild-type animals (cf. Noonan and De Fabo, 1992). Other studies have also implicated TNF-α in the immunosuppressive effect of UV radiation (cf. Meunier, 1999).

$\gamma\delta$ T Cells in the Immunological Host-Tumor Relationship

While more than 90% of T cells possess a T-cell receptor with α and β chains (Figures 19.10 and 19.11), about 1% to 10% of T cells in the peripheral blood and lymphoid organs express γ and δ

Table 19.13 Effects of UVB Radiation on the Ability of
Langerhans Cells (LC) to Keyhole Limpet Hemocyanin
(KLH)-specific T_h1 and T_h2 Clones in Vitro

Experimental Condition	Responder Cells	T-Cell Proliferation
LC + KLH	Th1	+++++
UVB-LC + KLH	Th1	−
LC + KLH	Th2	+++
UVB-LC + KLH	Th2	+++

Adapted from Cruz, 1992, with permission of the author and publisher.

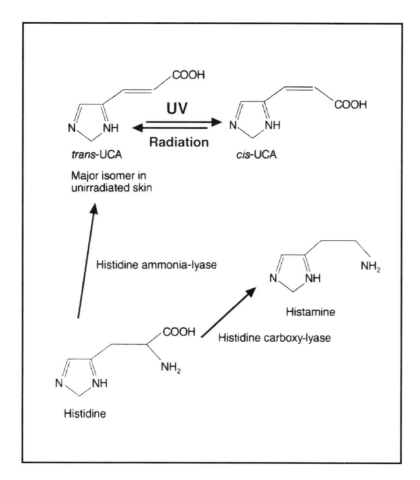

Figure 19.29 Initial reactions in histidine metabolism indicating the effect of ultraviolet radiation in the formation of *cis*-urocanic acid (UCA). (Adapted from Noonan and De Fabo, 1992, with permission of the authors and publisher.)

chains on their T-cell receptor. Their response to antigens is not restricted by classical MHC class I or class II antigen, but other MHC class I-related molecules such as CD1 may serve as antigen-presenting molecules for some γδ T cells (cf. Kabelitz, 1995). In a transgenic mouse system, immune resistance to acute T-cell leukemias depended on γδ T cells but was independent of MHC antigen or TAP-2 peptide transporter expression (Penninger et al., 1995). There is also evidence that γδ T cells may recognize various stress-induced or heat-shock antigens within neoplastic cells (cf. Kabelitz, 1995; Groh et al., 1999). Some γδ T cells functioning as dendritic antigen-presenting cells may serve to activate suppressor T lymphocytes (cf. Meunier, 1999). However, in most instances the percentage of γδ T cells that infiltrate various human carcinomas is relatively low, although an accumulation of up to 30% of intrahepatic lymphocytes from cancer patients may be γδ T cells (Seki et al., 1990). Thus, the actual role of γδ T cells in the immunological host-tumor relationship is not clear at this time, but there are clear suggestions that γδ T cells may contribute both to the host immune defense against neoplastic cells and the escape of neoplastic cells from the host immune system.

Upregulation of MHC Expression in Neoplastic Cells

As previously discussed (Table 19.10), several different factors were important in the downregulation of MHC expression in both normal and neoplastic cells. This included several virus infections as well as the expression of certain oncogenes, the latter making such cells prone to lysis by NK cells (Versteeg et al., 1989). However, it is also apparent that several cytokines are capable of upregulating the expression of MHC antigens in both normal and neoplastic cells. Perhaps the best-studied of such MHC modulators are the interferons. As we shall see below, interferons have been used in the immunotherapy of neoplasia and are particularly important in activating natural killer cells as well as macrophages (see above). Interferons, especially interferon-γ, act as transcriptional activators of MHC class I genes by inducing transactivating nuclear factors that bind specific interferon consensus sequences (cf. Tatake and Zeff, 1993). Interferon is capable of upregulating both class I and class II MHC antigens in normal and neoplastic cells, but there is significant diversity in this response in some melanomas (cf. Kappes and Strominger, 1988). In addition to inducing the expression of MHC antigens in some neoplasms that otherwise show essentially no expression, this cytokine can also induce the expression of such antigens in normal cells that express virtually no or very low levels of MHC class I antigens, as with cells in the central nervous system (Wong et al., 1984; Neumann et al., 1995).

In addition to interferons, tumor necrosis factor α may enhance the expression of both class I and class II MHC antigens, although reportedly, unlike interferon, this cytokine does not induce class I expression in class I–negative neoplasms (Singer and Maguire, 1990; Pfizenmaier et al., 1987).

A third example of the upregulation of MHC antigens that is presumably relevant to the immunological host–tumor relationship is the finding that expression of the hepatitis B virus X gene in both human and murine cell lines is associated with an upregulation of MHC antigen (Hu et al., 1990; cf. Rossner, 1992). The relevance of this to the development of hepatocellular carcinomas in patients with chronic hepatitis B virus infections is not clear at this time. However, the fact that MHC class I and class II antigens may be upregulated or induced by cytokines and possibly viral products indicates that such agents are capable of overcoming the subversion of the immune response by neoplastic cells that do not normally express HLA antigens in vivo.

AUTOIMMUNITY AND THE HOST–TUMOR RELATIONSHIP

Although Paul Ehrlich (Ehrlich and Morgenroth, 1957) argued that the organism should never react to its own tissues, during the last century a number of diseases resulting from immune reactions within the organism to its own or "self" antigens have now been described. A discussion of the development of autoimmune disease is beyond the scope of this text; however, the interested student may consider the following references: Schwartz, 1993; Eisenbarth and Bellgrau, 1994; Mayes, 1999; Bach, 1995. Interestingly, Prehn and Prehn (1987) have presented arguments that neoplasia, at least in part, should itself be considered an autoimmune disease. However, here are considered only an artificially induced autoimmune condition leading to neoplastic development and its potential application as well as some examples of autoimmunity stimulated in the host by antigens present in neoplasms. An artificial "autoimmune" disease has been induced in rodents by the production of "runt" disease resulting from a graft-versus-host (GVH) reaction in several mammalian species including the human. The basic requirements for a graft-versus-host reaction in vivo are (1) the graft must contain immunologically competent lymphocytes; (2) the host must be incapable of rejecting the graft either because of artificially induced immunological incompetence or because the host is tolerant to the engrafted cells; and (3) a degree of histoincompatibility must prevail between the graft and the host (cf. Seemayer et al., 1983).

The production of the GVH reaction resulting in runt disease is outlined in Figure 19.30; immunocompetent lymphoid and bone marrow tissues are removed from an adult animal that is genetically distinct from the recipient neonate. The cells from the adult survive within the neonatal animal because the donor cells do not produce a rejection reaction in the host, owing to

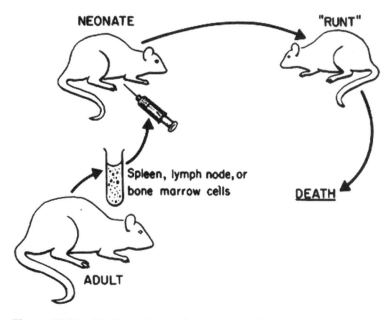

Figure 19.30 Classic method for the production of "runt" disease or a graft-versus-host reaction. Immunocompetent cells from the spleen, lymph node, or bone marrow are removed from an adult animal and inoculated into a neonate. Since the neonate is immunologically deficient, it will not react to the donor cells, but the donor cells will react to the host tissues, resulting in a graft-versus-host reaction and runt disease with ultimate death.

neonatal tolerance. However, the cells from the adult donor do react to the host tissues, producing both humoral and cell-mediated responses. Such a reaction of the donor cells damages the host tissues eventually to the point of death. During this process, the young animal does not grow—thus the term *runt*—and it may also exhibit other changes of the skin, tails, ears, and internal organs. A similar condition may be produced in the adult by making the recipient tolerant to a small number of cells, insufficient to produce runt disease, and subsequently administering a large number of immunocompetent cells from the same donor to the original recipient when this tolerant animal has grown to adulthood. This experimental model is analogous to several conditions found in the human under the general category of autoimmune diseases (Table 19.14), in which both humoral and cell-mediated immunity to the host's own tissues are produced by cellular populations within the host (cf. Theofilopoulos and Dixon, 1982).

One of the most interesting phenomena from such investigations was the description by Schwartz and André-Schwartz (1968) and Gleichmann et al. (1976) of the development of malignant lymphomas in recipient mice undergoing a chronic GVH reaction. In this instance the reaction is produced by the injection of the parent's spleen cells into its own neonatal offspring (F_1). The same sequence of events occurs as is seen in Figure 19.30; however, the genotype of the recipient is at least half identical to that of the donor. Therefore, the reaction in the host is relatively mild, and most of the recipients survive with relatively little runting. Later in life, however, many of these animals develop lymphomas. Gleichmann et al. (1976) have demonstrated that these lymphomas may develop from host cells, a mixture of host and donor cells, or donor cells only, although host-type lymphomas are seen most frequently. The initiation of lymphomagenesis in F_1 mice undergoing a chronic graft-versus-host reaction requires an immunological reaction of donor lymphocytes, probably T cells, to incompatible *H-2* gene products of the *I* region on cells of the F_1 recipient. In theory one would expect that the marked stimulation of the donor cells might ultimately lead to their neoplastic transformation. However, it is known that lymphoid cells of the host proliferate quite extensively in the GVH reaction, although the reason for this is not entirely understood. It would appear that the lymphomas resulting from these GVH reactions in genetically related animals are the result of chronic immunological stimulation of lymphoid cells, although some evidence has indicated a role for oncogenic RNA viruses in lymphoma production. Goh and Klemperer (1977) have presented cytogenetic evidence for the leukemic transformation of grafted bone marrow cells in the human.

Although the model system depicted above (Figure 19.30) has no real counterpart in the human, with possible rare exceptions, the model does mimic autoimmune disease seen in the

Table 19.14 Idiopathic Autoimmune Diseases in the Human in Association with Neoplasms

Autoimmune Disease	Neoplasm(s)	RR (Relative Risk)	Reference
Dermatomyositis	Various types	RR=1.8	Sigurgeirsson et al., 1992
Lupus erythematosus (systemic)	Various types	RR=2.0	Ramsey-Goldman et al., 1998
	Breast in Caucasians	RR=2.9	
Rheumatoid arthritis	non-Hodgkin lymphoma	RR=2.4	Mellemkjær et al., 1996
	Hodgkin lymphoma	RR=3.4	
Systemic sclerosis	Lung cancer	RR=4.9	Rosenthal et al., 1995
	Skin cancer (nonmelanoma)	RR=4.2	
	Liver cancer	RR=3.3	
Thyroiditis, chronic lymphocytic	Lymphomas/leukemias	RR=4.0	Holm et al., 1985

human and other animals with the difference that in such diseases all cells involved are of host or self origin. In Table 19.14 is seen a brief listing of some of the major idiopathic autoimmune diseases in the human and their association with neoplasia. As noted, the relative risks involved are not extremely great, but all are significant. In the case of dermatomyositis, a disease presenting as an inflammation of muscle and skin, the types of neoplasms found in patients with the disease parallel those observed in the general population but overall are at a higher percentage (Bernard and Bonnetblanc, 1993). In systemic lupus erythematosus, a disease affecting most tissues in the organism, the increased risk for various types of neoplasms in general was of the same order as that seen in dermatomyositis; however, a greater risk of breast cancer was seen in Caucasian women with lupus, while all women regardless of race also showed an increased risk of lung cancer (RR=3.1). In rheumatoid arthritis, a disease affecting joints, kidneys, and in later stages other tissues, lymphomas and leukemias were the most strikingly increased neoplasms (Mellemkjær et al., 1996). In systemic sclerosis or scleroderma, a disease affecting the skin and lungs, even higher incidences of specific carcinomas were noted, while lymphomas and leukemias were significantly associated with autoimmune thyroiditis.

While these autoimmune diseases are not considered neoplasms, they clearly, from our understanding of the immune process, have some of the characteristics of neoplasia. It is likely that clones of activated T and B cells act in a relatively autonomous manner to produce the reactions with self antigens, resulting in the disease pictures. Even more striking are some diseases of atypical lymphoid proliferation associated with autoimmune disease, such as "autoimmune disease–associated lymphadenopathy" and related diseases (cf. Koo et al., 1984) that may have the same biological basis as the idiopathic autoimmune diseases.

Already noted in Chapter 18 was the fact that neoplasms produce antigens to which the host mounts an immune response resulting in both humoral and cell-mediated reactions in target tissues. Similar "paraneoplastic" effects of antibodies and cell-mediated immunity induced by the production of antigens by neoplastic tissues include autoimmune hemolytic anemias occurring in association with a variety of carcinomas (Sokol et al., 1994) and chronic lymphocytic leukemia (cf. Kipps and Carson, 1993); autoimmune mucocutaneous disease associated with skin blistering and ulceration resulting from autoantibodies to keratin, also associated with lymphomas (Anhalt et al., 1990); and vasculitis resulting from antibodies to antigens within the vascular system (Carsons, 1997). It is estimated that 5% of patients with vasculitis have a malignancy. There have been suggestions that these autoimmune phenomena seen in the host–tumor relationship could actually be utilized to induce a self immunity to the neoplasm provided one could select the appropriate antigen as the target for the host immune system (cf. Nanda and Sercarz, 1995; Pardoll, 1999). However, a variety of other techniques have been utilized in an attempt to take advantage of the peculiar immunobiology of the host–tumor relationship in attempts to prevent, cure, or eliminate the neoplastic disease in the host.

IMMUNOTHERAPY

While we have seen both immune mechanisms for the successful destruction of neoplastic cells by the host as well as the ability of the neoplasms to escape such host immune mechanisms, the promise of utilizing this delicate immunological balance for the control and/or elimination of the neoplasm has not yet been realized. Our knowledge of immune mechanisms, both at the biological and molecular level, has increased exponentially during the last two or three decades. The use of immunotherapeutic measures, alone or in conjunction with other types of therapy, has only rarely led to a complete cure of the disease, while surgery, radiation, and chemotherapy have all been successful in eradication of neoplastic disease in hundreds of thousands of patients. Despite this failure, the search for a successful immunotherapeutic regimen leading to the cure of neoplastic disease continues at an even greater pace.

Vaccines

The first clinical use of a vaccine in the treatment of cancer was reported by Coley (1893) more than a century ago. The vaccine consisted of extracts of pyogenic bacteria with the object of stimulating a generalized immune response that would hopefully include the neoplasm. Since that time, and mostly in recent years, a number of other attempts have been made to produce a variety of vaccines aimed at inducing both cellular and humoral immunity toward antigens within specific neoplasms and also those that induce a more generalized enhancement of the immune response. Earlier studies simply utilized extracts or fractions of neoplastic cells, which were injected directly into the patient with or without various adjuvants. Adjuvants consisted of various simple or complex molecules known to enhance the immune response in general such as killed bacteria, complex polysaccharides, and certain lipids. More recently, however, cancer vaccines have become better defined and are used with specific targets or purposes, such as enhancing specific types of immunity. In Table 19.15 may be seen a listing of various types of acellular cancer vaccines and their targeted neoplasm or neoplastic condition.

Since neoplasms exhibit altered surface glycoproteins and gangliosides (Chapter 15), the potential for immunological responses to such structures is to be expected and has been demonstrated (cf. Livingston, 1992). Modification of autologous cancer cells and components with haptens, especially dinitrophenyl, produces altered proteins on the surface of such neoplastic cells, resulting, presumably, in immune reactions to both hapten-modified cells and unmodified cells. In this way, T-cell clones reactive to antigens on the surface of the neoplastic cell would be expected to occur (Berd et al., 1998). In certain neoplasms, especially lymphomas and myelomas producing excessive amounts of antibodies, use of the specific antibody produced by the neoplastic cells as an idiotype vaccine would be expected to produce antibodies and cell-mediated reactions to that specific antigen (Bianchi and Massaia, 1997). As was discussed earlier (Figure 19.20), some mucoproteins on neoplasms are underglycosylated and thus offer potential antigens for vaccination (Finn et al., 1995). Since specific peptide epitopes to antigens presented

Table 19.15 Cancer Vaccines—Noncellular

Vaccine Components	Potential Targets
Blood group–related carbohydrate antigens	Epithelial cancers, breast, etc.
Gangliosides	Melanoma
Hapten-modified vaccines	Metastatic melanoma
Idiotypic vaccines	Follicular lymphomas
Mucins, underglycosylated	Mucin-producing epithelial cancers
Peptide epitopes	Melanoma, mammary and lung carcinoma
Specific intracellular gene products	Prostate cancer in humans; transplanted cancers in mice
Proto-oncogenes	
Telomerase	
Tumor suppressor genes	
Stress (heat-shock) proteins	Various malignancies
Tumor-specific antigens	Melanoma
Viral antigens	Hepatitis B

by the MHC proteins of neoplastic cells have now been identified, such as those related to MAGE, GAGE, CEA, and others (Celis et al., 1995), it is possible to utilize such peptides as vaccines in association with various adjuvant or enhancement techniques (Rosenberg, 1996). Regressions of metastatic melanoma in patients treated with an antigen peptide encoded by the MAGE-3 gene presented by HLA-A1 in patients have been described (Marchand et al., 1999). Vaccines developed to proto-oncogene products, especially the *ras* family (Fenton et al., 1995; Halpern, 1997), and telomerase (Minev et al., 2000), a protein virtually absent in most adult cell types, have been used experimentally. Similarly, heat-shock proteins, when isolated from neoplastic cells, are usually complexed with a wide array of peptides. Such complexes have been utilized as vaccines in a variety of animal studies (Przepiorka and Srivastava, 1998). Vaccines against tumor-specific antigens have been employed predominantly against melanoma (Berd and Mastrangelo, 1993). By far the most successful preventive vaccines have been with virus-induced neoplasms, particularly hepatitis B in the human (Blumberg, 1997). Other known herpesviruses including the EBV and HSV-8 viruses are also potential candidates for the development of preventive vaccines (cf. Fischinger, 1992). Clinical trials are already under way with preventive and therapeutic vaccines for human papillomavirus-associated cervical cancers (Ling et al., 2000).

Recently, whole cells modified either by transfection, virus infection, or hybridization have been utilized as vaccines against specific neoplasms or more general enhancement of the host immune response. Cellular immunity in chimpanzees to human tumor-associated mucins has been effected by vaccination with Epstein-Barr virus–immortalized autologous B cells transfected with the MUC-1 cDNA (Pecher and Finn, 1996). In another experimental system, Newton et al. (2000) utilized a cell line for the formation of cell hybrids after fusion with patient-derived neoplastic cells. The hybrid cells were then irradiated to prevent their replication and inoculated as a vaccine into patients with melanoma or adenocarcinoma. Another method of cellular cancer vaccination is the transfection of neoplastic cells from the host with genes of specific antigens, cytokines, or costimulatory molecules involved in the interaction of T cells and neoplastic cells. In experimental systems, a variety of genes for different cytokines and costimulatory molecules have been transfected into specific neoplastic cells (cf. Forni et al., 1995). The rationale here is that the reinoculated cells will markedly stimulate the host-immune system to the neoplasm containing the transfected genes as well as the identical neoplasm in the host. A similar rationale has been used in transfecting specific antigens into neoplastic cells (e.g., Schweighoffer, 1996).

DNA Vaccines

The traditional cancer vaccines indicated above involve the use of protein, carbohydrate, and lipid macromolecules administered with the intent to stimulate specifically classical immune responses to the antigens employed. However, as discussed in earlier chapters (Chapters 5, 9, and 16), it is possible to transfect DNA directly into cells either as naked DNA, along with a carrier such as a liposome, as a component of the genetic apparatus of a virus whose genome is incorporated into the host DNA, or as part of the cellular metabolism. Based on our knowledge of the processes of antigen uptake, processing, and presentation (Figures 19.14 and 19.15), it appeared feasible to utilize DNA transfection in vivo as a method for vaccination against both pathogens and neoplastic cell antigens. In Figure 19.31 may be seen a diagram of the general technology utilized in DNA vaccination beginning with a neoplastic cell. Although this technology has thus far been utilized almost exclusively in animals for vaccination against viruses, bacteria, and parasites (Kowalczyk and Ertl, 1999), some human trials of DNA vaccines have also been undertaken, including those against specific human neoplasms (Koide et al., 2000). As noted in the

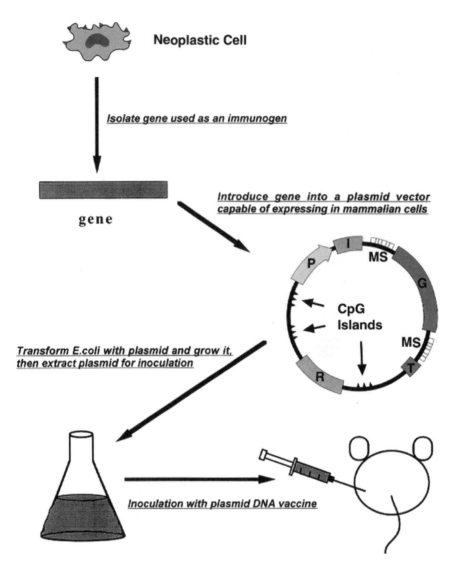

Figure 19.31 Schematic diagram of DNA vaccine technology utilized to produce vaccines against neoplastic cells. The symbols of the components making up the plasmid vector are as follows: G, the gene of interest taken from the neoplastic cell; MS, multicloning sites for restriction enzymes which facilitate insertion of the gene; T, termination signal; R, antibiotic resistance gene needed to amplify the plasma only in those bacteria that carry it; P, promoter sequence that initiates transcription of the gene; I, intron that enhances transcription of the gene of interest. The CpG island's function is discussed in the text. (Modified from Sasaki et al., 1999, with permission of the authors and publisher.)

figure, in addition to the gene of interest various other genes that allow the growth of the plasmid in bacteria are incorporated into the plasmid as well as CpG islands, which are unmethylated as they would be in bacteria in contrast to the methylation of such sequences seen in most vertebrate DNA (cf. Manders and Thomas, 2000). Such sequences have been shown to stimulate innate immunity because their structural characteristics are distinctly different from vertebrate CpG islands (cf. Krieg, 2000).

Administration of the DNA plasmid may be directly into the cell by using a variety of techniques such as "gene guns," intramuscular or intradermal injection, or an association with lipid molecules in the form of structures termed liposomes (cf. Lewis and Babiuk, 1999). The sequence of events then occurring in vivo is diagrammatically depicted in Figure 19.32 using the example of intramuscular administration of the naked DNA. However, DNA may be presented to other cells in the organism in vivo, or, as noted above, transfected in vitro and then implanted into the host, as in the case of dendritic cells (see above). The figure depicts the production of antigen by the DNA incorporated into the muscle cell genome. Presentation will be on the surface as with any other cell, with subsequent acquisition of such antigen by dendritic cells and specific activation of cytotoxic T lymphocytes. Also shown in the picture is the transfection of cytokine DNAs that recruit dendritic cells in order to enhance the immune response to the DNA-transfected gene, producing the antigen in the muscle cell (Giese, 1998; Biragyn et al., 1999). Although successful in animals, it may be some time before DNA vaccines will be realized for use in humans because of the potential dangers involved. These include transfection with contaminating DNA, leading to a variety of other potential problems including the neoplastic transformation and the possibility that DNA vaccines might induce autoimmune disease (Mor et al., 1997).

Another variant of DNA vaccination is to utilize viral vectors, i.e., viruses with modified genomes that include the gene of interest. Both potentially oncogenic viruses, such as the adenovirus (Hu and Garen, 2000), and nonpathogenic vaccinia viruses have been used for this purpose (Hareuveni et al., 1990; Tsang et al., 1995). In this instance, delivery to cells of the appropriate DNA would likely be more efficient because of the normal pathogenic mechanisms of the virus, but the potential for infection or even transformation may make this technique somewhat less desirable.

Vaccination with Adjuvants

Over the past 200 years, physicians have noted that, on rare occasions, cancer patients who went through a severe infection may have experienced a shrinkage and even an elimination of their neoplasm. Based on these occasional observations, Coley utilized preparations from bacteria to treat a variety of cancer patients (Coley, 1893). From these studies ultimately came the discovery of the tumor necrosis factor (Chapter 17). Coley's extensive series of well-documented cases of successful effects of this type of treatment is quite impressive even to this date (cf. Fiers, 1991). During the latter half of the last century, another form of such "vaccination" was utilized to treat a variety of animal and human neoplasms. This technique was vaccination with preparations consisting mostly of an attenuated strain of *Mycobacterium bovis* termed bacillus Calmette-Guérin, or BCG. Actually, the utilization of this bacterial preparation developed from its utilization as a vaccine for tuberculosis (Bast et al., 1974). The dramatic stimulation of the immune system by this preparation was noted, and it thus became a candidate for use in immunotherapy of neoplasia. While it was used in the immunotherapy of leukemias, melanoma, and some other neoplasms (Bast et al., 1974), its usefulness never achieved its anticipated promise. Furthermore, a variety of complications with its use have been described (Sparks, 1976), including the enhancement of neoplastic growth (Ishibashi et al., 1978). Other general immunostimulants that have been used experimentally include specific fractions of mycobacteria (McLaughlin et al., 1978) and *Corynebacterium parvum*, which has been used in humans (cf. Lutz, 1983).

More successful utilization of BCG has been reported in the past decade. This involves its use by installation in the bladders of patients with low-grade transitional cell carcinoma of the bladder. This technique has been used as a prophylaxis both against recurrence of multiple papillomas that are the usual finding in such patients and also for the regression of early lesions in

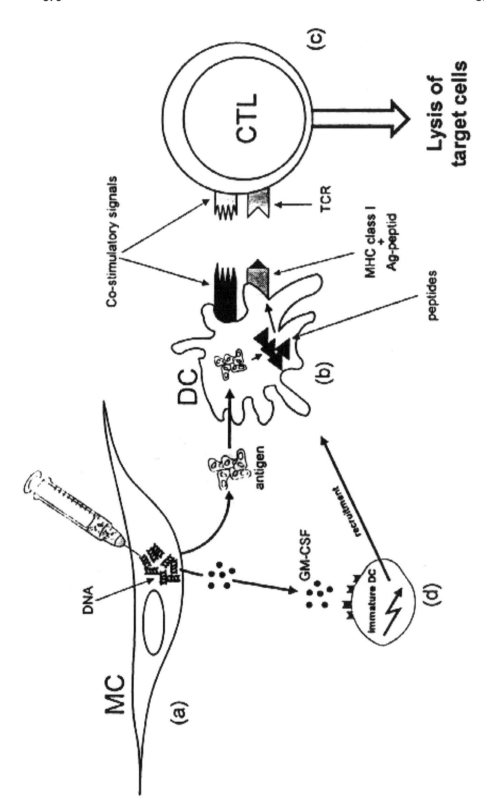

Figure 19.32 Diagram of effects of intramuscular injection of DNA plasmid vaccine. In this scenario, the vaccine also contains a gene for a cytokine, granulocyte-macrophage colony-stimulating factor (GM-CSF). Since muscle cells express little, if any, MHC molecules, dendritic cells acquire the antigen by secretion from or apoptosis of muscle cells, with subsequent presentation to appropriate cytotoxic T cells (CTL). In order to enhance or "cross-prime" the reaction, the GM-CSF produced by the muscle cell containing this gene after transfection recruits and stimulates dendritic cells to the site with enhancement of production of CTLs. (Adapted from Giese, 1998, with permission of the author and publisher.)

the bladder (Melekos, 1995). In general, however, nonspecific immunostimulation of the immune system has not found a major place in the immunotherapy of human neoplasia.

Antibody Therapy of Neoplasia

Although polyclonal antibodies had been raised against a variety of antigens from many neoplasms, their usefulness in therapy was never completely realized, primarily because the antibody source, usually an animal, disappeared with the death of the animal or the formation of multiple cross-reactive antibodies on repeated immunizations. In addition, the host response to the foreign antigen (antibody) usually prevented its use after a limited time period. It was not until the development of monoclonal antibodies that could be continuously produced in mice and/or tissue culture or even in human cells that the antibody therapy of neoplasia became more realistic. A diagram of the technique of producing monoclonal antibodies in mice is seen in Figure 19.33. Monoclonal antibodies specific for antigens on neoplastic cells can induce a variety of responses, including apoptosis, interference with ligand-receptor interactions, modulation of chemotherapeutic cytotoxic effects, and both complement-mediated and antibody-directed cytotoxicity (Weiner, 1999). While a number of clinical trials with various antibodies have been and are under study (cf. Scott and Welt, 1997), one of the most successful and presently clinically useful monoclonal antibodies is that directed toward the HER-2/*neu* cellular oncogene present on the surface of a variety of neoplastic cells. This molecule is a member of the epidermal growth factor receptor family and presumably functions as a growth factor receptor (cf. Disis and Cheever, 1997). Most normal tissues express this protein only slightly if at all, whereas up to 34% of breast cancers overexpress the molecule, many times probably owing to amplification (cf. Ross and Fletcher, 1999; Ménard et al., 2000). Although the use of this monoclonal antibody therapy is usually carried out according to standard therapy, up to 37% of patients treated with the antibody developed objective response and disease stabilization (cf. Ross and Fletcher, 1999).

Immune Conjugates in Antibody Therapy

Monoclonal antibodies to specific antigens on neoplastic cells may also be used as carriers for specific molecules that are toxic to the cell. In theory, this would then selectively eliminate the neoplastic cell carrying the antigen recognized by the monoclonal antibody. A diagram of such a system is seen in Figure 19.34. A variety of different toxins conjugated to monoclonal antibodies reactive with specific surface antigens have been studied (Kreitman, 1999).

In addition to the use of various toxins conjugated to monoclonal antibodies, radioactive elements and compounds have also been utilized. In a very similar manner, as noted in Figure 19.34, an antibody containing a conjugate of a radioactive element or compound is utilized in the same way. In this way the radioactivity enters the cell, thereby destroying it and the surrounding cells. In theory, the selectivity of this type of therapy should be quite high, and several different radioactive monoclonal antibody conjugates are now in clinical use (cf. DeNardo et al., 1998; White et al., 1999).

Adoptive Cellular Immunotherapy

As noted earlier in this chapter, several cellular populations, notably NK cells and macrophages as well as some dendritic cell populations, can exhibit effective immune responses against neoplasms. However, it was not until methods were developed to produce large populations of such cells that could be reinfused into the autologous donor that the use of cells in the immunotherapy

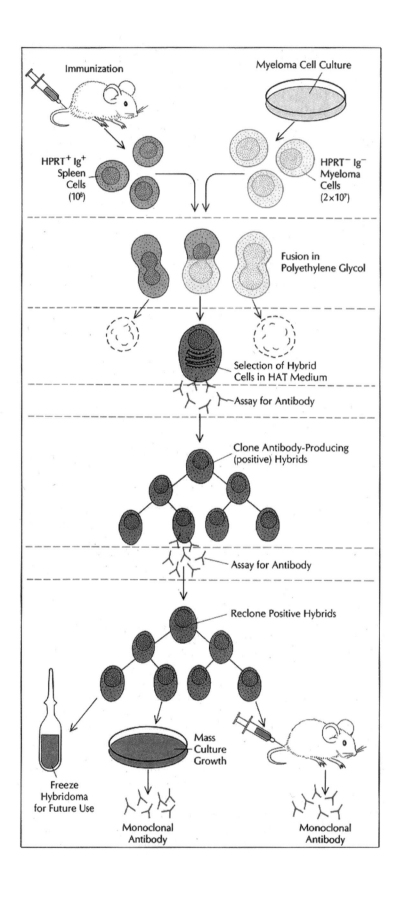

Immunization

Myeloma Cell Culture

HPRT⁺ Ig⁺ Spleen Cells (10^8)

HPRT⁻ Ig⁻ Myeloma Cells (2×10^7)

Fusion in Polyethylene Glycol

Selection of Hybrid Cells in HAT Medium

Assay for Antibody

Clone Antibody-Producing (positive) Hybrids

Assay for Antibody

Reclone Positive Hybrids

Freeze Hybridoma for Future Use

Mass Culture Growth

Monoclonal Antibody

Monoclonal Antibody

of neoplasia was realized. A major breakthrough in such techniques was the discovery of the cytokine, IL-2, originally known as T-cell growth factor (Morgan et al., 1976). This discovery allowed the expansion or growth of T cells and NK cells from relatively small numbers taken from the blood of the tumor-bearing host.

Lymphokine-Activated Killer Cells

The realization of the methodology mentioned above in both animals and humans came about within a decade of the discovery of T-cell growth factor. Mononuclear cells were isolated from blood by a continuous-flow cell separator, allowing the reinfusion of mononuclear cell–depleted blood back into the same patient. Some 10 to 14 L of whole blood could be processed from a patient within 4 hours (Rosenberg et al., 1987). These cells were then subjected to one of several schemes, an example of which is noted in Figure 19.35. The adherent lymphokine-activated killer (LAK) cells, which were adherent to the culture dish, were those expanded by growth in cell culture. These cells are predominantly derived from NK cells (cf. Whiteside and Herberman, 1990). Cumulative doses up to 1.5×10^{11} cells were administered intravenously over a period of 4 to 14 days together with IL-2 (Rosenberg et al., 1987). The principal neoplasms treated in this way were melanoma and renal cell carcinoma, with the average response from eight different studies of 16% and 22% respectively (Chang and Shu, 1992). Unfortunately, a variety of toxicities were associated with this type of therapy, and thus additional other modalities have been investigated.

Tumor-Infiltrating Lymphocytes

In an attempt to enhance the specificity of the LAK cell therapy, Rosenberg and colleagues studied a system in mice in which lymphocytes occurring directly within neoplasms, termed tumor-infiltrating lymphocytes (TILs), were cultured with IL-2 (Rosenberg et al., 1986). Their studies showed that in mice bearing micrometastases from various types of neoplasms, TILs are 50 to 100 times more effective in their therapeutic potency than are LAK cells. In humans, 60% to 70% of patients bearing a variety of different types of neoplasms allowed for the expansion of TIL successfully. Unfortunately, since it takes about 2 months to expand the population of TIL to therapeutic levels, the original neoplasm has usually grown significantly during this period in those cases in which this technique has been tried (cf. Schiltz et al., 1997). IL-2 is also adminis-

Figure 19.33 Basic steps in the production of a monoclonal antibody, beginning with the immunization of mice with the antigen of interest. Spleen cells that express the immunoglobulin (Ig^+) of interest as well as express an enzyme used for selection, hypoxanthine pyrophosphorylribosyltransferase ($HPRT^+$), are fused with malignant myeloma cells maintained in culture. The latter are $HPRT^-$ and Ig^-. Fusion of these cells results in self fusion of both myeloma and spleen cells seen on the right and left respectively, as well as a hybrid between the two cell types, seen in the middle. Utilization of a selection medium (HAT) containing both hypoxanthine and thymine as well as amethopterin allows the selection of myeloma hybrids that can bypass the amethopterin block by the presence of HPRT and thymidine kinase from the spleen cell. The fused myeloma cell is unable to do this and dies, while the fused spleen cells tend not to grow. One then clones the fused cell termed a hybridoma, each clone producing only a single antibody species for the reasons discussed earlier in this chapter. From this, one may obtain large amounts of monoclonal antibody by culture of the hybridoma cells or inoculation into mice as an ascites, which also produces large amounts of the monoclonal antibody. Hybridoma cells may be frozen for future use. (Adapted from Levy, 1985, with permission of the author and publisher.)

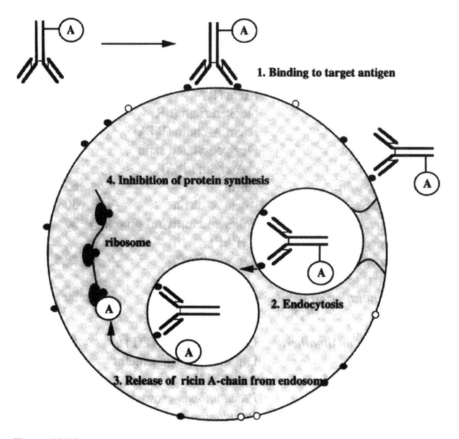

Figure 19.34 Diagrammatic representation of the mechanism of action of a monoclonal antibody to a specific antigen on the surface of a neoplastic cell. The antibody is conjugated to and is carrying a bacterial toxin, ricin A (A). The entire complex is endocytosed into the cell, and on degradation of the peptide the toxin is released intracellularly where it inhibits protein synthesis. (Adapted from Winkler et al., 1997, with permission of the author and publisher.)

tered together with TIL. A summary diagram of these two forms of cellular adoptive immunotherapy is seen in Figure 19.36.

Dendritic Cells for the Immunotherapy of Neoplasia

Methods for the expansion of dendritic cells and other antigen-presenting cells are not as effective as those for NK cells. However, it is possible to isolate such cells from both neoplasms and normal tissues and manipulate them in cell culture. In experimental systems, bone marrow–derived dendritic cells pulsed with synthetic peptides as epitopes presented on the surface of neoplastic cells have been used to elicit protective and therapeutic immunity to neoplasms in mice (Mayordomo et al., 1995). Phagocytosis of apoptotic cells from neoplasms by antigen-presenting cells (Henry et al., 1999) and fusion of dendritic and neoplastic cells (Gong et al., 1997) have also been methods tried with some success in experimental animals. A unique protocol that may have direct application in the human is the immunization of bone marrow transplantation donors with tumor antigens and the use of the transplant as adoptive therapy against the established

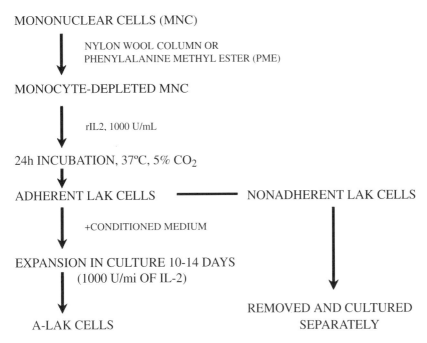

MONONUCLEAR CELLS (MNC)

NYLON WOOL COLUMN OR
PHENYLALANINE METHYL ESTER (PME)

MONOCYTE-DEPLETED MNC

rIL2, 1000 U/mL

24h INCUBATION, 37°C, 5% CO$_2$

ADHERENT LAK CELLS —————— NONADHERENT LAK CELLS

+CONDITIONED MEDIUM

EXPANSION IN CULTURE 10-14 DAYS
(1000 U/mi OF IL-2)

REMOVED AND CULTURED
A-LAK CELLS   SEPARATELY

Figure 19.35   A diagram of the preparation of human adherent lymphokine-activated killer (A-LAK) cells. Condition medium is obtained from 24-hour incubation cultures and is added back to A-LAK cells at a final concentration of 50% (v/v) in fresh IL-2–containing medium. A-LAK cells are grown in culture for 2 to 3 weeks, allowing for significant expansion of the cell population to the numbers utilized in therapy (see text). (Adapted from Whiteside and Herberman, 1990, with permission of the authors and publisher.)

neoplasm (Hornung et al., 1995). In fact, graft-versus-leukemia reactions can be induced in patients with hematological cancers by allogeneic stem cell and bone marrow transplantation and also have shown some success with renal cell carcinoma (Childs et al., 2000). In theory, such technologies may be an ideal way to produce dendritic cells specific for antigens in neoplasms (Björck, 1999; Fong and Engleman, 2000), but there are still a number of logistical problems to overcome.

Cytokine Immunotherapy of Neoplasia

The known number of hormone-like proteins affecting the immune system has increased exponentially during the last two decades. More than 18 interleukins are presently known, as well as a variety of other proteins directly affecting cells of the immune system (Table 19.4). Tumor necrosis factor and its family of ligands (Chapter 17) have already been discussed; below are several other important cytokines that have found some place in immunotherapy.

Interleukins

Of the 18 or more known interleukins, the one that has been found most effective in the therapy of neoplasia is interleukin-2 (IL-2). As noted above, IL-2, the T-cell growth factor, has been used in conjunction with cellular immunotherapy as well as by itself. In the latter instance, responses

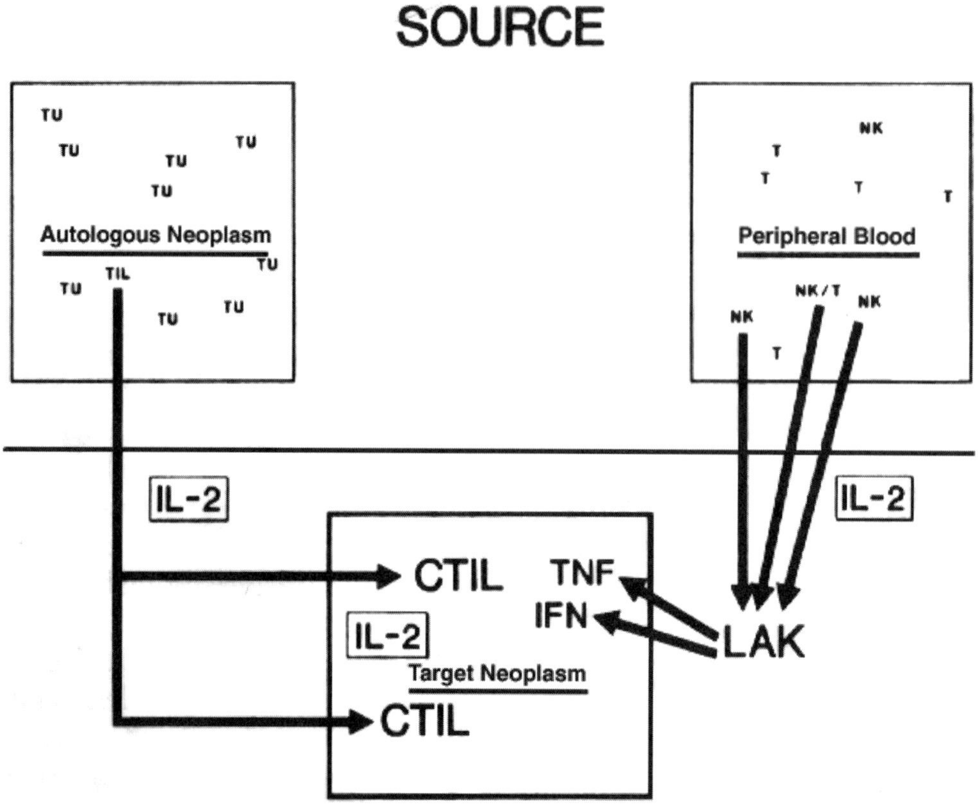

SOURCE

Figure 19.36   Diagrammatic model of immunotherapeutic interaction of LAK cells and TIL on a target neoplasm. TIL and LAK cells are obtained from the autologous neoplasm and peripheral blood of the patient, expanded as described above, and then reinoculated into the patient in the presence of interleukin-2 administered simultaneously. On the left, TIL are removed from fresh neoplasm obtained at surgery from the patient, expanded, and then reinfused together with interleukin-2 with subsequent reinfiltration of the target neoplasm. On the right, NK and T cells in peripheral blood are removed from leukapheresis and the LAK cells after expansion infused into the patient along with interleukin-2, many of the cells returning to the neoplasm where they in turn produce interferon-γ (IFN) and tumor necrosis factor (TNF). (Adapted from Atzpodien and Kirchner, 1990, with permission of the authors and publisher.)

of up to 40% have been seen (Oleksowicz and Dutcher, 1999) in metastatic renal cell carcinoma, while only a 13% response may be seen in the therapy of melanoma by IL-2 (cf. Bishop, 1996). IL-2 therapy, like a number of other immunotherapies, also has profound toxic effects in patients, probably because its effects are far more diverse than simply those of NK cells (Janssen et al., 1994). It should be noted that in a very small percentage of cases, 6% to 15% (Figlin et al., 1997; Oleksowicz and Dutcher, 1999), a complete remission was achieved, which remained for a number of years or as long as the study continued. Such effects are reminiscent of the "spontaneous" disappearance of neoplasms with no obvious explanation. The difficulty is determining the exact conditions within the individual that give rise to such complete responses. In addition to IL-2, IL-12 (Okuno et al., 1996) and IL-10 (Kundu and Fulton, 1997) have shown significant immunotherapeutic effects in both human and experimental situations.

As implied in the discussion above concerning transfection of genes into cells, attempts have also been made to transfect cytokine genes into neoplastic cells in vitro into the autologous host with the intention that such cells would stimulate an immune response in their immediate area, such a response being then translated to the primary and metastatic neoplasm of the host (Bubeník, 1993; Belli et al., 1997; Leong et al., 1997). Similar rationales have been utilized for transfecting hematopoietic growth factors, specifically granulocyte-macrophage colony-stimulating factor, with similar intent (Bubeník, 1999).

Interferons

The interferons are a family of glycoproteins made up of between 145 and 166 amino acids and having molecular weights ranging between 17,000 and 25,000. There are at least three different forms—alpha, beta, and gamma. Alpha interferon is produced primarily by activated leukocytes and appears within 4 to 6 hours after viral stimulation. Beta interferon is also rapidly induced by viral stimulation, but from fibroblasts. Gamma interferon is produced by lymphocytes and monocytes 2 to 3 days after these cells have been stimulated by exposure to antigens or mitogens. As noted earlier, interferon gamma activates macrophages and NK cells as well as inducing the expression of MHC antigens. Of these interferons, interferon alpha has been shown to have the most efficacy in treatment of a variety of neoplasms. Results of a large series is seen in Table 19.16. As noted from the table, while relatively large doses are required for effectiveness, some neoplasms—such as hairy cell leukemia, chronic myelogenous leukemia, and endocrine pancreatic neoplasms—appear to have a very reasonable response rate. As with other immunotherapeutic modalities, certain toxicities are seen with this type of therapy, many of them imitating a flu-like complex, but hematological, renal, and gastrointestinal toxicities have also been

Table 19.16 Interferon Alpha Treatment Results in Human Neoplasia

	Dose Schedule	Response Rates (Mean) %
Hematological malignancies		
Hairy cell leukemia	3 million IU/day	70–90 (80)
Chronic myelogenous leukemia	5 million IU/m^2/day	45–85 (58)
Lymphocytic lymphoma (low grade)	3–50 million IU/m^2/day or 3 times per week	9–67 (47)
Cutaneous T-cell lymphoma	3–50 million IU/m^2/day or 3 times per week	27–85 (48)
Multiple myeloma	5–12 million IU/m^2/day or 3 times per week	8–18 (15)
Solid neoplasms		
Malignant melanoma	5–20 million IU/m^2/day or 3 times per week	7–29 (18)
Renal cell carcinoma	5–20 million IU/m^2/day or 3 times per week	8–23 (15)
Kaposi sarcoma	3–50 million IU/m^2/day or 3 times per week	3–67 (30)
Endocrine pancreatic tumors	3–5 million IU/m^2/day or 3 times per week	33–77 (50)
Carcinoid tumors	12–24 million IU/m^2 3 times per weeks	20–40 (20)

Adapted from Hansen and Borden, 1992, with permission of the authors and publisher.

Table 19.17 Future Considerations for Successful Cancer Immunotherapy

Patient evaluation
  Size and location(s) of neoplasm
  MHC antigen expression on cells of the neoplasm
Debulking (removal) of the majority of the neoplasm
  Surgery
  Radiotherapy/chemotherapy
    Administration of cytokines and hematopoietic growth factors
Active immunotherapy
  Vaccines—DNA and cell
    Adjuvant support
    Suppressor cell inhibition
  Cytokines and related molecules
    Combinations
    Targeted delivery
Passive/adoptive immunotherapy
  LAK cell and TIL therapy

noted (Hansen and Borden, 1992). In general, however, interferon alpha has now become accepted as an immunotherapeutic agent not only for neoplasia but also for viral and other inflammatory diseases (Gutterman, 1994).

The Future of the Immunotherapy of Neoplasia

As may be noted from the length of this chapter, the immunobiology of the host–tumor relationship is one of the most active areas of investigation directed toward an ultimate effective therapy of neoplasia. However, a number of considerations must be taken into account if one is to be successful in utilizing the immunobiological host–tumor relationship for the therapy of cancer. Some of these are listed in Table 19.17. Of these various considerations, the selection of patients for immunotherapy on the basis of their immunological competence as well as the immunobiology of the neoplasm itself will be a major factor. Of equal or of greater importance is the removal by standard methods of the majority of the neoplasm from the host by surgery, radiotherapy, or chemotherapy. Immunotherapy has as its greatest potential the elimination of micrometastases and small masses of neoplastic cells that are completely available to the immune system. However, the patient must not be in an immunocompromised state when active and passive immunotherapy is undertaken. In fact, establishment of a normal immunocompetent state in a tumor-bearing host may be one of the greatest hurdles to overcome if immunotherapy is to be successful. As explained below, the immunobiology of the host–tumor relationship tends toward immunosuppression of the host as a result of the continued extension of the deterioration of the host–tumor relationship, as noted in Chapter 17 regarding the phenomenon of cachexia.

INFECTIOUS COMPLICATIONS OF NEOPLASTIC DISEASE

One of the characteristics of advanced cancer, especially neoplasms of the immune system, is a decrease in the host resistance to various infectious agents. This phenomenon appears to have three characteristics: (1) a decrease in mature granulocytes, seen in several lymphomas and leukemias, which may result in impaired phagocytosis; (2) an impaired cell-mediated immune response, commonly seen in several lymphomas and leukemias, especially Hodgkin disease; and (3) a decrease or alteration in circulating γ-globulin of host origin, occurring in a number of lymphomas and leukemias and resulting in an increased susceptibility to bacterial infections (Armstrong et al., 1971). In addition to the natural loss of host immunity resulting from the host-tumor relationship, chemotherapy itself may result in a marked suppression of the host immune response, leading to a number of infectious complications. In hematological neoplasms, infections may cause as many as 63% of the deaths in patients with these diseases (Nosari et al., 1991).

Many of the infectious processes that occur in patients with advanced cancer or in patients undergoing chemotherapy are the result of agents that normally do not cause disease in the host. Table 19.18 lists organisms that may cause severe infection in patients with neoplastic disease. The reader will note some familiar infectious agents such as *Salmonella* (typhoid), tuberculosis, measles, and varicella (chickenpox). But most of the agents listed in the table are relatively rare causes of disease in the normal human. These latter organisms can usually attack only the individual whose immune defenses are compromised. This is especially true of fungi (cf. Gold, 1984; Bow, 1998), which appear to be ubiquitous in the human population but rarely cause disease in the immunocompetent host. Earlier we saw that patients with progressive multifocal leukoencephalopathy (PML) were found to have a papovavirus infection within the central nervous system. It is likely that the virus causes PML, but predominantly in humans who exhibit significant immunosuppression associated with lymphomas and other debilitating diseases. In normal individuals the endogenous microbial flora (enteric bacteria) exist in a balanced symbiotic relation within the host. Nevertheless, 86% of the infections that occur in cancer patients arise from such endogenous flora (cf. Pizzo, 1981). Some 47% of the infecting organisms are acquired by patients during hospitalization. The relative malnutrition that accompanies cachexia may further decrease the immunocompetence of the host if the malnutrition is not treated aggressively (cf. Pizzo, 1981).

The extensive growth of tumors, predominantly but not exclusively those of the immune system, results in significant loss of immune resistance by the host, with the concomitant danger of an "opportunistic" infection by a variety of agents. On the other hand, heroic measures of therapy by chemicals and radiation may also leave the host immunosuppressed and vulnerable to infection. In many instances it is this infectious sequel of cancer or its therapy that leads to the ultimate demise of the patient.

Table 19.18 Organisms Causing Severe Infection in Patients with Neoplastic Disease

Bacterial	Fungal	Parasitic	Viral
Listeria monocytogenes	*Candida* spp.	*Pneumocystis carinii*	Cytomegalovirus
Salmonella spp.	*Cryptococcus neoformans*	*Toxoplasma gondii*	Varicella zoster virus
Nocardia asteroides	*Histoplasma capsulatum*		Herpes simplex virus
Mycobacterium tuberculosis	*Mucor* spp.		Vaccinia virus
Clostridium septicum	*Aspergillus* spp.		Rubella virus
Enteric bacteria	*Coccidioides immitus*		
	Sporotrichum schenkii		

After Armstrong et al., 1971, with permission of the authors and publisher.

REFERENCES

Abbas, A. K., and Janeway, C. A. Jr. Immunology: improving on nature in the twenty-first century. Cell, *100*:129–138, 2000.

Abbas, A. K., Murphy, K. M., and Sher, A. Functional diversity of helper T lymphocytes. Nature, *383*:787–793, 1996.

Abo, T. Extrathymic pathways of T-cell differentiation: a primitive and fundamental immune system. Microbiol. Immunol., *37*:247–258, 1993.

Algarra, I., Collado, A., and Garrido, F. Altered MHC class I antigens in tumors. Int. J. Clin. Lab. Res., *27*:95–102, 1997.

Angelopoulou, K., Rosen, B., Stratis, M., Yu, H., Solomou, M., and Diamandis, E. P. Circulating antibodies against p53 protein in patients with ovarian carcinoma. Cancer, *78*:2146–2152, 1996.

Anhalt, G. J., Kim, S., Stanley, J. R., Korman, N. J., Jabs, D. A., Kory, M., Izumi, H., Ratrie, H. III, Mutasim, D., Ariss-Abdo, L., and Labib, R. S. Paraneoplastic pemphigus. An autoimmune mucocutaneous disease associated with neoplasia. N. Engl. J. Med., *323*:1729–1735, 1990.

Antonia, S. J., Extermann, M., and Flavell, R. A. Immunologic nonresponsiveness to tumors. Crit. Rev. Oncog., *9*:35–41, 1998.

Apffel, C. A., and Peters, J. H. Tumors and serum glycoproteins. The "symbodies." Prog. Exp. Tumor Res., *12*:1–54, 1969.

Armstrong, D., Young, L. S., Meyer, R. D., and Blevins, A. H. Infectious complications of neoplastic disease. Med. Clin. North Am., *55*:729–745, 1971.

Arnon, R., and Teitelbaum, D. On the existence of suppressor cells. Int. Arch. Allergy Immunol., *100*:2–7, 1993.

Arvind, P., Papavassiliou, E. D., Tsioulias, G. J., Qiao, L., Lovelace, C. I. P., Duceman, B., and Rigas, B. Prostaglandin E$_2$ down-regulates the expression of HLA-DR antigen in human colon adenocarcinoma cell lines. Biochemistry, *34*:5604–5609, 1995.

Asano, Y., and Tada, T. Generation of T cell repertoire. Two distinct mechanisms for generation of T suppressor cells, T helper cells, and T augmenting cells. J. Immunol., *142*:365–373, 1989.

Atzpodien, J., and Kirchner, H. Cancer, cytokines, and cytotoxic cells: interleukin-2 in the immunotherapy of human neoplasms. Klin. Wochenschr., *68*:1–11, 1990.

Bach, J.-F. Organ-specific autoimmunity. Immunol. Today, *16*:353–355, 1995.

Baker, J. R., Jr., and Fosso, C. K. Immunological aspects of cancers arising from thyroid follicular cells. Endocr. Rev., *14*:729–746, 1993.

Bankhurst, A. D. The modulation of human natural killer cell activity by prostaglandins. J. Clin. Lab. Immunol., *7*:85–91, 1982.

Bast, R. C., Jr., Zbar, B., Borsos, T., and Rapp, H. J. BCG and cancer. N. Engl. J. Med., *290*:1413–1420, 1458–1469, 1974.

Basten, A. Basis and mechanisms of self-tolerance. *In*: The Autoimmune Diseases, 3rd ed., Chapter 2, pp. 9–27. New York: Academic Press, 1998.

Belli, F., Arienti, F., Sulé-Suso, J., Clemente, C., Mascheroni, L., Cattelan, A., Sanantonio, C., Gallino, G. F., Melani, C., Rao, S., Colombo, M. P., Maio, M., Cascinelli, N., and Parmiani, G. Active immunization of metastatic melanoma patients with interleukin-2–transduced allogeneic melanoma cells: evaluation of efficacy and tolerability. Cancer Immunol. Immunother., *44*:197–203, 1997.

Berd, D., Kairys, J., Dunton, C., Mastrangelo, M. J., Sato, T., and Maguire, H. C. Jr. Autologous, hapten-modified vaccine as a treatment for human cancers. Semin. Oncol., *25*:646–653, 1998.

Berd, H. C., and Mastrangelo, M. J. Treatment of human melanoma with a hapten-modified autologous vaccine. Ann. N.Y. Acad. Sci., *690*:147–152, 1993.

Bergman, Y. Allelic exclusion in B and T lymphopoiesis. Semin. Immunol., *11*:319–328, 1999.

Berke, G. The CTL's kiss of death. Cell, *81*:9–12, 1995.

Bernard, P., and Bonnetblanc, J.-M. Dermatomyositis and malignancy. J. Invest. Dermatol., *100*:128S–132S, 1993.

Bernards, R., Schrier, P. I., Houweling, A., Bos, J. L., van der Eb, A. J., Zijlstra, M., and Melief, C. J. M. Tumorigenicity of cells transformed by adenovirus type 12 by evasion of T-cell immunity. Nature, *305*:776–779, 1983.

Bianchi, A., and Massaia, M. Idiotypic vaccination in B-cell malignancies. Mol. Med. Today, *3*:435–441, 1997.

Biragyn, A., Tani, K., Grimm, M. C., Weeks, S., and Kwak, L. W. Genetic fusion of chemokines to a self tumor antigen induces protective, T-cell dependent antitumor immunity. Nature Biotechnol., *17*:253–258, 1999.

Bishop, J. A. N. Current immunotherapy for melanoma. Cancer Surv., *26*:321–333, 1996.

Björck, P. Development of dendritic cells and their use in tumor therapy. Clin. Immunol., *92*:119–127, 1999.

Blanchet, O., Bourge, J.-F., Zinszner, H., Israel, A., Kourilsky, P., Dausset, J., Degos, L., and Paul, P. Altered binding of regulatory factors to HLA class I enhancer sequence in human tumor cell lines lacking class I antigen expression. Proc. Natl. Acad. Sci. U.S.A., *89*:3488–3492, 1992.

Blumberg, B. S. Hepatitis B virus, the vaccine, and the control of primary cancer of the liver. Proc. Natl. Acad. Sci. U.S.A., *94*:7121–7125, 1997.

Boom, M., Pollock, R. E., Shenk, R. R., and Stanford, S. Tumor burden impairment of murine natural killer cell cytotoxicity. Invas. Metast., *8*:118–132, 1988.

Borecký, L. Cytokines: the fourth homeostatic system. Acta Virol., *37*:276–289, 1993.

Bow, E. J. Invasive fungal infections in patients receiving intensive cytotoxic therapy for cancer. Br. J. Haematol., *101*:1–4, 1998.

Brack, C., Hirama, M., Lenhard-Schuller, R., and Tonegawa, S. A complete immunoglobulin gene is created by somatic recombination. Cell, *15*:1–14, 1978.

Brandtzaeg, P. Molecular and cellular aspects of the secretory immunoglobulin system. APMIS (Acta Pathol. Microbiol. Immunol. Scand.), *103*:1–19, 1995.

Breit, T. M., and van Dongen, J. J. M. Unravelling human T-cell receptor junctional region sequences. Thymus, *22*:177–199, 1994.

Brennan, J., Takei, F., Wong, S., and Mager, D. L. Carbohydrate recognition by a natural killer cell receptor, Ly-49C. J. Biol. Chem., *270*:9691–9694, 1995.

Brodt, P. Tumor immunology—three decades in review. Annu. Rev. Microbiol., *37*:447–476, 1983.

Bubeník, J. IL-2 and gene therapy of cancer. Int. J. Oncol., *2*:1049–1052, 1993.

Bubeník, J. Granulocyte-macrophage colony-stimulating factor gene-modified vaccines for immunotherapy of cancer. Folia Biol. (Praha), *45*:115–119, 1999.

Burnet, F. M. The concept of immunological surveillance. Prog. Exp. Tumor Res., *13*:1–27, 1970.

Cai, X., and Garen, A. Anti-melanoma antibodies from melanoma patients immunized with genetically modified autologous tumor cells: selection of specific antibodies from single-chain Fv fusion phage libraries. Proc. Natl. Acad. Sci. U.S.A., *92*:6537–6541, 1995.

Carlsen, N. L. T. How frequent is spontaneous remission of neuroblastomas? Implications for screening. Br. J. Cancer, *61*:441–446, 1990.

Carsons, S. The association of malignancy with rheumatic and connective tissue diseases. Semin. Oncol., *24*:360–372, 1997.

Celis, E., Sette, A., and Grey, H. M. Epitope selection and development of peptide based vaccines to treat cancer. Semin. Cancer Biol., *6*:329–336, 1995.

Chang, A. E., and Shu, S. Immunotherapy with sensitized lymphocytes. Cancer Invest., *10*:357–369, 1992.

Chen, W., Peace, D. J., Rovira, D. K., You, S.-G., and Cheever, M. A. T-cell immunity to the joining region of p210[BCR-ABL] protein. Proc. Natl. Acad. Sci. U.S.A., *89*:1468–1472, 1992.

Chigira, M., Arita, S., and Watanabe, H. Myth of tumor immunology. Int. J. Oncol., *3*:645–654, 1993.

Childs, R., Chernoff, A., Contentin, N., Bahceci, E., Schrump, D., Leitman, S., Read, E. J., Tisdale, J., Dunbar, C., Linehan, W. M., Young, N. S., and Barrett, A. J. Regression of metastatic renal-cell carcinoma after nonmyeloablative allogeneic peripheral-blood stem-cell transplantation. N. Engl. J. Med., *343*:750–758, 2000.

Chouaib, S., Asselin-Paturel, C., Mami-Chouaib, F., Caignard, A., and Blay, J. Y. The host-tumor immune conflict: from immunosuppression to resistance and destruction. Immunol. Today, *18*:493–497, 1997.

Claman, H. N. The biology of the immune response. J.A.M.A., *268*:2790–2796, 1992.

Clarke, C. A. The prevention of Rh isoimmunization. Hosp. Pract., *8*:77–84, 1973.

Cohen, E. P., and Kim, T. S. Neoplastic cells that express low levels of MHC class I determinants escape host immunity. Semin. Cancer Biol., *5*:419–428, 1994.

Coley, W. B. The treatment of malignant tumors by repeated inoculations of erysipelas: with a report of ten original cases. Am. J. Med. Sci., *105*:487–511, 1893.

Cox, A. L., Skipper, J., Chen, Y., Henderson, R. A., Darrow, T. L., Shabanowitz, J., Engelhard, V. H., Hunt, D. F., and Slingluff, C. L. Jr. Identification of a peptide recognized by five melanoma-specific human cytotoxic T cell lines. Science, *264*:716–719, 1994.

Cruz, P. D. Jr. Langerhans cells are initiators of the immunosuppressive effect of ultraviolet B radiation. Springer Semin. Immunopathol., *13*:281–288, 1992.

Dalianis, T. Studies on the polyoma virus tumor-specific transplantation antigen (TSTA). Adv. Cancer Res., *55*:57–85, 1990.

David-Watine, B., Israël, A., and Kourilsky, P. The regulation and expression of MHC class I genes. Immunol. Today, *11*:286–292, 1990.

DeFranco, A. L. Tyrosine phosphorylation and the mechanism of signal transduction by the B-lymphocyte antigen receptor. Eur. J. Biochem., *210*:381–388, 1992.

DeFranco, A. L. Signaling pathways activated by protein tyrosine phosphorylation in lymphocytes. Curr. Opin. Immunol., *6*:364–371, 1993.

Delves, P. J., and Roitt, I. M. The immune system. N. Engl. J. Med., *343*:108–117, 2000.

DeNardo, G. L., O'Donnell, R. T., Oldham, R. K., and DeNardo, S. J. A revolution in the treatment of non-Hodgkin's lymphoma. Cancer Biother. Radiopharm., *13*:213–223, 1998.

De Plaen, E., Lurquin, C., Brichard, V., van der Bruggen, P., Renauld, J.-C., Coulie, P., Szikora, J.-P., Wölfel, T., Van Pel, A., and Boon, T. Cloning of genes coding for antigens recognized by cytolytic T lymphocytes. *In*: I. Lefkovits (Ed.), The Immunology Methods Manual, pp. 692–718. New York: Academic Press, 1997.

Desiderio, S. V., Yancopoulos, G. D., Paskind, M., Thomas, E., Boss, M. A., Landau, N., Alt, F. W., and Baltimore, D. Insertion of *N* regions into heavy-chain genes is correlated with expression of terminal deoxytransferase in B cells. Nature, *311*:752–755, 1984.

de Tribolet, N., and Carrel, S. Human glioma tumour-associated antigens. Cancer Immunol. Immunother., *9*:207–211, 1980.

Dhodapkar, M. V., Merlini, G., and Solomon, A. Biology and therapy of immunoglobulin deposition diseases. Hematol./Oncol. Clin. North Am., *11*:89–110, 1997.

Disis, M. L., and Cheever, M. A. HER-2/neu protein: a target for antigen-specific immunotherapy of human cancer. Adv. Cancer Res., *71*:343–371, 1997.

Dorf, M. E., and Benacerraf, B. I-J as a restriction element in the suppressor T cell system. Immunol. Rev., *83*:23–36, 1985.

Dorf, M. E., Kuchroo, V. K., and Collins, M. Suppressor T cells: some answers but more questions. Immunol. Today, *13*:241–243, 1992.

Du Pasquier, L. Origin and evolution of the vertebrate immune system. APMIS, *100*:383–392, 1992.

Dwyer, J. M. Manipulating the immune system with immune globulin. N. Engl. J. Med., *326*:107–116, 1992.

Early, P., Huang, H., Davis, M., Calame, K., and Hood, L. An immunoglobulin heavy chain variable region gene is generated from three segments of DNA: V_H, D and J_H.Cell, *19*:981–992, 1980.

Ehrlich, P., and Morgenroth, J. *In*: F. Himmelweit, M. Marquardt, and H. D. Dale (Eds.), The Collected Papers of Paul Ehrlich, pp. 205–212. London: Pergamon, 1957.

Eisenbarth, G. S., and Bellgrau, D. Autoimmunity. Sci. Am., *1*:38–47, 1994.

Ellem, K. A. O., Schmidt, C. W., Li, C.-L., Misko, I., Kelso, A., Sing, G., Macdonald, G., and O'Rourke, M. G. E. The labyrinthine ways of cancer immunotherapy—T cell, tumor cell encounter: "How do I lose thee? Let me count the ways." Adv. Cancer Res., *75*:203–249, 1998.

Evans, A. E., Gerson, J., and Schnaufer, L. Spontaneous regression of neuroblastoma. Natl. Cancer Inst. Monogr., *44*:49–54, 1976.

Fagarasan, S., and Honjo, T. T-independent immune response: new aspects of B cell biology. Science, *290*:89–92, 2000.

Fauve, R. M. Macrophages and cancer, 50th forum in immunology. Res. Immunol., *144*:265–298, 1993.

Fearon, D. T., and Locksley, R. M. The instructive role of innate immunity in the acquired immune response. Science, *272*:50–54, 1996.

Feizi, T., and Childs, R. A. Carbohydrate structures of glycoproteins and glycolipids as differentiation antigens, tumour-associated antigens and components of receptor systems. Trends Biochem. Sci., *10*:24–29, 1985.

Fenig, E., Nordenberg, J., Lurie, H., Angel, P., Feldman, M., and Eisenbach, L. Amplification of the expression of major histocomptibility class I antigens by inducers of differentiation and gamma interferon in murine and human solid tumor cell lines. Int. J. Oncol., *2*:279–282, 1993.

Fenton, R. G., Keller, C. J., Hanna, N., and Taub, D. D. Induction of T-cell immunity against ras oncoproteins by soluble protein or ras-expressing *Escherichia coli*. J. Natl. Cancer Inst., *87*:1853–1861, 1995.

Fiers, W. Tumor necrosis factor. Characterization at the molecular, cellular and in vivo level. FEBS Lett., *285*:199–212, 1991.

Figlin, R., Gitlitz, B., Franklin, J., Dorey, F., Moldawer, N., Rausch, J., deKernion, J., and Belldegrun, A. Interleukin-2-based immunotherapy for the treatment of metastatic renal cell carcinoma: an analysis of 203 consecutively treated patients. Cancer J. Sci. Am., *3*:S92–S97, 1997.

Finn, O. J., and Gendler, S. J. Mimic 1 of MUC1. Nature Biotechnol., *16*:236–237, 1998.

Finn, O. J., Jerome, K. R., Henderson, R., Pecher, G., Domenech, N., Magarian-Blander, J., and Barratt-Boyes, S. M. MUC-1 epithelial tumor mucin-based immunity and cancer vaccines. Immunol. Rev., *145*:61–89, 1995.

Fischinger, P. J. Prospects for reducing virus-associated human cancers by anti vaccines. J. Natl. Cancer Inst. Monogr., *12*:109–114, 1992.

Foley, E. J. Antigenic properties of methylcholanthrene-induced tumors in mice of the strain of origin. Cancer Res., *13*:835–837, 1953.

Fong, L., and Engleman, E. G. Dendritic cells in cancer immunotherapy. Annu. Rev. Immunol., *18*:245–273, 2000.

Forni, G., Cavallo, F., Consalvo, M., Allione, A., Dellabona, P., Casorati, G., and Giovarelli, M. Molecular approaches to cancer immunotherapy. Cytokines Mol. Ther., *1*:225–248, 1995.

Fraumeni, J. F., Jr., and Hoover, R. Immunosurveillance and cancer: epidemiologic observations. Natl. Cancer Inst. Monogr., *47*:121–126, 1977.

French, D. L., Laskov, R., and Scharff, M. D. The role of somatic hypermutation in the generation of antibody diversity. Science, *244*:1152–1157, 1989.

Fugmann, S. D., Lee, A. I., Shockett, P. E., Villey, I. J., and Schatz, D. G. The RAG proteins and V(D)J recombination: complexes, ends, and transposition. Annu. Rev. Immunol., *18*:495–527, 2000.

Garrido, F., Cabrera, T., Concha, A., Glew, S., Ruiz-Cabello, F., and Stern, P. L. Natural history of HLA expression during tumour development. Immunol. Today, *14*:491–499, 1993.

Gatenby, P. A., Basten, A., and Creswick, P. "Sneaking through": a T-cell-dependent phenomenon. Br. J. Cancer, *44*:753–756, 1981.

Gensler, H. L. Enhancement of chemical carcinogenesis in mice by systemic effects of ultraviolet irradiation. Cancer Res., *48*:620–623, 1988.

Gensler, H. L. Systemic modulation by ultraviolet irradiation of cutaneous *N*-methyl-*N'*-nitro-*N*-nitrosoguanidine-induced carcinogenesis. Cancer Lett., *61*:135–140, 1992.

Germain, R. N. MHC-dependent antigen processing and peptide presentation: providing ligands for T lymphocyte activation. Cell, *76*:287–299, 1994.

Giese, M. DNA-antiviral vaccines: new developments and approaches—a review. Virus Genes, *17*:219–232, 1998.

Girmann, G., Pees, H., Schwarze, G., and Scheurlen, P. G. Immunosuppression by micromolecular fibrinogen degradation products in cancer. Nature, *259*:399–401, 1976.

Gleichmann, E., Gleichmann, H., and Wilke, W. Autoimmunization and lymphomagenesis in parent-F_1 combinations differing at the major histocompatibility complex: model for spontaneous disease caused by altered self-antigens? Transplant. Rev., *31*:156–224, 1976.

Goh, K., and Klemperer, M. R. In vivo leukemic transformation: cytogenetic evidence of in vivo leukemic transformation of engrafted marrow cells. Am. J. Hematol., 2:283–290, 1977.

Gold, J. W. M. Opportunistic fungal infections in patients with neoplastic disease. Am. J. Med., *76*:458–463, 1984.

Goldman, J. N., and Goldman, M. B. The genetics of antibody production. J.A.M.A., *251*:774–787, 1984.

Gong, J., Chen, D., Kashiwaba, M., and Kufe, D. Induction of antitumor activity by immunization with fusions of dendritic and carcinoma cells. Nature Med., *3*:558–561, 1997.

Good, R. A. Disorders of the immune system. *In*: R. A. Good and D. W. Fisher (Eds.), Immunobiology, pp. 3–16. Sunderland, MA: Sinauer, 1971.

Gordon, J., and Stevenson, G. T. Antigenic modulation of lymphocytic surface immunoglobulin yielding resistance to complement-mediated lysis II. Relationship to redistribution of the antigen. Immunology, *42*:13, 1981.

Gordon, J., Abdul-Ahad, A. K., Hamblin, T. J., Stevenson, F. K., and Stevenson, G. T. Mechanisms of tumour cell escape encountered in treating lymphocytic leukaemia with anti-idiotypic antibody. Br. J. Cancer, *49*:547–557, 1984.

Grekou, A. N., Toliou, T., Stravoravdi, P., Patakiouta, F., Tsoukalas, T., Pinakidis, M., and Keramidas, G. Correlation of apoptosis with the distribution and composition of lymphocytic infiltrate in human breast carcinomas. Anticancer Res., *16*:3991–3996, 1996.

Groh, V., Rhinehart, R., Secrist, H., Bauer, S., Grabstein, K. H., and Spies, T. Broad tumor-associated expression and recognition by tumor-derived $\gamma\delta$ T cells of MICA and MICB. Proc. Natl. Acad. Sci. U.S.A., *96*:6879–6884, 1999.

Gumperz, J. E., and Parham, P. The enigma of the natural killer cell. Nature, *378*:245–248, 1995.

Güre, A. O., Stockert, E., Scanlan, M. J., Keresztes, R. S., Jäger, D., Altorki, N. K., Old, L. J., and Chen, Y.-T. Serological identification of embryonic neural proteins as highly immunogenic tumor antigens in small cell lung cancer. Proc. Natl. Acad. Sci. U.S.A., *97*:4198–4203, 2000.

Gutterman, J. U. Cytokine therapeutics: lessons from interferon α. Proc. Natl. Acad. Sci. U.S.A., *91*:1198–1205, 1994.

Halpern, M. Proto-oncogene products as target antigens for cancer vaccines. Int. J. Oncol., *11*:863–868, 1997.

Hanau, A. Erfolgreiche experimentelle Uebertragung von Carcinom. Fortschr. Med., 7:321–339, 1889.

Hanna, N. The role of natural killer cells in the control of tumor growth and metastasis. Biochim. Biophys. Acta, *780*:213–226, 1985.

Hansen, R. M., and Borden, E. C. Current status of interferons in the treatment of cancer. Oncology, 6:19–29, 1992.

Hanson, L. A., Dahlman-Höglund, A., Lundin, S., Karlsson, M., Dahlgren, U., Ahlstedt, S., and Telemo, E. Early determinants of immunocompetence. Nutr. Rev., *55*:S12–S20, 1997.

Hardy, K., and Chaudhri, G. Activation and signal transduction via mitogen-activated protein (MAP) kinases in T lymphocytes. Immunol. Cell Biol., *75*:528–545, 1997.

Hareuveni, M., Gautier, C., Kieny, M.-P., Wreschner, D., Chambon, P., and Lathe, R. Vaccination against tumor cells expressing breast cancer epithelial tumor antigen. Proc. Natl. Acad. Sci. U.S.A., *87*:9498–9502, 1990.

Hayes, C. E., and Klyczek, K. K. The I-J glycoprotein: genetic control, biochemistry, and function. Immunol. Rev., *83*:41–56, 1985.

Heim, M. H. The Jak-STAT pathway: cytokine signaling from the receptor to the nucleus. J. Recept. Signal Transduct. Res., *19*:75–120, 1999.

Heitger, A., and Ladisch, S. Gangliosides block antigen presentation by human monocytes. Biochim. Biophys. Acta, *1303*:161–168, 1996.

Hellström, K. E., and Hellström, I. Enhancement of tumor outgrowth by tumor-associated blocking factors. Int. J. Cancer, *23*:366–373, 1979.

Henry, F., Boisteau, O., Bretaudeau, L., Lieubeau, B., Meflah, K., and Grégoire, M. Antigen-presenting cells that phagocytose apoptotic tumor-derived cells are potent tumor vaccines. Cancer Res., *59*:3329–3332, 1999.

Herberman, R. B. Immunogenicity of tumor antigens. Biochim. Biophys. Acta, *473*:93–119, 1977.

Herman, A., Kappler, J. W., Marrack, P., and Pullen, A. M. Superantigens: mechanism of T-cell stimulation and role in immune responses. Annu. Rev. Immunol., *9*:745–772, 1991.

Heyman, B. The immune complex: possible ways of regulating the antibody response. Immunol. Today, *11*:310–313, 1990.

Hiserodt, J. C., Laybourn, K. A., and Varani, J. Laminin inhibits the recognition of tumor target cells by murine natural killer (NK) and natural cytotoxic (NC) lymphocytes. Am. J. Pathol., *121*:148–155, 1985.

Hoffmann, J. A., Kafatos, F. C., Janeway, C. A., Jr., and Ezekowitz, R. A. B. Phylogenetic perspectives in innate immunity. Science, *284*:1313–1318, 1999.

Holm, L.-E., Blomgren, H., and Löwhagen, T. Cancer risks in patients with chronic lymphocytic thyroiditis. N. Engl. J. Med., *312*:601–604, 1985.

Hoover, R., and Fraumeni, J. F., Jr. Risk of cancer in renal-transplant recipients. Lancet, *2*:55–57, 1973.

Hoover, S. K., Barrett, S. K., Turk, T. M. T., Lee, T.-C., and Bear, H. D. Cyclophosphamide and abrogation of tumor-induced suppressor T cell activity. Cancer Immunol. Immunother., *31*:121–127, 1990.

Hornung, R. L., Longo, D. L., Bowersox, O. C., and Kwak, L. W. Tumor antigen-specific immunization of bone marrow transplantation donors as adoptive therapy against established tumor. J. Natl. Cancer Inst., *87*:1289–1296, 1995.

Houbiers, J. G. A., Nijman, H. W., van der Burg, S. H., Drijfhout, J. W., Kenemans, P., van de Velde, C. J., Brand, A., Momburg, F., Kast, W. M., and Melief, C. J. In vitro induction of human cytotoxic T lymphocyte responses against peptides of mutated and wild type p53. Eur. J. Immunol., *23*:2072–2077, 1993.

Hu, K.-Q., Vierling, J. M., and Siddiqui, A. Trans-activation of HLA-DR gene by hepatitis B virus X gene product. Proc. Natl. Acad. Sci. U.S.A., *87*:7140–7144, 1990.

Hu, Z., and Garen, A. Intratumoral injection of adenoviral vectors encoding tumor-targeted immunoconjugates for cancer immunotherapy. Proc. Natl. Acad. Sci. U.S.A., *97*:9221–9225, 2000.

Irimura, T., Denda, K., Iida, S.-i., Takeuchi, H., and Kato, K. Diverse glycosylation of MUC1 and MUC2: potential significance in tumor immunity. J. Biochem., *126*:975–985, 1999.

Ishibashi, T., Yamada, H., Harada, S., Harada, Y., Takamoto, M., and Sugiyama, K. Inhibition and promotion of tumor growth by BCG. Int. J. Cancer, *21*:67–71, 1978.

Jacobs, H., Fukita, Y., van der Horst, G. T. J., de Boer, J., Weeda, G., Essers, J., de Wind, N., Engelward, B. P., Samson, L., Verbeek, S., de Murcia, J. M., de Murcia, G., te Riele, H., and Rajewsky, K. Hypermutation of immunoglobulin genes in memory B cells of DNA repair-deficient mice. J. Exp. Med., *187*:1735–1743, 1998.

Janeway, C. A., Jr., and Travers, P. Immunobiology. The Immune System in Health and Disease, 2nd Edition. New York: Garland, 1996.

Janssen, R. A. J., Mulder, N. H., The, T. H., and de Leij, L. The immunobiological effects of interleukin-2 in vivo. Cancer Immunol. Immunother., *39*:207–216, 1994.

Jenkins, M. K. The ups and downs of T cell costimulation. Immunity, *1*:443–446, 1994.

Jerne, N. K. Towards a network theory of the immune system. Ann. Immunol. (Paris), *125C*:373–389, 1974.

Jones, S. E. Autoimmune disorders and malignant lymphoma. Cancer, *31*:1092–1098, 1973.

Jurianz, K., Ziegler, S., Garcia-Schüler, H., Kraus, S., Bohana-Kashtan, O., Fishelson, Z., and Kirschfink, M. Complement resistance of tumor cells: basal and induced mechanisms. Mol. Immunol., *36*:929–939, 1999.

Justement, L. B. The B cell antigen receptor: consideration of structure and function. *In*: Handbook of B and T Lymphocytes, Chapter 12, pp. 289–319. New York: Academic Press, 1994.

Kabelitz, D. Role of γδ T cells in the immune response against tumor cells. Cancer J., *8*:190–194, 1995.

Kabelitz, D. Role of costimulation in tumor immunology. Cancer J., *10*:157–160, 1997.

Kabelitz, D., Wesch, D., and Hinz, T. γδ T cells, their T cell receptor usage and role in human diseases. Springer Semin. Immunopathol., *21*:55–75, 1999.

Kabelitz, D., Glatzel, A., and Wesch, D. Antigen recognition by human γδ T lymphocytes. Int. Arch. Allergy Immunol., *122*:1–7, 2000.

Kageshita, T., Hirai, S., Ono, T., Hicklin, D. J., and Ferrone, S. Down-regulation of HLA class I antigen-processing molecules in malignant melanoma. Am. J. Pathol., *154*:745–754, 1999.

Kaplan, J., Shope, T. C., Bollinger, R. O., and Smith, J. Human newborns are deficient in natural killer activity. J. Clin. Immunol., *2*:350–355, 1982.

Kapp, J. A., Pierce, C. W., and Sorensen, C. M. Antigen-specific suppressor T-cell factors. Hosp. Pract., *19*(8):85–98, August 1984.

Kappes, D., and Strominger, J. L. Human class II major histocompatibility complex genes and proteins. Annu. Rev. Biochem., *57*:991–1028, 1988.

Kawahara, K., Morishita, T., Nakamura, T., Hamada, F., Toyoshima, K., and Akiyama, T. Down-regulation of β-catenin by the colorectal tumor suppressor APC requires association with axin and β-catenin. J. Biol. Chem., *275*:8369–8374, 2000.

Khanna, R. Tumour surveillance: missing peptides and MHC molecules. Immunol. Cell Biol., *76*:20–26, 1998.

Killion, J. J., and Fidler, I. J. Therapy of cancer metastasis by tumoricidal activation of tissue macrophages using liposome-encapsulated immunomodulators. Pharmacol. Ther., *78*:141–154, 1998.

Kipps, T. J., and Carson, D. A. Autoantibodies in chronic lymphocytic leukemia and related systemic autoimmune diseases. Blood, *81*:2475–2487, 1993.

Klein, G. Tumor immunology. Transplant. Proc., *5*:31–41, 1973.

Klein, J. Homology between immune responses in vertebrates and invertebrates: does it exist? Scand. J. Immunol., *46*:558–564, 1997.

Klein, G., and Klein, E. Rejectability of virus-induced tumors and non-rejectability of spontaneous tumors: a lesson in contrasts. Transpl. Proc., *9*:1095–1104, 1977.

Koide, Y., Nagata, T., Yoshida, A., and Uchijima, M. DNA vaccines. Jpn. J. Pharmacol., *83*:167–174, 2000.

Komori, T., Okada, A., Stewart, V., and Alt, F. W. Lack of N regions in antigen receptor variable region genes of TdT-deficient lymphocytes. Science, *261*:1171–1175, 1993.

Koo, C. H., Nathwani, B. N., Winberg, C. D., Hill, L. R., and Rappaport, H. Atypical lymphoplasmacytic and immunoblastic proliferation in lymph nodes of patients with autoimmune disease (autoimmune-disease-associated lymphadenopathy). Medicine, *63*:274–290, 1984.

Koopman, L. A., van der Slik, A. R., Giphart, M. J., and Fleuren, G. J. Human leukocyte antigen class I gene mutations in cervical cancer. J. Natl. Cancer Inst., *91*:1669–1677, 1999.

Kowalczyk, D. W., and Ertl, H. C. J. Immune responses to DNA vaccines. Cell. Mol. Life Sci., *55*:751–770, 1999.

Kreitman, R. J. Immunotoxins in cancer therapy. Curr. Opin. Immunol., *11*:570–578, 1999.

Krieg, A. M. The role of CpG motifs in innate immunity. Curr. Opin. Immunol., *12*:35–43, 2000.

Kripke, M. L. Antigenicity of murine skin tumors induced by ultraviolet light. J. Natl. Cancer Inst., *53*:1333–1336, 1974.

Kripke, M. L. Immunology and photocarcinogenesis. J. Am. Acad. Dermatol., *14*:149–155, 1986.

Kumar, R. K., and Penny, R. Cell-mediated immune deficiency in Hodgkin's disease. Immunol. Today, *3*:269–273, 1982.

Kundu, N., and Fulton, A. M. Interleukin-10 inhibits tumor metastasis, downregulates MHC class I, and enhances NK lysis. Cell. Immunol., *180*:55–61, 1997.

Kurosawa, S., Harada, M., Matsuzaki, G., Shinomiya, Y., Terao, H., Kobayashi, N., and Nomoto, K. Early-appearing tumour-infiltrating natural killer cells play a crucial role in the generation of anti-tumour T lymphocytes. Immunology, *85*:338–346, 1995.

Ladisch, S., Li, R., and Olson, E. Ceramide structure predicts tumor ganglioside immunosuppressive activity. Proc. Natl. Acad. Sci. U.S.A., *91*:1974–1978, 1994.

Lanier, L. L. Follow the leader: NK cell receptors for classical and nonclassical MHC class I. Cell, *92*:705–707, 1998.

LeBien, T. W., and McCormack, R. T. The common acute lymphoblastic leukemia antigen (CD10)—emancipation from a functional enigma. Blood, *73*:625–635, 1989.

Le Bouteiller, P. HLA class I chromosomal region, genes, and products: facts and questions. Crit. Rev. Immunol., *14*:89–129, 1994.

Leder, P. The genetics of antibody diversity. Sci. Am., *246*(5):102–115, 1982.

Lee, K.-M., Chuang, E., Griffin, M., Khattri, R., Hong, D. K., Zhang, W., Straus, D., Samelson, L. E., Thompson, C. B., and Bluestone, J. A. Molecular basis of T cell inactivation by CTLA-4. Science, *282*:2263–2266, 1998.

Leong, C. C., Marley, J. V., Loh, S., Robinson, B. W. S., and Garlepp, M. J. The induction of immune responses to murine malignant mesothelioma by IL-2 gene transfer. Immunol. Cell Biol., *75*:356–359, 1997.

Levy, R. Biologicals for cancer treatment: monoclonal antibodies. Hosp. Pract., *20*:67–84, 1985.

Lewis, P. J., and Babiuk, L. A. DNA vaccines: a review. Adv. Virus Res., *54*:129–188, 1999.

Ling, M., Kanayama, M., Roden, R., and Wu, T.-C. Preventive and therapeutic vaccines for human papillomavirus-associated cervical cancers. J. Biomed. Sci., *7*:341–356, 2000.

Livingston, P. O. Construction of cancer vaccines with carbohydrate and protein (peptide) tumor antigens. Curr. Opin. Immunol., *4*:624–629, 1992.

Ljunggren, H.-G. Role of β2-microglobulin in cancer. Cancer J., *5*:308–314, 1992.

Lloyd, K. O. Tumor antigens known to be immunogenic in man. Ann. N.Y. Acad. Sci., *690*:50–58, 1993.

Lotzová, E. Definition and functions of natural killer cells. Nat. Immun., *12*:169–176, 1993.

Lowin, B., Krähenbühl, O., Müller, C., Dupuis, M., and Tschopp, J. Perforin and its role in T lymphocyte-mediated cytolysis. Experientia, *48*:911–920, 1992.

Lu, C. Y., and Unanue, E. R. Macrophage ontogeny: implications for host defence, T-lymphocyte differentiation, and the acquisition of self-tolerance. Clin. Immunol. Allergy, *5*:253–268, 1985.

Lutz, D. Immunotherapy of cancer: a critical review. Int. J. Clin. Pharmacol. Ther. Toxicol., *21*:118–129, 1983.

Manders, P., and Thomas, R. Immunology of DNA vaccines: CpG motifs and antigen presentation. Inflamm. Res., *49*:199–205, 2000.

Marchalonis, J. J., and Schluter, S. F. Development of an immune system. Ann. N.Y. Acad. Sci., *712*:1–12, 1994.

Marchand, M., van Baren, N., Weynants, P., Brichard, V., Dréno, B., Tessier, M.-H., Rankin, E., Parmiani, G., Arienti, F., Humblet, Y., Bourlond, A., Vanwijck, R., Liénard, D., Beauduin, M., Dietrich, P.-Y., Russo, V., Kerger, J., Masucci, G., Jäger, E., De Greve, J., Atzpodien, J., Brasseur, F., Coulie, P. G., van der Bruggen, P., and Boon, T. Tumor regressions observed in patients with metastatic melanoma treated with an antigenic peptide encoded by gene *MAGE-3* and presented by HLA-A1. Int. J. Cancer, *80*:219–230, 1999.

Marx, C., Wolkersdörfer, G. W., Brown, J. W., Scherbaum, W. A., and Bornstein, S. R. MHC class II expression—a new tool to assess dignity in adrenocortical tumours. J. Clin. Endocrinol. Metab., *81*:4488–4491, 1996.

Maschek, U., Pülm, W., and Hämmerling, G. J. Altered regulation of MHC class I genes in different tumor cell lines is reflected by distinct sets of DNase I hypersensitive sites. EMBO J., *8*:2297–2304, 1989.

Mason, D., and Powrie, F. Control of immune pathology by regulatory T cells. Curr. Opin. Immunol., *10*:649–655, 1998.

Matsuda, F., and Honjo, T. Organization of the human immunoglobulin heavy-chain locus. Adv. Immunol., *62*:1–29, 1996.

Maudsley, D. J., and Pound, J. D. Modulation of MHC antigen expression by viruses and oncogenes. Immunol. Today, *12*:429–431, 1991.

Max, E. E. Immunoglobulins. *In*: W. E. Paul (ed.), Fundamental Immunology, 3rd ed., pp. 315–382. New York: Raven Press, 1993.

Mayes, M. D. Epidemiologic studies of environmental agents and systemic autoimmune diseases. Environ. Health Perspect., *107*:743–748, 1999.

Mayordomo, J. I., Zorina, T., Storkus, W. J., Zitvogel, L., Celluzzi, C., Falo, L. D., Melief, C. J., Ildstad, S. T., Kast, W. M., Deleo, A. B., and Lotze, M. T. Bone marrow–derived dendritic cells pulsed with synthetic tumour peptides elicit protective and therapeutic antitumour immunity. Nature Med., *1*:1297–1302, 1995.

McBride, W. H. Phenotype and functions of intratumoral macrophages. Biochim. Biophys. Acta, *865*:27–41, 1986.

McKallip, R., Li, R., and Ladisch, S. Tumor gangliosides inhibit the tumor-specific immune response. J. Immunol., *163*:3718–3726, 1999.

McLaughlin, C. A., Strain, S. M., Bickel, W. D., Goren, M. B., Azuma, I., Milner, K., Cantrell, J. L., and Ribi, E. Regression of line-10 hepatocellular carcinomas following treatment with water-soluble, microbial extracts combined with trehalose or arabinose mycolates. Cancer Immunol. Immunother., *4*:61–68, 1978.

Melekos, M. D. Intravesical BCG or epirubicin prophylaxis in superficial bladder cancer. Cancer J., *8*:124–129, 1995.

Mellemkjær, L., Linet, M. S., Gridley, G., Frisch, M., Møller, H., and Olsen, J. H. Rheumatoid arthritis and cancer risk. Eur. J. Cancer, *32A*:1753–1757, 1996.

Ménard, S., Tagliabue, E., Campiglio, M., and Pupa, S. M. Role of HER2 gene overexpression in breast carcinoma. J. Cell. Physiol., *182*:150–162, 2000.

Mestecky, J. The common mucosal immune system and current strategies for induction of immune responses in external secretions. J. Clin. Immunol., *7*:265–276, 1987.

Mestecky, J., Schrohenloher, R. E., Kulhavy, R., Wright, G. P., and Tomana, M. Site of J chain attachment to human polymeric IgA. Proc. Natl. Acad. Sci. U.S.A., *71*:544–548, 1974.

Meunier, L. Ultraviolet light and dendritic cells. Eur. J. Dermatol., *9*:269–275, 1999.

Milgrom, F. Tissue-specific antigens and isoantigens. Ann. NY Acad. Sci., *129*:767–775, 1966.

Miller, J. F. A. P. The Croonian Lecture, 1992. The key role of the thymus in the body's defence strategies. Phil. Trans. R. Soc. Lond. B., *337*:105–124, 1992.

Minev, B., Hipp, J., Firat, H., Schmidt, J. D., Langlade-Demoyen, P., and Zanetti, M. Cytotoxic T cell immunity against telomerase reverse transcriptase in humans. Proc. Natl. Acad. Sci. U.S.A., *97*:4796–4801, 2000.

Möller, P., and Hämmerling, G. J. The role of surface HLA-A,B,C molecules in tumour immunity. Cancer Surv., *13*:101–126, 1992.

Moore, M., and Hughes, L. A. Circulating antibodies in human connective tissue malignancy. Br. J. Cancer, *28*:175–184, 1973.

Mor, G., Singla, M., Steinberg, A. D., Hoffman, S. L., Okuda, K., and Klinman, D. M. Do DNA vaccines induce autoimmune disease? Hum. Gene Ther., *8*:293–300, 1997.

Mora, P. T. The immunopathology of SV40-induced transformation. Springer Semin. Immunopathol., *5*:7–32, 1982.

Morgan, D. A., Ruscetti, F. W., and Gallo, R. C. Selective *in vitro* growth of T lymphocytes from normal human bone marrow. Science, *193*:1007–1009, 1976.

Mostoslavsky, R., Kirillov, A., Ji, Y.-H., Goldmit, M., Holzmann, M., Wirth, T., Cedar, H., and Bergman, Y. Demethylation and the establishment of κ allelic exclusion. Cold Spring Harbor Symp. Quant. Biol., *64*:197–206, 1999.

Muramatsu, M., Kinoshita, K., Fagarasan, S., Yamada, S., Shinkai, Y., and Honjo, T. Class switch recombination and hypermutation require activation-induced cytidine deaminase (AID), a potential RNA editing enzyme. Cell, *102*:553–563, 2000.

Nanda, N. K., and Sercarz, E. E. Induction of anti-self-immunity to cure cancer. Cell, *82*:13–17, 1995.

Naukkarinen, A., and Syrjänen, K. J. Quantitative immunohistochemical analysis of mononuclear infiltrates in breast carcinomas—correlation with tumour differentiation. J. Pathol., *160*:217–222, 1990.

Naume, B., and Espevik, T. Immunoregulatory effects of cytokines on natural killer cells. Scand. J. Immunol., *40*:128–134, 1994.

Neuberger, M. S., and Milstein, C. Somatic hypermutation. Curr. Opin. Immunol., *7*:248–254, 1995.

Neumann, H., Cavalié, A., Jenne, D. E., and Wekerle, H. Induction of MHC class I genes in neurons. Science, *269*:549–552, 1995.

Newton, D. A., Romano, C., and Gattoni-Celli, S. Semiallogeneic cell hybrids as therapeutic vaccines for cancer. J. Immunother., *23*:246–254, 2000.

Noonan, F. P., and De Fabo, E. C. Immunosuppression by ultraviolet B radiation: initiation by urocanic acid. Immunol. Today, *13*:250–254, 1992.

Normann, S. J. Macrophage infiltration and tumor progression. Cancer Metast. Rev., *4*:277–291, 1985.

North, R. J. Down-regulation of the antitumor immune response. Adv. Cancer Res., *45*:1–43, 1985.

Nosari, A., Barberis, M., Landonio, G., Magnani, P., Majno, M., Oreste, P., and Sozzi, P. Infections in haematologic neoplasms: autopsy findings. Haematologica, *76*:135–140, 1991.

Nowinsky, M. Zur Frage über die Impfung der krebsigen Geschwulste. Zentralbl. Med. Wissensch., *14*:790–791, 1876.

Oettinger, M. A. V(D)J recombination: on the cutting edge. Curr. Opin. Cell Biol., *11*:325–329, 1999.

Okuno, K., Jinnai, H., Lee, Y. S., Kaneda, K., and Yasutomi, M. Interleukin 12 augments the liver-associated immunity and reduces liver metastases. Hepatogastroenterology, *43*:1196–1202, 1996.

Old, L. J., and Stockert, E. Immunogenetics of cell surface antigens of mouse leukemia. Annu. Rev. Genet., *11*:127–160, 1977.

Old, L. J., Boyse, E. A., Clarke, D. A., and Carswell, E. A. Antigenic properties of chemically induced tumors. Ann. N.Y. Acad. Sci., *101*:80, 1962.

Old, L. J., Stockert, E., Boyse, E. A., and Kim, J. H. Antigenic modulation—loss of TL antigen from cells exposed to TL antibody. Study of the phenomenon *in vitro*. J. Exp. Med., *127*:523, 1968.

Oleksowicz, L., and Dutcher, J. P. A phase II trial of dose-intensive interleukin-2 in metastatic renal cell carcinoma. J. Cancer Res. Clin. Oncol., *125*:101–108, 1999.

Ollert, M. W., David, K., Schmitt, C., Hauenschild, A., Bredehorst, R., Erttmann, R., and Vogel, C.-W. Normal human serum contains a natural IgM antibody cytotoxic for human neuroblastoma cells. Proc. Natl. Acad. Sci. U.S.A., *93*:4498–4503, 1996.

Pardoll, D. M. Inducing autoimmune disease to treat cancer. Proc. Natl. Acad. Sci. U.S.A., *96*:5340–5342, 1999.

Pardoll, D. M., Kruisbeek, A. M., Fowlkes, B. J., Coligan, J. E., and Schwartz, R. H. The unfolding story of T cell receptor γ. FASEB J., *1*:103–109, 1987.

Parham, P. Alien antigens return to the fold. Immunol. Today, *10*:206–212, 1989.

Park, S.-H., Chiu, Y.-H., Jayawardena, J., Roark, J., Kavita, U., and Bendelac, A. Innate and adaptive functions of the CD1 pathway of antigen presentation. Semin. Immunol., *10*:391–398, 1998.

Paul, P., Rouas-Freiss, N., Khalil-Daher, I., Moreau, P., Riteau, B., Le Gal, F. A., Avril, M. F., Dausset, J., Guillet, J. G., and Carosella, E. D. HLA-G expression in melanoma: a way for tumor cells to escape from immunosurveillance. Proc. Natl. Acad. Sci. U.S.A., *95*:4510–4515, 1998.

Peace, D. J., Smith, J. W., Disis, M. L., Chen, W., and Cheever, M. A. Induction of T cells specific for the mutated segment of oncogenic p21ras protein by immunization in vivo with the oncogenic protein. J. Immunother., *14*:10–14, 1993.

Pecher, G., and Finn, O. J. Induction of cellular immunity in chimpanzees to human tumor-associated antigen mucin by vaccination with MUC-1 cDNA-transfected Epstein-Barr virus-immortalized autologous B cells. Proc. Natl. Acad. Sci. U.S.A., *93*:1699–1704, 1996.

Penn, I. Tumors after renal and cardiac transplantation. Hematol./Oncol. Clin. North Am., *7*:431–445, 1993.

Penninger, J. M., Wen, T., Timms, E., Potter, J., Wallace, V. A., Matsuyama, T., Ferrick, D., Sydora, B., Kronenberg, M., and Mak, T. W. Spontaneous resistance to acute T-cell leukaemias in TCRVγ1.1Jγ4Cγ4 transgenic mice. Nature, *375*:241–244, 1995.

Pfizenmaier, K., Scheurich, P., Schluter, C., and Kronke, M. Tumor necrosis factor enhances HLA-ABC and HLA-DR gene expression in human tumor cells. J. Immunol., *138*:975–980, 1987.

Pizzo, P. A. Infectious complications in the child with cancer. I. Pathophysiology of the compromised host and the initial evaluation and management of the febrile cancer patient. J. Pediatr., *98*:341–354, 1981.

Prehn, R. T. Cancer and immune response. Proc. Inst. Med. Chicago, *29*:339–345, 1973.

Prehn, R. T. Immunostimulation of the lymphodependent phase of neoplastic growth. J. Natl. Cancer Inst., *59*:1043–1049, 1977.

Prehn, R. T., and Prehn, L. M. The autoimmune nature of cancer. Cancer Res., *47*:927–932, 1987.

Prigozy, T. I., Naidenko, O., Qasba, P., Elewaut, D., Brossay, L., Khurana, A., Natori, T., Koezuka, Y., Kulkarni, A., and Kronenberg, M. Glycolipid antigen processing for presentation by CD1d molecules. Science, *291*:664–667, 2001.

Przepiorka, D., and Srivastava, P. K. Heat shock protein-peptide complexes as immunotherapy for human cancer. Mol. Med. Today, *4*:478–484, 1998.

Putnam, F. W. Immunoglobulin structure: variability and homology. Science, *163*:633–644, 1969.

Raffeld, M., Neckers, L., Longo, D. L., and Cossman, J. Spontaneous alteration of idiotype in a monoclonal B-cell lymphoma. N. Engl. J. Med., *312*:1653–1658, 1985.

Rammensee, H.-G., and Klein, J. Complexity of the *histocompatibility-3* region in the mouse. J. Immunol., *130*:2926–2929, 1983.

Ramsey-Goldman, R., Mattai, S. A., Schilling, E., Chiu, Y.-L., Alo, C. J., Howe, H. L., and Manzi, S. Increased risk of malignancy in patients with systemic lupus erythematosus. J. Invest. Med., *46*:217–222, 1998.

Rao, V. S., and Bonavida, B. Detection of soluble tumor-associated antigens in serum of tumor-bearing rats and their immunological role *in vivo*. Cancer Res., *37*:3385–3389, 1977.

Raulet, D. H. The structure, function, and molecular genetics of the γ/δ T cell receptor. Annu. Rev. Immunol., *7*:175–207, 1989.

Raulet, D. H. Development and tolerance of natural killer cells. Curr. Opin. Immunol., *11*:129–134, 1999.

Raz, A., Goldman, R., Yuli, I., and Inbar, M. Isolation of plasma membrane fragments and vesicles from ascites fluid of lymphoma-bearing mice and their possible role in the escape mechanisms of tumors from host immune rejection. Cancer Immunol. Immunother., *4*:53–59, 1978.

Reyburn, H., Mandelboim, O., Valés-Goméz, M., Sheu, E. G., Pazmany, L., Davis, D. M., and Strominger, J. L. Human NK cells: their ligands, receptors and functions. Immunol. Rev., *155*:119–125, 1997.

Rinaldo, C. R. Jr. Modulation of major histocompatibility complex antigen expression by viral infection. Am. J. Pathol., *144*:637–650, 1994.

Ritts, R. E., and Neel, H. B. An overview of cancer immunology. Mayo Clinic Proc., *49*:118–131, 1974.

Robertson, M. J., and Ritz, J. Biology and clinical relevance of human natural killer cells. Blood, *76*:2421–2438, 1990.

Robey, E., and Allison, J. P. T-cell activation: integration of signals from the antigen receptor and costimulatory molecules. Immunol. Today, *16*:306–308, 1995.

Robins, R. A., and Baldwin, R. W. Immune complexes in cancer. Cancer Immunol. Immunother., *4*:1–3, 1978.

Rodey, G. E. Anti-idiotypic antibodies and regulation of immune responses. Transfusion, *32*:361–376, 1992.

Roffo, A. H. Cancer y Sol. Bol Inst de med exper para el estud y trat del cancer, *10*:417–439, 1933.

Roitt, I. M. Essential Immunology, 3rd ed. London: Blackwell, 1977.

Romagnani, S. T_H1 and T_H2 subsets of CD4$^+$ T lymphocytes. Sci. Am. Sci. Med., *1*:68–77, 1994.

Röpke, M., Hald, J., Guldberg, P., Zeuthen, J., Nørgaard, L., Fugger, L., Svejgaard, A., Van Der Burg, S., Nijman, H. W., Melief, C. J. M., and Claesson, M. H. Spontaneous human squamous cell carcinomas are killed by a human cytotoxic T lymphocyte clone recognizing a wild-type p53-derived peptide. Proc. Natl. Acad. Sci. U.S.A., *93*:14704–14707, 1996.

Rosenberg, S. A. Development of cancer immunotherapies based on identification of the genes encoding cancer regression antigens. J. Natl. Cancer Inst., *88*:1635–1644, 1996.

Rosenberg, S. A., Spiess, P., and Lafreniere, R. A new approach to the adoptive immunotherapy of cancer with tumor-infiltrating lymphocytes. Science, *233*:1318–1321, 1986.

Rosenberg, S. A., Lotze, M. T., Muul, L. M., Chang, A. E., Avis, F. P., Leitman, S., Linehan, W. M., Robertson, C. N., Lee, R. E., Rubin, J. T., Seipp, C. A., Simpson, C. G., and White, D. E. A progress report on the treatment of 157 patients with advanced cancer using lymphokine-activated killer cells and interleukin-2 or high-dose interleukin-2 alone. N. Engl. J. Med., *316*:889–897, 1987.

Rosenthal, A. K., McLaughlin, J. K., Gridley, G., and Nyrén, O. Incidence of cancer among patients with systemic sclerosis. Cancer, *76*:910–914, 1995.

Ross, J. S., and Fletcher, J. A. The HER-2/*neu* oncogene: prognostic factor, predictive factor and target for therapy. Semin. Cancer Biol., *9*:125–138, 1999.

Ross, S. R. Mouse mammary tumor virus and the immune system. Adv. Pharmacol., *39*:21–46, 1997.

Rossner, M. T. Review: Hepatitis B virus *X*-gene product: A promiscuous transcriptional activator. J. Med. Virol., *36*:101–117, 1992.

Rubin, E., and Farber, J. L. Pathology. Philadelphia: Lippincott, 1988.

Rusch, H. P., Kline, B. Z., and Bauman, C. A. Carcinogenesis by UV rays with reference to wavelength and energy. Arch. Pathol., *371*:135–146, 1941.

Sahin, U., Türeci, Ö., and Pfreundschuh, M. Serological identification of human tumor antigens. Curr. Opin. Immunol., *9*:709–716, 1997.

Sakaguchi, S. Regulatory T cells: key controllers of immunologic self-tolerance. Cell, *101*:455–458, 2000.

Salinas, F. A., Wee, K. H., and Silver, H. K. B. Immune complexes and human neoplasia. Biomedicine, *37*:211–218, 1983.

Sasaki, S., Inamura, K., and Okuda, K. Genes that induce immunity—DNA vaccines. Microbiol. Immunol., *43*:191–200, 1999.

Schiltz, P. M., Beutel, L. D., Nayak, S. K., and Dillman, R. O. Characterization of tumor-infiltrating lymphocytes derived from human tumors for use as adoptive immunotherapy of cancer. J. Immunother., *20*:377–386, 1997.

Schrier, P. I., and Peltenburg, L. T. C. Relationship between *myc* oncogene activation and MHC class I expression. Adv. Cancer Res., *60*:181–246, 1993.

Schwartz, R. S. Autoimmunity and autoimmune diseases. *In*: W. E. Paul (Ed.), Fundamental Immunology, 3rd ed., pp. 1033–1097. New York: Raven Press, 1993.

Schwartz, R. S., and André-Schwartz, J. Malignant lymphoproliferative diseases: interactions between immunological abnormalities and oncogenic viruses. Annu. Rev. Med., *19*:269–282, 1968.

Schweighoffer, T. Tumor cells expressing a recall antigen are powerful cancer vaccines. Eur. J. Immunol., *26*:2559–2564, 1996.

Scott, A. M., and Cebon, J. Clinical promise of tumour immunology. Lancet, *349*:19–22, 1997.

Scott, A. M., and Welt, S. Antibody-based immunological therapies. Curr. Opin. Immunol., *9*:717–722, 1997.

Sedlacek, H. H. Vaccination for treatment of tumors: a critical comment. Crit. Rev. Oncog., *5*:555–587, 1994.

Seebach, J. D., and Waneck, G. L. Natural killer cells in xenotransplantation. Xenotransplantation, *4*:201–211, 1997.

Seemayer, T. A., Gartner, J. G., and Lapp, W. S. The graft-versus-host reaction. Hum. Pathol., *14*:3–5, 1983.

Seki, S., Abo, T., Masuda, T., Ohteki, T., Kanno, A., Takeda, K., Rikiishi, H., Nagura, H., and Kumagai, K. Identification of activated T cell receptor γδ lymphocytes in the liver of tumor-bearing hosts. J. Clin. Invest., *86*:409–415, 1990.

Shipp, M. A., Vijayaraghavan, J., Schmidt, E. V., Masteller, E. L., D'Adamio, L., Hersh, L. B., and Reinherz, E. L. Common acute lymphoblastic leukemia antigen (CALLA) is active neutral endopeptidase 24.11 ("enkephalinase"): direct evidence by cDNA transfection analysis. Proc. Natl. Acad. Sci. U.S.A., *86*:297–301, 1989.

Shiraki, K., Tsuji, N., Shioda, T., Isselbacher, K. J., and Takahashi, H. Expression of Fas ligand in liver metastases of human colonic adenocarcinomas. Proc. Natl. Acad. Sci. U.S.A., *94*:6420–6425, 1997.

Shu, S., Plautz, G. E., Krauss, J. C., and Chang, A. E. Tumor immunology. J.A.M.A., *278*:1972–1981, 1997.

Sigurgeirsson, B., Lindelöf, B., Edhag, O., and Allander, E. Risk of cancer in patients with dermatomyositis or polymyositis. A population-based study. N. Engl. J. Med., *326*:363–367, 1992.

Simon, J. C., Cruz, P. D., Jr., Bergstresser, P. R., and Tigelaar, R. E. Low dose ultraviolet B-irradiated Langerhans cells preferentially activate CD4$^+$ cells of the T helper 2 subset. J. Immunol., *145*:2087–2091, 1990.

Singer, D., and Maguire, J. Regulation of the expression of class I MHC genes. Crit. Rev. Immunol., *10*:235–257, 1990.

Smith, R. T. Cancer and the immune system. Pediatr. Clin. North Am., *41*:841–850, 1994.

Sokol, R. J., Booker, D. J., and Stamps, R. Erythrocyte autoantibodies, autoimmune haemolysis, and carcinoma. J. Clin. Pathol., *47*:340–343, 1994.

Solari, R., and Kraehenbuhl, J.-P. The biosynthesis of secretory component and its role in the transepithelial transport of IgA dimer. Immunol. Today, *6*:17–20, 1985.

Sotomayor, E. M., Borrello, I., and Levitsky, H. I. Tolerance and cancer: a critical issue in tumor immunology. Crit. Rev. Oncog., *7*:433–456, 1996.

Sparks, F. C. Hazards and complications of BCG immunotherapy. Med. Clin. North Am., *60*:499–509, 1976.

Spina, M., Vaccher, E., Carbone, A., and Tirelli, U. Neoplastic complications of HIV infection. Ann. Oncol., *10*:1271–1286, 1999.

Starzl, T. E., and Zinkernagel, R. M. Antigen localization and migration in immunity and tolerance. N. Engl. J. Med., *339*:1905–1913, 1998.

Staveley-O'Carroll, K., Sotomayor, E., Montgomery, J., Borrello, I., Hwang, L., Fein, S., Pardoll, D., and Levitsky, H. Induction of antigen-specific T cell anergy: an early event in the course of tumor progression. Proc. Natl. Acad. Sci. U.S.A., *95*:1178–1183, 1998.

Steerenberg, P. A., Korenromp, E. L., van Loveren, H., Mol, D. Q., Geerse, L., and de Gruijl, F. R. Natural killer cell activity during UVR-induced skin tumor formation in the Skh hairless mouse. Photochem. Photobiol., *65*:150–154, 1997.

Stevenson, F. K. Tumor vaccines. FASEB J., *5*:2250–2257, 1991.

Storb, U. The molecular basis of somatic hypermutation of immunoglobulin genes. Curr. Opin. Immunol., *8*:206–214, 1996.

Storkus, W. J., and Dawson, J. R. Target structures involved in natural killing (NK): characteristics, distribution, and candidate molecules. Crit. Rev. Immunol., *10*:393–416, 1991.

Strand, S., and Galle, P. R. Immune evasion by tumours: involvement of the CD95 (APO-1/Fas) system and its clinical implications. Mol. Med. Today, *4*:63–68, 1998.

Streilein, J. W., Taylor, J. R., Vincek, V., Kurimoto, I., Shimizu, T., Tie, C., and Golomb, C. Immune surveillance and sunlight-induced skin cancer. Immunol. Today, *15*:174–179, 1994.

Stutman, O. Spontaneous tumors in nude mice: effect of the viable yellow gene. Exp. Cell Biol., *47*:129–135, 1979.

Sulitzeanu, D. Immunosuppressive factors in human cancer. Adv. Cancer Res., *45*:247–267, 1985.

Sutherland, J. C., and Mardiney, M. R. Jr. Immune complex disease in the kidneys of lymphoma-leukemia patients: the presence of an oncornavirus-related antigen. J. Natl. Cancer Inst., *50*:633–644, 1973.

Talmadge, J. E., Meyers, K. M., Prieur, D. J., and Starkey, J. R. Role of natural killer cells in tumor growth and metastasis: C57BL/6 normal and beige mice. J. Natl. Cancer Inst., *65*:929–935, 1980.

Tatake, R. J., and Zeff, R. A. Regulated expression of the major histocompatibility complex class I genes. Proc. Soc. Exp. Biol. Med., *203*:405–417, 1993.

Teillaud, J.-L., Desaymard, C., Giusti, A. M., Haseltine, B., Pollock, R. R., Yelton, D. E., Zack, D. J., and Scharff, M. D. Monoclonal antibodies reveal the structural basis of antibody diversity. Science, *222*:721–726, 1983.

Theofilopoulos, A. N., and Dixon, F. J. Autoimmune diseases. Immunopathology and etiopathogenesis. Am. J. Pathol., *108*:321–365, 1982.

Thiers, B. H., Maize, J. C., Spicer, S. S., and Cantor, A. B. The effect of aging and chronic sun exposure on human Langerhans cell populations. J. Invest. Dermatol., *82*:223–226, 1984.

Thomas, L. Reactions to homologous tissue antigens in relation to hypersensitivity. *In*: H. S. Lawrence (Ed.), Cellular and Humoral Aspects of the Hypersensitivity Status, pp. 529–534. New York: Hoeber-Harper, 1959.

Trial, J., and McIntyre, B. W. Suppressor cell clones specific for ultraviolet radiation-induced tumors. J. Immunol., *145*:2044–2049, 1990.

Tsang, K. Y., Zaremba, S., Nieroda, C. A., Zhu, M. Z., Hamilton, J. M., and Schlom, J. Generation of human cytotoxic T cells specific for human carcinoembryonic antigen epitopes from patients immunized with recombinant vaccinia-CEA vaccine. J. Natl. Cancer Inst., *87*:982–990, 1995.

Uchida, A. The cytolytic and regulatory role of natural killer cells in human neoplasia. Biochim. Biophys. Acta, *865*:329–340, 1986.

Unanue, E. R., and Cerottini, J.-C. Antigen presentation. FASEB J., *3*:2496–2502, 1989.

van den Broek, M. F., Kägi, D., Zinkernagel, R. M., and Hengartner, H. Perforin dependence of natural killer cell-mediated tumor control *in vivo*. Eur. J. Immunol., *25*:3514–3516, 1995.

van den Broek, M. F., Kägi, D., and Hengartner, H. Effector pathways of natural killer cells. Curr. Top. Microbiol. Immunol., *230*:123–131, 1998.

Van den Eynde, B. J., and Boon, T. Tumor antigens recognized by T lymphocytes. Int. J. Clin. Lab. Res., *27*:81–86, 1997.

Van den Eynde, B. J., and van der Bruggen, P. T cell defined tumor antigens. Curr. Opin. Immunol., *9*:684–693, 1997.

Vandeputte, M. Immunopathology of polyoma-induced tumors. Springer Semin. Immunopathol., *4*:317–332, 1982.

Versteeg, R., Peltenburg, L. T. C., Plomp, A. C., and Schrier, P. I. High expression of the *c-myc* oncogene renders melanoma cells prone to lysis by natural killer cells. J. Immunol., *143*:4331–4337, 1989.

Vink, A. A., Moodycliffe, A. M., Shreedhar, V., Ullrich, S. E., Roza, L., Yarosh, D. B., and Kripke, M. L. The inhibition of antigen-presenting activity of dendritic cells resulting from UV irradiation of murine skin is restored by *in vitro* photorepair of cyclobutane pyrimidine dimers. Proc. Natl. Acad. Sci. U.S.A., *94*:5255–5260, 1997.

Viñuela, J. E., Rodriguez, R., Gil, J., Coll, J., De La Concha, E. G., and Subiza, J. L. Antigen shedding *vs.* development of natural suppressor cells as mechanism of tumor escape in mice bearing Ehrlich tumor. Int. J. Cancer, *47*:86–91, 1991.

von Boehmer, H., and Kisielow, P. How the immune system learns about self. Sci. Am., *265*:74–81, 1991.

Walker, T. M., Yurochko, A. D., Burger, C. J., and Elgert, K. D. IA$^-$ macrophages and cytokine networks contribute to tumor-induced suppression of CD4$^+$ autoreactive T cells. Immunol. Invest., *22*:169–187, 1993.

Walter, R. J., Danielson, J. R., Van Alten, P. J., and Powell, W. J. Defects in monocyte chemotaxis in patients with neoplastic disease. J. Surg. Res., *41*:215–224, 1986.

Weijzen, S., Velders, M. P., and Kast, W. M. Modulation of the immune response and tumor growth by activated Ras. Leukemia, *13*:502–513, 1999.

Weiner, L. M. Monoclonal antibody therapy of cancer. Semin. Oncol., *26*:43–51, 1999.

Weiss, A. T lymphocyte activation. *In*: W. E. Paul (Ed.), Fundamental Immunology, 3rd ed., Chapter 13, pp. 467–504. New York: Raven Press, 1993.

Weissman, I. L. Developmental switches in the immune system. Cell, *76*:207–218, 1994.

Wheelock, E. F., and Robinson, M. K. Endogenous control of the neoplastic process. Lab. Invest., *48*:120–139, 1983.

White, C. A., Larocca, A., and Grillo-López, A. J. Anti-CD20 monoclonal antibodies as novel treatments for non-Hodgkin's lymphoma. Pharm. Sci. Tech. Today, *2*:95–101, 1999.

Whiteside, T. L., and Herberman, R. B. Characteristics of natural killer cells and lymphokine-activated killer cells. Immunol. Allergy Clin. North Am., *10*:663–704, 1990.

Whitworth, P. W., Pak, C. C., Esgro, J., Kleinerman, E. S., and Fidler, I. J. Macrophages and cancer. Cancer Metast. Rev., *8*:319–351, 1990.

Winkler, U., Barth, S., Schnell, R., Diehl, V., and Engert, A. The emerging role of immunotoxins in leukemia and lymphoma. Ann. Oncol., *8*:S139–S146, 1997.

Wojtowicz-Praga, S. Reversal of tumor-induced immunosuppression: a new approach to cancer therapy. J. Immunother., *20*:165–177, 1997.

Wong, G. H. W., Bartlett, P. F., Clark-Lewis, I., Battye, F., and Schrader, J. W. Inducible expression of H-2 and Ia antigens on brain cells. Nature, *310*:688–691, 1984.

Yokoyama, W. M. Natural killer cell receptors specific for major histocompatibility complex class I molecules. Proc. Natl. Acad. Sci. U.S.A., *92*:3081–3085, 1995.

Yoshikai, Y. γ/δ T cell receptor. Microbiol. Immunol., *35*:493–506, 1991.

Yoshinaga, S. K., Whoriskey, J. S., Khare, S. D., Sarmiento, U., Guo, J., Horan, T., Shih, G., Zhang, M., Coccia, M. A., Kohno, T., Tafuri-Bladt, A., Brankow, D., Campbell, P., Chang, D., Chiu, L., Dai, T., Duncan, G., Elliott, G. S., Hui, A., McCabe, S. M., Scully, S., Shahinian, A., Shaklee, C. L., Van, G., Mak, T. W., and Senaldi, G. T-cell co-stimulation through B7RP-1 and ICOS. Nature, *402*:827–832, 1999.

Zeid, N. A., and Muller, H. K. S100 positive dendritic cells in human lung tumors associated with cell differentiation and enhanced survival. Pathology, *25*:338–343, 1993.

Zheng, B., Xue, W., and Kelsoe, G. Locus-specific somatic hypermutation in germinal centre T cells. Nature, *372*:556–559, 1994.

20

Some Basic and Applied Principles of Cancer Chemotherapy

Although our understanding of the basic molecular nature of the neoplastic transformation is still relatively primitive, significant advances have been made during the past three decades in the successful treatment of neoplasms that were not curable by surgery and/or radiation alone prior to 1970. The principal modality (used alone or in combination) that has resulted in significant improvement in treating a number of neoplasms, many of which are in persons less than 30 years of age (Chapter 1), is chemotherapy, by use of an increased spectrum of drugs, hormones, and other natural products.

Chemotherapy may be defined as the treatment of disease through the use of chemicals. This includes infectious as well as neoplastic disease. Cancer chemotherapy specifically is the treatment of cancer by chemicals that maximize the killing of neoplastic cells while minimizing the killing of most or all other cells of the host. With most malignant neoplasms, the greatest danger to the host results from dissemination of the disease throughout the organism. By definition, a malignant neoplasm is capable of metastatic growth, making successful surgery an impossibility unless carried out prior to successful metastatic dissemination of the neoplasm. Similarly, for radiotherapy, control of localized disease is quite reasonable, but anything less than whole-body irradiation would be unsatisfactory for the treatment of metastatic disease. The complications of whole-body radiation make this in most cases an untenable mode of therapy. As with infectious diseases, systemic treatment is absolutely necessary if one is to have any hope of eradicating disseminated disease. Such an ideal state has not been achieved for most neoplasms in the human. However, cancer chemotherapy, by eliminating small foci of metastatic disease, has been instrumental in increasing the survival of many patients with a variety of neoplasms. This curative effect of cancer chemotherapy has been most common in children; it has also been successful with a few selected neoplasms in adults (Table 20.1). Chemotherapy has also been combined with other therapeutic modalities to achieve both cures and dramatic, life-prolonging responses (see below).

HISTORY AND RATIONALES OF CANCER CHEMOTHERAPY

The term *chemotherapy* as well as a significant number of its basic concepts originated in the work of Paul Ehrlich, who coined the term in referring to the systemic treatment of both infectious disease and neoplasia. Ehrlich developed a system that allowed the transplantation of neoplasms in rodents, on which he could test the effectiveness of drugs in slowing or eliminating neoplastic development. Many of Ehrlich's concepts have formed the basis for modern chemo-

Table 20.1 Neoplasms Curable by Chemotherapy in Their Advanced Stages

Choriocarcinoma	Wilms tumor
Acute lymphocytic leukemia (in children and adults)	Burkitt's lymphoma)
Hodgkin disease	Embryonal rhabdomyosarcoma
Diffuse large-cell lymphoma	Ewing sarcoma
Lymphoblastic lymphoma (in children and adults)	Peripheral neuroepithelioma
Follicular mixed lymphoma	Neuroblastoma
Testicular cancer	Small-cell cancer of the lung
Acute myelogenous leukemia	Ovarian cancer

Adapted from DeVita, 1989, with permission of author and publisher.

therapy. Although the concept of treating cancers with drugs may be traced back several centuries, there were no examples of truly successful cancer chemotherapy in the whole organism until the 1940s (Donehower et al., 1995). During World War II, an explosion on a ship containing mustard gas resulted in the exposure of a number of people to this agent. It was noted at that time that exposed individuals exhibited a significant degree of bone marrow and lymphoid hypoplasia (Infield, 1971). As a result of this serendipitous finding, Gilman and Philips (1946) studied and reported the first clinical trial of nitrogen mustard in patients with malignant lymphomas at Yale University. Their results, which demonstrated dramatic although somewhat transient regression of lymphomas, may be considered as the beginning of modern chemotherapy.

Prior to 1960, the rationale for the therapy of neoplasia by drugs was derived largely from the successful treatment of a number of different neoplasms. Since that time, there has been not only an increasing number of drugs used for chemotherapy of cancer but also an increased understanding of their mechanism of action. Figure 20.1 gives a historical indication of the time of introduction of a variety of drugs in the chemotherapy of human cancer. The mechanism of action of many of these chemicals is considered further on, but it is important to point out that most of them exert their cytotoxic and/or cytostatic effects during one or more phases of the cell cycle (see below).

Most neoplasms for which chemotherapy has been most successful exhibit the similar biological characteristic of rapid growth. Neoplasms that are less susceptible or nonsusceptible to chemotherapy include many slowly growing malignant tumors such as colorectal cancer, renal cancer, melanoma, and carcinoma of the liver (see below). In many instances, drug responsiveness is related to the growth fraction—i.e., the percentage of cells in the neoplasm undergoing division at any one time. Where the growth fraction is large, rapid growth results, but the greater proportion of the cell population is susceptible to the effects of cytocidal and cytostatic drugs. Conversely, neoplasms having a small growth fraction are not affected significantly by most drugs used in cancer treatment. Some examples of growth fractions, labeling indices, and cell loss are given in Table 20.2.

More recently, considerable evidence has indicated that many chemotherapeutic agents—in addition to or as part of their primary mechanism of cell killing—induce apoptosis (cf. Schmitt and Lowe, 1999; Hannun, 1997; Martin et al., 1997). The mechanisms of programmed cell death or apoptosis (Figure 7.11) have previously been considered, and are not treated here. In addition to inhibiting cell replication through alteration in DNA synthesis or damaging the DNA template, drugs may also alter the intracellular levels of adenosine triphosphate (cf. Berger, 1986; Martin et al., 1997) and alter or disrupt a variety of signal transduction pathways, as exemplified by the responsiveness of a number of neoplasms to hormonal therapy (cf. Gulliford and Epstein, 1996). A number of chemotherapeutic agents whose action is associated with

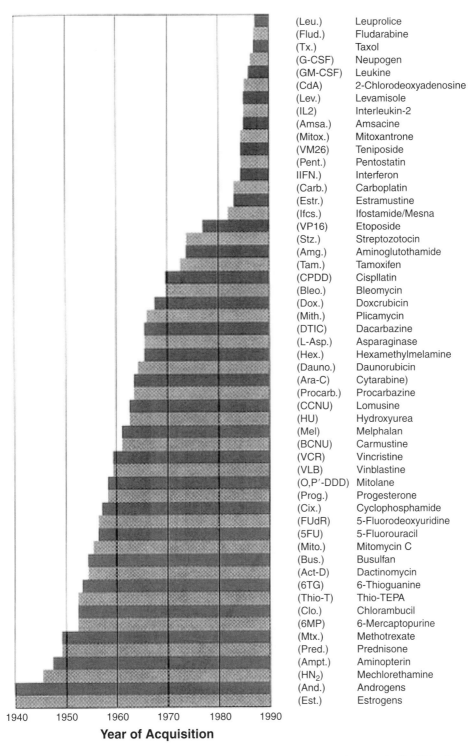

(Leu.)	Leuprolice
(Flud.)	Fludarabine
(Tx.)	Taxol
(G-CSF)	Neupogen
(GM-CSF)	Leukine
(CdA)	2-Chlorodeoxyadenosine
(Lev.)	Levamisole
(IL2)	Interleukin-2
(Amsa.)	Amsacine
(Mitox.)	Mitoxantrone
(VM26)	Teniposide
(Pent.)	Pentostatin
IIFN.)	Interferon
(Carb.)	Carboplatin
(Estr.)	Estramustine
(Ifcs.)	Ifostamide/Mesna
(VP16)	Etoposide
(Stz.)	Streptozotocin
(Amg.)	Aminoglutothamide
(Tam.)	Tamoxifen
(CPDD)	Cispllatin
(Bleo.)	Bleomycin
(Dox.)	Doxcrubicin
(Mith.)	Plicamycin
(DTIC)	Dacarbazine
(L-Asp.)	Asparaginase
(Hex.)	Hexamethylmelamine
(Dauno.)	Daunorubicin
(Ara-C)	Cytarabine)
(Procarb.)	Procarbazine
(CCNU)	Lomusine
(HU)	Hydroxyurea
(Mel)	Melphalan
(BCNU)	Carmustine
(VCR)	Vincristine
(VLB)	Vinblastine
(O,P'-DDD)	Mitolane
(Prog.)	Progesterone
(Cix.)	Cyclophosphamide
(FUdR)	5-Fluorodeoxyuridine
(5FU)	5-Fluorouracil
(Mito.)	Mitomycin C
(Bus.)	Busulfan
(Act-D)	Dactinomycin
(6TG)	6-Thioguanine
(Thio-T)	Thio-TEPA
(Clo.)	Chlorambucil
(6MP)	6-Mercaptopurine
(Mtx.)	Methotrexate
(Pred.)	Prednisone
(Ampt.)	Aminopterin
(HN$_2$)	Mechlorethamine
(And.)	Androgens
(Est.)	Estrogens

Year of Acquisition

Figure 20.1   Acquisition of new anti-cancer drugs, 1940–90. (Adapted from Krakoff, 1991, with permission of the author and publisher.)

Table 20.2   Mean Kinetic Parameters of Various Histological Types of Human Neoplasms

Histological Type	Doubling Time (days)	Labeling Index (%)	Growth Fraction (%)	Cell Loss Factor (%)	Radiosensitivity (mean tumor control dose in Gy)	Chemosensitivity
Embryonal tumors	27	30	90	93	25–30	++
Malignant lymphomas	29	29	90	93	35–45	++
Mesenchymal sarcomas	41	4	11	68	85	–
Squamous cell carcinomas	58	8	25	89	60–70	+
Adenocarcinomas	83	2	6	71	60–80	±

Adapted from Tubiana, 1989, with permission of author and publisher.

the induction of apoptosis in neoplastic cells are listed in Table 20.3. The table also indicates those neoplasms susceptible to the induction of apoptosis by one or more of the agents listed.

Chemical Agents Utilized in Human Cancer Chemotherapy

On the basis of the rationales for cancer chemotherapy given above, as well as by a certain amount of serendipity, a variety of different chemicals have been developed and found to be effective in the treatment of human cancer. The listing in Figure 20.1 gives a relatively complete picture of most of the drugs utilized today for the treatment of cancer as well as a number that

Table 20.3   Chemotherapeutic Agents Associated with the Induction of Apoptosis in Specific Types of Neoplasms

	Some Agents Associated with Apoptosis	Cancer Types Susceptible to Apoptosis
Etoposide	Camptothecin	Lymphoma
VM26	Hydroxyurea	Leukemia
m-AMSA	Ara-C	Breast carcinoma
Dexamethasone	5-Azacytidine	Ovarian carcinoma
Vincristine	Nitrogen mustard	Colon carcinoma
cis-Platinum	Methotrexate	Prostate cancer
Cyclophosphamide	Chlorambucil	Miscellaneous adenocarcinomas
Adriamycin	Bleomycin	Seminoma
Paclitaxel	BCNU	Malignant glioma
5′-Fluorouracil	Actinomycin D	
5′-Fluorodeoxyuridine	Melphalan	
Ionizing radiation		
Hyperthermia		
Hormone withdrawal		

Modified from Hannun, 1997, with permission of author and publisher.

have been found successful in the past but have been superseded by other, more effective agents. Some of these agents, listed by their classification on a functional and descriptive basis, are shown in Table 20.4. In many but not all instances, the mechanism of action of these drugs on cellular pathways and components is known. Alkylating agents are highly reactive chemicals capable of alkylating DNA and other macromolecules directly, just as the ultimate forms of chemical carcinogens alkylate DNA (Chapter 3). Some alkylating agents are bifunctional, e.g., bisulfan, and are thus capable of crosslinking the two strands of the DNA double helix. Another group of highly effective crosslinking agents are the platinum complexes based on the original structure cis-Pt(II)(NH$_3$)$_2$Cl$_2$, which is now known as the drug cisplatin. A more recently developed derivative is carboplatin, having a dicarboxylcyclobutane complex to two of the four coordinate covalent sites of the platinum complex (Figure 20.2). Such crosslinking prevents the replication of these alkylated molecules by preventing their separation during DNA synthesis. Melphalan similarly induces interstrand, intrastrand, or DNA protein crosslinks, as does cyclophosphamide (Donehower et al., 1995). Nitrosoureas directly alkylate DNA with the formation of specific adducts. The antibiotics listed are complex natural products acting by several different mechanisms. Actinomycin D (dactinomycin) and plicamycin form complexes with DNA, effectively inhibiting transcription of most genetic information, while daunorubicin binds to DNA by intercalation between base pairs, thus inhibiting both DNA and RNA synthesis (cf. Donehower et al., 1995). Bleomycin is a mixture of polypeptides, some or all of which bind to DNA, causing strand scission (cf. Black and Livingston, 1990). Antimetabolites effectively used in chemotherapy generally prevent the formation or the utilization of normal cellular metabolites essential for the synthesis of nucleic acids, either directly or indirectly. In addition, 5-azacytidine inhibits the methylation of DNA cytosines as well (Glover and Leyland-Jones, 1987).

Although the ability to induce differentiation of neoplastic cells in vitro has been known for a number of years (Friend et al., 1971; Sachs, 1978), only relatively recently have such ther-

---

Table 20.4 Classification and Examples of Drugs Useful in Clinical Cancer Chemotherapy

---

Alkylating agents: Bi- or monofunctional, chemically highly reactive:
   Melphalan, nitrosoureas, bisulfan, cyclophosphamide, carboplatin
Antibiotics: Complex natural products, acting by various mechanisms:
   Actinomycin D, duanorubicin, bleomycin, plicamycin
Antimetabolites: Slow-acting. Resemble normal metabolites in structure and compete with them for an enzyme, thus preventing further utilization of the normal metabolites:
      Antifolics: Methotrexate
      Antipurines: 6-Mercaptopurine, 6-thioguanine
      Antipyrimidines: 5-Fluorouracil, FUdR, cytosine arabinoside, 5-azacytidine
Differentiating agents: Induce differentiation of neoplastic cells
   All-*trans* retinoic acid
Enzymes: Asparaginase
Hormones: Estrogens, androgens, progestins, corticosteroids, antiestrogens, antiandrogens, gonadotropin-releasing hormone/agonists
Miscellaneous: Procarbazine, hydroxyurea, o,p'-dichlorodiphenyldichloroethane
Plant alkaloids: Colchicine, vinblastine, vincristine, maytansine, taxol
Topoisomerase inhibitors:
   Topoisomerase I (catalyzes DNA unwinding) Camptothecin, innotecan (CPF-11), topotecan
   Topoisomerase II (regulates 3D structure of DNA by binding to DNA, cleaving both strands and subsequent religation)
   Teniposide, etoposide, amsacrine

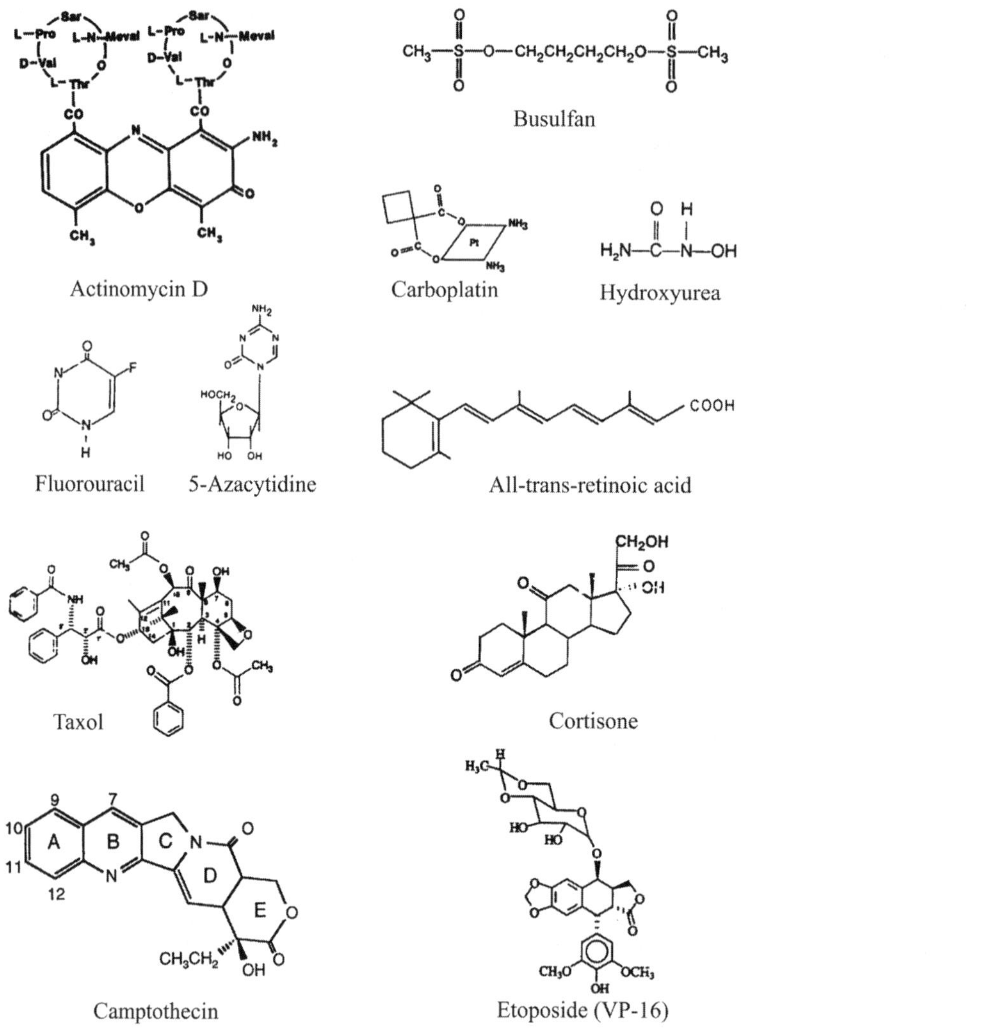

Fig. 20.2 Chemical structures of representative chemotherapeutic agents useful in clinical cancer chemotherapy.

apies been shown effective in the treatment of neoplastic disease. The principal effective agent is all-*trans*-retinoic acid (ATRA), which has been found especially effective in the treatment of acute promyelocytic leukemia (Fenaux et al., 1997). Unfortunately, this differentiation therapy with retinoids has not been very effective in other types of neoplasms, but it has shown some degree of efficacy as one of a number of retinoids effective in chemoprevention. In addition to specific chemicals, both synthetic and natural, several different enzymes have also been utilized in the chemotherapy of neoplasia, based at least in part on their ability to metabolize and eliminate specific metabolites, usually amino acids, essential for the growth of specific neoplastic cells (Chapter 8). Primary among these agents is the enzyme produced by *Escherichia coli*, L-asparaginase, which catalyzes the conversion of the amino acid L-asparagine to aspartic acid. By its catalytic action, the enzyme rapidly and completely depletes circulating pools of L-asparagine in the organism, thus compromising any cells that are unable or ineffective in synthesizing

L-asparagine. By a similar rationale, bacterial glutaminase and methioninase have been utilized both experimentally and in the clinic (Spiers and Wade, 1976; Tan et al., 1996). The efficacy of these other agents has not yet been suitably tested.

The usefulness of hormonal and antihormonal therapy in cancer dates back to the century-old observation by Beatson (1896) of the regression of metastatic breast cancer after oophorec-tomy. Nearly 50 years later, Huggins and Hodges (1941) demonstrated the effects of castration and of estrogens in inducing regression of prostatic neoplasia (cf. Figure 20.1). Since that time, a number of natural and synthetic hormones as well as antihormones have found use in the therapy of specific histogenetic types of neoplasms, predominantly those of endocrine origin or those from tissues exhibiting a relatively high degree of sensitivity to endocrine hormones. As noted in Chapter 18, for sex hormones to be effective in the treatment of specific neoplastic disease, the receptor for the therapeutic hormone or antihormone as a target must be present in the neoplastic cells. Mutations in steroid receptors have been associated causally with resistance of some neo-plasms to the effects of hormones and antihormones (Sluyser, 1994), but in most instances the presence of substantial amounts of receptor is indicative of a potential favorable response to its hormonal ligand. The exact mechanism of tumor regression by such agents, since they do not directly affect DNA synthesis or structure, is not clear. Because these agents exert their effects through signal transduction pathways (Chapters 3 and 7), it is likely that one of the mechanisms for inducing tumor regression is the induction of apoptosis in the hormonally responsive neo-plastic cell (Gulliford and Epstein, 1996). Apoptosis is induced in normal endocrine responsive tissues by removal of the appropriate trophic hormone (cf. Walker et al., 1989).

Several drugs effective in cancer chemotherapy are not easily classified in the listing of Table 20.4. An example is hydroxyurea, which has a relatively specific action in inhibiting one of the subunits of ribonucleotide reductase, thereby inactivating the enzyme (Yarbro, 1992). This eliminates the production of deoxyribonucleotides, thus indirectly inhibiting DNA synthesis and producing cell death in the S phase of the cell cycle and some synchronization of surviving cells that are also at risk for the development of gene amplification and chromosomal abnormalities owing to the dramatic alteration in the deoxyribonucleotide pool sizes (D'Anna et al., 1986). A number of plant alkaloids have also been found to be effective in cancer chemotherapy. Several of these, including colchicine (the first of many such compounds), vinblastine, vincristine, and most recently the taxanes (paclitaxel and docetaxel), are effective in the chemotherapy of a vari-ety of different neoplasms. These agents have in common a mechanism involving binding to microtubules and interruption of a variety of cellular functions, especially mitosis, cell migra-tion, and polarization. The topoisomerase inhibitors also represent a large class of naturally oc-curring compounds that have been found effective in the therapy of a variety of neoplasms. Topoisomerases are enzymes involved in the replication and stabilization of DNA by catalyzing breakage and reannealing of DNA strands to allow replication to occur as well as in relaxation and alteration of the structure of the DNA molecule (Rothenberg, 1997). Topoisomerase inhibi-tors prevent the religation of DNA after cleavage by the normal enzyme (Rothenberg, 1997; Pommier et al., 1996). In so doing, they disrupt DNA synthesis dramatically, leading to cell death or in many cases clastogenic effects. Figure 20.2 shows representative examples of chemo-therapeutic agents from each of the representative classes listed in Table 20.4.

DEVELOPMENT OF CHEMOTHERAPEUTIC DRUGS

It was Paul Ehrlich who first initiated a systematic screening program in the search for chemo-therapeutic agents. In his work, the agents were directed toward the treatment of several sys-temic parasitic diseases. Initially, the search for new drugs to be used in the chemotherapy of cancer followed a similar program. Figure 20.3 lists the stages in the development of drugs to be used in the chemotherapy of cancer. It should be noted that this formulation is not unique to cancer chemotherapy, but is also utilized in the development of a variety of other pharmaceuticals. At certain stages, as noted in the figure, decisions must be made whether to continue to study a particular drug. Thus, although a large number of compounds may be selected in the acquisition stage, relatively few survive to make an impact on general medical practice.

Acquisition or selection of the compounds to be tested may be done as a purely random screening of synthetic chemicals or biologicals. The results of this approach have been disappointing with respect to the yields of new classes of active compounds. Other approaches, such as rational synthesis and analog development, have been used with good results (cf. Goldin and Carter, 1982). When a compound is known to be somewhat effective in the treatment of neoplasia in either animal or human systems, closely related compounds with structural modifications of the parent compound are developed for testing. By this mechanism, one may be able to improve on the efficacy of the original compound. The development of certain antimetabolites has proceeded on the basis of our knowledge of specific metabolic pathways within the living cell. The development of 5-fluorouracil was one of the prime examples of this method for the selection of compounds used in drug development (cf. Heidelberger, 1975). A third method, one of the most popular for selecting compounds to be screened for activity against neoplastic growth, is the testing of compounds obtained from antibiotic fermentation of beers and plant products. Several highly active compounds have been isolated and characterized from a large number of naturally produced materials that have been screened. Some of these are presently in use. Products of such testing have been the taxanes, vinblastine, and the topoisomerase inhibitors.

After selection of the compounds to be tested, efficacy against neoplasia is analyzed in several systems, usually in the mouse. Originally, the primary system was the L-1210 leukemia in mice, but at present the primary screening system is the P-388 mouse leukemia. The screening procedure currently used at the National Cancer Institute in the United States is outlined in Figure 20.4. A list of other animal neoplasms that have been used as test systems in various screen-

Development of Chemotherapeutic Drugs

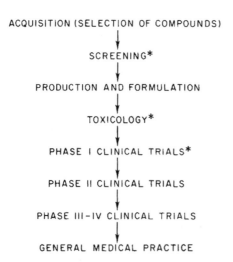

Figure 20.3 Listing of the stages involved in new drug development at the National Cancer Institute. The asterisks designate stages at which decisions are made as to further development of the drug.

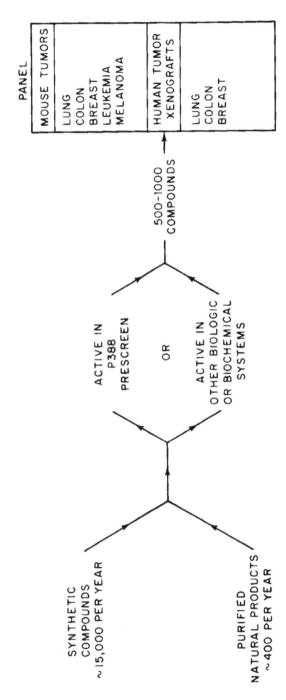

Figure 20.4 Outline of the currently employed standard screening design employed at the Division of Cancer Treatment at the National Cancer Institute.

ing programs is given in Table 20.5. Some of these have been used in the secondary panel screen, as seen in Figure 20.4. Within the last decade, human neoplasms grown in immunologically deficient animals—for example, the nude mouse—constitute a major component of this secondary panel. In addition, drugs have also been screened for their efficacy in tissue culture systems, a number of which are derived from human cells.

After the evaluation of a drug in a variety of animal tumor systems, toxicological and pharmacological evaluations of the drugs are undertaken (cf. Goldin and Carter, 1982). Purity, physicochemical characteristics (including solubility), and acute toxicity in animals—leading to

Table 20.5   Test Systems for Screening Chemotherapeutic Drugs

Mouse tumors
  Transplantable
    Lymphoid leukemia L-1210
    Adenocarcinoma 755
    Cloudman melanoma (S91)
    Ehrlich ascites
    Hepatoma 129
    Lewis lung carcinoma
    Osteogenic sarcoma HE 10734
    Sarcoma 180
    P388 leukemia
    L5178Y leukemia
    B16 melanoma
    LPC1 plasma cell
  Primary and transplantable
    AKR virus leukemia
    Moloney virus leukemia
    Rauscher virus leukemia
    Friend virus leukemia
    C3H mammary tumor
Rat tumors
  Dunning leukemia
  Murphy-Sturm lymphosarcoma
  Walker 256
Hamster tumors
  Adenocarcinoma of duodenum
  Adenocarcinoma of endometrium
  Adenocarcinoma of small bowel
  Melanotic melanoma
Chicken tumor
  Rous sarcoma
Carcinogen-induced tumors in rodents
  3-Methylcholanthrene–induced mammary adenocarcinoma
  Dimethylbenzanthracene-induced mammary adenocarcinoma
  Dibenzo[a,i]pyrene-induced fibrosarcoma
Tumors in heterologous hosts
  HS-1 in conditioned rats
  HEP-3 in conditioned rats
  DBA/2 mouse lymphatic leukemia in conditioned hamsters
  Human amelanotic melanoma in conditioned hamsters

systemic and local tissue damage from acute and cumulative doses—are determined. These tests are often extended from rodents to other species, including primates. Usually included in these investigations are specific studies related to the pharmacokinetics of the drugs, including determination of blood and tissue levels, and the metabolism and excretion of the drug (Workman, 1993).

When all of these studies are completed, clinical trials are initiated in several phases, the first (phase I) being in patients with advanced cancer, usually after all conventional therapeutic measures have failed. The evaluation of drugs in these patients includes a variety of studies on the pharmacology of the drug—its toxicity to the bone marrow, gastrointestinal tract, and other tissues—from which the maximally tolerated dose is determined. In order for a drug to continue to the next phase of clinical trial, an objective response need not necessarily be obtained in these patients. These studies are carried out with a specific protocol approved by the local committee on human experimentation as well as the National Cancer Institute (Freireich, 1979). The National Cancer Institute sponsors a large number of cooperative clinical trials which, prior to 1988, had more than 30,000 entries (Friedman and Cain, 1990). Today many more such trials are active but face a variety of problems, including their integration into the changing health care delivery system in this country as well as a number of ethical concerns that have emerged from a number of these trials (Durant, 1990). Only a limited number of institutions are allowed to participate in these studies. If a tolerated dose has a toxicity that is predictable, controllable, and reversible, the trial of the drug extends into the second phase, which is directed toward determining clinical activity against a variety of cancers in the human. The required and optional panel of neoplasms in human patients against which a potentially useful drug may be tested is given in Figure 20.5. If the efficacy of the drug is shown in phase II trials, then it is finally evaluated in controlled phase III clinical trials and in combination with other drugs. The National Cancer Institute officials estimate that fewer than 1 in 15,000 drugs ever reach the final stage of clinical trials. Despite this limited chance of success, over 40 drugs are effective in the treatment of one or more human cancers.

VARIABLES IN THE CHEMOTHERAPY OF CANCER

Although a variety of specific drugs are used in the chemotherapy of cancer, their effects can be quite variable from patient to patient and even within the same patient at different periods of the treatment regimen. Such variability involves different factors, some of which we have discussed above and others of which are noted in Figure 20.6. In this figure, the overall pharmacological-therapeutic process from a drug dose to its therapeutic effect is depicted. However, since neoplasia is a somewhat specific situation involving cell growth as well as specific humoral effects of the neoplasm on the host (Chapters 17 and 18), other variable factors come into play, some of which are considered here.

Therapeutic Index

It is already obvious that drugs used in the chemotherapy of cancer have a variety of toxic effects in the host that may or may not be directly related to its effect on the neoplasm. Thus, in any such situation, the toxicity to normal tissues and the organism as a whole becomes a limiting factor in the dose of drugs that can be given for effective therapy without inducing excessive toxicity. Some of the more commonly seen toxicities to the patient are seen in Table 20.6. A number of the toxicities noted in Table 20.6 occur predominantly at high doses or high doses given for extended periods of time. In addition to the toxicities noted there in the table, gonadal

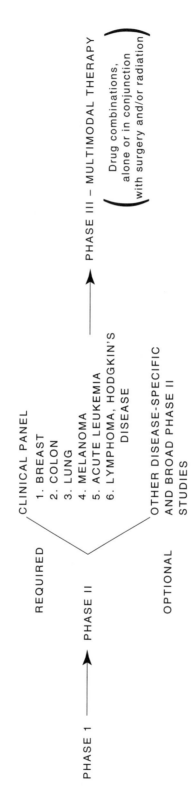

Figure 20.5 Outline of the flow of clinical trials in the early phases of testing of new drugs for potential use in cancer chemotherapy.

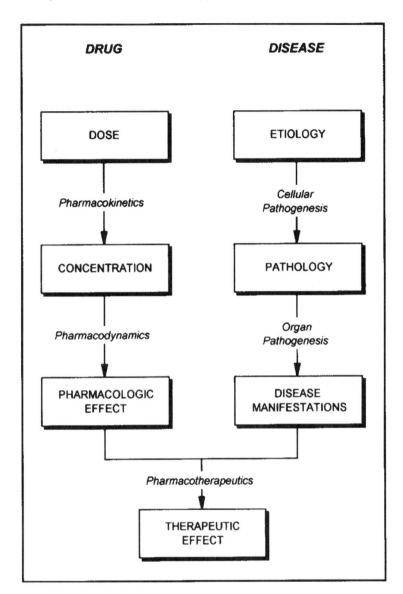

Figure 20.6 Scheme outlining the overall pharmacologic-therapeutic process from drug dose to a therapeutic effect, which in cancer chemotherapy is destruction and/or elimination of neoplastic cells. (Adapted from Bjornsson, 1996, with permission of the author and publishers.)

dysfunction, hypersensitivity reactions, and dermatological complications as well as alopecia (loss of hair) occur not uncommonly as toxic manifestations of a number of chemotherapeutic regimens.

The relationship between the probability of some biological or toxic effect of a drug and the dose administered to induce antineoplastic efficacy may be seen in Figure 20.7. As noted, if the drug is to be useful, the "antitumor effect" curve, ideally giving complete clinical remission, should be displaced toward lower doses compared with the curve describing the probability of significant toxicity to normal tissue. The therapeutic index (or therapeutic ratio) may be defined

Table 20.6 Some Toxic Effects of Chemotherapy

Organ System	Effect	Drugs Inducing These Effects[a]
Hematopoietic	Bone marrow depression	DNA reactive drugs, e.g. alkylating agents,
	Thrombosis and bleeding	antimetabolites, antibiotics, etc.
Gastrointestinal	Nausea and vomiting	Alkylating agents, enzymes, antibiotics, etc.
	Diarrhea and constipation	Vinca alkyloids, 5-fluorouracil (5-FU),
		some antibiotics
Cardiac	Cardiomyopathy	Doxorubicin (Adriamycin) and related
		antibiotics
Hepatic	Impaired liver function	Methotrexate, cyclophosphamide
Neurological	Peripheral neuropathy	Vincristine, cisplatin
	Cerebellar dysfunction	Cisplatin, 5-FU
	Encephalopathy	Methotrexate
	Epilepsy	Bisulfan, ifosfamide
Pulmonary	Fibrosis	Bleomycin
		Alkylating agents
Renal	Tubular damage	Cisplatin
	Renal failure	Mitomycin

[a]The list of drugs inducing these effects is not entirely complete. The reader is referred to the paper by
  Lowenthal and Eaton (1996) for further details of some of these toxicities.

from such relationships as the ratio of the dose required to produce a given probability of toxicity and of an antitumor effect. The therapeutic index seen in Figure 20.7 is represented as a ratio of the 5% level of probability to severe toxicity (referred to as toxic dose 05 or TD-05) and the 50% probability of an antineoplastic effect, referred to as the effective dose 50 or ED-50. The appropriate end points of neoplastic response and toxicity will depend on the limiting toxicity of the drug, the intent of the treatment (i.e., cure versus palliation), and whether treatment is given to a patient or an experimental animal. It should be noted, however, that dose-response curves similar to those of Figure 20.7 have rarely been obtained for drug effects in humans (Tannock, 1992).

Obviously, improvement in the therapeutic index of a drug is the goal of chemotherapy, whether experimental or clinical. Any method whereby the antineoplastic effect of a drug can be shifted such that the ED-50 gives very little if any normal tissue toxicity is to be the ultimate goal. Improvement in the therapeutic index still requires that any treatment modification leading to increased killing of neoplastic cells in experimental systems must be assessed for its effects on critical normal tissues prior to therapeutic trials.

Remission Versus Cure in Cancer Chemotherapy

It is now well established that the "curability" of cancer by chemotherapy is related to the body burden of viable neoplastic cells present at the time chemotherapy is initiated. Although treatment of the neoplasm in the patient may result in the disappearance of all clinical and laboratory findings pointing toward the presence of neoplastic cells in the patient, almost half of the cases of treated neoplasia in the United States recur after some period of time. Thus, it is more appropriate to use the term *remission* to indicate the clinical situation of a patient who has been treated, apparently successfully, for a neoplastic condition. While it is now possible by a variety of technologies (Pantel et al., 1999; Lambrechts et al., 1998) to detect extremely low levels of neoplastic cells remaining in the organism after apparently successful therapy, for most solid

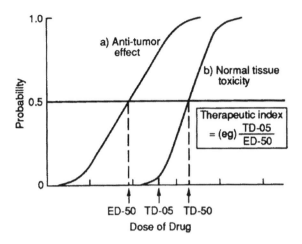

Figure 20.7   Schematic relation between the dose of a drug and (a) the probability of a given measure of antineoplastic effect, and (b) the probability of a given measure of normal-tissue toxicity. Although the therapeutic index might be defined as the ratio of doses to give 50% probabilities of normal tissue damage and antineoplastic effects, when the endpoint toxicity is severe, a more appropriate definition of the therapeutic index should be at a lower probability of toxicity as noted in the box. (Adapted from Tannock, 1992, with permission of the author and publisher.)

neoplasms the limit of clinical and/or radiological detection is of the order of 1 g of tissue or about 10^9 cells. If these 10^9 cells are scattered throughout the organism rather than in a single locus, obviously there will be no clinical detection of the neoplastic disease. The question of how many neoplastic cells could remain in the host before a cure was effected was answered several decades ago in experiments using rodents.

The L-1210 Leukemia Model and Chemotherapy

In 1965, Howard Skipper reported investigations on the therapy of experimental leukemia in mice. Skipper demonstrated that in this system it was necessary to kill every leukemic cell in the host (regardless of the total number, their anatomical distribution, or metabolic heterogeneity) in order to effect a cure, since one single, viable L-1210 cell could grow, proliferate, and kill the mouse. Obviously, the major problem in this investigation was associated with the killing of a relatively small but persistent fraction of leukemic cells that survived the maximum tolerated therapy because of the relative efficacy of the drug, drug resistance, or anatomical compartmentalization.

A hypothetical illustration of the possible importance of drug level and schedule in attempts to achieve a total cure in experimental leukemia in animals is seen in Figure 20.8. As indicated in the figure, if one initially administers 10^5 leukemic cells to a mouse, one finds that the cells, after a 2-day lag, proliferate logarithmically until the mouse is killed when 10^9 cells are present in the body. Therefore, the time of survival is inversely related to the number of leukemic cells in the mouse at any one time. Line A in the figure represents the number of leukemic cells in untreated animals as a function of days after inoculation of the cells. Line B, representing the daily drug treatment, termed *low-level, long-term* (until death), is plotted to show a daily 50% "drug kill" of the leukemic cell population in the animal together with a daily quadrupling of the surviving leukemic cells. The percentage of cells killed by a given dose of a given active drug is constant or, in other words, a constant fraction of cells is killed with each dose. This phenomenon is termed the *first-order kinetics of killing*. Line C, representing the daily drug treatment that is termed *moderate-level, long-term*, is plotted to show a daily 75% drug kill of the animal's leukemic cell population. Theoretically, this can result in a different host survival rate, assuming that cumulative drug toxicity and development of drug resistance or compartmentalization, such as in the central nervous system, do not occur. Line D, representing the daily drug treatment that is termed *high-level, short-term*, is plotted to show a daily 99% drug kill of the animal's leukemic cell population and, barring other complications, a "cure" of a 10^5 cell inoculum.

With this model, it is possible to devise drug schedules, usually intermittent, in which all tumor cells are killed and the mice cured, by allowing time for normal dividing cells to recover from toxicity. Although this model has potentially interesting implications, many cancer chemotherapeutic drugs kill only dividing cells (cf. Skipper and Schabel, 1982). Therefore, the L-1210 leukemia model has found its greatest applicability in the human in acute leukemias (cf. Frei, 1984), where most of the cells are dividing. Other studies have indicated that logarithmic decreases in tumor cell survival, resulting from drugs affecting dividing cells, require logarithmic rather than linear increases in dosages.

The application of Figure 20.8 to the situation in the human in the case of most solid neoplasms is seen in Figure 20.9. In this figure, the decreases noted in the number of neoplastic cells occurs to the point where there is a clinical "complete remission." However, at this point there are still more than 10^8 viable neoplastic cells remaining in the patient. At a later time these continue to grow and even in the face of continued therapy may have developed some resistance in the patient by a variety of mechanisms, some of which we will discuss now. Takahashi and Nishioka (1995) have also argued that significant gain in survival may occur without actual reduction in the amount of neoplasm by cell death or other such mechanisms. They have argued that, especially in solid neoplasms, the survival times of most patients depend more on an induced cytostatic phase rather than loss of tumor mass. This concept may be important in the prolonged survival sometimes noted with other means of therapy, such as immunotherapy.

Drug Resistance in Neoplastic Cells

In his early experiments, Skipper (1965) believed that the primary cause of death in leukemia in the face of continued daily treatment was the relatively rapid selection of a mutant, drug-resistant leukemia cell population. This result was especially notable when only single drugs were used at low or moderate levels. It is now evident that a variety of different mechanisms of drug resistance of neoplastic cells exist involving mutations, chromosomal abnormalities, gene amplification, and alternate metabolic pathways. A summary of several of the molecular mechanisms involved in resistance to chemotherapeutic drugs in neoplastic cells is seen in Figure 20.10.

The Multidrug-Resistance Phenotype

Some three decades ago, a number of descriptions demonstrating that neoplastic cell lines display a resistance to multiple different chemotherapeutic drugs was reported. The drugs involved showed no obvious strong chemical similarity but later were found to have similar physical properties in that they are relatively hydrophobic. Some of the drugs to which cells with the multidrug resistance (MDR) phenotype exhibit resistance include actinomycin D, etoposide, paclitaxel, and vinblastine (Bellamy, 1996). More recent investigations have demonstrated that a common feature of many of these drug-resistant lines is the existence of the P-glycoprotein, a specific protein in the plasma membrane of such cells. The function of this glycoprotein is an energy-dependent outward drug efflux from the cell, such that cells exhibiting the MDR phenotype fail to accumulate drugs (Gottesman, 1993). In the membrane, the molecule has 12

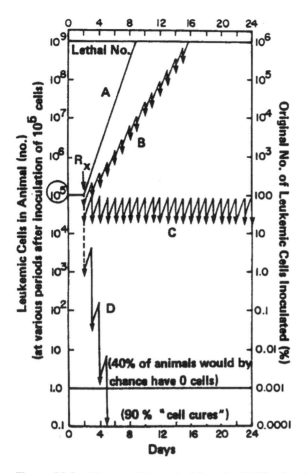

Figure 20.8 Diagram of drug schedule and cell killing in mice inoculated with the L-1210 leukemia. At day 0 the animal is inoculated with 10^5 cells. The subsequent four conditions (A, B, C, and D) represent the growth curves of the cells under several different drug regimens as described in the text. (After Skipper, 1965, with permission of the author and publisher.)

transmembrane regions as well as two large intracytoplasmic components. A diagram of its appearance and possible mechanism of action is seen in Figure 20.11. In the figure a cationic drug, such as doxorubicin, is shown entering the plasma membrane and subsequently a "pore" of the P-glycoprotein either within the membrane or from the cytoplasm. Such transport back to the outside of the cell requires energy, as noted in the figure (Gottesman, 1993). The P-glycoprotein occurs in normal tissues, especially those involved in major physiological transport mechanisms such as the liver, intestine, kidney, and brain (Schinkel, 1997). In these tissues, especially in the gut, the presumed function is to remove potentially deleterious exogenous materials from the cell rapidly. In neoplasms, expression of high levels of the P-glycoprotein usually is associated with a poor prognosis with a variety of different neoplasms (cf. Bellamy, 1996; Dicato et al., 1997).

The P-glycoprotein is one member of a large superfamily of similar transport protein complexes termed the *ABC superfamily* (Bellamy, 1996). Several transport proteins involving non-P-glycoprotein–mediated multidrug resistance have also been described (cf. Bellamy, 1996; Ya-

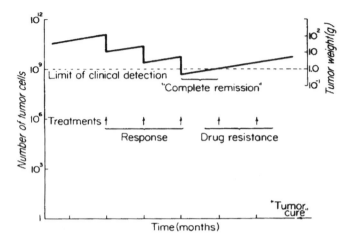

Figure 20.9 Relationship between remission of a neoplasm and a complete cure as a function of the remaining numbers of neoplastic cells in the host. In this hypothetical example, treatment is initiated when there are about 100 g (10^{11} cells) present in the host. Each treatment, given at monthly intervals, eliminates 90% of the cells present, leading to complete disappearance of any clinical evidence of the neoplasm in the host or a "complete remission." However, more than 10^8 viable cells are present, many of which have now become resistant to the therapy utilized, with subsequent regrowth requiring alternate methods of therapy or ultimately leading to demise of the patient. Note that despite the attainment of a complete remission or clinical response, more than 10^8 viable neoplastic cells remain and that the reduction in cell numbers is small compared to that required for a cure. (Adapted from Tannock, 1992, with permission of the author and publisher.)

mada et al., 1997; Baggetto, 1997). However, a variety of agents that are capable of modulating the function of the P-glycoprotein have been described (Kavallaris, 1997), but as yet it does not appear feasible to employ such agents together with the effective chemotherapeutic drugs that are transported by this protein.

Modified Availability of Drug Targets (Gene Amplification and Karyotypic Instability)

Some 25 years ago, Terzi (1974) pointed out that drug-resistant mutants of some cell lines were characterized by karyotypic instability, a high reversion frequency, and low plating efficiency. Subsequent studies have supported these initial observations in demonstrating alteration of response to drug therapy in cells by induced DNA rearrangements (Schnipper et al., 1989), hypoxia-inducing genetic instability in neoplastic cells (Teicher, 1994), and the importance of tumor heterogeneity resulting from karyotypic instability in the response of neoplasms to specific drugs (Simpson-Herren et al., 1988). Another closely related mechanism of drug resistance was initially described by Schimke, who demonstrated that cells resistant to the antifolate methotrexate exhibited a dramatic amplification of the gene to which the drug dihydrofolate reductase was targeted (Schimke, 1984). Subsequent to those studies, a number of examples of drug-induced gene amplification in karyotypically unstable cells have been reported (Table 20.7). In addition to the examples listed in the table, examples of induced gene amplification of topoisomerase II by etoposide in human melanoma cell lines (Campain et al., 1995) and the amplification of metallothionein genes by metals (Gick and McCarty, 1982) and potentially by alkylating agents (Kelley et al., 1988) have been reported.

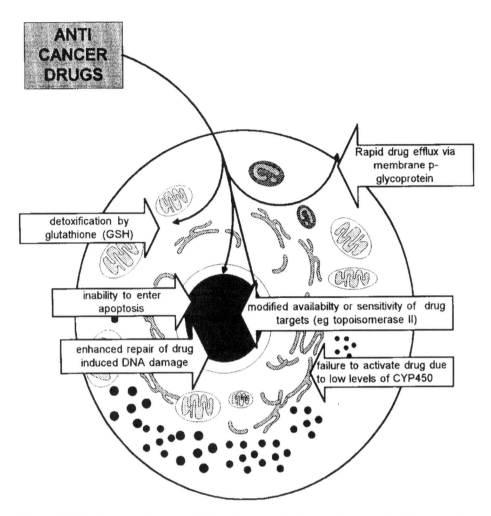

Figure 20.10 A schematic representation of some molecular mechanisms of resistance to chemotherapeutic agents within a neoplastic cell. (After Harrison, 1995, with permission of the author and publisher.)

In addition to induced gene amplification altering the DNA target, a variety of mechanisms resulting in resistance to the topoisomerase inhibitors have also been described, only some of which involve these mechanisms (cf. Skovsgaard et al., 1994). Alteration of the DNA target by hypermethylation induced by chemotherapeutic agents, resulting in altered responses to such drugs, has also been reported (Nyce et al., 1993).

Pharmacogenetics of Drug Resistance

A number of chemotherapeutic agents require "bioactivation" to produce pharmacologically active, cytotoxic species (cf. Sladek, 1987). Both phase I and phase II enzymes (Chapter 3) have been identified as responsible both for differential sensitivity of individuals to chemotherapeutic agents as well as the response of neoplastic cells themselves to specific agents (cf. Iyer and Ratain, 1998; Graham et al., 1991; Chang et al., 1994). Cyclophosphamide and ifosfamide are alkylating agents that require bioactivation by phase I enzymes, although such bioactivation oc-

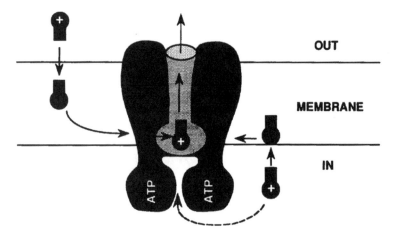

Figure 20.11 Proposed mechanism of action of P-glycoprotein as a "hydrophobic vacuum cleaner." As noted in the model, the multidrug transporter may remove drugs directly from the plasma membrane or from the cytoplasm through a single transport channel, as illustrated. (After Gottesman, 1993, with permission of the author and publisher.)

curs predominantly in the liver. While it is possible that some other chemotherapeutic agents requiring phase I metabolic activation may do so at very reduced rates in neoplastic cells, thus leading to drug resistance, it appears that the changes in the phase I enzymes, especially those involved in glutathione metabolism, are probably the most important in this potential mechanism of drug resistance (cf. Graham et al., 1991; cf. Iyer and Ratain, 1998).

DNA Repair Mechanisms and Cellular Resistance to Chemotherapeutics

As noted in Chapter 3, the cell contains a variety of mechanisms responsible for the repair of damaged DNA. Closely related to this fact is also the finding that a large number of neoplasms exhibit mutations in genes whose products are involved in the recovery of cells from DNA damage, such as the p53 gene. In examining the various types of DNA repair noted in Table 3.4, there is ample evidence that the O^6-alkylguanine-DNA alkyltransferase (AGAT) enzyme, when expressed at high levels, enhances the resistance of a cell, normal or neoplastic, to alkylating agents that produce O^6-alkylguanine. Transgenic mice expressing increased levels of AGAT

Table 20.7 Gene Amplification Induced by Chemotherapeutic Drugs

Drug	Gene (fold amplification)	Reference
Difluoromethylornithine	Ornithine decarboxylase (?)	Leinonen et al., 1987
Hydroxyurea	Ribonucleotide reductase (6–20)	Srinivasan et al., 1987
Methotrexate	Dihydrofolate reductase (100–1000)	Schimke, 1984
Nitrogen mustards	Glutathione S-transferase (4–8)	Lewis et al., 1988
	γ-Glutamyl transpeptidase (3.6)	
Phosphonacetyl-L-aspartate (PALA)	CAD gene (10–48) pyrimidine biosynthesis	Sharma and Schimke, 1994
Vincristine	P-glycoprotein (40–45)	Teeter et al., 1986

were found to be protected from alkylating agent treatment having a specificity for the tissues in which the AGAT transgene was expressed (Liu et al., 1996). The complexity of the mechanism of excisional DNA repair involving both short and long patches (Chapter 3) suggests that resistance mechanisms in this pathway would also be complex. At least some of the proteins of this pathway, namely, DNA polymerase β when overexpressed in neoplastic cells, result in a phenotype resistant to the effects of drugs causing alkylation and/or single strand breaks. Increased levels of nucleotide excision repair of interstrand crosslinks have been reported in cells resistant to a variety of DNA-damaging agents (cf. Barret and Hill, 1998). In addition, the expression of ERCC1 and ERCC2, genes whose products are involved in excisional DNA repair, are found to be increased by two- to threefold in neoplasms exhibiting a clinical resistance to therapy with platinum compounds (Dabholkar et al., 1992). There is also significant evidence that mismatch repair deficiency may mediate the resistance of human neoplasms to specific chemotherapeutic agents (Brown, 1999). While in some instances the exact proteins involved in resistance to DNA damaging agents are not certain, the increased activity of at least one important protein involved in DNA repair, poly(ADP) ribose polymerase, has been reported in some examples of drug resistance to both alkylating agents and chemotherapeutic antibiotics (Urade et al., 1989; Chen et al., 1994). Evidence for the involvement of double-strand DNA break repair in resistance to chemotherapeutics is rare, but there is a suggestion that decreased mismatch repair may contribute to the resistance of some chemotherapeutic drugs (cf. Barret and Hill, 1998). Thus, while this is an important area for potential drug resistance, the exact mechanisms involved in resistance of various chemotherapeutics, especially alkylating agents involving DNA repair mechanisms, needs considerable further investigation.

Drug Resistance and the Inhibition of Apoptosis

As noted previously (Figure 7.14), the process of apoptosis involves numerous potential inducing agents as well as a number of pathways within cells capable of modulating the apoptotic response to various agents. Primary among these are receptor-mediated events, many of which involve tumor necrosis factor alpha (TNF-α) and related pathways. These are transduced by specific receptors including the Fas antigen, the TNF receptors, and a variety of others (Nagata, 1997). Interaction with the appropriate ligand, e.g., TNF-α or the Fas ligand, can result in apoptosis mediated through signal transduction pathways. Resistance to such apoptotic mechanisms has been demonstrated in malignant lymphoid cells that are also resistant to certain chemotherapeutic drugs, such as doxorubicin or mitoxantrone (Landowski et al., 1997). An example of such an association is seen in Figure 20.12, where increasing concentrations of anti-Fas antibody, a surrogate for the Fas ligand, cause a rapid decrease in survival, which is completely absent in cells resistant to doxorubicin. However, resistance to Fas-mediated apoptosis does not select for drug resistance (Landowski et al., 1999).

Another major component of the apoptotic regulatory pathway is the bcl-2 gene, which occurs in the mitochondrial compartment and regulates the permeability of this organ system and interacts with specific proteins to inhibit apoptosis during potential apoptotic events (Kroemer, 1997; Reed, 1997). A large number of human neoplasms exhibit overexpression of the bcl-2 gene, as noted in Table 20.8. Overexpression of this gene does confer resistance to apoptosis on the cell, as discussed earlier in Chapter 6 in reference to the 14-18 translocation, resulting in an enhanced expression of bcl-2 in large-cell lymphomas (Figure 6.8). More recently, Voehringer and Meyn (1998) have suggested that bcl-2 also mediates its effects through alterations in glutathione metabolism. In an experimental system, they have demonstrated that depletion in glutathione in bcl-2–expressing cells restores apoptosis and reverses drug resistance.

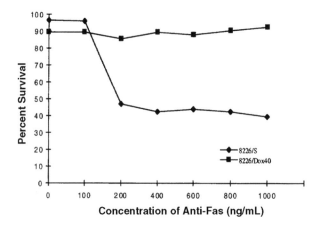

Figure 20.12   Dose response of the effects of an anti-Fas antibody on apoptosis (cell survival) in sensitive and doxorubicin (S and Dox40 respectively) in cell culture. (Adapted from Landowski et al., 1997, with permission of the authors and publisher.)

This finding further establishes and relates apoptosis resistance as a mechanism of drug resistance to the alterations in glutathione metabolism that are similarly related to drug resistance.

Glutathione and Related Enzymes in Multidrug Resistance

As noted in Chapter 8, glutathione and the enzyme glutathione peroxidase play important roles in the inhibition of active oxygen radical–induced alterations in cellular metabolism. These reactions appear to play a similar role in the metabolism and resistance to some chemotherapeutic agents (Morrow and Cowan, 1990). But perhaps more important in drug resistance is the family of glutathione S-transferases. These are phase II (Chapter 3) enzymes involved in the conjugation of a variety of substrates, many of which include drugs used in the chemotherapy of cancer or their metabolites. A listing of these is seen in Table 20.9, adapted from the review by O'Brien and Tew (1996). A variety of human neoplasms exhibit altered levels of glutathione-metabolizing enzymes, as can be noted from Table 20.10.

Table 20.8   Evaluation of the Frequency of bcl-2 Overexpression in Different Cancers

Primary	Percentage
Colon-rectum	92
Nasopharynx	85
Myeloma	80
Breast	70
NHL	65–70
Stomach	60–70
Prostate	30–60
Neuroblastoma	30–35
Lung (SCLC)	20 (80)

Adapted from Desoize, 1994, with permission of the author and publisher.

Table 20.9 Known Anticancer Drugs
and Metabolites That Are GST Substrates

Chlorambucil	Thiotepa
Melphalan	Ethacrynic acid
Cyclophosphamide	Base propenals
Acrolein	Hydroxyalkenals
BCNU[a]	Hydroperoxides

[a]BCNU, 1,3-bis(2-chloroethyl)-1-nitrosourea.
  Hydroxyalkenals, base propenals, and DNA hy-
  droxyperoxides are generated from DNA free
  radical damage.
Adapted from O'Brien and Tew, 1996, with permission of authors and publisher.

Like phase I enzymes, the glutathione S-transferases may also be regulated in their expression by a variety of different drugs and hormones. However, in the neoplasms listed in Table 20.10, the increased glutathione S-transferase activity is stable and not significantly altered by external factors. Furthermore, a number of the glutathione conjugates formed with chemotherapeutic drugs or their metabolites are removed by membrane pump proteins of the MDR family; thus, in a number of instances of resistance, increases in both the MDR p-glycoprotein or related proteins as well as GSTs may be seen (cf. O'Brien and Tew, 1996). This same review also discusses the suggestion that genetic polymorphisms in the GSTs may alter their response to chemotherapy in specific disease conditions. In any event, it is clear that glutathione and specific aspects of its metabolism, especially conjugation with reactive forms and elimination of active oxygen radicals, play significant roles in drug metabolism and resistance. Furthermore, while this discussion has concentrated on isolating specific drug resistance mechanisms and discussing each separately, both the possibility and reality of multiple pathways of drug resistance in neoplastic cells presently exist.

The Cell Cycle and Chemotherapy

Although many of the drugs used in chemotherapy eliminate neoplastic cells by effects during cell division, some drugs also have relatively specific effects during individual stages of the cell cycle. A schema of the relationship of the specific action of various cytostatic and cytotoxic drugs to the various periods of the cell cycle is seen in Figure 20.13. Chapter 9 presented a discussion of the doubling times of neoplastic cells as well as some of the characteristics of their growth. A better knowledge of such variables, as well as their determination in the individual patient, is the goal toward which the methods of chemotherapy are directed. The number of cells in each of the various phases of the cell cycle at any one time in a neoplasm is dependent on a variety of factors. During the logarithmic growth, a greater proportion of the cells are in the S phase, whereas later in the natural history of the neoplasm, more neoplastic cells may be seen in the G_1 or even G_0 stage of the cell cycle. This latter situation is the rule with relatively slowly growing solid neoplasms, whereas rapidly growing embryonal neoplasms and acute leukemias have a much greater proportion of cells entering the S phase during most of their natural history. Not all cells of a neoplasm or a normal tissue have the capacity to replicate indefinitely. In normal tissues there occur cells, termed *stem cells*, that have extensive cell-renewal capacity extending throughout the whole or most of the life span of the organism (Chapter 14; Trott, 1994). Similarly, it appears that neoplasms have stem cells, which are those cells capable of continued

Table 20.10 Altered GSH-Metabolizing Enzymes in Various Tumor Types

Tumor Type	GST Activity	Increased Isozyme Expression	Other Altered Expression
Ovarian		π	
	+		
	+		+GSH +GSH Px activity[a]
Breast	+		+GSH +GSH Px activity
	+		
Lymphocytes			
ALL		π	
CLL-chlorambucil resistant	+		
Bladder			+GSH Px activity +Catalase activity
Lung			
Mixed histologies-cisplatin resistant			+GR +GSH Px activity
Non-small cell lung carcinoma	+		+GSH +GSH Px activity
Colorectal	+	π	
	+		

[a]GSH Px, glutathione peroxidase; GR, glutathione reductase. Elevated enzyme activity represented by (+) symbol. π denotes the specific isozyme, the π form, of glutathione S-transferase (GST).
Adapted from O'Brien and Tew, 1996, with permission of authors and publisher.

replication as long as the neoplasm grows within the host. Under ideal circumstances, the delineation of stem cells in the neoplastic population and of cells in the nonproliferating compartment is critical for successful drug therapy aimed at killing such populations.

A method that has been utilized to isolate in part and determine the effects of drugs on the tumor stem cell population is the human tumor stem cell assay originally described by Salmon et al. (1978). The assay, depicted in Figure 20.14, is carried out by obtaining individual neoplastic cells from a surgical specimen of the neoplasm under study through mechanical dissociation, followed by the incubation of such cell preparations in the presence or absence of a specific test drug and subsequent plating in soft agar. Malignant "stem" cells from the neoplasm will form individual colonies in the soft agar, such as has been described for cells transformed in culture (Chapter 14). One may then monitor the effect of the drug on colony formation and growth. This assay has proved valuable in the in vitro phase II (Figure 20.3) studies of new agents and in the initial screening of new analogs. One of its most notable accomplishments has been in establishing patterns of cross-resistance and sensitivity in relapsing patients as well as monitoring the development of clinical drug resistance through the use of serial tumor biopsies (cf. Bellamy, 1992). As might be expected, however, a variety of technical difficulties prevent the use of this assay in routine clinical diagnosis and management of neoplastic therapy. Such difficulties include (1) a low plating efficiency of freshly isolated human neoplasms, limiting the number of neoplasms that will form colonies for the assessment of drug effects; (2) potential selection of only a portion of the stem cells from the original sample; (3) difficulties in obtaining pure suspensions of single cells that have not been damaged by the technology; (4) potential for significant errors in assessment of "response" rates in both the assay and in patients; and (5) not all neoplasms have stem cells capable of growth in soft agar, as predicted from our discussions in

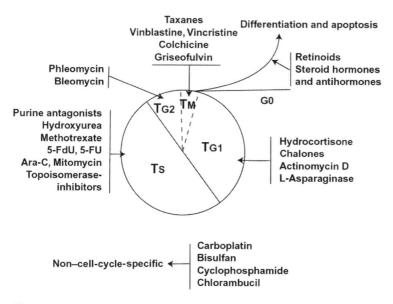

Figure 20.13   The effectiveness of chemotherapeutic drugs at various phases of the cell cycle.

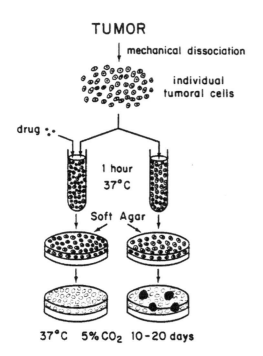

Figure 20.14   Steps involved in the establishment of the clonogenic (human tumor stem cell) assay of human neoplasms for the purpose of testing drug sensitivity and resistance of neoplastic stem cells. (Adapted from Riou and Bernard, 1982, with permission of the authors and publisher.)

Chapter 14. Despite these problems, there is some evidence for a correlation between clinical response and the in vitro response of neoplastic cells in the human tumor stem cell assay. These findings include the observation that cells from human neoplasms of a given histologic type have a response in vitro to therapeutic drug administration that is similar to the known clinical responses of such neoplasms and in particular the patient's clinical response (cf. Bellamy, 1992). Perhaps more important is that the assay has an extremely high capability (85%) to predict clinical resistance to the drug being studied (Von Hoff et al., 1983).

Unfortunately, the human tumor stem cell assay tells nothing about cells in the G_1 or G_0 phase of the cell cycle. However, a number of drugs (Figure 20.13) are effective during these phases, and a number of drugs appear to be non–cell-cycle-specific in their action. Thus, it is clear that the use of a single drug in the chemotherapy of neoplasia is doomed to failure both because of specific actions during the cell cycle and the development of drug resistance by the neoplastic cell through the variety of mechanisms discussed above (Figure 20.12). The apparent solution to this problem has been to use multiple drug combinations composed of chemicals active during different phases of the cell cycle. In some instances, attempts have been made either to synchronize neoplastic cells in vivo with subsequent administration of the drugs at the most sensitive times in relation to the synchronization of certain nonneoplastic tissues. This type of therapy has been termed *chronotherapy*, in which the peak of cell proliferation of neoplastic and normal cells during the daily cycle is determined by a variety of methods, with subsequent therapy administered at time periods giving appropriate and maximal differences between sensitivity of the neoplastic cells and resistance of the normal cells (Focan, 1995). An example of the different 24-hour patterns of DNA synthesis (S phase) in cells of bone marrow and a lymphoid neoplasm in the human is seen in Figure 20.15 (cf. Hrushesky and Bjarnason, 1993). Therapy

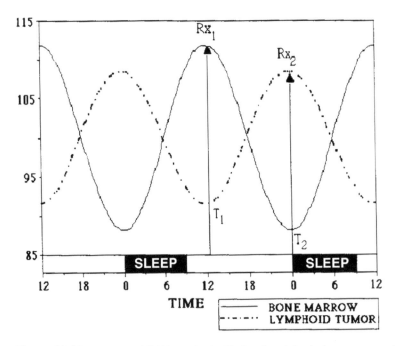

Figure 20.15 Patterns of DNA synthesis (S phase) activity in bone marrow (solid line) or malignant lymphoma (dashed line) sampled through two consecutive 24-hour periods. The curves represent best-fitting cosigned functions to the raw S phase data expressed as a predictable variation around the 24-hour mean (100%). (Adapted from Hrushesky and Bjarnason, 1993, with permission of the authors and publisher.)

with a drug active during the DNA synthesis phase (Figure 20.13) would expose a much higher proportion of neoplastic cells when given near 12 A.M. than bone marrow cells, which have a significantly lower number of cells in S phase at that time. Halberg (1977) was one of the first individuals to suggest taking advantage of differences in circadian rhythmicity for more effective therapy of not only cancer but other diseases as well (Belanger, 1993). However, unless careful analyses of parameters within the neoplasm compared with the host are undertaken, difficulties in results may occur (e.g., Adler et al., 1994). By combining knowledge of cell kinetics as applied to the human disease, differences in endogenous parameters such as seen in circadian rhythms, and the use of multiple drugs affecting different phases of the cell cycle, a rationale for therapy of both leukemias and solid neoplasms has been developed.

CHEMOTHERAPY REGIMENS FOR THE TREATMENT OF LEUKEMIAS AND SOLID NEOPLASMS

With the expansion of the knowledge base for modern chemotherapy of cancer, the efficacy as well as the rationale of the use of combinations of drugs for the therapy of neoplasia became of paramount importance. The ideal situation in which application of the basic knowledge developed to the present time is seen with rapidly growing neoplasms, particularly leukemias, in which neoplastic cells occur systemically but with easy access to the therapeutic agents through the vascular circulation. Here are considered examples of this more idealized treatment as well as the therapy of solid neoplasms, where delivery of the drug to the neoplastic cell becomes a major therapeutic hurdle.

Treatment of Leukemias

Many "protocols" have been devised, that is, therapeutic regimens for the treatment of specific neoplastic conditions, and more are being studied. Figure 20.16 shows an older example of such a protocol, termed the L-2 protocol by Clarkson and Fried (1971). The entire protocol extends over approximately 4 months, during which various combinations of drugs are given interspersed with several rest periods. These latter intervals are necessary in order to allow the host to recover from the toxic effects of the various chemicals given. Obviously, during these rest periods the neoplastic population expands. The estimated changes in cellular populations during the course of therapy are seen in the upper portion of the figure. The assumption is made that the initial size of the leukemic population is 3×10^{12} cells, which is the approximate cell number found in many severe, untreated cases of acute lymphoblastic leukemia in children. The choice of the drugs given at the various periods is made partly on the basis of their mechanism of action, their toxicity, and their known efficacy from past experience in producing remissions in the disease. The reader is referred to the original publication (Clarkson and Fried, 1971) for a more detailed discussion of the protocol.

Several major challenges still remain in the treatment of acute lymphoblastic leukemia in children despite the fact that more than 70% of those treated today by regimens somewhat similar to that seen in Figure 20.16 (Rivera et al., 1993) will be cured of their disease. Those children who relapse must be identified early in their disease and receive more effective therapy; children who respond well and in whom a cure can be expected should be identified so that their treatment may be modified to decrease short- and long-term toxicity (Holcenberg and Camitta, 1981). Today most acute lymphoblastic leukemias are of the pre-B type (approximately 85%), while most of the remaining are of the T-cell variety. The cure rate for children with the pre-B immunophenotype exhibit a cure rate in excess of 70% (Camitta et al., 1997; Rivera et al., 1993). However, cures in B-cell leukemias are relatively rare, while children with T-cell leuke-

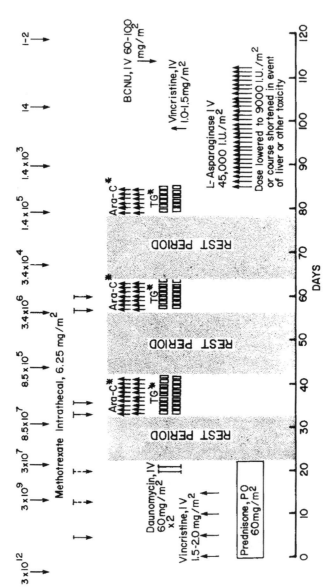

Figure 20.16 Part I of the intensive treatment protocol (L-2) used in the treatment of acute lymphoblastic leukemia. The numbers associated with the vertical arrows at the top of the figure indicate the theoretic leukemic cell number in the patient at that particular time. (Modified from Clarkson and Fried, 1971, with permission of the authors and publisher.)

mias may have cure rates in excess of 40% when aggressive chemotherapy regimens employing high doses of rotating chemotherapeutic agents are employed (cf. Amylon, 1990). Follow-up of patients exhibiting complete remission for extended periods of time can now be monitored by molecular techniques in which residual leukemic cells can be detected in bone marrow (Campana et al., 1991; Roberts et al., 1997).

In adults over 40 years of age, chemotherapy for leukemia generally is not nearly so effective as in children (cf. Freireich, 1984). On the other hand, the chemotherapy of acute myelogenous leukemia in adults has advanced to the stage at which a significant number of patients have been in remission from the disease for more than 5 years; such individuals represent true cures of this disease (Lister and Rohatiner, 1982; Hoelzer, 1994). Much greater success has been achieved with combination chemotherapy for Hodgkin disease, originally using a multidrug regimen of nitrogen mustard, vincristine, procarbazine, and prednisone (MOPP). This regimen (DeVita et al., 1980) has resulted in a cure rate for all stages of Hodgkin disease of up to 70% or better at 10 years. Addition of radiotherapy to combination chemotherapy may result in 10-year survivals of up to 95% in some series (Prosnitz and Roberts, 1992). Treatment of acute leukemia in adults has also included the use of bone marrow transplantation in patients given lethal doses of radiation and/or chemotherapy to eliminate all neoplastic cells in the bone marrow and organism as a whole (cf. Thomas, 1992; Geller, 1993). Treatment of children with non-Hodgkin lymphoma by combination chemotherapy with or without combined radiotherapy results in a very high rate of cure, in excess of 80% (Link et al., 1997). Therapy for the non-Hodgkin lymphomas may be quite effective in adults as well, where in certain cell types of this disease a 5-year cure rate of 60% to 80% has been produced (cf. Armitage, 1993; Lilleyman and Pinkerton, 1996).

Unfortunately, the efficacy of these various therapeutic regimens is not without some risk. At least two of the agents in the MOPP protocol, procarbazine and nitrogen mustard, are alkylating agents. It is now apparent that a significant number of patients treated with these compounds, especially those given radiation as well, later develop second malignancies, one of the most common of which is acute myeloid leukemia. The incidence of this latter neoplasm may be as high as 5% in patients treated for Hodgkin disease with MOPP and radiation (Grünwald and Rosner, 1982). In some series the risk of a second malignancy after treatment for Hodgkin disease may be in excess of 15% 15 years after the therapy itself (Tucker et al., 1988; Robinson et al., 1994). As pointed out in Chapter 11, secondary neoplasms have also been reported after chemotherapy and radiation therapy for a number of different types of human neoplasms, including carcinomas, myelomas, and even nonneoplastic diseases (Boffetta and Kaldor, 1994). On the other hand, one must recall that patients having had one cancer are at a greater risk of developing a second malignancy than are members of the population never exhibiting clinical neoplasia (Carter, 1984), and the highly significant increase in secondary malignancy seen in Hodgkin's disease may in part be related to the abnormal immune function see in these patients (cf. Chapter 19).

Chemotherapy of Solid Neoplasms (Other Than Lymphomas)

Although many of the conclusions drawn on the basis of the L-1210 leukemia model and the combination therapy, especially the latter, also apply to the treatment of solid tumors, it is clear that a rapidly dividing, continuously circulating cell population such as that seen in leukemias is significantly different from a slowly growing neoplasm, with variable doubling times and with erratic growth. In addition, unlike the growth characteristics of leukemias, in most solid neoplasms the cell growth is most rapid at the periphery of the neoplasm, with necrotic regions in the center and an intermediate zone in which cells are viable but nondividing. Some neoplasms, especially scirrhous tumors or neoplastic cells embedded in radiation-induced fibrous tissue, may represent difficult anatomical sites for drugs to permeate, leading to "compartmentaliza-tion" of some neoplastic cells within the host.

Some model experimental neoplasms have been studied (cf. Looney et al., 1977). How-ever, no specific test system like those mentioned above for leukemias has been devised or stud-ied in an attempt to establish new strategies of treatment of solid tumors. The human tumor stem cell assay (HTSCA) has been useful in predicting negative responses of individual neoplasms to chemotherapy. On the other hand, several solid neoplasms in both children and adults have been effectively treated with chemotherapy as the principal therapeutic modality. In children suffering from Wilms tumor, there is now a greater than 80% expectation of cure with a combination of surgery, radiation, and chemotherapy (D'Angio et al., 1991). Chemotherapy of breast cancer in adults has been largely carried out after primary surgical and/or radiotherapy (Bonadonna and Valagussa, 1983; Carbone, 1981). During the last two decades, cytotoxic and hormone therapy of metastatic breast cancer has shown some evidence of effectiveness for specific regimens (Fos-sati et al., 1998), and the endocrine treatment of breast cancer in women has been used exten-sively with a variety of different modalities (Santen et al., 1990). Postsurgical treatment of breast cancer with antiestrogens, particularly tamoxifen, has been most efficacious in reducing the risk of recurrence and death from breast cancer as well as offering some effective palliation for pa-tients with metastatic breast cancer (Osborne, 1998). In addition, tamoxifen given together with surgery and/or radiation therapy is effective in the treatment of very early breast cancer, espe-cially preventing the development of invasive neoplasia (Fisher et al., 1999). In a similar vein, combination chemotherapy has been found effective in the treatment of advanced and metastatic colorectal cancer with relatively nontoxic combinations of fluorouracil, leucovorin, and levami-sole. In this combination, leucovorin, a normal metabolite of folic acid, augments the activity and toxicity of fluorouracil, while levamisole appears to augment the immune system (Moertel, 1994). The treatment of small-cell lung cancer, which has an extremely poor prognosis, has been improved by combination chemotherapy, allowing for remissions of a year or more in a signifi-cant number of patients (Bunn and Carney, 1997). Even greater success has been achieved in the chemotherapy of choriocarcinoma (Lewis, 1980) and testicular cancer (Einhorn, 1990), in which 80% to 90% of patients are cured by chemotherapy in the former case, and over 50% in the latter. A variety of techniques for chemotherapy, including intraarterial and intracavitary chemo-therapy, chemotherapy in combination with hyperthermia, and a variety of drug delivery systems are being used (cf. Markman, 1984). A unique therapy for osteogenic sarcoma in younger indi-viduals involved the administration of high, essentially lethal doses of methotrexate, with subse-quent rescue by the administration of leucovorin, the reduced form of the normal vitamin (folic acid) (Rosenberg et al., 1979). This single-drug therapeutic regimen combined with surgery ap-peared to result in cure rates of up to 40% to 50% in such individuals. More recently, the use of combination chemotherapy involving several drugs has resulted in 5-year survival rates of more than 70% of patients with nonmetastatic osteogenic sarcoma (cf. Grem et al., 1988).

Unfortunately, the problem of destroying every single tumor cell within the host is much more difficult in solid tumors than in leukemias, largely because of the low growth fraction and because most effective chemotherapeutic agents hit cells only during DNA synthesis and mito-sis, as well as the barriers to drug delivery to the neoplastic cell placed by the static environment of the tissue itself. Nonetheless, with a better understanding of the dose and scheduling in multi-stage cancer chemotherapy (Sweetenham, 1995) and the development of new chemotherapeutic agents (e.g., Hanauske, 1996), as well as the potential for individualizing chemotherapy to par-ticular patients or small groups of patients (Cree and Kurbacher, 1997), there is still room for progress to be made in combination drug therapy of neoplasia.

Combinations of Chemotherapy with Other Therapies

At the present time, with the exception of the few neoplasms mentioned in Table 20.1, chemotherapy is used either when the principal cancer therapies of surgery and radiotherapy have not been effective or in conjunction with one or both of these modalities. We have already noted the effectiveness of combining radiotherapy with chemotherapy in the treatment of Hodgkin disease. Today in many instances, even when the primary surgical or radiotherapies are thought to be reasonably successful, chemotherapy will be used in addition as "adjuvant" therapy. This course of action is seen not infrequently in the treatment of breast, colon, prostate, and a number of other neoplasms more commonly seen in older age groups. Such adjuvant therapy has been extremely useful in extending the life span and even achieving complete cures with breast cancer (Olivetto et al., 1994) and to a lesser extent with colon cancer (Shulman and Schilsky, 1995). Since the adjuvant therapy is designed toward cytotoxic and/or cytostatic effects on any neoplastic cells that might remain in the host after surgery and/or radiotherapy, the difficulties with potential side effects and subsequent toxic consequences, even to the development of secondary neoplasms, must be considered. Theoretically, the ideal adjuvant therapy for neoplasia after removal of the majority of neoplastic cells within the host (debulking) is the use of immunotherapy, which depends to a great extent on the immune system of the host itself augmented with external, immunologically active agents. This subject was discussed more fully in Chapter 19, where it was pointed out that immunotherapy has the best chance of eliminating all neoplastic cells if the host recognizes them as foreign antigens. Thus, the combination of immunotherapy and chemotherapy should prove to be one of the most effective means of treating neoplasms to obtain complete cures. Some human neoplasms, particularly choriocarcinomas in females and Burkitt lymphoma, are highly antigenic and can be consistently cured by chemotherapy. This effectiveness probably occurs through a mechanism whereby the drug kills the majority of neoplastic cells and the immune response then destroys the remainder of the neoplastic population. A variety of potential mechanisms for such therapeutic activity by the combination of chemotherapy and immunotherapy have been suggested by Talmadge (1992). These are listed in Table 20.11. Note from the table that these mechanisms involve alteration of suppressor cell activity, cytokine and lymphokine enhancement of normal stem cell development, and responses to neoplastic cells, as well as an interesting suggestion that stimulation of tumor cell growth may occur with a subsequent increase in the sensitivity to chemotherapeutic agents. Kedar and Klein (1992) have also pointed out that chemotherapeutic agents may potentiate immunotherapy by increasing the sensi-

Table 20.11 Potential Mechanism of Therapeutic Activity by Chemoimmunotherapy

---

1. Reduction in tumor burden by cytoreductive agents resulting in a tumor burden more amenable to immunotherapy
2. Decreased suppressor cell activity resulting in an increased T cell adjuvant activity induced by agents such as rl1 IL-2
3. Increased therapeutic activity of two cytoreductive-cytostatic modalities such as a chemotherapeutic agent and tumor necrosis factor or interferon
4. Accelerated myeloid restoration due to increased stem cell activity, thereby allowing more aggressive doses of chemotherapy and reduced neutropenia
5. Addition of agents that stimulate stem cell cycling and accelerate myeloid restoration in conjunction with autologous bone marrow following aggressive cytoreductive therapy
6. Stimulation of tumor cell growth and subsequent increase in sensitivity to chemotherapeutic agents

---

After Talmadge (1992) with permission of the author and publisher.

tivity of neoplastic cells to immunological attack, imposing antigenic changes on the cells by acting as a hapten, and potentiating the stimulation of effector cells as a consequence of massive
release of tumor antigens by induced apoptosis. Thus, as we learn more of the mechanisms involved in the immunobiological aspects of the host–tumor relationship and develop more effective
chemotherapeutic agents, the combination of the two offer perhaps the best hope to ultimately successfully eliminate the "last remaining neoplastic cell" in the host, which effects an absolute cure.

RECENT MODALITIES IN AND POTENTIAL FOR CANCER CHEMOTHERAPY

Until recent years, the principal direction of cancer chemotherapy has been toward newer and better
drugs aimed at affecting cell replication as well as by endocrine-active drugs. A very significant
portion of the drugs presently in use were discovered as a result of serendipity or their efficacy is
directly related to serendipitous findings. With the dramatic increase in our knowledge of the cellular and molecular biology of living tissues, both normal and neoplastic, it is now reasonable to devise chemotherapeutic agents on the basis of several rationales. Several of these are discussed below.

Signal Transduction Pathways as Targets for Chemotherapy

With a dramatic increase in our knowledge of molecular mechanisms involved in signal transduction and its aberrations in neoplasia, components of this pathway have been suggested as
possible targets for chemotherapy (Powis, 1994). Although there are many possibilities, certain
specific sites have been targeted by agents developed specifically for such effects. A diagram of
the Ras/MAP kinase cascade is seen in Figure 20.17. In the figure are indicated sites at which
drug intervention has been developed and attempted.

Growth Factor Receptor Targets

While a variety of growth factors are involved in the development of neoplasia, predominantly
during the stage of promotion but continuing into the stage of progression, reagents—both drugs
and natural products—have been developed in an attempt to selectively alter or modulate such
functions. The epidermal growth factor family has been one target by use of inhibitors of the
tyrosine kinase function of the receptor, which has interesting potential, as well as interfering
with ligand-receptor interactions (Davies and Chamberlin, 1996). The latter approach has been
relatively successful and is now in clinical trials through the use of specific monoclonal antibodies directed toward members of the epidermal growth factor receptor family that are expressed
on many highly malignant neoplastic cells (cf. Disis and Cheever, 1997). Investigations have
also attempted to utilize modulation of the receptor to alter drug resistance (cf. Davies and
Chamberlin, 1996). In addition, in a recent study (Wosikowski et al., 1997) with cell lines and
computer analysis of cytotoxicity patterns, several compounds were identified as inhibitors of
the epidermal growth factor receptor pathway, probably by modulating phosphorylation. Some
studies have also demonstrated that both natural and synthetic agents may modulate the expression of growth factors on neoplastic cells (Tagliaferri et al., 1994).

Protein Kinase Inhibitors

As noted above, some disruption of the epidermal growth factor pathway may be effected by
inhibiting the tyrosine kinase component of the receptor. A large number of other protein kinase
inhibitors have also been synthesized and utilized, primarily in in vitro systems (cf. Boutin,
1994). A variety of structures of such inhibitors can be seen in Figure 20.18. Some of these are

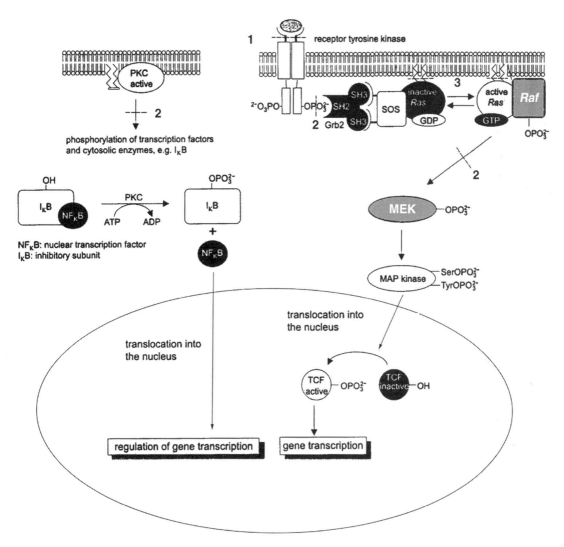

Figure 20.17 Signal transduction pathways by the Ras/MAP kinase cascade as well as via protein kinase C and subsequent activation of the nuclear transcription factor $NF_\kappa B$. The student is referred to earlier figures (7.6, 7.7, 7.8) giving some details of the specific pathways. Inhibitory actions of drugs and natural products are noted by the numbers within circles adjacent to the reaction and its product. (1) Growth factor-receptor inhibition; (2) inhibition of protein kinases; (3) inhibition of prenylation of G proteins. (Modified from Hinterding et al., 1998, with permission of the authors and publisher.)

relatively selective for the epidermal growth factor receptor such as DAPH-1 (cf. Patrick and Heimbrook, 1996). Inhibitors of the protein kinase C family of serine/threonine protein kinases have involved both the use of active-site-directed inhibitors targeting both peptide substrate and nucleotide binding sites. However, cell-penetration problems remain as important factors in the use of these agents. Nucleotide binding-site-directed inhibitors include H-7 and staurosporine, while R0 32-0432 is an ATP-competitive inhibitor of some members of the protein kinase C family (cf. Patrick and Heimbrook, 1996). Inhibitors of the raf serine/threonine protein kinase and the mitogen activated kinases (MEK, MAP) have also been described affecting several mem-

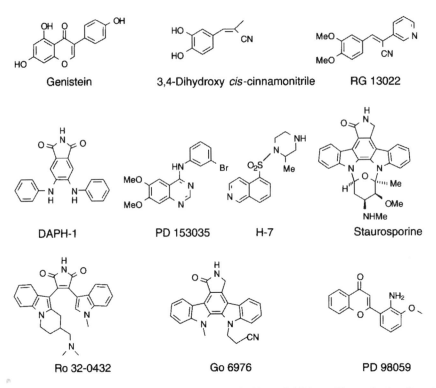

Figure 20.18 Structural features of some protein kinase inhibitors. The reader is referred to the original reference (Patrick and Heimbrook, 1996) and the text for further details. (Adapted from Patrick and Heimbrook, 1996, with permission of the authors and publisher.)

bers of this pathway. The example from Figure 20.18 is PD 98059, which inhibits both the MEK-kinase or raf-dependent activation of MEK but does not seem to affect raf autophosphorylation (cf. Patrick and Heimbrook, 1996). In addition to inhibitors of signal transduction kinases, there are also being developed chemotherapeutic agents capable of altering the function of cyclin-dependent kinase inhibitors that may have important usefulness in chemotherapy (Kaubisch and Schwartz, 2000). Despite the extensive work in this area and the large involvement of protein kinase activities in signal transduction pathway, one must remember that all of these pathways function in normal cells, and thus the differential between effective treatment in neoplasia and lack of toxicity in normal tissues (therapeutic index, see above) may be less than desired in many instances.

Protein Prenylation as a Target for Chemotherapy

As noted in Figure 20.17, the ras protein is shown bound to the plasma membrane through a lipid moiety, farnesyl, which is covalently linked to a cysteine sulfhydryl of the protein, forming a thioether bond. As briefly discussed in Chapter 7, this interaction of these G proteins with the cell membrane is required for normal signal transduction. Inhibitors of the formation of isoprenoids, especially farnesyl and geranyl moieties and/or their linkage to the protein, can result in inhibition of signal transduction pathways. This has been demonstrated by the rational design of peptidomimetics of the carboxyl terminal tetrapeptide farnesylation site on ras (Lerner et al., 1997; Moasser et al., 1998). The resulting agents are capable of inhibiting ras processing, selectively antagonizing oncogenic signaling, and suppressing neoplastic growth in mouse models with relatively small side effects. While there are a number of key problems that still must be overcome in order for such agents to enter clinical trials, other inhibitors of isoprenoid synthesis may become effective additions to the chemotherapeutic armamentarium (Waddick and Uckun, 1998).

On the other hand, the variety of signal transduction pathways extending all the way into nuclear factors and mechanisms may be amenable to attack by the use of structure-based strategies by drug design and discovery (Kuntz, 1992). The modern technologies involving combinatorial chemistry as well as detailed structural knowledge of the protein targets, especially their active sites, can lead to the development of drugs extremely specific in their site of action with a much greater potential for an effective therapeutic index (Lam, 1997). One potential target for such strategies would be the nuclear factor κB, which affects cell survival and determines the sensitivity of neoplastic cells to cytotoxic agents as well as to ionizing radiation (Waddick and Uckun, 1999). In Figure 20.17, this pathway may be noted as being related to a cytoplasmic factor, IκB, which normally maintains NFκB as a complex but when phosphorylated by protein kinase C releases the active NFκB to become involved in specific gene transcription within the nucleus. A recent example of the use of such technologies is the synthesis of monastrol, an agent that specifically inhibits the motility of a mitotic motor protein required for normal spindle structure (Mayer et al., 1999). It is very likely that, as more basic knowledge of the structural characteristics of specific proteins within signal transduction pathways become known, specific drugs can be exquisitely tailored to interact and alter the effectiveness of these gene products within neoplastic cells.

Induced Differentiation of Neoplastic Cells

As discussed in earlier chapters (Chapters 6, 10, and 14), the chemical induction of differentiation of neoplastic cells has been achieved in systems studied in vitro. Lotem and Sachs (1981) and Honma et al. (1997) have reported the inhibition of leukemia development and the prolongation of survival time of mice inoculated with myeloid leukemia by the administration of various chemical inducers of differentiation. In the human in vivo, the principal example of the effectiveness of induced differentiation in the treatment of specific neoplasia is the use of all-*trans*-retinoic acid in the treatment of acute promyelocytic leukemia (cf. Tallman et al., 1997). These and other studies have demonstrated the effectiveness of all-*trans*-retinoic acid in inducing or maintaining remission and improving overall survival when compared with chemotherapy alone. Other examples of effects of differentiating agents in vivo include high-dose methylprednisolone in children with acute promyelocytic leukemia (Hiçsönmez et al., 1993) and the use of tetradecanoylphorbol acetate, an effective skin tumor–promoting agent, in patients with myelocytic leukemia (Han et al., 1998). The theoretical potential for this modality is great, especially since little or no toxicity is associated with the therapy; but in the examples thus far studied in both humans and animals, the effects require continued administration of the differentiating agent. The usual history in the human is that eventually neoplasms will escape the differentiating effect for a variety of mechanistic reasons (Early and Dmitrovsky, 1995). In addition, the theoretical combination of multiple differentiating agents may prove to be effective in the future (Taimi et al., 1998).

Antiangiogenesis as an Approach to Chemotherapy of Cancer

As noted in Chapter 18, the importance of a vascular supply for the viability of solid neoplasms is well documented. Investigation of this critical component of neoplastic growth with an aim toward therapy was initiated by Folkman and associates in experimental situations almost three decades ago (Folkman et al., 1971). Since that time, and especially during the past few years, a large number of antiangiogenic agents have entered clinical trial, the number being in excess of 30 and exhibiting a variety of mechanisms either directly or indirectly associated with angiogenesis of neoplasia (Thompson et al., 1999). The directly acting agents, such as angiostatin and endostatin, inhibit endothelial cell proliferation directly (O'Reilly et al., 1997). Other agents are directed toward inhibiting the signal transduction pathway regulated by the vascular endothelial growth factor (VEGF) (Salven et al., 1998; Veikkola and Alitalo, 1999). Both antibodies directed toward the growth factor and direct antagonists of smaller molecular structure have been utilized in clinical trials (Thompson et al., 1999). In theory, this approach offers great promise, since it does not involve a direct attack on the neoplastic cell itself but rather on host cells that the neoplasm requires for maintenance and growth (Boehm et al., 1997; Gastl et al., 1997). Although these agents are not without side effects, it might be anticipated that they are much less toxic than a number of the chemotherapeutic agents in standard use (Thompson et al., 1999), and thus the potential for this type of therapy as primary therapy or as an adjunct to other therapies appears to be very great at the present time.

Gene Therapy of Neoplasia

As our capability for the direct transfer of genetic information into cells increases, the use of gene therapy in neoplasia has become a realistic potential in modern-day chemotherapy. Transfection of a normal tumor suppressor gene that is defective in neoplastic cells, such as the p53 gene (El-Deiry, 1998), would be an obvious target for gene therapy. However, a number of other potentials include the use of gene transfer vectors to provide high concentration of antiangiogenic proteins within organs (Kong and Crystal, 1998), methods to modify methylation of introduced genes (Szyf, 1996), and the specific stimulation of the immune system, thereby enhancing immunity to specific neoplasms in the form of DNA vaccines, as discussed in Chapter 19.

A variety of gene transfer methods affording introduction of specific genes into target cells have been utilized. A number of these methods are listed in Table 20.12. Such gene transfer may

Table 20.12 Gene Therapy: Gene Transfer Methods

Methods	Applications		
	Ex Vivo Use	In Vivo Use	Expression
Viral			
Adeno-associated virus	+	+	S
Adenovirus	+/−	+	T
Baculovirus	+/−	−	T
Herpesvirus	+/−	+	T
HIV-derived vector	+/−	−	S
Poliovirus	+/−	+	T
Poxvirus	+/−	+	S
Retroviruses	+	+	S
Sindbis and other RNA viruses	+/−	+	T
Vacciniavirus	+/−	+	T
Nonviral			
Ca-phosphate precipitation	+/−	−	S/T
Direct DNA injection	−	+	T
Ligand DNA conjugate	−	+	T
Lipofection	+/−	+	T
Polyethylenimine	+	+	T

Key: + = frequent, +/− = occasional, − = rare; expression: S = stable, T = transient.
Adapted from Blum et al., 1997, with permission of the authors and publisher.

Table 20.13 Potential Contributions of Gene Therapy to Overcome Obstacles for Curing Cancer

1. All tumours are *genetically unstable* and thus they are extraordinarily adaptable to environmental changes.

   Gene transfer of DNA repair or cell cycle checkpoint genes that restore DNA stability and cell susceptibility to therapeutic insults.

2. Tumours are heterogeneous in many respects, including genetic mutations, expression of oncoproteins, immunogenicity, response to environmental changes, etc.

   Targeting of genetically homogeneous and stable tissues, such as the tumour vasculature and stroma; genetic immunopotentiation; chimeric vectors.

3. As a consequence of obstacles 1 and 2, tumours have, or acquire, *resistance* to cellular toxins and to many other therapeutically induced cellular insults.

   Strategies above, associated with chemotherapy or radiotherapy or with the transfer of additional genes that sensitise tumour cells to drugs or radiation.

4. Tumours can have a low *cellular growth fraction*; therefore, they are less susceptible to mitotic toxins and to gene transfer vectors that require dividing cells.

   Use of vectors that do not require cellular division for gene delivery and expression (adenovirus, herpesvirus, lentivirus, chimeric vectors); repeated administration of non-immunogenic vectors.

5. Tumours form *metastases*, which have to be reached systemically to eradicate the tumour completely.

   Use of targetable, injectable vectors (tropism-modified viruses, cellular vehicles, liposomes); genetic immunopotentiation.

6. Tumours do not express specific tumour antigens or immune costimulatory molecules; alternatively, tumours down-regulate antigen-presentation, induce *immunological tolerance*, or inhibit the effector mechanisms of the immune response.

   Transfer of genes encoding costimulatory molecules and cytokines; genetic modification of antigen-presenting cells; induce inflammatory reactions that activate antigen presentation; transfer of genes blocking tumour-secreted inhibitors of the immune response.

7. The *spontaneous* behaviour of human tumours is somewhat different from that of malignant cells *in vitro*, and from that of experimental tumours in animal models.

   Development of better animal models, including tumour models in transgenic mice.

8. Tumours are diagnosed in *advanced stages*, when billions of tumour cells exist in the body, frequently widely disseminated.

   Development of amplification vector systems (replicative viral vectors and exploitation of bystander effects); use of targetable, injectable vectors; genetic immunopotentiation.

9. The understanding and treatment of cancer requires the contribution of very *diverse fields* of basic knowledge, biotechnology, and medical practice.

   De facto multidisciplinary recruitment of gene therapy researchers.

After Gómez-Navarro et al. (1999), with permission of authors and publisher.

be carried out in cells in vitro, such cells then being administered to the host, or a cell-free direct gene transfer into cells in vivo. When administered in vivo, viral vectors may be used, a number of which have been attempted (cf. Roth and Cristiano, 1997), but DNA in liposomes or some other complex that is readily taken up by cells allowing entrance of the DNA into the nucleus have also been used. Although it is likely that only a few neoplastic cells may take up specific genes in these therapeutic regimens, the "bystander" effect, mediated to a significant degree by connexins (Freeman et al., 1993; Mesnil et al., 1996), may prove an effective mediator of such gene therapies.

As pointed out by Gómez-Navarro et al. (1999), there are a variety of obstacles in cancer therapy for which potential contributions of gene therapy may be effective. A list of these, taken from their recent article, is seen in Table 20.13, which is relatively self-explanatory. As noted, many of the potential contributions of gene transfer may not be realized until well into the future; however, with the continuing increase in knowledge and technology, the future for specific gene therapy of neoplasia is bright.

REFERENCES

Adler, S., Lang, S., Langenmayer, I., Eibl-Eibesfeldt, B., Rump, W., Emmerich, B., and Hallek, M. Chronotherapy with 5-fluorouracil and folinic acid in advanced colorectal carcinoma. Cancer, *73*:2905–2912, 1994.

Amylon, M. D. Treatment of T-lineage acute lymphoblastic leukemia. Hematol. Oncol. Clin. North Am., *4*:937–948, 1990.

Armitage, J. O. Treatment of non-Hodgkin's lymphoma. N. Engl. J. Med., *328*:1023–1030, 1993.

Baggetto, L. G. Non P-glycoprotein novel proteins involved in human cancer multidrug resistance. Bull. Cancer, *84*:385–390, 1997.

Barret, J.-M., and Hill, B. T. DNA repair mechanisms associated with cellular resistance to antitumor drugs: potential novel targets. Anticancer Drugs, 9:105–123, 1998.

Beatson, G. T. On the treatment of inoperable cases of carcinoma of the mamma: suggestions for a new method of treatment, with illustrative cases. Lancet, 2:104–107, 162–165, 1896.

Belanger, P. M. Chronopharmacology in drug research and therapy. Adv. Drug Res., *24*:1–80, 1993.

Bellamy, W. T. Prediction of response to drug therapy of cancer. A review of *in vitro* assays. Drugs, *44*:690–708, 1992.

Bellamy, W. T. P-Glycoproteins and multidrug resistance. Annu. Rev. Pharmacol. Toxicol., *36*:161–183, 1996.

Berger, N. A. Cancer chemotherapy: new strategies for success. J. Clin. Invest., *78*:1131–1135, 1986.

Bjornsson, T. D. A classification of drug action based on therapeutic effects. J. Clin. Pharmacol., *36*:669–673, 1996.

Black, D. J., and Livingston, R. B. Antineoplastic drugs in 1990. A review (part II). Drugs, *39*:652–673, 1990.

Blum, H. E., Wieland, S., von Weizsäcker, F. Gene therapy: basic concepts and applications in gastrointestinal diseases. Digestion, *58*:87–97, 1997.

Boehm, T., Folkman, J., Browder, T., and O'Reilly, M. S. Antiangiogenic therapy of experimental cancer does not induce acquired drug resistance. Nature, *390*:404–407, 1997.

Boffetta, P., and Kaldor, J. M. Secondary malignancies following cancer chemotherapy. Acta Oncol., *33*:591–598, 1994.

Bonadonna, G., and Valagussa, P. Chemotherapy of breast cancer: current views and results. Int. J. Radiat. Oncol. Biol. Phys., 9:279–297, 1983.

Boutin, J. A. Tyrosine protein kinase inhibition and cancer. Int. J. Biochem., *26*:1203–1226, 1994.

Brown, R. Mismatch repair deficiency, apoptosis, and drug resistance. *In*: J. A. Hickman and C. Dive (Eds.), pp. 69–85, Apoptosis and Cancer Chemotherapy. Totowa, NJ: Humana Press, 1999.

Bunn, Jr., B. A., and Carney, D. N. Overview of chemotherapy for small cell lung cancer. Semin. Oncol., *7*:S7-69–S7-74, 1997.

Camitta, B. M., Pullen, J., and Murphy, S. Biology and treatment of acute lymphocytic leukemia in children. Semin. Oncol., *24*:83–91, 1997.

Campain, J. A., Slovak, M. L., Schoenlein, P. V., Popescu, N. C., Gottesman, M. M., and Pastan, I. Acquisition of multiple copies of a mutant topoisomerase IIα allele by chromosome 17 aneuploidy is associated with etoposide resistance in human melanoma cell lines. Somatic Cell Mol. Genet., *21*:451–471, 1995.

Campana, D., Coustan-Smith, E., and Behm, F. G. The definition of remission in acute leukemia with immunologic techniques. Bone Marrow Transplant., *8*:429–437, 1991.

Carbone, P. P. Options in breast cancer therapy. Hosp. Pract., Hosp. edn., *16*(2):53–61, Feb., 1981.

Carter, S. K. The carcinogenic potential of cytotoxic chemotherapy and its implications for therapeutic decision making. Cancer Chemother. Pharmacol., *1*:67–69, 1984.

Chang, T. K. H., Chen, G., and Waxman, D. J. Role of individual human liver P450s and other enzymes in anti-cancer drug metabolism: drug activation and drug resistance mechanisms. *In*: M. C. Lechner (Ed.), Cytochrome P450. 8th International Conference, pp. 103–108. Paris: John Libbey Eurotext, 1994.

Chen, G., and Zeller, W. J. Increased poly(ADP-ribose) formation in cisplatin-resistant rat ovarian tumor cells. Anticancer Res., *14*:1462–1468, 1994.

Clarkson, B. D., and Fried, J. Changing concepts of treatment in acute leukemia. Med. Clin. North Am., *5*:561, 1971.

Cree, I. A., and Kurbacher, C. M. Individualizing chemotherapy for solid tumors—is there any alternative? Anticancer Drugs, *8*:541–548, 1997.

Dabholkar, M., Bostick-Bruton, F., Weber, C., Bohr, V. A., Egwuagu, C., and Reed, E. ERCC1 and ERCC2 expression in malignant tissues from ovarian cancer patients. J. Natl. Cancer Inst., *84*:1512–1517, 1992.

D'Angio, G. J., et al. Wilms' tumor: status report, 1990. By the National Wilms' Tumor Study Committee. J. Clin. Oncol., *9*:877–887, 1991.

D'Anna, J. A., Church, V. L., and Tobey, R. A. Changes in H1 content, nucleosome repeat lengths and DNA elongation under conditions of hydroxyurea treatment that reportedly facilitate gene amplification. Biochim. Biophys. Acta, *868*:226–237, 1986.

Davies, D. E., and Chamberlin, S. G. Targeting the epidermal growth factor receptor for therapy of carcinomas. Biochem. Pharmacol., *51*:1101–1110, 1996.

Desoize, B. Anticancer drug resistance and inhibition of apoptosis. Anticancer Res., *14*:2291–2294, 1994.

DeVita, V. T. Principles of chemotherapy. *In*: V. T. DeVita, S. Hellman, and S. A. Rosenberg (Eds.), Cancer—Principles and Practice of Oncology, Vol. 1, 3rd ed., pp. 276–300. Philadelphia: Lippincott, 1989.

DeVita, V. T., Simon, R. M., Hubbard, S. M., Young, R. C., Berard, C. W., Moxley, J. H. III, Frei, E. III, Carbone, P. P., and Canellos, G. P. Curability of advanced Hodgkin's disease with chemotherapy. Ann. Intern. Med., *92*:587–595, 1980.

Dicato, M., Duhem, C., Pauly, M., and Ries, F. Multidrug resistance: molecular and clinical aspects. Cytokines, Cell. Mol. Ther., *3*:91–100, 1997.

Disis, M. L., and Cheever, M. A. HER-2/neu protein: a target for antigen-specific immunotherapy of human cancer. Adv. Cancer Res., *71*:343–371, 1997.

Donehower, R. C., Abeloff, M. D., and Perry, M. C. Chemotherapy. *In*: M. D. Abeloff, J. O. Armitage, A. S. Lichter, and J. E. Niederhuber (Eds.), Clinical Oncology, pp. 201–218. New York: Churchill Livingstone, 1995.

Durant, J. R. Overview: current status of clinical trials. Cancer, *65*:2371–2375, 1990.

Early, E., and Dmitrovsky, E. Acute promyelocytic leukemia: retinoic acid response and resistance. J. Invest. Med., *43*:337–344, 1995.

Einhorn, L. H. Treatment of testicular cancer: a new and improved model. J. Clin. Oncol., *8*:1777–1781, 1990.

El-Deiry, W. S. The p53 pathway and cancer therapy. Cancer J., *11*:229–236, 1998.

Fenaux, P., Chomienne, C., and Degos, L. Acute promyelocytic leukemia: biology and treatment. Semin. Oncol., *24*:92–102, 1997.

Fisher, B., Dignam, J., Wolmark, N., Wickerham, D. L., Fisher, E. R., Mamounas, E., Smith, R., Begovic, M., Dimitrov, N. V., Margolese, R. G., Kardinal, C. G., Kavanah, M. T., Fehrenbacher, L., and Oishi, R. H. Tamoxifen in treatment of intraductal breast cancer: National Surgical Adjuvant Breast and Bowel Project B-24 randomised controlled trial. Lancet, *353*:1993–2000, 1999.

Focan, C. Circadian rhythms and cancer chemotherapy. Pharmacol. Ther., *67*:1–52, 1995.

Folkman, J., Merler, E., Abernathy, C., and Williams, G. Isolation of a tumor factor responsible for angiogenesis. J. Exp. Med., *133*:275–288, 1971.

Fossati, R., Confalonieri, C., Torri, V., Ghislandi, E., Penna, A., Pistotti, V., Tinazzi, A., and Liberati, A. Cytotoxic and hormonal treatment for metastatic breast cancer: a systematic review of published randomized trials involving 31,510 women. J. Clin. Oncol., *16*:3439–3460, 1998.

Freeman, S. M., Abboud, C. N., Whartenby, K. A., Packman, C. H., Koeplin, D. S., Moolten, F. L., and Abraham, G. N. The "bystander effect": tumor regression when a fraction of the tumor mass is genetically modified. Cancer Res., *53*:5274–5283, 1993.

Frei, E. III. Acute leukemia in children. Model for the development of scientific methodology for clinical therapeutic research in cancer. Cancer, *5*:2013–2025, 1984.

Freireich, E. J. Ethical considerations in cancer chemotherapy. Ann. Rev. Pharmacol. Toxicol., *1*:547–557, 1979.

Freireich, E. J. Acute leukemia. A prototype of disseminated cancer. Cancer, *5*:2026–2033, 1984.

Friedman, M. A., and Cain, D. F. National Cancer Institute sponsored cooperative clinical trials. Cancer, *65*:2376–2382, 1990.

Friend, C., Scher, W., Holland, J., and Sato, T. Hemoglobin synthesis in murine erythroleukemia cells *in vitro*: stimulation of erythroid differentiation by dimethylsulfoxide. Proc. Natl. Acad. Sci. U.S.A., *68*:378–382, 1971.

Gastl, G., Hermann, T., Steurer, M., Zmija, J., Gunsilius, E., Unger, C., and Kraft, A. Angiogenesis as a target for tumor treatment. Oncology, *54*:177–184, 1997.

Geller, R. B. Role of autologous bone marrow transplantation for patients with acute and chronic leukemias. Hematol. Oncol. Clin. North Am., *7*:547–575, 1993.

Gick, G. G., and McCarty Sr., K. S. Amplification of the metallothionein-I gene in cadmium- and zinc-resistant Chinese hamster ovary cells. J. Biol. Chem., *257*:9049–9053, 1982.

Gilman, A., and Philips, F. S. The biological action and therapeutic applications of β-chloroethyl amines and sulfides. Science, *103*:409–411, 1946.

Glover, A. B., and Leyland-Jones, B. Biochemistry of azacitidine: a review. Cancer Treat. Rep., *71*:959–964, 1987.

Goldin, A., and Carter, S. K. Screening and evaluation of antitumor agents. *In*: J. F. Holland and E. Frei, III (Eds.), Cancer Medicine, 2nd ed., pp. 633–663. Philadelphia: Lea & Febiger, 1982.

Gómez-Navarro, J., Curiel, D. T., and Douglas, J. T. Gene therapy for cancer. Eur. J. Cancer, *35*:867–885, 1999.

Gottesman, M. M. How cancer cells evade chemotherapy: Sixteenth Richard and Hinda Rosenthal Foundation Award Lecture. Cancer Res., *53*:747–754, 1993.

Graham, M. A., Riley, R. J., and Kerr, D. J. Drug metabolism in carcinogenesis and cancer chemotherapy. Pharmacol. Ther., *51*:275–289, 1991.

Grem, J. L., King, S. A., Wittes, R. E., and Leyland-Jones, B. The role of methotrexate in osteosarcoma. J. Natl. Cancer Inst., *80*:626–656, 1988.

Grünwald, H. W., and Rosner, F. Acute myeloid leukemia following treatment of Hodgkin's disease. Cancer, *5*:676–683, 1982.

Gulliford, T., and Epstein, R. J. Endocrine treatment of cancer. J. R. Soc. Med., *89*:448–453, 1996.

Halberg, F. Implications of biologic rhythms for clinical practice. Hosp. Pract., *12*(1):139–149, 1977.

Han, Z. T., Zhu, X. X., Yang, R. Y., Sun, J. Z., Tian, G. F., Liu, X. J., Cao, G. S., Newmark, H. L., Conney, A. H., and Chang, R. L. Effect of intravenous infusions of 12-O-tetradecanoylphorbol-13-acetate (TPA) in patients with myelocytic leukemia: preliminary studies on therapeutic efficacy and toxicity. Proc. Natl. Acad. Sci., U.S.A. *95*:5357–5361, 1998.

Hanauske, A.-R. The development of new chemotherapeutic agents. Anticancer Drugs, *7*:29–32, 1996.

Hannun, Y. A. Apoptosis and the dilemma of cancer chemotherapy. Blood, *89*:1845–1853, 1997.

Harrison, D. J. Molecular mechanisms of drug resistance in tumours. J. Pathol., *175*:7–12, 1995.

Heidelberger, C. Fluorinated pyrimidines and their nucleosides. *In*: A. C. Sartorelli and D. G. Johns (Eds.), Handbuch der Experimentellen Pharmakologie (Handbook of Pharmacology), New Series, Vol. XXXVIII/2, pp. 193–231. Berlin: Springer Verlag, 1975.

Hiçsönmez, G., Tuncer, A. M., Güler, E., Tan, E., and Tekelioglu, M. The potential role of high-dose methylprednisolone on the maturation of leukemic cells in children with acute promyelocytic leukemia (APL). Exp. Hematol., *21*:599–601, 1993.

Hinterding, K., Alonso-Díaz, D., and Waldmann, H. Organic synthesis and biological signal transduction. Angew. Chem. Int. Ed., *37*:688–749, 1998.

Hoelzer, D. Treatment of acute lymphoblastic leukemia. Semin. Hematol., *31*:1–15, 1994.

Holcenberg, J. S., and Camitta, B. M. Recent approaches to the treatment of acute lymphocytic leukemia in childhood. Annu. Rev. Pharmacol. Toxicol., *2*:231–249, 1981.

Honma, Y., Tobe, H., Makishima, M., Yokoyama, A., and Okabe-Kado, J. Induction of differentiation of myelogenous leukemia cells by humulone, a bitter in the hop. Leukemia Res., *22*:605–610, 1998.

Hrushesky, W. J. M., and Bjarnason, G. A. Circadian cancer therapy. J. Clin. Oncol., *11*:1403–1417, 1993.

Huggins, C., and Hodges, C. V. Studies on prostatic cancer. I. The effect of castration of estrogen and the androgen injection on serum phosphatases in metastatic carcinoma of the prostate. Cancer Res., *1*:293–297, 1941.

Infield, G. B. Disasters at Bari. Macmillan, New York, 1971.

Iyer, L., and Ratain, M. J. Pharmacogenetics and cancer chemotherapy. Eur. J. Cancer, *34*:1493–1499, 1998.

Kaubisch, A., and Schwartz, G. K. Cyclin-dependent kinase and protein kinase C inhibitors: a novel class of antineoplastic agents in clinical development. Cancer J., *6*:192–212, 2000.

Kavallaris, M. The role of multidrug resistance-associated protein (MRP) expression in multidrug resistance. Anticancer Drugs, *8*:17–25, 1997.

Kedar, E., and Klein, E. Cancer immunotherapy: are the results discouraging? Can they be improved? Adv. Cancer Res., *59*:245–322, 1992.

Kelley, S. L., Basu, A., Teicher, B. A., Hacker, M. P., Hamer, D. H., and Lazo, J. S. Overexpression of metallothionein confers resistance to anticancer drugs. Science, *241*:1813–1815, 1988.

Kong, H.-L., and Crystal, R. G. Gene therapy strategies for tumor autoangiogenesis. J. Natl. Cancer Inst., *90*:273–286, 1998.

Krakoff, I. H. Cancer chemotherapeutic and biologic agents. CA, *41*:264–278, 1991.

Kroemer, G. The proto-oncogene Bcl-2 and its role in regulating apoptosis. Nature Med., *3*:614–620, 1997.

Kuntz, I. D. Structure-based strategies for drug design and discovery. Science, *257*:1078–1082, 1992.

Lam, K. S. Application of combinatorial library methods in cancer research and drug discovery. Anticancer Drug Design, *12*:145–167, 1997.

Lambrechts, A. C., van't Veer, L. J., and Rodenhuis, S. The detection of minimal numbers of contaminating epithelial tumor cells in blood or bone marrow: use, limitations and future of RNA-based methods. Ann. Oncol., *9*:1269–1276, 1998.

Landowski, T. H., Gleason-Guzman, M. C., and Dalton, W. S. Selection for drug resistance results in resistance to Fas-mediated apoptosis. Blood, *89*:1854–1861, 1997.

Landowski, T. H., Shain, K. H., Oshiro, M. M., Buyuksal, I., Painter, J. S., and Dalton, W. S. Myeloma cells selected for resistance to CD95-mediated apoptosis are not cross-resistant to cytotoxic drugs: evidence for independent mechanisms of caspase activation. Blood, *94*:265–274, 1999.

Leinonen, P., Alhonen-Hongisto, L., Laine, R., Jänne, O. A., and Jänne, J. Human myeloma cells acquire resistance to difluoromethylornithine by amplification of ornithine decarboxylase gene. Biochem. J., *242*:199–203, 1987.

Lerner, E. C., Hamilton, A. D., and Sebti, S. M. Inhibition of Ras prenylation: a signaling target for novel anti-caner drug design. Anticancer Drug Design, *12*:229–238, 1997.

Lewis, A. D., Hickson, I. D., Robson, C. N., Harris, A. L., Hayes, J. D., Griffiths, S. A., Manson, M. M., Hall, A. E., Moss, J. E., and Wolf, C. R. Amplification and increased expression of alpha class glutathione S-transferase-encoding genes associated with resistance to nitrogen mustards. Proc. Natl. Acad. Sci. U.S.A., *85*:8511–8515, 1988.

Lewis, J. L. Jr. Choriocarcinoma: a success story for chemotherapy. Int. J. Radiat. Oncol. Biol. Phys., *6*:897–898, 1980.

Lilleyman, J. S., and Pinkerton, C. R. Lymphoblastic leukaemia and non-Hodgkin's lymphoma. Br. Med. Bull., *52*:742–763, 1996.

Link, M. P., Shuster, J. J., Donaldson, S. S., Berard, C. W., and Murphy, S. B. Treatment of children and young adults with early-stage non-Hodgkin's lymphoma. N. Engl. J. Med., *337*:1259–1266, 1997.

Lister, T. A., and Rohatiner, A. Z. S. The treatment of acute myelogenous leukemia in adults. Semin. Hematol., *1*:172–192, 1982.

Liu, L., Lee, K., Wasan, E., and Gerson, S. L. Differential sensitivity of human and mouse alkyltransferase to 0^6-benzylguanine using a transgenic model. Cancer Res., *56*:1880–1885, 1996.

Looney, W. B., Trefil, J. S., Hopkins, H. A., Kovacs, C. J., Ritenour, R., and Schaffner, J. G. Solid tumor models for assessment of different treatment modalities: therapeutic strategy for sequential chemotherapy with radiotherapy. Proc. Natl. Acad. Sci. U.S.A., *7*:1983–1987, 1977.

Lotem, J., and Sachs, L. *In vivo* inhibition of the development of myeloid leukemia by injection of macrophate- and granulocyte-inducing protein. Int. J. Cancer, *28*:375–386, 1981.

Lowenthal, R. M., and Eaton, K. Toxicity of chemotherapy. Hematol. Oncol. Clin. North Am., *10*:967–990, 1996.

Markman, M. New techniques in cancer chemotherapy. Dis. Mon., 30(10):1–48, 1984.

Martin, D. S., Stolfi, R. L., and Colofiore, J. R. Perspective: the chemotherapeutic relevance of apoptosis and a proposed biochemical cascade for chemotherapeutically induced apoptosis. Cancer Invest., *15*:372–381, 1997.

Mayer, T. U., Kapoor, T. M., Haggarty, S. J., King, R. W., Schreiber, S. L., and Mitchison, T. J. Small molecule inhibitor of mitotic spindle bipolarity identified in a phenotype-based screen. Science, *286*:971–974, 1999.

Mesnil, M., Piccoli, C., Tiraby, G., Willecke, K., and Yamasaki, H. Bystander killing of cancer cells by herpes simplex virus thymidine kinase gene is mediated by connexins. Proc. Natl. Acad. Sci. U.S.A., *93*:1831–1835, 1996.

Moasser, M. M., Sepp-Lorenzino, L., Kohl, N. E., Oliff, A., Balog, A., Su, D.-S., Danishefsky, S. J., and Rosen, N. Farnesyl transferase inhibitors cause enhanced mitotic sensitivity to taxol and epothilones. Proc. Natl. Acad. Sci., U.S.A. *95*:1369–1374, 1998.

Moertel, C. G. Chemotherapy for colorectal cancer. N. Engl. J. Med., *330*:1136–1142, 1994.

Morrow, C. S., and Cowan, K. H. Glutathione *S*-transferases and drug resistance. Cancer Cells, *2*:15–22, 1990.

Nagata, S. Apoptosis by death factor. Cell, *88*:355–365, 1997.

Nyce, J., Leonard, S., Canupp, D., Schulz, S., and Wong, S. Epigenetic mechanisms of drug resistance: drug-induced DNA hypermethylation and drug resistance. Proc. Natl. Acad. Sci. U.S.A., *90*:2960–2964, 1993.

O'Brien, M. L., and Tew, K. D. Glutathione and related enzymes in multidrug resistance. Eur. J. Cancer, *32A*:967–978, 1996.

Olivotto, I. A., Bajdik, C. D., Plenderleith, I. H., Coppin, C. M., Gelmon, K. A., Jackson, S. M., Ragaz, J., Wilson, K. S., and Worth, A. Adjuvant systemic therapy and survival after breast cancer. N. Engl. J. Med., *330*:805–810, 1994.

O'Reilly, M. S., Boehm, T., Shing, Y., Fukai, N., Vasios, G., Lane, W. S., Flynn, E., Birkhead, J. R., Olsen, B. R., and Folkman, J. Endostatin: an endogenous inhibitor of angiogenesis and tumor growth. Cell, *88*:277–285, 1997.

Osborne, C. K. Tamoxifen in the treatment of breast cancer. N. Engl. J. Med., *339*:1609–1618, 1998.

Pantel, K., Cote, R. J., and Fodstad, Ø. Detection and clinical importance of micrometastatic disease. J. Natl. Cancer Inst., *91*:1113–1124, 1999.

Patrick, D. R., and Heimbrook, D. C. Protein kinase inhibitors for the treatment of cancer. DDT, *1*:325–330, 1996.

Pommier, Y., Fesen, M. R., and Goldwasser, F. Topoisomerase II inhibitors: the epipodophyllotoxins, *m*-AMSA, and the ellipticine derivatives. *In*: B. A. Chabner and D. L. Longo (Eds.), Cancer Chemotherapy and Biotherapy, 2nd ed., pp. 435–461. Philadelphia: Lippincott-Raven, 1996.

Powis, G. Recent advances in the development of anticancer drugs that act against signalling pathways. Tumori, *80*:69–87, 1994.

Prosnitz, L. R., and Roberts, K. B. Combined chemotherapy and radiotherapy for Hodgkin's disease. Oncology, *6*:113–128, 1992.

Reed, J. C. Double identity for proteins of the Bcl-2 family. Nature, *387*:773–776, 1997.

Riou, G., and Bernard, J. The culture of human tumour stem cells. Clinical prospects in cancer chemotherapy. Trends Pharmacol. Sci., *3*:78–80, 1982.

Rivera, G. K., Pinkel, D., Simone, J. V., Hancock, M. L., and Crist, W. M. Treatment of acute lymphoblastic leukemia. 30 years' experience at St. Jude Children's Research Hospital. N. Engl. J. Med., *329*:1289–1295, 1993.

Roberts, W. M., Estrov, Z., Ouspenskaia, M. V., Johnston, D. A., McClain, K. L., and Zipf, T. F. Measurement of residual leukemia during remission in childhood acute lymphoblastic leukemia. N. Engl. J. Med., *336*:317–323, 1997.

Robinson, B. A., Colls, B. M., Fitzharris, B. M., and Atkinson, C. H. Second malignant neoplasms in patients with Hodgkin's disease. Aust. N.Z. J. Med., *24*:368–373, 1994.

Rosenberg, S. A., Chabner, B. A., Young, R. C., Seipp, C. A., Levine, A. S., Costa, J., Hanson, T. A., Head, G. C., and Simon, R. M. Treatment of osteogenic sarcoma. I. Effect of adjuvant high-dose methotrexate after amputation. Cancer Treat. Rep., *6*:739–751, 1979.

Roth, J. A., and Cristiano, R. J. Gene therapy for cancer: what have we done and where are we going? J. Natl. Cancer Inst., *88*:21–39, 1997.

Rothenberg, M. L. Topoisomerase I inhibitors: review and update. Ann. Oncol., *8*:837–855, 1997.

Sachs, L. Control of normal cell differentiation and the phenotypic reversion of malignancy in myeloid leukaemia. Nature, *274*:535–539, 1978.

Salmon, S. E., Hamburger, A. W., Soehnlen, B., Durie, B. G. M., Alberts, D. S., and Moon, T. E. Quantitation of differential sensitivity of human-tumor stem cells to anticancer drugs. N. Engl. J. Med., *298*:1321–1327, 1978.

Salven, P., Lymboussaki, A., Heikkilä, P., Jääskela-Saari, H., Enholm, B., Aase, K., von Euler, G., Eriksson, U., Alitalo, K., and Joensuu, H. Vascular endothelial growth factors VEGF-B and VEGF-C are expressed in human tumors. Am. J. Pathol., *153*:103–108, 1998.

Santen, R. J., Manni, A., Harvey, H., and Redmond, C. Endocrine treatment of breast cancer in women. Endocr. Rev., *11*:221–265, 1990.

Schimke, R. T. Gene amplification, drug resistance, and cancer. Cancer Res., *44*:1735–1742, 1984.

Schinkel, A. H. The physiological function of drug-transporting P-glycoproteins. Semin. Cancer Biol., *8*:161–170, 1997.

Schmitt, C. A., and Lowe, S. W. Apoptosis and therapy. J. Pathol., *187*:127–137, 1999.

Schnipper, L. E., Chan, V., Sedivy, J., Jat, P., and Sharp, P. A. Gene activation by induced DNA rearrangements. Cancer Res., *49*:6640–6644, 1989.

Sharma, R. C., and Schimke, R. T. The propensity for gene amplification: a comparison of protocols, cell lines, and selection agents. Mutat. Res., *304*:243–260, 1994.

Shulman, K., and Schilsky, R. L. Adjuvant therapy of colon cancer. Semin. Oncol., *22*:600–610, 1995.

Simpson-Herren, L., Noker, P. E., and Wagoner, S. D. Variability of tumor response to chemotherapy. II. Contribution of tumor heterogeneity. Cancer Chemother. Pharmacol., *22*:131–136, 1988.

Skipper, H. E. The effects of chemotherapy on the kinetics of leukemic cell behavior. Cancer Res., *25*:1544–1550, 1965.

Skipper, H. E., and Schabel, F. M., Jr. Quantitative and cytokinetic studies in experimental tumor systems. *In*: J. F. Holland and E. Frei III (Eds.), Cancer Medicine, 2nd ed., pp. 663–685. Philadelphia: Lea & Febiger, 1982.

Skovsgaard, T., Nielsen, D., Maare, C., and Wassermann, K. Cellular resistance to cancer chemotherapy. Int. Rev. Cytol., *156*:77–157, 1994.

Sladek, N. E. Oxazaphosphorines. *In*: G. Powis and R. A. Prough (eds.), Metabolism and Action of Anti-Cancer Drugs, pp. 48–90. London: Taylor & Francis, 1987.

Sluyser, M. Hormone resistance in cancer: the role of abnormal steroid receptors. Crit. Rev. Oncog., *5*:539–554, 1994.

Spiers, A. S. D., and Wade, H. E. Bacterial glutaminase in treatment of acute leukaemia. Br. Med. J., *1*:1317–1319, 1976.

Srinivasan, P. R., Tonin, P. N., Wensing, E. J., and Lewis, W. H. The gene for ornithine decarboxylase is co-amplified in hydroxyurea-resistant hamster cells. J. Biol. Chem., *262*:12871–12878, 1987.

Sweetenham, J. W. The importance of dose and schedule in cancer chemotherapy: haematological cancer. Anticancer Drugs, 6:7–15, 1995.

Szyf, M. The DNA methylation machinery as a target for anticancer therapy. Pharmacol. Ther., 70:1–37, 1996.

Tagliaferri, P., Caraglia, M., Muraro, R., Pinto, A., Budillon, A., Zagonel, V., and Bianco, A. R. Pharmacological modulation of peptide growth factor receptor expression on tumor cells as a basis for cancer therapy. Anticancer Drugs, 5:379–393, 1994.

Taimi, M., Chen, Z.-X., and Breitman, T. R. Potentiation of retinoic acid-induced differentiation of human acute promyelocytic leukemia NB4 cells by butyric acid, tributyrin, and hexamethylene bisacetamide. Oncol. Res., 10:75–84, 1998.

Takahashi, Y., and Nishioka, K. Survival without tumor shrinkage: re-evaluation of survival gain by cytostatic effect of chemotherapy. J. Natl. Cancer Inst., 87:1262–1263, 1995.

Tallman, M. S., Andersen, J. W., Schiffer, C. A., Appelbaum, F. R., Feusner, J. H., Ogden, A., Shepherd, L., Willman, C., Bloomfield, C. D., Rowe, J. M., and Wiernik, P. H. All-*trans*-retinoic acid in acute promyelocytic leukemia. N. Engl. J. Med., 337:1021–1028, 1997.

Talmadge, J. E. Development of immunotherapeutic strategies for the treatment of malignant neoplasms. Biotherapy, 4:215–236, 1992.

Tan, Y., Xu, M., Guo, H., Sun, X., Kubota, T., and Hoffman, R. M. Anticancer efficacy of methioninase *in vivo*. Anticancer Res., 16:3931–3936, 1996.

Tannock, I. F. Experimental Chemotherapy. *In*: I. F. Tannock and R. P. Hill (Eds.), The Basic Science of Oncology, 2nd ed., pp. 338–359. New York: McGraw-Hill, 1992.

Teeter, L. D., Atsumi, S.-i., Sen, S., and Kuo, T. DNA amplification in multidrug, cross-resistant Chinese hamster ovary cells: molecular characterization and cytogenetic localization of the amplified DNA. J. Cell Biol., 103:1159–1166, 1986.

Teicher, B. A. Hypoxia and drug resistance. Cancer Metast. Rev., 13:139–168, 1994.

Terzi, M. Chromosomal variation and the origin of drug-resistant mutants in mammalian cell lines. Proc. Natl. Acad. Sci. U.S.A., 71:5027–5031, 1974.

Thomas, E. D. Bone marrow transplantation: past experiences and future prospects. Semin. Oncol., 19:3–6, 1992.

Thompson, W. D., Li, W. W., and Maragoudakis, M. The clinical manipulation of angiogenesis: pathology, side-effects, surprises, and opportunities with novel human therapies. J. Pathol., 187:503–510, 1999.

Trott, K. R. Tumour stem cells: the biological concept and its application in cancer treatment. Radiother. Oncol., 30:1–5, 1994.

Tubiana, M. Tumor cell proliferation kinetics and tumor growth rate. Rev. Oncol., 2:113–121, 1989.

Tucker, M. A., Coleman, C. N., Cox, R. S., Varghese, A., and Rosenberg, S. A. Risk of second cancers after treatment for Hodgkin's disease. N. Engl. J. Med., 318:76–81, 1988.

Urade, M., Sugi, M., Mima, T., Ogura, T., and Matsuya, T. High induction of poly(ADP-ribose) polymerase activity in bleomycin-resistant HeLa cells. Jpn. J. Cancer Res., 80:464–468, 1989.

Veikkola, T., and Alitalo, K. VEGFs, receptors and angiogenesis. Semin. Cancer Biol., 9:211–220, 1999.

Voehringer, D. W., and Meyn, R. E. Reversing drug resistance in bcl-2-expressing tumor cells by depleting glutathione. Drug Resistance Updates, 1:345–351, 1998.

Von Hoff, D. D., Clark, G. M., Stogdill, B. J., Sarosdy, M. F., O'Brien, M. T., Casper, J. T., Mattox, D. E., Page, C. P., Cruz, A. B., and Sandbach, J. F. Prospective clinical trial of a human tumor cloning system. Cancer Res., 43:1926–1931, 1983.

Waddick, K. G., and Uckun, F. M. Innovative treatment programs against cancer. I. Ras oncoprotein as a molecular target. Biochem. Pharmacol., 56:1411–1426, 1998.

Waddick, K. G., and Uckun, F. M. Innovative treatment programs against cancer. II. Nuclear factor-κB (NF-κB) as a molecular target. Biochem. Pharmacol., 57:9–17, 1999.

Walker, N. I., Bennett, R. E., and Kerr, J. F. R. Cell death by apoptosis during involution of the lactating breast in mice and rats. Am. J. Anat., 185:19–32, 1989.

Workman, P. Pharmacokinetics and cancer: successes, failures and future prospects. Cancer Surv., 17:1–26, 1993.

Wosikowski, K., Schuurhuis, D., Johnson, K., Paull, K. D., Myers, T. G., Weinstein, J. N., and Bates, S. E. Identification of epidermal growth factor receptor and c-erbB2 pathway inhibitors by correlation with gene expression patterns. J. Natl. Cancer Inst., *89*:1505–1515, 1997.

Yamada, T., Endo, R., Gotoh, M., and Hirohashi, S. Identification of semaphorin E as a non-MDR drug resistance gene of human cancers. Proc. Natl. Acad. Sci. U.S.A., *94*:14713–14718, 1997.

Yamamoto, H., Fujimoto, J., Okamoto, E., Furuyama, J.-i., Tamaoki, T., and Hashimoto-Tamaoki, T. Suppression of growth of hepatocellular carcinoma by sodium butyrate *in vitro* and *in vivo*. Int. J. Cancer, *76*:897–902, 1998.

Yarbro, J. W. Mechanism of action of hydroxyurea. Semin. Oncol., *19*:1–10, 1992.

Epilogue
Cancer: Tomorrow and the Future

In the 15 years since the publication of the third edition of this textbook, a veritable explosion of knowledge has occurred in the fields of cell and molecular biology, genetics, computer technology and bioinformatics, and many other basic and applied fields. Simultaneously, there has been an explosion in our knowledge of neoplasia. This knowledge has possibly led to some concrete results in that the overall death rate from cancer in the United States decreased by 3% during the period 1990–1995 (Cole and Rodu, 1996) and in the European Union by about 7% between 1988 and 1996 (Levi et al., 2000). However, as was the case 15 years ago, there is still no "magic bullet" to cure cancer, unlike the antibiotics that are able to cure the majority of bacterial infections in the human. Just as it was 15 years ago, despite the explosion in knowledge, medical science continues to be frustrated in its effort to establish a truly effective therapy for the most common forms of malignant neoplasms in the human, such as lung, breast, prostate, and gastrointestinal tract. The elusive "answer to cancer" appears to be just over the hill and beyond, despite the many truly striking discoveries that have been made in biology in this past decade and a half.

As in the earlier editions of this text, and at the suggestion of several reviewers, we proposed several areas of oncology that might hold promise for a control of this disease. Review of the epilogue to the third edition indicates that progress has been made in the areas suggested at that time: cancer prevention, the natural history of development and the nature of the cancer cell, and the therapy of neoplasia itself. This epilogue is not prophetic, but is more of an update and suggests some directions for investigation that might be taken in the future. They are necessarily biased and thus open to considerable criticism. An old colleague of mine, Dr. Vladimir Shapot of the former Soviet Union, once remarked in a seminar he gave at the McArdle Laboratory, "Each investigator doing cancer research is completely convinced that his or her direction is leading to a better understanding of the disease and its control." The truth in this statement is self-evident, since investigators in the field would not be undertaking their studies unless, at least in the back of their minds, they were convinced that their approach was the way to go. If such optimism exists and continues, then we hope one day to control neoplasia.

CANCER PREVENTION

Just as our knowledge of the nature of the chemical induction of cancer increased dramatically prior to the publication of the third edition of this text, our knowledge and application of such knowledge to the viral causation of neoplasia have increased rapidly in the past 15 years. Even more rapidly, perhaps, has the field of the genetics of cancer development expanded, as well as our understanding of the molecular mechanisms involved in the genetic induction of neoplasia. In fact, much of our present knowledge of the basic molecular nature of the cancer cell itself in comparison with its normal counterpart has developed from these latter two areas. Such information offers enormous potential in the area of cancer prevention. The vaccine against the hepatitis B virus is very effective in preventing infection by the virus and, when given early in life, prevents the chronic hepatitis that can so readily result when the infection develops in young children. It is the chronic infection that leads to hepatocellular carcinoma. Vaccines for the papilloma virus, which may cause at least as many cases of neoplasia in humans as hepatitis B, are already being tested. A vaccine for the Epstein-Barr virus is also quite feasible, and since viral and other infectious causes of neoplasia are probably associated with 15% or more of all human neoplasms worldwide, prevention by active vaccination could lead within a few decades to a dramatic decrease in several types of neoplasms if public health systems were to function at reasonable efficiency in all countries.

It is now possible to determine by molecular technologies the presence of mutations in specific tumor suppressor genes that lead to heritable neoplasms, but various social requirements for privacy, as well as the fear of individuals that they may carry a defective gene, have not allowed us to realize the promise that cancer genetics holds. Perhaps with the elucidation of the DNA sequence of the entire human genome, and with it the identification of the numerous other "modifier" genes that are probably far more important, the genetic mechanisms leading to neoplasia will be made clear. The use of genetic information to prevent the development of cancer in specific individuals may then be brought closer to fruition.

The "passive" prevention of neoplasia by abstinence from tobacco use, moderate consumption of alcohol, and healthy dietary practices is beginning to alter in a favorable way both the incidence and the death rate of specific neoplasms such as those of the lung, stomach, and, in some populations, liver. The potential for cancer prevention through such passive means is enormous. Epidemiological studies have shown that smoking, diet, reproductive mores, infectious agents, alcoholic beverages, and industrial contaminants are factors in more than two-thirds of neoplasias in the human. Almost all the epidemiological studies of the causes of human neoplasia are supported by numerous scientific investigations in the laboratory. It is hoped that, in the future, a major priority of our society will be the prevention of cancer caused by these various agents through educational, governmental, and behavioral-modification modalities. Ultimately, however, cancer prevention must be an individual and societal decision. Hopefully, such decisions will be based on solid scientific grounds. Although gerontologists tell us that the elimination of cancer as a disease would increase the expected lifetime of each of us by only a few years, the collective fear of cancer in our society is still reflected in the words of former University of Wisconsin President Glenn Frank (quoted on page 1).

THE NATURAL HISTORY OF NEOPLASTIC DEVELOPMENT AND THE NATURE OF THE CANCER CELL

That the natural history of neoplastic development occurs in stages in a multistep manner is virtually an accepted fact. In both animals and humans, substantial evidence for the existence of distinct cell types occurring in the stages of promotion and progression has been elucidated (Chapters 7, 9, and 10). Most of the factors causing the two-thirds of preventable human cancer are promoting agents or have as their major component promoting agents. The action of promoting agents may be eliminated by their removal from the environment of the individual or by the simultaneous administration of chemopreventive agents that will antagonize or completely prevent the action of the promoting agent even if exposure continues. The majority of so-called "nongenotoxic" carcinogens (Table 9.11) are promoting agents and thus, from our knowledge of the characteristics of promoting agents (Chapter 7), pose a risk to the general population that is significantly different from that from complete carcinogens. Hopefully, future regulatory actions taken by governments in an attempt to reduce the cancer risk of humans exposed to such agents will be based on the distinctive known characteristics of promoting agents rather than on treatment of all carcinogens as mechanistically identical.

There have been considerable advances in the methods used to detect the early development of neoplasia, through a variety of radiological devices such as the CAT scan, nuclear magnetic resonance, and nuclear medical techniques for identifying and localizing preneoplasia and early neoplasia. Such techniques have already been utilized in the early control and cure of major human neoplasms such as those of the breast, gastrointestinal tract, and lymphoid system. In the future such technologies may become almost routine in evaluation of patients at potential risk for the development of neoplasia long before the disease becomes clinically apparent.

It would appear that our basic knowledge of the stage of progression has become both a blessing and a curse with respect to the ultimate control of cancer as a disease. Molecular biology has allowed us to define and describe numerous molecular changes in neoplastic cells and identify an ever-expanding number of proto-oncogenes and tumor suppressor genes as well as many of the basic mechanisms involved in the regulation of cell replication. Although this enormous amount of work has described in ever-increasing detail the molecular characteristics of neoplastic cells—even to the point of the changes in expression of thousands of genes now measured on "chips" and "gene screens"—the information derived has still not allowed us a basic understanding of the mechanism of evolving karyotypic instability, the critical characteristic of the stage of progression. In fact, the latter could be the curse behind the elusiveness of the "magic bullet" to control cancer after its evolution to successful metastatic spread. If we cannot control the karyotypic evolution of the neoplastic cell by some reasonably selective means, we may not be able to control the disease when it is first apparent to physicians in many cancer patients. The optimistic view of this conundrum is that molecular technologies and knowledge of the neoplastic cell itself will ultimately reveal the mechanistic nature of karyotypic evolution, allowing for a rational therapeutic elimination of all neoplastic disease.

THE FUTURE OF CANCER THERAPY

Only two facets of the therapy of neoplasia are considered in this text: chemotherapy and immunotherapy. However, most students of oncology are vitally interested in—and usually have acquired a significant amount of knowledge about—the types of therapy used in the treatment of human cancer. In the past, the principal therapies to treat neoplasia were surgery, radiotherapy, and chemotherapy, as well as, although it has not been highly successful, immunotherapy. Since the publication of the third edition of this text, there have been considerable refinements in radiotherapy, chemotherapy, and immunotherapy. Advances in radiotherapy have been concerned primarily with the ability to treat an exact volume of tissue with a specific dose by using a variety of sophisticated instrumentations. In particular, this has led to decreased morbidity and, in a number of instances, to increased therapeutic effectiveness. Several new families of chemotherapeutic drugs have become available, such as the taxols and topoisomerase inhibitors discussed in Chapter 20. One of the most exciting and potentially effective chemotherapeutic modalities being extensively investigated is the group of chemicals, growth factors, and related agents that prevent the growth or alter or destroy the vasculature of the growing neoplasm (Chapter 18). Although the efficacy of such agents has been clearly demonstrated only in animal systems thus far, this type of therapy, since it does not attack the neoplastic cell directly and therefore is not influenced by the karyotypic instability of the neoplastic cell, could potentially be a true "magic bullet" against malignant neoplasms.

As emphasized in Chapter 19, the role of immunotherapy in preventing the development of early neoplasia and in curing advanced neoplasms that have previously been treated by the standard methods of surgery, radiotherapy, or chemotherapy has not yet been realized. With the advances in vaccine technology, antigen identification and characterization, and immune-cell therapy, immunotherapy should play a greater role both in preventing early disease and in eliminating micrometastases and residual neoplasms after "debulking" of the primary neoplasms and major metastases in the patient. However, unlike the attack on the vascular system of the neoplasm, which is indirect, the direct effect of immunotherapy on the neoplastic cell must still contend with karyotypic evolution in the stage of progression.

The induced differentiation of neoplastic cells, which has been shown to occur both in vivo and in vitro, has also not yet been successfully used in the therapy of most neoplasms. The induced differentiation of cells of acute promyelocytic leukemia by retinoids (Chapter 6) is the best example of successful differentiation therapy of neoplasia, although it does not lead to a lasting cure in the human patient. Since a large number of "differentiating agents" that induce the differentiation of neoplastic cells both in vivo and in vitro has been developed in animal systems, their potential for the treatment of human disease still remains a significant possibility.

As the population of the world increases, so will the incidence of neoplastic disease in both the young and the old unless we can apply in much stricter ways our knowledge of the prevention of neoplasia and develop effective curative therapies for cancer in all age groups. Let us hope that present and future generations will strive to achieve the goals of effective prevention and cure of cancer toward which this text is directed.

REFERENCES

Cole, P., and Rodu, B. Declining cancer mortality in the United States. Cancer, _78_:2045-2048, 1996.

Levi, F., Lucchini, F., Negri, E., and La Vecchia, C. The decline in cancer mortality in the European Union, 1988-1996. Eur. J. Cancer, _36_:1965-1968, 2000.

Glossary

This glossary is not meant to be exhaustive, but rather to assist the student who is unfamiliar with some of the terms used in the text. A number of the following definitions were modified from *Stedman's Medical Dictionary*, 24th edition, Lippincott Williams & Wilkins, Philadelphia, 1982.

acidosis   the result in an organism of an actual or relative decrease in the pH of body fluids.

adduct   in chemical terms, used here to denote the product of the reaction between an electrophilic chemical and a nucleophilic molecule, usually one of biological importance such as a protein or a nucleic acid or their components.

ad libitum   literally, in accordance with one's wishes. Used with reference to dietary or other administration in the sense of being available without limitation.

agglutinin   a substance that causes the clumping of cells with which it interacts.

alkylating agent   a chemical that reacts with a second chemical nonenzymically to substitute an alkyl group for a hydrogen atom.

allotypic   pertaining to one of the genetically determined antigenic structures that distinguish among members of a given class of immunoglobulins.

analgesic   an agent capable of relieving pain without altering consciousness.

anaplasia   loss of positional, organizational, or structural differentiation of cells and/or tissues.

anastomosis   a connection, natural or induced, between two blood vessels or other tubular structures.

anemia   a condition characterized by a lower than normal concentration of red blood cells or hemoglobin in the blood of an organism.

anergy   the absence of a sensitivity reaction in an individual to materials that would be antigenic (immunogenic, allergenic) in the majority of other individuals.

aneuploidy   the state of possessing an abnormal number of chromosomes—one that is not a whole-number multiple of the haploid set—or in which a demonstrable chromosomal structural change is present.

anorexia   decreased appetite or acquired aversion to food.

anorexia nervosa   a personality disorder manifested by extreme aversion to food, usually occurring in young women. The disorder is characterized by extreme weight loss, amenorrhea, and other constitutional disorders.

antibiotic   a chemical substance that may be synthetic or derived from a mold or bacteria and that exhibits the ability to inhibit the growth of other microorganisms.

antibody   a globular serum protein produced during an immune response, the specific synthesis of which is evoked in most vertebrate species by exposure of appropriate cells to a specific antigen.

anticarcinogen   an agent that, when administered simultaneously with a complete carcinogen, inhibits its carcinogenic action, usually by altering the process of initiation.

antigen   any substance that, after contact with appropriate cells of a vertebrate organism, induces a state of sensitivity to infectious or toxic substances following a latent period and that reacts in a measurable way with tissues and/or specific antibodies of the sensitized subject in vivo or in vitro.

antigenic determinant   the portion of an antigen that reacts with an antibody specific for that antigen.

antimetabolite   a chemical substance, usually exhibiting structural similarities to a normal metabolite, that competes with, replaces, or antagonizes its normal counterpart.

antioxidant   any substance that, when present at low concentrations compared with those of an oxidizable substrate, delays or inhibits oxidation of that substrate to a significant degree.

apoptosis   death of individual cells within a tissue as a result of the normal cell turnover within a tissue or of the toxicity of an environmental agent.

arteriosclerosis   a disease resulting from the thickening of arterial walls because of fibrosis, lipid deposition, calcification, cell proliferation, and/or inflammation.

arthralgia   pain, usually severe, in a joint, generally in the absence of inflammation.

asthenia   weakness or debility.

autosomal   pertaining to any chromosome other than a sex chromosome.

cachexia the sum of those effects in the host produced by neoplasms, such effects not being due to the immediate result of mechanical interference with recognizable structures (see Chapter 17).

calcification deposition of calcium salts as a replacement for necrotic cells or within intercellular spaces.

cancer a malignant neoplasm.

canceremia the presence of malignant cells circulating in the blood vascular system.

carcinoembryonic antigen (CEA) a glycoprotein constituent of embryonic endodermal epithelium that is generally absent from adult normal cells but may be present in some carcinomas derived from endoderm.

carcinoma a malignant neoplasm of endodermal or ectodermal origin exhibiting a morphological pattern distinguished from sarcomas by light microscopy. Some carcinomas are so classified because of their morphological epithelial cell pattern rather than their embryological derivation, e.g., renal cell carcinoma.

chemoprevention the inhibition, retardation, or reversal of the neoplastic process and of degenerative or other diseases by the use of dietary, pharmacological, or other chemical agents.

chromatid each of the two nucleoprotein strands formed by longitudinal duplication of a chromosome that become visible during prophase of mitosis or meiosis; the two chromatids are joined by the still undivided centromere, but after the centromere divides at metaphase and the two chromatids have separated, each chromatid develops into a chromosome.

chromosome a structure within the cell nucleus of eukaryotes, consisting of DNA in association with proteins and other molecules.

clone a colony or group of cells derived from a single cell by asexual reproduction, all the cells having identical characteristics.

cocarcinogen any agent that enhances the action of a complete carcinogen when given simultaneously with the latter.

complete carcinogen a carcinogen capable of both initiating and promoting carcinogenesis.

contact inhibition the inhibition of cell movement and/or replication as a result of cell-to-cell contact.

Cori cycle the cyclic conversion of glycogen to lactate and back to glycogen, the complete metabolic cycle being formed only in the liver.

cotermination a term referring to the completion of transcription of an exon involved in the production of several transcripts, all of which terminate at the same nucleotide.

C-terminal related to a free carboxyl group at one end of a polypeptide chain.

cytophilic antibody antibody having an affinity for certain kinds of cells, such affinity being unrelated to the specific affinity of the antibody for the antigen by which it was induced.

derepression a biochemical mechanism for the regulation of enzyme production through interference with the action of a repressor in the same system.

diagnosis determination of the nature of a disease.

dysplasia abnormal tissue development.

ectopic an organ out of place, or a function attributed to cells or tissues not normally possessing the capability for such function.

electrophilic relating to an electron-attracting atom or chemical compound in an organic reaction.

electrophoresis the movement of particles in an electric field toward the anode or the cathode.

endogenous pertaining to the origination or production of a substance within an organism.

endomitosis replication of the chromosomes of a cell without accompanying formation of a spindle or cytokinesis, resulting in a polyploid nucleus.

endoreduplication a form of polyploidy characterized by chromosome doubling, resulting in four-stranded chromosomes during prophase and metaphase.

enteric relating to the intestine.

enzyme an organic catalyst, usually protein in nature, that catalyzes chemical reactions while in most cases remaining chemically unchanged.

euploidy the state of a cell in which the number of chromosomes is a whole-number multiple of the haploid number normal for that species.

exogenous pertaining to the origination or production of a substance outside an organism.

exon a portion of DNA that is transcribed but not excised during mRNA maturation, the transcript subsequently being translated in the mature mRNA in most cases.

fetal relating to the unborn, intrauterine young of a mammal.

fibrosis the formation of fibrous tissue as part of a reparative or reactive process.

free radical a neutral or charged atom or compound possessing an unpaired electron.

genome the total gene complement present in the normal chromosome or set of chromosomes characteristic of an organism.

glucocorticoid a steroid hormone, produced by the adrenal cortex or a synthetic analog, that enhances gluconeogenesis in the organism.

gluconeogenesis the metabolic formation of glucose from noncarbohydrate sources, e.g., protein.

glycolysis the fermentation of glucose to lactic acid.

gnotobiotes animals living in the absence of contaminating internal or external microorganisms.

goitrogens agents that induce or cause goiter, a chronic enlargement of the thyroid gland that is not due to a neoplastic process.

granuloma a nodular inflammatory lesion, usually chronic, consisting of a chronic inflammatory infiltrate (lymphocytes, monocytes, plasma cells, and the like) with accompanying fibrosis and/or necrosis.

gynecomastia excessive development of the mammary glands in the male.

hapten an incomplete or partial antigen that is incapable, by itself, of causing the production of antibodies but is capable of combining with antibodies having a specificity for the chemical nature of the hapten.

hemopoiesis the process of formation and development of various formed elements of the blood cells.

heterokaryon a cell hybrid resulting from the fusion of cells from two different species.

heterozygous relating to the state of having different allelic genes at one or more paired loci in homologous chromosomes.

histogenetic relating to the origin, formation, and development of the tissues of an organism.

homeobox an evolutionarily conserved DNA-sequence motif of about 180 basepairs found in insects and vertebrates. This DNA sequence is involved in the control of morphogenesis and contains a homeodomain of about 60 basepairs that is involved in the coding of DNA-binding domains of proteins containing such sequences.

homeostasis the natural state of equilibrium in an organism with respect to various physiological functions and to the chemical compositions of its fluids and tissues.

homologous recombination inter- or intrachromosomal events involving DNA strand exchange (breakage and reunion of strands) involving extensive sequence identity between the DNA duplexes that are recombined. Homologous recombination occurs at rates dependent on both the length of "homologous" sequences and the degree to which they are identical.

homozygous having identical genes at one or more paired loci in homologous chromosomes.

homokaryon a cell hybrid resulting from fusion of cells from the same animal or the same species.

horizontal transmission transmission of infectious agents from one individual to another in a nonhereditary manner.

hormesis   a dose–response relationship in which there is a stimulatory or efficacious response at low doses but an inhibitory or toxic response at high doses, resulting in a U- or inverted U–shaped dose response.

hormone   a biochemical substance, usually formed in one organ or tissue of an organism, carried in the blood or lymph throughout the organism, and exhibiting specific effects in altering the functional activity and/or structure of one or more organs and tissues.

hybridoma   cells resulting from the fusion of malignant B cells, usually plasmacytoma cells, and specific antibody-producing normal cells to form a cell hybrid with unlimited growth potential whose ultimate progeny may synthesize a homogeneous species of antibody originally produced by the normal cell.

hydroxylase   enzyme catalyzing the formation of hydroxyl groups through the addition of an oxygen atom to the substrate.

hyperalimentation   the administration of nutrients in excess of normal requirements.

hypercalcemia   an abnormally high concentration of calcium ions in the blood.

hyperlipemia   an abnormally high concentration of lipids in the blood.

hyperplasia   a numerical increase in one or more constituents of a living organism, usually referring to an increased number of cells within a tissue or organ, but also relating to the number of specific organelles within cells or the number of functional cellular units such as renal nephrons, pulmonary alveoli, or glandular acini.

hypertrophy   increase in the bulk of an organelle, cell, tissue, or organ within a living system. This term is distinct from *hyperplasia* in that it refers to an increase in size rather than in number.

hypophysectomy   the surgical removal of the pituitary gland.

idiotype   an antigenic determinant that confers on an immunoglobulin molecule an antigenic "individuality" that is analogous to the "individuality" of the molecule's antibody activity.

incomplete carcinogen   an agent capable only of initiation of carcinogenesis.

initiation   a heritable change in a cell resulting from the action of an initiating agent, such change most likely being the result of a direct alteration in the molecular structure of the genome of the cell (see Chapter 7).

internal milieu   the environment within the body of an organism.

intron   portion of DNA between two exons that is transcribed into RNA, but is then excised and not present in mature RNA.

isoschizomer   a restriction endonuclease whose ability to cleave specific sequences in DNA depends on the presence or absence of methylated nucleic acid bases in the target sequence.

isozyme (isoenzyme) one of a group of enzymes with measurably different physical properties that exhibit similar, if not identical, catalytic properties.

ketosis the enhanced production of ketones (ketone bodies) in an organism.

kwashiorkor severe malnutrition usually seen in young children in less developed areas of the world, owing to dietary deficiency of protein or of one or more essential amino acids.

latency period the period of time between the application of an agent to a living organism and a demonstrable effect of such application.

lectin a protein of plant or animal source that effects agglutination, precipitation, or other related cell-to-cell interaction through its surface reactivity with carbohydrate moieties in glycoproteins.

lesion a pathological change in a cell, tissue, organ, or body of a living organism.

linear energy transfer the transfer of energy from energetic particles to the surrounding medium or tissue.

lymphopoiesis formation of lymphocytes.

malignancy a synonym for cancer.

marasmus a cachectic state of malnutrition resulting from a prolonged deficiency of protein and calories.

mastectomy excision or removal of the breast.

metabolic cooperation the direct exchange of molecules between two cells in contact with each other. Such exchange is thought to proceed through gap junctions in the apposed membranes of the two cooperating cells.

metaplasia the conversion in vivo of an adult, fully differentiated tissue of one morphological type into a differentiated tissue of another morphological type.

metastasis the dissemination and/or growth of cells originating from a primary neoplasm at another site.

microfilament the smallest of the fibrous cytoskeletal elements; they have diameters between 30 and 60 Ångstroms, lack periodicity, and are chemically related to actins.

microtubule a widely occurring cylindrical cytoplasmic element 200 to 270 Ångstroms in diameter and of variable length, increasing in number during mitosis.

mitogenic pertaining to a substance that stimulates mitosis.

modality any form of physiological or medical therapeutics.

morphology   the science concerned with the configuration and/or structure of animals and plants and their constituents.

mutation   a change in the structure and/or expression of a gene that is perpetuated in subsequent progeny of the cell in which it first occurs. Germ-line mutations occur in the germ cells (eggs or sperm) and are thus transmitted from generation to generation within a species. Somatic mutation refers to a mutation within a somatic cell and all its progeny within an individual organism.

necrosis   the pathological death of one or more cells, of a portion of a tissue, or of an organ, usually resulting from irreversible damage to the affected cell(s).

neoplasm   a heritably altered, relatively autonomous growth of tissue.

neoplastic transformation   the conversion of a normal to a neoplastic cell.

neuropathy   any disorder affecting a component(s) of the nervous system, usually spinal and/or peripheral.

nevus   a benign localized growth of melanin-forming cells in the skin, usually in early life.

N-terminal α amino group, not in peptide linkage, at one end of a polypeptide chain.

oligosaccharide   a relatively short polymeric form of one or several carbohydrates.

paleopathologist   one who studies the science of disease as revealed in archeological artifacts such as bones, mummies, etc.

papilloma   a circumscribed benign epithelial tumor projecting from a body surface.

paroxysmal   relating to the sudden onset of a symptom or disease, e.g., spasm or convulsion.

pharmacokinetics   relating to the disposition (change in availability with time) of drugs in the body.

phosphorylation   the addition of a phosphoryl group to an organic compound with the formation of a phosphate ester or phosphamate.

plasmid   an extrachromosomal genetic element containing DNA.

polycythemia   an abnormal increase in the number of red cells in the blood.

polymorphic   occurrence in more than one morphological form.

polymyositis   inflammation of a number of muscles.

polyp   a mass of tissue that bulges or projects outward or upward from a normal tissue surface, such as the skin or lining of the colon, lung, or genital organs.

polytenization   formation of many filaments of chromatin within a single chromosome.

preneoplastic lesion   any lesion that, while itself not neoplastic, exhibits a high propensity for development into a neoplastic lesion.

procarcinogen   a carcinogen that is ineffective without metabolic modification.

prognosis   the forecasting of the outcome of a disease process.

progression   the stage of neoplastic development characterized either by demonstrable changes in the number and/or arrangement of genes (as evidenced by nucleic acid sequence and/or hybridization studies) or by visible karyotypic alterations (as evidenced by light microscopic techniques) within a majority of the neoplastic cells that make up the tumor. These alterations are in turn associated with increased growth rate, increased invasiveness, metastases, and alterations in biochemical and morphological characteristics of the neoplasm (see Chapter 9).

promotion   the stage of neoplastic development characterized by a change in the expression of genetic information, resulting from the action of a promoting agent (see Chapter 6).

protocol   a plan, usually detailed, for the study of a problem or for a regimen of therapy.

proximate carcinogen   a metabolite of a carcinogen intermediate in the conversion to an ultimate carcinogen.

rad   an absorbed dose of ionizing radiation equivalent to 100 ergs/g tissue.

redox cycling   the univalent reduction of a chemical to a radical intermediate by intracellular enzymes. The radical intermediate then transfers an electron to O_2, producing O_2^- and regenerating the parent compound.

relative biological effectiveness (RBE)   the relative effects on tissues of absorbed doses of various ionizing radiations.

rem   the amount of ionizing radiation that causes an effect equivalent to 1 rad of x- or gamma-radiation.

repression   in biochemical terms, the inhibition of enzyme synthesis by the action of an intracellular effector (repressor) in combination or not with an extracellular mediator molecule.

restriction enzymes   enzymes, mostly endonucleases, that cleave DNA at specific nucleotide sequences.

RNA editing   the transcriptional or posttranscriptional modification of an RNA molecule that changes its coding specificity by a process other than RNA splicing.

sarcoma   a malignant neoplasm of tissues derived from the embryonic mesoderm.

sister chromatid exchange   the morphological reflection of an interchange between DNA molecules at homologous loci within a replicating chromosome.

somatic cell hybridization (cell fusion)   the coalescence of two cells to form a single cell that ultimately becomes mononuclear.

stroma   the supportive tissue or framework, usually made of connective tissue, of an organ or neoplasm.

symbiotic   relating to an intimate association between two species, usually with the viability and/or replication potential of each dependent on this relation with the other.

syndrome   the signs and symptoms of a pathological process that, taken in the aggregate, define the disease.

therapeutic   relating to the treatment of disease.

3T3 cells   a series of aneuploid cell lines selected from mouse embryos.

threshold   the level of an agent below which no physiological, biochemical, or pathological effect can be measured.

thrombus   a clot formed within the vascular system during life.

tissue   a collection of morphologically and biochemically similar cells and the intercellular substances surrounding them.

tolerance (immunological)   specific failure of the immune mechanism to respond to exposure to a given antigen.

total parenteral nutrition   nutrition administered entirely by intravenous, subcutaneous, intramuscular, or related means.

transformation (phenotypic)   alteration of the morphological appearance and of certain biochemical characteristics of cells in culture to cells that may exhibit neoplasia in vivo.

transfection   introduction of DNA molecules into living cells.

transition   conversion of a purine or pyrimidine base in the DNA chain to another purine or pyrimidine base, respectively.

transversion   conversion of a purine base into a pyrimidine base, or vice versa, within the DNA chain.

trophic   hormones or related agents that stimulate cell replication in tissues and cells responsive to their action.

tumor   any swelling or mass of tissue occupying a volume of space.

ultimate carcinogen   the form of a carcinogen that directly interacts with a cell constituent (presumably DNA) to initiate carcinogenesis.

urothelium   epithelial lining and related structures of the genitourinary system.

vasculature   the network of blood vessels of an organ or organism.

vena cava   the major vein returning blood from the head and arms (superior vena cava) and from the trunk and lower extremities (inferior vena cava) to the heart.

vertical transmission   hereditary characteristics transmitted to the offspring through the egg or sperm.

xenobiotic   a pharmacologically active drug, hormone, or toxic substance not produced endogenously by the organism.

zygote   the diploid cell or individual resulting from the union of a sperm and an ovum (egg).

Index